Haematology and Blood Transfusion
Hämatologie und Bluttransfusion 40

**Springer-Verlag Berlin Heidelberg GmbH**

T. Büchner  W. Hiddemann  B. Wörmann
G. Schellong  J. Ritter  U. Creutzig (Eds.)

# Acute Leukemias VIII

Prognostic Factors and Treatment Strategies

With 276 Figures and 211 Tables

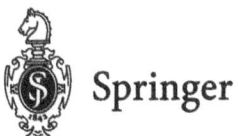 Springer

Prof. Dr. T. Büchner
Department of Internal Medicine A

Prof. Dr. J. Ritter
Prof. Dr. U. Creutzig
Prof. Dr. G. Schellong
Department of Pediatrics
University of Münster
Albert-Schweitzer-Straße 33
48149 Münster
Germany

Prof. Dr. med. W. Hiddemann
Department of Internal Medicine III
University Hospital Großhadern
Ludwig-Maximilians-University
Marchioninistr. 15
81377 München
Germany

Prof. Dr. B. Wörmann
Dept. of Internal Medicine
University of Göttingen
Robert-Koch-Str. 40
37075 Göttingen
Germany

ISBN 978-3-540-41123-9

Library of Congress Cataloging-in-Publication Data

Acute leukemias VIII: prognostic factors and treatment strategies / T. Büchner ... [et al.], (eds.).
    p. cm. – (Haematology and blood transfusion = Hämatologie und Bluttransfusion,
    ISSN 0949-7021 ; 40)
    Includes bibliographical references and index.
    ISBN 978-3-540-41123-9    ISBN 978-3-642-18156-6 (eBook)
    DOI 10.1007/978-3-642-18156-6

    1. Leukemia. 2. Leukemia-Prognosis. I. Title: Acute leukemias 8. II. Title: Acute leukemias eight. III.
Büchner, Th. IV. Hämatologie und Bluttransfusion; 40.
    [DNLM: 1. Leukemia-Therapy. 2. Acute Disease. 3. Monitoring, Physiologic. 4. Opportunistic Infec-
tions-prevention & control. 5. Prognosis. WH 250 A1895 2001]
    RC643 .A3175 2001
    616.99'419–dc21

© Springer-Verlag Berlin Heidelberg 2001
Originally published by Springer-Verlag Berlin Heidelberg in 2001

Cover design: *design & production* GmbH, Heidelberg
Typesetting: cicero Lasersatz, Dinkelscherben
Printed on acid-free paper  –  SPIN: 10709575     21/3130   5 4 3 2 1 0

# Preface

Thirteen years after the appearance of the first volume in the series »Acute Leukemias«, this 8th volume once again presents the rapid progress in our understanding of the biology of leukemia and in the identification of more effective and novel therapeutic approaches. The main issues are:

- Chromosome translocations: mechanisms and molecular background, transcription factors, recurrent gene mutations
- Monitoring minimal residual disease
- Karyotype and prognosis, risk-adapted versus randomized treatment
- Antileukemic drugs: pharmacodynamics, interactions and modulations
- Acute promyelocytic leukemia: the role of ATRA and arsenic trioxide
- Cellular immunotherapy using non-myeloablative allogeneic transplantation
- Angiogenesis in AML
- Targeted therapy
- Supportive care: more effective antimicrobial agents and strategies, platelet support
- Antileukemic treatment and quality of life

First-hand reports from leading leukemia study groups worldwide provide the latest updates of their multicenter trials. Outstanding authors combine to present an invaluable review of the state of the art.

The editors wish to thank Beate Kosel for her excellent contribution as principal coordinator of the editorial work.

T. BÜCHNER, W. HIDDEMANN, B. WÖRMANN, J. RITTER, U. CREUTZIG,
G. SCHELLONG

# Table of Contents

**Recent Antileukemic Strategies**

X

XI

## ALL in Children

## ALL in Adults

## AML in Children

## AML in Elderly Patients

## Allogeneic and Autologous Transplantation

# Authors and Institutions

AHLMANN, M.
  Department of Pediatric Hematology/Oncology, Westfälische Wilhelms-University, Albert-Schweizter-Straße 33, 48129 Münster, Germany

AIVADO, M.
  Clinic for Hematology, Oncology, and Clinical Immunology, Heinrich-Heine-Universität, Moorenstraße 5, 40225 Düsseldorf, Germany

ALBRECHT, O.
  Department of Medicine, Hematology/Oncology, Westfälische Wilhelms-University, Albert-Schweitzer-Straße 33, 48129 Münster, Germany

ANNALORO, C.
  Department of Bone Marrow Transplantation, Ospedale Maggiore di Milano, Via Francesco Sforza 35, 20122 Milano, Italy

APLAN, P.D.
  Department of Pediatrics, Roswell Park Cancer Institute, Buffalo, NY 14263, USA

AUL, C.
  Department of Hematology, Oncology, and Clinical Immunology, Heinrich-Heine-University of Düsseldorf, Moorenstraße 5, 40225 Düsseldorf, Germany

BAERSCH, G.
  Department of Pediatric Hematology/Oncology, Westfälische Wilhelms-University, Albert-Schweitzer-Straße 33, 48129 Münster, Germany

BASSAN, R.
  Department of Hematology, Ospidali Riuniti di Bergamo, Azienda Ospedaliera, 24128 Bergamo, Largo Barozzi, 1, Italy

BEHRE, G.
  Department of Medicine III, University Hospital Großhadern, Ludwig-Maximilians-University, Marchioninistraße 15, 81377 Munich, Germany

BERER, A.
  Department of Internal Medicine I, Division of Hematology, University of Vienna, Waehringer Guertel 18-20, 1090 Vienna, Austria

BEYER-SEHLMEYER, G.
Department of Hematology/Oncology, University of Göttingen,
Robert-Koch-Straße 40, 37075 Göttingen, Germany

BLOOMFIELD, C.
Arthur G. James Cancer Hospital and Richard J. Solove Research Institute,
A455 Tarling-Loving Hall, 320 West 10th Avenue, Columbus, OH 43210-
1240, USA

BORNHÄUSER, M.
Medical Clinic I, University Hospital Carl Gustav Carus, Technical
University of Dresden, Fetscherstraße 74, 01307 Dresden, Germany

BRENDEL, C.
Medical Clinic I, University Hospital Carl Gustav Carus, Technical
University of Dresden, Fetscherstraße 74, 01307 Dresden, Germany

BÜCHNER, T.
Department of Medicine, Hematology/Oncology, Westfälische Wilhelms-
University, Albert-Schweitzer-Straße 33, 48129 Münster, Germany

CHEN, Z.
Department of Hematology/Oncology, Shainghai Institute of Hematology,
Rui Jin Hospital, Shanghai Second Medical University, 197 Rui Jin Road II,
Shanghai 200025, China

CHOMIENNE, Ch.
Institute of Hematology, Laboratoire de Biologie Cellulaire Hémato-
poisétique, Hôpital Saint-Louis, 1 avenue Claude Vellefaux, 75010 Paris,
France

CHYBICKA, A.
Department of Pediatric Hematology and Oncology, University of
Wroclaw, ul. Bujwida 44, 50-345 Wroclaw, Poland

CREUTZIG, U.
Department of Pediatric Hematology/Oncology, Westfälische Wilhelms-
University, Albert-Schweitzer-Straße 33, 48129 Münster, Germany

CURTIS, J.E.
Windsor Regional Cancer Centre, 2220 Kildare Road, Windson,
ON, N8W-2X3, Canada

DÖHNER, K.
Department of Internal Medicine V, University of Heidelberg,
Hospitalstraße 3, 69115 Heidelberg, Germany

DONSKA, S.
Department of Pediatric Oncology/Hematology, Kiev Regional Oncologic
Dispensary, Baggovutovska Street 1, 04107 Kiev, Ukraine

DREYLING, M.H.
Department of Medicine III, University Hospital Großhadern,
Ludwig-Maximilians-University, Marchioninistraße 15, 81377 Munich,
Germany

EBENER, U.
Department of Hematology and Oncology, Clinic of Pediatrics III,
Johann-Wolfgang-Goethe-University, Theodor-Stern-Kai 7,
60590 Frankfurt/M., Germany

ESTEY, E.H.
Department of Leukemia, Division of Medicine, The University of Texas,
M.D. Anderson Cancer Center, 1515 Holcombe Blvd., Houston, Texas
77030, USA

FEKETE, S.
Szent Laszlo Korhaz, Gyali u. 5/7, 1097 Budapest, Hungary

FIÈRE, D.
Hôpital Edouard Herriot, Service d'Hématologie, Pav. E bis,
Place d'arsonval, 69437 Lyon, Cedex 03, France

FLEGE, S.
Department of Pediatric Hematology/Oncology, Westfälische Wilhelms-
University, Albert-Schweitzer-Straße 33, 48129 Münster, Germany

FLEISCHHACK, G.
Department of Pediatric Haematology/Oncology, University of Bonn,
Adenauerallee 119, 53113 Bonn, Germany

FRÖHLING, S.
Department of Medicine V, University Hospital Heidelberg,
Hospitalstraße 3, 69115 Heidelberg, Germany

GIAGOUNIDIS, A.A.N.
Clinic for Hematology, Oncology, and Clinical Immunology,
Heinrich-Heine-Universität, Moorenstraße 5, 40225 Düsseldorf, Germany

GIESELER, F.
Department of Hematology and Oncology, Clinic of Internal Medicine,
Christian-Albrechts-University of Kiel, Schittenhelmstraße 12, 24105 Kiel,
Germany

HAARMAN, E.G.
Department of Pediatric Hematology/Oncology, University Hospital Vrije
Universiteit, De Boelelaan 1117, 1081 HV, Amsterdam, NL

HANN, I.M.
Haematology Department, Camelia Botnar Laboratories, Great Ormond
Street Hospital for Children NHS Trust, Great Ormond Street,
London WC1N 3JH, UK

HAROUSSEAU, J.L.
Department of Hematology, Hôtel-Dieu, University of Nantes,
Place Alexis Ricordeau, B.P. 1005, 44093 Nantes, Cedex 01, France

HAUS, O.
Department of Genetics, Medical Academy, Marcinkowskiego 1,
50-368 Wroclaw, Poland

HEUSSEL, C.P.
Department of Internal Medicine III, Clinic for Radiology, Johannes-
Gutenberg-University, Langenbeckstraße 1, 55131 Mainz, Germany

HIDDEMANN, W.
Department of Medicine III, University Hospital Großhadern, Ludwig-
Maximilians-University, Marchioninistraße 15, 81377 Munich, Germany

HÖCHSMANN, B.
Department of Internal Medicine III, University of Ulm,
Robert-Koch-Straße 8, 89081 Ulm, Germany

HORN, P.A.
Department of Internal Medicine III, Clinic I for Internal Medicine,
University of Cologne, Joseph-Stelzmann-Straße 9, 50924 Cologne,
Germany

KAHL, C.
Department of Medicine, Division of Hematology/Oncology,
Otto-von-Guericke-University of Magdeburg, Leipziger Straße 44,
39120 Magdeburg, Germany

KAISER, U.
Department of Hematology/Oncology, Philipps-University Marburg,
Baldinger Straße, 35033 Marburg, Germany

KARTHAUS, M.
Ev. Johannes Krankenhaus, Schildescher Straße 101, 33611 Bielefeld,
Germany

KERN, W.
Department of Medicine III, University Hospital Großhadern, Ludwig-
Maximilians-University, Marchioninistraße 15, 81377 Munich, Germany

KOLB, H.-J.
Department of Medicine III, University Hospital Großhadern, Ludwig-
Maximilians-University, Marchioninistraße 15, 81377 Munich, Germany

KRAUTER, J.
Department of Hematology and Oncology, Hannover Medical School,
OE 6860, 30625 Hannover, Germany

LANGE, B.J.
Division of Oncology, The Children's Hospital of Philadelphia,
34th Civic Center Blvd., 19104 Philadelphia, PA, USA

LANGER, Th.
Department of Immunology and Oncology, University Clinic for Children, Friedrich-Alexander-University, Loschgestraße 15, 91054 Erlangen, Germany

LARSON, R.A.
Section of Hematology/Oncology, University of Chicago Medical Center, 5841 S. Maryland Avenue, MC2115, Chicago IL 60637-1470, USA

LEMEZ, P.
Department of Hematology and Blood Transfusion, Hospital Jihlava, Vrchlického 59, 58600 Jihlava, Czech Republic

LERCHENMÜLLER, C.
Department of Medicine, Hematology/Oncology, Westfälische Wilhelms-University of Münster, Albert-Schweitzer-Straße 33, 48129 Münster, Germany

LIE, S.O.
Department of Pediatrics, National Hospital of Norway, Pilestredet 32, 0027 Oslo, Norway

LO COCO, F.
Department of Cellular Biotechnologies and Hematology, University La Sapienza of Rome, Via Benevento 6, 00161 Rome, Italy

LÖWENBERG, B.
Dr. Daniel Den Hoed Cancer Center, Radio-Therapeutic Institute, P.O. Box 5201, 3008 AE Rotterdam, NL

MALINOWSKA, I.
Department of Paediatric Haematology and Oncology, Medical University of Warsaw, Marszalkowska 24, 00-576 Warsaw, Poland

MARMONT, F.
Department of Hematology, San Giovanni Battista Hospital, Corso Bramante 88, 10126 Torino, Italy

MIZUKI, M.
Department of Medicine, Hematology/Oncology, Westfälische Wilhelms-University Münster, Albert-Schweitzer-Straße 33, 48129 Münster, Germany

MUSSO, M.
Department of Hematology, University of Palermo, Via del Vespro No 129, 90127 Palermo, Italy

NACHMANN, J.B.
400 E Randolph St. Apt. 913, Chicago, IL 60601-7305, USA

NIEGEMANN, E.
Department of Hematology and Oncology, Clinic of Pediatrics III, Johann-Wolfgang-Goethe-University, Theodor-Stern-Kai 7, 60590 Frankfurt/M., Germany

OLSHANSKAYA, Yu. V.
Department of Hematological Oncology and BMT, National Center for Hematology, Novozykovsky pr. 4a, 125167 Moscow, Russia

PADRO, T.
Department of Medicine, Hematology/Oncology, Westfälische Wilhelms-University Münster, Albert-Schweitzer-Straße 33, 48129 Münster, Germany

PROCTOR, St.
Department of Haematology, School of Clinical and Laboratory Sciences, Royal Victoria Infirmary, University of Newcastle, Newcastle upon Tyne, NE1 4LP, UK

PUI, C.-H.
St. Jude Children's Research Hospital, 332 North Lauderdale St., Memphis, TN 38105-2729, USA

RAVINDRANATH, Y.
Division of Hematology/Oncology, Department of Pediatrics, Children's Hospital of Michigan, Wayne State University School of Medicine, 3901 Beaubien Boulevard, Detroit, Michigan 48201, USA

REICHLE, A.
Department of Hematology and Oncology, University of Regensburg, Franz-Josef-Strauß-Allee 11, 93042 Regensburg, Germany

REUTER, Ch.W.M.
Department of Hematology and Oncology, University Hospital Ulm, Robert-Koch-Straße 8, 89081 Ulm, Germany

ROLSTON, K.V.I.
Section of Infectious Diseases, The University of Texas, M.D. Anderson Cancer Center, 1515 Holcombe Blvd. (Box 47), Houston, Texas 77030, USA

ROKICKA-MILEWSKA, R.
Department of Paediatric Haematology and Oncology, University Medical School of Warsaw, Marszalkowska 24, 00-576 Warsaw, Poland

RUPPERT, V.
Department of Hematology, Oncology and Tumor Immunology, Robert-Rössle-Clinic, Charité, Humboldt-University of Berlin, 13125 Berlin, Germany

RYZHAK, O.
Department of Pediatric Oncology/Hematology, Kiev Regional Oncologic Dispensary, Baggovutovska Street 1, 04107 Kiev, Ukraine

SAVCHENKO V.
Department of Hematological Oncology and BMT, National Research
Center for Hematology, Novozykovsky pr. 4a, 125167 Moscow, Russia

SCHAISON, G.
Saint Louis Hospital, Av. Vellefaux, 75010 Paris, France

SCHLENK, R.F.
Department of Medicine V, University of Heidelberg, Hospitalstraße 3,
69115 Heidelberg, Germany

SCHNITTGER, S.
Department of Medicine III, University Hospital Großhadern, Ludwig-
Maximilians-University, Marchioninistraße 15, 81377 Munich, Germany

SCHOCH, C.
Department of Medicine III, University Hospital Großhadern, Ludwig-
Maximilians-University, Marchioninistraße 15, 81377 Munich, Germany

SCHUI, D.K.
Department of Hematology/Oncology, Medical Hospital III, Johann-
Wolfgang-Goethe-University, Theodor-Stern-Kai 7, 60590 Frankfurt/M.,
Germany

SCHUMACHER, A.
Department of Medicine, Hematology/Oncology, Westfälische Wilhelms-
University, Albert-Schweitzer-Straße 33, 48129 Münster, Germany

SIKORSKA-FIC, B.
Department of Paediatric Haematology and Oncology, University Medical
School of Warsaw, Marszalkowska 24, 00-576 Warsaw, Poland

SILLING, G.
Department of Medicine, Hematology/Oncology, Westfälische Wilhelms-
University, Albert-Schweitzer-Straße 33, 48129 Münster, Germany

SLAVIN, S.
Department of Bone Marrow Transplantation, Cancer Immunotherapy &
Immunobiology, Research Program, Hadassah University Hospital, POB
12000, Jerusalem 91120, Israel

SNYDER, D.S.
Department of Hematology / Bone Marrow Transplantation, City of Hope
National Medical Center, 1500 E. Duarte Road, Duarte, CA 91010, USA

SPECCHIA, A.
Department of Hematology, Hematology University Policlinic;
Piazza Giulio Cesare, Bari, Italy

STAIB, P.
Department of Internal Medicine III, Clinic I for Internal Medicine, University of Cologne, Joseph-Stelzmann-Straße 9, 50924 Cologne, Germany

STEVENS, R.F.
  Manchester Children's Hospital, Hospital Road, Pendlebury,
  Manchester M27 4HA, UK

STOCKSCHLÄDER, M.
  Department of Hematology and Oncology, University Hospital
  of the Albert-Ludwigs-University, Hugstetter Straße 55, 79106 Freiburg,
  Germany

STONE, R.M.
  Harvard Medical School, Leukemia Program, Dana-Farber Cancer Institute, 44 Binney Street, Boston, MA 02115, USA

SZATROWSKI, T.
  Division of Hematology-Oncology, Weill Medical College of Cornell Uni-
  versity, New York Presbyterian Hospital, 1300 York Avenue C-606,
  New York, N.Y. 10021, USA

TALLMAN, M.S.
  Division of Hematology/Oncology, Department of Medicine,
  Northwestern University Medical School, Robert H. Lurie Comprehensive
  Cancer Center, 233 East Erie Street, # 700, Chicago, IL, 60611, USA

THOMAS, X.
  Service d'Hématologie, Hôpital Edouard Herriot, 69437 Lyon Cedex 03,
  France

VERHOEF, G.
  Department of Haematology, University Hospital Leuven, Herestraat 49,
  3000 Leuven, Belgium

VORWERK, P.
  Department of Pediatric Oncology, Otto-von-Guericke-University
  Magdeburg, Halberstaedter Straße 13, 39112 Magdeburg, Germany

WAGIEL, E.
  Department of Paediatric Haematology and Oncology, University Medical
  School of Warsaw, Marszalkowska 24, 00-576 Warsaw, Poland

WANDT, H.
  Medical Clinic 5, Institute for Medical Oncology/Hematology,
  Prof. Ernst-Nathan-Straße 1, 90340 Nürnberg, Germany

WEHNER, S.
  Department of Hematology and Oncology, Clinic of Pediatrics III,
  Johann-Wolfgang Goethe-University, Theodor-Stern-Kai 7,
  60590 Frankfurt/M., Germany

WESSEL, T.
  Department of Pediatric Hematology/Oncology, Westfälische Wilhelms-
  University, Albert-Schweitzer-Straße 33, 48129 Münster, Germany

WILCZEK, H.E.
Department of Transplantation Surgery, Karolinska Institute, Huddinge
Hospital, Halsovigin 1, B 56, 14186 Stockholm, Sweden

WILHELM, M.
Department of Medicine, University of Würzburg, Klinikstraße 6-8,
97070 Würzburg, Germany

WITHERSPOON, R.P.
Division of Clinical Oncology, Fred Hutchinson Cancer Research Center,
1100 Fairview Avenue N FM804, PO Box 19024, Seattle, WA 98109-1024,
USA

ZARITSKEY, A.
Oncohaematological Department for Adults, BMT Center, City Hospital
N32, pr. Dinamo 3, 197042 St. Petersburg, Russia

ZIMMERMANN, U.
Department of Internal Medicine II, Friedrich-Schiller-University of Jena,
Erlanger Allee 101, 07747 Jena, Germany

ZWAAN, Ch.M.
Department of Pediatric Hematology/Oncology, University Hospital Vrije
Universiteit, De Boelelaan 1117, 1007 MB Amsterdam, NL

**Leukemia Cell Biology**
**Monitoring and Prognosis**

# Mechanisms of Chromosomal Translocation Breakpoints

P. D. Aplan and M. Stanulla

ABSTRACT. Recurrent, non-random chromosomal translocations are causal events for many forms of acute leukemia. The clinical relevance of these non-random translocations is underscored by the use of these translocations in developing risk-directed therapy for many forms of acute leukemia. However, the demonstration that the translocations can be causal events for leukemia immediately raises an important, related question regarding the pathogenesis of leukemia. The essence of this question can be summarized as "if the translocation causes leukemia, what causes the translocation?" We and others have studied several potential mechanisms for the generation of these non-random balanced translocations. These mechanisms include
1. illegitimate V(D)J recombination,
2. homologous recombination between Alu repeats,
3. the recombinogenic potential of alternate "Z" DNA structures, and
4. illegitimate recombination caused by treatment with topoisomerase (topo) II religation inhibitors.

The last mechanism listed deserves special attention given the development of secondary, or therapy-related acute myeloid leukemia (t-AML) following the therapeutic use of topo II religation inhibitors such as the epipodophyllotoxins and the anthracyclines for a primary malignancy.

## 1. Introduction

Since the discovery of the Philadelphia chromosome in leukemic cells of patients with chronic myelogenous leukemia (CML) in 1962 (Nowell PC and Hungerford DA, 1960), it has become apparent that many leukemias and lymphomas are associated with non-random chromosomal abnormalities including deletions, inversions, and translocations (Rabbitts TH, 1994). Several general themes have emerged over the past three decades regarding the clinical and biological significance of chromosomal translocations.

First, specific translocations are often associated with specific types of leukemia. For instance, the t(15;17) is associated with acute promyelocytic leukemia and not other forms of leukemia (Grignani F et al., 1994). Similarly, the t(1;19) translocation is associated with pre-B acute lymphoblastic leukemia, and not other forms of leukemia (Hunger SP, 1996). Of course, there are exceptions to this generalization; the t(9;22) is associated with both CML and acute lymphoblastic leukemia (ALL), and the t(8;14) is associated with both Burkitt's lymphoma and aggressive transitions of follicular lymphoma (Rabbitts TH, 1994). Nonetheless, the association of specific translocations with a specific phenotype has strengthened the suspicion that these translocations are causal events during leukemogenesis.

A second theme relates to the molecular consequences of the translocations. In general, translocations either fuse two distinct genes, with the resultant production of a

This work was supported in part by grants from the Roswell Park Alliance Foundation, the NIH (CA73773) and from the Deutsche Forschungsgemeinschaft. PDA is a Scholar of the Leukemia Society of America. MS is the recipient of a "Kind Philipp-Rückkehrstipendium" through the "Stifterverband der Deutschen Wissenschaft", Essen, Germany.

fusion protein such as the bcr-abl fusion protein associated with CML, or deregulate a normal gene product such as bcl2 deregulation caused by the t(14;18) associated with follicular lymphoma) (Rabbitts TH, 1994; Thandla S and Aplan PD, 1997). A variety of murine experimental models, including transgenic mice and bone marrow reconstitution experiments, have verified that overexpression of many of these presumptive oncoproteins leads to leukemia and/or lymphoma in mice (Korsmeyer SJ, 1992).

The clinical relevance of these non-random chromosomal translocations has been underscored by the use of chromosomal rearrangements in devising risk-appropriate treatment strategies. Retrospective studies have demonstrated that patients with AML whose leukemic cells show certain translocations, for instance t(8;21) have a superior clinical outcome when compared to AML patients without a t(8;21) (Grimwade D et al., 1998). In contrast, pediatric ALL patients whose leukemic cells display a t(4;11) or t(9;22) have a poorer clinical outcome compared to those without these abnormalities; therefore, these patients are selected for intensive therapies, including allogeneic bone marrow transplant in first remission (Rubnitz JE et al., 1996).

## 2. Mechanisms of Chromosomal Translocations

If non-random chromosomal translocations are causal events in leukemogenesis, then a better understanding of the molecular genesis of these translocations would seem to be important in order to understand the more general causes of leukemias (i.e., the translocation may cause the leukemia, but what caused the translocation?). In addition, it is not clear at this point in time whether these non-random chromosomal translocation breakpoints represent sites within the genome that are "fragile", and highly susceptible to breakage and religation, or whether these simply represent sites near growth promoting proto-oncogenes, whose deregulation gives cells which have undergone the translocations a proliferative advantage. Our laboratory has recently become interested in these questions. As a general approach to understanding

mechanisms which underlie these translocations, an initial step is simply to clone and sequence the translocated alleles, as well as their germline counterparts. This approach has provided clues as to the mechanisms which may cause these non-random translocations. Several potential mechanisms for chromosomal translocations have been proposed. These include

i) illegitimate V(D)J recombination,
ii) homologous recombination mediated by *Alu* elements,
iii) *translin* activity,
iv) purine/pyrimidine repeat regions, and
v) DNA topoisomerase II poisons. Each of these potential mechanisms will be discussed in more detail below.

## 3. Chromosomal Translocations Mediated via Illegitimate V(D)J Recombination

In many cases, a powerful argument can be made that a chromosomal translocation is the result of mistakes in normal V(D)J recombinase action (Tycko B and Sklar J, 1990). Most commonly, the translocations attributed to illegitimate V(D)J recombination juxtapose a proto-oncogene to a gene which codes for an antigen receptor (either immunogolobulin or T-cell receptor). The proto-oncogene then becomes activated through immunoglobulin or T-cell receptor gene regulatory regions. The hypothesis that these translocations are the result of illegitimate V(D)J recombinase activity is strengthened by the identification of the hallmarks of normal V(D)J recombinase activity at the translocation breakpoints (Grawunder U et al., 1998; Roth DB and Craig NL, 1998). These features include site-specific DNA cleavage at cryptic heptamer sequences, non-templated "N" region nucleotide addition, and exonucleolytic deletion of germline nucleotides. There are several specific examples of chromosomal translocations where some or all of these features are present (for review see Tcyko and Sklar, 1990).

Furthermore, the most common chromosomal rearrangement leading to proto-oncogene activation in T-cell acute lymphoblastic leukemia (T-ALL) is a site-specific recombination event between the *SIL* and *SCL* (*tal-1,*

TCL5) genes (Bash RO et al., 1993). This recombination event replaces the *SCL* promoter region with the *SIL* promoter, and results in inappropriate expression of *SCL*, under the control of *SIL* regulatory elements, in thymocytes (Aplan PD et al., 1991). Although neither *SIL* nor *SCL* encode antigen receptor genes, the *SIL/SCL* recombination event displays all of the hallmarks of normal V(D)J recombination, including site-specific cleavage at heptamer sequences, "N" region nucleotide addition, and a variable amount of exonucleolytic deletion at the breakpoint junctions (Aplan PD et al., 1990; Brown L et al., 1990).

## 4. Chromosomal Translocations Mediated via alu Elements

Homologous recombination between repetitive *Alu* elements is generally considered to be a common mechanism of recombination in meiotic cells. In some cases, it seems likely that imperfect exchange during meiosis may be responsible for adenosine deaminase deficiency (Markert ML, 1994) or lipoprotein lipase deficiency (Devlin RH et al., 1990). *Alu*-mediated exchange has been implicated in the etiology of some chromosomal translocations, particularly complex translocations involving the *BCR* and *ABL* loci (Jeffs AR et al., 1998). However, the majority of BCR-ABL translocations do not seem to recombine within *Alu* elements (Zhang JG et al., 1995).

Perhaps the most convincing evidence for *Alu*-mediated rearrangement in leukemic cells is the partial tandem duplication of *MLL*, a recent series demonstrated that seven of nine patients with a partial tandem duplication had undergone a rearrangement within *Alu* elements (Strout MP et al., 1998).

## 5. Translin Binding Sequences and Chromosomal Translocations

The *Translin* protein was cloned by virtue of its ability to bind to nucleotide sequences (GCAGA[A/T]C and CCCA[C/G]GAC) that are sometimes found at translocation breakpoints (Aoki K et al., 1995). Subsequently, *translin* has been shown to bind single-strand

DNA ends as well as single-strand RNA (Kasai M et al., 1997), and potential *translin* binding sites have been identified at the breakpoints of a number of chromosomal translocations in solid tumors such as liposarcomas and rhabdomyosarcomas as well as leukemias. However, a mechanism by which *translin* binding might lead to chromosomal translocations remains unknown.

## 6. Chromosomal Translocations and Z-DNA

Regions of alternating purine and pyrimidine residues occur throughout the genome and have the potential to form an unusual left-handed helical structure known as Z-DNA (Drew HR et al., 1988). This unusual DNA structure is preferentially located in internucleosomal regions of the genome, presumably because of the energy cost of compacting Z-DNA into the histone-rich nucleosomes (Garner MM and Felsenfeld G, 1987). Therefore, it is conceivable that these inter-nucleosomal regions have an increased susceptibility to double-strand DNA cleavage compared to histone-bound nucleosomal DNA. Several chromosomal translocation breakpoints (Aplan PD et al., 1992; Boehm T et al., 1989; Thandla SP et al., 1999) associated with ALL have been mapped within or near extended (200+ consecutive bp) tracts of alternating purine and pyrimidine residues (Pu/Py tracts) (Fig. 1). It has been speculated that these regions of potential Z-DNA structure are susceptible to DNA recombination events. This speculation is supported by the observations that these repeat regions are susceptible to "slippage" during DNA replication both in vitro and in vivo (Dutreix M, 1997; Samadashwily GM et al., 1997).

## 7. Chromosomal Translocations Caused by DNA Topoisomerase II Poisons

Over the past decade, treatment-related AML (t-AML) following chemotherapy with DNA topoisomerase (topo) II poisons has been recognized with increasing frequency (Pedersen-Bjergaard J et al., 1995; Smith MA et al., 1996). The topo II poisons that have been

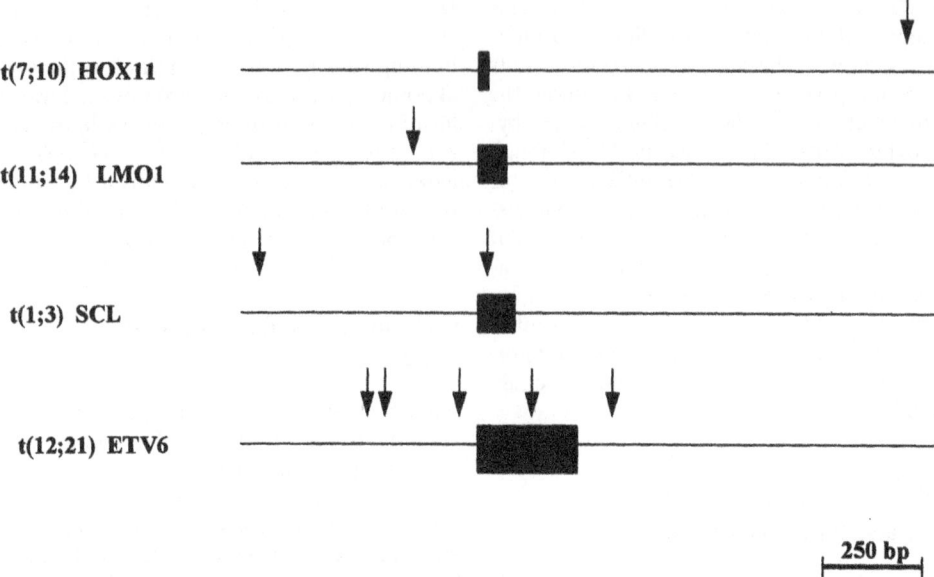

**Fig. 1. Translocation breakpoints near purine/pyrimidine (Pu/Py) repeats.** Four loci (HOX11, LMO1, SCL, ETV6) with known breakpoints near pu/py repeats are shown. Solid box indicates pu/py repeat region; downward arrows represent cloned breakpoints. The scale is shown as base-pairs.

most highly associated with these t-AMLs are the epipodophylotoxins etoposide (VP-16) and teniposide (VM-26) (Smith MA et al., 1994), although the anthracyclines daunorubicin and doxorubicin have also been implicated in t-AML (Felix CA, 1998; Smith MA et al., 1996; Thirman MJ and Larson RA, 1996). In contrast to t-AML associated with alkylating agent chemotherapy, which often demonstrate clonal deletions of 7q or 5q, t-AML associated with topo II poison treatment generally demonstrate balanced chromosomal translocations involving one of a few loci. The most common chromosomal region involved is 11q23, although recurrent breakpoints involving 21q22, and 17q21 have also been reported following topo II poison therapy; rare breakpoints at other loci, such as 16p13 and 11p15 have also been reported. The 11q23 translocations disrupt the *MLL* (also known as *ALL-1* or *HRX*) gene; the breakpoints generally lie within a 8.3 kb breakpoint cluster region (bcr) (Thirman MJ et al., 1993). The consistent association of t-AML, *MLL* translocation breakpoints, short latency periods, and prior exposure to a topo II poison have led many investigators to speculate that

treatment with topo II poisons can directly cause *MLL* translocations and a resultant t-AML (Aplan PD et al., 1996; Smith MA et al., 1994). This speculation is supported by the observation that treatment of peripheral blood lymphocytes in vitro with etoposide can induce chromosomal translocations (Maraschin J et al., 1990).

Our working hypothesis linking topo II inhibitors, chromosomal translocations, and t-AML asserts that topo II poisons induce DNA breaks, many of which are repaired, allowing the cell to proceed through the cell division cycle. Rarely, DNA double strand breaks induced by topo II poisons are repaired improperly, with re-ligation occurring between strands from two distinct chromosomes, resulting in a chromosomal translocation. Certain translocations induced in this manner will give the cell a proliferative advantage, and result in a leukemia. If this hypothesis is true, then the important target cell in t-AML is a normal hematopoietic progenitor cell. Of course, the possibility remains that the individual who suffers a t-AML has a genetic predisposition to malignancy (perhaps through a undiagnosed defect in an enzyme involved in

DNA repair?) and the "normal" hematopoietic precursor which undergoes the translocation is not truly normal.

## 7.1 Topo II Subunit Exchange Model

Topo II normally catalyzes a multi-step reaction consisting of DNA double strand cleavage, strand passage, and religation (Wang JC, 1996). The reaction involves a topo II homodimer, and the half-life of a transient intermediate consisting of topo II monomers covalently bound to the DNA phosphodiester backbone is dramatically increased by topo II poisons. It is thought that these transient intermediates (cleavable complexes) are recognized as damaged DNA, and this recognition triggers the cell to undergo an apoptotic death. It has been speculated that topo II monomeric subunits, covalently bound to DNA, may exchange partners leading to a chromosomal translocation (Baguley BC and Ferguson LR, 1998) (Fig. 2). While DNA rearrangements consistent with this hypothesis have been detected in vitro (Bae Ys et al., 1988), and in hamster cells treated with eto-

poside (Zhou RH et al., 1997), there are as yet no reports of t-AML patients having undergone chromosomal translocations consistent with this process. Arguing against the likelihood of a topo II subunit exchange is the observation that topo II dimers are highly stable in solution (Tennyson RB and Lindsley JE, 1997). The general applicability of this model as a mechanism for t-AML associated with topo II poisons can only be tested through sequence analysis of both germline alleles and both derivative alleles of t-AML patients with balanced translocations.

## 7.2 Site-Specific DNA Cleavage and a DNA-Damage Repair Model

An alternative model to explain the chromosomal translocations induced by topo II poisons has recently been proposed (Reichel M et al., 1998). In this model, the chromosomal translocations are initiated by double-strand DNA cleavage, and created by improper DNA repair. In support of this model, chromosomal translocations from patients with t(4;11) translocations have been cloned and sequen-

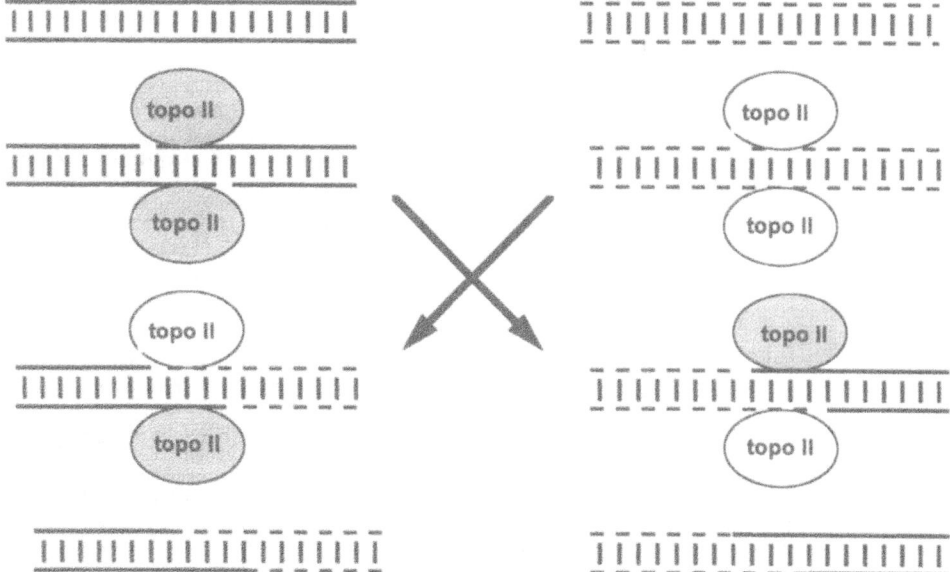

**Fig. 2. Topoisomerase II subunit exchange model.** Two DNA double helices from separate chromosomes are shown as horizontal solid or dotted lines, base pairs are represented by vertical lines. Topoisomerase II subunits are shown as filled or open ovals. Exchange of topoisomerase II subunits produces a reciprocal translocations between two chromosomes, represented by solid and dotted lines.

ced; DNA sequences flanking the breakpoints have been duplicated, deleted, and inverted during the translocation process (Reichel M et al., 1998).

Additionally, our lab and others have demontrated a site near *MLL* exon 9, within the *MLL* breakpoint cluster region (bcr), that is uniquely susceptible to DNA double-strand cleavage induced by treatment with topo II inhibitors (Aplan PD et al., 1996; Strissel PL et al., 1998). Moreover, it has been shown that an identical form of site-specific *MLL* cleavage can be induced in vivo by a wide variety of apoptotic stimuli, and in vitro by DNAse I (Stanulla M et al., 1997; Strissel PL et al., 1998). Taken together, these observations suggest that this site within the *MLL* bcr delineates a region of DNA uniquely susceptible to DNA double strand cleavage. Although it remains to be shown that double strand DNA cleavage at this site is truly an initiating event for chromosomal translocations, there is a recent report (Super HG et al., 1997) of an *MLL* translocation and associated deletion which is consistent with a mechanism whereby the translocation was initiated by cleavage at the exon 9 site, followed by deletion of ~200 nucleotides at each chromosomal end, and religation to chromosome 9, creating the translocation (Fig. 3).

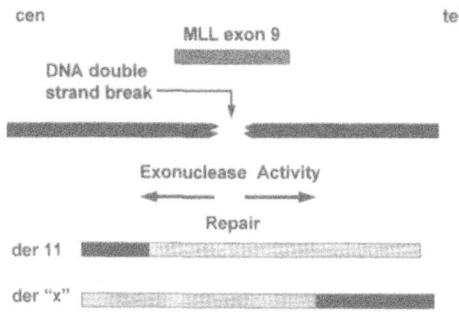

**Fig. 3. DNA break/repair model.** A DNA double strand break occurs at the cleavage site within *MLL* exon 9, followed by processing of the ends by cellular exonucleases, and repair by religation to a non-homologous chromosome ("X" in this example). Note that a corollary of this model is that the translocation would not be perfectly balanced, but rather a translocation/deletion event.

# 8. Summary

Non-random chromosomal translocations have clearly been shown to be causal events for the development of many forms of leukemia; the clinical utility of these translocations is underscored by their use in devising risk-appropriate treatment strategies. However, the mechanisms which cause these recurrent, non-random translocations remain elusive. A more complete understanding of the mechanisms which cause these translocations should be expedited by characterizing large series of breakpoints, and by developing in vitro and/or in vivo model systems which reproducibly recapitulate these translocations.

# References

Aoki K, Suzuki K, Sugano T, Tasaka T, Nakahara K, Kuge O, Omori A, and Kasai M (1995). A novel gene, translin, encodes a recombination hotspot binding protein associated with chromosomal translocations. Nature Genetics *10*, 167-174.

Aplan PD, Chervinsky DS, Stanulla M, and Burhans WC (1996). Site-specific DNA cleavage within the MLL breakpoint cluster region induced by topoisomerase II inhibitors. Blood *87*, 2649-58.

Aplan PD, Lombardi DP, Ginsberg AM, Cossman J, Bertness Vl, and Kirsch IR (1990). Disruption of the human SCL locus by »illegitimate« V-(D)-J recombinase activity. Science *250*, 1426-9.

Aplan PD, Lombardi DP, and Kirsch IR (1991). Structural characterization of SIL, a gene frequently disrupted in T-cell acute lymphoblastic leukemia. Molecular & Cellular Biology *11*, 5462-9.

Aplan PD, Raimondi SC, and Kirsch IR (1992). Disruption of the SCL gene by a t(1;3) translocation in a patient with T cell acute lymphoblastic leukemia. Journal of Experimental Medicine *176*, 1303-10.

Bae Ys, Kawasaki I, Ikeda H, and Liu Lf (1988). Illegitimate recombination mediated by calf thymus DNA topoisomerase II in vitro. Proceedings of the National Academy of Sciences of the United States of America *85*, 2076-80.

Baguley BC, and Ferguson LR (1998). Mutagenic properties of topoisomerase-targeted drugs. Biochimica et Biophysica Acta *1400*, 213-22.

Bash RO, Crist WM, Shuster JJ, Link MP, Amylon M, Pullen J, Carroll AJ, Buchanan GR, Smith RG, and Baer R (1993). Clinical features and outcome of T-cell acute lymphoblastic leukemia in childhood with respect to alterations at the TAL1 locus: a Pediatric Oncology Group study. Blood *81*, 2110-7.

Boehm T, Mengle-Gaw L, Kees Ur, Spurr N, Lavenir I, Forster A, and Rabbitts Th (1989). Alternating purine-pyrimidine tracts may promote chromosomal translocations seen in a variety of human lymphoid tumours. EMBO Journal *8*, 2621-31.

Brown L, Cheng JT, Chen Q, Siciliano MJ, Crist W, Buchanan G, and Baer R (1990). Site-specific recombination of the tal-1 gene is a common occurrence in human T cell leukemia. EMBO Journal 9, 3343-51.

Devlin RH, Deeb S, Brunzell J, and Hayden MR (1990). Partial gene duplication involving exon-Alu interchange results in lipoprotein lipase deficiency. American Journal of Human Genetics 46, 112-9.

Drew HR, McCall MJ, and Calladine CR (1988). Recent studies of DNA in the crystal. Annual Review of Cell Biology 4, 1-20.

Dutreix M (1997). (GT)(n) repetitive tracts affect several stages of RecA-promoted recombination. Journal of Molecular Biology 273, 105-113.

Felix CA (1998). Secondary leukemias induced by topoisomerase-targeted drugs. Biochimica et Biophysica Acta Gene Structure & Expression 1400, 233-255.

Garner MM, and Felsenfeld G (1987). Effect of Z-DNA on nucleosome placement. Journal of Molecular Biology 196, 581-90.

Grawunder U, West RB, and Lieber MR (1998). Antigen receptor gene rearrangement. Current Opinion in Immunology 10, 172-180.

Grignani F, Fagioli M, Alcalay M, Longo L, Pandolfi PP, Donti E, Biondi A, Lo Coco F, Grignani F, and Pelicci PG (1994). Acute promyelocytic leukemia: from genetics to treatment. Blood 83, 10-25.

Grimwade D, Walker H, Oliver F, Wheatley K, Harrison C, Harrison G, Rees J, Hann I, Stevens R, Burnett A, and Goldstone A (1998). The importance of diagnostic cytogenetics on outcome in AML - analysis of 1,612 patients entered into the MRC AML 10 trial. Blood 92, 2322-2333.

Hunger SP (1996). Chromosomal translocations involving the E2A gene in acute lymphoblastic leukemia: clinical features and molecular pathogenesis. Blood 87, 1211-24.

Jeffs AR, Benjes SM, Smith TL, Sowerby SJ, and Morris CM (1998). The Bcr gene recombines preferentially with Alu elements in complex Bcr-Abl translocations of chronic myeloid leukaemia. Human Molecular Genetics 7, 767-776.

Kasai M, Matsuzaki T, Katayanagi K, Omori A, RT, M., Strominger JL, Aoki K, and Suzuki K (1997). The translin ring specifically recognizes DNA ends at recombination hot spots in the human genome. Journal of Biological Chemistry 272, 11402-11407.

Korsmeyer SJ (1992). Chromosomal translocations in lymphoid malignancies reveal novel proto-oncogenes. Annual Review of Immunology 10, 785-807.

Maraschin J, Dutrillaux B, and Aurias A (1990). Chromosome aberrations induced by etoposide (VP-16) are not random. International Journal of Cancer 46, 808-12.

Markert ML (1994). Molecular basis of adenosine deaminase deficiency. Immunodeficiency 5, 141-57.

Nowell PC, and Hungerford DA (1960). A minute chromosome in human chronic granulocytic leukemia. Science 132, 1497-1499.

Pedersen-Bjergaard J, Pedersen M, Roulston D, and Philip P (1995). Different genetic pathways in leukemogenesis for patients presenting with therapy-related myelodysplasia and therapy-related acute myeloid leukemia. Blood 86, 3542-52.

Rabbitts TH (1994). Chromosomal translocations in human cancer. Nature 372, 143-9.

Reichel M, Gillert E, Nilson I, Siegler G, Greil J, Fey GH, and Marschalek R (1998). Fine structure of translocation breakpoints in leukemic blasts with chromosomal translocation t(4;11): the DNA damage-repair model of translocation. Oncogene 17, 3035-44.

Roth DB, and Craig NL (1998). V(D)J recombination - a transposase goes to work. Cell 94, 411-414.

Rubnitz JE, Behm FG, and Downing JR (1996). 11q23 rearrangements in acute leukemia. Leukemia 10, 74-82.

Samadashwily GM, Raca G, and Mirkin SM (1997). Trinucleotide repeats affect DNA replication in vivo. Nature Genetics 17, 298-304.

Smith MA, McCaffrey RP, and Karp JE (1996). The secondary leukemias: challenges and research directions. Journal of the National Cancer Institute 88, 407-18.

Smith MA, Rubinstein L, and Ungerleider RS (1994). Therapy-related acute myeloid leukemia following treatment with epipodophyllotoxins: estimating the risks. Medical & Pediatric Oncology 23, 86-98.

Stanulla M, Wang J, Chervinsky DS, Thandla S, and Aplan PD (1997). DNA cleavage within the MLL breakpoint cluster region is a specific event which occurs as part of higher-order chromatin fragmentation during the initial stages of apoptosis. Molecular & Cellular Biology 17, 4070-9.

Strissel PL, Strick R, Rowley JD, and Zeleznik-Le NJ (1998). An in vivo topoisomerase II cleavage site and a DNase I hypersensitive site colocalize near exon 9 in the MLL breakpoint cluster region. Blood 92, 3793-803.

Strout MP, Marcucci G, Bloomfield CD, and Caligiuri MA (1998). The partial tandem duplication of ALL1 (MLL) is consistently generated by Alu-mediated homologous recombination in acute myeloid leukemia. Proceedings of the National Academy of Sciences of the United States of America 95, 2390-2395.

Super HG, Strissel PL, Sobulo OM, Burian D, Reshmi SC, Roe B, Zeleznik-Le NJ, Diaz MO, and Rowley JD (1997). Identification of complex genomic breakpoint junctions in the t(9;11) MLL-AF9 fusion gene in acute leukemia. Genes, Chromosomes & Cancer 20, 185-95.

Tennyson RB, and Lindsley JE (1997). Type II DNA topoisomerase from Saccharomyces cerevisiae is a stable dimer. Biochemistry 36, 6107-14.

Thandla S, and Aplan PD (1997). Molecular biology of acute lymphocytic leukemia. Seminars in Oncology 24, 45-56.

Thandla SP, Ploski JE, Raza-Egilmez SZ, Chhalliyil PP, Block AW, de Jong PJ, and Aplan PD (1999). ETV6-AML1 translocation breakpoints cluster near a purine/pyrimidine repeat region in the ETV6 gene. Blood 93, 293-299.

Thirman MJ, Gill HJ, Burnett RC, Mbangkollo D, McCabe NR, Kobayashi H, Zieminvanderpoel S, Kaneko Y, Morgan R, Sandberg AA, Chaganti RSK, Larson RA, Lebeau MM, Diaz MO, and Rowley JD (1993). Rearrangement of the MLL gene in acute lymphoblastic and acute myeloid leukemias with 11q23 chromosomal translocations. New England Journal of Medicine 329, 909-914.

Thirman MJ, and Larson RA (1996). Therapy-related myeloid leukemia. Hematology Oncology Clinics of North America 10, 293-320.

Tycko B, and Sklar J (1990). Chromosomal translocations in lymphoid neoplasia: a reappraisal of the recombinase model. Cancer Cells 2, 1-8.

Wang JC (1996). DNA topoisomerases. Annual Review of Biochemistry 65, 635-692.

Zhang JG, Goldman JM, and Cross CNP (1995). Characterization of genomic BCR-ABL breakpoints in chronic myeloid leukaemia by PCR. British Journal of Haematology 90, 138-146.

Zhou RH, Wang P, Zou Y, Jackson-Cook CK, and Povirk LF (1997). A precise interchromosomal reciprocal exchange between hot spots for cleavable complex formation by topoisomerase II in amsacrine-treated Chinese hamster ovary cells. Cancer Research 57, 4699-4702.

# Hematologic Malignancies Following Organ Transplantation

H. E. WILCZEK and C. BRATTSTRÖM

Organ transplantation and the subsequent life-long immunosuppression increases the risk of developing a malignancy after transplantation. This is well in accordance with the assumption that an impaired immune system permits carcinogenic factors to act uncontrolled. Several studies have demonstrated an overall cancer incidence of 6%, ranging from 4–18%, which is 3–5 times higher than that of the general population [1, 2].

Posttransplant malignancies occur in age group younger than the general population and are often more aggressive.

## Risk of malignancy

An extremely high relative risk (10–30 times that in the general population) has been observed for non-Hodgkin lymphomas, skin/lip cancer, cancer of the vulva and vagina and endocrine gland tumors [3]. Elevated risks (2–5 times that in the general population) are seen for cancers of the colon, recturn, larynx, lung, kidney and bladder, melanomas, brain and central nervous system tumors as well as leukemia [3]. The commonest malignancies involve the skin and lips (37% of all tumors), with the incidence varying proportionally with the amount of exposure to sunshine.

## Time of cancer occurrence after transplantation

Some cancers quite consistently develop soon after transplantation, while others manifest themselves later. The early-occurring cancers, include the lymphomas, Kaposi_s sarcoma and cancer of the endocrine glands. Kaposi_s sarcoma is the first to develop, at an average of 21 months (range 2–225 months), lymphomas are found at an average of 32 months (range 1–254 months) [1] after transplantation while cancer of the viscera, breast and blood tend to occur later, with mean times of diagnosis at 7–8 years. If all cancers are considered, the average time of their appearance is 61 months (range 1–298 months) [1].

## Hematologic malignancies

Hematologic malignancies after organ transplantation are predominantly made up by the lymphomas. These tumors are second only to cutaneous neoplasms in their frequency. The incidence varies with the organ transplanted, ranging from approximately 1% of renal transplant recipients, to 2.7% of hepatic allograft recipients, 4–6% of heart or heart-lung transplant recipients and 19% of intestinal transplant recipients [4–8]. The lymphomas comprise 57% and 47%, respectively, of all posttransplant malignancies in hepatic and cardiac transplant recipients compared to 12% in renal transplant recipients [1, 9]. Hepatic and cardiac transplant recipients are given more intensive immunosuppressive medication to prevent rejection. The difference in lymphoma incidence most probably reflects the more intensive immunosuppression given. The lymphomas in the hepatic transplant population appeared earlier (median 6 months) than after renal transplantation (median 26 months).

Department of Transplantation Surgery, Karolinska Institute, Huddinge Hospital, Stockholm, Sweden

Only 2–3% of the lymphomas after transplantation are cases of Hodgkin_s disease, whereas it comprises 10–14% of lymphomas in the general population [1, 6]. Similarly, myeloma and plasmacytoma comprise <4% of cases compared with an approximately 20% incidence among lymphoproliferative disorders in the general population [1, 6]. The overwhelming majority of the posttransplant lymphomas consist of non-Hodgkin lymphomas (approximately 93–94%) of the total, compared to only 65% in the general population. The incidence of non-Hodgkin lymphomas is estimated to be 28–49 fold over that seen in age-matched controls [1, 10]. 87% of the non-Hodgkin lymphomas have been shown to be of B-cell origin, approximately 12.6 are of T-cell origin and 0.4% are of null cell origin [11].

Posttransplant lymphoproliferative disorders show an even stronger dominance in pediatric recipients compared to adults. Lymphomas comprised 53% of malignancies in transplanted children, compared with 15% in adult recipients [1, 12]. On reason that lymphomas are commoner in pediatric transplant patients is that children have more lymphoid tissue, which may become the site of these neoplasms. In addition, primary infections with Epstein-Barr virus are more common in children than in adults, and under immunosuppression this is more likely to mutate into posttransplant lymphoproliferative disease.

## Epstein-Barr virus as risk factor for developing posttransplant lymphoproliferative disorder

Studies have demonstrated that 90–95% of posttransplant lymphoproliferative disorders are positive for Epstein-Barr virus [13]. One significant risk factor is a seronegative status at the time of transplantation, which may result in primary EBV infection after transplantation is carrying a significant risk for the development of posttransplant lymphoproliferative disease. Some investigators found that as many as 11% seronegative pediatric and 5% of seronegative adult recipients developed lymphomas in contrast to only 0% and 2% in seropositive transplant recipients [14]. The relative incidence ratio has been found to be 76 times higher in seronegative than in seropositive patients [15].

## Localization of posttransplantation lymphomas and clinical presentation

Between 51–53% of posttransplant lymphomas involve multiple organs or sites, and 47–49% are localized to a single organ or site [1, 6]. Seventy percent of posttransplant lymphomas develop in extranodal locations in contrast to lymphomas in the general population which frequently involve lymph nodes (52–76%) [6]. The organs most often affected are the liver (25%), lungs (21%), central nervous system (21%), intestines (19%), kidneys (18%) and spleen (12%) [6]. The central nervous system, often the brain parenchyma, is affected in about 26% in contrast to only 1% in the general population [1, 6]. Clinical symptoms may be very variable. In cases with renal dysfunction the diagnosis has sometimes been mistaken for rejection. Patients may be asymptomatic or present with a picture resembling infectious mononucleosis. If the transplanted organ is affected a palpable mass may be felt. Other symptoms are usually related to the organ(s) affected. A suspicion of CNS lymphoma be aroused whenever a transplant patient develops neurologic symptoms. Symptoms are usually more prominent if the disease manifests itself early after transplantation, while lymphomas that develop late (>1 year after transplantation) often run a more gradual course with less dramatic systemic symptoms.

## Morbidity and mortality in patients developing malignancies after transplantation

In general, posttransplant malignancies prove to be aggressive. The occurrence of malignancy after kidney transplantation significantly affect the patient_s survival: survival of transplant patients with cancer was 77% at 5 years, 59% at 10 years and 44% at 20 years versus 87%, 80%, and 72% respectively, in patients without cancer [15]. In a series of 26 patients who developed posttransplant lymphoproliferative disorders after solid organ transplantation during a 27 year period, 21 (81%) patients died (median survival time 14 months) despite aggressive treatment including reduction in immunosuppressive therapy [17].

## Treatment and prevention of posttransplant lymphomas

Multimodality therapy is often used. A large proportion of more extensive malignant lesions have partially or completely regressed after reduction or discontinuation of immunosuppressive therapy, which often seems to be the treatment of choice. Localized lesions may be available for surgical excision or treatment with radiation therapy. Other therapeutic options are trials with acyclovir, interferon and anti-B-cell antibodies. Chemotherapy can be necessary in selected cases, but should be regarded as a treatment of last resort for posttransplant lymphoproliferative disease refractory to reduction in immunosuppression. Once the posttransplant lymphoproliferative disease has regressed, immunosuppression may be resumed in small doses. Recurrence of posttransplant lymphoproliferative disease occurs in <5% of cases [18]. Retransplantation should not be considered until at least 1 year or more after complete remission [19].

## Leukemia

Although lymphomas are the most common of the hematologic malignant neoplasms, myelogenous leukemias have also been encountered. Acute and chronic leukemia have a slightly increased incidence in transplanted patients on immunosuppressive therapy [20]. Compared with the general population (incidence 3–4/100000), the incidence in the transplant population is estimated to be approximately 5-fold increased (incidence 5/25000) [21]. Chronic granulocytic leukemia is the most common leukemia observed after organ transplantation [22]. Chronic myelomonocytic leukemia and acute myeloid leukemia following renal transplantation has also been reported [23, 24]. Chronic granulocytic leukemia in the transplanted

patient seems to develop rapidly. The warning signals seen in these patients usually consists of a progressive leukocytosis in the absence of fever, and the leukocytosis in disproportionate to the amount maintenance steroid dose given [22, 25]. Often there is also thrombocytosis and no splenomegaly. The clinical course of chronic granulocytic leukemia after transplantation appears to be similar to that seen in the general population and it seems to respond to similar therapies.

## Summary

In the transplanted population, lymphomas constitute the second largest group of cancers, exceeded only by cancers of skin and lips. Leukemias also occur with an increased frequency but to a much lesser extent. Lymphomas are best treated by the reduction or cessation of immunosuppression, and for leukemias standard antileukemic treatment is used.

## References

1. Penn I. Tumours after renal and cardiac transplantation. Hematology/Oncology Clinics of North America, 7: 431–445, 1993.
2. Penn I. Malignant neoplasia in the immunosuppressed patient. In Cooper DKC, Novitsky D eds. The transplantation and replacement of thoracic organs. The presents status of biological and mechanical replacement of the heart and lungs. Dordrecht, Kluwer Academic Publishers, 1990; p 183.
3. Penn I. The effect of immunosuppression on pre-existing cancers. Transplantation 55 (4): 742–747, 1993.
4. Nalesnik MA, Makowka L, Starzl TE. The diagnosis and treatment of posttransplant lymphoproliferative disorders. Curr Probl Surg, 25: 367–472, 1988.
5. Armitage JM, Kormos RL, Stuart RS, Fricker FJ, Griffith BP, Nalesnik M, Hardsty RL. Dummer JS. Posttransplant lymphoproliferative disease in thoracic organ transplant patients: ten years of cyclosporine-based immunosuppression. J Heart Lung Transplant 10: 877–886, 1991.
6. Penn I. De novo cancers in organ allograft recipients. Curr Opinion in Organ Transpl, 3: 188–196, 1998.
7. Nalesnik MA. Clinicopathologic features of post-transplant lymphoproliferative disorders. Ann Transplant 2: 33–40, 1997.
8. Nalesnik MA, Locker, Jaffe R, Reyes J, Cooper M, Fung J, Starzl TE. Experience with posttransplant lymphoproliferative disorders in solid organ transplant recipients. Clin Transpl 6: 249–252, 1992.

9. Penn I. Posttransplantation de novo tumors in liver allograft recipients. Liver Transpl Surg 2 (1): 52–59, 1996.

10. Kinlen LJ. Incidence of cancer in rheumatoid arthritis and other disorders after immunosuppressive treatment. Am J Med (1A): 44, 195.

11. Penn I. Malignancy. Surg Clin N Am, 74 (5): 1247–1257, 1994.

12. Penn I. Posttransplant malignancies in pediatric organ transplant recipients. Transplant Proc 26 (5): 2763–2765, 1994.

13. Hanto DW. Classification of Epstein-Barr virus-associated posttransplant lymphoproliferative diseases: Implications for understanding their pathogenesis and developing rational treatment strategies. Annual Rev Med 46: 381–394, 1995.

14. Ho M, Jaffe R, Miller G, Breinig MK, Dummer JS, Makowka L, Atchison RW, Karrer F, Nalesnik MA, Starzl TE. The frequency of Epstein-Barr virus infection and associated lymphoproliferative syndrome after transplantation and its manifestations in children. Transplantation 45: 719–727, 1988.

15. Walker RC, Paya CV, Marshall WF, Strickler JG, Wiesner RH, Velosa JA, Haberman TM, Daly RC, McGregor CG. Pretransplantation seronegative Epstein-Barr virus status is the primary risk factor for posttransplantation lymphoproliferative disorder in adult heart, lung and other solid organ transplantation. J Heart Lung Transplant 14: 214–221, 1995.

16. Hiesse C, Kriaa F, Rieu P, Larue JR, Benoit G, Bellamy J, Blanchet P, Charpentier B. Incidence and type of malignancies occurring after renal transplantation in conventionally and cyclosporine-treated recipients: analysis of a 20-year period in 1600 patients. Transplant Proc 27 (1): 972–974, 1995.

17. Morrison VA, Dunn DL, Manivel JC, Gajl Peczalska KJ, Peterson BA. Clinical characteristics of post-transplant lymphoproliferative disorders. Am J Med 97 (1): 14–24, 1994.

18. Wu TT, Swerdlow SH, Locker J, Bahier D, Randhawa PS, Yunis E, Dickman PS, Nalesnik MA. Recurrent Epstein-Barr virus-associated lesions in organ transplant recipients. Hum Pathol 27: 157–164, 1996

19. Penn I. Risks of recurrence of posttransplant lymphoproliferative disease, Hodgkin_s disease or Kaposi_s sarcoma after retransplantation. In Touraine JL, Traeger J, Bétuel H, Dubernard JM, Revillard JP, Dupuy C eds. Retransplantation. Dordrecht, Kluwer Academic Publishers, pp 45–53, 1997.

20. Brunner FP, Landais P, Selwood H. Malignancies after renal transplantation: the EDTA-ERA registry experience. Nephrol Dial Transplant 10 (1): 74–80, 1995.

21. Penn I. Recent results in cancer research. N.Y., Springer-Verlag Inc., 69: 7–13, 1979.

22. Kirchner KA, Files JC, Didlake R, Seshadri R, Krueger RP. Chronic granulocytic leukemia after renal transplantation. Arch Intern Med, 143: 1984–1987, 1983.

23. Shima T, Oku N, Goto H, Inaba T, Murakami S, Itoh K, Fujita N, Shimazaki C, Misawa S, Nakagawa M. Chronic myelomonocytic leukemia and esophageal cancer developed in a renal allograft recipient. Rinsho Ketsueki (Japanese Journal of Clinical Hematology), 34 (7): 842–846, 1993.

24. Hand MF, Anderton JL. Acute myeloid leukaemia following renal transplantation and previous Wilms_ tumour. Nephr Dialysis Transpl, 7 (7): 653, 1992.

25. Adler KR, Lempert N, Scharfman WB. Chronic granulocytic leukemia following successful renal transplantation. Cancer 41: 2206–2208, 1978.

# Molecular Cytogenetic Characterization of a Critical Region in Bands 7q35–q36 Commonly Deleted in Malignant Myeloid Disorders

K. Döhner[1], U. Hehmann[1], J. Brown[1], C. Hetzel[1], J. Stewart[2], G. Lowther[2], C. Scholl[1], S. Fröhling[1], A. Cuneo[3], L.C. Tsui[4], P. Lichter[5], S.W. Scherer[4] and H. Döhner[1]

## Introduction

Cytogenetic studies have shown loss of chromosome 7 (-7) or deletions of the long arm (7q-) in various tumor types. These findings suggest that chromosome 7 harbours tumor suppressor genes which play a role in the pathogenesis of these malignancies (Atkin et al. 1993; Zenklusen et al. 1996). In particular, in myeloid disorders loss of -7/7q- are among the most frequent chromosome abnormalities. These aberrations are associated with myelodysplastic syndrome (MDS) and acute myeloid leukemia (AML), in particular with therapy-related MDS/AML (t-MDS/t-AML) following therapy with alkylating agents or secondary MDS/AML after occupational exposure to chemical mutagens (Le Beau et al. 1986).

Furthermore, -7/7q- occur in MDS/AML that develop in patients with constitutional disorders (eg, Fanconi's anemia, Kostmann's syndrome, neurofibromatosis type 1, familial monosomy 7) (Luna-Fineman et al. 1995). Clinically, myeloid leukemias exhibiting -7/7q- have been associated with high susceptibility to infections, poor response to chemotherapy, and short survival times (Bloomfield and de la Chapelle 1987). Based on chromosome banding analysis, two critical regions have been identified, one in band 7q22, and another in bands 7q32-q35. The association of -7/7q- with myeloid leukemia suggests that these regions contain novel tumor suppressor gene(s), whose loss of function contribute to leukemic transformation or tumor progression. The molecular delineation of the proximal critical region in 7q22 has been focus of attention of several investigators. Using fluorescence in situ hybridization (FISH) and loss of heterozygosity (LOH) studies, distinct critical regions in bands 7q22-q31.1 have been identified which are shown to be commonly deleted or contain translocation/inversion breakpoints in myeloid disorders (Kere et al. 1989a; Lewis et al. 1996; Le Beau et al. 1996; Johnson et al. 1996; Fischer et al. 1997). In contrast, only scarce data are available on the molecular characterization of the distal critical region (Döhner et al. 1998; Koike et al. 1999).

In the present study, we analyzed samples from 15 patients with myeloid leukemia exhibiting deletions or translocations affecting bands 7q31-qter by FISH. As probes we selected representative yeast artificial chromosome (YAC) clones from a physical map encompassing bands 7q31-qter (Cohen et al. 1993; Kunz et al. 1994; Scherer et al. 1992). Because overlapping YACs were used, it was possible to systematically delineate the extent of the deletions and to locate the breakpoint of one reciprocal translocation at the molecular level.

## Delineation of 7q31-qter Aberrations Using Chromosome Banding Analysis

In myeloid disorders loss of the whole chromosome 7 represents the most common abnormality, thus the delineation of a com-

[1]Department of Internal Medicine V, University of Heidelberg, Hospitalstraße 3, 69115 Heidelberg, Germany
[2]Duncan Guthrie Institute of Medical Genetics, Glasgow, Scotland
[3]Dipartimento di Scienze Biomediche e Terapie Avanzate Univerista Degli Studi di Ferrara, Italy
[4]The Department of Genetics, The Hospital for Sick Children, Toronto, Canada
[5]Department „Organisation of Complex Genomes", German Cancer Research Center, Im Neuenheimer Feld 280, Heidelberg, Germany

monly deleted segment on 7q has been more difficult than that of deletions of other chromosomes. Fewer myeloid tumors are available for analysis which exhibit an interstitial or a terminal deletion. Furthermore, deletions/translocations involved in the distal critical region are scarce and occur in only approximately 20% of myeloid tumors exhibiting 7q aberrations. In a study of 54 patients with MDS and AML by Rodrigues Pereira Velloso et al. (1996), 7q22 and 7q32 were the most commonly deleted bands in the proximal and distal critical region, respectively. Le Beau et al. (1996) reported on 16 cases with de novo MDS/AML and t-MDS/t-AML exhibiting deletions involving the distal part of 7q. All deletions were interstitial with the proximal and the majority of distal breakpoints localized to 7q31 or 7q32 and 7q36, respectively. The commonly deleted segment in this study was defined to bands 7q32-q33.

In our study (Döhner et al. 1998), we analyzed bone marrow and blood samples from 13 patients with myeloid leukemia [de novo MDS, n=3; de novo AML, n=9; t-AML, n=1]. As determined by chromosome banding analysis, 11 of the 13 cases had aberrations involving bands 7q31-qter. The remaining two cases could only be characterized by FISH. In contrast to the studies reported by Rodrigues Pereira Velloso et al. (1996) and Le Beau et al. (1996) we localized the commonly deleted segment of these deletions to chromosomal bands 7q35-qter. Interestingly, one case which exhibited a balanced translocation t(3;7) with a breakpoint in band 7q34 or q35 also had a monosomy 7. This patient had received total body irradiation and high-dose cyclophosphamid followed by autologous bone marrow transplantation for stage IV follicular lymphoma. Two years after transplantation the patient developed t-MDS which rapidly progressed to t-AML. Cytogenetic analysis of phytohemagglutinin (PHA)-stimulated blood at the time of diagnosis of the t-AML showed a normal karyotype.

## Delineation of 7q31-qter Aberrations by Molecular Cytogenetics (FISH)

To the present day, only scarce data are available on the molecular delineation of the distal critical region and no tumor suppressor gene of pathogenetic signifiance has yet been identified.

FISH using contiguously mapped DNA probes is a very powerful tool to delineate commonly deleted segments at the molecular level more precisely (Johnson et al. 1996; Le Beau et al. 1996; Fischer et al. 1997). We previously reported on a series of 13 patients with various myeloid leukemias (Döhner et al. 1998). We now have extended this series to 15 tumors which on chromosome banding analysis exhibited deletions, or in one case a reciprocal translocation of bands 7q31-qter. For the metaphase and interphase FISH experiments we selected representative clones from a panel of YAC clones (Fig.1) that were previously mapped to chromosome bands 7q31.1-qter including a set of contiguously mapped YACs in bands 7q35-q36. Detailed information on the YACs is available at:http://www.genet.sickkids.on.ca/chromosome7/ and http://www.ceph.fr/ceph-genethon-map.html.

The results of the deletion/translocation mapping by FISH are given in Fig.1. In the 15 cases exhibiting 7q31-qter deletions, unbalanced translocations, or monosomy 7 within a complex karyotype, we identified a commonly deleted segment in bands 7q35-q36. This commonly deleted segment extended from YAC HSC7E124 in the distal part of 7q35 to YAC C_724_G_5 in the proximal part of band 7q36 (Fig.1). This region comprises approximately 4 to 5 Mb. The proximal and distal boundaries of this segment were defined by 3 cases each (nos. 5, 6, 7 and nos. 1, 5, 7, respectively). The breakpoint of the t(3;7)(p13;q34 or q35) was mapped to a 1300 kb genomic segment encompassed by YAC C_945_H_1 in band 7q35. This genomic segment is located near the proximal boundary of the commonly deleted region. Based on the available physical map the distance between the translocation breakpoint and the commonly deleted region is estimated to be in the range of 2 to 3 Mb. Interestingly, in this case chromosome 7 was homozygously affected by somatically acquired rearrangements, one homolog was lost (-7) and the second exhibited the t(7q34 or 7q35). One possible interpretation of the significance of this translocation breakpoint is that – by analogy to the proxi-

| Chromosome 7 | YAC | Band | MDS | | | | AML | | | | | | | | | | t-AML |
|---|---|---|---|---|---|---|---|---|---|---|---|---|---|---|---|---|---|
| | | | 1 | 2 | 3 | 4 | 5 | 6 | 7 | 8 | 9 | 10 | 11 | 12 | 13 | 14 | 15 |
| | HSC7E481 | 7q21.1-q21.3 | | | | di | di | di | | | di | di | di | di | di | di | di | |
| | HSC7E506 | 7q22 | | di | | | di | di | del | | di | di | di | di | di | di | di | di |
| | HSC7E161 | 7q22.3-q31.1 | | | di | di | di | | del | | di | di | di | | di | di | del | di |
| | HSC7E132 | 7q22.3-q31.1 | | | | del | | | del | | | | | di | di | del | | di |
| | HSC7E589 | 7q22.3-q31.1 | | | di | | | | | | | | | del | del | del | del | del |
| | HSC7E222 | 7q31.3-q32.1 | | | di | del | | | | | | | | del | del | | | di |
| | HSC7E648 | 7q33-q34 | | di | del | del | | di | di | del | di | di | del | del | del | del | del | di |
| | HSC7E1175 | 7q33-q35 | | di | del | del | | di | | del | di | di | del | del | del | del | del | di |
| | HSC7E116 | 7q33-q35 | di | del | del | del | di | di | di | del | di | del | del | del | del | del | del | di |
| | HSC7E190 | 7q34-q35 | del | del | del | del | di | di | di | del | del | del | del | del | del | del | del | di |
| | HSC7E248 | 7q35-q36 | del | del | del | del | di | di | di | del | del | del | del | del | del | del | del | di |
| | HSC7E630 | 7q35 | del | del | del | del | di | di | di | del | di | di | del | del | del | del | del | di |
| | C_940_A_12 | 7q34-q35 | del | del | del | del | di | di | di | del | del | del | del | del | del | del | del | di |
| | C_761_H_5 | 7q34-q35 | del | del | del | del | di | di | di | del | del | del | del | del | del | del | del | di |
| | C_745_G_6 | 7q33-q35 | del | del | del | del | di | di | di | del | del | del | del | del | del | del | del | di |
| | C_945_H_1 | 7q33-q35 | del | del | del | del | di | di | di | del | del | del | del | del | del | del | del | t |
| | HSC7E162 | 7q34-q35 | di | di | | | di | di | di | del | del | | del | del | | del | del | di |
| | C_932_D_12 | 7q35-q36 | di | di | | del | di | di | di | | del | | | | | | | di |
| | HSC7E124 | 7q35 | | | | | di | di | di | del | del | del | del | del | del | | | di |
| | HSC7E131 | 7q36 | | | | | | di | di | di | del | di | di | del | del | | | di |
| | C_868_G_5 | 7q35-q36 | | | | | | del | di | di | del | di | del | del | del | del | del | di |
| | C_880_B_7 | 7q35-q36 | del | di | | | | del | di | di | di | di | del | del | del | del | del | di |
| | HSC7E113 | 7q36 | di | di | di | di | di | di | di | di | di | di | del | del | del | del | del | di |
| | C_724_G_5 | 7q36 | | | | | di | | | | | | | | | | | |
| | HSC7E802 | 7q36 | | | | del | | del | di | di | del | del | del | del | del | del | di | di |
| | HSC7E224 | 7q36 | | del | | | | del | di | di | di | di | del | del | del | del | del | di |
| | HSC7E769 | 7q36 | di | di | del | | | di | di | di | di | di | del | del | del | del | del | di |
| | HSC7E526 | 7q36.3 | di | di | di | di | di | di | di | di | di | di | | | del | del | del | |

HSC7E-YACs are from the chromosome 7-specific YAC library and the C_row_plate_column YACs are from the CEPH-Généthon collection del = deletion (only one fluorescence signal); t = translocation breakpoint; di = disomy (two fluorescence signals indicating retention of both alleles) empty boxes = not done; light grey boxes indicate the extent of the deletion, dark grey boxes the commonly deleted segment Clones HSC7E248 to HSC7E113 recognize a contiguous genomic fragment in chromosome bands 7q35-q36

17

mal critical region in 7q22-q31.1 – there is heterogeneity of the translocation and deletion breakpoints. More than one gene in either critical region of chromosome 7 could be involved. So far, only the gene encoding *ras homologue enriched in brain 2* (*RHEB*) has been mapped to the commonly deleted region (Mizuki et al. 1996). None of the genes that are located in the distal part of 7q and may be good candidates based on their protein function such as *NEDD2*, *XRCC2*, and *TIM* map to the commonly deleted region or to the genomic segment containing the translocation breakpoint. Recently, Koike et al. (1999) studied a series of 26 patients with AML using LOH analysis with 15 different polymorphic microsatellite markers. The critical region in their study was localized to 7q33-q34 (D7S498, D7S505). Interestingly, D-Marker D7S505 maps to the critical region identified in our study, whereas D-Marker D7S498 is located proximal. However, the resolution of the deletion map in their study was limited because the applied probes were scattered along a large genomic region.

## Conclusion

Using FISH with contiguously mapped DNA probes we defined a genomic fragment in chromosome bands 7q35-q36 that is commonly affected in malignant myeloid disorders. Furthermore, we mapped the translocation breakpoint of a balanced translocation to a 1300 kb sized genomic fragment that is located close to the proximal border of the commonly deleted region. In analogy to the proximal critical region these data show heterogeneity of 7q35-q36 deletion/translocation breakpoints in myeloid leukemias. One possible interpretation is that in analogy to the proximal critical region more than one gene in either critical region of chromosome 7 could be involved. The genomic fragment identified in this study provides the first step for the identification of candidate gene(s) from the critical region by using positional cloning strategies. Moreover, refinement of the critical region by the analysis of additional tumor samples together with the growing data from the human chromosome 7 map-

ping and sequencing project will facilitate the identification of the relevant disease gene(s). Once candidate genes from the critical region are identified, it will be necessary to analyze MDS/AML tumors associated with 7q35-q36 deletions for mutations of the remaining allele.

*Acknowledgements.* This work is supported by the Forschungsförderungsprogramm of the Medical Faculty, University of Heidelberg, the Medical research Council (MRC) of Canada and the Deutsche Forschungsgemeinschaft (Fi 659/1-2).

## References

Atkin NB, Baker MC (1993): Chromosome 7q deletions: observation on 13 malignant tumors. Cancer Genet Cytogenet 67:123-125

Bloomfield CD and de la Chapelle A (1987) Chromosome abnormalities in acute nonlymphocytic leukemia: Clinical and biological significance. Semin Oncol 14:372-383

Cohen D, Chumakov I, Weissenbach J (1993) A first generation physical map of the human genome. Nature 366:698-701

Le Beau MM, Albain KS, Larson RA, Vardiman JW, Davis EM, Blough RR, Golomb HM, Rowley JD (1986) Clinical and cytogenetic correlation in 63 patients with therapy-related myelodysplastic syndromes and acute myeloid leukemias: further evidence for characteristic abnormalities of chromosome no. 5 and 7. J Clin Oncol 3:325-345

Döhner K, Brown J, Hehmann U, Hetzel C, Stewart J, Lowther G, Scholl C, Fröhling S, Cuneo A, Tsui LC, Lichter P, Scherer SW, Döhner H (1998) Molecular cytogenetic characterization of a critical region in bands 7q35-q36 commonly deleted in malignant myeloid disorders. Blood 92:4031-4035

Fischer K, Fröhling S, Scherer SW, McAllister Brown J, Scholl C, Stilgenbauer S, Tsui LC, Lichter P, Döhner H (1997) Molecular cytogenetic delineation of deletions and translocations involving chromosome band 7q22 in myeloid leukemias. Blood 89:2036-2041

Fourth International Workshop on Chromosomes in Leukemia 1982 (1984) Abnormalities of chromosome 7 resulting in monosomy 7 or in deletion of the long arm (7q-): review of translocations, breakpoints and associated abnormalities. Cancer Genet Cytogenet 11:300-303

Johnson EJ, Scherer SW, Osborne L, Tsui LC, Oscier D, Mould S, Cotter FE (1996) Molecular definition of a narrow interval at 7q22.1 associated with myelodysplasia. Blood 87:3579-3586

Kere J, Ruutu T, Davis KA, Roninson IB, Watkin PC, Winqist R, de la Chapelle A (1989a) Chromosome 7 long arm deletion in myeloid disorders: a narrow breakpoint region in 7q22 defined by molecular mapping. Blood 73:230-234

Kiuru-Kuhlefelt S, Kristo P, Ruutu T, Knuutila S, Kere J (1997) Evidence for two molecular steps in the pathogenesis of myeloid disorders associated with deletion of chromosome 7 long arm. Leukemia 11:2097-2104

Koike M, Tasaka T, Spira S, Tsuruoka N, Koeffler HP (1999) Allelotyping of acute myelogenous leukemia: loss of heterozygosity at 7q31.1 (D7S486) and 7q33-q34 (D7S498, D7S505). Leuk Res. 23:307-310

Kunz J, Scherer SW, Klawitz I, Soder S, Du YZ, Speich N, Kalff-Suske M, Heng HHQ, Tsui LC, Grzeschik KH (1994) Regional localization of 725 human chromosome 7-specific yeast artificial chromosome clones. Genomics 22:439-448

Le Beau MM, Espinosa III R, Davis EM, Eisenbart JD, Larson RA, Green ED (1996) Cytogenetic and molecular delineation of a region of chromosome 7 commonly deleted in malignant myeloid diseases. Blood 88:1930-1935

Lewis S, Abrahamson G, Boultwood J, Fidler C, Potter A, Wainscoat JS (1996) Molecular characterization of the 7q deletion in myeloid disorders. Br J Haematol 93:75-80

Liang H, Fairman J, Claxton DF, Nowell PC, Green ED, Nagarajan L (1998) Molecular anatomy of chromosome 7q deletions in myeloid neoplasms: Evidence for multiple critical loci. Proc Natl Acad Sci USA 95:3781-3785

Luna-Fineman S, Shannon KM, Lange BJ (1995) Childhood monosomy 7: Epidemiology, biology, and mechanistic implications. Blood 85:1985-1999

Mizuki N, Kimura M, Ohno S, Miyata S, Sato M, Ando H, Ishihara M, Goto K, Watanabe S, Yamazaki M, Ona A, Taguchi S, Okumura K, Nogami M, Taguchi H, Ando A, Onoko H (1996) Isolation of cDNA and genomic clones of a human RAS-related GTP binding protein gene and its chromosomal localization to the long arm of chromosome 7, 7q36. Genomics, 34:114-118

Neuman WL, Rubin CM, Rios RB, Larson RA, Le Beau MM, Rowley JD, Vardiman JW, Schwartz JL, Farber R (1992) Chromosomal loss and deletion are the most common mechanisms for loss of heterozygosity from chromosomes 5 and 7 in malignant myeloid disorders. Blood 79:1501-1510

Rodrigues Pereira Velloso E, Michaux L, Ferrant A, Hernandez JM, Meeus P, Dierlamm J, Criel A, Louwagie A, Verhoef G, Boogaerts M, Michaux JL, Bosly A, Mecucci C, Van den Berghe H (1996) Deletions of the long arm of chromosome 7 in myeloid disorders: loss of band 7q32 implies worst prognosis. Br J Haematol 92:574-581

Scherer SW, Tompkins BJF, Tsui LC (1992) A human chromosome 7-specific genomic DNA library in yeast artificial chromosomes. Mammal Genome 3:179-181

Zenklusen JC, Conti CJ (1996) Cytogenetic, molecular, and functional evidence for novel tumor suppressor genes on the long arm of human chromosome 7. Mol Carcinog 15:167-175

19

# Molecular Characterization of the Translocation (10;11)(p13;q14): *MLL* and *CALM* are Fused to *AF10* in Morphologically Different Subsets of Acute Leukemia

M. H. Dreyling[1,2], K. Schrader[3], V. Muschinsky[4], C. Fonatsch[5], B. Schlegelberger[6], D. Haase[3], C. Schoch[1], W.-D. Ludwig[7], W. Hiddemann[1] and S. K. Bohlander[4]

ABSTRACT. The t(10;11)(p13;q14) is a recurring translocation that has been observed in acute lymphoblastic as well as acute myeloid leukemia. A previous study revealed a *MLL/AF10* fusion in all cases of AML with t(10;11) and various breakpoints on chromosome 11 ranging from q13 to q23. In contrast, we recently cloned *CALM* (Clathrin Assembly Lymphoid Myeloid leukemia gene), another fusion partner of *AF10* located at 11q14, in the monocytic cell line U937. To further define the role of these genes in acute lymphoblastic and acute myeloid leukemia, we analyzed 10 patient samples (9 AML, 1 ALL) with cytogenetically identified t(10;11)(p12-14;q13-21) and well characterized morphology and immunophenotype. Interphase fluorescence *in situ* hybridization (FISH) was performed using YAC probes flanking the breakpoint regions. In all cases with simple t(10;11) tested, *AF10* was involved whereas in 2 cases with complex translocations, no rearrangement of *AF10*, *MLL* or *CALM* was detected. In 4 cases including one secondary AML (1 AML-M0, 2 AML-M1, 1 ALL), the signals of the *CALM* YACS were separated in interphase cells indicating a translocation breakpoint within the *CALM* region. In all of these cases, RT-PCR revealed *CALM/AF10* fusions containing virtually the whole coding region of *CALM* and *AF10*. In 2 of 4 cases different splice variants were identified. The reciprocal *AF10/CALM* fusion was detected in all 3 cases of AML, but not in the one ALL patient. FISH identified a *MLL* rearrangement in 3 cases (2 AML-M2, 1 AML-M5). In one additional case (AML-M5), RT-PCR detected a fusion product between *MLL*/exon 7 and *AF10*. The different morphology of AML with either *CALM* (immature phenotype) or *MLL* (myelomonocytic differentiation) rearrangement corresponded to a characteristic immunophenotype. We conclude that *CALM* and *MLL* rearrangement identify morphologically different subsets of acute leukemia with t(10;11)(p13;q14). However, functional studies are necessary to elucidate the biological role of the fusion products in leukemogenesis.

## Introduction

The chromosomal translocation t(10;11) is a recurring translocation in acute leukemia (Mitelman 1994). Cytogenetically, two different types can be distinguished:
- the t(10;11)(p12;q23) is found in acute myeloid leukemia (AML) and results in the fusion of the *MLL* gene at 11q23 to the putative transcription factor *AF10* at 10p12 (Chaplin *et al.*, 1995a; Chaplin *et al.*, 1995b; Saha *et al.*, 1995; Thirman *et al.*, 1993).
- the t(10;11)(p13;q14) has been observed in AML as well as acute lymphoblastic leukemia (ALL) (Berger *et al.*, 1989; Berger *et al.*, 1995; Heim *et al.*, 1989; Sait *et al.*, 1987). In a recent study of 10 AML-M4 and M5 with t(10;11) and various breakpoints on 11q (11q12 – 11q23), all cases showed an

[1] Dept of Medicine III, University Hospital Großhadern, Munich, Germany
[2] GSF, Institute of Hematology, Munich, Germany
[3] Dept. of Hematology/Oncology, University of Göttingen, Germany
[4] Institute of Human Genetics, University of Göttingen, Germany
[5] Institute of Medical Biology, University of Vienna, Austria
[6] Institute of Human Genetics, University of Kiel, Germany
[7] Dept. of Hematology/Oncology, Robert-Rössle-Clinic, University of Berlin, Germany

*AF10/MLL* fusion as identified by fluorescence *in situ* hybridization (Beverloo *et al.*, 1995). The various cytogenetic breakpoints are the result of rather complicated rearrangements including inversions of 11q in all cases which are not always resolved on the cytogenetic level. In contrast, the molecular characterization of the t(10;11)(p13;q14) in the myelomonocytic cell line U937 revealed a different breakpoint on 11q, involving the previously unknown gene *CALM* (Clathrin Assembly Lymphoid Myeloid leukemia gene) (Dreyling *et al.*, 1996). Interestingly, both translocations t(10;11) have the same fusion partner on chromosome 10, the putative transcription factor *AF10* (Chaplin et al. 1995a; Dreyling et al. 1996; Saha et al. 1995).

To further delineate the role of these three genes (*AF10*, *CALM* and *MLL*) in acute lymphoblastic and acute myeloid leukemia, we analyzed 10 patient samples (9 AML, 1 ALL) with cytogenetically identified t(10;11)(p12-14;q13-21) and well characterized morphology and immunophenotype.

## Material and Methods

### Patients samples

Based on the cytogenetic data and the availability of material, 9 AML and 1 ALL with t(10;11)(p12-14;q14-21) were collected from the major German cytogenetic centers (Table 1). All cases were morphologically classified according to the French-American-British (FAB) criteria by a reference hematologist (Bennett *et al.*, 1976). Immunophenotyping was performed according to the consensus protocol for hematopoietic malignancies (Rothe *et al.*, 1996).

### FISH

Only fixed cells stored in Carnoy's solution for up to several years were available for this study. Therefore, an interphase fluorescence *in situ* hybridization approach was chosen. Non-chimeric YACs from the genomic region of the three genes were selected. A transloca-

tion was assumed, when one of the YAC signals was split resulting in 3 hybridization signals in a diploid interphase nucleus.

YAC-derived probes were generated by sequence-independent amplification (SIA) or nick translation (Bohlander *et al.*, 1994b; Rowley *et al.*, 1992):

### AF10

YAC 807b3 (CEPH library), that spans the breakpoint region on 10p, was described previously (Dreyling et al. 1996).

### MLL

A pool of two YACS (785c6, 856b9) was used that spans the *MLL* gene and approximately 1.0 mega-bp of distally flanking sequences, because 11q23 translocations are often associated with interstitial deletions (Cherif *et al.*, 1994).

### CALM

YACS of the *CALM* region were evaluated by FISH for chimerism (hybridization with normal peripheral blood cells) and mapped relative to the *CALM* breakpoint. Two YACS (proximal 785c1, distal 914d9) were chosen for two color analysis of the *CALM* breakpoint region.

Dual color FISH was performed with the two *CALM* probes as well as the *AF10* or the *MLL* probe and the corresponding centromere probe as previously described (Dreyling et al. 1996).

### RT-PCR

Total RNA was isolated from fixed cells using a commercially available kit (RNeasy, Quiagen) and transcribed with random hexamer primers (Superscript, Gibco). PCR of the putative breakpoint regions was performed using previously published primers of the encoding regions of *AF10*, *MLL* and *CALM* (Chaplin et al. 1995b; Dreyling et al. 1996). In case of a positive amplification product, PCR

**Table 1.** Characterization of Acute Leukemias with t(10;11)

| No | Sex | Age | Morphology | Karyotype |
|----|-----|-----|------------|-----------|
| 1 | M | 51 | AML-M5a | 46, XY, t(10;11)(p13;q14) |
| 2 | F | 46 | AML-M2 | 48, XX, +6, +8, t(10;11)(p12-13;q14-21) |
| 3 | F | 39 | AML-M2 | 45, X, -X, der(10) t(10;11)(p12-13;q13) inv(11)(q13q23), der(11)t(10;11)(p12-13;q13) |
| 4 | M | 2 | AML-M5 | 46,XY, t(10;11)(p12;q21) |
| 5 | F | 37 | AML-M1 | 46, XX, der(10)t(10;11)(p12-13;q21), der(11)t(10;11;11;16)(p12-13;q21;p14-15;q13-22)del(11)(p13), del(12)(p11) |
| 6 | F | 74 | AML-M5 | 46, XX, t(10;11;17)(p13;q13;q23) |
| 7 | M | 19 | AML-M1 | 46,XY, t(10;11)(p13;q14) |
| 8 | M | 47 | AML-M0 | 48,XY, +3, add(7)(q33-35), der(9), der(9), +der(9), t(10;11)(p13;q21), der(12)t(12;18)(p11;q11), -18, +mar |
| 9 | F | 21 | AML-M1 | 47,XX, +19, t(10;11)(p13-14;q14-21) |
| 10 | M | 31 | ALL | 46,XY, del(7)(q34-35), i(9)(q10), t(10;11)(p1?4;q14), der(17)t(1;17)(p13;p11) |

aliquots were cloned and sequenced as previously described (Bohlander et al., 1994a).

## Results

### Cytogenetics

The t(10;11) was the only structural abnormality in 6 cases indicating an early event in malignant transformation (Table 1).

### FISH

AF10 was involved in all simple t(10;11) tested (Table 2). In contrast, no rearrangement of AF10, CALM, or MLL was detected in 2 complex translocations.

MLL was rearranged in 3 AML cases (Figure 1 D–F). All cases showed a myelomo-nocytic differentiation beyond the promyelocyte stage according to the FAB classification (M2 or M5). This homogenity is reflected by a characteristic immunophenotype: CD4+, CD13-, CD33+, CD65s+ (Table 2).

CALM was rearranged in 1 ALL as well as 3 AML with a rather immature phenotype (M0 or M1, Figure 1 A–C, Table 2).

### RT-PCR

In all cases with CALM rearrangement and one case with exclusive AF10 involvement detected by FISH (No 4, Table 2), the quality of the available material was sufficient for further RNA analysis. In the latter case, RT-PCR revealed a MLL/CALM fusion which was missed by FISH probably because of a larger interstitial deletion of the telomeric MLL sequences (Table 2, Figure 2).

**Table 2.** Molecular Analysis of t(10;11)(p13:q14-21) in acute leukemia

| t(10;11) | No | Morphology | Immunophenotype | FISH AF10 | FISH CALM | FISH MLL | RT-PCR |
|----------|----|-----------:|-----------------|------|------|-----|--------|
| AF10/MLL | 1 | AML-M5a | CD4+, CD13-, CD33+, CD65s+ | SPLIT | N | SPLIT | nd |
| | 2 | AML-M2 | CD4+, CD13-, CD33+, CD65s+ | nd | N | SPLIT | nd |
| | 3 | AML-M2 | CD4+, CD13-, CD33+, CD65s+ | nd | N | SPLIT | nd |
| | 4 | AML-M5 | CD4-, CD13-, CD33+, CD65s+ | SPLIT | N | N | AF10/MLL |
| complex | 5 | AML-M1 | CD4-, CD13+, CD33-, CD65s+ | N | N | N | nd |
| rearrangement | 6 | AML-M5 | CD4+, CD13-, CD33+, CD65s+ | nd | N | nd | nd |
| AF10/CALM | 7 | AML-M1 | CD4-, CD13+, CD33-, CD65s- | SPLIT | SPLIT | N | AF10/CALM |
| | 8 | AML-M0 | CD4nd, CD13+, CD33+, CD65nd | SPLIT | SPLIT | N | AF10/CALM |
| | 9 | AML-M1 | nd | SPLIT | SPLIT | N | AF10/CALM |
| | 10 | T-ALL | CD4+ | nd | SPLIT | N | AF10/CALM |

N: NOT SPLIT; nd: not done

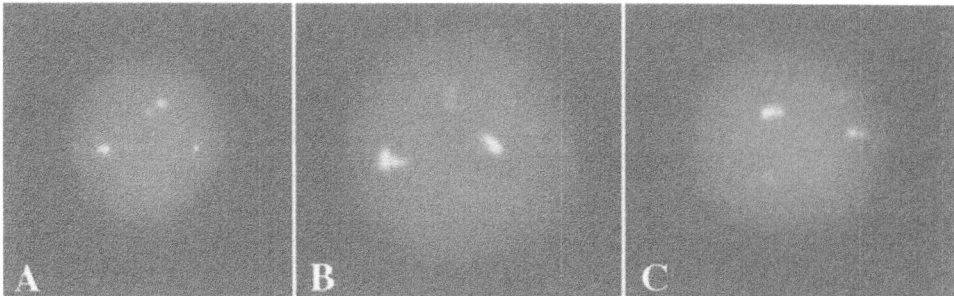

**Fig. 1A–C.** AML with *AF10* and *CALM* Rearrangement. Three AF-10 signals (arrow), indicating a split of one YAC signal, and two centromere 10 signals (triangle) are detectable (panel A). One proximal (arrow) and one distal *CALM* YAC (triangle) are separated, indicating a breakpoint within this genomic region (panel B). Two *MLL* signals (arrow) and two centromere 11 signals (triangle) merely exclude a rearrangement of the *MLL* region (panel C).

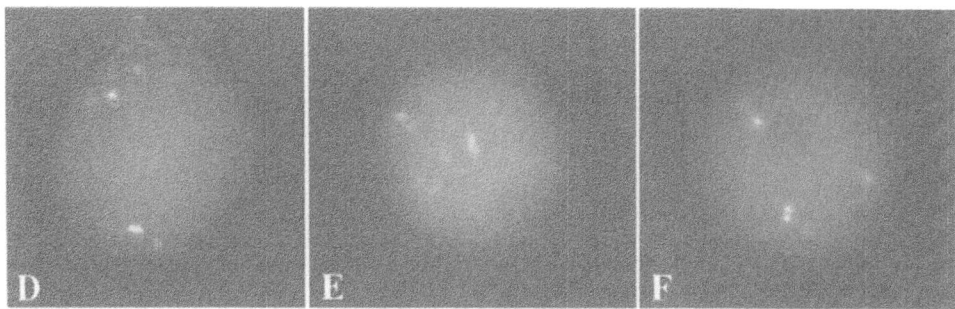

**Fig. 1D–F.** AML with *AF10* and *MLL* Rearrangement. Three AF-10 signals (arrow), indicating a split of one YAC signal, and two centromere 10 signals (triangle) are detectable (panel D). The proximal (arrow) and the distal CALM YACs (triangle) are colocalized excluding a breakpoint within that genomic region (panel E). Three MLL signals (arrow), indicating a split of one YAC signal, and two centromere 11 signals (triangle) are shown (panel F).

A *CALM/AF10* fusion was amplified in the other 4 cases identified by FISH. The reciprocal *AF10/CALM* fusion could be detected in the three AML cases but not in the ALL sample. However, in this case the internal *AF10* control RT-PCR was negative as well, suggesting a lower *AF10* expression in lymphoid cells or poor RNA quality. In addition, different splice variants of the *CALM* breakpoint were detected in 2 AML (No. 7 and 9, data not shown).

## Discussion

The translocation t(10;11)(p13;q14) is a recurring chromosomal abnormality that has been observed in acute lymphoblastic as well as acute myeloid leukemia (Berger et al. 1989;

Berger et al. 1995; Heim et al. 1989; Sait et al. 1987). On the molecular level, two types of t(10;11)(p13;q13-q21) have been characterized so far, both of them involve the putative transcription factor *AF10* on 10p13. One type results in a *MLL/AF10* fusion, the other one causes a *CALM/AF10* fusion (Chaplin et al. 1995a; Dreyling et al. 1996). We performed this study to define the relevance of *MLL* and *CALM* rearrangements in acute leukemia with t(10;11)(p13;q13-21). Both types of rearrangements were detected with similar frequency and represented all cases with simple translocation t(10;11). Interestingly, the two different rearrangements represented two distinct morphological subsets of AML. In accordance with the previous reports, all four cases with t(10;11) and a *MLL* rearrangement showed a monocytic morphology or a myelo-

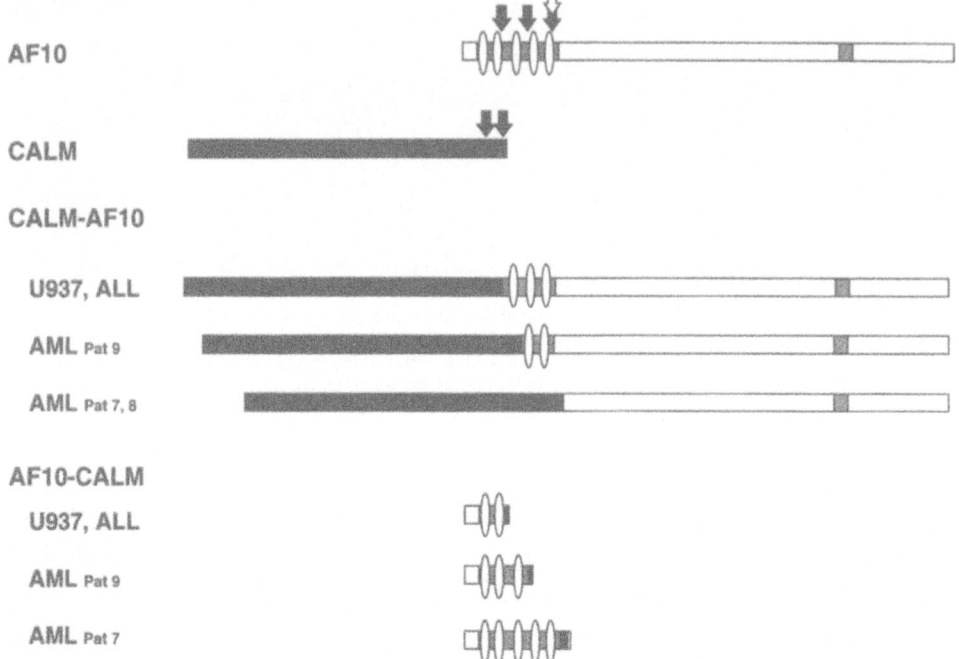

**Fig. 2.** *AF10/ CALM* Breakpoints in the Cell Line U937, 1 ALL AND 3 AML. Black arrows: *AF10 /CALM* breakpoints. White arrow: *AF10/MLL* breakpoint. Shown are the *AF10* domains (5 zinc fingers and the leucin zipper motif, light grey) and the *ap-3* homologous regions (dark grey) of *CALM* .

id maturation beyond the promyelocyte stage (Berger *et al.*,1995a; Chaplin *et al.*,1995c; Thirman *et al.*,1993). Similarly, in three of the four cases a previously described characteristic immunophenotype was identified: CD4+, CD 13-, CD33+, CD65s+ (Creutzig *et al.*, 1995). However, as these markers are panmyeloid markers that are rather broadly expressed we do not consider them leukemia-specific.

*CALM* was rearranged in AML with a rather immature phenotype as well as in ALL suggesting that the *CALM/AF10* fusion may play a critical role in the transformation of early progenitor/ stem cells before either myeloid or lymphoid differentiation takes place. Interestingly, *MLL/AF10* and *CALM/AF10*, although representing morphologically different subtypes of AML, share some of the breakpoints in *AF10* (Figure 2). Similarly, there was no evident difference between the *CALM/AF10* fusion products in ALL and AML.

Both fusion RNAs (*CALM/AF10* and *AF10/CALM*) were detected in the 3 AML.

However, we think that the *CALM/AF10* fusion is critical for malignant transformation. This conclusion is based on two observations:

– The *CALM/AF10* fusion combines almost the complete coding sequences of *CALM* and of *AF10*.
– The *CALM/AF10* fusion can be compared to the *MLL/AF10* fusion. Since the reciprocal *AF/MLL* fusion is not formed due to the complex cytogenetic rearrangements, the *MLL/AF10* must be the critical fusion protein in these cases (Beverloo et al. 1995; Tanabe *et al.*, 1996). In accordance with the one case published so far, we could identify different *CALM/AF10* splice variants (Silliman *et al.*, 1998).

*CALM* has a very high homology to ap-3, a murine clathrin assembly protein (Morris *et al.*, 1993). So far, CALM is the only protein interacting with clathrin that has been found to be involved in malignant transformation. It is still speculative by which mechanism the fusion product may promote malignant transformation. In T-lymphocytes, assembly of clathrin is proliferation-dependent and regulated by growth factors (Fox et al., 1992). It is thus conceivable that alterations in clathrin-mediated receptor endocytosis are caused by the *CALM/AF10* fusion protein. Alternatively, AF10 nuclear localization signals may cause the *CALM/AF10* fusion to be translocated to the nucleus where a recently characterized transactivation domain of *CALM* would interfere with normal *AF10* function (Bohlander and Bartels 1997). However, further functional studies are necessary to define the precise mechanism by which the *CALM/AF10* fusion contributes to malignant transformation.

*Acknowledgements.* We thank H. Döhner for generously providing the *MLL* YACs.

# References

Bennett JM, Catovsky C, Daniel MT, Flandrin G, Galton DAG, Gralnick HR, and Sultan C (1976) Proposals for the classification of the acute leukemias. Br J Haematol 33: 451

Berger R, Le Coniat M, Derre J, Vechione D, and Chen SJ (1989) Chromosomal rearrangement on chromosome 11q14-q21 in T-cell acute lymphoblastic leukemia. Leukemia 3: 560-562

Berger R, Le Coniat M, Flexor M-A, and Leblanc T (1995) Translocation t(10;11) involving the MLL gene in acute myeloid leukemia. Importance of fluorescence in situ hybridization (FISH) analysis. Ann Genet 39: 147-151

Beverloo HB, Le Coniat M, Wijsman J, Lillington DM, Bernard O, de Klein A, van Wering E, Welborn J, Young BD, Hagemeijer A, and Berger R (1995) Breakpoint heterogeneity in t(10;11) translocation in AML-M4/M5 resulting in fusion of AF10 and MLL is resolved by fluorescent in situ hybridization analysis. Cancer Res 55: 4220-4224

Bohlander SK, and Bartels S (1997) Identification and mapping of a transcriptional activation domain in CALM, the fusion partner of AF10 in the t(10;11)(p13;q14) found in the monocytic cell line U937. Med Genet 9: 44

Bohlander SK, Dreyling M, Hagos F, Sveen L, Le Beau MM, Olopade OI, and Díaz MO (1994a) Mapping the critical region of the tumor suppressor gene on chromosome 9 bands p21-22 with microdissection probes. Genomics 24: 211-217

Bohlander SK, III RE, Fernald AA, Rowley JD, Le Beau MM, and Diaz M (1994b) Sequence-independent amplification and labeling of yeast artificial chromosomes for fluorescence in situ hybridization. Cytogenet Cell Genet 65: 108

Chaplin T, Ayton P, Bernard OA, Saha V, Della Valle V, Hillion J, Gregorini A, Lillington D, Berger R, and Young BD (1995a) A novel class of zinc finger/leucine zipper genes identified from the molecular cloning of the t(10;11) translocation in acute leukemia. Blood 85: 1435-1441

Chaplin T, Bernard O, Beverloo HB, Saha V, Hagemeijer A, Berger R, and Young BD (1995b) The t(10;11) translocation in acute myeloid leukemia (M5) consistently fuses the leucine zipper motif of AF10 onto the HRX gene. Blood 86: 2073-2076

Cherif D, Bernard O, Paulien S, James MR, Le Paslier D, and Berger R (1994) Hunting 11q23 deletions with fluorescence in situ hybridization. Leukemia 8: 578

Creutzig U, Harbott J, Sperling C, Ritter J, Zimmermann M, Löffler H, Riehm H, Schellong G, and Ludwig W-D (1995) Clinical significance of surface antigen expression in children with acute myeloid leukemia: results of study AML-BFM-87. Blood 86: 3097-3108

Dreyling MH, Martinez-Climent JA, Zheng M, Mao J, Rowley JD, and Bohlander SK (1996) The t(10;11)(p13;q14) in the U937 cell line results in the fusion of the AF10 gene and CALM, a new member of the AP-3 clathrin assembly protein family. Proc Natl Acad Sci (USA) 93: 4804-4809

Fox FE, Capocasale RJ, Ford HC, Lamb RJ, Moore JS, and Nowell PC (1992) Transforming growth factor-beta inhibits human T-cell proliferation through multiple targets. Lymphokine Cytokine Res 11: 299-305

Heim S, Bekassy A, Garwicz S, Heldrup J, Kristoffersson U, Mandahal N, Wiebe T, and Mitelmann F (1989) Bone marrow karyotypes in 94 children with acute leukemia. Eur J Hematol 44: 227-233

Mitelman F. (1994). *Catalog of chromosome aberrations in cancer*, Alan. R. Liss, New York.

Morris SA, Schroder S, Plessmann U, Weber K, and Ungewickell E (1993) Clathrin assembly protein AP180: Primary structure, domain organization and identification of a clathrin binding site. EMBO 12: 667-675

Rothe G, Schmitz G, Adorf D, Barlage S, Gramatzki M, Hanenberg H, Höffkes HG, Janossy G, Knüchel R, Ludwig WD, Nebe T, Nerl C, Orfao A, Serke S, Sonnen R, Tichelli A, and Wörmann B (1996) Consensus protocol for the flow cytometric immunophenotyping of hematopoietic malignancies. Leukemia 10: 877-895

Rowley JD, Diaz MO, Espinosa III R, Patel YD, van Melle E, Ziemin S, Taillon-Miller P, Lichter P, Evans GA, Kersey JH, Ward DC, Domer PH, and Le Beau MM (1992) Mapping chromosome band 11q23 in human acute leukemia with biotinylated probes: identification of 11q23 translocation breakpoints with a yeast artificial chromosome. Proc Natl Acad Sci (USA) 87: 9358-9362

Saha V, Chaplin T, Gregorini A, Ayton P, and Young BD (1995) The leukemia-associated-protein (LAP) domain, a cysteine-rich motif, is present in a wide range of proteins including MLL, AF10, and MLLT proteins. PNAS 92: 9735-9741

Sait SNJ, Dal Cin P, and Sandberg AA (1987) Recurrent involvement of 11q13 in acute nonlymphocytic leukemia. Cancer Cytogenetics Cytogenetics 26: 351-354

Silliman CC, Mc Gavran L, Wei Q, Miller LA, Li S, and Hunger SP (1998) Alternative splicing in wild type AF10 and CALM cDNAs and in AF10-CALM and CALM-AF10 fusion cDNAs produced by the t(10;11)(p13-14;q14-q21). Leukemia 12: 1404-1410

Tanabe S, Bohlander SK, Vignon CV, EspinosaIII R, Zhao N, Strissel PL, Zeleznik-Le N, and Rowley JD (1996) AF10 is split by MLL and HEAB, a human homolog to a putative caenorhabditis elegans ATP/GTP-binding protein in an inv ins(10;11) (p12;q23q12). Blood 88: 3535-3545

Thirman MJ, Gill HJ, Burnett RC, Mbangkollo D, McCabe NR, Kobayashi H, Ziemin-van der Poel S, Kaneko Y, Morgan R, Sandberg AA, Chaganti RSK, Larson RA, Le Beau MM, Diaz MO, and Rowley JD (1993) Rearrangement of the MLL gene in acute lymphoblastic and acute myeloid leukemias with 11q23 chromosomal translocations. N Engl J Med 329: 909-914

# MLL-Duplications are Rare and Associated with Poor Prognosis in Acute Myeloid Leukemia

S. Schnittger, U. Kinkelin, C. Schoch, D. Haase, T. Haferlach, T. Büchner, B. Wörmann, W. Hiddemann and F. Griesinger

*Abstract.* Partial tandem duplications (PTD) within the MLL-gene have been described in a limited number of patients with acute myeloid leukemia (AML). In this study a systematic screening of 387 unselected AML was performed to evaluate the real frequency and prognostic relevance of this molecular marker. The frequency of PTD in the analyzed 387 unselected patients at the RNA and DNA level was of 3.4%. Most but not all patients were karyotypically normal. It was never found in patients with t(15;17), t(8;21), inv(16), other AML specific reciprocal translocations, or complex karyotypes. All PTD positive cases revealed a very bad outcome. Thus PTD may be an early event in leukemia that defines a specific AML subgroup.

## 1. Introduction

The characterization of chromosome alterations in AML has allowed to establish biological and prognostic subgroups. However, nearly 50% of AML reveal normal karyotypes and lack molecularly detectable genetic markers. Rearrangements within the MLL-gene localizing in 11q23 are well described in AML and ALL. Recently, a direct partial tandem duplication within the MLL gene has been described in AML patients with trisomy 11 and also in karyotypically normal AML [1-9]. This rearrangement leads to fusion of a portion of the putative protooncogene with itself, and this seems to represent a new genetic mechanism for leukemogenesis. Thus the PTD was thought to be a very promising new molecular marker for AML studies. In order to test the incidence and prognostic significance of this molecular marker, we have retrospectively analyzed 8 cases of AML with trisomy 11 and prospectively 387 unselected consecutive cases with AML for partial duplications of the MLL gene. Patients with normal karyotypes and those with various chromosome aberrations were included. De novo as well as secondary leukemias including all FAB subtypes were analyzed. Thus the aims of this study were:

1. to analyze the frequency of MLL-duplications in 387 unselected cases of AML;
2. to correlate MLL-duplication with karyotype, FAB subtype and age;
3. to investigate the outcome of patients with MLL-duplications.

## 2. Materials and methods

### 2.1 Patient samples

Within a two year period fresh blood or bone marrow samples from 387 consecutive patients were analyzed. All cases were diagnosed as having AML according to standard French-American-British (FAB) classification [9,10] and were referred to our lab for cytogenetic analysis. With the exception of one child all patients were adults. De novo as well as secondary AML after MDS or treatment of a previous malignant disease (t-AML) were included. Additionally, 8 patients with a known trisomy 11 were retrospectively included in the analysis.

1 Department of Internal Medicine, Hematology/Oncology, Georg- August-University, Göttingen, Germany
2 Department of Internal Medicine III, University Hospital Grosshadern, Ludwig-Maximilians-University, München, Germany
3 Department A of Internal Medicine, University of Münster, Münster, Germany

## 2.2 Treatment protocol

Six patients (cases # 4, 7, 8, 10, 14, and 16) were treated according to the AMLCG92 protocol as published [11]. Six patients (cases # 1, 2, 3, 6, 12, 15) were not included within the AMLCG92 study but were treated with analogous protocols or even with more intensive chemotherapy (HAM) (cases #3 and #12). Patients were either put on maintenance therapy or received S-HAM for late consolidation (case #4). Three adult patients (# 5, 9, 13) did not receive chemotherapy due to bad performance status, 1 child (case #11) was treated according to the German Pediatric AML protocol and subsequently underwent allogeneic BMT.

## 2.3 Cytogenetics

Cytogenetic G-banding analysis was performed with standard methods. The definition of a cytogenetic clone and descriptions of karyotypes followed the International System for Human Cytogenetic Nomenclature [12].

## 2.4 Molecular genetic analysis

### 2.4.1 Nucleic acid purification
DNA was extracted with a salting out procedure [13] from fresh bone marrow or peripheral blood cells after ficoll separation of mononucleated cells. From the same specimens total RNA was isolated with RNeasy (Quiagen) following manufacture's instructions.

### 2.4.2 RT-PCR
One μg of total RNA was reverse transcribed with 200 U Superscript (Gibco/BRL) in a 40 μl reaction using random primers. An equivalent quantity of 25 ng RNA amplified for 35 cycles (1' 94°C, 1' 63°C, 1' 72°C), in 50 μl with each 10 pmol of forward primer *6.1:* 5'GTC-CAGAGCAGAGCAAACAG3' (bp 4013-4032, numbering according to [14]) and reverse primer *E3AS:* 5'ACACAGATGGATCTGA-GAGG3' (bp 567-586), 10 mmol dNTPs, and 1.25 units of Taq polymerase (Gibco/BRL) in the buffer shipped by the supplier. For nested PCRs primers *3.C1* 5'AGGAGAGAGTTTACC-

TGCTC3' (bp 821-840), and *MLLint:* 5'CTTC-CAGGAAGTCAAGCAAGCAGGT3' (bp 3869-3892) were used in the primary reaction and a 1μl aliquot of these reaction was further amplified for additional 35 cycles with primers *6.1* and *E3AS*. For each RNA sample an ABL specific RT-PCR was performed to control the integrity of RNA using primers *abl5':* 5'GGCCAGTAGCATCTGACTTTG3' and *abl3':* 5'ATGGTACCAGGAGTGTTTCTCC3'. Water instead of cDNA was included as a blank sample in each experiment. Amplification products were analyzed on 2% agarose gels stained with ethidium bromide.

### 2.4.3 Sequencing
All RT-PCR products were sequenced to identify the involved exons and the extent of the duplication. To this end, the amplified fragments were cut from the agarose gels and isolated with Quiaex II (Quiagen) following the manufactures instructions. Approximately 100 ng of purified RT-PCR products were directly sequenced with 3.3 pmol of primer *6.1* for forward and *E3AS* for reverse reactions using the Dye Terminator Cycle Sequencing Kit (Perkin Elmer). After initial denaturation at 95°C for 5 minutes, 25 cycles at 94°C for 15 seconds and 60°C for 4 minutes were performed. Sequence analysis was performed on 6% polyacrylamid gels on an ABI 373 sequencer.

### 2.4.5 Southern blot analysis
DNA from all patients that revealed MLL-duplication by PCR were reevaluated by Southern blot analysis. In addition, some duplication negative patients were included. Each 5-10 μg DNA was digested with the restriction enzymes BamHI and EcoRI overnight. Completely digested DNA was size fractionated on 0.7% agarose gels and transferred to nylon membranes (SureBlot, Oncor). A diogixin-dUTP labelled MLL cDNA probe (Oncor) containing exons 8-15 was used for hybridization. The membrans were washed under high stringency (0.1 x SSC for 2 x 15 min at 65°C). Detection was performed with an anti-digoxin antibody (Boehringer) and CSPD (Boehringer).

### 2.5 Nomenclature

We use the new MLL exon nomenclature according to Nilson et al. 1996 [15] that differs from the widespread older nomenclature.

## 3. Results

### 3.1 Incidence of MLL-duplication in 395 AML patients

395 AML patients were analyzed for the presence of a MLL duplication. The patients were divided into two subgroups.

### 3.1.1 PTD in patients with trisomy 11

Eight cases were retrospectively analyzed because of a trisomy 11 . Two had +11 as sole karyotypic aberration, three had +11 and one or two additional chromosomal changes, and three had +11 in the context of komplex karyotype. PTD was found in three of these patients (37.5%). One had +11 as sole karyotypic abnormality (case #1), one had del(13)(q12q14) (case #2) and one del(5)(q15q33) (case #3) in addition to trisomy 11 (table 1).

### 3.1.2 PTD in unselected AML

387 consecutive cases were prospectively analyzed. All FAB subtypes were included, and no selection was performed according to de novo or secondary leukemia or karyotype. The primary screening was performed using RT-PCR (fig. 1). The specificity of each PCR fragment was confirmed by nucleotide sequencing and the PTD was confirmed at the genomic level by southern blot analysis. In total 3.4% (13/387) of the unselected AML patients were found to have a PTD (table 1). Ten of these had a normal karyotype (cases #4-9, #12-14, #16). Three cases revealed chromosome aberrations: a del 7(q22) (case # 11), a t(1;16)(q21;q22) (case #10), and a del(9)(q22) (case #15), respectively (table 1). Thus, MLL-duplications are not restricted to karyotypically normal AML.

### 3.2 MLL-duplications as marker for follow up studies

Case #3 and Case #4 relapsing at 7 months and 2 months were monitored by RT-PCR for the PTD. Relapse samples showed the same MLL exon fusions as at diagnosis. In case #4 cytogenetics revealed a normal karyotype at diagnosis and gains of chromosomes 8, 13, and 19 at relapse. Case #3 revealed additional structural alterations presenting as del(17)(q23) and add(7)(q3?4) at relapse 7 months after diagnosis. Thus, MLL-duplication may represent an early event in the malignant transformation process, which seems to be a stable molecular marker and may therefor be helpful to distinguish true relapse from a secondary leukemia.

### 3.3 Correlation of MLL-duplication positive cases with FAB-subtype

Within the control cohort of 217 cases on which total clinical data were available, 6 cases were AML M0 (2.8%), 32 AML M1 (14.7%), 60 AML M2 (27.6%), 16 AML M3

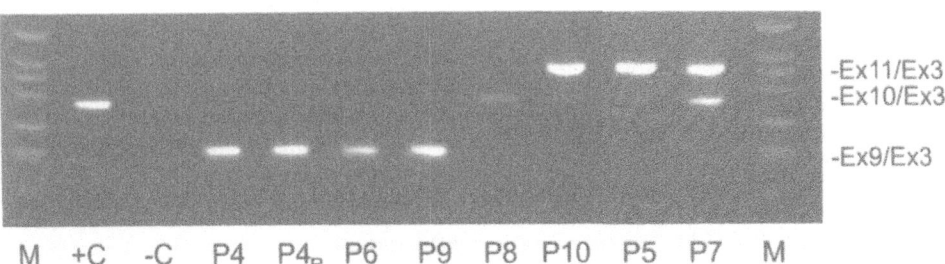

**Fig. 1.** RT-PCR amplification of the MLL-duplication transcripts presented on an ethidium bromide stained agarose gel. M: molecular weight standard VI (Boehringer), +C: sample with known MLL-duplication, -C: blank control containing water instead of cDNA, P: patient numbers corresponding to the numbers in table 1. All products were sequenced to determine the exons involved in the fusion. Kinds of the respective fusions are indicated at the right.

**Table 1.** Characteristics of Patients with PTD

| case | sex/age | FAB | karyotype | fusion (old nomenclature) | fusion (new nomenclature) |
|------|---------|-----|-----------|---------------------------|---------------------------|
| #1 | m/61 | M4 | 46,XY [8]/47,XY,+11[15] | e7/e2 | e10/e3 |
| #2 | m/66 | M1 | 47,XY,+11[10]/47,XY,+11,del(13)(q12q14)[5] | e8/e2 | e11/e3 |
| #3 | f/53 | M2 | 47,XX,del(5)(q15q33),+11[20] | e8/e2 + e7/e2 | e11/e3 + e10/e3 |
| | | Relapse | 47,XX,del(5)(q15q33)+11[9]/ 47,idem,del(17)(q23)[9]/47,idem,add(7)(q3?4)[2] | e8/e2 + e7/e2 | e11/e3 + e10/e3 |
| #4 | m/55 | M2 | 46,XY[25] | e6/e2 | e9/e3 |
| | | Relapse | 49,XY,+8,+13,+19[20] | e6/e2 | e9/e3 |
| #5 | m/72 | M2 | 46,XY[25] | e8/e2 | e11/e3 |
| #6 | m/50 | M2 | 46,XY[25] | e6/e2 | e9/e3 |
| #7 | m/59 | M2 | 46,XY[22] | e8/e2 + e7/e2 | e11/e3 + e10/e3 |
| #8 | f/56 | M4 | 46,XX[20] | e6/e2 | e9/e3 |
| #9 | f/68 | M5b | 46,XX[27] | e7/e2 | e10/e3 |
| #10 | m/63 | M1 | 46,XY,der(16)t(1;16)(q21;q22)[11]/47,idem,+6[6]/ 46,XY[2] | e8/e2 | e11/e3 |
| #11 | f/9 | t-M2 | 46,XX,del(7)(q22)[19] | e8/e2 + e7/e2 | e11/e3 + e10/e3 |
| #12 | m/54 | M4 | 46,XY[25] | e6/e2 | e9/e3 |
| #13 | f/73 | t-M4 | 46,XX[25] | e6/e2 | e9/e3 |
| #14 | m/60 | M4 | 46,XY[20] | e8/e2 + e7/e2 | e11/e3 + e10/e3 |
| #15 | m/72 | s-M2 | 46,XY,del(9)(q22)[7]/46,XY[17] | e7/e2 | e10/e3 |
| #16 | m/73 | t-M0 | 46,XY[25] | e6/e2 | e9/e3 |

(7.4%), 40 AML M4 (18.4%), 20 AML M4eo (9.2%), 21 AML M5 (9.7%), 7 AML M6 (3.2%), 2 M7 (0.9%), and 13 cases (6%) were not classified. Twenty six cases (12%) were known to have s-AML after MDS or treatment for a previous malignant disease (t-AML) and 10 (4.6%) were AML relapses. The PTD was present in different FAB subtypes. Of the 16 cases, 1 was M0 (6.3%), 2 M1 (12.5%), 7 M2 (43.8%), 5 M4 (31.25%), 1 M5b (6.3%) (table 1). Thus, the majority of PTD positive cases were observed in M2 and M4.

### 3.4 Incidence of MLL-duplication in cytogenetically defined subgroups

Of the control cohort of 217 cases, 105 (49.4%) were karyotypically normal and 112 (51.6%) showed various common or uncommon chromosome aberrations. Within this cohort, 7 cases (#4-10, #12) were PTD positive (3.2%). The percentage of positive cases is slightly higher with 4.3% (7/164) if AML with typical rearrangements like inv(16), t(15;17), t(8;21), t(3;21), and t(6;9) (46 cases) were excluded, because none of those cases was positive for the PTD. If only AML with normal karyotype are regarded PTD positivity increases to 5.7% (6/105).

### 3.5 Outcome of adult patients with MLL-duplication positive AML

Of the 15 adult patients with MLL-duplication, 3 patients did not receive treatment. Of the 12 patients receiving therapy, 3 did not achieve complete remission after the first TAD9 induction course. Of the 9 remitters, 2 did not get any further therapy, one received an additional course of TAD9, 6 patients received 1 or two high-dose Ara-C/Mitoxantrone courses. Of the 9 remitters, 8 have relapsed: 4 patients with early relapse at 2, 4, 4, and 5 months (cases #2, #6, #10, and #14 respectively) and 4 patients with later relapses at 8, 8, 9, 11 months (cases #3, #4, #15, #12, respectively). One patient died in aplasia with complete blast clearance in the bone marrow (case #8). The only childhood case achieved CR and died of complications of allo-BMT at 10 months. The median survival of all cases was 5 months, the median relapse free interval of responders was 4 months.

## 4 Discussion

The screening for the MLL duplication in 395 cases of AML revealed a total of 16 positive cases. Three duplication positive cases were observed in 8 AML patients selected based on the presence of trisomy 11. The frequency of MLL-duplication was 13 of 387 unselected AML. Both frequencies are well below the incidence reported in previous publications (table 2). Some explanations of the different frequencies reported in different studies, are as follows:

1. Regional or genetic population differences as have been reported for the t(15;17)/PML-RARa can not be ruled out.
2. It is possible, that the different RT-PCR studies for the detection of MLL-duplication transcripts were performed at different sensitivity levels. As previously reported [16] MLL-duplication transcripts are observed in virtually all healthy individuals at a level of 1/5000-10000 cells. Sensitivity of RT-PCR in our screening was set in a way that fusion transcripts in healthy donors were not detected by a one step RT-PCR with 35 cycles. In addition, all RT-PCR results were confirmed at the genomic level. From intensity of rearranged hybridization fragments of Southern blots we conclude that at least 20% of cells carry the duplication. Other studies did not quantify the amount of duplication positive cells.
3. In most of the previous studies, only restricted AML-types, such as karyotypi-

cally normal AML or AML FAB M2 subtypes, were analyzed. In contrast, we have analyzed unselected AML cases. If frequencies in our analysis are calculated only for karyotypically normal cases (5.7%) or for AML FAB M2 including t(8;21) (6.7%) or exluding t(8;21) (7.8%), they approach the incidences reported by other groups. In addition, our analysis included AML patients irrespectively of treatment protocol. Thus our cohort may be more representative for the biological spectrum of AML.

In accordance with previous studies the MLL-duplication was not found to be restricted to a specific FAB subtype, but there was a tendency towards a higher incidence within the M2 subtype, as 7/16 (43.8%) duplication positive cases were M2 whereas only 60/217 (27.6%) in the control group were M2 (table 3). This is in contrast to translocations involving MLL which predominantly occur in the myelomonocytic (M4) or monocytic (M5) subtypes. As the MLL-duplication has been found in M0, M1, M2, M4, M5 the molecular event does not seem to be restricted to a specific stage of differentiation or lineage commitment within the myeloid compartment.

**Table 2.** Frequencies of MLL-duplication. Summary of reported studies.

| Reference | total (n) | type of selection | MLL-duplication n | % |
|---|---|---|---|---|
| Caligiuri et al., 95 Cancer Research | 4 | trisomy 11 | 3 | 75 |
| Bernard et al., 95, Leukemia | 3 | trisomy 11 | 2 | |
| Caligiuri et al., 96, Cancer Research | 11 | trisomy 11 | 10 | 91 |
| Yu et al., 96, Leukemia | 34 | normal karyotype, de novo | 7 | 21 |
| Schichman et al., 94, PNAS | 19 | normal karyotype | 2 | 10.5 |
| Caligiuri et al., 94, Cancer Research | 21 | normal karyotype | 2 | 9.5 |
| Caligiuri et al., 94, Cancer Research | 33 | 21 normal karyotype 2 with t(9;11) 10 with various alterations de novo and secondary | 2 | 6.1 |
| So et al., 97, Cancer Research | 56 | de novo FAB M4/M5 | 1 | 1.8 |
| Caligiuri et al., 98, Cancer Research | 98 | normal karyotype de novo | 9* (11) | (9.2)* 11.2 |

* MLL rearrangements were found by Southern blot in 11 cases, but only in 9 cases a duplication was confirmed.

**Table 3.** Frequency of PTD in single FAB-subtypes

| FAB-subtype | total number analyzed n=217 | | cases with MLL-duplication n=16 | |
|---|---|---|---|---|
| | n | % | n | % |
| M0 | 6 | 2.8 | 1 | 6.3 |
| M1 | 32 | 14.7 | 2 | 12.5 |
| M2 | 60 | 27.6 | 7 | 43.8 |
| M3 | 16 | 7.4 | – | – |
| M4 | 40 | 18.4 | 5 | 31.25 |
| M4eo | 20 | 9.2 | – | – |
| M5 | 21 | 9.7 | 1 | 6.3 |
| M6 | 7 | 3.2 | – | – |
| M7 | 2 | 0.9 | – | – |

MLL-duplications were observed in cases with relatively frequent cytogenetic markers, such as del(7)(q22) (case#11), del(9)(q22) (case #15), and together with rare aberrations (case #10). Whether these alterations are primary or secondary to the MLL-duplication is unclear. However, two patients were analyzed in relapse. Case #3 revealed further structural alterations, such as del(17)(q23) and add(7)(q3?4), and case #4 showed gains of chromosomes 8, 13, and 19 at relapse. The duplication fusion transcripts remained constant in these cases, suggesting that MLL-duplication may represent an early, if not the initiating event, in the leukemic transformation.

MLL-duplication were not observed in association with frequent and prognostically favorable alterations, such as t(15;17); t(8;21), or inv(16), nor were MLL-duplications found in the prognostically unfavorable subgroup with complex karyotypes, suggesting a certain mechanism for transformation in MLL-duplication positive leukemia.

MLL-duplications may represent a potential unique molecular marker for a subset of AML cases which are otherwise not amenable for detection of minimal residual disease by cytogenetics or FISH. However, as published [16], MLL-duplications frequently occur in normal hematopoiesis in a subset of 1/5000-10000 cells and are easily detectable by nested RT-PCR. The biological significance of this finding is still unclear, but renders nested RT-PCR for MLL-duplications unsuitable for MRD monitoring.

The prognostic relevance of complex karyotypes as well as of the „favorable" t(8;21), inv(16) and t(15;17) have been established by several groups, although treatment variables as well as the still unresolved impact of additional chromosomal alterations still hamper definitive statements [17;18]. However, risk factors within the prognostically intermediate group with normal karyotype are lacking and eagerly awaited. Previous publications with limited numbers of patients have suggested that the presence of an MLL-duplication may have an unfavorable impact on survival [7, 8, 19, 20]. In addition to these cases our data confirm the notion, that MLL-duplication heralds a bad prognosis.

*Acknowlegdement.* This work was supported by a program grant of the Deutsche Forschungsgemeinschaft and (SFB500, project A1).

## References

1. Caligiuri M, Schichman SA, Strout MP, Mrozek K, Baer MR, Frankel SR, Barcos M, Herzig GP, Croce CM, Bloomfield CD (1994) Molecular rearrangement of the ALL-1 gene in acute myeloid leukemia without cytogenetic evidence of 11q23 chromosomal translocations. Cancer Res 54:370
2. Schichman SA, Caligiuri M, Strout M, Carter S, Gu Y, Canaani E, Bloomfield C, Croce C (1994) ALL-1 tandem duplication in acute myeloid leukemia with a normal karyotype involves homologous recombination between ALU elements. Cancer Res 54:4277
3. Schichman S, Caligiuri M, Gu Y, Strout M, Canaani E, Bloomfield C, Croce C (1994) ALL-1 partial duplication in acute leukemia. PNAS 91:6236
4. Bernard OA, Romana SP, Schichman SA, Mauchauffe M, Jonveaux P, Berger R (1995) Partial duplication of HRX in acute leukemia with trisomy 11. Leukemia 9:1487
5. Schichman S, Canaani E, Croce C: Self-fusion of the ALL1 gene (1995) A new genetic mechanism for acute leukemia. JAMA 273:571
6. Caligiuri MA, Strout MP, Schichman SA, Mrozek K, Arthur DC, Herzig GP, Baer MR, Schiffer CA, Heinonen K, Knuutila S, Nousiainen T, Ruutu T, Block AW, Schulman P, Pedersen BJ, Croce CM, Bloomfield CD (1996) Partial tandem duplication of ALL1 as a recurrent molecular defect in acute myeloid leukemia with trisomy 11: Cancer Res 56: 1418
7. Yu M, Honoki K, Andersen J, Paietta E, Nam DK, Yunis JJ (1996) MLL tandem duplication and multiple splicing in adult acute myeloid leukemia with normal karyotype. Leukemia 10:774
8. Caligiuri MA, Strout MP, Lawrence D, Arthur DC, Baer MR, Yu F, Knuutila S, Mrozek K, Oberkircher AR, Marcucci G, de, la, Chapelle, A, Elonen E, Block AW, Rao PN, Herzig GP, Powell BL, Ruutu T, Schiffer

CA, Bloomfield CD (1998) Rearrangement of ALL1 (MLL) in acute myeloid leukemia with normal cytogenetics. Cancer Res 58:55

9. Bennett J, Catovsky D, Daniel M-T, Flandrin G, Galton D, Gralnick H, Sultan C (1996) Proposals for the classification of acute leukemias, a report of the French-American-British Cooperative Group. Br J Haematol 33:451

10. Bennett J, Catovsky D, Daniel M-T, Flandrin G, Galton D, Gralnick H, Sultan C (1985) Criteria for the diagnosis of acute leukemias of mega-karyocyte lineage(M7), a report of the French-American-British Cooperative Group. Ann Intern Med 103:460

11. Büchner T, Hiddemann W, Wörmann B (1996) Intensive consolidation versus prolonged maintenance following intensive induction and conventional consolidation in primary AML: a study by AMLCG. Blood 88, Suppl I:214 A

12. ISCN: Guidelines for cancer cytogenetics. Basel, Karger, 1995

13. Miller S (1988) A simple salting out procedure for extracting DNA from nucleated cells. Nucl. Acid. Res. 16:1215

14. Gu Y, Nakamura T, Alder H, Prasad R, Canaani O, Cimino G, Croce C, Canaani E (1992) The t(4;11) chromosome translocation of human acute leukemias fuses the ALL-1 gene, related to drosophila trithorax to the AF-4 gene. Cell 71:701

15. Nilson I., Löchner K., Siegler G., Greil J., Beck D.J., Fey G.H., Marschaleck R (1996) Exon/Intron structure of the human ALL-1 (MLL) gene involved in translocations to chromosomal region 11q23 and acute leukemias. British Journal of Haematology 93:966-972

16. Schnittger S, Wörmann B, Hiddemann W, Griesinger F (1998) Partial tandem duplications of the MLL gene are detectable in peripheral blood and bone marrow of nearly all healthy donors. Blood 92:1728

17. Bloomfield C, Lawrence D, Byrd J, Carroll A, Pettenati M, Tantravahi R, Patil S, Davey F, Berg D, Schiffer C, Arthur D, Mayer R (1998) Frequency of prolonged remission duration after high-dose cytarabine intensification in acute myeloid leukemia varies by cytogenetic subtype. Cancer Res 58:4173

18. Schlenk R, Fischer K, Del Valle F, Harmann F, Pralle H, Fischer J, Gunzer U, Pezzutto A, Weber W, Grimminger W, Preiss J, Göckel F, Haase R, Döhner H: Stratification of postremission therapy in adult acute myeloid leukemia according to the karyotype-preliminary results of a multicenter treatment trial AML HD93, in Hiddemann W, Büchner T, Wörmann B, Ritter J, Creutzig U, Keating M, Plunkett W (eds): Acute Leukemias VII: Experimental approaches and novel therapies, vol. 39. Berlin, Heidelberg, Springer, 1998, p 867

19. So CW, Ma ZG, Price CM, Dong S, Chen SJ, Gu LJ, So CK, Wiedemann LM, Chan LC: (1997) MLL self fusion mediated by Alu repeat homologous recombination and prognosis of AML-M4/M5 subtypes. Cancer Res 57:117

20. Strout M, Marcucci G, Bloomfield C, Caligiuri M (1998) The partial tandem duplication of ALL1 (MLL) is consistently generated by Alu-mediated homologous recombination in acute myeloid leukemia. Proc Natl Acad Sci USA 95:2390

# Real-Time RT-PCR for the Detection and Quantification of AML1/MTG8 Fusion Transcripts in Patients with t(8;21) Positive AML

J. Krauter[1], M. P. Wattjes[1], S. Nagel[1], O. Heidenreich[2], U. Krug[1], S. Kafert[1], D. Bunjes[3], L. Bergmann[3], A. Ganser[1] and G. Heil[1]

*Abstract.* AML1/MTG8 was quantified relative to the expression of the GAPDH house-keeping gene by real-time RT-PCR in 22 patients with t(8;21) positive AML at initial diagnosis and in seven of these patients also during/after chemotherapy and allogeneic bone marrow transplantation. Real-time PCR was able to specifically detect and quantify AML1/MTG8 over a 5 log range. The detection limit for t(8;21) positive cells was a dilution of $1:10^5$. The AML1/MTG8 expression varied considerably among the 22 AML patients at initial diagnosis with a ratio AML1/MTG8:GAPDH of $0,5135 \pm 0,536$ (range 0,1 to 2,14, median 0,318). In six patients with t(8;21) positive AML a marked decline of AML1/MTG8 could be induced by chemotherapy. These patients are in ongoing complete hematological remission (CR) with a constant low-level AML1/MTG8 expression. In another patient, a rapid rise of AML1/MTG8 transcripts could be detected in CR after allogeneic bone marrow transplantation transplantation and the patient relapsed ten weeks later. In conclusion, real-time RT-PCR is a suitable approach for the quantification of AML1/MTG8 transcripts in the monitoring of AML-patients with t(8;21) during/after chemotherapy and can provide data of prognostic relevance.

blastic leukemia (AML). It fuses the 5'-part of the AML1-gene on chromosome 21 to the almost complete MTG8 gene on chromosome 8. The AML1 gene encodes for a transcription factor essential for normal hematopoiesis, whereas the function of MTG8 is still unknown [1]. In all t(8;21) positive patients a constant AML1/MTG8 fusion mRNA can be detected by reverse transcriptase polymerase chain reaction (RT-PCR) [2,3]. The presence of a t(8;21) is associated with a high complete remission rate. However, the impact of this chromosomal aberration on long-term prognosis remains controversial [4-7]. RT-PCR for AML1/MTG8 can be used as a sensitive tool for the detection of residual t(8;21) positive cells in these patients [8]. However, in several studies using RT-PCR for the detection of minimal residual disease most of the patients remained positive for AML1/MTG8 even in long-term complete hematological remission [8-10]. Preliminary data using quantitative competitor PCR suggest, that quantification of the AML1/MTG8 transcripts might be able to detect patients with a high risk of relapse [11,12]. We used a novel quantitative PCR assay, real-time PCR, for the prospective quantification of AML1/MTG8 transcripts in patients with t(8;21) positive AML at initial presentation and after intensive induction and consolidation chemotherapy.

## 1 Introduction

The translocation t(8;21)(q22;q22) is one of the most common structural chromosomal aberrations in patients with acute myelo-

[1] Department of Hematology and Oncology, Hannover Medical School
[2] Department of Molecular Biology, Institute of Cell Biology, University of Tübingen
[3] Department Internal Medicine III, University of Ulm

## 2 Patients and Methods

### 2.1 Generation of an AML1/MTG8 standard plasmid

A 338bp DNA-fragment spanning the AML1/MTG8 fusion site was generated by 35 cycles of standard PCR with cDNA from the t(8;21) positive Kasumi-1 cell line as described [3]. This fragment was cloned into the pCR2.1 vector. After UV-quantification, this plasmid was used for the generation of the AML1/MTG8 standard-curves.

### 2.2 Real-Time PCR for AML1/MTG8

The probe and primers for the AML1/MTG8 real-time PCR (table 1) were designed with the PRIMER-EXPRESS" software (Perkin-Elmer). FAM (6-carboxyfluorescein) was used as the reporter and TAMRA (6-carboxy-tetra-methyl-rhodamine) as the quencher dye. The reaction was carried out in 50µl with 1 × Taqman buffer A, 8,5mmol $MgCl_2$, nucleotides 200µmol, probe 150nmol, primers 300 nmol each, 0,25U AmpliTaq-Gold Polymerase (Perkin Elmer) and 1µl cDNA-template. The reaction conditions were 95°C 10min and then 40 cycles of 15s 95°C followed by 60s 59°C. All experiments were carried out in triplicate and several negative controls were included. Fluorescence spectra were continously monitored and analysed by a SDS 7700 system (Applied Biosystems).

### 2.3 Real-time PCR for GAPDH

GAPDH expression was quantified with a 5´-JOE-(2,7-dimethoxy-4,5-dichloro-6-carboxy-fluorescein)-labelled probe (GAPDH control reagents kit, Perkin Elmer). The reaction was carried out in 50µl with 1 × Taqman buffer A, 5,5mmol $MgCl_2$, nucleotides 200µmol, probe 100nmol, primers 200 nmol each, 0,25U AmpliTaq-Gold Polymerase (Perkin Elmer)

and 1µl cDNA-template. The reaction conditions were 95°C 10min and then 40 cycles of 15s 95°C followed by 60s 60°C. A serial dilution of Raji-cDNA with a defined number of GAPDH copies from $10^6$ to $10^2$ was used for the generation of a standard curve.

### 2.4 Kasumi-1 dilution series

Kasumi-1 cells positive for t(8;21) were serially diluted in t(8;21) negative HL60 cells from 1:0 to $1:10^5$. Total cellular RNA was extracted from $10^7$ cells of this dilution series using the Trizol-method (GibcoBRL). cDNA was synthesised for 1 hour at 37°C using 2µg RNA, random primers (1µmol/l) and murine Moloney virus reverse transcriptase in a total volume of 20µl.

### 2.5 Detection of AML1/MTG8 transcripts by real-time PCR in patient samples

After informed consent was given, bone marrow samples were taken from 22 patients with t(8;21) positive AML at initial diagnosis (≥80% blasts in the bone marrow). Prior to analysis, the mononuclear cells were enriched by a Ficoll-Isopaque gradient (1,077g/ml). RNA-extraction, cDNA-synthesis and real-time PCR for AML1/MTG8 were performed as described above. AML1/MTG8 was quantified relative to the GAPDH expression in the samples analysed. In seven of the patients also bone marrow samples at various time points during/after chemotherapy were analysed to detect minimal residual disease. These patients were treated with two cycles of induction chemotherapy consisting of standard dose AraC, VP16 and idarubicine. After that, they received a first consolidation cycle of intermediate dose AraC (1g/m², 8 doses) and daunorubicin. For late consolidation, the patients were treated with high dose AraC (3g/m², 12 doses) and daunorubicine [5].

**Table 1.** Primers and probe for AML1/MTG8 real-time PCR

| AML1-Primer | 5'-AATCACAGTGGATGGGCCC -3' |
|---|---|
| MTG8-Primer | 5'-TGCGTCTTCACATCCACAGG-3' |
| AML1/MTG8-probe | 5'-*FAM*-CTGAGAAGCACTCCACAATGCCAGACT-*TAMRA*-3' |

# 3 Results

## 3.1 AML1/MTG8 standard curve

A serial dilution from $10^6$ to $10^2$ molecules/ml of the AML1/MTG8 plasmid was used as a template for real-time PCR. A specific increase in reporter fluorescence could be detected in the AML1/MTG8 probes but not in samples with a control plasmid or cDNAs from normal bone marrow or t(8;21) negative AMLs. There was a linear decrease of the threshold cycle in proportion to the log of the starting copy number with a correlation coefficient of 0,97 to 0,99 in various repetitions of the experiment (Fig. 1).

## 3.2. Sensitivity of AMI1/MTG8 real-time PCR

Real-time PCR was able to quantify the number of AML1/MTG8 transcripts in the cDNA probes from pure Kasumi-1 cells to a $1:10^5$ dilution and displayed a linear correlation of the $C_T$ and the log of the Kasumi-1 cell number in the sample over a five log range.

## 3.3. Quantification of AML1/MTG8 Expression in t(8;21) positive AMLs

AML1/MTG8 expression was quantified in 22 patients with t(8;21) positive AMLs at initial diagnosis. The AML1/MTG8 expression was quantified relative to the expression of the GAPDH housekeeping gene. The ratio AML1/MTG8:GAPDH in the patients was $0,5135\pm0,536$ (range 0,1 to 2,14, median 0,318). The mean ratio of AML1/MTG8: GAPDH in repeated experiments with the Kasumi-1 cell-line was 0,684.

## 3.4. Detection and quantification of minimal residual disease in patients with t(8;21) positive AML by real-time PCR

In seven patients with t(8;21) positive AML, AML1/MTG8 was quantified relative to GAPDH during and after chemotherapy by real-time PCR (Fig. 2a and b).

Three patients (no. 1-3) were analysed in aplasia after the first induction cycle. Despite good response to chemotherapy without detectable blasts in the microscopic analysis, they showed only a modest decline in the ratio AML1/MTG8:GAPDH. However, after additional chemotherapy, the patients displayed a 3-4 log decrease in AML1/MTG8 expression. Also, three patients (no. 4-6) who were analysed after completion of the induction chemotherapy and after consolidation showed a similar decline of AML1/MTG8 (Fig. 2a). All six patients are in ongoing complete hematological remission with constant low-level AML1/MTG8 expression or a nega-

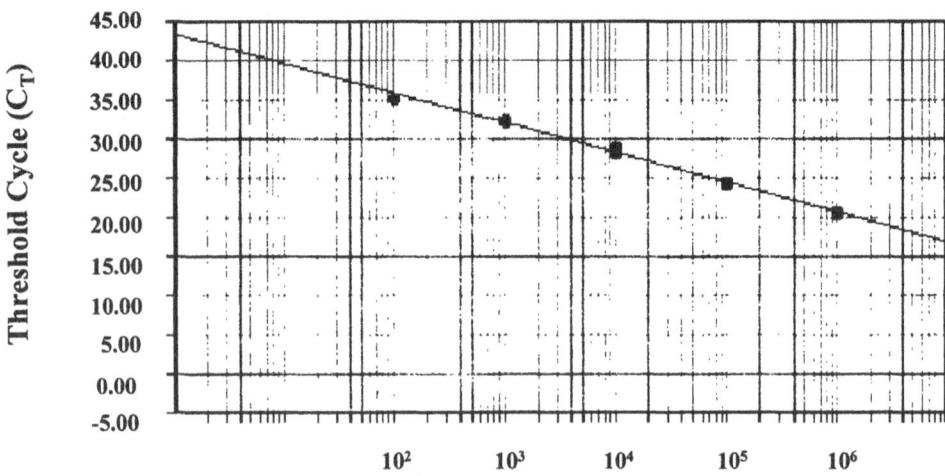

**Fig. 1.** AML1/MTG8 standard curve. The $C_T$-values for a known amount of starter molecules are used for the calculation of a standard curve.

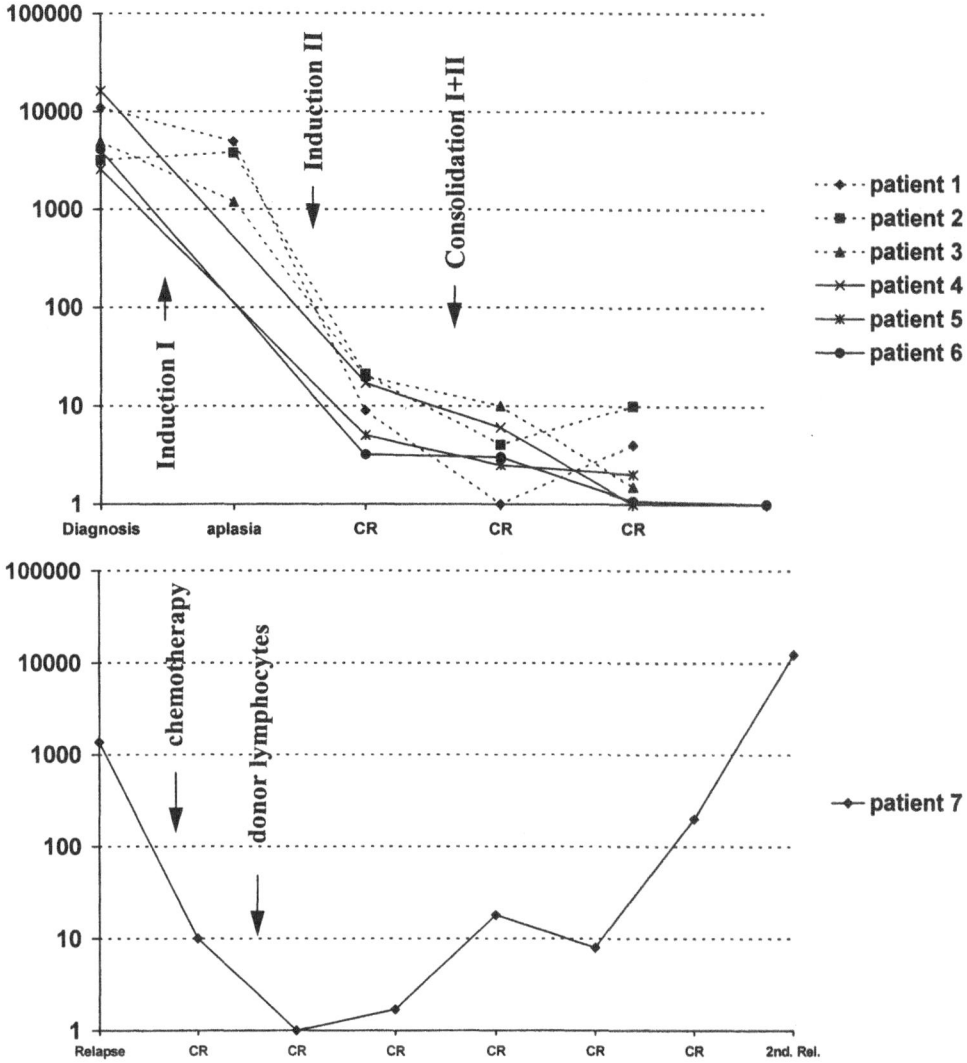

**Fig. 2a,b.** Quantification of residual disease by AML1/MTG8 real-time PCR. AML1/MTG8 was quantified relative to GAPDH in seven patients with t(8;21) positive AML at initial diagnosis and at various time points during and after chemotherapy. For graphical reasons (log scale) a normalised ratio AML1/MTG8:GAPDH ([copy number of AML1/MTG8] : [copy number GAPDH] × 10000 + 1) on the vertical axis is plotted against the clinical course of the patients. The horizontal axis displays the clinical state of the patient at the time of analysis.

tive PCR result. One patient, who relapsed after allogeneic bone marrow transplantation, showed a decrease in AML1/MTG8 expression after chemotherapy and became PCR negative after additional donor lymphocyte infusions (figure 2b). Subsequently she showed a rapid rise of the AML1/MTG8 transcripts and relapsed again ten weeks later.

## 4 Discussion

We used real-time PCR for the detection and quantification of AML1/MTG8 transcripts in t(8;21) positive AML at initial presentation as well as during and after chemotherapy. This technique has been shown to be equally accurate and sensitive as standard competitor PCR [13] and preliminary data indicate, that it can be used for the sensitive quantification of tumor specific DNA- and RNA-targets in a variety of hematological diseases [14-17]. To analyse the sensitivity of our real-time PCR assay, we used not only an AML1/MTG8 plasmid but also a cellular dilution series of t(8;21) positive Kasumi-1 cells in HL60. Since we found, that the AML1/MTG8 expression of Kasumi-1 cells is in the same range as in native t(8;21) positive AML blasts, this dilution series can be used as an accurate model for the clinical situation of minimal residual disease (MRD) and we were able to detect t(8;21) positive cells with a sensitivity of $1:10^5$. We found a considerable heterogeneity of the AML1/MTG8 expression level in 22 patients with newly diagnosed, untreated AML with t(8;21): The ratio AML1/MTG8: GAPDH varied over the range from 0,1 to 2,14 although the material analysed contained ≥80% blasts in all cases under study. Further studies are necessary to analyse if the AML1/MTG8 expression level correlates with certain phenotypes of these leukemias and if it can be modulated by stimulation of the blasts with certain cytokines, e.g. interferon-α as reported for PML/RARα expression in t(15;17) positive AML [18,19]. In this context it would be of special interest to know if the intracellular AML1/MTG8 expression level is indicative of disease progression in patients in complete hematological remission from whom we know that at least a certain proportion harbours t(8;21) positive multipotent progenitor cells [20]. Irrespectively of the underlying mechanisms this heterogeneity in AML1/MTG8 expression has to be taken into account if MRD is assessed by qualitative or quantitative PCR since it greatly influences the sensitivity of a PCR assay in individual AML-patients. In addition to the analysis at initial presentation, six patients with t(8;21) positive AML were analysed during and after an identical chemotherapy and one patient after allogeneic bone marrow transplantation. In contrast to a recent report [16], we found a relatively uniform pattern of AML1/MTG8 expression after chemotherapy: All six patients showed a marked decline of AML1/MTG8 after the completion of the induction and consolidation chemotherapy and all these patients are in ongoing hematological CR. On the other hand, one further

patient, who was analysed after allogeneic bone marrow transplantation, had a rapid rise in AML1/MTG8 ten weeks prior to clinical relapse confirming previous reports which also showed by competitor based quantitative PCR that an increase in AML1/MTG8 transcripts heralds disease progression [11,12]. Taken together, real-time quantitative PCR allows the accurate and reliable quantification of AML1/MTG8 transcripts over a five log range. It is a suitable approach to monitor the leukemic burden during and after chemotherapy. In addition, it can provide decisive information about the mechanisms involved in the control and/or elimination of residual leukemic cells.

*Acknowledgements.* Supported by grants from the Dr. Wilhelm Kempe Foundation and the Deutsche Krebshilfe (10-1217-He).

The authors wish to thank Kerstin Görlich, Elvira Lux and Dagmar Reile for their excellent technical assistance.

# References

1. Okuda T, van Deursen J, Hiebert SW, Grosveld G, Downing JR: (1996) AML1, the target of multiple chromosomal translocations in human leukemia, is essential for normal fetal liver hematopoiesis. Cell 84:321-330
2. Miyoshi H, Kozu T, Shimizu K, Enomoto K, Maseki N, Kaneko Y, Kamada N, Ohki M: (1993) The t(8;21) translocation in acute myeloid leukemia results in production of an AML1-MTG8 fusion transcript. EMBO J 12:2715-2721
3. Krauter J, Peter W, Pascheberg U, Heinze B, Bergmann L, Hoelzer D, Lübbert M, Schlimok G, Arnold R, Kirchner H, Port M, Ganser A, Heil G: (1998) Detection of karyotypic aberrations in acute myeloblastic leukemia: A prospective comparison between PCR/FISH and standard cytogenetics in 140 patients with de novo AML. Br J Haematol 103:72-78
4. Grimwade D, Walker H, Oliver F, Wheatley K, Harrison C, Harrison G, Rees J, Hann I, Stevens R, Burnett A, Goldstone A: (1998) The importance of diagnostic cytogenetics on outcome in AML: analysis of 1612 patients entered into the MRC AML 10 trial. Blood 92:2322-2333
5. Heil G, Krauter J, Raghavachar A, et al (1997) Risk-adapted induction and consolidation therapy including autologous peripheral blood stem cell transplantation (PBSCT) in adult de-novo AML patients. Blood 90:508a (Abstract)
6. Bloomfield CD, Lawrence D, Byrd JC, Carrol A, Pettenati MJ, Tantravahi R, Patil SR, Davey FR, Berg DT, Schiffer CA, Arthur DC, Mayer RJ: (1998) Frequency

of prolonged remission duration after high-dose cytarabine intensification in acute myeloid leukemia varies by cytogenetic subtype. Cancer Res 58:4173-4179

7. Fenaux P, Lai JL, Preudhomme C, Jouet JP, Deminatti M, Bauters F: (1990) Is translocation (8;21) a »favorable« cytogenetic rearrangement in acute myeloid leukemia? Nouv Rev Fr Hematol 32:179-182

8. Kusec R, Laczika K, Knobl P, Friedl J, Greinix H, Kahls P, Linkesch W, Schwarzinger I, Mitterbauer G, Purtscher B, Haas O, Lechner K, Jaeger K: (1994) AML1/ETO fusion mRNA can be detected in remission blood samples of all patients with t(8;21) acute myeloid leukemia after chemotherapy or autologous bone marrow transplantation. Leukemia 8:735-739

9. Nucifora G, Larson RA, Rowley JD: (1993) Persistence of the 8;21 translocation in patients with acute myeloid leukemia type M2 in long-term remission. Blood 82:712-715

10. Jurlander J, Caligiuri MA, Ruutu T, Baer MR, Strout MP, Oberkircher AR, Hoffmann L, Ball ED, Frei Lahr DA, Christiansen NP, Block AM, Knuutila S, Herzig GP, Bloomfield CD: (1996) Persistence of the AML1/ETO fusion transcript in patients treated with allogeneic bone marrow transplantation for t(8;21) leukemia. Blood 88:2183-2191

11. Tobal K, Yin JA: (1996) Monitoring of minimal residual disease by quantitative reverse transcriptase-polymerase chain reaction for AML1-MTG8 transcripts in AML-M2 with t(8; 21). Blood 88:3704-3709

12. Muto A, Mori S, Matsushita H, Awaya N, Ueno H, Takayama N, Okamoto S, Kizaki M, Ikeda Y: (1996) Serial quantification of minimal residual disease of t(8;21) acute myelogenous leukemia with RT-competitive PCR assay. Br J Haematol 95:85-94

13. Desjardin LE, Chen Y, Perkins MD, Teixeira L, Cave MD, Eisenach KD: (1998) Comparison of the ABI 7700 system (TaqMan) and competitive PCR for quantification of IS6110 DNA in sputum during treatment of tuberculosis. J Clin Microbiol 36:1964-1968

14. Mensink E, van de Locht A, Schattenberg A, Linders E, Schaap N, Geurts van Kessel A, De Witte T: (1998) Quantitation of minimal residual disease in Philadelphia chromosome positive chronic myeloid leukemia using real-time quantitative RT-PCR. Br J Haematol 102:768-774

15. Gerard CJ, Olsson K, Ramanathan R, Reading C, Hanania EG: (1998) Improved quantitation of minimal residual disease in multiple myeloma using real-time polymerase chain reaction and plasmid-DNA complementarity determinig region III standards. Cancer Res 58:3957-3964

16. Marcucci G, Livak KJ, Bi W, Strout MP, Bloomfield CD, Caligiuri MA: (1998) Detection of minimal residual disease in patients with AML1/ETO-associated acute myeloid leukemia using a novel quantitative reverse transcription polymerase chain reaction assay. Leukemia 12:1482-1489

17. Pongers-Willemse MJ, Verhagen OJ, Tibbe GJ, Wijkhuijs AJ, de Haas V, Roovers E, van der Schoot CE, van Dongen JJ: (1998) Real-time quantitative PCR for the detection of minimal residual disease in acute lymphoblastic leukemia using junctional region specific TaqMan probes. Leukemia 12:2006-2014

18. Nason Burchenal K, Gandini D, Botto M, Allopenna J, Seale JR, Cross NC, Goldman JM, Dmitrovsky E, Pandolfi PP: (1996) Interferon augments PML and PML/RAR alpha expression in normal myeloid and acute promyelocytic cells and cooperates with all-trans retinoic acid to induce maturation of a retinoid-resistant promyelocytic cell line. Blood 88:3926-3936

19. Seale JR, Varma S, Swirsky DM, Pandolfi PP, Goldman JM, Cross NC: (1996) Quantification of PML-RAR alpha transcripts in acute promyelocytic leukemia: explanation for the lack of sensitivity of RT-PCR for the detection of minimal residual disease and induction of the leukemia-specific mRNA by alpha interferon. Br J Haematol 95:95-101

20. Miyamoto T, Nagafuji K, Akashi K, Harada M, Kyo T, Akashi T, Takenaka K, Mizuno S, Gondo H, Okamura J, Dohy H, Niho Y: (1996) Persistence of multipotent progenitors expressing AML1/ETO transcripts in long-term remission patients with t(8;21) acute myelogenous leukemia. Blood 87:4789-4796

# Combined Cytogenetic, FISH and RT-PCR Technique in Detection of t(15;17) and Monitoring of Minimal Residual Disease in Acute Promyelocytic Leukemia

Yu.V. Olshanskaya, I.A. Demidova, N.G. Tiurina, A.I. Udovitchenko, L.A. Vodinskaia, A.B. Sudarikov, R.G. Kuliev, E.N. Parovitchnikova, E.V. Domratcheva and V.G. Savchenko

## Introduction

Detection of the t(15;17) or PML/RARa rearrangment is important for analysis of clinical trials involving patients with suspected acute promyelocytic leukemia (APL). According to the majority of reports the translocation t(15;17)(q22;q12-21) is detected in 70% to 100% of cases [1]. PML/RARa fusion transcript from add(15q) is beleived to play crucial role in leukemogenesis of this type of leukemia [2]. It's presence remains the predictor of favourable prognosis and good response to modern modalities of therapy, especially ATRA [3].

We evaluated the relative efficacy of conventional cytogenetics, fluorescence in situ hybridization (FISH) method and RT-PCR in order to identify the translocation in patients with APL at admission and during treatment. Cytogenetic evaluations were dependent on finding of an adequate number of metaphases with sufficient quality to identify the translocation while the quality of bone marrow cultures of patients with APL was usually poor. A potentially more effective method is FISH which can be used for the chromosome analysis of both interphase and methaphase cells. RT-PCR can be performed rapidly from a small amount of sample.

RT-PCR and FISH technique allow to reveal minimal residual disease during remission [4]. It is known that detection of PML/RARa fusion transcript predicts relaps however the relaps can appear in spite of several RT-PCR negative assays. The sensitivity of FISH method is lower than RT-PCR, but persistence of PML/RARA fusion gene in dividing cells means forthcoming relaps in most cases. The role of different methods such as RT-PCR, quantitative RT-PCR and FISH in diagnosis of minimal residual disease is still under investigation [5,6].

## Materials and methods

We performed t(15;17) detection in bone marrow samples of 19 patients with APL (M3) at the diagnosis. The M3 variant of AML was confirmed by morphological evaluation and cytochemistry. Ten patients were evaluated for minimal residual disease using FISH and PCR techniques. All patients recieved chemotherapy and in seven of them chemotherapy was combined with ATRA. In eight patients first evaluation was performed after first month of treatment.

Chromosome analysis was performed on metaphases from direct and short-term (24h, 48h) cultures of bone marrow without mitogen stimulation using trypsine-Wrights banding technique. Chromosomes were classified according to the ISCN [7].

Interphase FISH was performed using the Vysis LSI PML/RARA translocation probe on the same samples following the procedure recommended by Vysis Protocol. 200 cells were evaluated routinely. In negative cases up to 800 cells were investigated. From ten of the normal specimens, we calculated a normal cutoff of 10% for interphase cells.

m RNA for RT-PCR was isolated using standard guanidine-isotiocyanate method. The reverse transcription and double round nested amplification was performed on 1 microgram of total RNA as described by Castagne et al [8] with slight modifications ("hot start" nested PCR). Two types of fusion transcript sized as 212 and 402 b.p. were visualized in 2% agarose gel via UV illumination.

## Results

Conventional cytogenetics was available in 14 of 19 pts. Typical t(15;17) was revealed in 10 cases of 19 pts at the diagnosis as the sole aberration. In three cases t(15;17) was accompanied by trisomy 8, ider(17q), and trisomy 8 with del(9q) respectively. In five cases G-band analysis failed because of poor quality of metaphases. One patient demonstrated normal karyotype.

FISH analysis on interphase cells showed the presence of PML/RARa fusion in all cases with t(15;17) revealed by G-band and in 4 of 5 cases where G-band was not available. One case with normal karyotype was positive for PML/RARA by FISH.

Twelve patients at diagnosis were evaluated using RT-PCR technique. Eleven of them showed typical PML/RARa fusion transcript. Nine patients demonstrated S-type (bcr3) of transcript and one – L-type (bcr1). In one

**Table 1.** Detection of PML/RARA using FISH and RT-PCR techniques in 10 patients with APL during follow-up

| Pt No | Percent of positive cells by FISH/ type of transcript by PCR at the diagnosis | Presence of detectable PML/RARA during follow-up (percent of positive cells by FISH and detection of transcript) Horizontal line represents a period of follow-up (in months) | Karyotype at diagnosis |
|---|---|---|---|
| 1. | 90% / 0 / bcr3 | 5% (1mo) / neg ————— (10mo) neg ————— (24mo) | 46,XX,t(15;17) |
| 2. | 96% / 0 / bcr3 | ————— (14mo) 6,8% / neg ——— (20mo) 8% / neg ——— (48mo) | 46,XY,t(15;17) |
| 3. | 84% / 0 / bcr3 | 12% (1mo) / bcr3 ——— 13% (2mo) ——— (5mo, relapse, died) | 46,XX,t(15;17) |
| 4. | 95% / 0 / bcr1 | 13% (1mo) / bcr1 ——— (5mo) pos 9,8% ——— (12mo) 9% ——— (16mo) neg ——— (19mo) neg | ND |
| 5. | 76% / 0 / bcr3 | 8% (1mo) ————— (8mo) 9,7% / neg ————————— (17mo) neg | 46,XX,t(15;17)/ 46,XX,t(15;17), ider(17)t(15;17) |
| 6. | 62% / 0 / bcr3 | 4,3% (1mo) / pos ————— (8mo) 7% / neg ————— (16mo) | 46,XY,t(15;17) |
| 7. | 94% / 0 / bcr3 | 7,3% (1mo) / neg ——— (4mo) 7,7% / neg ————————— (12mo) | 46,XX,t(15;17) |
| 8. | 97% / 0 / bcr3 | 31% (1mo) / pos ——— (4mo) 4,5% / neg ——— (6mo) 5,7% / neg ——— (12mo) | 46,XY,t(15;17) |
| 9. | 83% / 0 / bcr3 | 12% (1mo) / pos ——— (3mo, died, sepsis) | ND |
| 10. | 70% / 0 / bcr3 | 6% (3mo) / neg ——— (10mo) 4,5% / neg ——— (15 mo) 9% / neg ——— (18mo) neg ——— (20mo, relapse) | 47,XY,+8,t(15;17)/ 47,XY,+8,t(15;17), del(9)(q12q22) |

patient both FISH and RT-PCR assays were negative for PML/RARA.

Ten patients were evaluated for minimal residual disease (MRD) using FISH and eight of them – with PCR technique during treatment. The data of patients included in investigation is summarized in Table 1. Five patients demonstrated PML/RARA positivity after first course of induction chemotherapy (ATRA and 7+3) while complete remission was estimated by morphology. Three of them turn into negative during subsequent chemotherapy. One of them died of progressive leukemia and the other of infection during consolidation. Seven patients are in complete remission with duration from 8 to 42 months. All of them are negative by FISH and RT-PCR for PML/RARA. One patient was PML/RARA negative by RT-PCR but relapsed after 20 months of remission in two months after last investigation.

## Discussion

Karyotype is a key indicator of prognosis in AML. The presence of t(15;17) is thought to be linked closely to M3 phenotype and predict good response to differentiation therapy with ATRA and relatively favourable outcome. However, the morphological evaluation sometimes is not sufficient for therapy determination. Therefore the identification of this translocation or PML/RARA rearrangement is very important for stratification [9].

The results of our study demonsrated that frequency of t(15;17) was about 94% in morphologicaly proved APL cases at diagnosis. This data are correlated with data of other investigations [10,11,12,13]. FISH was very useful in detection of PML/RARA in those patients were the conventional cytogenetic failed to find out this translocation. One case with typical morphological features of M3 at diagnosis lacked t(15;17) by conventional cytogenetics, FISH and RT-PCR analysis, and during next investigation after achievement of remission karyotype 46,XX,del(3)(q23q25) [3]/46,XX,inv(3)(q21q26[5]/46,XX[3] was revealed. The absence of PML/RARA, confirmed by different methods, allows to suggest some other mechanism of leukemic formation.

Evaluation of minimal residual disease was performed using FISH and RT-PCR. We find out good correlation between both the methods used and proved that FISH and RT-PCR are equally useful to evaluation of gene rearrangement. It seems to be more rational to use RT-PCR for routine monitoring of minimal residual disease. However, the absense of detectable PML/RARA transcript in one patient closely to time of relapse supposes that even the negative results can not exclude the probability for disease recurrence. Of the special concern seems to be the fact that this patient had two clones revealed by conventional cytogenetics at the diagnosis (47,XY,+8,t(15;17)/47,XY,+8,t(15;17), del(9)(q12q22)). Additional chromosome aberrations are not rare events in patients with APL, but influence of relative clones on achievement of remission and prognosis of disease is still under investigation [13]. Probably the existence of two relative clones suggests clonal evolution as sighn of tumor progression and can predict negative prognosis.

The data of some investigators proposed some prognostic value of transcript type (L or S) [14]. We are not able yet to confirm these findings.

In future the development of FISH and more sensitive methods such as quantitative PCR will help to find out the impact of PML/RARA detection on prognosis of leukemia course.

## References

1. Rowley JD, Golomb HM, Dougherty C. 15/17 translocation, a consistent chromosomal change in acute promyelocytic leukemia. Lancet 1977, 1:549-550.
2. Mitelman F, Heim S. Cancer cytogenetics. Second edition. New-York, Wiley-Liss, 1995.
3. Petkovich M, Brand NJ, Krust A, et al. A human retinoic acid receptor which belongs to the family of nuclear receptors. Nature 1987, 30:444-450.
4. Schad CR, Hanson CA, Paietta E et al. Efficacy of fluorescence in situ hybridization for detecting PML/RARA gene fusion in treated and untreated acute promyelocytic leukemia. Mayo Clinic Proceedings 1994, 69(11)1047-1053.
5. Grimwade D, Howe K, Langabeer S et al. Establishing the presence of the t(15;17) in suspected acute promyelocytic leukaemia: cytogenetic, molecular and PML immunofluorescence assessment of patients entered into the M.R.C. ATRA trial. British Journal of Haematology, 1996, 94:557-573.

6. Grignani F, Pelicci PG. Pathogenetic role of the PML/RAR alpha fusion protein in acute promyelocytic leukemia. Current Topics in Microbiology and Immunology. 1996; 211: 269-278.

7. ISCN (1995) Recommendations of the International Standing Committee on Human Cytogenetic Nomenclature. Mitelman F.(ed), Basel, S Karger 1995.

8. Castaigne S, Balitrand N, de The H et al. A PML/Retinoic acid receptor a fusion transcript is constantly detected by RNA-based polymerase chain reaction in acute promyelocytic leukemia. Blood 1992, 79(12):3110-3115.

9. Warell RP, Frankel SR, Miller WH et al. Differentiation therapy for acute promyelocytic leukemia with tretinoin (all-trans retinoic acid). 1991 New England Journal of Medicine 324:1385-1392.

10. Larson RA, Kondo K, Vardiman JW et al. Evidence for a 15/17 translocation in every patient with promyelocytic leukemia. American Journal of Medicine 1984, 76:827-841.

11. Heim S, Mitelman F. Secondary chromosome aberrations in the acute leukemias. Cancer Genetics and Cytogenetics 1986, 22:331-338.

12. Berger R, Le Coniat M, Derre J et al. Cytogenetic studies in acute promyelocytic leukemia: A survey of secondary chromosomal abnormalities. Genes, Cromosomes, Cancer. 1991, 3:332-337.

13. Schoch C, Haase D, Haferlach T et al. Incidence and implication of additional chromosome aberrations in acute promyelocytic leukaemia with translocation t(15;17)(q22;q21): a report on 50 patients. British Journal of Haematology 1996, 94:493-500.

14. Gallagher RE, Willman CL, Slack JL et al. Association of PML-RAR alpha fusion mRNA type with pretreatment hematologic characteristics but not treatment outcome in acute promyelocytic leukemia: an intergroup molecular study. Blood. 1997; 90(4): 1656-1663.

# RT-PCR in Diagnostics and Monitoring of Acute Myeloid

S. Schnittger[1,2], C. Schoch[1,2], F. Griesinger[1], T. Büchner[3], H. Löffler, T. Haferlach[1,2] and W. Hiddemann [1,2]

*Abstract.* Since the characterization of specific fusion genes in some AML subtypes, RT-PCR is an upcoming tool in diagnosis and subclassification of AML as well as in follow up studies. In our lab PCR analysis was indicated for one third of all AML cases at diagnosis. The most frequent fusion transcripts found in AML are AML1-ETO, PML-RARα, CBFβ-MYH11 but others like different MLL-transcripts are gaining importance for diagnosis and follow up studies. The importance of PML-RARα specific PCR in remission samples of M3/M3v patients is well established. The relevance of RT-PCR-positivity of other AML specific fusion transcripts still has to be established and needs more quantitative methods than high sensitive nested PCR.

dual therapy containing ATRA which leads to a highly improved prognosis. In addition, prognostic factors can be deduced from PCR-negativity or -positivity during and after therapy. The importance of persistend PCR-positivity of AML1-ETO- and MYH11-CBFβ is less clear and more quantitative studies are needed to correlate the kinetics of these transcripts with prognosis.

In addition, we used PCR diagnosis for various MLL-fusions and for rare fusion transcripts in AML like DEK-CAN [t(6;9)], BCR-ABL [t(9;22)], MOZ-CBP [t(8;16)] and AML1-MDS/EAP/EVI1 [t(3;21)] to confirm cytogenetics and to evaluate the importance and usefullness of these markers for follow up studies.

## 1 Introduction

Since the characterization of specific fusion genes in some subtypes of acute myeloid leukemia, RT-PCR is an upcoming tool in diagnosis and subclassification of AML as well as in follow up studies. During the last 18 month we have used RT-PCR for diagnosis and follow up studies in addition to cytogenetics and cytomorphology. Within a total cohort of 561 unselected consecutive AML we have performed RT-PCR for the most frequent fusion transcripts like MYH11-CBFβ in cases with inv(16)/t(16;16) (FAB M4eo), PML-RARα in cases with t(15;17) (FAB M3/M3v), and AML1-ETO in cases with t(8;21) (M1/M2). Diagnosis of M3/M3v is most important because these AML are subjected to an indivi-

## 2 Material and methods

### 2.1 Patient samples

Fresh blood or bone marrow samples were analyzed. All were diagnosed as having AML according to standard French-American-British (FAB) classification (Bennett 1976, Bennett 1985) and were referred to our lab for central AML diagnosis. 50% were included within the German AMLCG study.

### 2.2 Cytogenetics

All patients with a specific fusion transcript shown by RT-PCR were also positive for the correlating cytogenetic rearrangement.

1 Department of Internal Medicine, Hematology/Oncology, Georg- August-University, Göttingen, Germany
2 Department of Internal Medicine III, University Hospital Grosshadern, Ludwig-Maximilians-University, München, Germany
3 Department A of Internal Medicine, University of Münster, Münster, Germany

Cytogenetic G-banding analysis was performed with standard methods. The definition of a cytogenetic clone and descriptions of karyotypes followed the International System for Human Cytogenetic Nomenclature (ISCN, 1995).

## 2.3 RT-PCR

### 2.3.1 RT-PCR at diagnosis
Total RNA was isolated with RNeasy (Quiagen) following the manufacture´s instructions. One µg of total RNA was reverse transcribed with 200 U Superscript (Gibco/BRL) in a 40 µl reaction using random primers. For diagnosis an equivalent quantity of 25 ng RNA amplified for 35 cycles (1' 94°C, 1' 60°C, 1' 72°C), in 50 µl with each 10 pmol of forward primer and reverse primer, 10 mmol dNTPs, and 1.25 units of Taq polymerase (Gibco/BRL) in the buffer shipped by the supplier.

### 2.3.2 RT-PCR for MRD detection
For follow up studies equivalents of 50 ng, 250 ng, and 1250 µg of RNA were amplified as indicated above. 1 µl of these primary reactions were submitted to a nested PCR with additional 35 cycles with internal („nested") primers. Each experiment was performed in duplicate with two different enzymes (BRL, Quiagen). For each RNA sample a c-ABL specific RT-PCR was performed to control the integrity of RNA. Water instead of cDNA was included as a blank sample in each experiment. Oligonucleotides for specific PCR priming were used in accordance to Evans et al. (1995), Repp et al. (1995), and Schnittger et al. (1998).

### 2.3.3 Estimation of sensitivity of RT-PCR experiments
The sensitivity of single specific PCR systems for the detection of fusion transcripts in normal cell populations was estimated by limited dilution experiments. For this purpose a defined number of leukemic cells was diluted in normal controls and RT-PCR performed as described above. The sensitivity was 1 in $10^{-3}$ - $10^{-4}$ cells for PML-RARα, $10^{-5}$ -$10^{-6}$ for AML1-ETO, $10^{4}$-$10^{-5}$ for CBFβ-MYH11, and $10^{-4}$ -$10^{-5}$ for MLL-AF9 and each two logs more for nested PCR.

## 3 Results

### 3.1 PML-RARa fusion transcripts

Acute promyelocytic leukemia with t(15;17)(q21;q11) is characterized by a hypergranular (FAB M3) or microgranular (FAB M3v) morphology. The translocation results in the fusion of the PML gene with the RARα gene. While 17q breakpoints invariably occur in the second intron of the RARα gene, three different breakpoints may occur in the PML gene on 15q: in PML intron 6 reffered to as bcr1 or L-form; in PML exon 6 reffered to as bcr2 or V-form; or in PML intron 3, reffered to as the bcr3 or S-form of the fusion transcript (Fig.1).

Analysis of 561 unselected AML revealed APL with translocation t(15;17) and PML-RARa fusion transcripts in 38 cases (6.8 %). Of these 18 cases revealed bcr1 (L-form), one case bcr2 (V-form), and 19 case bcr3 (S-form) transcripts.

For 26 cases PCR follow ups for MRD detection were performed at 1-6 time points within a range of up to 17 month. With a PCR sensitivity of $10^{-3}$-$10^{-4}$ most cases remained positive for 4-8 weeks and converted to negativity after 6-8 weeks. Only one case was still positive after 12 weeks died of persistence of leukemia.

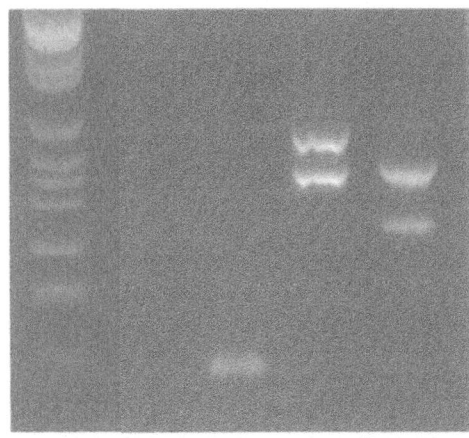

M    -C    bcr3    bcr1    bcr2

**Fig. 1.** RT-PCR for detection of PML-RARα fusion transcripts. M: molecular weight standard (Boehringer VI); -C: negative control; bcr3, bcr1, bcr2: different fusion transcripts, corresponding to S-type, L-type, and V-type, respectively.

## 3.2 AML1-ETO fusion transcripts

More than 90% of the cases with t(8;21)(q22;q22) translocation with the underlying gene fusion of AML1 with ETO were classified as M2 by French-American-British (FAB) classification, with the remainder classified as M1. In 50% of cases needle-like Auer rods, dysgranulopoiesis and eosinophilia are detectable. Other features include a tendency to form tumor masses outside the bone marrow, and a frequent loss of sex chromosome. Genomic breakpoints within the AML1 and ETO genes are relatively uniform resulting in a single AML1-ETO fusion transcript that can consistently be detected in all AML patients with t(8;21).

We have detected t(8;21) and AML1-ETO transcripts in 30/561 (5.4%) unselected AML. PCR follow ups were performed in 14 of these cases. Two cases converted to PCR negativity after 8 and 11 month, respectively. All other cases remained PCR positive, even after up to one year in complete remission.

## 3.3 CBFβ-MYH11 fusion transcripts

The inv(16)((p13q22) or the rare variant t(16;16)(p13;q22) can be found in nearly 100% of patients with acute myelomonocytic leukemia with abnormal bone marrow eosi-

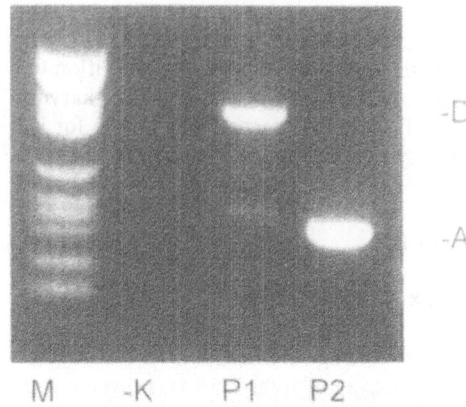

**Fig. 3.** RT-PCR for detection of CBFβ-MYH11 fusion transcripts. M: molecular weight standard; -K: negative control; P1: patient with type D transcript; P2: patient with the most common type A transcript.

nophilic precursors (FAB M4eo). The molecular correlate of both cytogenetic aberrations is the fusion of the CBFβ gene in 16q22 with the MYH11 gene in 16p13. The molecular heterogeneity of CBFβ-MYH11 fusion transcripts in different patient samples is striking, and arises from variable genomic breakpoints in both genes and alternative splicing. About 90% of all patients positive for CBFβ-MYH11 have been reported to express type A fusion transcripts and the remaining 10% to show rare transcripts. Eight different CBFβ-MYH11 transcripts named B-H and one further fusion transcript have been described.

We have detected CBFβ-MYH11 transcripts in 41/561 (7.3%) of all AML at diagnosis. In contrast to some findings in the literature this gene rearrangement was specifically associated with FAB M4eo and inv(16) (39 cases) and t(16;16) (2 cases). PCR follow ups were performed in 16 of these cases. Similar to AML with AML1-ETO most patients remained PCR positive even in CR. Three patients were still positive after 12 month in CR. Only one patient converted to negativity after 6 month.

## 3.4 CBFβ-MYH11 rearrangements in de novo versus secondary AML M4eo

The AML M4eo is a typical primary AML but can also occur in cases secondary to treat-

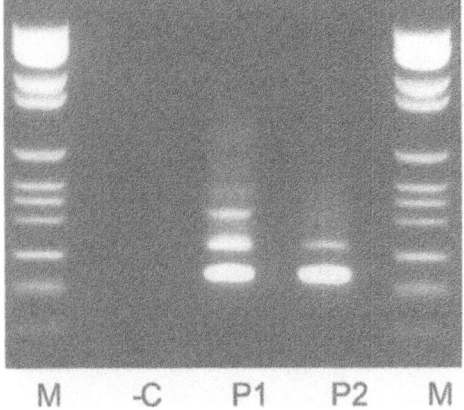

**Fig. 2.** RT-PCR for detection of AML1-ETO fusion transcripts. M: molecular weight standard; -K: negative control; P1 and P2: patients with AML1-ETO fusion transcripts. Alternative splice products are visible as a ladder above the main transcript of 338 bp.

**Table 1.** Most frequent rearrangements in AML at diagnosis

| chromosomal rearrangement | fusion transcript | morphology | frequency in unselected AML |
|---|---|---|---|
| inv(16)(p13q22); t(16;16)(p13;q22) | CBFβ-MYH11 | M4eo | 7.3 % |
| t(15;17)(q21;q11) | PML-RARα | M3, M3v | 6.8 % |
| t(8;21)(q22;q22) | AML1-ETO | (M1), M2 | 5.4 % |
| not visible | DUP-MLL | M0, M1, M2, M4, M5 | 3.4 % |
| t(9;11)(p22;q23) | MLL-AF9 | M5b | 0.7 % |

ment of a preceeding malignancy. As indicated above many different CBFβ-MYH11 transcripts have been described. Whether these different fusion transcripts have variable biologic and clinical significance remains to be determined. It has been suggested that rare CBFβ-MYH11 transcripts are more commonly found in therapy related M4eo (Dissing et al., 1998). We have analyzed 41 cases with M4eo for their type of fusion transcript. All cases were positive for a single CBFβ-MYH11 fusion transcript. Thirty-six cases (87.8%) revealed a common A-type fusion. In 5/41 (12.2%) cases rare fusion transcripts of 4 different types were detected. Five of 41 AML M4eo cases were therapy related AML (after breast cancer, cervical cancer, lung cancer, testicular cancer, M. Hodgkin). Two of these five t-AML revealed rare transcripts (40%). These two patients had preceeding testicular cancer or M. Hodgkin, respectively and were treated with topoisomerase II inhibitors. In contrast, only 3/36 (8.33%) of the primary AML expressed rare fusion transcripts.

### 3.5 MLL-AF9 fusion transcripts

Lymphoblastic as well as myeloid leukemia with rearrangements of the MLL gene are usually classified as unfavourable risk groups. However, recent data (Mrozek et al., 1997) indicated that AML with t(9;11)(p22;q23) and MLL-AF9 fusion gene shoud be regarded differently as they probably have a better prognosis than various other MLL rearrangements. In order to evaluate the molecular response of this AML subgroup, we performed RT-PCR specific for MLL-AF9 in cytological remission of 4 adult patients (28, 33, 36, and 48 years). Three patients had de novo AML and one was secondary after PEI treatment for testicular carcinoma. All 4 patients were

classified as AML M5 and all revealed a t(9;11)(p22;q23) at diagnosis. In all diagnostic samples MLL-AF9 fusion transcripts were detectable. Three of the patients had a common MLL exon 6/AF9 nt 1321 fusion. One patients revealed a MLL exon 6/AF9 nt 1627 fusion. Performing nested RT-PCR on bone marrow remission controls in two patients no fusion transcripts were detectable 9 weeks and in one eight weeks after initial therapy with one course of TAD and still remained in remission for 6, 6, and 12 month. One patient obtained allogenenic bone marrow transplantation and is in molecular remission for 12 month. These data reveal a good molecular response of AML with MLL-AF9 rearrangement and support the hypothesis of a relatively good prognosis of patients with MLL-AF9 fusion.

### 3.6 Partial tandem duplications within the MLL gene

About 40-50% of AML reveal normal karyotypes and lack molecularly detectable genetic markers. Thus, it is indicated to define new molecular markers for better genetic characterization of these AML. MLL-duplication represents a molecular marker in AML which lacks a cytogenetical correlate. We have analyzed 395 unselected cases with AML for partial duplications of the MLL gene. Performing a one step RT-PCR partial tandem duplications of the MLL-gene were demonstrated in 16/395 (4.05%) cases. The duplications were confirmed by Southern blot hybridization. Ten of these cases were karyotypically normal, three had a trisomy 11, one had a karyotype 46,XX,del(7)(q22), one 46,XY,der(16) t(1;16)(q21;q22)+6, and one 46,XY,del(9)(q22). Twelve of the duplication-positive cases were de novo myeloid leukemia, one had a

MDS prephase, and three were secondary to preceeding malignanccies. FAB classification was M0 (1 case), M1 (2 case), M2 (7 cases), M4 (4 cases), M5b (1 case), and one was not classified. The mean age was relatively high with 62.3 years versus 50.1 year in the control group.

## 4 Discussion

From our results we confirm that RT-PCR is indicated at diagnosis to confirm cytogenetics and morphology and thus complete the diagnosis of a specific AML subtype. In addition, this ascertains the subtype of fusion transcript and gives a basis for follow up studies in the individual patients. Especially the detection of t(15;17) and/or PML-RARα fusion transcripts is essential for all clinically suspected APL cases, because these patients derive therapeutic benefit from ATRA induction therapy.

RT-PCR at different times during and after therapy is usefull to control minimal residual disease (MRD) status. Molecular monitoring in FAB M3 follow up studies is well established. All studies performed at a sensitivity of $10^{-3}$-$10^{-4}$, demonstrated that persistence of PCR positivity or conversion to positivity after negativity resulted in a great risk for relapse and has clinical consequences. MRD monitoring by RT-PCR in patients with t(8;21) and inv(16) has been discussed controversial. As many of the patients reveal PCR positivity during months or even years in complete clinical remission the importance and diagnostic significance of PCR positivity is unclear. In future, exact quantification of these fusion transcripts by „real time PCR" is necessary in follow up samples to analyse the kinetics of transcript disappearence in remission and thus distinguish patients who are in pending relapse and who require further therapeutic intervention.

Within our cohort of inv(16) patients we have detected a relatively high frequency of rare transcript-types in therapy related M4eo in comparison to de novo M4eo. This distribution of specific fusion types may suggest different underlying molecular mechanisms for the different fusion transcripts.

Besides, mainly two differerent rearrangements of the MLL gene seem to be of impor-

tance in AML. The t(9;11)(p22;q23) was found in 5 cases (0.8%) and seems to be correlated with early disappearance of the MLL-AF9 fusion transcript and a relatively good prognosis. With the systematical screening for MLL partial tandem duplication in 395 consecutive AML cases we have established a new subgroup in a subset (3.36%) of AML that is cytogenetically or cytomorphologically not differentiable. Thus, the detection of new molecular markers may be important to establish new AML subgroups and to make MRD-detection possible in more patients that lack cytogenetic markers.

## References

Bennett JM, Catovsky D, Daniel MT, Flandrin G, Galton DAG, Gralnick HR, Sultan C (1982) Proposals for the classification of the myelodysplastic syndromes. Br. J. Haematol. 51: 189-199

Bennett JM, Catovsky D, Daniel MT, Flandrin G, Galton DAG, Gralnick HR, Sultan C (1985) Proposed revised criteria for the classification of acute myeloid leukaemia. Annals Int. Med. 103: 620-625

Dissing M, Le Beau MM, Pedersen-Bjergaard J (1998) Inversion of chromosome 16 and uncommon rearrangements of the CBFB and MYH11 genes in therapy-related acute myeloid leukemia: rare events related to DNA-topoisomerase II inhibitors. J. Clin Oncology 16: 1890-1896

Evans P, Jack A, Short M, Haynes A, Shiach C, Owen R, Johnson R, Morgan GJ: (1995) A single tube nested RT-PCR for detecting the common myeloid specific chromosomal translocations. Leukemia 9: 1285-1290

ISCN (1995). Guidelines for cancer cytogenetics. In: Mitelman F., ed. Supplement to an international system for human cytogenetic nomenclature. Basel: Karger, 1995.

Mrozek K, Heinonen K, Lawrence D, Carroll AJ, Koduru PR, Rao KW, Strout MP, Hutchison RE, Moore JO, Mayer RJ, Schiffer CA, Bloomfield CD: Adult patients with de novo acute myeloid leukemia and t(9; 11)(p22; q23) have a superior outcome to patients with other translocations involving band 11q23: a cancer and leukemia group B study. Blood 90:4532, 1997

Repp R, Borkhard A, Haupt E, Kreude J, Brettreich S, Hammermann J, Nishida K, Harbott J, Lampert F (1995) Detection of four different 11q23 chromosomal abnormalities by multiplex-PCR and fluorescence-basedautomatic DNA-fragment analysis. Leukemia 9:210-215

Schnittger S, Kinkelin U, Schoch C, Haase D, Haferlach T, Büchner T, Wörmann B, Hiddemann W, Griesinger F (1998) Partial tandem duplications of the MLL gene are detectable in peripheral blood and bone marrow of nearly all healthy donors. Blood 92: 1728-1734

# Chromosome Aberrations in Primary and Secondary Acute Myeloblastic Leukemia (AML)

O.Haus[1,2], M.Czarnecka[1], S.Kotlarek-Haus[1], K.Kuliczkowski[1], E.Duszenko[1] and I.Makowska[1]

*Abstract.* The aim of the study was a comparative analysis of the presence of clonal chromosome aberrations in primary (p-AML) and secondary, MDS-related, AML (MDS-AML), in relation to hematologic and clinical status of patients. Cytogenetic analyses were performed in 85 untreated patients; 64 with primary, and 21 with secondary AML. The studies were carried out on at least 20 GTG-banded mitoses, obtained after 24-hour unstimulated culture of bone marrow cells. All but two MDS-AML patients showed cytogenetic changes at diagnosis and among 64 pAML patients 31 had chromosome aberrations (p<0.005). There were no typical AML translocations in MDS-AML. The most frequent aberrations in this group of patients were –5/5q- and 7q-, followed by various translocations, deletions and monosomies. The aberrations in MDS-AML group were significantly more often complex and unbalanced than those in pAML group (p<0.01 and p<0.05, respectively). In the pAML group chromosome aberrations were more frequently observed in patients with occupational mutagenic exposure prior to the onset of disease (p<0.05). In this group aberrations typical of FAB subtypes were mainly observed. Patients with MDS-AML were significantly older, did not achieve complete remission and had a slightly shorter survival time than the patients with pAML. Patients with pAML and atypical aberrations also were older and had shorter survival time than pAML patients with typical aberrations.

## Introduction

Traditionally, the term „secondary acute myeloblastic leukemia" is used to describe cases that arise secondary to:

1. chemotherapy or radiotherapy (treatment-related leukemia = t-AML),
2. documented environmental or occupational exposure to mutagenetic agents such as benzene, petroleum, organic solvents, and arsenic pesticides,
3. antecedent myelodysplasia. [1].

Recently, the first description is the most often used. The third one stands for a basis of a newly proposed clasification of AML: myelodysplasia related (MDS-related = MDR-AML or MDS-AML) and True De Novo AML [5]. The former group includes i.a. t-AML and, also AML in the elderly.

Chromosome aberrations are distinct in primary and secondary (strictly: MDS-related) AML. In the primary one (pAML), balanced translocations, such as t(8;21), t(15;17), and other balanced aberrations [inv(16)] are the main changes. Disease development and its clinical course depends in these cases on genes fusion, which change their „morphology" and function [2]. The aberrations in secondary AML (sAML) are mainly unbalanced (e.g. -5/5q-, -7/7q-, +8) and often complex [9,12]. There are some differences in the characteristics of patients suffering from primary and secondary leukemia: the latter are older, and they are more frequently exposed to mutagenic factors before the onset of the disease, less frequently achieve a complete remission (CR), and their survival time is

---

[1] Department of Haematology, Medical University, Wroclaw, Poland.
[2] Department of Genetics, Medical University, Bydgoszcz, Poland.

shorter than that of patients with pAML. Hematological data also are less favourable in s-AML patients [4].

In this paper we present an analysis of cytogenetic, hematologic and clinical diffe-rences between a group of patients with AML preceded by MDS (called here MDS-AML) and a group of patients with AML not prece-ded by MDS (called pAML). The patients > 60 year old and the patients with occupational mutagenic exposure were included in both groups.

## Material and methods

### Patients

Cytogenetic examinations were performed in 85 untreated patients with AML, hospitalized in Department of Hematology. 64 had pri-mary AML, defined as not preceded by MDS, and 21 the secodary one = MDS-related AML. The general data about the first group, pre-viously described [3], are as follows: The group consisted of 64 patients; 31 women and 33 men, aged 17-75 years. 18 among them were occupationally exposed to mutagenic agents. They had various AML FAB subtypes: M1 (6 patients), M2 (16 pts), M3 (7 pts), M4 (22 pts), M5 (5 pts), M6 (2 pts), M7 (2 pts), AML/ALL (4 pts). Their mean Hb level was 8.94 g%, range 2.8-12.9, WBC 44.5 G/l, range 0.2-442, platelet count 63.0 G/l, range 3.0-249.0, % of blasts in bone marrow (BM) 71.7, range 30-100. Their mean survival time (ST) was 8.0 months (median - 5.75 mo), range 0.1-30 mo. Detailed data concerning the patients from the second group, together with cytogenetic results, are collected in Table 1.

**Table 1.** The detailed data of patients with myelodysplastic syndrome-related AML (group II).

| No | Age | Sex | Expo | ST [mo] | Hb level [G/l] | WBC [g%] | Plts [G/l] | BM Blasts [%] | FAB type | Karyotype |
|---|---|---|---|---|---|---|---|---|---|---|
| 1. | 59 | F | + | 16 | 8.8 | 20.7 | 234.0 | 77 | M4 | 47,XX,+6, t(7;13)(q36;q14) |
| 2. | 59 | F | - | 15 | 7.3 | 35.5 | 152.0 | 73 | M4 | 46,XX,del(5)(q15q33) |
| 3. | 77 | M. | + | 5 | 14.0 | 27.8 | 208.0 | 41 | M4 | 46,XY,+13,-17 |
| 4. | 25 | M. | + | 14 | 5.2 | 14.5 | 170.0 | 41 | M4 | 94,XXYY,+7,+8/46,XY |
| 5. | 40 | M. | + | 7 | 8.6 | 0.8 | 266.0 | 30 | M4 | 46,XY,inv(20)(p12q12)del(20)(q12) |
| 6. | 74 | F | - | 9 | 9.3 | 2.6 | 27.0 | 83 | M6 | 45,XX,del(16)(q22),-20/46,XX |
| 7. | 76 | F | + | 1 | 7.1 | 1.5 | 94.0 | 83 | M2 | 46,XX,del(5)(q13q33), del(21)(q11)/46,XX |
| 8. | 43 | F | + | 4 | 6.7 | 8.1 | 47.0 | 96 | M1/ M2 | 46,XX |
| 9. | 38 | M. | + | 4+ | 8.7 | 1.7 | 35.0 | 50 | M6 | 46,XY |
| 10. | 75 | M. | + | 1 | 8.3 | 13.5 | 8.0 | 45 | M5 | 47,XY,+8 |
| 11. | 67 | M. | - | 1 | 8.4 | 4.0 | 4.0 | 61 | M4 | 46,XY,del(3)(p21),del(3)(q21), del(5)(q13q31),-12 |
| 12. | 63 | M. | + | 1 | 7.3 | 175.0 | 65.0 | 59 | M4 | 45-50,del(X)(q22)Y,+1,+2,del(5)(q13q35), del(6)(q21q23),del(7)(q22),-9, add(15)(qter),-17, -18,+21,+1-4mar[cp] |
| 13. | 47 | F | - | 1 | 5.5 | 1.3 | 4.0 | 78 | M4 | 47,XXX,del(5)(q12q33),-7,-12, t(7;12)(q22;q13), der(17),+2mar |
| 14. | 55 | M. | - | 2 | 10.5 | 5.8 | 219.0 | 74.5 | M4 | 47,XY,+mar |
| 15. | 36 | F | + | 1 | 8.8 | 1.6 | 132.0 | 41 | AML/ ALL | 46,XX,inv(8)(p21q22) |
| 16. | 63 | F | - | 5 | 10.4 | 1.8 | 87.0 | 31 | M4 | 43,XX,-5,-12,+dic(5;12)(p13;p11), del(7)(q22), -15,-21,+i(21q) |
| 17. | 63 | M. | + | 3 | 9.8 | 0.9 | 115.0 | 64 | M4 | 47,XY,+21/46,XY |
| 18. | 62 | F | - | 2 | 8.9 | 3.2 | 70.0 | 45 | M2 | 47,XX,add(4)(qter),-5,+8,t(13;15),+i(17q),-21, +mar |
| 19. | 71 | M. | - | 1 | 8.5 | 1.1 | 105.0 | 34 | M2 | 46,XY,t(1;?)(q21;?),t(1;2)(p23;p32), del(5)(q22q35),del(7)(q22) |
| 20. | 60 | M. | + | 5 | 9.6 | 6.6 | 5.0 | 42 | M2 | 42-44,XY,-5,-7,+dic(7;17),-8,add(9)(q22),t(8;9),t(9;12),t(11;14)(q13;p11, der(12),-13,-14,-17,-18,+mar[cp] |
| 21. | 71 | F | - | 11 | 8.0 | 4.0 | 117.0 | 62 | M0 | 45,XX,+der(1),der(8),der(10),t(17;19),-21,-22 |

Legend:Expo=exposition to mutagenic agents, ST=survival time, Plts=platelet count,BM blasts [%]=% of blasts in bone marrow.

The most frequent FAB type in both groups was M4, followed by M2.

By means of t-Student test, Wilcoxon test, chi-square test, and others, a comparison between cytogenetic, hematologic and clinical data between the patients of both groups was done. The following data were analysed:

1. cytogenetic: the presence of chromosome aberrations in general, the presence of certain types of chromosome aberrations and a complex or a simple karyotype,
2. hematologic: Hb level, leukocyte count, platelet count, blasts percentage in bone marrow, FAB type,
3. clinical: age, sex, occupational or medical exposure to mutagenic agents (without those mentioned above), complete remission rate (CRR), survival time (ST).

## Methods

Cytogenetic examinations were performed on bone marrow cells from 24 h unstimulated cultures at 37∞ C under 5% $CO_2$. A culture medium was RPMI 1640, supplemented with 15% FCS and antibiotics. Cells were harvested with colcemid, treated with hypotonic KCl (0.075M) and fixed with 75% methanol/ 25% acetic acid. Five-day-old air-dried slides were treated with trypsin solution and stained with Giemsa stain. At least 20 GTG-banded metaphases were analysed according to ISCN'91 and ISCN'95 [7,8].

## Results

Results of cytogenetic examination.

In 31 among 64 patients of group I clonal chromosome aberrations were found. There were typical structural aberrations in 12: t(8;21) – in 4 pts, t(15;17) – in 2 pts, inv/del(16) – in 2 pts, and atypical aberrations in 19 patients. The atypical aberrations were as follows: del(11)(q21) – in 2 patients, and t(2;10)(p11;q11), add(2)(q37), add(14) (q32), t(9;?;4)(p24;?;q12), t(1;13)(p13;p11), t(11;14)(q13;p11), add(17)(p13), add(11) (p15), t(3;5;7)(p21;p15;q11), inv(7)(q11qter), add(9)(q34), add(13)(q34), add(14)(q32) – in single patients. Numerical aberrations were found in 14 patients; trisomy 8 in 6 patients, trisomies 3, 7, 9, 21, 22, and monosomies 13, 14, 16, and a lack of X and of Y – in single cases. Summing up; complex karyotypes were found in 8 patients, simple aberrant karyotypes in 23, unbalanced in 20, balanced aberrant karyotypes in 11. Structural aberrations of chromosomes 5 and 7 were found twice [t(3;5;7), inv (7)(q11qter)]. They were not typical of MDS. Numerical aberration of 7 – trisomy 7 also atypical of MDS was found once.

Among 21 patients with MDS-AML 19 had chromosome aberrations, detailed in table 1. There were 13 complex aberrant karyotypes, versus 6 simple aberrant karyotypes, 18 unbalanced karyotypes, versus 1 balanced aberrant karyotype. –5/5q- was found in 8 patients, 7q- in 4 patients.

Results of comparison of clinical, hematologic and cytogenetic data.

The results of comparison of both groups of patients are presented in Table 2.

Among the patients with pAML a comparison between various subgroups was done, (detailed description in [3]). Chromosome aberrations were more frequently observed in patients with occupational mutagenic exposure before the onset of disease, than in unexposed patients (p<0.05). Patients with pAML and atypical aberrations were older and had shorter survival time than that of patients with only typical aberrations.

Additionally, a comparison of data of MDS-AML patients (II group) with or without aberrations (monosomies and deletions) of chromosomes 5 and 7, the most frequent aberrations in this group, was done. There were not statistically significant differences, with one exception: patients with –5/5q- had only M2 (4x) and M4 (3x) FAB type AML. These patients were generally older (62.6 mo, versus 56.1 mo), and had less favourable hematological parameters: Hb 7.74 g%, v. 9.23, WBC 32G/l, v. 7.7, Plt 85G/l, v. 104, however without statistical significance, than the patients without these aberrations. Their mean (and median) ST was ~ 2 months shorter. Patients with 7q- did not generally differ from those without this aberration, as to clinical and hematologic data.

**Table 2.** The comparison of clinical, hematologic and cytogenetic data between the patients with de novo AML (group I), and MDS-related AML (group II).

| Feature | t-Student test (median value) I group : II group [mean (median) value] | Chi-square test No of patients with/without a feature (or with 1st/2nd feature) in I group : II group | P value |
|---|---|---|---|
| Age | 49.4 (52.5) : 58.3 (62.0) | (-) | 0.032 |
| Sex F/M. | (-) | 31/33 : 10/11 | NS |
| Mutagenic exposure +/- | (-) | 18/46 : 10/11 | NS |
| Hb level [g%] | 8.94 (9.15) : 8.73 (8.60) | (-) | NS |
| WBC [G/l] | 44.5 (9.9) : 15.8 (4.0) | (-) | 0.021 |
| Platelets [G/l] | 63.0 (52.0) : 98.3 (87.0) | (-) | NS |
| % of bone marrow blasts | 71.7 (77.0) : 57.6 (59.0) | (-) | 0.011 |
| FAB M4/others | (-) | 22/42 : 11/10 | NS |
| Complete remission | (-) | 17/47 : 0/21 | (-) |
| Survival time [months] | 8.0 (5.75) : 6.75 (5.0) | (-) | NS |
| Chromosome aberrations +/- | (-) | 31/33 : 19/2 | 0.0014 |
| Karyotype complex/simple | (-) | 8/23 : 13/6 | 0.00762 |
| Karyotype unbalanced/balanced | (-) | 20/11 : 18/1 | 0.0182 |
| -5/5q- +/- | (-) | 0/31 : 8/11 | (-) |
| -7/7q- +/- | (-) | 0/31 : 4/15 | (-) |

## Discussion

The overall cytogenetic findings presented here are similar to those presented by others [6,9,12]. Chromosome aberrations were significantly most frequent in MDS-AML (present in 90% of cases), than in pAML (48%). A relative risk of presence of aberrations in MDS-AML group was 1.9x higher than in pAML group. The most common changes in MDS-AML were −5/5q-, 7q-, absent in pAML. Complex and unbalanced karyotypes also were significantly more frequent in this group. These changes, followed by a complete lack of genetic balance, may cause unfavourable clinical course. The patients with MDS-AML did not achieve complete remission and their survival time was slightly (1.25 mo) shorter than that of the patients in pAML group. This very small difference in ST might have been a result of a broad dispersion of individual ST values and also of a difference in the number of patients in either group. Similar clinical findings were also stressed by others [4,6]. Poor clinical outcome may be a result of the fact that unbalanced and complex chromosome aberrations in MDS-AML are the „secondary" ones. It means, in this context, that they are secondary to a cytogenetically undetectable initiating event, which might appear many months or years earlier, sometimes induced by a mutagenic agent [9]. It may also account for mean older age of patients with these changes in both groups and other differences between the groups. Probably, after an initial genetic event (e.g. instability) a disease smoldered, to burst after an appearance of cytogenetic changes. The presence of atypical and complex chromosome aberrations and the worse clinical course in the elderly has been already described [10,11]. AML of the elderly strongly resembles secondary AML, regardless it is appearing after an mutagenic exposure and MDS or not [1,3].

## References

1. Appelbaum FR, Le Beau MM, Willman CL (1996) Secondary Leukemia. In: Hematology 1996, Educational Program ASH, pp33-47.
2. Appelbaum FR, Gilliland DG, Tallman MS (1998) The biology and treatment of Acute Myeloid Leukemia. In: Hematology 1998, Educational Program ASH, pp 15-43.
3. Czarnecka M, Haus O, Kuliczkowski K, Duszeńko E, Makowska I, Rybczyńska H, Kotlarek-Haus S (1999) Chromosome aberrations in de novo acute myeloid leukemia in adults. Acta Haemat Pol (submitted).
4. Greef GE de, Hagemeijer A (1996) Molecular and cytogenetic abnormalities in acute myeloid leukaemia and myelodysplastic syndromes. Bailliere's Clinical Hematology, 9: 1-55.
5. Head DR (1996) Revised classification of acute myeloid leukemia. Leukemia, 10: 1826-1831.
6. Heim S, Mitelman F (1991) Cancer, 70 suppl: 1701-1709.

7. ISCN (1991) Guidelines for Cancer Cytogenetics, Supplement to An International System for Human Cytogenetic Nomenclature. Mitelman F (ed). S.Karger, Basel.

8. ISCN (1995) An International System for Human Cytogenetic Nomenclature. Mitelman F (ed), S. Karger, Basel.

9. Johansson B, Mertens F, Mitelman F (1996) Primary versus secondary neoplasia associated chromosomal abnormalities – balanced rearrangements vs. genomic imbalance ? Gene Chromosome Cancer, 16: 155-163.

10. Karp JE (1998) Molecular pathogenesis and targets for therapy in myelodysplastic syndrome (MDS) and MDS-related leukemias. Current Opinion Oncol, 10: 3-9.

11. Leith CP, Kopecky KJ Godwin J, McConnell T, Slovak ML, Chen I-M., Head DR, Appelbaum FR, Willman CL (1997) Acute myeloid leukemia in the elderly: assessment of multidrug resistance (MDR1) and cytogenetics distinguishes biologic subgroups with remarkably distinct responses to standard chemotherapy. A Southwest Oncology Group study. Blood, 89: 3323-3329.

12. Mrózek K, Heinonen K, de la Chapelle A, Bloomfield CD (1997) Clinical significance of cytogenetics in acute myeloid leukemia. Semin Oncol, 1: 17-31.

# Are there Two Main Categories of de Novo Acute Myeloid Leukemias with a Normal Karyotype?

P. Lemež[1], J. Gáliková[1] and T. Haas[2]

*Abstract.* Patients with de novo acute myeloid leukemias (AML) and a normal karyotype are considered to be associated with an intermediate prognosis. The aim of the study was to determine the influence of erythroid and/or megakaryocytic dysplasia (EMD) in diagnostic bone marrow smears of patients under 65 years with de novo AML and a normal karyotype on their response to therapy and prognosis. EMD was diagnosed when more than 25% erythroblasts and/or 50% megakaryocytes exhibited dysplastic features evaluated according to the FAB criteria. Twenty-three patients with AML and a normal karyotype were diagnosed between 02/1991–05/1995. Ten cases, 21–65 (median 47) years old, were categorized without EMD, eleven patients 34–63 (median 56) years old with EMD, and two patients were not evaluable for EMD. One cycle of therapy consisting of 3–4 doses of daunorubicin (DNR) 45 mg/m$^2$/d and cytosine arabinoside (AraC) 150-200 mg/m$^2$/12-h for 7 days induced 8 complete (CR) and 2 partial remissions in 10 cases without EMD but in 8 cases with EMD one CR, 6 non-responses and one induction death (p=0.015). However, six of seven patients with EMD reached CR with high doses of AraC 2,000 mg/m$^2$/12-h x 10 plus 2 doses of DNR.. Median event–free survival in patients without EMD was 25.1 months and 3.5 months in cases with EMD (p=0.08). Our data have shown a probable existence of two different categories of AML with a normal karyotype distinguished by the presence of EMD. These categories seem to differ in the response to classical induction chemotherapy 3+7 and prognosis.

## Introduction

De novo acute myeloid leukemia (AML) is a very heterogeneous group of malignant clonal diseases characterized by acquired nonrandom DNA rearrangements that, in most cases, can be detected by cytogenetic and/or molecular biological methods. More than 30 different primary cytogenetic abnormalities involving different genes were described in AML patients some of which represented well defined distinctive morphologic, immunologic and cytogenetic (MIC) AML types with different responses to therapy and prognosis [1–5]. A specific therapy for each AML type, defined by a specific DNA abnormality, would seem to be optimal similarly like all-trans retinoic acid treatment for patients with acute promyelocytic leukemia - AML M3 [6–7].

However, the proof of a primary clonal DNA abnormality in AML is usually not available at diagnosis for the choice of therapy at most hospitals and even it is not detected at all in 45% – 22% of adults with AML diagnosed with "a normal karyotype" [1, 3, 4]. Patients with de novo AML and "a normal karyotype" are considered to have an intermediate prognosis [1, 3, 4]. In the study we have shown that the presence of erythroid and/or megakaryocytic dysplasia is a strong predictor of response of such patients to classical induction chemotherapy and prognosis.

## Patients and Methods

Between February 1991 and May 1995 induction treatment of 23 consecutive patients with

---

[1] Department of Hematology and Blood Transfusion, Hospital Jihlava, Jihlava,
[2] Institute of Biophysics, 1st Medical Faculty, Charles University, Prague, Czech Republic

de novo AML M1, M2, M4, M5 under 65 years old and "a normal karyotype" was started according to the ÚHKT-911 study at the Institute of Hematology and Blood Transfusion in Prague. Informed consent was obtained from all patients. Patients with secondary AML after prior myelodysplasia or after chemotherapy for another cancer were not eligible for the study.

The French-American-British (FAB) classification [8, 9] and standard cytochemical methods, in some cases supplemented with immunophenotyping or tissue cultivation methods [10] were used for establishing the diagnosis of AML. Morphologic dysplastic features of erythroblasts, megakaryocytes and granulocytes in diagnostic bone marrow smears of the patients were evaluated according to the criteria of the FAB group [11] independently by two experienced hematologists.

Erythroid and/or megakaryocytic dysplasia (EMD) was diagnosed when at least 25% of 50–200 evaluable erythroblasts had to show dyserythropoietic features (DysE, Table 1) and/or when 50% or more of at least 5 megakaryocytes (DysMg) were dysplastic. Dysgranulopoiesis (DysG) was diagnosed when 50% or more of 50–200 neutrophilic metamyelocytes, stabs and segments were dysplastic [12].

Furthermore, as controls for EMD, we evaluated diagnostic bone marrow smears with 100–200 evaluable erythroblasts from 7 patients (4 men, 3 women) aged 17–70 (mean 45) years with acute hypergranular promyelocytic leukemia (AML M3) who had been treated in other studies at the Institute in this period [13].

Chromosomal preparations were made from 24–hours unstimulated cultures of patients' bone marrow cells [14]. At least 20 metaphases, when available, G–banded by Wright's stain were examined and the ISCN (1995) nomenclature was used [15].

Induction chemotherapy consisted of these treatment types:
a) standard (S): 3–4 doses of daunorubicin (DNR) (Rubomycin, Medexport, Russia) 45 mg/m$^2$/d and cytosine arabinoside (AraC) (Alcysten, Spofa, Czech Republic) 150–200 mg/m$^2$/3–h infusion every 12 hours for 7 days.

b) HD: high doses of AraC 2,000 mg/m$^2$/3–h infusion every 12 hours for 5 days (10 doses) and DNR 45 mg/m$^2$/d on days 4 and 5.

c) EMi: etoposide (Vepesid, Bristol-Myers, Germany) 100 mg/m$^2$/d for 5 days and mitozantrone (Refador, Spofa, Czech Republic) 10–12 mg/m$^2$/d on days 1, 3, and 5.

One cycle of standard chemotherapy was given as the first induction therapy. One patient No. 19 (Table 1.) with an impaired cardiac function was given standard induction with only two doses of daunorubicin (2/7 cycle) and two patients (Nos. 19 and 20, Table 1.) received the HD cycle as the first induction therapy.

Consolidation therapy consisting of 1–3 HD cycles and one EMi cycle was given and patients in CR received 2–4 consolidation cycles according to the patient´s tolerance of chemotherapy.

The standard criteria were used to define complete (CR) and partial (PR) remission [16]. Non–response (NonR): < 50 % reduction of bone marrow blasts.

Statistical analysis. Comparisons of CR rate in categories with and without EMD were performed by the two–sided Fisher's exact test. Comparisons of hematological data and the necessary doses of cytostatics for CR induction were done by the Mann-Whitney test. Overall survival (OS) was calculated from the first day of therapy until the date of death. Event-free survival (EFS) was calculated from the date of achieving CR and events were relapse, death or failure to reach CR. Patients who underwent allogeneic bone marrow transplantation (BMT) were censored at the date of their decision for BMT which had changed their therapy. The Kaplan-Meier method was performed to determine survival function of OS and EFS to October 1, 1998, when the minimal follow-up of surviving patients was longer than 46 (46–80) months. The comparison of OS or EFS in two categories of patients with or without EMD was carried out by the Mantel-Cox log-rank test. BMDP programs were used for the analysis.

**Table 1.** Patients characteristics and response to therapy

| Pt | Age/Sex Yrs | FAB | Blood WBC x10⁹/L | Bl % | Bone marrow Bl % | Bone marrow Erb % | DysE % | DysMg | DysG % | 1.TH | Outcome | 2.TH | Outcome | Event-free survival months | Overall survival months |
|---|---|---|---|---|---|---|---|---|---|---|---|---|---|---|---|
| **Patients without EM – dysplasia** | | | | | | | | | | | | | | | |
| 1 | 30/m | M4 | 93.6 | 90 | 81 | 0 | NE | 2/5 | 89 | S | CR | | | 4.4 | 5.4 |
| 2 | 54/m | M2 | 109.0 | 87 | 75 | 2 | 8 | 1/3 | 80 | S | CR | | | +45.5 | +46.6 |
| 3 | 49/m | M5 | 74.6 | 84 | 66 | 2 | 11 | 1/6 | 31 | S | CR | | | +58.3 | +59.4 |
| 4 | 65/m | M1 | 1.0 | 0 | 57 | 25 | 11 | 4/10 | 8 | S | CR | | | 3.6 | 4.9 |
| 5 | 37/f | M2 | 112.0 | 95 | 87 | 9 | 13 | 1/2 | 42 | S | CR | | | 15.6 | +20.0 |
| 6 | 60/f | M2 | 26.2 | 66 | 91 | 2 | 15 | 0/3 | 49 | S | CR | | | +59.0 | +60.1 |
| 7 | 47/m | M4 | 162.0 | 99 | 91 | 1 | 19 | 0/2 | 65 | S | CR | | | +68.4 | +69.4 |
| 8 | 47/m | M1 | 1.6 | 1 | 80 | 2 | 19 | 7/18 | 51 | S | CR | | | +2.0 | +3.0 |
| 9 | 46/f | M2 | 4.0 | 24 | 78 | 12 | 16 | 3/10 | 80 | S | PR | HD | CR | 32.7 | 65.4 |
| 10 | 21/f | M2 | 36.6 | 75 | 69 | 4 | 5 | 0/5 | 60 | S | PR | S | Death | 0 | 1.8 |
| **Patients with EM – dysplasia** | | | | | | | | | | | | | | | |
| 11 | 63/f | M2 | 6.5 | 70 | 67 | 25 | 45 | 2/7 | 90 | S | CR | HD | CR | +79.3 | +80.3 |
| 12 | 39/m | M4 | 31.8 | 70 | 78 | 3 | 23 | 19/30 | 43 | S | NonR | HD | CR | 2.7 | 5.4 |
| 13 | 34/m | M1 | 4.3 | 58 | 39 | 18 | 33 | 11/20 | 69 | S | NonR | HD | CR | 17.4 | +22.0 |
| 14 | 41/f | M4 | 2.8 | 42 | 80 | 6 | 34 | 13/20 | 59 | S | NonR | HD | PR | +4.0 | +6.0 |
| 15 | 56/f | M4 | 15.0 | 67 | 83 | 7 | 29 | 2/11 | 79 | S | NonR | HD | | 4.6 | 10.5 |
| 16 | 59/f | M1 | 1.3 | 12 | 49 | 20 | 31 | 3/9 | 23 | S | NonR | | | 0 | 1.0 |
| 17 | 41/f | M4 | 100.0 | 86 | 91 | 1 | 32 | 15/25 | 25 | S | NonR | S | NonR | 0 | 2.3 |
| 18 | 57/m | M4 | 99.0 | 38 | 64 | 4 | 32 | 3/5 | 88 | S | Death | | | 0 | 0.4 |
| 19 | 47/m | M4 | 17.9 | 66 | 67 | 1 | 61 | 0/0 | 52 | 2/7 | PR | HD | CR | 5.0 | 13.7 |
| 20 | 60/m | M4 | 56.6 | 77 | 84 | 2 | 36 | 10/14 | NE | HD | CR | | | 1.1 | 3.2 |
| 21 | 59/m | M2 | 6.7 | 70 | 66 | 25 | 44 | 32/40 | 23 | HD | CR | | | 22.0 | 29.4 |
| **Patients non-evaluable for EM – dysplasia** | | | | | | | | | | | | | | | |
| 22 | 35/m | M2 | 18.5 | 84 | 94 | 0 | NE | 0/0 | NE | S | PR | HD | CR | 10.5 | +14.0 |
| 23 | 25/f | M5 | 174.0 | 97 | 96 | 0 | NE | 0/1 | 42 | S | Death | | | 0 | 0.2 |

Pt: the number of the patient. 1.TH, (2.TH): the 1st, (2nd ) induction therapy.
Bl: myeloblasts, promyelocytes and promonocytes. Erb: erythroblasts. DysE: dysplastic erythroblasts. DysMg: number of megakaryocytes with dysplasia of the total number of examined megakaryocytes. DysG: dysplastic granulocytes. NE: not evaluable. Percentages were rounded off .
S – standard induction: 3 - 4 doses of daunorubicin 45 mg/m²/d and cytosine arabinoside 200 mg/m²/3-h infusion every 12 h for 7 days.
HD: 10 doses of cytosine arabinoside 2,000 mg/m²/d and daunorubicin 45 mg/m²/d on days 4 and 5.
2/7: the same cycle like the standard induction with only 2 doses of daunorubicin.
CR: complete remission. PR: partial remission. NonR: non-response.
+45.5: plus before 45.5 denotes censored (alive or transplanted) patients.

## Results

Bone marrow smears of 7 patients with AML M3 exhibited dysplastic features in 9.5 – 21.0% (median 12.5%) of erythroblasts and in 3 of 22 megakaryocytes.

Twenty-three patients (13 men, 10 women) with de novo AML, except AML M3, and a normal karyotype treated in the ÚHKT-911 study were 21-65 (median 47) years old.

### Patients without EMD

Ten patients (No. 1-10, Table 1.) were categorized without erythroid and/or megakaryocytic dysplasia (EMD). Their diagnostic bone marrow smears exhibited 5-19% (median 13%) dysplastic erythroblasts and less than 50% of dysplastic megakaryocytes. They were 21-65 (median 47) years old. One cycle of standard induction chemotherapy induced 8 complete and 2 partial remissions in them. The patient No. 9 reached CR with the HD cycle while the patient No. 10 died of sepsis after the second standard induction. Four patients (Table 1.) have been living in their $1^{st}$ CR after chemotherapy for 45-68 months. The fifth patient (No. 8) has been living for 77 months in his $1^{st}$ CR after sibling HLA-matched bone marrow transplantation (BMT) which has been carried out at 2 months of his $1^{st}$ CR (Table 1., censored). The patient No. 5 died of sepsis following sibling HLA-matched BMT carried out in her $2^{nd}$ CR (Table 1., censored at 20 months for OS). The median overall and event-free survival with the appropriate interquartile range (IR: lower quartile–upper quartile) was 36.5 (IR 5.1 – not reached) months and 25.1 (IR 3.9 – not reached) months, respectively.

### Patients with EMD

Eleven patients (Nos. 11–21, Table 1.) were categorized with EMD. Their diagnostic bone marrow smears exhibited dysplastic features in 23-61% (median 33%) of erythroblasts and more than 50% of dysplastic megakaryocytes in 6 of them including the only one patient (No. 12, Table 1.) with the number of dysplastic erythroblasts under the 25% limit.

Patients with EMD were 34–63 (median 56) years old. Standard induction therapy given to 8 of them lead to only one complete remission, 6 non–responses and one induction death. Three of four non–responders to standard induction therapy achieved CR and one PR after the cycle with high doses of cytosine arabinoside (HD cycle) as well as the patient No. 19 with PR after the 2/7 cycle. Two patients (Nos. 20 and 21) with EMD were initially treated with the HD cycle and both reached complete remission. Thus six of seven patients with EMD reached CR after the cycle with high doses of AraC. The patient (No. 16) with a PR after the HD cycle achieved eventually CR after the cycle with etoposide and mitozantrone. Altogether 8 of 11 (73%) patients with EMD reached CR.

Only one patient No. 11 is a long-term survivor of patients with EMD. The patient No. 14 underwent related allogeneic BMT in her $1^{st}$ CR and the patient No. 13 unrelated BMT in his $2^{nd}$ CR (both censored in the Table 1.) but both died of septic complications and their real survival was 13.5 and 26.1 months, respectively. The median overall survival of patients with EMD was 7.5 (IR 2.0–21.1) months and their median event–free survival was 3.5 (2.0–13.8) months.

### Patients non–evaluable for EMD

Two patients (No. 22 and 23, Table 1.) were not evaluable for EMD, because very low numbers of erythroblasts and megakaryocytes were found in their bone marrow smears. The patient No. 23 died during the standard induction therapy. The patient No. 22 has been living for 55 months after unrelated BMT carried out in his $2^{nd}$ CR.

### Comparison of patients with and without EMD

Complete remission after standard induction chemotherapy was significantly more frequently reached (p=0.015) in patients without EMD (8 of 10) in comparison to patients with EMD (1 of 8). The median dose of AraC to reach CR was 2,800 (IR 2,800–3,600) mg/m² in patients without EMD, significantly lower than in patients with EMD who needed a

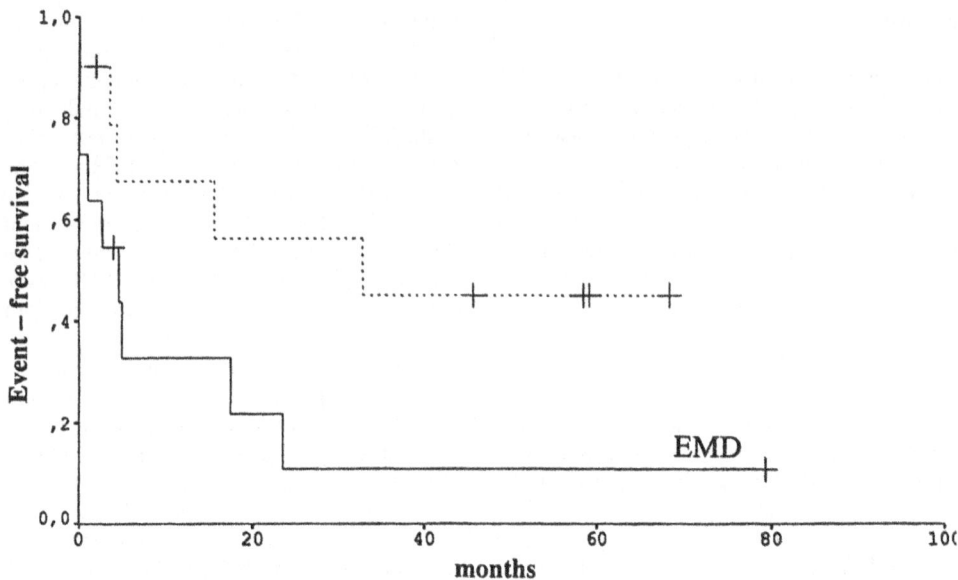

**Fig. 1.** Event-free survival of patients under 65 years with de novo AML and a normal karyotype without (10 cases) or with (11 cases) EMD, p=0.08

median dose of 22,800 (IR 20,000–22,800) mg/m² of AraC to reach CR (p=0.009). Two of 10 patients without EMD were classified as AML M4 in the FAB classification in comparison to 7 of 11 patients with EMD (p=0.08). The median of white blood cells was 55.6 x 10⁹/L in patients without EMD and 15.0 x 10⁹/L in cases with EMD but this difference was not statistically significant (p=0.324) probably due to the great variability of WBC values and small numbers of patients in both categories. The other characteristics as sex, age, percentage of bone marrow blasts or erythroblasts and the DNR dose needed for CR were not significantly different between patients with EMD and without EMD.

When transplanted patients were censored there was a trend (log-rank test, p=0.08) to a better event–free survival of patients without EMD in comparison to those with EMD (Fig. 1.) The difference became significant (p<0.05) when transplantation results were included.

## Discussion

Leukemic cells of most de novo AML are considered as a clonal expansion of a single transformed cell. Two main broad categories of de novo AML according to the leukemic transformation at two different stages of myeloid differentiation can be distinguished. The first one are AML originating from granulocyte-macrophage progenitors CFU-GM in which only cells of these two lineages are parts of leukemic population and the remaining erythroblasts and megakaryocytes are normal [17-20]. De novo AML of the other category originate from transformation of myeloid pluripotent progenitor cells CFU-GEMM when parts of leukemic population are cells of granulocytic, monocytic, erythroblastic and megakaryocytic lineages [17-20]. These two categories differ by involvement of erythroid and megakaryocytic lineages into the leukemic clone that could be detected in them by the finding of the same chromosomal abnormality [17, 18], by the proof of clonality [19, 20] or by increase of morphologic abnormalities (dysplasia) in these lineages.

In the study we used the evaluation of morphologic dysplastic features in erythroid and megakaryocytic lineages to distinguish these two main categories of AML. The first problem was to set up distinctive quantitative criteria for dysplasia in these lineages because bone marrow of healthy persons had shown dysplastic features in up to 10% of erythroblasts and in up to two megakaryocytes [21]. From this point of view the criterion for dysplasia in the megakaryocytic lineage (DysMg) requiring at least three (or 50% of 5 or more) dysplastic megakaryocytes [12] was arbitrarily well defined.

Dyserythropoiesis (DysE) in AML had to be diagnosed when more than 25% of erythroblasts showed dysplastic features [12]. The value of this criterion was confirmed by our finding of 9.5–21% dysplastic erythroblasts in 7 patients with AML M3 because erythroblasts in AML M3 are not a part of leukemic clone [22]. The use of these criteria enabled us to distinguished two different categories of de novo AML with a normal karyotype exhibiting different response to classical induction therapy and prognosis. Dyserythropoiesis present in more than 25% erythroblasts was found in 10 of 23 (44%) our patients while it was found in 54% [23] and 61% [24] in patients with de novo AML regardless of cytogenetics. We diagnosed megakaryocytic dysplasia (DysMg) in 6 of 23 (26%) patients which was a similar finding to 23% [23], 30% [24] or 31% [25] in other series of patients with de novo AML. Megakaryocytic dysplasia has been associated with a significantly lower CR rate [23, 26] after standard chemotherapy. These data support the prognostic value of our EMD categorization.

Dysgranulopoiesis may be found in AML originating from myeloid pluripotent progenitors CFU-GEMM as well as in AML from granulocyte-macrophage progenitors CFU-GM because the differentiation of leukemic clone may be aberrant [8, 9, 22]. We found more than 50% of dysplastic granulocytes in 6 of 10 patients without EMD as well as in 6 of 10 patients with EMD (Table 1.) The examination of dysgranulopoiesis in de novo AML M0-M5 seems not to be a useful discriminating factor between the two categories of AML but it may be so in acute erythroleukemias (M6) or megakaryoblastic leukemias (M7).

Patients with de novo AML and trilineage (granulocytic, erythroid, and megakaryocytic) myelodysplasia (AML-TMDS) were delineated as a special category of de novo AML with a significantly lower remission rate [12,

23, 24, 27]. Survival of patients with AML-TMDS was shorter [27] or insignificantly different from AML without TMDS [12, 23, 24]. We diagnosed 3 (13%) patients with AML–TMDS (Table 1.) in our series, a comparable percentage to 17% AML–TMDS in the original study [12]. AML-TMDS category was defined only according to strict morphologic criteria without the relationship to two main biologic categories of AMLs. AML-TMDS is a subgroup of our AML with EMD category in which dyserythropoietic and/or dysmegakaryopoietic features may point to the origin of all these AMLs from myeloid pluripotent progenitors. The EMD categorization may reflect better than the TMDS categorization the biological differences of de novo AMLs with relevant clinical consequences. EMD in de novo AML patients seems to be an independent prognostic factor for CR rate after classical chemotherapy and survival not only in patients with »a normal karyotype« but in de novo AML regardless of karyotypic findings, too [28]. De novo AML with EMD might represent a poor–risk category and AML without EMD a good–risk category.

The determination of EMD was feasible in 21 of 23 (91%) our patients. It required experience in morphology and technically well prepared and stained bone marrow smears, which are necessary for the diagnosis of AML as well [8, 9]. However, myelodysplastic features in AML may not only represent the leukemic clone itself but may be caused by other diseases affecting the same patient like anemias due to iron, folic acid or vitamin B12 deficiency, anemias of chronic disease, etc. [17]. These possible causes of EMD in AML should be kept in mind and could be excluded by patient's personal history and if necessary by a further laboratory examination. Although, the examination of EMD is subjective and thus prone to observer error, the agreement between two independent hematologists was in 20 out of 23 (87%) patients.

In conclusion we stress the need of a precise characterization of DNA abnormalities in AML by all available cytogenetic and molecular–biologic methods which could provide the best specification of each MIC AML type. The involvement of erythroid and/or megakaryocytic lineages into the leukemic clone, as demonstrated by the finding of EMD, was an independent prognostic factor for CR rate and event–free survival in de novo AML with a normal karyotype. The evaluation of EMD seems to be useful for the best choice of induction treatment in individual AML patients. A large prospective trial with risk–targeted therapy for patients with de novo AML with a normal karyotype plus EMD seems to be needed.

*Acknowledgments.* Supported in part by grants Nos. 0029–3 and 1912–4 from the Internal Grant Agency of the Ministry of Health of the Czech Republic.

The results of cytogenetic examinations were kindly provided by Prof. Ing. K. Michalová, Ph.D., and RNDr. Z. Zemanová, Ph.D.

We thank Miss Zdena Baláková for her help in preparing the manuscript.

# References

1. Fourth International Workshop on Chromosomes in Leukemia, 1982 (1984) A prospective study of acute nonlymphocytic leukemia. Cancer Genet Cytogenet 11: 249-360.
2. Yunis JJ, Brunning RD, Howe RB, Lobell M (1984) High-resolution chromosomes as an independent prognostic indicator in acute nonlymphocytic leukemia. N Engl J Med 311: 812-818.
3. Second MIC Cooperative Study Group (1988) Morphologic, immunologic and cytogenetic (MIC) working classification of the acute myeloid leukaemias. Br J Haemat 68: 487-494.
4. Mrózek K, Heinonen K, de la Chapelle A, Bloomfield CD (1997) Clinical significance of cytogenetics in acute myeloid leukemia. Semin Oncol 24: 17-31
5. Caligiuri MA, Strout MP, Gilliland DG (1997) Molecular biology of acute myeloid leukemia. Semin Oncol 24: 32-44.
6. Huang M-E, Ye Y-C, Chen S-R, et al (1988) Use of all-trans retinoic acid in the treatment of acute promyelocytic leukemia. Blood 72: 567-572.
7. Fenaux P, Chomienne C, Degos L (1997) Acute promyelocytic leukemia: biology and treatment. Semin Oncol 24: 92-102.
8. Bennett JM, Catovsky D, Daniel M-T, et al (1985) Proposed revised criteria for the classification of acute myeloid leukemia. Ann Intern Med 103: 620-624.
9. Bennett JM, Catovsky D, Daniel M-T, et al (1991) Proposal for the recognition of minimally differentiated acute myeloid leukaemia (AML-M0). Br J Haemat 78: 325-329.
10. Lemež P, Jelínek J, Michalová K, et al (1994) Near-tetraploid poorly differentiated acute myeloid leukemia M0 diagnosed by short-term cultures with a phorbol ester TPA. Leuk Res 18: 493-497.
11. Bennett JM, Catovsky D, Daniel M-T, et al (1982) Proposals for the classification of the myelodysplastic syndromes. Br J Haemat 51: 189-199.
13. Leme P, Schwarz J, Jelínek J, et al (1994) Late and slow diagnosis of acute promyelocytic leukemia - main cause of early deaths. Vnitø Lék 40: 654-659.
14. Michalová K, Musilová J, Zemanová Z (1991) Consecutive chromosomal studies in patients with myelodysplastic syndromes (MDS). Ann Génet 34: 212-218.
15. ISCN. An International System for Human Cytogenetic Nomenclature (1995) Mitelman F (ed) Karger, Basle, 114 pp.
16. Cheson BD, Cassileth PA, Head DR, et al (1990) Report of the National Cancer Institute-sponsored workshop on definitions of diagnosis and response in acute myeloid leukemia. J Clin Oncol 8: 813-819.
17. Krogh Jensen M, Killmann S-A (1971) Additional evidence for chromosome abnormalities in the erythroid precursors in acute leukaemia. Acta Med Scand 189: 97-100.
18. Blackstock AM, Garson MO (1974) Direct evidence for involvement of erythroid cells in acute myeloblastic leukaemia. Lancet 2: 1178-1179.
19. Fialkow PJ, Singer JW, Adamson JW, et al (1981) Acute nonlymphocytic leukemia: heterogeneity of stem cell origin. Blood 57: 1068-1073..
20. Fialkow PJ, Singer JW, Raskind WH, et al (1987) Clonal development, stem-cell differentiation, and clinical remissions in acute nonlymphocytc leukemia. N Engl J Med 317: 468-473.
21. Bain BJ (1996) The bone marrow aspirate of healthy subjects. Br J Haemat 94: 206-209.
22. Berger R, Bernheim A, Daniel M-T, et al (1982) Cytologic characterization and significance of normal karyotypes in t(8;21) acute myeloblastic leukemia. Blood 59: 171-178.
23. Estienne MH, Fenaux P, Preudhomme C, et al (1990) Prognostic value of dysmyelopoietic features in de novo acute myeloid leukaemia: a report on 132 patients. Clin Lab Haemat 12: 57-65.
24. Goasguen JE, Matsuo T, Cox C, Bennett JM (1992) Evaluation of the dysmyelopoiesis in 336 patients with de novo acute myeloid leukemia: major importance of dysgranulopoiesis for remission and survival. Leukemia 6: 520-525.
25. Gahn B, Haase D, Unterhalt M, et al (1996) De novo AML with dysplastic hematopoiesis: cytogenetic and prognostic significance. Leukemia 10: 946-951.
26. Jinnai I, Tomonaga M, Kuriyama K, et al (1987) Dysmegakaryocytopoiesis in acute leukaemias: its predominance in myelomonocytic (M4) leukaemia and implication for poor response to chemotherapy. Br J Haemat 66: 467-472.
27. Kuriyama K, Tomonaga M, Matsuo T, et al (1994) Poor response to intensive chemotherapy in de novo acute myeloid leukaemia with trilineage myelodysplasia. Br J Haemat 86: 767-773.
28. Leme P, Gáliková J (1998) Erythroid and/or megakaryocytic dysplasia in de novo acute myeloid leukaemias is a valuable indicator for inclusion of high doses of cytosine arabinoside in induction chemotherapy (abstract). Histochem J 30: 842.

# Asynchronous Expression of AC133 on CD34-Negative Leukemic Blast Cells in Childhood B-Cell Precursor ALL

G. Baersch, M. Baumann, J. Ritter, H. Jürgens and J. Vormoor

Abstract. Expression of AC113 was studied in the bone marrow of 17 patients with B-cell precursor ALL and 4 normal controls. 11 of 17 patients (65%) expressed AC133 on 1% to 99% of the leukemic blast cells. 6 patients (35%) had no AC133 expression detectable within the leukemic clone. Interestingly and in contrast to normal bone marrow, 6 patients showed an asynchronous expression of AC133 on CD19$^+$CD34$^-$ blasts. There was no correlation between the expression of AC133 and CD34 within the leukemic cell clone or the expression of AC133 and the immunological ALL subtype. This abnormal expression pattern of AC133 may be useful in monitoring minimal residual disease.

## Introduction

In 1997, a novel stem cell marker was identified on immature CD34$^+$ cells, detected by the monoclonal antibody AC133 [5, 8]. AC133 has been shown to be expressed on immature CD34$^+$ cells from adult bone marrow, cord blood and fetal liver [8]. The AC133$^+$ cell fraction is enriched for *in vitro* clonogenic progenitor cells, including multilineage CFU-GEMM [8], longterm culture-initiating cells [3], NOD/SCID mouse repopulating cells [3] and fetal sheep engrafting cells [8]. Thus, AC133 appears to be expressed on primitive repopulating human hematopoietic stem cells as well as myeloid progenitor cells. AC133 is a member of a newly identified family of 5 transmembrane cell surface glycoproteins that includes mouse kidney prominin [2, 6]. Its exact function is still unkown.

Samples from 4 normal bone marrow aspirates and 17 children with B-cell precursor ALL were characterized by 4-color flow cytometry to compare the expression pattern of AC133 in normal and leukemic human hematopoiesis.

## Materials and Methods

Bone marrow aspirates resp. peripheral blood (1 patient, UPN #1) were obtained from 16 children and one adult with B-cell precursor ALL at diagnosis. Normal bone marrow aspirates were available from 4 patients who received diagnostic bone marrow punctures to exclude malignant disease.

Immunophenotyping was performed applying four-color flow cytometry as described before [1, 7]. For time delay calibration APC beads (Calibrite APC, Becton Dickinson Immunocytometry systems (BDIS)) were used according to the manufacturer's instructions. Calibration and compensation were performed with unstained and anti-CD19-FITC, anti-CD19-PE, anti-CD19-PerCP or anti-CD19-APC single stained leukemic cells of the respective patient or with unstained and anti-CD34-FITC, anti-CD34-PE, anti-CD34-PerCP or anti-CD34-APC single stained normal bone marrow cells.

1 x 10$^6$ cells were incubated with saturating amounts of the antibodies anti-CD34-FITC, anti-AC133-PE, anti-CD45-PerCP and anti-CD19-APC for 20 minutes at room temperature. Subsequently, red cells were lysed and the samples washed twice with PBS buffer. Data acquisition and analysis was performed on a 2-laser (488 and 633nm) FACSCalibur

Department of Pediatric Hematology/Oncology, University of Münster, Germany

(BDIS) using CellQuest and Paint-A-Gate-Pro software (BDIS). 30.000 ungated events were acquired for all samples. Matched isotype controls were always included.

## Results

First, expression of AC133 was analysed in 4 normal control bone marrow samples. Approximately 50% of primitive CD34$^+$CD19$^-$ cells expressed AC133. There was a correlation between the expression of CD34 and AC133 with the CD34$^{bright}$ cells displaying the highest

levels of AC133. Only few B-lineage committed CD34$^+$CD19$^+$ progenitor cells expressed AC133 while all other mature cells, including CD19$^+$CD34$^-$ B-lymphocytes lacked expression of AC133.

In addition, 17 patients with B-cell precursor ALL were analysed for AC133 expression within the leukemic cell clone. As shown in table 1, in 7 children (41%) a high percentage of the leukemic blast cell population (> 20%) expressed AC133, in 4 children (24%) only a small subpopulation within the leukemic cell clone (< 20%) was positive for AC133, while in 6 patients (35%) no expression of AC133 could be detected. Interestingly, in 6 patients an asynchronous expression of AC133 was observed on CD19$^+$CD34$^-$ leukemic blast cells (Fig. 1). There was no correlation between the expression of AC133 and CD34 within the leukemic cell clone (Fig. 2). There was also no correlation between the expression of AC133 and the immunological ALL subtype (Table 1).

**Table 1.** Expression of CD34 and AC133 on the leukemic cell clone of pediatric B-cell precursor ALL

| patients | ALL subtype | CD34 | AC133 |
|----------|-------------|------|-------|
| UPN# 1 | pre-pre-B ALL | 1 % | 0% |
| UPN# 2 | c ALL | 95 % | 1 % |
| UPN# 4 | c ALL | 28 % | 42 % |
| UPN# 5 | c ALL | 0 % | 99 % |
| UPN# 6 | c ALL | 19 % | 40 % |
| UPN# 8 | c ALL | 94 % | 18 % |
| UPN# 9 | c ALL | 97 % | 0 % |
| UPN# 10 | c ALL | 84 % | 4 % |
| UPN# 11 | c ALL | 7 % | 0 % |
| UPN# 14 | pre-B ALL | 35 % | 1 % |
| UPN# 16 | pre-B ALL | 83 % | 28 % |
| UPN# 19 | pre-B ALL | 57 % | 90 % |
| UPN# 20 | pre-B ALL | 70 % | 0 % |
| UPN# 21 | B ALL | 0 % | 0 % |
| UPN# 22 | ALL relapse | 1 % | 97 % |
| UPN# 23 | ALL relapse | 83 % | 90 % |
| UPN# 24 | ALL relapse | 1 % | 0 % |

## Discussion

In accordance with published data [3, 5, 8] the highest levels of AC133 expression in normal bone marrow were seen on primitive CD34$^{bright}$ cells. Only few B-lingeage committed CD19$^+$CD34$^+$ progenitor expressed AC133, while mature cells lacked expression of AC133 altogether.

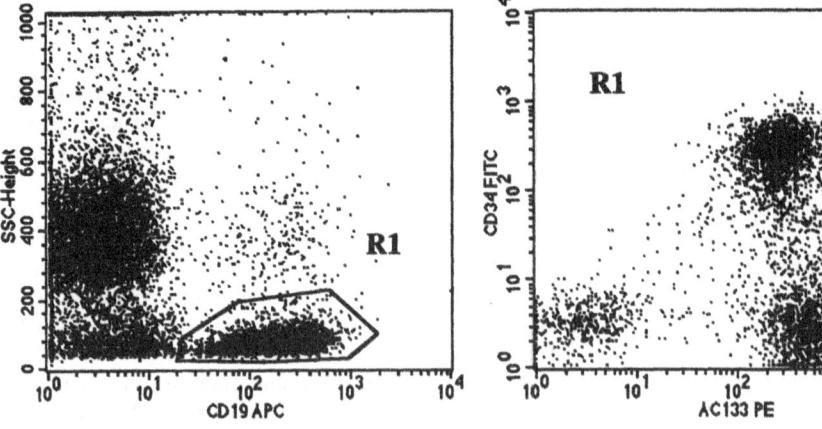

**Fig. 1.** Asynchronous expression of AC133 on CD34-negative leukemic blast cells in a patient with B-cell precursor ALL. A gate was set on the CD19$^+$ leukemic cell population (left dot plot). A large CD34$^+$AC133$^+$ cell population was seen within the CD19$^+$ leukemic cell clone (right dot plot).

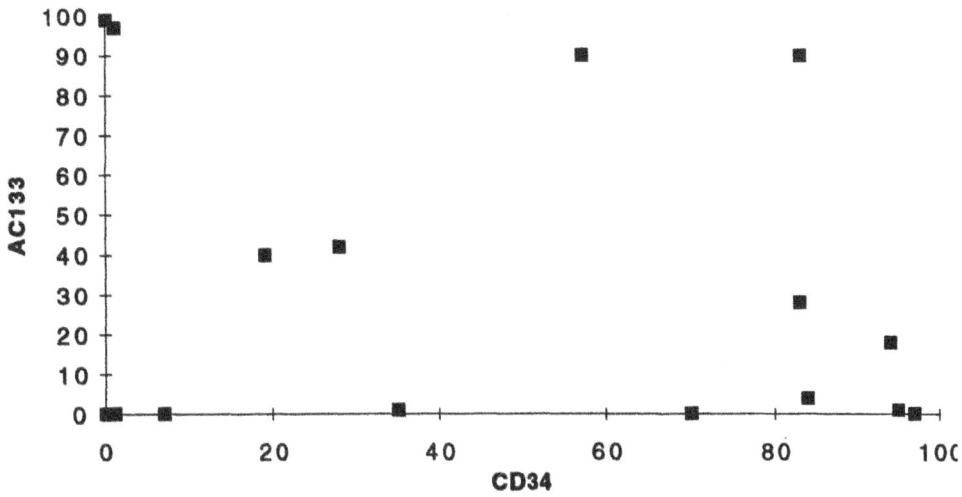

**Fig. 2.** Absent correlation between the expression of CD34 and AC133 within the leukemic cell clone.

11 of 17 children (65%) with B-cell precursor ALL expressed AC133 on a variable fraction (1–99%) of the leukemic cell clone. Interestingly, there was no correlation between the expression of CD34 and AC133 and in contrast to normal bone marrow expression of AC133 could also be detected on CD34⁻ leukemic blast cells. This is similar to what has recently been described for acute myeloid leukemia [4]. If expression of AC133 on CD34⁻ leukemic blast cells reflects an abnormal differentiation or is merely consequence of a gene dysregulation within the malignant cell clone remains unclear. However, this abnormal pattern of AC133 may be useful for monitoring minimal residual disease.

## References

1. Baersch G, Baumann M, Meltzer J, Möllers T, Ritter J, Jürgens H, Vormoor J (1996) Durchflußzytometrische Charakterisierung von Reifungsvorgängen und stammzellnahen Zellpopulationen bei der B-Vorläuferzell-ALL im Kindesalter. Klin. Pädiatr. 208: 160 - 167
2. Corbeil D, Roper K, Weigmann A, Huttner WB (1998) AC133 hematopoietic stem cell antigen: human homologue of mouse kidney prominin or distinct member of a novel protein family. Blood 91: 2625 - 2626
3. de Wynter EA, Buck D, Hart C, Heywood R, Coutinho LH, Clayton A, Rafferty JA, Burt D, Guenechea G, Bueren JA, Gagen D, Fairbairn LJ, Lord BI, Testa NG (1998) CD34+AC133+ cells isolated from cord blood are highly enriched in long-term culture-initiating cells, NOD/SCID-repopulating cells and dendritic cell progenitors. Stem Cells 16: 387 - 396
4. Kratz-Albers K, Zühlsdorf M, Leo R, Berdel WE, Büchner T, Serve H (1998) Expression of AC133, a novel stem cell marker, on human leukemic blasts lacking CD34-antigen and on a human CD34+ leukemic cell line: MUTZ-2. Blood 92: 4485 - 4487
5. Miraglia S, Godfrey W, Yin AH, Atkins K, Warnke R, Holden JT, Bray RA, Waller EK, Buck DW (1997) A novel five-transmembrane hematopoietic stem cell antigen: isolation, characterization, and molecular cloning. Blood 90: 5013 - 5021
6. Miraglia S, Godfrey W, Buck D (1998) A response to AC133 hematopoietic stem cell antigen: human homologue of mouse kidney prominin or distinct member of a novel protein family. Blood: 91, 4390 - 4391
7. Vormoor J, Baersch G, Baumann M, Ritter J, Jürgens H (1998) Flow cytometric identification of candidate normal stem cell populations in CD45-negative B-cell precursor acute lymphoblastic leukaemia (ALL). Br. J. Haematol. 100: 501 - 508
8. Yin AH, Miraglia S, Zanjani ED, Almeida-Porada G, Ogawa M, Leary AG, Olweus J, Kearney J, Buck DW (1997) AC133, a novel marker for human hematopoietic stem and progenitor cells. Blood 90: 5002 - 5012

# Expression of AC133 in Childhood Acute Leukemia

U. Ebener, S. Wehner, A. Brinkmann, E. Niegemann and B. Kornhuber

*Abstract.* The antigen AC133 is a novel 5-transmembrane cell surface molecule with a molecular weight if 117–120 kD. It is selectively expressed on a subset of CD34$^+$ human hematopoietic stem and progenitor cells. The monoclonal antibodies ACV133/1 and AC133/2 recognize early progenitor cells derived from peripheral blood and bone marrow and provide an alternative to conventionally applied anti-CD34 antibodies used for the selection and characterization of cells necessary for short- and long term engraftment in transplant situation.

In the present study we analysed bone marrow of leukemic blast cells at the time of initial diagnosis and in relapse (n = 28; 19 ALLs, 9 AMLs) just as various leukemia derived cell lines (i.e. KG1, KG1a, Molt-4, Jurkat) using flow cytometry.

Additionally we evaluated the expression of AC133 bs. CD34 in umbilical cord blood (UCB, n = 43), peripheral blood (PB) from healthy donors (n = 10) and peripheral blood from patients (neuroblastoma, rhabdomyosarcoma and leukemia) undergoing mobilization with the cytokine G-CSF (n = 34) and from leukapheresis products (n = 15) as well as CD34$^+$- or AC133$^+$-selected cell populations (n = 6) following MiniMACS- or Vario-MACS-System (Miltenyi Biotec, Bergisch Gladbach, Germany). Cells were stained with the MoAbs anti-AC133-PE (Miltenyi Biotec) and anti-CD34-PE/-FITC (clone HPCA-2/BD Heidelberg).

Our results so far obtained by standard flow cytometry demonstrate that only CD34$^+$ stem- and progenitor cells originated from different sources were exclusively positive for AC133 antigen. In contrast to this observation we found in acute leukemias with CD34$^+$-phenotype (74%) high or partial coexpression of AC133 in 13/19 cases (68%). These data have shown, that about 30% of the phenotyped acute leukemias had no detectable levels of AC133 molecules as well as for the myeloid leukemia cell line KG1a (CD34$^+$/AC133$^+$).

On the basis of our results we believe than the usage of anti-AC133 applying positive selection with MACS-technology proves to be of great benefit in order to separate contaminating CD34$^+$/AC133$^+$ tumor cells from leukapheresis harvests.

## Introduction

The CD34 antigen, a 110–115 kD cell surface molecule, is expressed by all hematopoietic stem and progenitor cells [1–3]. The physiological function of this highly glycosilated antigen suggests a role for the CD34 antigen in intercellular contact [4]. This stem cell antigen CD34 is encoded by a gene located and mapped to a region in the long arm of chromosome 1 (1q32) [5, 6]. The recently developed techniques to identify and characterize stem cells by function and specific surface molecules [7] have provided an access to stem cell biology in normal hematopoiesis and malignant disorders [8, 9].

Stem cells excess a cell surface antigen defined as CD34 [10]. With increasing maturation process the expression of CD34 gets lost. Immunological classification of acute leukemias is based on the comparison of leukemic blast cells with their presumed normal

J. W. Goethe University, Clinic of Pediatrics III, Department of Hematology and Oncology, D-60590 Frankfurt/M., Germany counterparts [3, 11–16]. Therefore CD34 is an important antigen for leukemia and lymphoma typing [15].

Analysis of CD34 expression by leukemic blasts in 230 pediatric and 251 adult patients with *de novo* AML enrolled in two large multicenter trials (AML-BFM-87 and AMLCG) has shown that approximately 45% of all AML cases were positive to this marker [13, 14].

The use of monoclonal antibodies (moAb) against the CD34 antigen [17, 18] permits flow cytometric quantitation of the size of this cell pool, which appears to be an important parameter in assessing the quality of a hematopoietic graft [1]. The quantitation of CD34+ cells will depend on the epitope recognized by the CD34 antibody used.

Applying antibodies directed against class II/-III epitopes of CD34 antigen is recommended [12]. Investigations of commercially available moAbs designated BIRMA-K3 (DAKO, Hamburg/Germany) and HPCA-2 (BD, Heidelberg/Germany) with reactivity to class III epitope resulted in a clear cut-off staining with strong correlation [19].

It is consensus that the determination of the number of CD34 expressing cells may help to estimate numbers of the hematopoietic progenitor cells as defined by in vitro culture [20].

The AC133 antigen has been developed recently in human hematopoietic stem- and progenitor cells [21, 22]. It is a novel cell surface molecule with a molecular weight of 117–120 kD. This glycosylated polypeptide consisting of 865 amino acids (aa) has a predicted size of 97 kD and contains five transmembraneous (5-TM) domains with an extracellular N-terminus and a cytoplasmic C-terminus [21, 22]. This 5-TM type of structure containing intracellular and extracellular aa-loops represents a new class of 5-TM receptors (Fig. 1).

AC133 is selectively expressed on immature hematopoietic stem cells and progenitors. The antibodies specific for the surface marker AC133 stain about 30–60% of all CD34+ cells including CD34bright, CD38dim/neg, HLA-DR, CD90+ and CD117+ cells [21].

AC133 antigen may be the human homologue of the mouse protein called prominin. It was recently identified and shown to be expressed on neuroepithelial and epithelial cells in mice [23, 24].

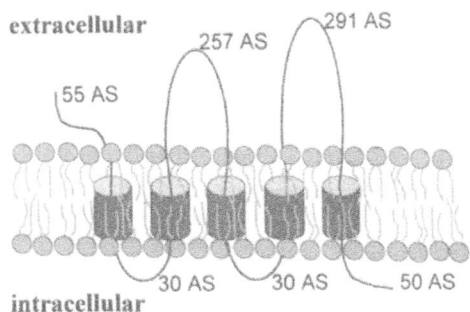

**Fig. 1.** Structure of the proposed Model of AC133

The AC133 molecule is also expressed on two retinoblastoma cell lines, also on a teratoma [21] and on a human CD34+ cell line derived from AML designated »MUTZ-2« [25].

The group of David Buck was the first to describe a monoclonal antibody (moAb), directed against AC133 and recognizing only CD34bright cells in bone marrow, fetal liver, cord blood and peripheral blood [22]. The commercially, available antibodies specific for AC133 antigen (AC133/1, AC133/2, Miltenyi Biotec, Bergisch Gladbach/Germany) stain 30–60% of all CD34+ population including CD34bright, CD38ncg/dim, HLA-DR, CD90+ (Tny-1) and CD117+ (c-kit) cells [21, 22]. AC133 is expressed on lineage non-committed stem- and progenitor cells, e.g. long-term repopulating (LTRC), LTCIC and CFU-GEMM as well as on CFU-GM [8, 26].

## Objective

In the present study our intention was the investigation of AC133 antigen expression, i.e. in umbilical cord blood (UCB), in peripheral blood (PB) from healthy donors and G-CSF mobilized PB to proof qualitative and quantitative extent of AC133 coexpression in CD34+-stem cell/-progenitors of hematopoietic system.

Our primary interest was to study the expression of these surface markers in acute leukemic blast cells at the onset of diagnosis demonstrating mainly CD34+-phenotype. We intend to answer the question, if leukemic blasts do simultaneously express the new discovered antigen AC133 on cellular surface membrane. Maybe an absence of AC133 will result in consequences with respect to peripheral blood stem cell transplantation (PBSCT) due to alternative purging strategies.

## Material and Methods

### Cell Sources

Umbilical cord blood (UCB) samples were obtained from Centre of Gynaecology (clinic of J. W. Goethe University of Frankfurt/M.) and processed within 12 h after birth. 43 specimens were analysed in a flow cytometer (FACScan/BD Heidelberg, Germany). The peripheral blood (PB) samples in this report were maintained from 10 different healthy donors.

34 peripheral blood samples derived from oncological/hematological pediatrics in our clinic (neuroblastoma, rhabdomyosarcoma, acute leukemia) undergoing administration with rhG-CSF were included to our investigation.

Analyses of the leukapheresis harvests (LP, n = 15) collected from selected patients for autologous transplantation were also included to the present study.

Bone marrow (BM) aspirates were obtained from twenty eight children with acute leukemias (ALL/AML), diagnosed according to the French-American-British (FAB) criteria and to the immunological classification scheme [11] of the »European Group for Immunological Characterisation of Leukemias (EGIL). All specimens were investigated for expression of CD34 (HPCA-2/BD Heidelberg/Germany) and AC133 (AC133-PE/Miltenyi Biotec, Bergisch Gladbach/Germany).

### Cell Lines

Molt-4, Jurkat, KG1 and KG1a cell lines used for this study were obtained from »German Collection of Microorganisms and Cell Cultures« (Braunschweig/Germany) and maintained in RPMI 1640 with 10% FCS, 2 mmol/L-glutamine in a 5% $CO_2$ humidified atmosphere.

### Flow Cytometric Analysis

Two-, or three-color FACS analysis was used for antigen screening, determination of AC133 and CD34 antigen expression in several hematological specimens. Monoclonal antibodies (mo-Abs) used in the present study (CD45, CD14, CD10, CD19, CD79a, HLA-DR, CD1a, CD7, CD13, CD33, CD34, CD38, CD90, CD117, TdT, AC133-1-/-2-PE and isotype matched moAbs as a negative control, were purchased from different companies. In order to proof various combinations of moAbs for multiparametric flow cytometry (FACScan/BD Heidelberg, Germany) antibodies were directly conjugated by fluorescent dyes (FITC, RPE, PerCP, PhycoCy5).

### Data Acquisition

All data were acquired on a FASCan equipped with an 488-nm argon ion laser for excitation of FITC, RPE, PerCP and PhycoCy5 fluorochromes.

For each sample, between 10.000 and 50.000 events were acquired in list mode files, applying Cell Quest software (BD/Heidelberg, Germany). Forward scatter, orthogonal light scatter and fluorescence signals were estimated for each cell.

### Leukapheresis Products

Selected children, who were candidates for high-dose chemotherapy followed by stem cell rescue, were enrolled to this study. The patients received 10 µg/kg rhG-CSF (Neupogen; Amgen/Munich, Germany) per day subcutaneously beginning day 1 after the end of a chemotherapy course. Autologous progenitor cells were harvested by a Fenwal CS 3000 plus (Baxter/Munich, Germany).

### Immunomagnetic Isolation of CD34+ or AC133+ Cells

For isolation and purification of peripheral stem-/progenitor cells, we applied CD34 Multisort Kit and/or AC133 Cell Isolation Kit (Miltenyi Biotec GmbH/Bergisch Gladbach,

Germany in combination with Mini-/Vario-MACS-System (MS+ column, Lot.-No. 0452) likewise available by Miltenyi Biotec [27, 28]. In accordance with standardized isolation protocols CD34+- or AC133+-enriched stem cells [29–31] were maintained and subsequently analysed using flow cytometry [12, 32–35].

as on unselected and positiv selected (MACS-System) apheresis products as demonstrated previously [33, 34].

Our results referring to flow cytometric cell marker analyses in order to quantify CD34 and AC133 antigens on stem cells and progenitors are summarized in Table 1–3.

## Results and Discussion

In view of the large impact of determining CD34 expressing cells in the setting of autologous blood stem- and progenitor cells support and by immunophenotyping of acute leukemias [13, 14, 16, 20, 35, 36] we tried to compare the expression of CD34 antigen with the novel hematopoietic marker AC133.

In this study, we evaluated the frequency and intensity of AC133 vs. CD34 expression as defined by reactivity with the anti-AC133-PE conjugated antibody and anti-CD34-FITC or -PE antibody in different types of childhood leukemia (ALL and AML) as well as on umbilical cord blood and peripheral blood, as well

**Table 1.** Expression of AC133 vs CD34 on Cell Surface of Hematopoietic Cells

| Specimen | n | CD34 [%] | AC133 [%] |
|---|---|---|---|
| UCB | 43 | 0,385 ± 0,156 | 0,29 ± 0,165 |
| PB (volunteer) | 10 | 0 – 0,15 | 0 – 0,05 |
| PB (G.CSF-administration) | 34 | 0,1 – 3,94 | 0,1 – 3,51 |
| Leukapheresis harvests | 15 | 0,8 – 5,4 | 0,55 – 4,4 |
| CD34+-cell fraction*) | 5 | 92,6 ± 4,6 | 88,07 ± 7,01 |
| AC133+-cell fraction**) | 1 | 94,3 | n.t. |

UCB umbilical cord blood
PB peripheral blood
n.t. not tested
*) CD34+ separation (Mini-/VarioMACS)
**) AC133+ separation (Mini-VarioMACS)

**Table 2.** Expression of AC133 vs. CD34 in Childhood Acute Lymphoblastic Leukemia (ALL)

| Immunophenotype | n | f / m | age | CD34 [%] | AC133 [%] |
|---|---|---|---|---|---|
| cALL | 9 | 2 / 7 | 1 – 17 | 67 – 94 | 21 – 88 |
| My+ cALL | 2 | 1 / 1 | 3 – 10 | 74 – 78 | 20 – 41 |
| pre-pre B-ALL | 1 | 1 / 0 | <1 | 21 | 95 |
| My+ cALL, cALL | | | | | |
| T-ALL | 4 | 0 / 4 | 9 | 23 – 85 | 0 |
| cALL, T-ALL | 3 | 0 / 3 | 9 | 0 | 0 |

ALL acute lymphoblastic leukemia    f female    n number
My+ coexpression of myeloid antigen(s)    m male    CD Cluster of Differentiation

**Table 3.** Expression of AC133 vs. CD34 in Childhood Acute Myeloid Leukemia (AML)

| FAB-classification | I/R | f/m | age | CD34 [%] | AC133 [%] |
|---|---|---|---|---|---|
| AML-M6 | R | m | 6 years | 48 | 59 |
| AML-M2 | R | m | 15 years | 69 | 0 |
| Ly+-AML | I | m | 8 days | 89 | 0 |
| AML-M3 | I | f | 10 months | 0 | 0 |
| AML-M6 | I | m | 18 months | 0 | 0 |
| AML-M4 | I | m | 18 months | 0 | 0 |
| Ly+ AML-M4 | R | f | 7 years | 0 | 0 |
| AML-M6 | R | m | 6,5 years | 0 | 0 |
| AML-M7 | I | m | 9 months | 0 | 0 |

AML acute myeloid leukemia    I initial diagnosis    f female
Ly+ coexpression of lymphatic antigen(s)    R relapse    m male
FAB French-American-British cooperative group

In peripheral blood AC133+-stem-/-progenitor cells are normally available in only very small concentrations (<0,05%). Cells stained with the moAbs AC133-PE remain to be exclusively cells, expressing simultaneously CD34+ (<0,15%).

In comparison to peripheral blood (PB) from healthy donors, umbilical cord blood (UCB) established more prominent compartment of AC133+-cells in UCB (0,29ë 0,165%/AC133+ vs. 0,385ë 0,156%/CD34+). Due to the demonstration of likewise coexpression of classical stem cell marker CD34, it seems to be a subpopulation of progenitor cells (Table 1).

In peripheral blood from pediatric oncological patients, following hematological growth factor rhG-CSF treatment, a temporal increasing in the concentration of AC133+/CD34+-stem cells is verifiable depending on the duration of application of this factor (Figure 2).

Using MACS-technology CD34+-selected cell fractions as well as AC133+-cells could be enriched in high concentrations from UCB in a purity of 92% for CD34+ compared to AC133+ with an extend of 88%.

Since the availability of monoclonal antibodies directed against the molecule AC133 we have flow cytometrically analysed bone marrow aspirates from 28 acute leukemias (ALLs': n = 19; AMLs: n = 9).

11 cases with »common« ALL subtype (cALL) showed high expression of both, CD34 and AC133 antigen. In one case of pre-pre-B ALL we observed a clearly higher expression of AC133 vs. CD34. In 4 cases of different subtypes of ALL with CD34 phenotype we could not detect any expression of AC133 on the blast cells. In the group of ALLs we found a minority of cases (n = 3) as well not showing an expression neither for AC133- nor for CD34 antigen

In the group of 9 AMLs (newly diagnosed untreated AML: n = 5; relapse: n = 4) we could detect in only one case a coexpression of CD34 and AC133 as demonstrated in Table 3.

6 of 9 cases showed no reaction with both antibodies anti-CD34 and anti-AC133/1.

All leukemias investigated in the small group of ALLs and AMLs lacking from CD34-positivity were also negative for AC133 antigen.

In this study we have also investigated the expression of AC133 antigen in various cell lines derived from leukemic specimens. None of the investigated cell lines (i.e. Molt-4, Jurkat, KG1 and the CD34+ cell line KG1a) showed any expression of AC133. Till now, in literature are published only two human retinoblastoma cell lines (Y79.1 and WERI-Rb-1) as well as one teratocarcinoma-derived cell line (NT2), showing positive reaction with the antibody AC133 [21]. Actually there was a short report about the identification of AC133 on human leukemic CD34+ cell line, which is called MUTZ-2 [25].

Our results to be demonstrated correspond to first indication given in literature [21, 22]. As shown by us and other groups, there is a considerable percentage [>30%] of acute leukemias with CD34+-phenotype not expressing AC133 antigen [22, 25, 37–40]. These leukemic blast cells can therefore be separated in an effective way from AC133+-stem/and -precursor cells applying appropriate MACS-technology in combination with AC133-MicroBeads [41].

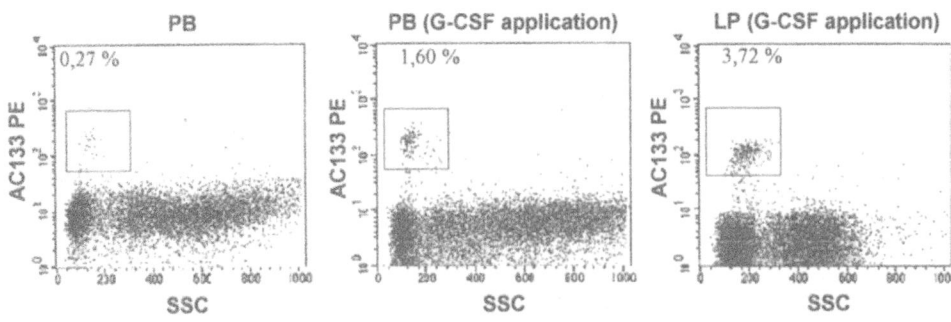

**Fig. 2.** Flowcytometric Detection of AC133-Antigen-Expression in Various Specimens

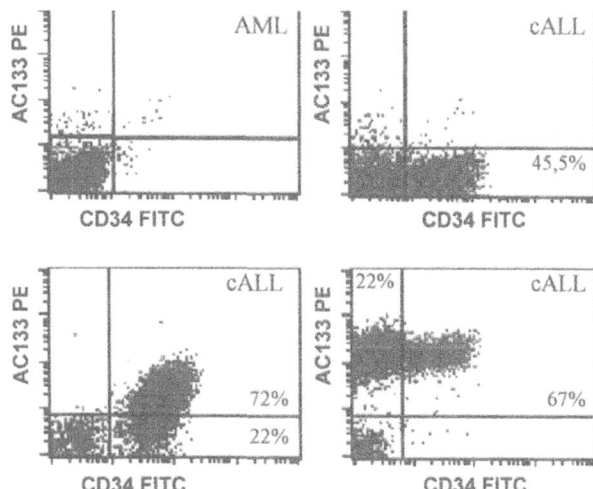

**Fig. 3.** Flowcytometric Analysis of Antigen-Expression in Childhood Acute Leukemias (AC133 vs. CD34)

Consequently likewise patients suffering from acute leukemias with CD34+-/AC133-phenotype not reacting in compliance with therapeutic regimens, will obtain the possibility of an autologous PBSCT, not covered by contaminations caused by tumor cells within the transplant.

*Acknowledgment.* This work was supported by »Hilfe für Krebskranke Kinder Frankfurt/M. e.V.«

# References

1. Bender JG, Lum L, Unverzagt KL, Lee W, Van Epps D, George S, Coon J, Ghalie R, McLeod B, Kaizer H, Williams SF (1994) Correlation of colony-forming cells, long-term culture initiating cells and CD34+ cells in aphresis products from patients mobilized for peripheral blood progenitors with different regimens. Bone Marrow Transpl 13 (4): 479–485

2. Civin CI, Strauss LC, Brovall C, Fackler MJ, Schwartz JF, Shaper JH (1984) Antigenic analysis of hematopoiesis. III. A hematopoietic progenitor cell surface antigen defined by a monoclonal antibody raised abainst KG-1a cells. J Immunol 133 (1): 157–165

3. Strauss LC, Rowley SD, La Russa VF, Sharkis SJ, Stuart RK, Civin CI (1986) Antigenic analysis of hematopoiesis. V. Characterization of My-10 antigen expression by normal lymphohematopoietic progenitor cells. Exp Hematol 14 (9): 878–886

4. Majdic O, Stockl J, Pickl WF, Bohuslav J, Strobl H, Scheinecker C, Stockinger H, Knapp W (1994) Signaling and induction of cytoadhesiveness via the hematopoietic progenitor cell surface molecule CD34. Blood 83 (5): 1226–1234

5. Molgaard HV, Spurr NK, Greaves MF (1989) The hemopoietic stem cell antigen CD34+, is encoded by a gene located on chromosome 1. Leukemia 31 (1): 773–776

6. Satterthwaite AB, Burn TC, Le Beau MM, Tenen DG (1992) Structure of the gene encoding CD34, a human hematopoietic stem cell antigen Genomics 12 (4): 788–794

7. Krause DS, Fackler MJ, Civin CI, May WS (1996) CD34: Structure, biology, and clinical utility. Blood 87 /1): 1–13

8. Sutherland HJ, Lansdorp PM, Henkelman DH, Eaves AC, Eaves CJ (1990) Functional characterization of individual human hematopoietic stem cells cultured at limiting dilution on supportive marrow stromal layers. Proc Natl Acad Sci USA 87 (9): 3584–3588

9. Falkenburg JH, van-Luxenburg-Heijs SA, Zijlman JM, Fibbe WE, Kluin-Nelemans JC, Kanhai HH, Willemze R (1993) Separation, enrichment, and characterization of human hematopoietic progenitor cells from umbilical cord blood. Ann Hematol 67 (5): 231–236

10. Dercksen MW, Daams GM, Haas de M (1995) Characterization of the CD34 cluster. In Schlossmann SF, Boumsell L, Golks W et al (eds) Leucocyte Typing V. Oxford University press, Oxford, New York, Tokio, Vol 1: 850

11. Bene MC, Castoldi G, Knapp W, Ludwig WD, Matudes E, Orfao A, van't Veer MB (1995) Proposals for the immunological classification of acute leukemias. European Group for the Immunological Characterization of Leukemias (EGIL). Leukemia 9 (10): 1783–1786

12. Rothe G, Schmitz Ge, Adorf D, Barlage S, Gramatzki M, Hanenberg H, Höffkes HG, Janossy G, Knüchel R, Ludwig WD, Nebe T, Nerl C, Orfao A, Serke S, Sonnen R, Tichello A, Wörmann B (1996) Consensus protokol for the flow cytometric immunophenotyping of hematopoietic malignancies. Working Group on Flow Cytometry and

Image Analysis. Leukemia 10 (5): 877–895

13. Sperling C, Buechner T, Sauerland C, Fonatsch C, Thiel E, Ludwig WD (1993) CD34 expression in de novo acute myeloid leukaemia. Br J Haematol 85 (3): 635–637

14. Sperling C, Büchner T, Creutzig U, Ritter J, Harbott J, Fonatsch C, Sauerland C, Mielcarek M, Maschmeyer G, Löffler H, Ludwig WD (1995) Clinical, Morphologic, Cytogenetic and Prognostic Implications of CD34 Expression in Childhood and Adult de novo AML. Leukemia & Lymphoma 17 (5–6): 417–426

15. Pui CH, Hancock ML, Head DR, Rivera GK, Look AT, Sandlund JT, Behm FG (1993) Clinical significance of CD34 Expression in Childhood Acute lymphoblastic Leukemia. Blood 82 (3): 889–894

16. Haase D, Feuring-Buske M, Schoch C, Schäfer C, Griesinger F, Troff C, Gahn B, Hiddemann W, Wörmann B (1998) Involvement of CD34+ Stem Cells in Malignant Transformation on AML and MDS-Genetic Analysis of Sorted Subpopulations by Classical and Molecular Cytogenetics. Acute Leukemias VII. Experimental Approaches and Novel Therapies. Hiddemann W, Büchner T, Wörmann B, Ritter J, Creutzig U, Keating M, Plunkett (eds). Springer-Verlag, p 19–28

17. Greaves MF, Brown J, Molgaard HV, Spurr NK, Robertson D, Delia D, Sutherland DR (1992) Molecular features of CD34: A hematopoietic progenitor cell-associated molecule. Leukemia 6 (Suppl 1): 31–36

18. Sutherland DR, Stewart AK, Keating A (1993) CD34 antigen: molecular features and potential clinical applications. Stem Cells 11(Suppl 3): 50–57

19. Höffkes HG, Lowe JA, Pederson RO, Schmidtke G, McDonald DF (1996) BIRMA-K3, a new monoclonal antibody for CD34 immunophenotyping and stem and progenitor cell assay. J Hematotherapy 5 (3): 261–270

20. Serke S, Huhn D (1996) Expression of Class I, II, and III Epitopes of the CD34 Antigen by Normal and Leukemic Hemopoietic Cells. Cytometry 26 (2): 154 g20.   Serke S, Huhn D (1996) Expression of Class I, II, and III Epitopes of the CD34 Antigen by Normal and Leukemic Hemopoietic Cells. Cytometry 26 (2): 154–160

21. Yin AH, Miraglia S, Zanjani ED, Almeida-Porada G, Ogawa M, Leary AG, Olweus J, Kearney J, Buck DW (1997) AC133, a novel marker for human hematopoietic stem and progenitor cells. Blood 90 (12): 5002–5012

22. Miraglia S, Godfrey W, Yin AH, Atkins K, Warnke R, Holden JT, Bray RA, Waller EK, Buck D (1997) A novel 5-transmembrane hematopoietic stem cell antigen: Isolation, Characterization, and molecular cloning. Blood 90 (12): 5013–5021

23. Corbeil D, Roper K, Weigmann A, Huttner WB (1998) AC133 hematopoietic stem cell antigen: Human homologue of mouse kidney prominin or distinct member of a novel protein family? Blood 91 (7): 2625–2627

24. Weigmann A, Corbeil D, Hellwig A, Huttner WB (1997) Prominin, a novel microvilli specific polytopic membrane protein of the apical surface of epithelial cells, is targeted to plasmalemmal protrusions of non-epithelial cells. Proc Natl Acad Sci USA 94 (23): 12425–12430

25. Kratz-Albers K, Zülsdorf M, Leo R, Berdel WE, Büchner Th, Serve H (1998) Identification of AC133 on human leukemic CD34-Blasts and on human CD34+ cell ine: MUTZ-2. Annals of Hematology, Supplement II, Vol 77 (abstract No. 575)

26. Srour EF, Brandt JE, Briddell RA, Grigsby S, Leehmhuis T, Hoffman R (1993) Long-term generation and expansion of human primitive hematopoietic progenitor cells in vitro. Blood 81 (3): 661–669

27. Miltenyi S, Müller W, Weichel W, Radbruch A (1990) High Gradient Magnetic Cell Separation with MACS. Cytometry 11 (2): 231–238

28. Kato K, Radbruch A (1993) Isolation and characterization of CD34+ hematopoietic stem cells from human peripheral blood by high-gradient magnetic cell sorting. Cytometry 14 (4): 384–392

29. Handgretinger R, Lang P, Schumm M, Taylor G, Neu S, Koscielnak F, Niethammer D, Klingebiel T (1998) Isolation and transplantation of autologous peripheral CD34+ progenitor cells highly purified by magnetic-activated cell sorting. Bone Marrow Transpl 21 (10): 987–993

30. Neu S, Geiselhart A, Kuci S, Baur F, Niethammer D, Handgretinger R (1996) Isolation and phenotypic characterization of CD117-positive cells. Leukemia Res 20 (11–12): 963–971

31. de Wynter E, Hart C, Heywood R, Testa NG (1998) Characteristics of MACS isolated CD34+AC133 +AC133+ hematopoietic progenitor cells. MACS & more: Vol 2: 8–9

32. Sutherland DR, Keating A, Nayar R, Anania S, Stewart AK (1994) Sensitive detection and enumeration of CD34+ cells in peripheral and cord blood by flow cytometry. Exp Hematol 22 (10): 1003–1010

33. Ebener U, Hakuba S, Wehner S, Stegmüller M, Niegemann E, Kornhuber B, Schwabe D (1998) Phenotypic characterization of various CD34+ cell populations using anti-AC133. Annals of Hematology, Supplement II, Vol 77 (abstract No. 606)

34. Ebener U, Wehner S, Niegemann E, Kornhuber B, Schwabe D (1999) Expression of AC133 in acute childhood leukemia. Annals of Hematology, Supplement II, Vol 78 (abstract No. 103)

35. Cassens U, Fischer J, Fritsch G, Fruehauf S, Garritsen HSP, Gebauer W, Haas R, Höffkes HG, Humpe A, Kleine HD, Moog R, Riggert J, Rothe G, Schlenke P, Schmitz G, Tonn T, Wörmann B, Ziegler BL (1996) Durchflußzytometrische Analyse CD34-exprimierender Zellen in Blut und Zytapherese-produkten (Konsensusprotokoll). Infusionstherapie Transfusionsmed 23 (2): 2–23

36. Wells SJ, Bray RA, Stempora LL, Farhi DC (1996) CD117/CD34 Expression in Leukemic Blasts. Am J Clin Pathol 106 (2): 192–195

37. Horn PA, Tesch H, Staib P, Kube D, v. Bergwelt M, Schultes H, Voliotis D (1998) Expression of CD34 and AC133, a novel hematopoietic precursor antigen, on acute myeloid leukemia cells. Annals of Hematology, Supplement II, Vol 77 (abstract No. 567)

38. Horn PA, Tesch H, Staib P, Schoch C, Kube D, Diehl V, Voliotis D (1999) Significance of AC133 and CD34 expression on acute myeloid cells. Annals of

Hematology, Supplement II, Vol 78 (abstract No. 128)

39. Baersch G, Baumann M, Ritter J, Jürgens J, Vormoor J (1999) Expression of AC133 and CD117 on CD34-positive subpopulations in childhood B-cell precursor acute lymphoblastic leukemia (BCP-ALL). Annals of Hematology, Supplement II, Vol 78 (abstract No. 102)

40. Scheding S, Bühring HJ, Kanz L, Brugger W (1998) Mobilization of AC133 positive hematopoietic progenitor cells in normal PBPC donors and cancer patients. Annals of Hematology, Supplement II, Vol 77 (abstract No. 609)

41. Viehmann K, von Neuhoff N, Schmitz N, Dreger P (1998) Purging of autografts from patients with CLL by positive selection via the AC133 antigen. Preclinical data. Annals of Hematology, Supplement II, Vol 77 (abstract No. 156)

# CD10 Expression in T-Lineage Adult Acute Lymphoblastic Leukemia

X. Thomas[1], C. Charrin[2], J.-P. Magaud[2] and D. Fière[1]

*Abstract.* Fifty-five adult patients with newly diagnosed T-lineage acute lymphoblastic leukemia (ALL) were analysed for CD10 expression on leukemic cells. CD10 was expressed on 18/55 (33%) cases. There were no differences between CD10+ and CD10- cases in clinical features or karyotypic patterns, except for white blood cell (WBC) counts that were higher in CD10+ patients. CD10 positivity was significantly associated with the expression of CD1 (p = 0.0001), and tend to be associated with that of CD4 and CD8. CD10 negativity tend to be associated with CD34 expression. After intensive induction chemotherapy according to LALA protocols, 50 of the 55 patients (91%, 95% confidence interval [CI]: 80–97%) achieved a complete remission (CR). The median disease-free survival (DFS) and the median overall survival were 26 and 36 months respectively with 2-year survival rates of 40% and 47%. Relapse was observed in 21 cases (42% of patients achieving CR). Despite better results in CD10+ cases, no statistical differences were seen between CD10+ and CD10- patients in terms of CR rates, DFS and overall survival. We conclude that this lack of statistical difference could be related to the use of adapted therapy involving cytarabine and cyclophosphamide. However, a trend for a better outcome in CD10+ patients warrants a more intensive form of therapy in patients with CD10- expression.

## Introduction

The neutral endopeptidase 24.11/CD10 antigen (initially known as cALLA), a 95 to 100 kDa glycoprotein, was identified as one of the earliest markers expressed by leukemic cells of the lymphoblastic lineage (Greaves et al. 1975). It belongs to a large family of exopeptidases expressed in a variety of tissues and mostly involved in the activation or deactivation of peptides through the removal of terminal amino acids. On leukemic cells, the CD10 could hydrolyse peptides that regulate cell proliferation (Tran-Paterson et al. 1990). CD10 expression on leukemic cells is a useful subclassification tool for B-lineage leukemias (Boucheix et al. 1994), but it can also be found on other types of leukemic cells such as T-lineage leukemic cells. Numerous studies have evaluated the prognostic significance of CD10 expression in childhood ALL (Pui et al. 1993, Vannier et al. 1989, Shuster et al. 1990, Greaves et al. 1981, Dowell et al. 1987, Gomez et al. 1991), while less studies have evaluated the clinical importance of CD10 expression in adult ALL (Boucheix et al. 1994). In general, CD10 expression has been linked to a more favourable prognosis.

Our intention in this study was to reassessed the prevalence of CD10 expression in T-lineage adult ALL and to relate its presence to initial clinical and biological features and treatment outcome.

## Patients and Methods

### Patients

Fifty-five patients (42 males and 13 females) aged more than 15 years (median age 25 years, range 16–73) with newly diagnosed T-lineage ALL, seen in our department between August 1982 and March 1998 and tested for

---

[1] Service d'Hématologie, Hôpital Edouard Herriot, Lyon, France.
[2] Laboratoire Central d'Hématologie et de Cytogénétique, Hôpital Edouard Herriot, Lyon, France.

CD10 expression, entered this study. Diagnosis of ALL was based on May-Grünwald-Giemsa (MGG) smears of the bone marrow aspirates. Leukemic cells were classified according to the French-American-British (FAB) morphological and cytochemical criteria (Bennett et al. 1976). Immunophenotyping of leukemic cells was attempted in patients to classify ALL and to define T-cell subtypes. The percentage of positive cells was calculated by counting the number of positive cells comparatively to the controls. The criteria for antigen positivity was expression of surface antigens by at least 20% of the leukemic cells as previously described (Thomas et al. 1995a). Based on the pattern of reactivity, lymphoblasts were classified as T1 (CD7+, CD5+, CD2+, CD1-, CD3-), T2 (CD7+, CD5+, CD2+, CD1+, CD3-), or T3 (CD7+, CD5+, CD2+, CD1-, CD3+) (Boucheix et al. 1994). In case of coexpression or non-adequate expression, the most differentiated marker was considered for the classification. Myeloid-antigen-positive (My+) ALL was defined as coexpression of lymphoid markers and at least two myeloid-lineage-associated antigen (CD13 / CD14 / CD15 / CD33) on $\geq$ 20% of the lymphoblasts. Cytogenetic analysis was performed in 53 patients on bone marrow or seldom on peripheral blood cells before initiation of therapy, using short unstimulated cultures and RHG banding. Karyotypes were analyzable in 48 patients and chromosomal abnormalities were classified according to the International System for Human Cytogenetic Nomenclature (ISCN 1991). 14q11 rearrangements were observed in 9 cases, 9p abnormalities in 6 cases, and 7q32-q36 rearrangements in 3 cases. In order to establish correlation between karyotypes of ALL and the expression of CD10, patients were grouped according to the presence or absence of normal metaphases (NN/AN/AA).

## Treatment

Our patients were enrolled in 6 successive therapy studies based on therapeutic schedules of LALA protocols (Fiere et al. 1987, Fiere et al. 1989, Fiere et al. 1993, Thomas et al. 1995, Dombret et al. 1998, Delannoy et al. 1997). Induction chemotherapy consisted of an anthracycline, prednisone, vincristine and cyclophosphamide combination. Marrow response status was determined by bone marrow aspirates on day 28 of induction chemotherapy. Patients who did not achieve CR in one course of chemotherapy as evaluated by the persistence of blast in day 28 bone marrow aspirate, received salvage therapy with combinations of either amsacrine and cytarabine, or anthracycline, cytarabine and asparaginase, or mitoxantrone and cytarabine, or prednisone, anthracycline, vincristine and cyclophosphamide according to the protocol design in which they were included. Patients with CR after induction or salvage were given consolidation chemotherapy. As post-induction therapy, 36 patients followed a chemotherapy program, while 10 patients underwent allogeneic bone marrow transplantation and 3 patients received autologous transplantation. One patient, although in CR, did not receive post-induction chemotherapy because of severe aspergillosis.

## Evaluation of therapy

Complete remission was defined according to the CALGB criteria as less than 5% blasts in bone marrow aspirates with evidence of maturation of cell lines and restoration of peripheral blood counts (Ellison et al. 1968). Patients failing induction therapy were categorized as failures and divided into
(i) death during induction (death occurred while the patient was receiving induction therapy), and
(ii) resistant (the patient survived induction but resistant leukemia redeveloped).

Survival was defined as time from diagnosis to death. Disease-free survival (DFS) was calculated from the first CR to the time of relapse or death from any cause. Hematological relapse was considered when more than 5% blasts were seen in two bone marrow aspirates obtained at a 15-day interval (Ellison et al. 1968).

## Statistical analysis

Expression of CD10 antigen was often given as a percent of positive cases in addition to the average percent of labeled leukemic cells per case. According to standard criteria, samples were considered positive when the percentage of stained cells exceeded that of the control by at least 20%. In the statistical analysis of correlation with other markers, CD10 antigen expression and other antigen expressions, were considered as a continuous variable, rather than arbitrarily positive or negative. The relationships between expression of CD10 and characteristics of patients were studied using non-parametric statistics based on the Kruskal-Wallis test or the Spearman rank correlation test. The 95% confidence intervals on proportions of CR patients were calculated using a binomial formula. Survival and DFS curves were estimated by the Kaplan-Meier method. For analysis of overall survival and DFS, patients receiving allogeneic or autologous bone marrow transplantation in first CR were censored at the time of transplantation. Differences were assessed for statistical significance using the log-rank test. All p values indicated are two-tailed and reported as statistically significant if $< 0.05$. Computations were performed using BMDP PC-90 statistical program (BMDP Statistical Software, Los Angeles, CA, USA).

## Results

### Expression of CD10 by T-lineage lymphoblastic leukemic cells

CD10 antigen was expressed on >20% of blast cells in 18 of the 55 cases tested (33%). None of the initial clinical and biologic features differed between CD10+ and CD10- cases, except for lower levels of WBC counts in the CD10+ cases (median 41.6 G/l versus 102.5; p $< 0.05$) (Table 1). Expression of CD10 did not correlate with FAB subtype. No statistical dif-

**Table 1.** Presenting clinical and biological features according to CD10 expression in adult with T-lineage ALL

| Feature | CD10- (n = 37) | CD10+ (n = 18) |
|---|---|---|
| Age | 28 (17 - 73)* | 24 (16 - 65) |
| Sex (male/female) | 28 / 9 | 14 / 4 |
| WHO performance status (0/1/2/3/ND) | 15/17/3/1/1 | 5/8/3/0/2 |
| Tumoral syndrome (yes/no) | 35 / 2 | 16 / 2 |
| Adenopathies (yes/no) | 33 / 4 | 15 / 3 |
| Mediastinal adenopathies (yes/no) | 12 / 25 | 6 / 12 |
| Splenomegaly (yes/no) | 17 / 20 | 9 / 9 |
| Hepatomegaly (yes/no) | 14 / 23 | 7 / 11 |
| CNS involvement (yes/no) | 1 / 36 | 1 / 17 |
| "Blastic fever" (yes/no) | 11 / 26 | 2 / 16 |
| Coagulopathy (yes/no) | 4 / 33 | 3 / 15 |
| LDH (units/l) | 1647 (207 - 18000) | 1025 (230 - 5990) |
| Hemoglobin (g/l) | 120 (53 - 176) | 94 (51 - 165) |
| WBC counts (G/l) | 102.5 (1.12 - 660) | 41.6 (0.8 - 100) |
| Platelets (G/l) | 57 (8 - 210) | 85 (13 - 250) |
| PB blast cells (%) | 82 (1 - 99) | 80 (5 - 100) |
| BM blast cells (%) | 95 (55 - 100) | 93 (22 - 98) |
| Morphology (L1,L2,undif., unclas.) | 22/10/2/3 | 9/8/0/1 |
| Karyotype (NN/AN/AA/ND) | 12/16/6/3 | 6/8/0/4 |
| CD1 (%) | 1 (0 -85) | 82 (0 -96) |
| CD3 (%) | 9 (0 - 97) | 25 (0 - 96) |
| CD4 (%) | 18 (0 - 96) | 77 (1 - 95) |
| CD8 (%) | 23 (0 - 97) | 84 (3 - 95) |
| CD11b (%) | 9 (0 - 87) | 0 (0 - 0) |
| CD15 (%) | 3 (0 - 17) | 0 (0 - 4) |
| CD21 (%) | 0 (0 - 95) | 2 (0 - 91) |
| CD34 (%) | 7 ( 0 - 97) | 0 (0 - 89) |

* median (range); ND: not determined; undif.: undifferentiated; unclas.: unclassified.

ferences in CD10 expression were found regarding T-cell immunological subtypes. There were no differences regarding karyotypic patterns. Expression of CD10 was significantly associated with that of CD1 (p = 0.0001). While it was not statistically significant, the expression of CD10 tend to be associated with that of CD4 and CD8. CD10 negativity tend to be associated with CD34 expression. No relationship was found between the expression of CD10 and those of any B-lineage and myeloid markers.

## Relationship between expression of CD10 and evolution of the disease

All patients were evaluable for response to therapy, with 50 patients entering CR (91%, 95% CI: 80–97%). 44 patients (80%) entered CR after one course chemotherapy. Two patients died during induction therapy. Nine were resistant. 6 of the 8 patients (75%) receiving salvage therapy achieved CR. The median DFS and overall survival of the entire cohort were of 26 months and 36 months respectively with 2-year survival rates of 40% and 47%. There was no statistical difference in overall survival and DFS between CD10+ and CD10- ALL cases. However, there was a trend for a better prognosis with CD10+ T-lineage ALL (Figure 1 and Figure 2). With a median follow-up of 26 months, relapse was observed in 21 cases (42% of patients achieving CR).

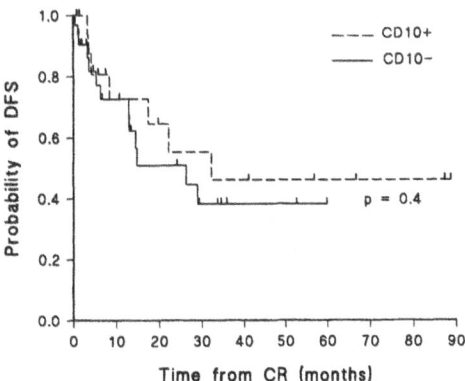

**Fig. 1.** DFS according to CD 10 expression in T-lineage ALL

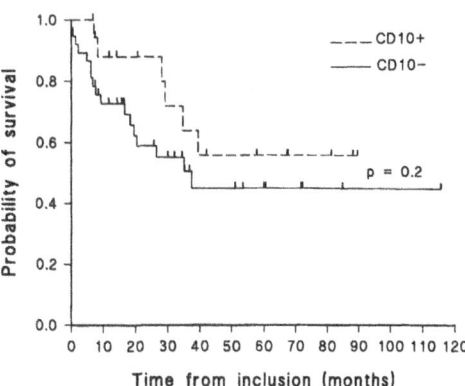

**Fig. 2.** Overall survival according to CD 10 expression in T-lineage ALL

## Discussion

Studies of the prognostic significance of CD10 expression in T-lineage ALL have yielded conflicting results. However, CD10- cases are generally recognised having a higher risk of failure than CD10+ T-lineage ALL. In our series CD10 positive expression was observed in 33% of T-cell ALL patients. This is in accordance to previous papers showing an expression of CD10 ranging from 29% to 35% of cases (Boucheix et al. 1994, Pui et al. 1990). Our study found no significant difference in the presenting clinical and biological features between CD10+ and CD10- ALL, except for WBC counts higher in CD10- cases. We did not confirm here previous reports in childhood ALL that described a relationship between CD10 negative expression and CNS involvement (Pui et al. 1993). However, our findings confirm that T-cell ALL is an heterogeneous disease. The different patterns of cell surface antigen expression by CD10+ and CD10- cases suggest biologically distinct leukemias. CD10+ cases have a higher frequency of CD1, CD4, and CD8 antigen expression (Pui et al. 1993) and are less likely to express CD34 (Thomas et al. 1995b). However, we did not find in those patients a higher expression of CD21 or a lower frequency of CD3 expression as it has been previously described (Pui et al. 1993). Despite a striking similarity between adult and childhood T-lineage ALL regarding clinical and biological characteristics of CD10+ and CD10- cases, the results of treatment of childhood T-cell ALL have been different to the treatment of what appears to be the same disease in adults. Indeed lack of CD10 expression was significantly associated with an adverse prognosis in childhood T-lineage ALL, while there were only a trend for a favourable outcome of patients with CD10+ T-lineage ALL in adults. With the introduction of more intensive chemotherapy, we observed a progressive improvement in the clinical outcome of patients with CD10- T-lineage immunophenotype. Results for adult T-lineage ALL have improved with CR rates up to 95% and DFS of up 40 to 60% (Fiere et al. 1993, Hoelzer et al. 1992). In vivo and in vitro evidence has accumulated that the inclusion in therapeutic schedules of agents such as cyclophosphamide and cytarabine are mainly responsible for this improvement (Lauer et al. 1987, Clarkson et al. 1990, Schiffer et al. 1992).

Much remains to be discovered regarding the physiological role of CD10, its functions or lack of activity on leukemic cells. The present study shows that although immunophenotypes help us in understanding the biological heterogeneity of ALL, they have also prognostic implications depending on therapy schedules. The CD10 surface marker appears to confer a better outcome than do T-cell subsets without the antigen. The prognostic influence of CD10 expression is variably diminished or lost in protocols featuring aggressive multiagent chemotherapy. In our study, the expression of CD10 on leukemic cells from T-lineage immunophenotype showed no important impact on the outcome pattern. This demonstrate the loss of adverse prognostic factor by T-lineage ALL submitted to a large program of intensive chemotherapy developed over the past decade.

# References

Bennett JM, Catovsky D, Daniel MT, Flandrin G, Galton DAG, Gralnick HR, Sultan C (1976) Proposals for the classification of acute leukaemias. Br J Haematol 33:451-458

Boucheix C, David B, Sebban C, Racadot E, Bené MC, Bernard A, Campos L, Jouault H, Sigaux F, Lepage E, Hervé P, Fiere D for the French Group on Therapy for Adult Acute Lymphoblastic Leukemia (1994) Immunophenotype of adult acute lymphoblastic leukemia, clinical parameters, and outcome: An analysis of a prospective trial including 562 tested patients (LALA87). Blood 84:1603-1612

Clarkson B, Gaynor J, Little C, Berman E, Kempin S, Andreeff M, Gulati S, Cunningham I, Gee T (1990) Importance of long-term follow-up in evaluating treatment regimens for adults with acute lymphoblastic leukemia. Haematol Blood Transfus 33:397-408

Delannoy A, Sebban C, Cony-Makhoul P, Cazin B, Cordonnier C, Bouabdallah R, Cahn JY, Dreyfus F, Sadoun A, Vernant JP, Gay C, Broustet A, Michaux JL, Fiere D (1997) Age-adapted induction treatment of acute lymphoblastic leukemia in the elderly and assessment of maintenance with interferon combined with chemotherapy. A multicentric prospective study in forty patients. Leukemia 11:1429-1434

Dombret H, Thomas X, Blaise D, Huguet F, Boiron JM, Buzyn A, Stamatoulas A, Delannoy A, Bradstock K, Boucheix C, Charrin C, Gabert J, Lebbé G, Lhéritier V, Fiere D, for the LALA Group (1998) Intensive therapy in 100 patients with Ph1 and/or BCR-ABL positive acute lymphoblastic leukemia (ALL): First interim analysis of the French-Belgian-Australian LALA-94 trial. Br J Haematol 102:270

Dowell BL, Borowitz MJ, Boyett JM, Pullen DJ, Crist WM, Quddus FF, Russell EC, Falletta JM, Metzgar RS (1987) Immunologic and clinicopathologic features of common acute lymphoblastic leukemia antigen-positive childhood T-cell leukemia: A Pediatric Oncology Group Study. Cancer 59:2020-2026

Ellison RR, Holland JF, Weil M, Jacquillat C, Boiron M, Bernard J, Sawitsky A, Rosner F, Gussoff B, Silver RT, Karanas A, Cuttner J, Spurr CL, Hayes DM, Blom J, Leone LA, Haurani F, Kyle R, Hutchison JL, Forcier RJ, Moon JH (1968) Arabinosyl cytosine: a useful agent in the treatment of acute leukemia in adults. Blood 32:507-523

Fiere D, Archimbaud E, Extra JM, Marty M, David B, Witz F, Sotto JJ, Rochant H, Gastaut JA, LePrise PY (1987) Treatment of adult acute lymphoblastic leukemia. Preliminary results of a trial from the French Group. In: Büchner T, et al. (eds) Acute leukemias. Prognostic factors and treatment strategies. Springer-Verlag, Berlin Heidelberg New York, pp 125-129

Fiere D, Brouset A, Leblond V, et al. (1989) Comparison of chemotherapy and autologous and allogeneic transplantation as postinduction regimen in adult acute lymphoblastic leukemia: a preliminary multicentric study. In: Büchner T, et al. (eds) Acute leukemias II. Prognostic factors and treatment strategies. Springer-Verlag, Berlin Heidelberg New York, pp 409-412

Fiere D, Lepage E, Sebban C, Boucheix C, Gisselbrecht C, Vernant JP, Varet B, Broustet A, Cahn JY, Rigal-Huguet F, Witz F, Michaux JL, Michallet M, Reiffers J, for the French Group on Therapy for Adult Acute Lymphoblastic Leukemia (1993) Adult acute lymphoblastic leukemia: a multicentric randomized trial testing bone marrow transplantation as postremission therapy. J Clin Oncol 11:1990-2001

Gomez E, San Miguel JF, Orfao A, Canizo MC, Moraleda JM, Lopez Borrasca A (1991) The value of the immunological subtypes and individual markers compared to classical parameters in the prognosis of acute lymphoblastic leukemia. Hematol Oncol 9:33-42

Greaves MF, Brown C, Rapson NT, Lister TA (1975) Antisera to acute lymphoblastic leukemia cells. Clin Immunol Immunopathol 4:67-84

Greaves MF, Janossy G, Peto J, Kay H (1981) Immunologically defined subclasses of acute lymphoblastic leukemia in children: their relationship to presentation features and prognosis. Br J Haematol 48:179-197

Hoelzer D, Thiel E, Ludwig WD, Löffler H, Büchner T, Freund M, Heil G, Hiddemann W, Maschmeyer G, Volkers B, Aydemir U, for the German Adult ALL Study Group (1992) The German multicentre trials for treatment of acute lymphoblastic leukemia in adults. Leukemia 6:175-177

ISCN (International System for Human Cytogenetic Nomenclature) (1991) Guidelines for Cancer Cytogenetics. In: Mitelman F (ed) Supplement to an International System for Human Cytogenetic Nomenclature. Karger, Basel, pp 1-53

Lauer SJ, Pinkel D, Buchanan GR, Sartain P, Cornet JM, Krance R, Borella LD, Casper JT, Kun LE, Hoffman RG, Camitta BM (1987) Cytosine arabinosine/cyclophosphamide pulses during continuation therapy for childhood acute lymphoblastic leukemia. Cancer 60:2366-2371

Pui CH, Behm FG, Singh B, Schell MJ, Williams DL, Rivera GK, Kalwinsky DK, Sandlund JT, Crist WM, Raimondi SC (1990) Heterogeneity of presenting features and their relation to treatment outcome in 120 children with T-cell acute lymphoblastic leukemia. Blood 75:174-179

Pui CH, Rivera GK, Hancock ML, Raimondi SC, Sandlund JT, Mahmoud HH, Ribeiro RC, Furman WL,

Hurwitz CA, Crist WM, Behm FG (1993) Clinical significance of CD10 expression in childhood acute lymphoblastic leukemia. Leukemia 7:35-40

Schiffer CA, Larson RA, Bloomfield CD (1992) Cancer and Leukemia Group B (CALGB) studies in adult acute lymphocytic leukemia. Leukemia 6(suppl.2): 171-174

Shuster JJ, Falletta JM, Pullen DJ, Crist WM, Humphrey GB, Dowell BL, Wharam MD, Borowitz M (1990) Prognostic factors in childhood T-cell acute lymphoblastic leukemia: a Pediatric Oncology Group Study. Blood 75:166-173

Thomas X, Archimbaud E, Charrin C, Magaud JP, Fiere D (1995a) CD34 expression is associated with major adverse prognostic factors in adult acute lymphoblastic leukemia. Leukemia 9:249-253

Thomas X, Danaïla C, Bach QK, Dufour P, Christian B, Corront B, Bosly A, Bastion Y, Gratecos N, Leblay R, Sebban C, Archimbaud E, Fiere D (1995b) Sequential induction chemotherapy with vincristine, daunorubicin, cyclophosphamide, and prednisone in adult acute lymphoblastic leukemia. Ann Hematol 70:65-69

Tran-Paterson R, Boileau G, Giguère V, Letarte M (1990) Comparative levels of CALLA/neutral endopeptidase of normal granulocytes, leukemic cells, and transfected COS-1 cells. Blood 76:775-782

Vannier JP, Bené MC, Faure GC, Bastard C, Garand R, Bernard A (1989) Investigation of the CD10 (cALLA) negative acute lymphoblastic leukaemia: further description of a group with a poor prognosis. Br J Haematol 72:156-160

# Acute Lymphoblastic Leukemia in Childhood with an Unusual Immunophenotype (CD7 +/CD56 +/CD33 +)

U. Ebener, S. Wehner, E. Niegemann and B. Kornhuber

*Abstract.* We have identified and characterized an unusual and unrecognized type of acute leukemia with features of T-lymphoid, myeloid and natural killer cell (NK) associated markers in a five year old girl with morphologically and cytochemically undifferentiated acute leukemic blast cells.

The bone marrow and peripheral blood smears showed ALL FAB-L1/2 morphology with immunological features of CD7 +, CD33 +, CD56 + myeloid/natural killer cell precursor type. The marker analysis exhibited the coexpression pattern of cyCD3, CD34, CD38, CD45, CD54, CD71 and HLA-DR antigens just as the neutrophil marker CD11b. In 50% of the blast cells cytoplasmic CD3 was detectable but on the other hand this leukemic entity failed to express other NK associated antigens (e.g. CD16/CD57) additionally no other expressions of T- and B-cell lineage associated markers could be observed. The blasts expressing the stem cell marker CD34 failed to express AC133 and CD117.

This unusual phenotype seems to be very similar to the recently by Scott et al. [24] and by Suzuki et al. [20] proposed »myeloid/NK cell precursor acute leukemia« entity in adults. In comparison to our case the Scott's type was characterized by mature myeloid morphology with MPO reactivity but without information about the expression of CD7. Their cases were described to be exclusively negative for HLA-DR. The phenotype of our case seems to be more identical to the recently reported entity by Suzuki et al. (1997), with exception of MPO expression and missing cyCD3 positivity in their cases of adults. CD7 is a T-cell marker which is expressed in immature NK cell progenitors and was a feature of the myeloid/NK cell precursor acute leukemia in our and Suzukius' cases.

## Introduction

Acute leukemias are traditionally classified according to their morphological and cytochemical features. However, some acute leukemia cases lack characteristic that are currently important to be diagnostic parameters for ALL or AML within the morphological French-American-British (FAB)-classification system [1–4]. Diagnostic importance has increased with the development and usage of immunological techniques. Since the recent availability of highly specific monoclonal antibodies (MoAbs) recognizing differentiation antigens (CD cluster code) the diagnostic precision for leukemic cells and various tumor cell types has increased. The application of morphology, cytochemistry and immunological methods in combination with selective antibodies makes it possible to subclassify of leukemic blast cells.

Flow cytometry has become the preferred technique for the lineage assignment (T- and B-lineage ALL) and maturational analysis of malignant cells in acute leukemias and lymphomas. Furthermore, the multiparametric immunophenotyping allows the detection of aberrant antigen coexpressions (i.e. ALL coexpression of myeloid antigens: My +-ALL, or AML with coexpression of lymphoid markers: Ly +-AL) [5–8].

J. W. Goethe-University, Clinic of Pediatrics-III, Department of Hematology and Oncology, Theodor-Stern-Kai 7, 60590 Frankfurt/Main, Germany

Despite these advances, the lineage of the leukemic blasts may still remain uncertain in a minority of acute leukemia (AL) cases. This is due to the lack membraneous expression of some lymphoid and myeloid antigens or to the expression of an atypically marker constellation on the same cells.

In the last few years, it has become apparent that at least a proportion of the unclassifiable AL (AUL) cases can be meticulously classified by analysing cytoplasmic expressions of early T, B and myeloid antigens such as CD3, CD22, CD13, MPO as well as nuclear TdT [6, 9–13].

The »European Group for the Immunological Characterization of Leukemias« (EGIL) recognised a rare subtyp of acute leukemias in which the leukemic blast cells do not express lineage specific markers [14]. At the present time, the nature of this rare entity can not be clarified by immunophenotyping.

Here we report a child case of acute leukemia fitting into neither of standardized categories. We describe the immunological findings in an acute lymphoblastic leukemia with the immunophenotype of a putative precursor cell common to the T-/NK and myeloid cell.

## Case report

A 5 1/2 year old girl was admitted to our clinic of pediatrics-III in november 1997, in order to clarify the diagnosis hematological malignancy.

Examination of peripheral blood (PB) displayed 4,70 g/dl hemoglobin, a platelet count of 59 x 10 $^3$/µl and leukocyte count about 11.100/µl. PB-white blood cells could be subdevided to neutrophils (21%), lymphocytes (34%), monocytes (1%) and pathological blast cells (42%). Bone marrow (BM) smears disclosed leukemic blast cell population of nearly 100%. The blasts consisted of two different morphological features fulfilling criteria of FAB-ALL-L1/L2.

The major population reflects mainly lymphoblastic morphology (66%), while the remaining 34% showed rather undifferentiated myeloblastic signs but lacking of azurophilic granules.

Cytochemical staining of leukemic blasts in bone marrow did usually not reveal POX or PAS reactivity, consistent with an acute undifferentiated leukemia. All of the pathological blast cells were negative for tested Esterase, too. Acid phosphatase was demonstrated to be negative as well in most cells; only a few blasts were diffuse positive, some seemed to be positive in a polar manner. Immunological profile is reported below. DNA-index of blast cell population was shown to be diploid.

To the child a chemotherapeutic regimen according to the ALL-protocol (ALL-BFM-95) was administered. On day 8 following starting with therapy, PB demonstrated remaining 25% pathological blast cells. No peripheral blast cells were detectable on day 15. At this time bone marrow aspirates showed participation of still 83% blast cells. Remission was achieved on day 28. Till now the reported child is shown to be in complete remission.

## Materials and Methods

Bone marrow (BM) aspirates were obtained from a five year old girl with de novo acute leukemia. BM smears were staind with panoptical May-Gruenwald-Giema dyes according to Pappenheim, cytochemistry stainings (i.e. Peroxidase, alpha-naphthyl butyrate esterase, and periodic acid Schiff_s reagents, acid phosphatase) respectively to standard procedures.

Morphological diagnosis was made according to the FAB classification system [1 –4]. Immunological characterization of leukemic blast cells in terms to their lineage commitment and differentiation stage was done by multiparametric flow cytometry [8, 12].

### Flow Cytometry (FACS)

FACS analysis was carried out in a standard manner applying whole lysed blood procedure [8, 12]. A large panel of monoclonal antibodies as listed in Table 1 was used. Detailed information is given in Table 1 as well.

The expression of antigens on blast cells was assessed by direct immunofluorescence using appropriate double and triple staining combinations with the following flurochromes; fluorescein isothiocyanate (FITC), phy-

**Table 1.** Antigenic Pattern of Monoclonal Antibodies used in the present study

| | **T-Lineage** | | **My-Lineage** |
|---|---|---|---|
| CD1a | cortical thymocytes | CD13 | monocytes, granulocytes |
| CD2 | T cells, NK cells | CD14 | monocytes |
| CD3 | mature T cells | CD15 | granulocytes, monocytes |
| CD4 | helper/inducer T cells, monocytes, macrophages | CD33 | myeloid progenitor cells, monocytes |
| CD5 | T cells, B cell subset | MPO | myeloperoxidase |
| CD7 | T cells | glycophorin A | erythroblasts, erythrocytes |
| CD8 | cytotoxic/suppressor T cells, NK cells | CD41 a, b | platelets, megakaryocytes |
| TCR $\alpha/\beta$ | alpha/beta chain of T cell receptor | CD61 | platelets, megakaryocytes |
| TCR $\gamma/\delta$ | gamma/delta chain of T cell receptor | CD64 | monocytes |
| | | CD65 | neutrophils |
| | **B-Lineage** | | **Non-Lineage specific** |
| CD10 | (CALLA), pre B cells, granulocytes | CD11b | granulocytes, monocytes, NK cells |
| CD19 | B cells | CD34 | hematopoietic progenitor cells |
| CD20 | B cells | CD38 | activated T cells, plasma cells |
| CD22 | B cells | CD45 | leukocytes |
| CD24 | B cells; granulocytes | HLA-DR | B cells, activated T cells |
| CD79a | B cells | CD71 | proliferating cells |
| | | TdT | terminale deoxinucleotidyl transferase |
| | | CD117 | progenitor cells |
| | **NK-associated** | | |
| CD16 | NK cells, macrophages, granulocytes | | |
| CD56 | NK cells | | |
| CD57 | NK cells, T cell subsets | | |

CD Cluster of Differentiation

coerythrin (PE) and either PerCP or PE-Cyanin5. The fluorescence signal was evaluated on FACScan flow cytometer (Becton Dickinson, Heidelberg, Germany), equipped with an argon ion laser. For data acquisition and following analysis of list mode files Cell Quest software (Becton Dickinson, Heidelberg, Germany) was used. Calibration of the instrument was done using fluorescence coated beads. As a negative control, cells were stained with fluorescence labeled isotype specific control antibodies.

## Immunocytochemistry

Smears of mononucleated leukemic blast cells were prepared and stored in a refrigerator at –20°C as described previously [15]. Retrospectively we analysed these preparations of leukemic blasts performing alkaline phosphatase anti-alkaline phosphatase (APAPP)-complex technique (DAKO, Hamburg, Germany) with new monoclonal antibodies AC133-1/-2 (Miltenyi Biotec, Bergisch Gladbach, Ger-

many) raised against AC133, a novel hematopoietic stem cell antigen [16, 17].

## Results

### Flow cytometric immunophenotyping

The clinical feature and outlined hematological profile of the young girl is demonstrated as followed. The leukemic blast cells showed immature morphologic appearance with FAB-ALL-L1/-L2 criteria without MPO reactivity but with the phenotype of a CD56 + natural killer cell [18]. As summarized in Table 2, the unique antigen profile of the analysed blast cells showed coexpression of CD7, cyCD3, CD33, CD34, CD38, CD45, CD56, CD71, HLA-DR and partial expression of sCD3 and CD2.

Immunophenotyping of bone marrow (BM) was negative for the B-cell lineage markers CD10, CD19, CD20, CD22 and mature T-cell markers CD3, CD4, CD8. The NCAM antigen CD56 was strongly positive but no other

**Table 2.** Results of Multiparametric FACS-Analysis

| T-Lineage | B-Lineage | My-Lineage | NK-associated | non-Lineage |
|---|---|---|---|---|
| | | **positive marker expression** | | |
| | | | | CD11b $^+$ |
| | | | | CD34 $^+$ |
| CD3cy $^+$ | | | | CD38 $^+$ |
| CD7 $^+$ | CD33 $^1$ | CD56 $^+$ | | CD45 $^+$ |
| | | | | HLA-DR $^+$ |
| | | | | CD71 $^+$ |
| | | **partial marker expression** | | |
| CD3s ( $^+$ ) | CD79a ( $^+$ ) | CD13 ( $^+$ ) | | |
| | | **antigens not expressed** | | |
| | | CD14 – | | |
| | | CD15 – | | |
| CD1a – | CD19 – | MPO – | | |
| CD4s –, CD4cy – | CD20 – | Glyc A – | CD16 – | CD117 – |
| CD8s –, CD8cy – | CD22 – | CD31a, b – | CD57 – | AC133 – |
| TCR α/β | CD10 – | CD61 – | | |
| TCR γ/δ | | CD64 – | | |
| | | CD65 – | | |

CD Cluster of Differentiation

NK-associated cell markers (CD16/CD57) exhibited positive reaction nor partial coexpression. The CD56 positive blasts displayed coexpression of CD34, CD33, HLA-DR, CD7 and cyCD3 with low partial expression of CD79a and CD13. The marker profile of the presented case does not fulfill existing criteria for classification of acute leukemia [14], we therefore provisional included it to the group of unclassified acute leukemia (AUL) [11, 19].

Retrospective analysis with the moAb AC133 applying the APAAP-technique [15] to the CD34-positive blasts showed no positive staining results.

The entire results of multimarker flow cytometric analysis are given in Table 2 and presented in Figure 1.

## Discussion

In the present study we have described a case of acute lymphoblastic leukemia in childhood with an unusual phenotype which seems to be very similar to recently by Suzuki et al. (1997) proposed »Myeloid/NK cell precursor acute leukemia« entity in adults [20]. Our immunological results revealed a unique phenotype: it was positive for CD7, cytoplasmic CD3, NK cell antigen CD56, myeloid antigen CD33 and a low percentage of the B cell antigen CD79a. Being positive for CD56, an isoform of the neural cell adhesion molecule (NCAM), pathological blast cells seem to distinguish the NK cells from T cells [21 –23].

Natural killer (NK) cells differentiate from immature thymocytes under appropriate conditions in vitro and in vivo, and share some surface antigens with T cells, indicating a close relationship with T-lineage. NK and T cells are developmentally related and probably share a common progenitor cell [18].

Recently, it is reported that NK cells are developed from a cell population expressing CD34 $^+$-, CD33 $^+$-antigens but still lacking CD56-antigen [22]. Suzuki et al. described seven cases of acute leukemias characterized by the antigen expression of CD7 $^+$ and CD56 $^+$ myeloid/NK cell precursor acute leukemia as a distinct hematolymphoid disease entity. The leukemic cells showed immature morphologic appearance without MPO reactivity but coexpression of CD34, CD33 and frequently HLA-DR [20]. Scott et al. [24] reported an acute leukemia with NK cell mediated cytotoxicity, with CD33 $^+$, CD56 $^+$, HLA-DR phenotype and cytochemically positive staining for MPO but without investigation of the T cell antigen CD 7.

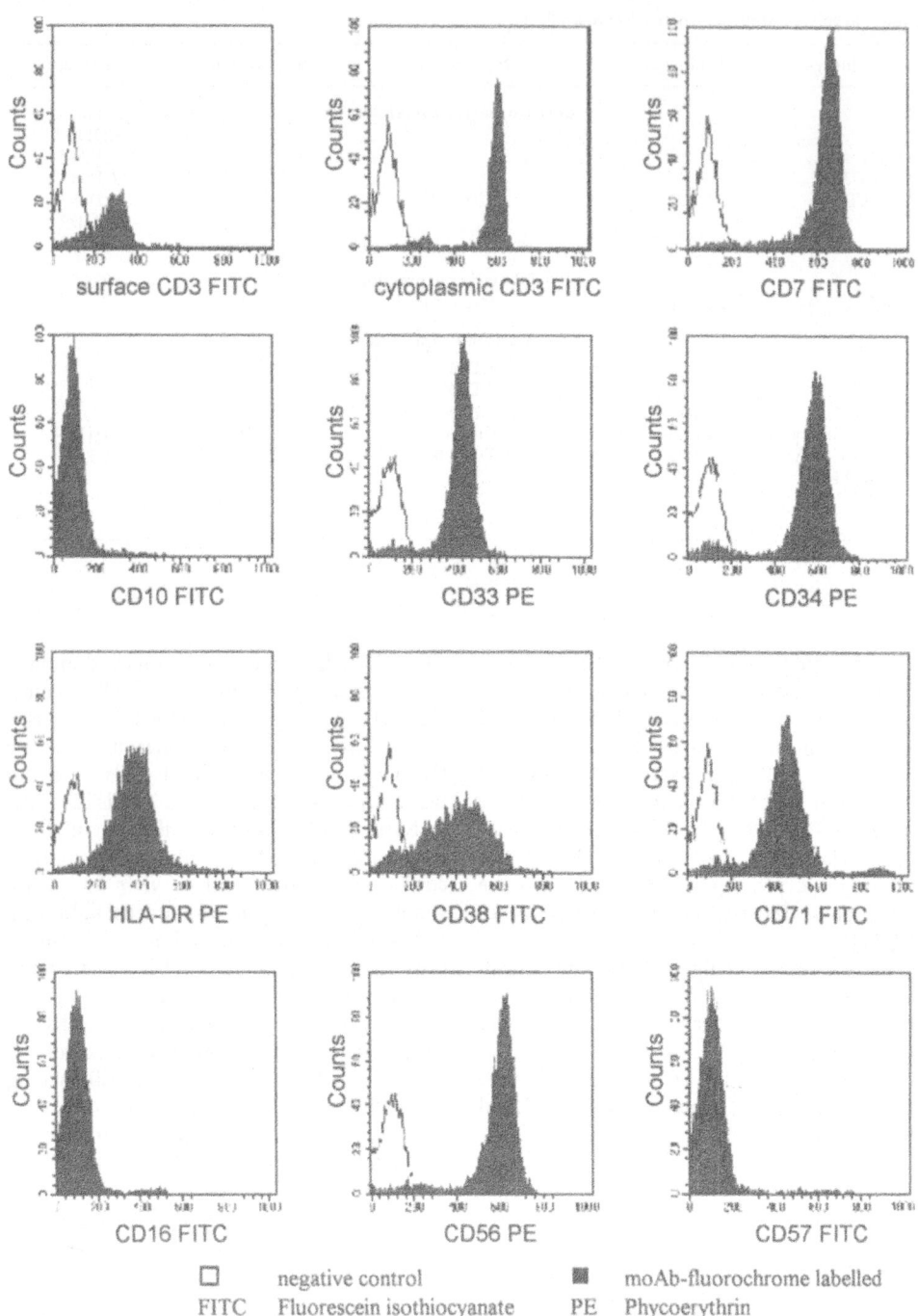

**Fig. 1.** Immunophenotype of Patients' Leukemic Blast Cells (FACS-Analysis)

CD7, an antigen, also expressed in immature NK cell progenitors [21 –23] was a common immunological feature of the myeloid/NK cell precursor acute leukemia in our and Suzuki's CD7 is a 40 kD glycoprotein found on mature T- and NK-cells. The function of this molecule is unknown, although it has been postulated to play a role in adhesion and cell activation [25, 26]. CD34 +/CD7 + immature precursors have been identified on both, acute lymphoblastic and acute myeloid leukemias [27]. It is demonstrated that the small CD34 +/CD7 + population may be an uncomitted progenitor, still capable of myeloid differentiation to granulocytes after long-term culture [28]. Miller et al. [28] hypothesized that a CD34 +/CD7+ progenitor may also be a direct intermediate in NK cell differentiation.

Most of the patients with similar phenotypic under tumor cells (CD56 +) as described in literature reported about an aggressive clinical course [20, 29 –33]. In comparison to this young girl, described in the recent study, was treated with chemotherapy according to ALL-BFM-95 protocol and has achieved a complete remission till now.

As comprehensive cytometric multimarker analysis is employed and additional similar cases are recognized, characterized and evaluated, this kind of entity will be better understood and defined.

*Acknowlegdement.* This work was supported by »Hilfe für Krebskranke Kinder Frankfurt e.V.«

# References

1. Bennett JM, Catovsky D, Daniel MT, Flandrin G, Galton DA, Gralnick HR, Sultan C (1976) Proposals for the classification of the acute leukemias. French-American-British (FAB) co-operative group. Br J Haematol 33 (4): 451 –458
2. Bennett JM, Catovsky D, Daniel MT, Flandrin G, Galton DA, Gralnick HR, Sultan C (1985) Proposed revised criteria for the classification of acute myeloid leukemia. A report of the French-American-British Cooperative Group. Ann Int Med 103 (4): 620 –625
3. Bennett JM, Catovsky D, Daniel MT, Flandrin G, Galton DA, Gralnick HR, Sultan C (1985) Criteria for the diagnosis of acute leukemia of megakaryocyte lineage (M7). A report of a the French-American-British Cooperative Group. Ann Int Med 103 (3): 460 –461
4. Bennett JM, Catovsky D, Daniel MT, Flandrin G, Galton GA, Gralnick HR, Sultan C (1991) Proposal for the recognition of minimally differentiated acute myeloid leukemia (AML-M0). Br J Haematol 78 (3): 325 –329
5. Catovsky D, Matutes E (1992) The classification of acute leukemia. Leukemia 6 (Suppl 2): 1 –6
6. Knapp W, Strobl H, Majdic O (1994) Flow cytometric analysis of cell-surface and intracellular antigens in leukemia diagnosis. Cytometry 18 (4): 187 –194
7. Matutes E, Buccheri V, Morilla R, Shetty V, Dyer M, Catovsky D (1993) II. Phenotypic heterogeneity in acute leukemias: Immunological characterization and clinical relevance. Immunological, ultrastructural and molecular features of unclassifiable acute leukemia. Recent Results in Cancer Research 131: 41 –52
8. Rothe G, Schmitz G, Adorf D, Barlage S, Gramatki M, Hanenberg H, Höffkes HG, Janossy G, Knüchel R, Ludwig WD, Nebe T, Nerl C, Orfao A, Serke S, Sonnen R, Tichelli A, Wörmann B (1996) Consensus protocol for the flow cytometric immunophenotyping of hematopoietic malignancies. Leukemia 10 (5): 877 –895
9. Drexler HG, Thiel E, Ludwig WD (1991) Review of the Incidence and Clinical Relevance of Myeloid Antigen-positive Acute Lymphoblastic Leukemia. Leukemia, 5 (8): 637 –645
10. Meckenstock G, Heyll A, Schneider EM, Hildebrandt B, Runde V, Aul C, Bartram CR, Ludwig WD, Schneider W (1995) Acute leukemia coexpressing myeloid, B- and T-lineage associated markers: Multiparameter analysis of criteria defining lineage commitment and maturational stage in a case of undifferentiated leukemia. Leukemia 9 (2): 260 –264
11. Bernier M, Massy M. Deleeuw N, Bron D, Debuscher L, Stryckmans P (1995) Immunological definition of acute minimally differentiated myeloid leukemia (MO) and acute undifferentiated leukemia (AUL). Leukemia & Lymphoma, 18 Suppl 1, 13 –17
12. Bassan R, Biondi A, Benvestito S, Tini ML, Abbate M, Viero P, Barbui T, Rambaldi A (1992) Acute undifferentiated leukemia with CD7 + and CD13 + immunophenotype. Lack of molecular lineage commitment and association with poor prognostic features. Cancer 69 (2): 396 –404
13. van_t Veer MB (1992) The diagnosis of acute leukemia with undifferentiated or minimally differentiated blasts. Ann Hematol 64 (4): 161 –165
14. Bene MC, Castoldi G, Knapp W, Ludwig WD, Matutes E, Orfao A, van't Veer MB (1995) Proposal for the immunological classification of acute leukemias. European Group for the Immunological Characterization of Leukemias (EGIL): Leukemia 9 (10): 1783 –1786
15. Ebener U, Hauser S, Wehner S, Kornhuber B (1989) Retrospective marker analyses performed with blood and bone marrow smears using an immunoenzyme procedure (alkaline phosphatase-antialkaline phosphatase technic). Klinische Pädiatrie 201 (4). 242 –246
16. Yin AH, Miraglia S, Zanjani ED, Almeida-Porada G, Ogawa M, Leary AG, Olweus J, Kearney J, Buck DW (1997) AC133, a novel marker for human

hematopoietic stem and progenitor cells. Blood 90 (12): 5002 –5012

17. Miraglia S, Godfrey W, Yin AH, Atkins K, Warnke R, Holden JT, Bray RA, Waller EK, Buck D (1997) A novel 5-transmembrane hematopoietic stem cell antigen: Isolation, Characterization, and molecular cloning. Blood 90 (12): 5013 –5021

18. Lanier LL, Testi R, Bindl J, Phillips JH (1989) Identity of Leu-19 (CD56) leukocyte differentiation antigen and neural cell adhesion molecule. J Exp Med 169 (6): 2233 –2238

19. Reuss-Borst MA, Jaschonek K, Muller CA (1996) Acute undifferentiated leukemia with an unusual CD7 $^+$, CD56 $^+$, CD33 $^+$ immunophenotype of NK progenitors (letter). Leukemia 10 (5): 923 –924

20. Suzuki R, Yamamoto K, Seto M, Kagami Y, Ogura M, Yatabe Y, Suchi T, Kodera Y, Morishima Y, Takahashi T, Saito H, Ueda R, Nakamura S (1997) CD7 $^+$ and CD56 $^+$ myeloid/natural killer cell precursor acute leukemia: A distinct hematolymphoid disease entity. Blood 90 (6): 2417 –2428

21. Kaplan J, Ravindranath Y, Inoue S (1986) T-cell acute lymphoblastic leukemia with natural killer cell phenotype. Am J Hematol 22 (4): 355 –364

22. Sanchez MJ, Muench MO; Roncarolo MG, Lanier LL, Phillips JH (1994) Identification of a common T/natural killer cell progenitor in human fetal thymus. J Exp Med 180 (2): 569 –576

23. Jaffe ES (1996) Classification of Natural Killer (NK) Cell and NK-Like T-Cell Malignancies. Blood 87 (4): 1207 –1210

24. Scott AA, Head DR, Kopecky KJ, Appelbaum FR, Theil KS, Grever MR, Chen IM, Whittaker MH, Griffith BB, Licht JD, Waxman S, Whalen MM, Bankhurst AD, Richter LC, Grogan TM, Willman CL (1994) HLA-DR⁻, CD33⁺, CD56⁺, CD16⁻ myeloid/natural killer cell acute leukemia: a previously unrecognized form of acute leukemia potentially misdiagnosed as French-American-British acute myeloid leukemia-M3. Blood 84 (1): 244 –255

25. Terstappen LW, Huang S, Picker LJ (1992) Flow cytometric assessment of human T-cell differentiation in thymus and bone marrow. Blood 79 (3): 666 –677

26. Miller JS, Alley KA, McGlave P (1994) Differentiation of natural killer (NK) cells from human primitive marrow progenitors in a stroma-based long-term culture system: identification of a CD34⁺ 7⁺ NK progenitor. Blood 83 (9): 2594 –2601

27. Kondo S, Okamura S, Harada N, Ikematsu W, Kawasaki C, Fukuda T, Kubota A, Shimoda K, Harada M, Shibuya T (1992) CD7-positive acute myeloid leukemia: further evidence of cellular immaturity. J Cancer Res Clin Oncol 118 (5): 386 –388

28. Chabannon C, Wood P, Torok-Storb B (1992) Expression of CD7 on normal human myeloid progenitors. J Immunol 149 (6): 2110 –2113

29. Fernandez LA, Pope B, Lee C, Zayed E (1986) Aggressive natural killer cell leukemia in an adult with establishment of a NK cell line. Blood 67 (4): 925 –930

30. Gentile TC, Uner AH, Hutchinson RE, Wright J, Ben-Ezra J, Russell EC, Loughran TP Jr. (1994) CD3⁺, CD56⁺ Aggressive Variant of Large Granular Lymphocyte Leukemia. Blood 847 (7): 2315 –2321

31. Imamura N, Kusunoki Y, Kajihara H, Okada K, Kuramoto A (1988) Aggressive natural killer cell leukemia/lymphoma with N901-positive surface phenotype: evidence for the existence of a third lineage in lymphoid cells. Acta Haematologica 80 (3): 121 –128

32. Kern WF, Spier CM, Miller TP, Grogan TM (1993) NCAM (CD56)-positive malignant lymphoma. Leuk Lymphoma 12: 1

33. Dunphy CH, Gregowicz AJ, Rodriguez G Jr. (1995) Natural killer cell acute leukemia with myeloid antigen expression. A previously undescribed form of acute leukemia. American Journal of Clinical Pathology 104 (2): 212 –215

# Expression of IGFBP-rP2 / CTGF is Specific for Malignant Lymphoblasts of Children with Acute Lymphoblastic Leucemia (ALL)

P. Vorwerk[1], J. Elsner[1], K. Mohnike[1], Y. Oh[2], R.G. Rosenfeld[2] and U. Mittler[1]

## Introduction

The role of insulin-like growth factors (IGF) and their specific binding proteins (IGFBP) has been shown to be an integral part of the growth promotion in a number of neoplasms. IGFBPs are a family of homologues proteins that regulate the biological activities of the IGFs, and may also be capable of IGF-independent actions [1,2]. Proceeding from our previous reports on expression of IGFs and IGFBPs in human leucemic lymphoblasts, we studied the gene expression of IGFBP-rP2/CTGF (connective tissue growth factor) in acute lymphoblastic leucemia [3, 4].

CTGF has been identified as a major chemotactic and mitogenic factor for connective tissue cells. It has platelet-derived growth factor (PDGF)-related biological and immunological activities [5]. The amino acid sequence shares an overall 28-38% identity to IGFBPs and contains critical conserved sequences including the common IGFBP motif. It could be demonstrated that human CTGF binds specifically IGFs with a low affinity [6]. IGFBP-rP2/CTGF is considered to be a new member of the IGFBP superfamily that regulates cell growth through both IGF-dependent and IGF-independent actions [6]. The CTGF gene encodes a 38-kDa prepeptide containing 349 amino acids [5]. Northern blot analysis of various normal human tissues showed expression of CTGF mRNA at high levels in spleen, ovary, gastrointestinal tract, prostate, heart, and testis. No expression was found in peripheral blood leukocytes, liver and brain [6].

## Material and Methods

### Patient samples

Blood or bone marrow samples from 107 patients (age 1.22-21.93 years, median 6.0 years) with childhood acute lymphoblastic leucemia (ALL) at time of diagnosis (B-precursor ALL, n=15; B-ALL, n=2; T-ALL, n=22; c-ALL, n= 66; not classified, n=2) were obtained. None of the ALL-patients received any drugs before the first blood or bone marrow sample was drawn. From 43 of these patients (B-precursor ALL, n=6; B-ALL, n=2; T-ALL, n=8; c-ALL, n= 26; not classified, n=1) samples were also obtained at day 33 after the onset of chemotherapy according the ALL-BFM 90/95 protocol of the German Society of Pediatric Oncology and Hematology [7]. All 43 patients were in full hematological remission at day 33. In addition blood or bone marrow samples from 57 patients (age 6.37- 83.98 years, median 47.85 years) with chronic myeloid leucemia (CML), 120 blood samples from 47 children (age 1.85-15.8 years, median 10.95) with insulin dependent diabetes mellitus (IDDM) at various time points and 200 cord blood samples from healthy newborns were investigated.

For separation of lymphoid progenitor cells 10 ml blood from a patient with Ewing's sarcoma before chemotherapy were used.

### Separation of mononuclear cells (MNC)

MNC were separated using gradient centrifugation with Ficoll-Paque (Pharmacia) at 400 xg.

---

[1] Otto-von-Guericke-University Magdeburg/Germany, Department Pediatric Hematology and Oncology
[2] Oregon Health Sciences University, Portland, OR (USA), Department Pediatrics

At the time of diagnosis, the tumor clones generally represented 50-90% of MNC fraction.

## Separation of CD34+/CD38+ lymphoid stem cells

CD34+ /CD38+ progenitor cells were stained from blood and separated by standard methods using a FACScalibur with FACSort equipment (Becton Dickinson). Approx. 60.000 cells were separated and used for extraction of RNA.

## RNA isolation and cDNA synthesis

Total RNA was extracted using TRIzol reagent (Gibco BRL) following the manufacturers protocol. The RNA was stored at -80°C until use. 2μg of total RNA were reverse transcribed into 40μl cDNA by AMV reverse transcriptase (Reverse Transcription System, Bioproducts) as recommended by the manufacturer.

## Enzymatic amplification of cDNA

A 2μl aliquot of the cDNA reaction mixture was directly used for enzymatic amplification, which was performed in 50μl of reaction buffer containing 1x reaction buffer mixture (Prime Zyme, Biometra), 1 unit of *Taq*-polymerase (Biometra) and 0.2 pmol of gene specific primers in a Hybaid Gene Thermocycler (Hybaid). Initial denaturation at 95°C for 5 min was followed by 35 cycles with denaturation at 95°C for 1 min, annealing at 62°C for 1 min and elongation at 72°C for 0.5 min. The final elongation step was extended to 15 min. One-fifth of the reaction mix was loaded onto a 1,75% agarose gel, separated by electrophoresis at 5 V cm$^{-1}$ in TAE buffer and stained with ethidium bromide. The b-actin amplification as a control was carried out using the same protocol (figures 1,2) [3, 4].

IGFBP-RP2/CTGF forward primer: *CAA CTG CCT GGT CCA GAC C*
corresponding to nucleotide number 371-389 IGFBP-RP2/CTGF reverse primer: *CAC TCT CTG GCT TCA TGC C*

corresponding to nucleotide number 842-824 of the human CTGF-mRNA, GenBank accession number U14750 [5]; the resulting PCR product is 471 bp long.

β-actin forward primer: TCA AAC ATG ATC TGG GTC AT
β-actin reverse primer: CCC AGG CAC CAG GGC GTG AT
The resulting amplification product is 260 bp long [4].

## Results

62.6% of the patients with ALL (67 out of 107) were positive for IGFBP-rP2/CTGF expression at diagnosis. In the group of CML patients only 3.5% (2 out of 57) were positive for IGFBP-rP2/CTGF expression and no IGFBP-rP2/CTGF expression was detected in neither diabetics nor cord blood samples.

From 43 patients with ALL we were able to investigate a second MNC sample from day 33 of chemotherapy. On this day all 43 patients had achieved hematological remission.

24 patients (55,8%) of these 43 ALL-patients expressed IGFBP-rP2/CTGF mRNA at diagnosis. 20 patients (83,3%) from these 24 initially IGFBP-rP2/CTGF positive patients

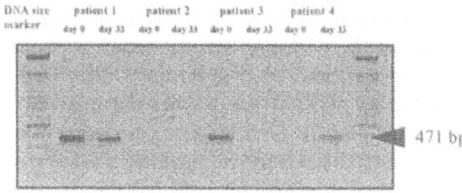

β-actin control

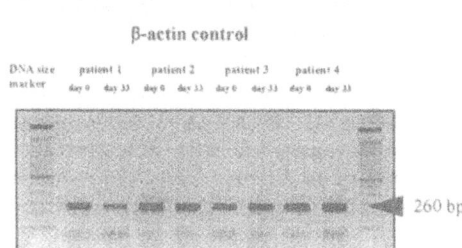

**Fig. 1.** IGFBP-rP2/CTGF expression in four different patients at diagnosis and day 33 of treatment according protocol ALL-BFM 90/95( upper panel). The lower panel shows the b-actin controls of the cDNA used for RT-PCR.

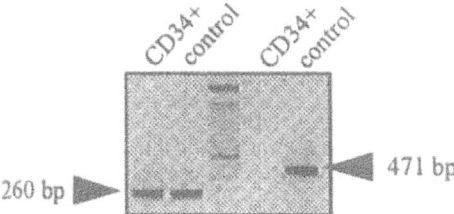

260 bp ▶
471 bp ◀

**Fig. 2.** β-actin and IGFBP-rP2 expression in CD 34+ / CD 38+ lymphoid progenitor cells from a patient with Ewin's sarcoma.

became negative for IGFBP-rP2/CTGF after the initial treatment, whereas 4 patients remained positive (16,6%). From the 19 out of 43 (44,2%) initially IGFBP-rP2/CTGF-negativ ALL patients 14 remained negative and 5 became positive for IGFBP-rP2/CTGF mRNA expression (Fig. 1).

CD34+/CD38+ positive lymphoid progenitor cells were separated for stem cell transplantation after chemotherapy from a patient with Ewing's sarcoma. These cells were also negative for IGFBP-rP2 expression in RT-PCR (Fig. 2).

## Discussion

Insulin-like growth factor binding proteins (IGFBPs) are a group of homologous proteins that regulate the biological activities of IGFs and may also be able to act in an IGF-independent way [1,2,8]. In addition to the six well-characterized IGFBPs with high affinity for IGF, at least five new binding proteins were described by structural relationship [6]. These proteins contain 16-18 conserved cysteins in the $NH_2$- and COOH-terminal regions and also the „IGFBP-motif" (GCGCCXXC). So far IGF-binding could be described to at least three new members of the predicted superfamily, IGFBP-rP1/MAC25, IGFBP-rP2/CTGF, and IGFBP-rP3/NOVH [6, 9, 10].

It is known that malignant diseases lead to alterations in the IGF signaling system. Proceeding from our previous reports on expression of insulin-like growth factors and their binding proteins in human leukemic lymphoblasts we studied the gene expression of new members of the IGFBP-superfamily in leucemia. Preliminary data suggested that in

contrast to IGFBP-rP1/MAC25, IGFBP-rP3/NOVH and IGFBP-rP4/CYR61, only IGFBP-rP2/CTGF is specifically expressed in leukemic lymphoblasts.

In the present study we demonstrate by RT-PCR that IGFBP-rP2/CTGF mRNA is specifically expressed in more than 62% of patients with acute lymphoblastic leukemia at time of diagnosis. In contrast to this findings, no expression of IGFBP-rP2/CTGF mRNA could be detected in neither peripheral blood lymphocytes from diabetics, nor myeloid leucemic cells of CML patients, nor in cord blood samples from healthy newborns.

Our data suggest, that malignant cells of B- and T-line in patients with ALL are able to express IGFBP-rP2/CTGF. The disappearance of gene expression after chemotherapy in the majority of initial IGFBP-rP2/CTGF positive patients may reflect the disappearance of the tumor cells itself. Despite all patients reached complete hematological remission at day 33 16,6% of all initial IGFBP-RP2/CTGF positive patients remained positive, and a number of initial IGFBP-rP2/CTGF negative patients expressed the gene at this time point.

The question, if the ability of this cell populations to express IGFBP-rP2/CTGF is a property of all lymphoid progenitors and not exclusive for tumor cells was addressed by investigating a clean CD34+/CD38+ cell population for expression of IGFBP-rP2/CTGF. Our data suggest that normal lymphoid progenitor cells do not express IGFBP-rP2. Further investigations of IGFBP-rP2/CTGF expression in malignant lymphoblasts, normal lymphoid progenitor cells, and other tumor specimens are necessary to answer this question.

*Acknowledgements.* This work was supported by »Deutsche Leukämie Forschungshilfe e.V.« and »Magdeburger Förderkreis krebskranker Kinder e.V.«. The authors thank Inga Handke and Bianka Hohmann for their excellent technical assistance.

## References

1. Rosenfeld RG, Pham H, Cohen P et al. (1994) Insulin-like growth factor binding proteins (IGFBP) and their regulation. Acta Paediatr Scand (Suppl), 399:415

2. Jones JL, Clemmons DR (1995) Insulin-like growth factors and their binding proteins: biological actions. Endocr Rev 16:3-30
3. Vorwerk P, Mohnike K, Kluba U et al. (1995) The expression of insulin-like growth factors and their binding proteins in human leucemic lymphoblasts. Third International Symposium on IGFBPs, Eberhard Karl University Tuebingen, 3/24
4. Wex H, Vorwerk P, Mohnike K et al. (1998) Elevated serum levels of IGFBP-2 found in children suffering from acute leukemia is accompanied by the occurrence of IGFBP-2 mRNA in the tumor clone. British J Cancer 78(4):515-520
5. Bradham DM, Igarashi A, Potter RL et al. (1991) Connective tissue growth factor: a cysteine-rich mitogen secreted by human vascular endothelial cells is related to the SRC-induced immediate early gene product CEF-10. J Cell Biol 114(6):1285-1294
6. Kim HS, Nagalla SR, Oh Y et al. (1997) Identification of a family of low-affinity insulin-like growth factor binding proteins (IGFBPs): Characterization of connective tissue growth factor as a member of the IGFBP superfamily. Proc Natl Acad Sci USA, 94:12981-12986.
7. Riehm H et al. (1990) Multizentrische Therapiestudie der Gesellschaft für Pädiatrische Onkologie und Hämatologie ALL-BFM 90 Hannover
8. Oh Y, Mueller HL, Lamson G, Rosenfeld RG (1993) Insulin-like growth factor (IGF)-independent action of IGF-binding protein-3 in Hs578T human breast cancer cells. J Biol Chem 268:14964-14971
9. Oh Y, Nagalla SR, Yamanaka Y, et al. (1996) Synthesis and Characterization of insulin-like growth factor binding protein (IGFBP-7). J Biol Chem 271:30322-30325
10. Burren CP, Wilson E, Oh Y, Rosenfeld RG (1998) IGF-binding demonstrated for NOVH, a member of the CTGF family and the IGFBP Superfamily. 80th Annual Meeting, New Orleans, The Endocrine Society, P2-306

# NM23-H1 Protein Expression as a New Prognostic Factor in Acute Lymphoblastic Leukemia

B. Höchsmann[1], E. Müller[1], G. Heil[3], N. Frickhofen[2] and L. Bergmann[1]

*Abstract.* Nm23-H1 is a candidate metastasis suppressor gene in solid tumors that was first identified in highly metastatic murine melanoma cell lines. The product of nm23-H1 has nucleoside diphosphate kinase activity. As a differentiation inhibitory factor the nm23 protein maintains proliferation and inhibits the induction of differentiation of several mouse and human cell lines. Block of differentiation may be associated with the aggressiveness of leukemia. In acute monocytic leukemia high nm23-H1 mRNA levels were reported to be correlated with a poor outcome of patients.

To elucidate the prognostic significance of nm23-H1 in acute lymphoblastic leukemia (ALL) we examined the nm23-H1 protein levels in bone marrow or peripheral blood mononuclear cells (PBMNC) of 55 patients with ALL at the time of initial diagnosis and in PBMNC of 15 healthy individuals by Western Blot Analysis. All ALL-patients were treated according to the German ALL therapy schedule. The results show a heterogenous nm23-H1 protein expression in the patient group, whereas homogenous low nm23-H1 protein levels are observed in the healthy control group. Statistical data of the patient group confirmed a significant correlation of nm23-H1 protein expression and clinicopathological parameters. Nm23-H1 protein overexpression correlates with a high relapse rate, a short relapse free survival and a short overall survival. 78% of the patients with with low nm23-H1 protein levels were relapse free 3 years after first complete remission (CR), while only 21% of the patients with nm23-H1 protein overexpression were still in remission in the same follow up period (p<0.0001). The 5-year probability of overall survival was 85% in the patient group with low nm23-H1 protein levels and only 19% in the patient group with nm23-H1 protein overexpression (p=0.0016). Our data indicate that nm23-H1 protein expression is a significant prognostic factor in ALL.

## Introduction

Nm23 was originally identified in highly metastatic murine melanoma cell lines [1]. So far four subgroups of human nm23 are known, nm23-H1, nm23-H2, Dr-nm23 and nm23-H4 [2–4]. All known members of the nm23 family encode proteins with nucleoside diphosphate kinase activity. The nm23-H1 and nm23-H2 genes are mapped on human chromosome 17q21.3 and encode a 17 kilodalton nuclear and cytoplasmatic protein of 152 amino acids[5, 6]. Four other important genes are clustered at this region: BRCA1, the early onset breast and ovarian cancer gene, c-erb, an oncogene known to be amplified in breast cancer, RARalpha, the retinoic acid receptor alpha gene recognized to be involved in the controll of cellular differentiation and MDC, a metalloprotease/disintegrin like gene [7]. Nm23-H1 was reported as a candidate metastasis suppressor gene in various solid tumors, exspecially data in breast cancer [8–10] and malignant melanoma [11] suggest an important role of nm23 in the mechanism of metastasis. This thesis was confirmed by

[1] Department of Internal Medicine III, University of Ulm, 89081 Ulm, Germany
[2] Department of Internal Medicine III, Dr. Horst-Schmidt-Kliniken, 65193 Wiesbaden, Germany
[3] Department of Hematology/ Oncology, Medizinische Hochschule Hannover, 30625 Hannover, Germany

transfection studies with reduced metastatic potential of nm23 cDNA transfectants in vivo and the ability of the cells to migrate in vitro [12, 13]. In neuroblastoma and pancreatic carcinoma the opposite trend with a correlation of high nm23-H1 expression and aggressive disease and high metastatic potential was observed [14, 15]. Therefore data in solid tumors are heterogenous and this contradictions are not solved yet.

Inspite of that, the few studies about the role of nm23 in hematopoietic malignancies are unified in the result of an association between a high nm23-H1 expression and the aggressiveness of the disease[16–19].

Lack of differentiation is one of the main characteristics of leukemias and a important factor of their aggressive behaviour. Normal hematopoietic differentiation is controlled by several negative and positive regulatory factors. Nm23-H1 was identified as a differentiation inhibitory factor of murine and human myeloid leukemia cell lines [20, 21]. Additionally an increased nm23-H1 expression during proliferation was observed [22]. Functional associations of the nm23 protein product, the nucleosid diphosphate kinase, with G-proteins or Ras has been described. Nm23-H2 is reported as a DNA-binding protein and as a transcription factor for c-myc in vitro [23, 24].

In summary these facts suggest, that nm23-H1 could play an important role in the growth and differentiation of normal and malignant hematopoietic cells.

To evaluate the importance of nm23-H1 as a prognostic factor in ALL, we compared in our present study the levels of nm23-H1 protein expression with remission rate, relapse rate, relapse free survival, overall survival and known prognostic factors in ALL by statistical analysis. The statistical data of this study indicate the nm23-H1 protein expression at the time of initial diagnosis as a significant prognostic factor in ALL.

## Methods

### Patient samples

Mononuclear cells of bone marrow (BMMNC) or peripheral blood (PBMNC) samples were obtained from 55 patients with ALL at the time of initial diagnosis. All patients were treated according to the German ALL therapy schedule for adults.

As control samples MNC of peripheral blood from 15 healthy volunteers and from three human ALL cell lines (MOLT-4, JURKAT, TOM-1) were obtained.

15 cell lines of hematopoietic malignancies (KASUMI-1; K-562, HL-60, MOLT-3, TOM-1, JURKAT, EHEB, KARPAS-299, HUT-78, DOHH-2, RAJI, U-937, JB-6, SU-DHL-1, HDLM-2) were tested.

### Cell lysis

Cell lysis was perforfmed in 0.01 Tris puffer pH 7.3, 0.15 M NaCl, 0.01 $MgCl_2$, 0.5% NP-40, 1 mM phenylmethylsulfonylfluoride and 20 µg/ml aprotinin (Bayer). Protein concentration of samples were measured by absorbance at 595 nm wave length using the protein assay dye reagent concentrate (Bio-rad).

### Western-Blot-Analysis

10 µg protein of each sample were seperated by sodium dodecyl sulfate polyacrylamide gel electrophoresis (SDS-PAGE) according to Lämmli et al. (1970) applying a multigel-long electrophoresis system (Biometra). Proteins were transfered to 0.45 µm PVDF-membranes (Milipore) by semi-dry blotting. Protein blots were incubated in phosphate buffered saline (PBS) containing 5% skim milk at 4°C overnight. For detection of nm23-H1 membranes were processed according to standard immunodetection protocolls with polyclonal primary antibody anti-nm23 (C-20, Santa Cruz) and HRP-conjugated secondary antibody anti-rabbit (Santa Cruz). Equal amounts of protein and the possibility of a semiquantification by ratio were assured by detection of actin as an internal control using a polyclonal primary antibody anti-actin (C11, Santa Cruz) and a HRP-conjugated secondary antibody anti-goat (Santa Cruz). The immobilized specific antigens were detected employing the ECL-system. Results of chemiluminescense were quantified by densiometry.

## Statistics

Overall survival (OS) was calculated from date of initial diagnosis until death, the relapse free survival (RFS) was calculated from time of first CR until diagnosis of first relapse. Treated patients were juged to have achieved CR when BM aspirates showed trilineage regeneration with less than 5% blasts by morphology in the presence of a regenerated peripheral blood count. Patients with allogenic transplantation, death caused by infection during aplasia after chemotherapy or death by suicide were censored at the date of event. The survival curves were estimated by the Kaplan-Meier method. The log-rank test was used to assess the significance of differences in OS and RFS. Chi-square were used to examine correlation of the nm23-H1 protein expression with CR-rate, relapse rate, age, sex, WBC and LDH.

## Results

### Expression of nm23-H1 protein in acute lymphoblastic leukemias

Nm23-H1 protein levels of 55 patients with newly diagnosed ALL were examined by Western-Blot-analysis. To normalize differences in protein loading, values of nm23-H1 protein expression were divided with values of actin protein expression of the individual samples. To define a base line for comparison we examined nm23-H1 protein levels in normal PBMNC of 15 healthy volunteers. These normal cells showed a homogenous low nm23-H1 protein expression with a median nm23-H1/actin-ratio of 1.0. Range for the nm23-H1/actin-ratio in this healthy control group was between 0.4 to 1.5 (Table 1). We

**Table 1.** nm23-H1 protein indices in normal PBMNC, hematopoietic cell lines and ALL-patients

| Diagnosis (n) | nm23-H1 protein index (median +/– SD) |
|---|---|
| Normal PBMNC (15) | 1,07 +/- 0,39 |
| Hematopoietic cell lines (15) | 21,76 +/- 12,84 |
| ALL (55) | 4,57 +/- 4,82 |

**Table 2.** Variability of nm23- H1 protein expression in ALL-patients

| nm23-H1 protein expression in ALL-patients | n (nm23-H1 protein index +/-SD) |
|---|---|
| nm23-H1 protein index $\leq 1,5$ | 14 (0,85 +/- 0,44) |
| nm23-H1 protein index $> 1,5 \leq 4,0$ | 20 (2,49 +/- 0,70) |
| nm23-H1 protein index $> 4,0 \leq 10,0$ | 15 (6,74 +/- 1,92) |
| nm23-H1 protein index $>10,0$ | 6 (14,72 +/- 6,64) |

selected the sample with the highest nm23-H1/actin-ratio as control for the following Western-Blot-analysis of the ALL samples and equated this ratio with 1. The nm23-H1 protein index was defined as the nm23-H1/actin-ratio in comparison to this control ratio.

The nm23-H1 protein expression of the ALL samples showed a remarkably heterogenity (Figure 1; Table 2). The median nm23-H1 protein index in the 55 ALL patient samples was 4.5 with a maximum of 27.78 and a minimum of 0.15. Inspite of that the 15 examined cell lines of hematopoietic malignancies showed homogenous high nm23-H1 protein expession with nm23-H1 protein indices between 5.31 and 43.10 and a median of 21.8 (Table 1). Therefore, we examined the relationship between nm23-H1 protein expression and clinical data. For statistical evaluation the patients were divided in two groups: normal

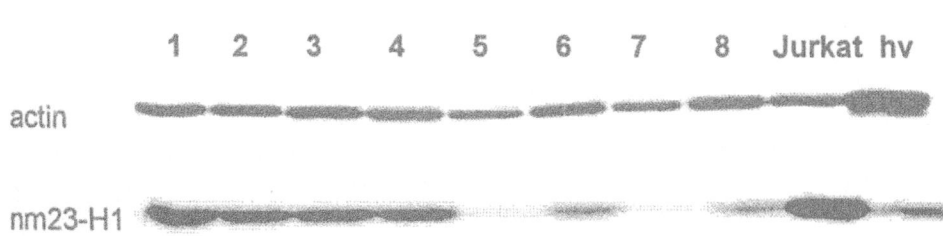

**Fig. 1.** Western Blot analysis of nm23-H1 and actin in ALL patient samples (lane 1-8). PBMNC of a healthy volunteer (hv) and MNC of the ALL cell line Jurkat were used as controlls.

**Table 3.** Relationship between nm23-H1 protein expression and clinicopathological factors

| Clinical Factor (number of patients) | median nm23-H1 protein index (± SD) | p |
|---|---|---|
| Age | | |
| ≤50 (49) | 4,54 ± 4,93 | |
| ≥50 (6) | 4,32 ± 3,24 | 0,796 |
| Sex | | |
| M (39) | 4,81 ± 5,19 | |
| F (16) | 3,97 ± 3,84 | 0,612 |
| LDH | | |
| ≤500 (28) | 4,41 ± 4,02 | |
| >500 (27) | 4,51 ± 5,63 | 0,891 |
| WBC | | |
| ≤30 G/l (29) | 4,99 ± 5,92 | |
| >30 G/l (26) | 3,86 ± 3,15 | 0,135 |
| Subgroups | | |
| C-ALL (30) | 5,15 ± 5,61 | |
| prae-prae-B-ALL (3) | 2,49 ± 1,16 | |
| prae-B-ALL (1) | 3,46 | |
| B-ALL (3) | 6,90 ± 3,83 | |
| prae-T-ALL (5) | 1,94 ± 2,23 | |
| T-ALL (13) | 3,52 ± 3,99 | 0,827 |
| Response to initial chemotherapy | | |
| CR (51) | 4,37 ± 4,87 | |
| NR (4) | 7,10 ± 3,72 | 0,634 |

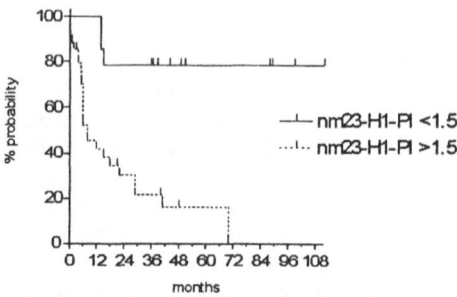

**Fig. 2.** Relapse free survival of ALL patients according to nm23-H1 protein index (nm23-H1-PI) prognostic score by Kaplan-Meier calculation. Patients undergoing a allogenic bone marrow transplantation, dying by infection in aplasia or by suizid were censored at time of the event.

expression with a nm23-H1 protein index ≤ 1.5 and overexpression with a nm23-H1 protein index > 1.5.

## Association of nm23-H1 protein expression and clinical data

We examined the correlation of nm23-H1 protein expression with age, sex, white blood cell counts (WBC), lactate dehydrogenase (LDH), ALL-subtypes, response to initial therapy, relapse rate, relapse free survival and overall survival. A summary of our statistical data in ALL patients is given in Table 3. No associations were obtained between nm23-H1 protein expression and age (p=0.769), sex (p=0.612), WBC (p=0.135) or LDH (0.891). There was no statistical correlation between the nm23-H1 protein expression and the ALL-subtypes (p=0.827), but all 3 B-ALL and the 1 pre-B-ALL showed nm23-H1 protein overexpression. Although there was no statistical correlation found between nm23-H1 protein expression and response to initial

therapy (p=0.634), all 3 patient who failed to achieve a remission showed high nm23-H1 protein indices.

High nm23-H1 protein indices correlate with a high relapse rate (p=0.0332). Therefore, we examined the relapse free survival and the overall survival of the ALL patients according to nm23-H1 protein expression based prognostic score by Kaplan-Meier calculation. Nm23-H1 protein expression correlates significantly with relapse free survival (p<0.0001). The 3-year probability of relapse free survival was 78% for patients with low nm23-H1 protein expression and 21% for patients with nm23-H1 overexpression in the same follow up period (Fig. 2). A statistical correlation (p=0.0016) was found between nm23-H1 protein expression and overall survival, too. The 5-year probability of survival was 85% in the patient group with normal nm23-H1 expression and only 19% in the patient group with nm23-H1 protein overexpression (Fig. 3).

## Discussion

Former studies identifying nm23 protein as a differentiation inhibitory factor in mouse myeloid leukemia M1 and WEHI-3BD+ and human erythroleukemia HEL, KU812 and K562 cell lines [19–21]. Nucleoside diphosphate kinase activity seems not to be involved in this differentiation inhibition as a mutant

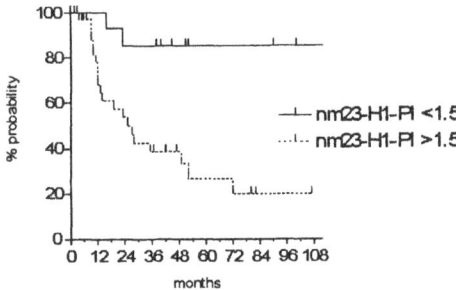

**Fig. 3.** Overall survival of ALL patients according to nm23-H1 protein index (nm23-H1-PI) prognostic score by Kaplan-Meier calculation. Patients undergoing a allogenic bone marrow transplantation, dying by infection in aplasia or by suizid were censored at time of the event.

nm23 protein with lack of NDPK-activity also inhibited the differentiation of human and mouse myeloid leukemia cells [25].

Additionally an increase of nm23-H1 levels during proliferation was observed [22]. The few studies focussing on the role of nm23 in hematopoietic malignancies indicate an association of nm23 expression and aggressiveness of disease [16–19].

In this study nm23-H1 protein has been shown to be overexpressed in the majority of the examined hematopoietic cell lines (15) and in patients with acute lymphoblastic leukemia (55). In contrast all samples of normal healthy donors (15) showed low nm23-H1 protein levels. These data confirm the thesis of the above described studies that nm23 protein is involved in the differentiation of leukemia cells and indicate a possible role of leukemogenesis, not only in myeloid leukemia cells but also in acute lymphoblastic leukemia.

Therefore we investigated the correlation of nm23-H1 protein expression in the examined ALL-samples with clinicopathological factors. In accordance with the data of Yokoyama et al. in acute myeloid leukemia on RNA level[17], our data in acute lymphoblastic leukemia indicate a correlation of nm23-H1 protein expression and prognosis. Regarding the relevance of nm23-H1 protein expression for survival, the present data show that initially high expression of nm23-H1 protein is significantly correlated with a worse long-term outcome in respect to relapse rate, relapse free survival and overall survival. No other correlations were obtained yet. Remarkably is, that all 3 patients who failed to achieve a remission showed high nm23-H1 protein indices, although there was no correlation observed between nm23-H1 protein expression and response to initial chemotherapy. Interestingly, in B-ALL and pre-pre-B-ALL, all 4 patients showed nm23-H1 protein overexpression and 3 of the 5 false positive results were found in this group. For a decision about the validity of nm23-H1 protein as a prognostic marker in this ALL-subgroup data should be controlled in a bigger collective of B-ALL samples.

In the context of various data in solid tumors the uniform data in hematopoietic malignancies suggest different functions of the nm23 gene depending on the respective tissue. This thesis of nm23 as a gene with tissue dependent functions could explain the correlation of reduced nm23 expression with increased metastatic potential and aggressive disease in human breast [8–10], hepatocellular [26], ovarian [27] and gastric carcinoma [28] and in malignant melanoma [11] as well as the opposite trend indicated by a correlation of nm23 overexpression with aggressiveness of disease and poor prognosis identified in neuroblastoma [14], pancreatic carcinoma [15] and the so far examined hematopoietic malignancies [17,18].

Although cause and effect in the functional and regulatory role of nm23 in hematology is not clarified yet, the collected data suggest an important part of nm23 in the growth and differentiation of normal and malignant hematopoietic cells. A hint for the pathophysiological relevance of nm23 may be the data of Okabe-Kado et al. and Honma et al. in mouse myeloid leukemia cells showing that differentiation-resistant M1 cells producing the differentiation inhibitory factor nm23 have higher leukemogenicity than the parent differentiation-sensitive cells and possess apparent differences in responsiveness to various regulatory molecules [20, 21, 29]. Additionally Yamashiro et al. showed alterations of nm23 gene expression during induced differentiation in several human leukemia cell lines [19] and Venturelli et al. identified in a CML blast-crisis cDNA library DR-nm23, which inhibits granulocyte differentiation and induces apoptosis in 32Dc13 myeloid cells [3]. Keim et al. detected increased nm23 protein expression in proliferation stimulated lymphocytes in comparison to unstimulated lymphocytes and in ALL patient samples [22].

Another potential link is the identification of nm23-H2 gene product as the c-myc transcription factor PuF [24]. Overexpression of c-myc is associated with inhibition of differentiation in human and mouse leukemia cells [30, 31], too. However, there was no correlation between nm23-H2 expression and c-myc expression in AML patients[32].

Although molecular alterations have been described for nm23 no association with prognosis has been found yet. As molecular aberrations of nm23 are rare events they do not give any approach to the multiple aspects of nm23 in differentiation, metastasis and oncogenesis.

On that background we presented our data of nm23-H1 protein expression in adult ALL patients and various hematopoietic cell lines including statistical analysis of nm23-H1 protein expression regarding to different clinical parameters of the patient group. The statistical analysis showed as result a significant correlation of nm23-H1 overexpression with a high relapse rate, a short relapse free survival and a short overall survival. The clinical relevance of determining nm23-H1 expression accompanying to cytogenetic analysis may be in a better identification of a high risk patient group with the aim of a more sufficient risk-stratified therapy.

In conclusion, the reported data indicate that nm23-H1 protein expression is a significant prognostic factor in ALL.

# References

1. Steeg PS, Bevilacqua G, Kopper L, et al. (1988) Evidance for a novel gene associated with low tumor metastatic potential. J Natl Cancer Inst 80: 200-204
2. Stahl JA, Leone A, Rosengard AM, et al. (1991) Identification of a second human nm23 gene, nm23-H2. Cancer Res 51: 445-449
3. Venturelli D, Martinez R, Melotti P, et al. (1995) Overexpression of Dr-nm23, a protein encoded by a member of the nm23 gene family, inhibits granulocyte differentiation and induces apoptosis in 32Dc13 myeloid cells. Proc Natl Acad Sci USA 92: 7435-7439
4. Milon L, Rosseau-Merck MF, Murnier A, et al. (1997) Nm23-H4, a new member of the family of human nm23/nucleosid diphosphate kinase genes localised on chromosome 16p13. Hum Genet 99: 550-557
5. Gilles AM, Presecan E, Lascu I, et al. (1991) Nucleoside diphosphate kinase from human erythrocytes. J of Biol Chem 266: 8784-8749
6. Backer JM, Mendola CE, Kovesdi I, et al. (1993) Chromosomal localization and nucleoside diphosphate kinase activity of human metastasis suppressor genes nm23-H1 and nm23-H2. Oncogene 8: 497-504
7. Chen H, Wang L and Banerjee S (1994) Isolation and characterization of the promoter region of human nm23-H1, a metastasis suppressor gene. Oncogene 9: 2905-2912
8. Steeg PS, De La Rosa A, Flatow U, et al. ( 1993) Nm23 and breast cancer metastasis. Breast Cancer Research and Treatment 25: 175-187
9. Steeg PS and Wagner PD (1998) Nm23 and tumor metastasis: biochemical and translational advances. Advances in Oncology 13: 3-9
10. Bevilacqua G, Sobel ME, Liotta LA, et al. (1989) Association of low nm23 RNA levels in human primary infiltrating ductal breast carcinomas with lymph node involvement and other histopathological indicators of high metastatic potential. Cancer Res 49: 5185-5190
11. Florenes VA, Aamdal S, Myklebost O, et al. (1992) Levels of nm23 mRNA in metastatic malignant melanomas: inverse correlation to disease progression. Cancer Res 52: 6088-6093
12. Leone A, Flatow U, King CR, et al. (1991) Reduced tumor incidence, metastatic potential and cytokine responsivness of nm23-transfected melanoma cells. Cell 65:65-70
13. Leone A, Flatow U, Steeg PS, et al. (1993) Transfection of human nm23-H1 into the human MDA-MB-435 breast carcinoma cell line: effects on tumor metastatic potential, colonization and enzymatic activity. Oncogene 8: 2325-2330
14. Leone A, Seeger RC, Hong CM, et al. (1993) Evidence for nm23 RNA overexpression, DANN amplification and mutation in aggressive childhood neuoblastomas. Oncogene 8:855-865
15. Nakamori S, Ishikawa O, Kimura N, et al. (1993) Expression of nukleoside diphosphate kinase/nm23 gene product in human pancreatic cancer: an association with lymph node metastasis and tumor invasion. Clin ExpMetast 11: 151-158
16. Wakimoto N, Yokoyama A, Mukai Y, et al. (1998) Elevated expression of differentiation inhibitory factor nm23 mRNA in monoblastic crisis of a patient with chronic myelogenous leukemia. Int J Hematol 67: 313-318
17. Yokoyama A, Okabe-Kado J, Wakimoto N, et al. (1998) Evaluation by multivariant analysis of the differentiation inhibitory factor nm23 as a prognostic factor in acute myelogenous leukemia and application to other hematologic malignancies. Blood 91: 1845-1851
18. Aryee D, Simonitsch I, Mosberger I, et al. (1996) Variability of nm23-H1/NDPK-A expression in human lymphomas and ist relation to tumor aggressiveness. Br J Cancer 74; 1693-1698

19. Yamashiro S, Urano T, Shiku H, et al. (1994) Alterations of nm23 gene expression during the induced differentiation of human leukemia cell lines. Oncogene 9: 2461-2468

20. Okabe-Kado J, Hayashi M, Honnma J, et al. (1985) Characterization of a differentiation-inhibitory activity from non differentiating mouse myeloid leukemia cells. Cancer Res 45: 4848-4857

21. Okabe-Kado J, , Kasukabe T, Hozumi M, et al. (1992) Identity of a differentiation inhibiting factor for mouse myeloid leukemia cells with nm23/nucleoside diphosphate kinase. Biochem Biophys Res Commun 182: 987-993

22. Keim D, Hailat N, Melhem R, et al. (1992) Proliferation-related expression of p19/nm23 nucleoside diphosphate kinase. J Clin Invest 89:919-924

23. Hildebrandt M, Lacombe ML, Veron M, et al. (1995) A human NDP-kinase B specifically binds single-stranded poly-pyrimidine sequences. Nucleic Acids Research 23: 3858-3864

24. Postel EH, Berberich SJ, Ferrone CA, et al. (1993) Human c-myc transcription factor PuF identified as nm23-H2 nucleoside diphosphate kinase, a candidate suppressor of tumor metastasis. Science 261: 478-480

25. Okabe-Kado J, Kasukabe T, Honma Y, et al. (1995) A new function of nm23/ NDP kinase as a differentiation inhibitory factor, which does not require ist kinase activity. FEBS Lett 363: 311-315

26. Nakayama T, Ohtsuru A, Nakao K, et al. (1992) Expression in human hepatocellular carcinoma of nucleoside diphosphate kinase, a homologue of the nm23 gene product. J Natl Cancer Inst 84: 1349-1399

27. Mandai M, Konishi I, Hiai H, et al. (1994) Expression of metastasis-related nm23-H1 and nm23-H2 genes in ovarian carcinomas: Correlation with clinicopathology, EGFR, c-erB-2, and c-arB-3 genes, and sex steroid receptor expression. Cancer Res 54:1825-1830

28. Nakayama H, Yasui W, Tahara E, et al. (1993) Reduced expression of nm23 is associated with metastasis in human gastric carcinomas. Jpn J Cancer Res 84: 184-189

29. Honma Y, Kasukabe T, Hozumi M (1978) Relationship between leukemogenicity and in vivo inducibility of normal differentiation in mouse myeloid leukemia cells. J Natl Cancer Inst 61: 837-843

30. Dmitrovsky E, Kuehl WM, Segal S, et al. (1986) Expression of a transfected human c-myc oncogene inhibits differentiation of mouse erythroleukemia cell line. Nature 322: 748-751

31. Prochownik EV, Kukowska J (1986) Deregulated expression of c-myc by murine erythroleukemia cells prevents differentiation. Nature 322: 748-751

32. Yokoyama A, Okabe-Kado J, Honma Y, et al. (1996) Differentiation inhibitory factor nm23 as a new prognostic factor in acute monocytic leukemia. Blood 88: 3555-3561

# Monitoring of Wilms' Tumor Gene Transcription in Leukemia Patients

E. Niegemann, S. Wehner, D. Schwabe and U. Ebener

*Abstract.* We examined the presence of WT1-specific mRNA in bone marrow aspirates or peripheral blood samples of 76 children suffered from acute leukemia at diagnosis and / or relapse. Samples were analyzed by RT-PCR. WT1-specific mRNA was detected in 79% of patients at diagnosis and in 90% of samples at time of relapse.

The WT1 expression in bone marrow was monitored during the clinical course of some patients. The prognostic value and qualification of WT1 expression for monitoring of MRD (minimal residual disease) during chemotherapy must be confirmed. In contrast to other tumor-specific markers the applicability of WT1 gene expression in most cases of acute leukemia is an important advantage.

## Introduction

The Wilms' tumor gene WT1 encodes a zinc-finger transcription factor, regulating the transcription of several growth factors and growth factor receptors (1–5). Depending on the presence or absence of wild type p53 the WT1 gene acts as a repressor or activator of gene transcription (6). WT1 itself is regulated in a strong time- and tissue-specific manner. As a result of alternative RNA splicing, the gene can be expressed as four proteins differing in just some amino acids (7). The expression of WT1 has been reported for various developing tissues and early CD34$^+$ hematopoietic progenitors, but it is also found in some human malignancies.

In the recent study we investigated the expression of WT1 in acute childhood leukemia by RT-PCR. Bone marrow aspirates or peripheral blood samples from seventy-six pediatric patients (61 at initial diagnosis, 20 at first or second relapse) were analyzed. Frequency of WT1 expression in different subtypes of acute leukemia and expression levels were compared with data reported on adult patients.

## Materials and Methods

### Patients

This study included 76 patients who were admitted between 1995 and 1999. Samples were taken from 61 children with acute leukemia at diagnosis (median age, 6 years) and 20 patients at first or second relapse (median age, 10 years). Acute leukemia was classified by morphological and immunological characteristics into B-precursor leukemia (n = 52), T-cell leukemia (n = 6), AMLs (n = 17), and one case of AUL (phenotyped as My$^+$/ NK-cell precursor ALL).

### Morphological, cytochemical and immunofluorescence analysis

Smears of each specimens were stained with May-Grünwald-Giemsa dye non-specific esterase, peroxidase (POX), acid phosphatase, and periodic acid-Schiff (PAS). The portion of blast cells in samples was estimated by morphological features. Acute leukemia was classified according to the criteria devised by the French-American-British (FAB) Committee. Immunophenotyping was performed on

Dedicated to Prof. Dr. Dr. h.c. Bernhard Kornhuber

Clinic of Pediatrics III, Department of Hematology and Oncology, J. W. Goethe-University, Frankfurt/Main, Germany

whole lysed PB/BM cells using a FACScan flow cytometer (Becton Dickinson, Heidelberg, Germany). The blast cells were subsequently analyzed for the presence of cell surface antigens with direct one and two color analysis using a panel of fluorecein-conjugated (FITC) or R-phycoerythrin-conjugated (R-PE) mouse monoclonal antibodies. Staining of cytoplasmic antigens e.g. cyMPO, cyCD3, cyCD22 and nuclear terminal deoxynucleotidyl transferase (TdT) were performed as described elsewhere [8]. Multiparameter analysis of gated cells was used to subclassify the leukemic blasts and to provide supplementary immunological information.

### Sample preparation

Heparinized PB cells or BM aspirates were centrifuged on Ficoll-Isopaque solution and washed with 50 ml of phosphate-buffered saline (PBS). Total RNA of $10^6$ to $10^7$ mononuclear cells was isolated according to the single-step extraction method described by Chomczynski and Sacchi, 1987.

### RT-PCR

5 µg total RNA was converted into cDNA by using SuperScript reverse transcriptase (Gibco) according to the manufacturer´s instructions. PCR was performed for 35 cycles amplifying a 857 bp fragment of the WT1 gene. The quality and the amount of RNA was analyzed by amplification of the β-actin gene (675 bp) as control.

For evaluating the detection limit of WT1 analysis by RT-PCR, known numbers of cells from line K562 were mixed with aliquotted mononuclear cells from PB of healthy volunteers. Between 1 to $10^5$ leukemic blast cells were added to $10^7$ cells in each case. The amplification products were separated by agarose gel electrophoresis and stained with ethidium bromide. Afterwards gels were photographed with ultraviolet illumination. For negative controls we analyzed mononuclear cells (MNC) from healthy individuals.

## Results and Discussion

48 (79 %) of the tested 61 acute leukemias showed WT1 gene expression at time of diagnosis, and 18 samples from 20 patients who had relapsed for first or second time were positive for the WT1 transcript. Table 1 summarizes the results of WT1 gene expression in various types of leukemia. Particularly, the WT1 transcript was found in 34 of 41 (83 %) samples of newly diagnosed B-precursor leukemia, in 1 of 5 T-ALLs, and in 12 of 14 cases (86 %) of AML (Table 1). These results meet the data to be found in adults up to now; high frequency of WT1 transcript in blast cells of acute myeloid leukemias and B-precursor acute lymphoblastic leukemias – low frequency in T cell acute leukemias [10–14]. Differences in the methods and the minor age of patients included in our study may account for the small variations.

Low levels of WT1 gene expression has also been observed in primitive hematopoietic cells bearing the CD34 positive phenotype [15] The WT1 gene expression detectable by our method is malignancy-associated in acute leukemias and not sensitive enough to show WT1 gene expression MNC from PB and BM of healthy volunteers. The high frequency in which the WT1 gene expression is detectable in leukemic blast cells, qualifies this feature as an important marker in acute childhood leukemias.

No striking differences between expression levels in acute leukemia at time of diagnosis and those at time of relapse were found. On the other hand, WT1 expression is detectable more often in relapsed cases (90 %)

**Table 1.** WT1 expression in acute childhood leukemias detected by RT-PCR

|  | newly diagnosed | relapsed | total |
|---|---|---|---|
| B-precursor ALL | 34/41 (83%) | 13 / 15 (87%) | 47/56 (84%) |
| T-lineage ALL | 1/5 (20%) | 1/1 | 2/6 (33%) |
| AML | 12/14 (86%) | 4/4 | 16/18 (89%) |
| AUL | 1 / 1 | – | 1 / 1 |
| summarized | 48 / 61 (79%) | 18 / 20 (90%) | |

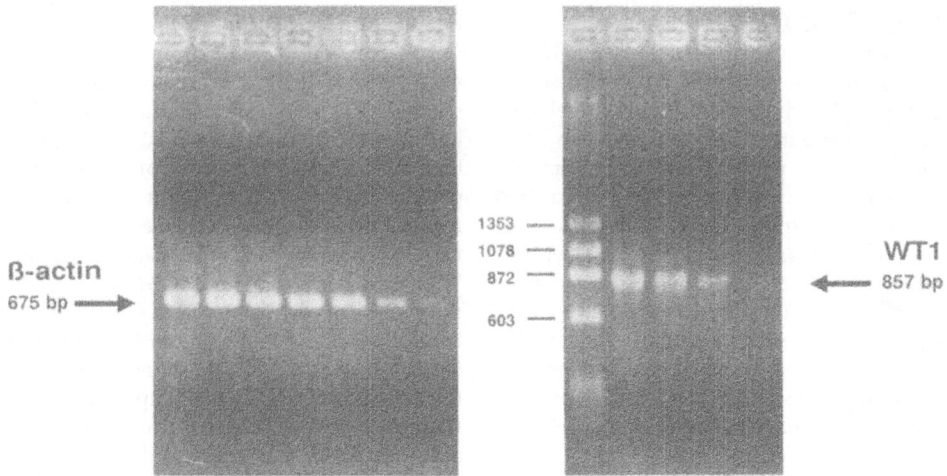

**Fig. 1.** Dilution series of cDNA from leukemic cell lineage K562 to define WT1 expression level examined by RT-PCR. The cDNA was diluted 1:10 usind diethyl pyrocarbonate-treated water in order to apply PCR ($10^0$, $10^{-1}$, $10^{-2}$, $10^{-3}$, $10^{-4}$, $10^{-5}$, $10^{-6}$, M, $10^0$, $10^{-1}$, $10^{-2}$, $10^{-3}$).

than at time of diagnosis (79 %) (Table 1). Maybe some patients, who showed low WT1 expression at time of relapse would have been negative in RT-PCR at time of diagnosis.

The detection limit of RT-PCR was experimentally evaluated by mixing of WT1 positive cells of lineage K562 with WT1 negative peripheral blood lymphocytes of healthy donors. The sensitivity of the method was detection of one leukemic cell in 10000 normal blood cells.

Furthermore we assessed relative levels of WT1 expression in 41 bone marrow aspirates. The degree of WT1 expression was determined by serial dilutions of cDNA, followed by PCR for WT1 and β-actin genes (Fig. 1). As shown in Fig. 2, patients with AML exhibited on an average higher rates of strong WT1 expression than those with ALL.

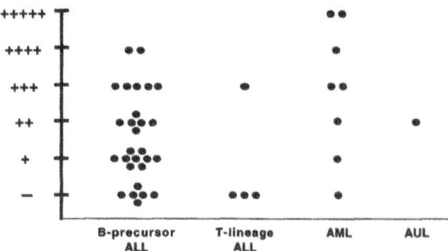

**Fig. 2.** Relative expression of WT1 gene in newly diagnosed acute childhood leukemia. Classification of WT1 expression was done by comparison of b-actin and WT1 PCR products.

Figure 3 shows the relationship between the levels of WT1 gene expression in the BM and the clinical course of five patients (shown for examples). The behavior of WT1 gene expression was quite heterogeneous. Similar results were reported for adult patients by Schmid et al. (1997). Typically the WT1 expression levels rapidly decreased during therapy and sometimes WT1 mRNA was not detectable by PCR after complete remission (e.g. patient No.2). Some patients who had no detectable WT1 mRNA at diagnosis showed WT1 gene expression at time of relapse (e.g. patient No.3), while two cases were still WT1 negative at time of relapse (e.g. patient No. 5). Because of the heterogeneous behavior of WT1 gene expression and from these limited data it is not useful to draw any conclusions concerning the predictive value of WT1 gene expression. The prognostic value and qualification of WT1 expression for monitoring minimal residual disease (MRD) during chemotherapy must be confirmed.

*Supported by „Hilfe für krebskranke Kinder Frankfurt e.V." and „Edith von Heyden Vermächtnis"*

### References

1. Gashler AL, Bonthron DT, Madden SL, Rauscher FJ III, Collins T, Sukhatme VP (1992) Human platelet-derived growth factor A chain is transcriptio-

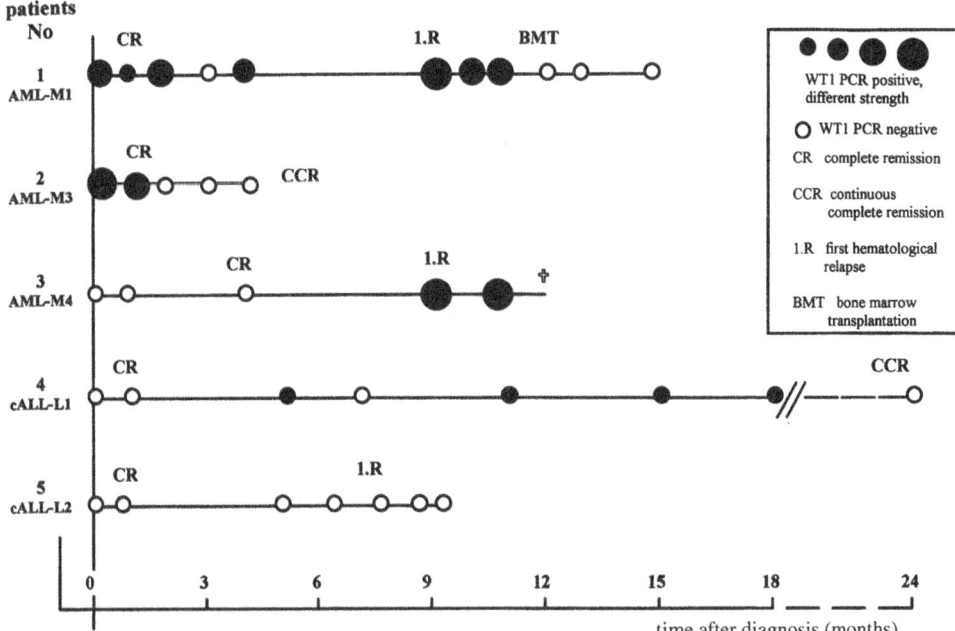

**Fig. 3.** Monitoring of WT1 gene expression in BM of patients.

time after diagnosis (months)

nally repressed by the Wilms' tumor suppressor WT1. Proc Natl Acad Sci USA 89:10984-10988

2. Harrington MA, Konicek B, Song A, Xia X, Fredricks WJ, Rauscher FJ III (1993) Inhibition of colony-stimulating factor-1 promoter activity by the product of the Wilms' tumor locus. J Biol Chem 268:21271-21275

3. Drummond IA, Madden SL, Rohwer-Nutter P, Bell GI, Sukhatme VP, Rauscher FJ III (1992) Repression of the insulin-like growth factor II gene by the Wilms' tumor suppressor WT1. Science 257:674-678

4. Dey BR, Sukhatme VP, Roberts AB, Sporn MB, Rauscher FJ III, Kim SJ (1994) Repression of the transforming growth factor-b1 gene by Wilms' tumor suppressor WT1 gene product. Endocrinology 8:595-602

5. Werner H, Shen-Orr Z, Rauscher FJ III, Morris JF, Roberts CT, Leroith D (1995) Inhibition of cellular proliferation by the Wilms' tumor suppressor WT1 is associated with suppression of insulin-like growth factor I receptor gene expression. Mol Cell Biol 15:3516-3522

6. Maheswaran S, Park S, Bernard A, Morris JF, Rauscher FJ III, Hill DE, Haber DA (1993) Physical and functional interaction between WT1 and p53 proteins. Proc Natl Acad Sci USA 90:5100-5104

7. Haber DA, Sohn RL, Buckler AJ, Pelletier J, Call KM, Housman DE (1991) Alternative splicing and genomic structure of the Wilms' tumor gene WT1. Proc Natl Acad Sci USA 88:9618-9622

8. Knapp W, Strobl H, Majdic O (1994) Flow cytometric analysis of cell-surface and intracellular antigens in leukemia diagnosis. Cytometry 18:187-198

9. Chomczynski P, Sacchi N (1987) Single-step method of RNA isolation by acid guanidium thio-cyanate-phenol-chloroform extraction. Anal Biochem 162:156-159

10. Miwa H, Beran M, Saunders GF (1992) Expression of the Wilms' tumor gene (WT1) in human leukemia. Leukemia 6:405-409

11. Brieger J, Weidmann E, Fenchel K, Mitrou PS, Hoelzer D, Bergmann L (1994) The expression of the Wilms' tumor gene in acute myelocytic leukemias as a possible marker for leukemic blast cells. Leukemia 8:2138-2143

12. Inoue K, Sugiyama H, Ogawa H, Nakagawa M, Yamagami T, Miwa H, Kita K, Hiraoka A, Masaoka T, Nasu K, Kyo T, Dohy H, Nakauchi H, Ishidate T, Akiyama T, Kishimoto T (1994) WT1 as a new prognostic factor and a new marker for the detection of minimal residual disease in acute leukemia. Blood 84:3071-3079

13. Menssen HD, Renkl H-J, Rodeck U, Maurer J, Notter M, Schwartz S, Reinhardt R, Thiel E (1995) Presence of Wilms' tumor gene (wt1) transcripts and the WT1 nuclear protein in the majority of human acute leukemias. Leukemia 9:1060-1067

14. Patmasiriwat P, Fraizer GC, Kantarjian H, Saunders GF (1996) Expression pattern of WT1 and GATA-1 in AML with chromosome 16q22 abnormalities. Leukemia 10:1127-1133

15. Baird PN, Simmons PJ (1997) Expression of the Wilms' tumor gene (WT1) in normal hemopoiesis. Exp Hematol 25:312-320

16. Schmid D, Heinze G, Linnerth B, Tisljar K, Kusec R, Geissler K, Sillaber C, Laczika K, Mitterbauer M, Zöchbauer S, Mannhalter C, Haas OA, Lechner K, Jäger U, Gaiger A (1997) Prognostic significance of WT1 gene expression at diagnosis in adult de novo acute myeloid leukemia. Leukemia 11:639-643

# Effect of Mutationally Activated Ras on the Ras to MAP Kinase Signaling Pathway and Growth Inhibition of Myeloid Leukemia Cells by Inhibitors of the MAP Kinase Cascade

CH. W. M. REUTER*, M. A. MORGAN and L. BERGMANN

## Summary

Ras proteins are small G-proteins that have been shown to play a key role in signal transduction, proliferation and malignant transformation. Mutations in the *ras* genes have been implicated in a large number of human cancers including myeloid leukemias (AML, CML, CMML, JCML). Transfection of mutationally activated Ras into NIH3T3 fibroblasts resulted in a transformed phenotype and activation of the MAP kinase signal transduction pathway (MAP kinase kinase activators, B-Raf and c-Raf-1 [5 fold and 17 fold], MAP kinase kinases, MEK-1 and MEK-2 [6-8 fold], and MAP kinases, ERK-1 and ERK-2 [3-12 fold]). The activation of the MAP kinase cascade was dependent on both the type and the expression level of the Ras proteins. Enhancement of the MAP kinase cascade was not observed in cells overexpressing wild-type c-H-Ras. Treatment of the cells with inhibitors of MAP kinase signaling (e.g. MEK and FTase inhibitors) resulted in a reversion of the Ras-induced transformed phenotype of these fibroblasts. In addition, 10 myeloid leukemia cell lines were tested for MAP kinase activation and the effect of these inhibitors on leukemia cell growth. In five cell lines MAP kinases ERK-1 and ERK-2 were found to be constitutively activated. Incubation with the MEK inhibitor resulted in a significant inhibition of the colony formation of these cell lines (60-100%). Maximal inhibition of cell growth was observed after 7 days of incubation and hematopoietic growth factor dependent cell lines were most sensitive to PD 098059. Most FTase inhibitors were less effective in the inhibition of myeloid leukemia growth; the FPTase inhibitor 3 inhibited growth of leukemic cells by 95-100%. These results support the potential role of inhibitors of the Ras to MAP kinase signaling pathway in the treatment of myeloid leukemias.

## Introduction

The deregulation of Ras function appears to be a common theme in the molecular pathogenesis of myeloid leukemias. Activating *ras* mutations were identified in up to 30% of both adult and childhood acute myeloid leukemia (AML) (Bos 1989, Clark & Der 1995). The mutations arise at codons 12, 13 and 61 of N-ras and occasionally K-ras. These mutations lead to the production of constitutively activated Ras proteins that cannot be switched off. Activating mutations of Ras may result in uncontrolled growth-factor-independent proliferation of hematopoietic progenitors and/or accumulation due to reduced levels of apoptosis (Byrne & Marshall, 1998). In addition, over-expression of all three *ras* genes due to mutations in the promotor region of *ras* has been implicated in the leukemogenesis of myeloid leukemias.

Deregulation of Ras in myeloid leukemias can also occur by expression of constitutively activated versions of normal proto-oncogenes and tumor suppressor genes. Philadelphia-chromosome positive chronic myelogeneous leukemia (CML) is a myeloproliferative condition characterized by the presence of a balanced translocation between chromosomes 9 and 22, t(9;22), which leads to the

Department of Hematology & Oncology, Section Molecular Biology, University of Ulm, Robert-Koch-Str. 8, 89081 Ulm, Germany.

expression of a BCR-Abl fusion tyrosine kinase. The expression of this deregulated chimeric protein results in cellular transformation by abrogation of growth factor dependence, blockade of differentiation and direct inhibition of apoptosis. The involvement of Ras has been demonstrated by the presence of increased levels of GTP-Ras in cells expressing BCR-Abl (Cortez et al. 1995).

Another fusion tyrosine kinase, which is the result of the t(5;12) translocation found in a subset of patients with chronic myelomonocytic leukemia (CMML), consists of Tel, a member of the Ets-family of transcription factors, and the platelet-derived growth factor receptor β (PDGF-R β). The constitutive activation of Ras is thought to be a result of the Tel-PDGF-R ß fusion protein dimerization in the absence of ligand (Golub et al. 1994).

Patients with juvenile chronic myeloid leukemia (JCML) commonly show activating *ras* mutations or loss of the neurofibromin type 1 (NF-1) gene. The NF-1 gene encodes a Ras GTPase activating protein which down-regulates Ras (Xu et al. 1990). This gene is also inactivated in the autosomal dominant condition neurofibromatosis type 1. Deletions of NF-1 lead to moderate but consistent elevation of GTP-Ras levels in leukemic cells from children with neurofibromatosis type 1 (Bollag et al. 1996).

Ras activation may also occur as a result of point mutations of receptor tyrosine kinases which are upstream of Ras. Mutation of c-Fms, the M-CSF receptor or the c-kit receptor activate proliferation of hematopoietic cells (Carlberg et al. 1994, Kitayama et al. 1995).

In the GTP-bound state, Ras interacts with various downstream effectors leading to cellular proliferation, differentiation or protection against apoptosis. These Ras effectors include the Raf protein kinases, phosphatidylinositol 3-OH kinase, PI(3)-K, and Ral-GDS (Marshall 1996, Byrne & Marshall 1998). The interaction of the Raf kinases (A-Raf, B-Raf, and c-Raf-1) with GTP-Ras results in the phosphorylation and activation of the MAP kinase kinases, MEK-1 and MEK-2, which in turn phosphorylate and activate the MAP kinases ERK-1 and ERK-2. These three sequential kinases are the core components of the Ras to MAP kinase signaling cascade

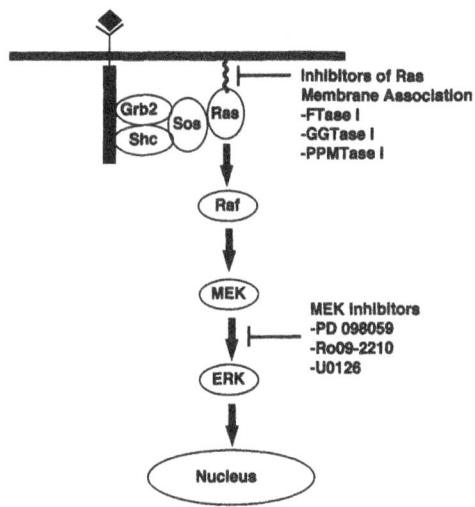

**Fig. 1.** Schematic diagram of the Ras to MAP kinase signaling pathway. The Ras to MAP kinase signaling cascade is activated by cytokines binding to their receptors at the cell surface. Inhibitors of the membrane association of Ras include farnesyl transferase (FTase) inhibitors, geranylgeranyl transferase (GGTase) inhibitors and prenylated protein methyltransferase (PPMTase) inhibitors. PD 098059, U0126 and Ro09-2210 are MEK inhibitors which block the activation of the MAP kinase kinases MEK-1 and MEK-2.

(Fig. 1). Activated ERKs translocate into the nucleus where they phosphorylate transcription factors such as ElK-1, c-Myc and CREB and thereby regulate gene expression.

The role of Ras in the pathophysiology of myeloid leukemias has considerable potential implications for a therapeutic approach which targets the Ras to MAP kinase signaling pathway. To address this issue we studied the effect of mutationally activated Ras on MAP kinase activation in NIH3T3 fibroblasts and the potential of inhibitors of the Ras to MAP kinase cascade to revert the Ras-induced, transformed phenotype. Furthermore, we demonstrate the constitutive activation of ERK-1 and ERK-2 in several human myeloid leukemia cell lines as well as growth inhibition of leukemia cells incubated with various inhibitors of the Ras to MAP kinase cascade. These results suggest a potential role of these inhibitors in the treatment of myeloid leukemias.

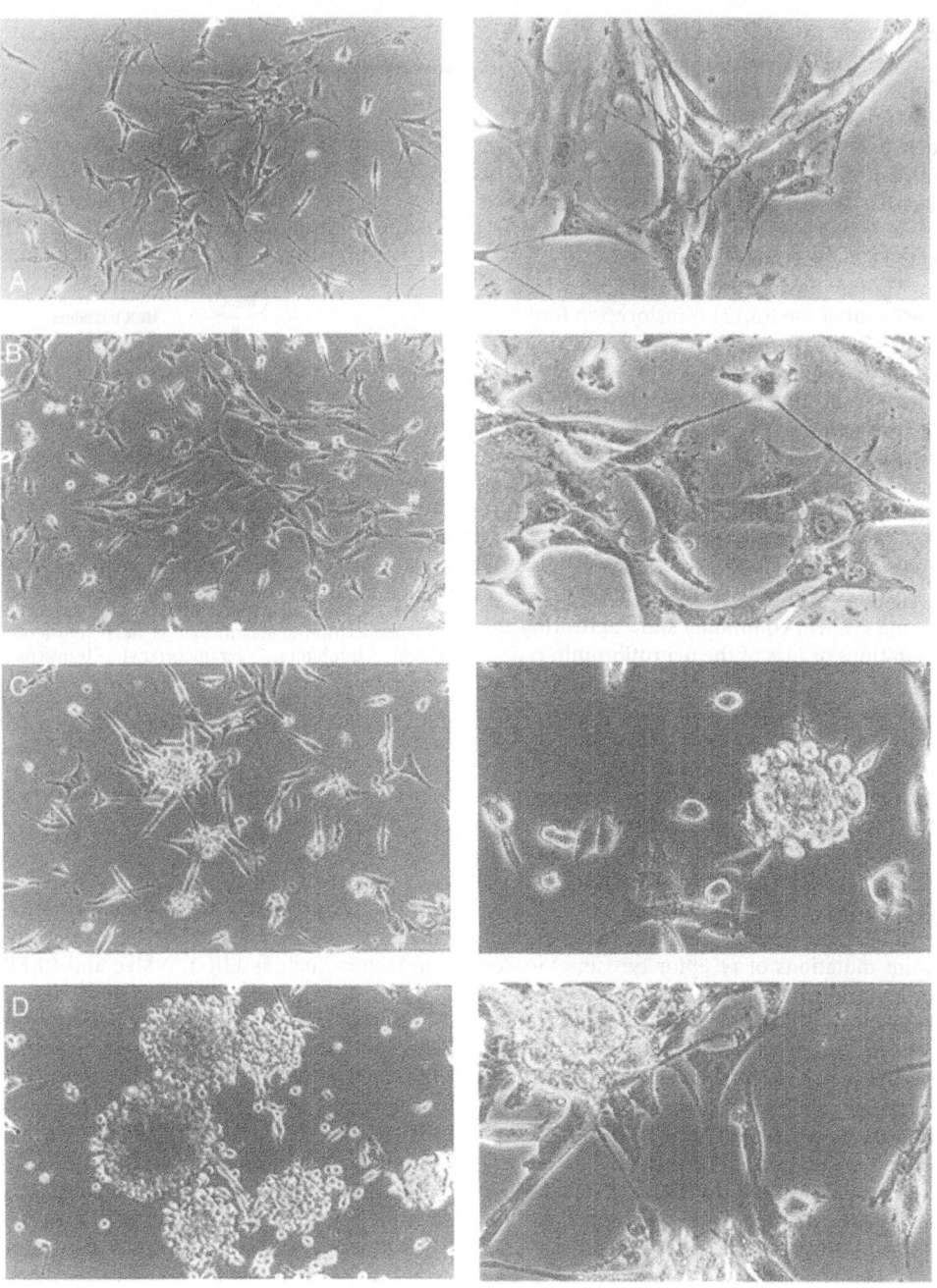

**Fig. 2.** Morphology of NIH3T3 fibroblasts expressing (A) wild-type c-H-Ras, (B) over-expressed wild-type c-H-Ras, (C) V12-H-Ras and (D) L61-H-Ras. Notice the round shape, the lack of adherent growth and the focus formation in V12-H-Ras and L61-H-Ras transformed fibroblasts.

## Material and Methods

### Cells and antibodies

All leukemia cell lines were from the German Collection of Microorganisms and Cell cultures (DSM, Braunschweig, Germany). Antibodies against MAP kinases ERK-1 and ERK-1, MAP kinase kinases, MEK-1 and MEK-2, B-Raf and c-Raf-1 were purchased from Santa Cruz Biotechnology Inc. (Santa Cruz, California). Recombinant GST/His6-MEK-1 and –MEK-2, purified recombinant kinase-defective K52R-ERK2 and the antibody against activated, phospho-ERK-1/2 were gifts from Michael J. Weber (University of Virginia, Charlottesville, Virginia).

### Western blot analysis

Cells were cultured in RPMI medium containing 10% heat-inactivated fetal calf serum (FCS), glutamine (292 µg/ml) and antibiotics (penicillin 60.2 mg/ml, streptomycin 133 µg/ml). Cell extracts were prepared by standard methods. Briefly, after washing in phosphate buffered saline (PBS) cells were lysed in 50 mM Tris/HCl pH 7.5, 100 mM NaCl, 1% Triton X-100, 5 mM EDTA, 1 mM PMSF, 50 mM NaF, 1 mM sodium ortho vanadate, 1 mM dithiothreitol (DTT) and 10 µg/ml pepstatin. Cellular debris and insoluble proteins were pelleted by centrifugation at 13,000 rpm for 15 min at 4° C. Supernatants were recovered and analyzed by SDS-PAGE after normalization of protein concentrations. Protein bands were visualized by Western blotting using the ECL kit (Amersham-Buchler, Braunschweig, Germany).

### Colony forming assays

Colony forming assays were done as described (Reuter et al. 1994).

### MAP kinase and MEK assays

MAP kinase and MEK assays were done as described recently (Reuter et al. 1995).

### Biochemical determinations

Cellular protein concentrations were determined using the Commassie dye-binding assay according to Bradford (1976) (Bio-Rad).

## Results

### Activation of the MAP kinase cascade by expression of mutationally activated H-Ras

To study the effect of mutationally activated Ras on the activity of the different members of the MAP kinase cascade, c-H-Ras, V12-H-Ras and L61-H-Ras were overexpressed in NIH3T3 fibroblasts (Jelinek et al. 1996). Expression of mutationally activated H-Ras but not wild-type c-H-Ras into NIH3T3 fibroblasts resulted in a transformed phenotype as shown by anchorage independent growth and

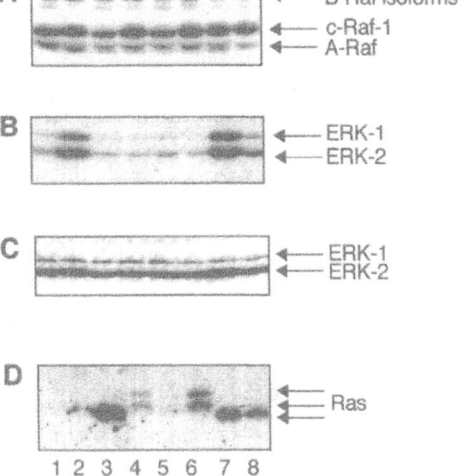

**Fig. 3.** Expression of mutated Ras proteins and activation of MAP kinases in whole cell extracts of NIH3T3 fibroblasts. (A) Western blot with C-terminal antibodies against A-Raf, B-Raf and c-Raf-1. (B) Western blot using an antibody against diphosphorylated, activated MAP kinases ERK-1 and ERK-2. (3) Western blot with antibodies against ERK-1 and ERK-2. (D) Western blot with a pan-Ras antibody. Lanes: 1, serum starved NIH3T3 fibroblasts; 2, serum-stimulated (5 min) NIH3T3 fibroblasts; 3, serum-starved NIH3T3 fibroblasts overexpressing c-H-Ras; 4-6, three different clones of serum-starved NIH3T3 fibroblasts overexpressing V12-H-Ras; 7-8, two clones of serum-starved NIH3T3 fibroblasts over-expressing L61-H-Ras.

focus formation in Fig. 2C and D. Strongest activation of the MAP kinase signal transduction pathway was observed in the L61-H-Ras mutants (Fig. 3, panel B). The activation of the MAP kinase pathway was dependent both on the type and the expression level of the mutated H-Ras proteins (Fig. 3, panels B and D). Cells transfected with L61-H-Ras showed a 5- and a 17-fold activation of B-Raf and c-Raf-1, which are the major MAP kinase kinase activators in these cells (Reuter et al. 1995). The activities of MAP kinase kinases MEK-1 and MEK-2 were increased 6-8 fold as compared to normal, serum-starved controls and the MAP kinases ERK-1 and ERK-2 were activated 3-12 fold (Fig. 4). Activated c-Raf-1 and B-Raf proteins were exclusively phosphorylated on serine residues (not shown).

### Effect of inhibitors of the Ras to MAP kinase cascade

Treatment with 50 µM of the MEK inhibitor PD 098059 and with 100 µM of the Ras farnesyl transferase inhibitor L739,749 resulted in a reversion of the phenotype of the Ras-transformed fibroblasts (Fig. 5A). Maximal inhibition was observed after 48 hours of incubation. Incubation with the MEK inhibitor PD 098059 led to a significant inhibition of the activity of ERK-1 and ERK-2. Inhibition of MAP kinase was observed as early as 30 min after incubation with PD 098059 (Fig. 5B).

### Effect of inhibitors of Ras to MAP kinase signaling on myeloid leukemia cell growth

It has previously been reported that 37 out of 73 (approximately 50%) cases of AML showed a constitutive activation of MAP kinases (Towatari et al. 1997). However, this study may be open to artifact since cross-reactive ERK antibodies were employed in MAP kinase band shift assays. In order to re-investigate the constitutive activation of the MAP kinase cascade in myeloid leukemia, ten myeloid leukemia cell lines were tested for activation of MAP kinases. Using a monoclonal antibody specific for diphosphorylated, activated ERK-1/2 we observed a strong constitutive activation of MAP kinases in 5 out of 10 myeloid leukemia cell lines: K562, MV4-11, ML-2, AML-OCI 2, and Mono-Mac. We also observed activation of MAP kinases in HL-60 and THP-1 cell lines, albeit to a lesser extent (Fig. 6, panel A). Using the cross-reactive ERK antibodies we demonstrate variable expression levels of MAP kinase ERK-1 in these cell lines. In contrast, ERK-2 levels were fairly consistent (Fig. 6, panel B). Activation of MAP kinases did not correlate with the MAP kinase double band observed with the cross-reactive ERK antibodies (Fig. 6). Incubation with the MEK inhibitor PD 098059 (50 µM) resulted in a significant reduction of cell viability and colony formation for all cell lines tested (60-100%). Maximal inhibition of cell growth was observed after 7 days of incubation (Fig. 7). Most FTase inhibitors including FTase inhibitors 1 and 2 and FPTase inhibitor 2 (100 µM) were less effective (0-25%) in inhi-

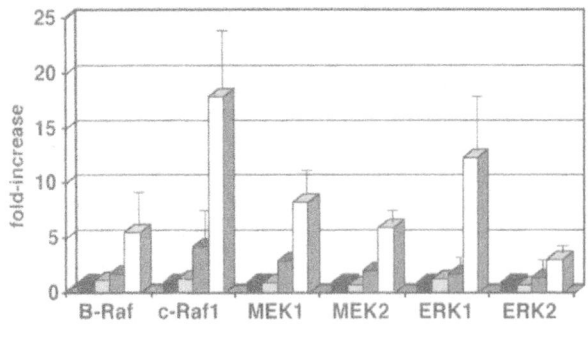

**Fig. 4.** Activation of the kinases of the Ras to MAP kinase signal transduction cascade in V12-H-Ras and L61-H-Ras transformed NIH3T3 fibroblasts. After serum-starvation for 16 hours cells were lysed and assayed for MEK-1/2 and ERK-1/2 activity (Reuter et al. 1995). B-Raf and c-Raf-1 activities were determined in a two-step MEK activation assay as described (Reuter et al. 1995).

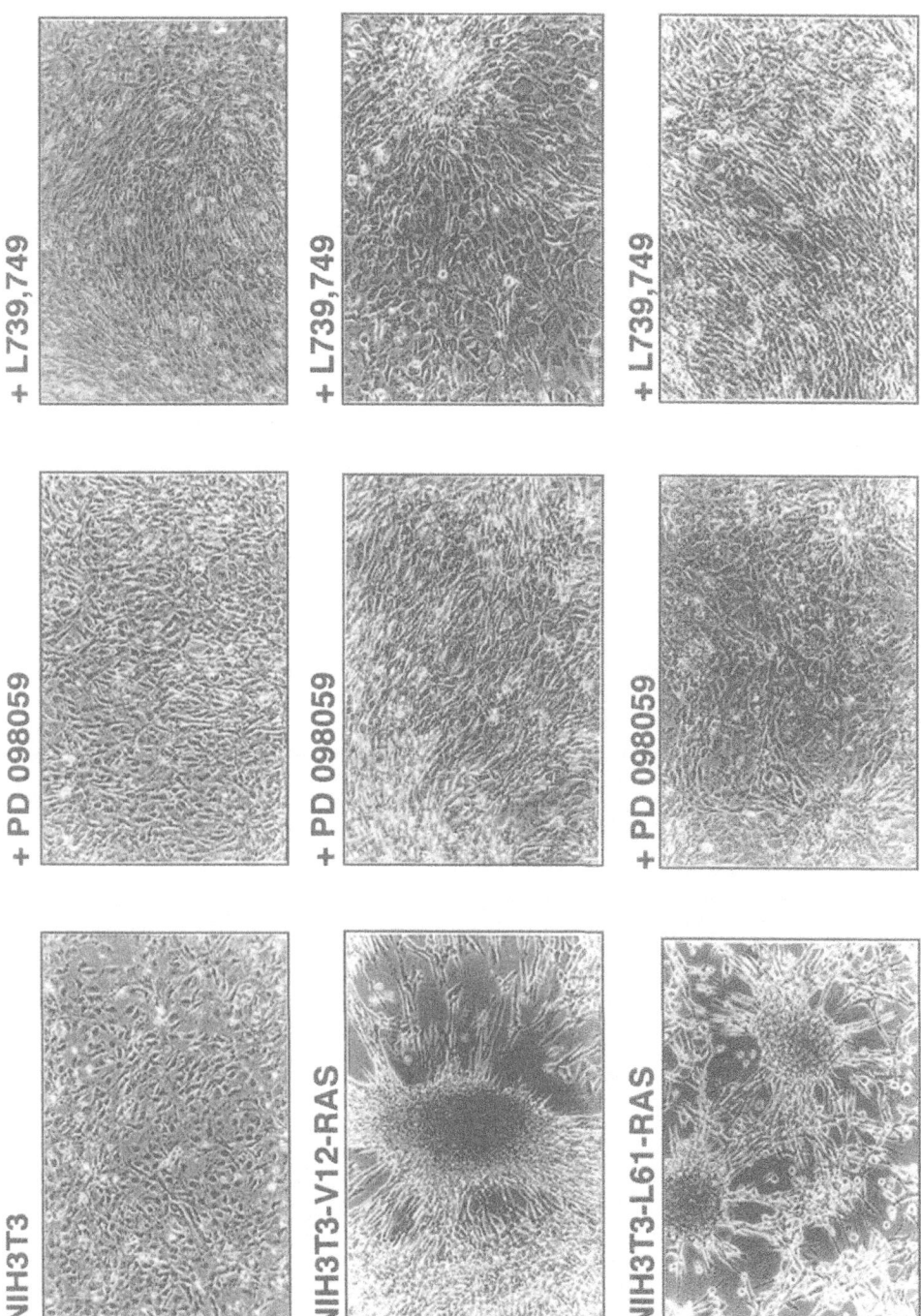

**Fig. 5.** (A) Morphology of normal, V12-H-Ras- and L61-H-Ras-transformed NIH3T3 fibroblasts after a 48-hour incubation with the MEK inhibitor PD 098059 (50 μM) or the FTase inhibitor L-739,749 (100 μM). (B) Activities of MAP kinase kinases MEK-1 and MEK-2 as well as MAP kinases ERK-1 and ERK-2 after a 30-min incubation with MEK inhibitor PD 098059.

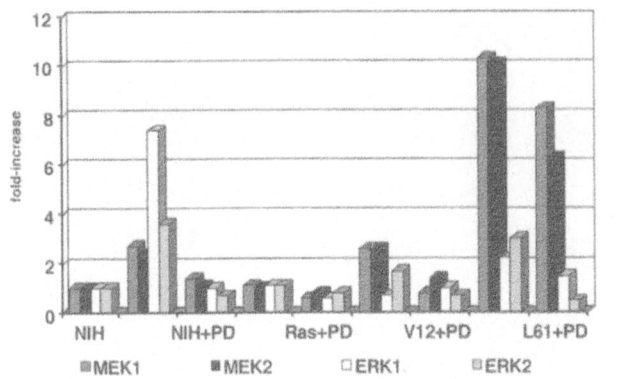

**Fig. 5b**

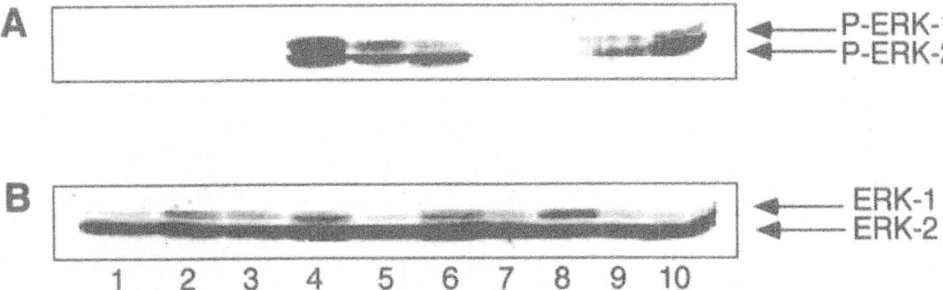

**Fig. 6.** Constitutive activation of MAP kinases ERK-1 and ERK-2 in myeloid leukemia cell lines. Western blots were done with a monoclonal antibody against diphosphorylated, activated MAP kinases (A) and an antibody specific for ERK-2 which cross-reacts with ERK-1 (B). Lanes: 1, Kasumi; 2, KG-1; 3, THP-1; 4, Mono-Mac-1; 5, ML-2; 6, K562; 7, HL-60; 8, RC2A; 9, AML-OCI-2; 10, MV4-11.

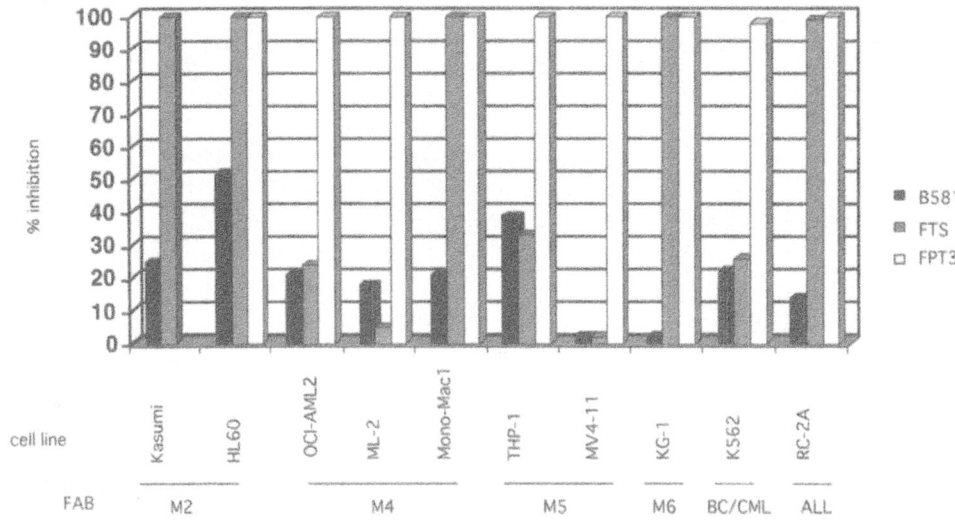

**Fig. 7.** Effect of MEK inhibitor PD 098059 on growth of myeloid leukemia cell lines.
Viability of leukemia cells was determined by trypan blue dye exclusion assays and colony formation assays. 2.5 x 10⁵ cells were incubated for 4 days with MEK inhibitor (50 μM).

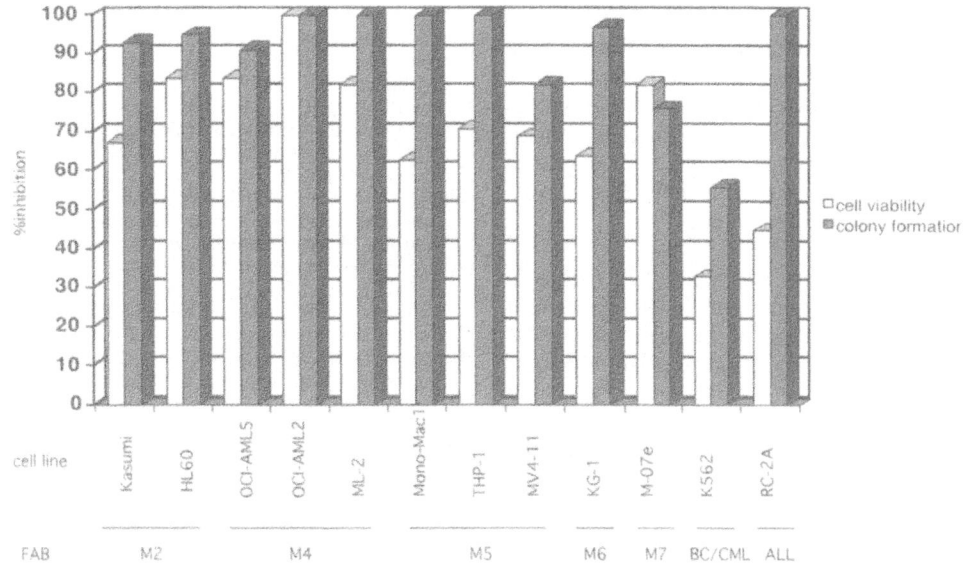

**Fig. 8.** Effect of FTase and PPTMase inhibitors on growth of myeloid leukemia cell lines. 2.5 x 10⁵ cells were incubated for 96 hours with FTase (100 μM) or PPMTase (25 μM) inhibitors.

biting the growth of myeloid leukemia cell lines. The FTase inhibitor 2, which was very effective in reverting the transformed phenotype of L61-H-Ras NIH3T3 fibroblasts, had only a minor effect on cell growth of the majority of leukemic cell lines tested, including those with activating N-Ras mutations. However, FPTase inhibitor 3 inhibited growth of several leukemic cells (e.g. THP-1) by 95-100% (Fig. 8).

## Discussion

There is accumulating evidence supporting the role of the deregulation of Ras function in the molecular pathogenesis of myeloid leukemias (Denny et al. 1994, Byrne et al. 1998). Elevated signaling through the Ras to MAP kinase cascade may lead to increased proliferation or inhibition of apoptosis. Using NIH3T3 fibroblasts as a model, we demonstrate that H-Ras-induced transformation and activation of the MAP kinase cascade are dependent upon both the expression levels and the type of the mutationally activated Ras proteins. Treatment with the MEK inhibitor PD 098059 resulted in a reversion of the Ras-

induced transformation and an inhibition of MAP kinases. This finding is consistent with earlier results showing reversion of the Ras-transformed phenotype in Balb3T3 mouse fibroblasts and rat kidney cells (Dudley et al. 1995). Moreover, we demonstrate a constitutive activation of the MAP kinase cascade in at least 5 out of 10 myeloid leukemia cell lines. This finding underscores the role of deregulated Ras to MAP kinase signaling in myeloid leukemias. Although leukemogenesis is a multi-step process involving different oncogenes and tumor suppressor genes, these observations are of considerable potential usefulness for therapy since the inhibition of oncogenic Ras function and signaling is a very promising pharmacological strategy (Gibbs & Oliff 1997, Omer & Kohl 1997, Heimbrook & Oliff 1998). We observed that treatment with MEK inhibitor PD 098059 resulted in a significant reduction in cell viability and colony formation in all leukemia cell lines tested. Most FTase inhibitors were less effective in the inhibition of leukemia cell growth. However, certain FTase inhibitors (e.g. FPTase inhibitor 3) and PPMTase inhibitor FTS showed strong inhibition of growth of several myeloid leukemia cell lines. This fin-

107

ding suggests a more specific mechanism of action of the inhibitors of post-translational modification of Ras than the MEK inhibitor PD 098059, which shows a strong, uniform inhibitory effect on all cell lines. In conclusion, our results suggest a potential role of inhibitors of Ras signaling in the future treatment of myeloid leukemias.

*Acknowledgments.* We thank Dr. Kristine A. Henningfeld for preparation of figures and for critical reading of the manuscript. We thank Natalja Möbius for excellent technical assistance.

This work was supported by a grant from the Deutsche Forschungsgemeinschaft (Re 864/4-1) and a grant from the University of Ulm (P.541).

# References

Bollag G, Clapp DW, Shih S, Adler F, Zhang YY, Thompson P (1996) Loss of NF1 results in activation of the Ras signalling pathway and leads to aberrant growth in haematopoietic cells. Nature Genetics 12: 144-148

Bos JL (1989) Ras oncogenes in human cancer: a review. Cancer Res. 49: 4682-4689

Bradford MM (1976) A rapid and sensitive method for the quantitation of microgram quantities of proteins utilizing the principle of protein-dye binding. Anal. Biochem. 72: 248-254

Byrne JL, Marshall CJ (1998) The molecular pathophysiology of myeloid leukemias: Ras revisited. Br. J. Haematol. 100: 256-264

Carlberg K, Rohrschneider L (1994) The effect of activating mutations on dimerization, tyrosine phosphorylation and internalization of the macrophage colony stimulating factor receptor. Mol. Cell. Biol. 5: 81-95

Clark GJ & Der CJ (1995) Ras proto-oncogene activation in human malignancy. In: Garrett CT, Sell S (eds) Cellular cancer markers. Humana Press, Totowa, New Jersey, pp 17-52

Cortez D, Kadlec L, Pendergast A (1995) Structural and signalling requirements for BCR-Abl mediated transformation and inhibition of apoptosis. Mol. Cell. Biol. 15: 5531-5541

Dudley DT, Pang L, Decker SJ, Bridges AJ, Saltiel AR (1995) A synthetic inhibitor of the mitogen-activated protein kinase cascade. Proc. Natl. Acad. Sci. U.S.A. 92: 7686-7689

Gibbs JB & Oliff A (1997) The potential of farnesyltransferase inhibitors as cancer chemotherapeutics. Annu. Rev. Pharmacol. Toxicol. 37: 143-166

Golub T, Barker G, Lovett M, Gilliland D (1994) Fusion of PDGF receptor beta to a novel ets-like gene, tel, in chronic myelomonocytic leukemia with t(5;12) chromosomal translocation. Cell 77: 307-316

Heimbrook DC & Oliff A (1998) Therapeutic intervention and signaling. Curr. Opin. Cell Biol. 10: 284-288

Kitayama H, Kanakura Y, Furitsu T, Tsujimura T, Oritani K, Ikeda H, Sugahara H, Mitsui H, Kanayama Y, Kitamura Y, Matsuzawa Y (1995) Constitutively activating mutations of c-Kit receptor tyrosine kinase confer factor-independent growth and tumorigenicity of factor-dependent hematopoietic cell lines. Blood 85: 790-798

Marshall CJ (1996) Ras effectors. Curr. Biol. 8: 197-204

Omer CA & Kohl NE (1997) CA1A2X-competitive inhibitors of farnesyltransferase as anti-cancer agents. TIBS 18: 437-444

Reuter C, Auf der Landwehr U I, Auf der Landwehr U II, Schleyer E, Zühlsdorf M, Ameling C, Rolf C, Wörmann B, Büchner T, Hiddemann W (1994) Modulation of intracellular metabolism of cytosine arabinoside in acute myeloid leukemia by granulocyte-macrophage colony stimulating factor. Leukemia 8: 217-225

Reuter CWM, Catling AD and Weber MJ (1995) Immune complex kinase assays for mitogen-activated protein kinase and MEK. Methods Enzymol. 205: 245-256

Reuter CWM, Catling AD, Jelinek T & Weber MJ (1995) Biochemical analysis of MEK activation in NIH3T3 fibroblasts. J. Biol. Chem. 270: 7644-7655

Sawyers CL, Denny CT (1994) Chronic myelomonocytic leukemia: Tel-a-kinase what ets all about. Cell 77: 171-173

Towatari M, Iida H, Tanimoto M, Iwata H, Hamaguchi M, Saito H (1997) Constitutive activation of mitogen-activated protein kinase pathway in acute leukemia cells. Leukemia 11: 479-484

Xu G, O'Connell P, Viskochil D, Cawthon R, Robertson M, Culver M, Dunn D, Stevens J, Gesteland R, White R, Weiss R (1990) The neurofibromatosis type 1 gene encodes a protein related to GAP. Cell 62: 599-608

# C-Jun is a JNK-Independent Coactivator of the PU.1 Transcription Factor

G. Behre[1,2], A. J. Whitmarsh[3], M. P. Coghlan[4], T. Hoang[5], C. L. Carpenter[4], D.-E. Zhang[2], R. J. Davis[3], W. Hiddemann[1] and D. G. Tenen[2]

The ETS domain transcription factor PU.1 is necessary for the development of monocytes and regulates, in particular, the expression of the monocyte-specific macrophage colony-stimulating factor (M-CSF) receptor, which is critical for monocytic cell survival, proliferation, and differentiation. The bZIP transcription fact c-Jun, which is part of the AP-1 transcription factor complex, is also important for monocytic differentiation, but the monocyte-specific M-CSF receptor promoter has no AP-1 consensus binding sites. We asked the question of whether c-Jun could promote the induction of the M-CSF receptor by collaborating with PU.1. We demonstrate that c-Jun enhances the ability of PU.1 to transactivate the M-CSF receptor promoter as well as a minimal thymidine kinase promoter containing only PU.1 DNA binding sites (Fig. 1). c-Jun does not directly bind to the M-CSF receptor promoter but associates via its basic domain with the ETS domain of PU.1 (Fig. 2). Consistent with our observation that AP-1 binding does not contribute to c-Jun coac-

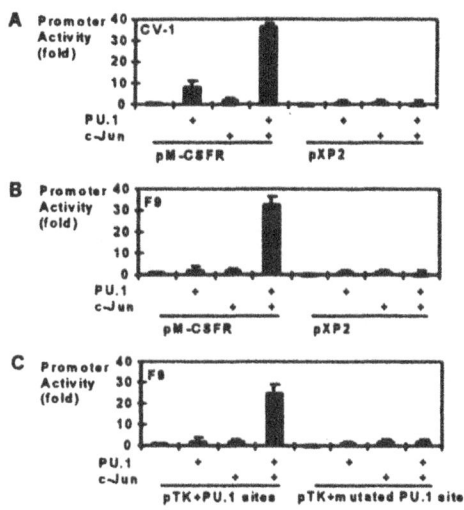

**Fig. 1**

tivation is the observation that the activation of PU.1 by c-Jun is blocked by overexpression of c-Fos (Fig. 3). Phosphorylation of c-Jun by c-Jun NJ2-terminal kinase on Ser-63 and -73

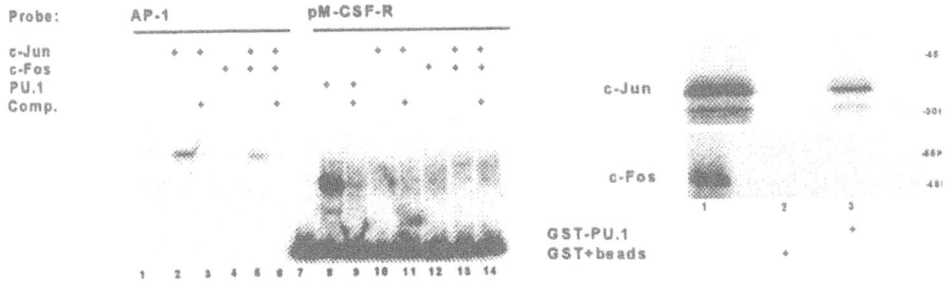

**Fig. 2**

[1]Med III, LMU University Hospital Grosshadern and KKG Leukemia, GSF, Munich, Germany
[2] Harvard Medical School and Divisions of Hematology/Oncology[2] and Signal Transduction[4], Beth Israel Deaconess Medical Center, Boston, MA, USA; Dept. of Biochemistry and Molecular Biology, University of Massachusetts Medical School, Worcester, MA, USA[3]; and the Clinical Research Institute of Montreal, Montreal, Quebec, Canada[5] (gbehre@gmx.de).

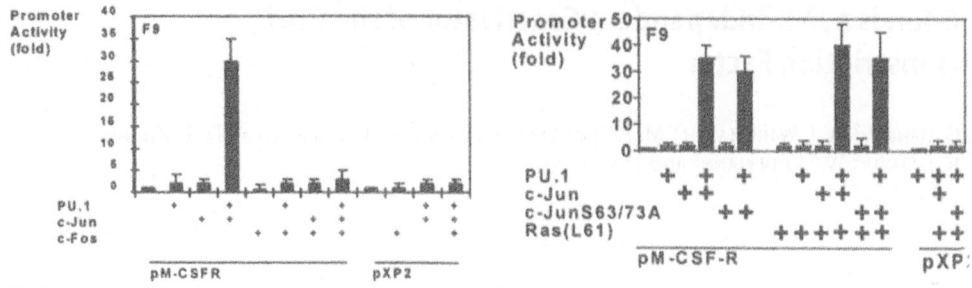

**Fig. 3**

**Fig. 4**

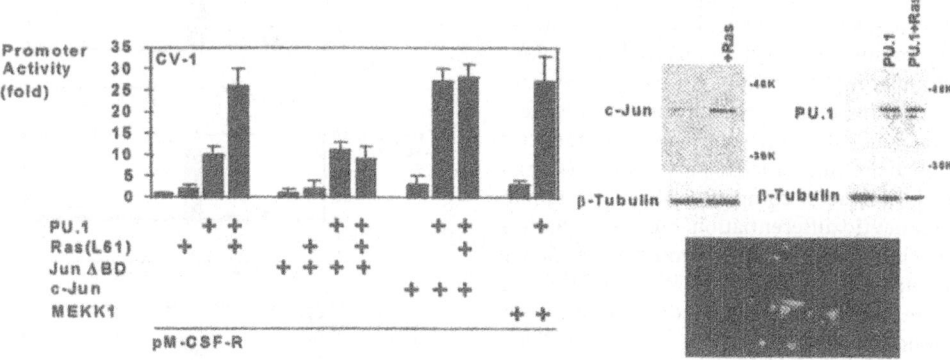

**Fig. 5**

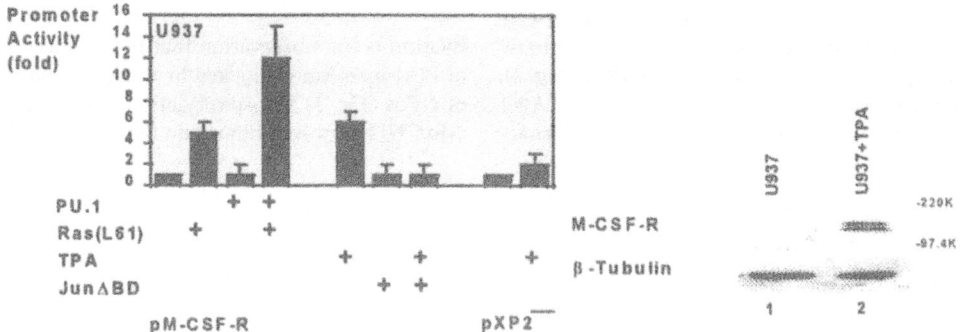

**Fig. 6**

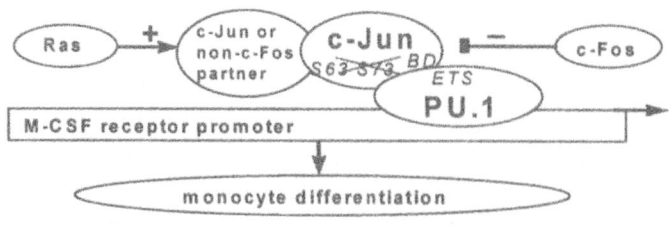

**Fig. 7**

does not alter the ability of c-Jun to enhance PU.1 transactivation (Fig. 4). Activated Ras enhances the transcriptional activity of PU.1 by up-regulating c-Jun expression without changing the phosphorylation pattern of PU.1 (Fig. 5). The activation of PU.1 by Ras is blocked by a mutant c-Jun protein lacking the basic domain (Fig. 5). The expression of this mutant form of c-Jun also completely blocks 12-O-tetradecanoylphorbol-13-acetate-induced M-CSF receptor promoter activity during monocytic differentiation (Fig. 6). We propose therefore that c-Jun acts as a c-Jun NH2-terminal kinase-independent coactivator of PU.1, resulting in M-CSF receptor expression and development of the monocyclic lineage (Fig. 7).

# CD7+ and CD56+ Acute Myelogenous Leukemia is a Distinct Biologic and Clinical Disease Entity

C.Kahl, A.Florschütz, S.Leuner, K. Jentsch-Ullrich, A.Franke, C.R. Bartram #
and H.-G.Höffkes

Abstract. The rapid progress of diagnostic tools contributes to better understanding of biology and management of acute myelogenous leukemia. Some reports described a high incidence of extramedullary manifestation and a significant shorter survival in patients (pts.) with CD7+ and CD56+ co-expression of AML-blasts. Thus, retrospectively 12 cases of myeloid/natural killer cell precursor phenotype AML diagnosed between 7/95 -3/98 were analysed (5 men and 7 women varying from 30 to 85 years of age, median 57,9 years). Extramedullary involvement was evident at initial presenting in 4 cases (one pts. sulcus coronaris penis, three involvement of CNS). Six of the pts. had a high leukocytes concentration (> 30 Gpt/l). At time of presentation the majority (11 pts.) of pts. had circulating blasts. According to the FAB classification 5 cases were classified as FAB M0 or M1. Expression of CD13/CD33/CD38/CD56/CD7 and HLA-DR without other NK-, T-cell and B-cell marker as well as MPO+/LF- was observed. Five out of the 12 pts. presented a germline configuration of the T-cell receptor β, γ, δ, and Ig heavy chain and Ig k gene by Southern blotting. Only five pts. were successfully treated with aggressive induction chemotherapy (cytarabine and anthracycline) and achieved complete or partial remission, whereas 7 pts. were refractory to induction chemotherapy. Median overall survival for the group was 4,5 month. The data presented suggest that the myeloid/natural killer cell precursor phenotype AML constitute a distinct biologic and clinical disease entity with worse clinical prognosis. It seems to be important to distinguish CD7/CD56 positive AML from other subtypes for the development of novel therapeutic approaches for this entity.

## Introduction

Exact diagnosis of acute myelogenous leukemia (AML) needs detailed information of morphology, immunophenotype and chromosomal alterations [20]. Karyotypic abnormalities such as t(8; 21) and t (15;17) are of prognostic importance to clinical outcome [20]. Immunophenotyping identifies lineage specifity and stage of maturation [11]. One of the most expressed so-called pan T-cell antigens by AML blasts is CD7 which appears at a very early stage of maturation and is thought to be originated from the immature hematopoetic stem cell [3]. This subtype has been described as CD7+ AML and is associated with leukocytosis, low response to chemotherapy and poor prognosis. Furthermore, expression of CD56 is a rare phenomenon in lymphoid malignancies and mostly restricted to malignancies of T/NK cell origin [21]. In AML, CD56 expression has been identified in approximately 20% of all cases [21] and is generally associated with cytogenetic abnormalities, like t(8; 21) or trisomy 8 [21, 22]. Because the CD56 antigen has been found to correspond to a neural cell adhesion molecule, its expression in leukemia or lymphoma cells is thought to play an important role in their extranodal localisation [8, 12, 21].

Recently, Suzuki et al. published a series of 7 cases of CD7+/CD33+/CD34+/CD56+ and frequently HLA-DR+ acute leukemia of con-

Division of Hematology/Oncology, Department of Medicine, Otto-von-Guericke-University of Magdeburg, Germany
# Institute of Humangenetics, University of Heidelberg, Germany

ceivable myeloid and NK cell precursor phenotype [23]. All patients have had an extramedullary involvement, represented by peripheral lymphadenopathy and/or mediastinal bulk masses. On the other hand CD56 is identical to a neural cell adhesion molecule (NCAM) and is expressed mainly on neural tissues [10]. Hatano et al. reported the rare case of acute myelogenous leukemia as an intracranial myeloblastoma, where the blasts expressed CD7/CD56 [8]. Thus, 12 cases of AML of conceivable myeloid/NK precursor phenotype (i.e., CD7/CD13/CD33/CD38/CD56/HLA-DR) with no NK-, T-cell or B-cell marker were re-analysed. At time of presentation the majority of patients (11 pts.) had peripheral blasts and extramedullary involvement was evident as primary symptom in 4 cases. Most of the patients were refractory to induction therapy (Ara-C and anthracycline) and the median overall survival was 4,5 month.

## Material and Methods

### Patients

During a period of 3 years (1995-1998) 12 cases of CD7/CD56 double positive myeloid/NK precursor acute leukaemia were diagnosed. These cases (8%) were identified from 150 cases of complete immunophenotyped acute leukaemias. The clinical records and pathologic findings of these cases were reported.

### Morphology

Bone marrow aspirates or peripheral blood cells underwent May-Grünwald-Giemsa (MG), MPO, alpha-naphthol AS-D chloroacetate esterase, alpha-naphthyl butyrate (BN) esterase and periodic acid-Schiff (PAS) staining. Biopsied tissues were fixed in 10% formaldehyde and embedded in paraffin. Section were cut at 5 mm and stained with hematoxylin and eosin, PAS MG.

### Immunophenotyping

Surface and intracytoplasmatic immunophenotyping were performed by flow cytometry using a broad panel of antibodies (see Table 1). Mononuclear cells were separated from heparinized bone marrow or blood samples using Ficoll-Hypaque centrifugation and cells were analyzed on FACSCalibur (Becton-Dickinson (BDIS), Germany). The antibody panel was CD33/CD65/CD13, CD34/CD117/HLA-DR, CD45/CD14/CD20, CD19/CD14/CD64, CD2/CD56/CD7 and intracytoplasmatic Myeloperoxydase/Lactoferrin [14].

**Table 1.** Antibody panel used for three colour immunophenotyping of acute myelogenous leukemia

| FITC | PE | PerCP/PeCy5 |
|---|---|---|
| CD45 (2 0 1) | CD14 (M j P 9) | CD20 (L 27) |
| CD34 (8 G 12) | CD38 (Hb-7) | HLA-DR (L243) |
| CDw65 (88 H7) | CD33 (P67 .6) | CD13 (WM-47) |
| CD15 (MMA) | CD117 (104 D2) | CD16 (3 G 8) |
| CD2 (MT910) | CD14 (M j P 9) | CD64 (32.2) |
| CD7 (4H9) | CD56 (My 31) | CD19 (SJ25C1) |
| IZMPO (H-43.5) | IZ lactoferrin (3C5) | |

### Cytogenetic analysis

Pretreatment bone marrow cells or peripheral blood cells were cultured in PRMI1640 supplemented with 20% fetal calf serum without mitogens for 72 hours and incubated with colcemid at a final concentration of 0,02 µg/ml KCL solution for 20 minutes at room temperature and fixed with methanol-acetic acid (3:1). Chromosomes were banded using the trypsin-Giemsa method.

### Southern blot analysis

High molecular weight DNA was isolated from cryopreserved leukemic cells and analyzed by Southern blotting using standard techniques. To demonstrated Ig gene rearrangements, BgIII and HindIII digests were hybridized with a 2.5 kb EcoRI-BgIII JH probe [24] and BamHI digest with a 5.7 kb BamHI-EcoRI Jk probe[9]. TCRβ genes were studied on EcoRI and BamHI digests with a

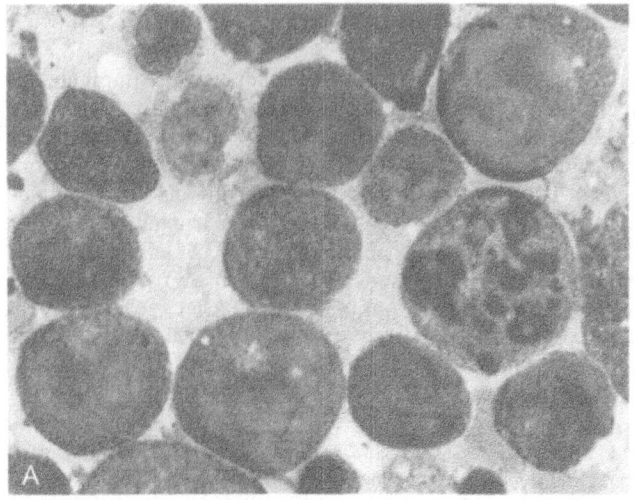

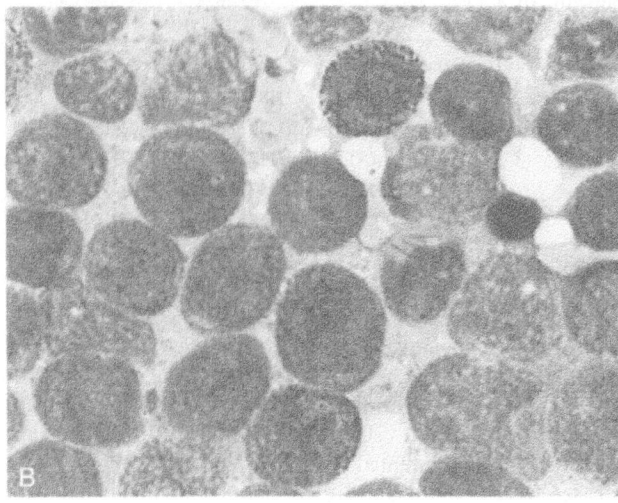

**Fig. 1.** Morphologic features of myeloid/NK cell precursor acute leukemia. MG-stained bone marrow smears of patient no. 12 (A). The leukemic cells show a variable nucleocytoplasmatic ratio, have a round or oval nucleus, the cytoplasm contains Auer rods. (B) Morphologic findings of patient 9 with AML-M3. The predominant cell is the highly abnormal promyelocyte. The cytoplasm is tightly packed with coarse red or purple granules.

0.7 kb BglII-PstI fragment containing Cβ1 segments, where TCRγ genes were investigated on EcoRI blots with a 1.0 kb PstI-EcoRI Jγ2 fragment hybridizing to both Jγ1 and Jγ2 segments. To investigate the TCRδ gene configuration, BglII and HindIII digest were hybridized to a 873 bp HindIII-EcoRI Jδ1 gene segment [4].

## Results

### Clinical features

The clinical features of the 12 patients are summarised in Table 2. Five men and seven women, aged from 30 to 85 years with a median of 57,9 years were included. Six of the pts. had initial high leukocytes (> 30 Gpt/l) counts. At time of diagnosis, circulating blast cells were observed in 11 pts, thrombocytopenia in 11 pts. and all pts. were anaemic (Hb < 7,0 mmol/l). Primary extramedullary involvement was observed in 4 pts. (nos. 1, 6, 9, 12), of which three showed central-nervous involvement. Patient No. 12 who had a primary intracranial manifestation of the acute myelogenous leukemia, manifesting with neurological impairment (impairment of visus and occurrence of double pictures). Cranial-computertomography showed an intracranial tumor and histological examination demon-

**Table 2.** Pretreatment Presentation of Patients with Myeloid/NK Cell Precursor Acute Leukemia

| No. | Age/Sex | Hb mmol/l | Ptl Gpt/l | WBC Gpt/l | Blasts % | extramedullary involvement |
|-----|---------|-----------|-----------|-----------|----------|----------------------------|
| 1.  | 39/F    | 5,5       | 91        | 171,2     | 91       | meningeosis leukemica      |
| 2.  | 69/M    | 6,0       | 38        | 1,7       | 0        | no                         |
| 3.  | 60/M    | 4,6       | 51        | 80,2      | 92       | no                         |
| 4.  | 75/F    | 5,6       | 124       | 2,8       | 26       | no                         |
| 5.  | 30/M    | 6,7       | 216       | 207,6     | 88       | no                         |
| 6.  | 73/F    | 4,3       | 19        | 91,03     | 1        | meningeosis leukemica      |
| 7.  | 59/F    | 6,9       | 70        | 194       | 98       | no                         |
| 8.  | 85/F    | 6,8       | 55        | 6,1       | 14       | no                         |
| 9.  | 47/M    | 6,5       | 57        | 1,1       | 21       | sulcus coronarius penis    |
| 10. | 66/M    | 5,7       | 43        | 139,1     | 98       | no                         |
| 11. | 39/F    | 6,0       | 47        | 5,9       | 22       | no                         |
| 12. | 53/F    | 5,8       | 55        | 5,3       | 54       | intracerebral tumor        |

strated myeloid blast cells. Patient No. 9 suffered from a balanoposthitis which did not respond to antibiotics and ambulatory treatment. The histological examination of tumor lesion showed blast cells as a first manifestation of AML.

## Morphology

The bone marrow or peripheral blood smears of all pts. showed blasts cells of various size. The blasts are large with a variable nucleocytoplasmatic ratio, they have a round or oval nucleus, one or more nucleoli and the cytoplasm contains Auer rods. The blasts are positive for MPO (Fig. 1A). Patients No. 9 had the typical morphology of AML-M3 with the predominant abnormal promyelocyte (Fig.1B). According to the FAB classification 5 cases

were M0 or M1 (Pts. no 4, 5, 6, 7, 8) and 4 Pts. had a myelomonocytic (M4) or monocytic (M5) (Pts. no 1, 3, 10, 11) one Pts. (Pts. no. 12) had a AML-M2 AML. One Pts. had a MDS RAEB-t (Pts. no 2) [2].

## Immunophenotyping

The immunophenotypes of all twelve cases are listed in Table 3. All cases expressed the natural-killer cell antigen CD56 and the T-cell lymphoid antigen CD7. In addition all pts. expressed two of the typical myeloid antigens CD13/CD33/CD65 (Fig. 2) and all were MPO+/LF- as well. Cytoplasmatic CD79a and CD3 were negative and all cases were negative for other B- or T-cell antigens (CD19, CD20, CD22, CD2, CD3, CD5).

**Table 3.** Immunophenotyping Findings in Patients with Myeloid/NK Cell Precursor Acute Leukemia (Value are expressed as percentage of cells for each marker)

| No. | CD7  | CD13 | CD33 | CD38 | CD56 | HLA-DR | MPO  |
|-----|------|------|------|------|------|--------|------|
| 1.  | 94,7 | 92,1 | 92,5 | 98,2 | 28,4 |        | 77,2 |
| 2.  | 77,1 | 76,2 | 77,7 | 96,4 | 78,5 | 62,8   | 64,2 |
| 3.  | 72,8 | 65,3 | 85,0 | 95,2 | 55,9 | 66,1   | 78,2 |
| 4.  | 82,9 | 70,8 | 69,2 | 92,2 | 45,5 | 68,6   | 1,8  |
| 5.  | 91,3 | 96,2 | 92,3 | 97,4 | 39,9 | ND     | 1,4  |
| 6.  | 18,6 | 19,0 | 95,4 | 97,5 | 92,3 | 11,2   | 92,7 |
| 7.  | 99,1 | 62,0 | 97,6 | 99,4 | 18,1 | 37,5   | 95,6 |
| 8.  | 75,9 | 53,2 | 43,6 | 93,2 | 51,7 | 48,0   | 46,0 |
| 9.  | 87,2 | 69,4 | 69,5 | 91,2 | 71,3 | 25,6   | 58,9 |
| 10. | 96,2 | 24,6 | 90,2 | 97,8 | 94,0 | 94,6   | 92,2 |
| 11. | 52,4 | 72,9 | 83,7 | 92,5 | 41,4 | 32,0   | 9,0  |
| 12. | 76,4 | 65,9 | 78,4 | 66,9 | 64,0 | 33,5   | 33,2 |

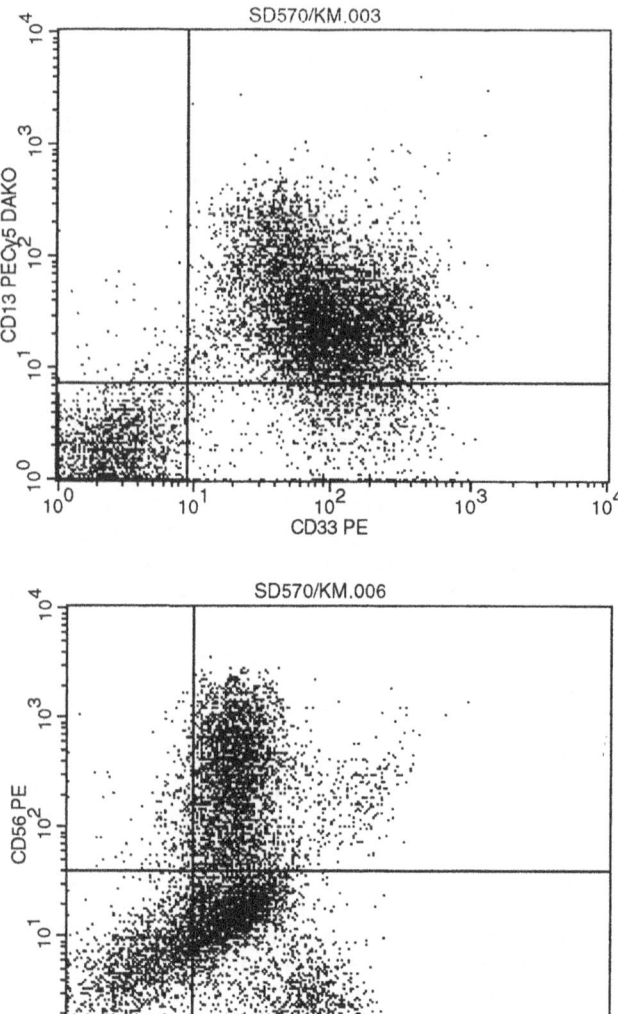

**Fig. 2.** Typical flow cytometric analysis of CD13/CD33/CD38/HLA-DR and CD7/CD56 in pts. with Myeloid/NK Cell Precursor Acute Leukemia (patient no. 12).

### Genotypic analysis

The results are listed in Table 4. In five out of the 12 pts. Southern blotting were done. No clonal rearrangements of the TCR β, γ and δ chain genes or the Ig H and the Ig k gene were detected.

### Cytogenetic analysis

The results of cytogenetic examinations are listed in Table 5. In 10 out of 12 pts. cytogene-

tic analysis was available (83,3%). Two of them have had a normal karyotype (no.4, 6), patient No.9 with AML FAB M3 showed the typical genetic aberration t(15,17). All other pts. have had complex cytogenetic aberration with trisome chromosomes, hyperploide or hypertetraploide metaphasis.

### Therapy and clinical course

Therapy, clinical response and overall survival (OS) are listed in Table 6. Majority of pts.

**Table 4.** Genotyping Findings in Patients with Myeloid/ NK Cell Precursor Acute Leukemia using Southern blotting

| Pts.-No | IgH | Ig κ | TCR β | TCR γ | TCR δ |
|---------|-----|------|-------|-------|-------|
| 1. | G | G | G | G | G |
| 2. | ND | ND | ND | ND | ND |
| 3. | ND | ND | ND | ND | ND |
| 4. | ND | ND | ND | ND | ND |
| 5. | ND | ND | ND | ND | ND |
| 6. | ND | ND | ND | ND | ND |
| 7. | G | G | G | G | G |
| 8. | ND | ND | ND | ND | ND |
| 9. | G | G | G | G | G |
| 10. | G | G | G | G | G |
| 11. | G | G | G | G | G |
| 12. | ND | ND | ND | ND | ND |

Abbreviations: IgH, Ig heavy chain, G; germline; TCR, t-cell receptor; ND not determinated

**Table 5.** Cytogenetic Findings in Patients with Myeloid/ NK Cell Precursor Acute Leukemia

1. 45, XX
2. n.d.
3. 45, XY, t(3;17)(q21; p13), -7, der(9)T(9;?)(q34;ß)
4. 46, XX
5. 47, XY,+8, t(9;22)(q34;q11)
6. 46, XX
7. 47, XX, +8, t(9,11)(p22,q23)[10]/46, XX,del7(q32),t(9;11)(p22,q23)[2]
8. n.d.
9. 46, XY,t(15,17)
10. 46, XY,t(11,14)(11q,14q),t(9p,11)
11. 46, XX , t(3,3)(q21;q26); inc[13], 46 XX; inc[1]
12. 46, XX[2], hypoploide, hyperploide, hypertetra-ploide

(10 pts.) received aggressive induction chemotherapy consisting of Ara-C and anthracycline (Ara-C 100 mg/m$^2$ /24h day 1-7; daunorubicine 45 mg/m$^2$ day 3-5, e.g. Ara-C 2g/m$^2$ day 1,3,5,7, idarubucine 12 mg/m$^2$ day 1-3) . Two pts. (no. 6, 8) received palliative chemotherapy (vepeside p.o. e.g. Ara-C s.c.). The patient (no. 9) suffering from AML-M3 was treated with ATRA and induction therapy. Two pts. (no. 9, 12) received local radiation because of centralnervous manifestation. Five pts. were successfully treated and achieved complete or partial remission (no. 3, 4, 9, 11, 12) whereas 7 pts. were refractory to chemotherapy and had refractory disease. Median overall survival for this group was 4,5 month.

## Discussion

In the present study the twelve described cases of acute myelogenous leukemia were characterized by distinct morphologic, immunophenotypic, genotypic and clinical features. All leukemic cells showed immature immunophenotypic appearance with typical expression of two myeloid antigens CD13/CD33/CD65 and were MPO+/LF- with co-expression of CD7/CD56. The phenotype of NK cell progenitor cells is considered to be CD34+, CD33+, CD7+, CD2+/-, CD56-, whereas mature NK cell are CD34-, CD33-, CD7-, CD2+/-, CD56+. The cases presented showed a different phenotype compared to the phe-

**Table 6.** Therapeutic Response and Clinical Outcome in Patients with Myeloid/NK Cell Precursor Acute Leukemia (abbreviation: CR-complete remission, PR partial remission, NC no change, PD progressive disease)

| No. | Age/Sex | FAB | Treatment | Response | Survival (month) |
|-----|---------|-----|-----------|----------|------------------|
| 1. | 39/F | M5a | Ara-C, idarubicine | PD | 0 |
| 2. | 69/M | MDS-RAEB-t | Ara-C, daunorubicine | NC | 6 |
| 3. | 60/M | M4 | Ara-C, daunorubicine | PR | 7 |
| 4. | 75/F | M1 | Ara-C, daunorubicine | CR | 12 |
| 5. | 30/M | M0 | Ara-C, idarubicine | PD | 0 |
| 6. | 73/F | M1 | Ara-C | PD | 0 |
| 7. | 59/F | M0 | Ara-C, daunorubicine | PD | 0 |
| 8. | 85/F | M0 | vepeside oral | NC | 7 |
| 9. | 47/M | M3 | ATRA, Ara-C, idarubicine | CR | 9 |
| 10. | 66/M | M5 | Ara-C, daunorubicine | PD | 1 |
| 11. | 39/F | M4 | Ara-C, idarubicine | CR | 5 |
| 12. | 53/F | M2 | Ara-C, idarubicine | CR | 8 |

notypes mentioned above. One of the main clinical features of this series is the high incidence of extramedullary involvement of the myeloid/NK precursor AML (central nervous involvement: n=3 and one patient with a balanoposthitis). These clinical, immunophenotypic and genotypic findings showed that the immunological myeloid/NK cell type of acute myelogenous leukemia appear to be a distinct clinicopathological entity.

Recently, Suzuki et al. described seven cases of myeloid/NK precursor AML which were CD7/CD33/CD34/CD56 and (frequently) HLA-DR positive [23]. Leukemic cells showed not rearrangement in the TCR-beta, TCR-gamma and IgH genes. The authors concluded that the blasts might be phenotypically identical to those of myeloid/NK cell precursor phenotype. The incidence of extramedullary involvement were high and the therapeutic response and therefore the clinical outcome were very limited. In this series, five pts. showed clinical response to induction chemotherapy and achieved a CR or PR. Nevertheless, overall survival (OS) was very short (4,5 month).

In the present series, five pts. have had features that classify the AML M0 or M1 according to FAB classification. AML FAB-M0 is charaterized by immature lymphoblastoid morphology, expression of myeloid antigens, lack of T- or B-cell antigens, complex karyotype and poor prognosis. CD7 was found in about 40% whereas CD56 expression has not been described [6, 26]. It is possible that some AML-M0 might be classifiable as myeloid/NK precursor acute leukemia but this needs further investigations.

Extramedullary involvement of AML is a rare complication, Kurtzberg et al. described a population of CD7+, CD4-, CD8- acute leukemias with high incidence of extramedullary involvement and poor prognosis but unfortunately CD56 co-expression was not investigated [15]. Suzuki et al. described seven cases of CD7/CD56 positive myeloid/NK cell precursor AML, again, with high incidence of extramedullary involvement [23].

CD56 is a cell adhesion molecule and therefore its expression on tumor cells is supposed to play an important role in extramedullary localisation of AML. In a review

Byrd et al. described CD56 as possible prognostic risk factor for extramedullary involvement [5] but other investigators did not confirm the findings [21, 25].

In this report, seven cases showed no clinical response to aggressive chemotherapy (Ara-C and anthracycline) and patients died within 0-7 month (median overall survival (OS) of 4,5 month). These results and the high incidence of extramedullary involvement support the clinicopathological concept of a myeloid/NK cell precursor acute leukemia and the need for alternative therapeutic concepts.

## References

1. Baer MR, Stewart CC, Lawrence D, Arthur DC, Mrozek K, Strout MP, Davey FR, Schiffer CA, Bloomfield CD (1998) Acute myeloid leukemia with 11q23 translocations: myelomonocytic immunophenotype by multiparameter flow cytometry. Leukemia 12(3), 317-325
2. Bennett JM, Catovsky D, Daniel MT, Flandrin G, Galton DAG, Gralnick M, Sultan C (1985) Proposed revised criteria for the classification of the acute leukemia: a report of the French-American-British group. Ann Intern Med 103: 626-629
3. Bradstock KF, Kirk J, Grimsey PG, Karbral A, Hughes WG (1989). Unusual immunophenotypes in acute leukemias: Incidence and clinical correlations. Br J Haematol 72: 512-518
4. Breit TM, Wolvers-Tettero IL, Beishuizen A, Verhoeven MA, van Wering ER, van Dongen JJ 1993 Southern blot patterns, frequencies, and junctional diversity of T-cell receptor-delta gene rearrangements in acute lymphoblastic leukemia. Blood 82: 3063-3074
5. Byrd JC, Edenfield WJ, Shields DJ, Dawson NA (1995). Extramedullary meyloid cell tumors in acute nonlymphocytic leukemia: A clinical review. J Clin Oncol 13: 1800-1816
6. Cadwell FJ, Burns P, Dick FR, Jones MP, Heckman KD, Weiner GJ, Goeken JA (1993) Minimally differentiated acute leukemia. Leuk Res 17: 199-206
7. Gale RP, Bassat IB (1988) Hybride acute leukemia. Br J Haematol 65: 261-264
8. Hatano Y, Miura I, Horiuchi T, Hoshi N, Nanjou, Masuda H, Miura AB (1997) Cerebellar myeloblastoma formation in CD7-positive, neural cell adhesion molecule (CD56)-positive acute myelogenous leukemia (M1). Ann Hematol 75: 125-128
9. Hieter PA, Minzel JV, Leder P (1982) Evolution of human immunoglobulin κ J region genes. J Biol Chem 257: 1516-1522
10. Iizuka Y, Aiso M, Kanemaru M, Kawamura M, Takeuchi J, Horikoshi A, Ohsima T, Mizoguchi H, Horie T (1992) Myeloblastoma formation in acute myeloid leukemia. Leuk Res 16: 665-671
11. Jennings CD, Foon KA. Recent advances in Flow Cytometry (1997) Application to the diagnostis of hematologic malignancy. Blood 90: 2863-2892

12. Kern WF, Spier CM, Hannemann EH, Miller TP, Matzner M, Grogan TM. Neural cell adhesion molecule-positive peripheral T-cell lymphoma (1992) A rare variant with a propensitiy for unusual sides of involvement. Blood 79: 2432-2437

13. Kita K, Miwa H, Nakase K, Kawakami K, Kobayashi T, Shirakawa S, Tanaka I, Ohta C, Tsutani H, Oguma S, Kyo T, Dohy H, Kamada N, Nasu K, Uchino H (1993) Clinical importance of CD7 expression in acute myelogenous leukemia. Blood 81: 2399-2405

14. Knapp W, Majdic O, Strobl H. Flow cytometric analysis of intracellular myeloperoxidase and lactoferrin in leukemia diagnosis. In: Recent Advances in Cell Biology of Acute Leukemia - Impact on Clinical Diagnosis and Therapy. Ludwig WD, Thiel E eds. Recent Results in Cancer Research, Springer Verlag Berlin Heidelberg; 131: 31-40

15. Kurtzberg J, Waldmann TA, Davey MP, Bigner SH, Moore JO, Hershfield MS, Haynes BF (1989) CD7+, CD4-, CD8- acute leukemia: A syndrome of malignant pluripotent lymphohematopoetic cells. Blood 73: 381- 390

16. Lo-Coco F, De Rossi G, Pasqualetti D, Lopez M, Diverio D, Latagliata R, Fenu S, Mangelli F (1989) CD7-positive acute myelogenous leukemia: a subtype associated with cell immaturity. Br J Haematol 73: 480-485

17. Loughran TP (1993) Clonal disease of large granular lymphocytes. Blood 82: 1-14

18. Reust-Borst MA, Steinke B, Waller HD, Buhring HJ, Muller CA (1992) Phenotypic and clinical heterogeneity of CD56-positive acute-non-lymphoblastic leukemia. Ann Hematol 64: 78-82

19. Scott AA, Head DR, Kopecky KJ, Appelbaum FR, Theil KS, Grever MR, Whittaker MH, Griffith BB, Licht JD, Grogan TM, Willmann CL (1994) HLA-DR-, CD33+, CD56+, CD16- myeloid/natural killer cell acute leukemia: A previously unrecognized form of acute leukemia potentially misdiagnosed as French-American-British acute myeloid leukemia-M3. Blood 84: 244-255

20. Second MIC Cooperative Study Group (1988) Morphologic, immunologic and cytogenetic (MIC) working classification of the acute myelogenous leukemias. Cancer Gen Cytogen 30: 1-15

21. Seymour JF, Pierce SA, Kantarjian HM, Keating MJ, Estey EH (1993) Neural cell adhesion molecule (CD56) is associated with FAB subtyp, cytogenetic and skin infiltration in acute myelogenous leukemia (AML). Blood 82 (suppl.1), 126a

22. Seymour JF, Pierce SA, Kantarjian HM, Keating MJ, Estey EH (1994) Investigation of karyotypic, morphological and clinical features in patients with Acute Myeloid Leukemia blast cells expressing the neural cell adhesion molecule (CD56). Leukemia 8: 823-826

23. Suzuki R, Yamamoto K, Seto M, Kagami Y, Ogura M, Yatabe Y, Suchi T, Kodera Y, MorishimaY, Takahashi T, Saito H, Ueda R, Nakamura S (1997) CD7+ and CD56+ myeloid/natural killer cell precursor acute leukemia: A distinct hematolymphoid disease entity. Blood 90: 2417-2427

24. Takahashi N, Nakai S, Honjo T (1980) Cloning of human immunoglobulin μ gene and comparison with mouse μ gene. Nucl Acids Res 8: 5983-5991

25. Thomas X, Vila L, Campos L, Sabido O, Archimbaud E (1995) Expression of N-CAM (CD56) on acute leukemia cells: Relationship with disease characteristics and outcome. Leuk Lymph 19: 295-300

26. Vendetti A, Poetea GD, Stasi R, Buccisano F, Aronica G, Bruno A, Cox C, Maffei L, Tamburini A, Papa G, Amadori (1996) Biological profile of 23 cases of minimally differntiated acute myeloid leukemia (AML-M0) and its clinical implications. Blood 87: 418-420 (letter)

27. Vidriales MB, Orfano A, Gonzales M, Hernandez JM, Lopez-Berges MC, Garcia MA, Canizo MC, Cabarello MD, Macedo A, Landolfi C (1993) Expression of NK and lymphoid-associated antigens in blast cells of acute myeloblastic leukemia. Leukemia 7: 2026-2029

# The Role of Apoptosis in the Course of Acute Leukemia in Children

A Chybicka, D Turkiewicz, B Rybka, R Ryczan and J Boguslawska-Jaworska

*Summary:* Apoptosis is the process of programmed cell death. Its disturbances are important part of cancer development. This study aimed at examining clinical and prognostic significance of spontaneous apoptosis level in leukemic population at diagnosis. The study included 33 children suffering from acute leukemia: 26 with acute lymphoblastic leukemia (8 LRG, 9 MRG, 8 HRG and one child classified to risk group C) and seven with acute myeloid leukemia. Apoptotic cells were identified by flow cytometric test with Annexin V and PI. No significant difference in apoptosis intensity among children stratified to different risk groups was noted. No correlation between early response to treatment and percentage of apoptotic cells among bone marrow MNCs was observed. Our data suggest that detection of spontaneous apoptosis among leukemic cells at diagnosis has no prognostic significance. Further studies upon clinical significance of induced apoptosis are necessary.

Apoptosis is the process of programmed cell death. It plays an essential role in the cell differentiation and proliferation control as well as in elimination of cells with major genome alternations that failed to be repaired [1]. Thus, disturbances of apoptosis are of great importance in cancer development, permitting transformed cells to proliferate and expand [5]. It is postulated that anticancer effect of chemotherapeutics may also depend upon induction of apoptosis in cancer cells [2].

In this study, we were interested in the differences in spontaneous apoptosis of leukemic cells among children with acute leukemia belonging to different risk groups. Another interesting question is if any correlation between percentage of apoptotic cells at diagnosis and early response to treatment was present.

## Materials

The study included 33 children, 19 boys and 14 girls, aged from 2 to 17 years, treated in our department from 1996 to 1999. In all of them acute leukemia was diagnosed, in twenty-three cases ALL and in seven cases AML. Among twenty-six ALL patients eight were stratified to LRG, 9 to MRG and 8 to HRG risk groups. One patient with mature B-ALL immunophenotype was classified as risk group C according to LMB protocol. Apoptosis was measured in mononuclear cells separated by density gradient centrifugation (Phicoll Paque, Pharmacia) from diagnostic bone marrow aspirates. Blast content in each sample exceeded 80% in ALL children and 50% in children with AML. Patients with acute lymphoblastic leukemia are characterized in Fig. 1.

## Methods

Apoptotoc cells were detected using Annexin V and PI according to manufacturer protocol (Annexin V kit, Genzyme). Briefly, mononuclear cells isolated from bone marrow were washed and incubated for 10 minutes with Annexin V conjugated with fluorescein. After incubation, the cells were washed twice with PBS and incubated with PI for at least 10

Department of Pediatric Hematology and Oncology, Wroclaw University of Medicine, Wroclaw Poland

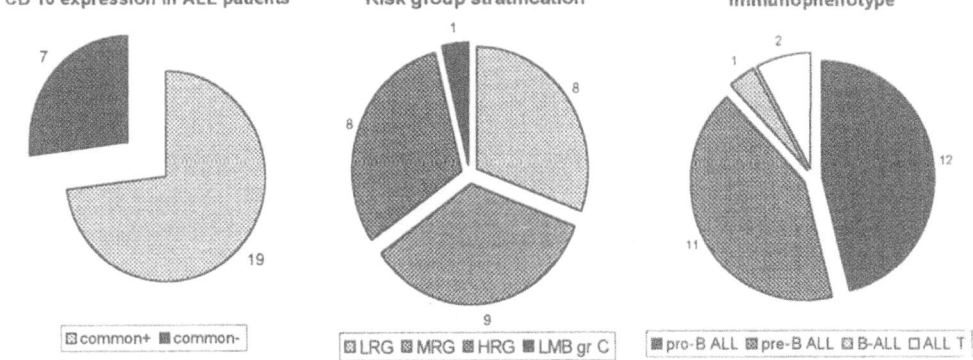

**Fig. 1.** Clinical characteristics of ALL patients.

minutes. Samples were then analyzed with EPIX XL flow cytometer (Coulter, FL). Apoptotic cells were described as excluding propidium iodide and binding Annexin V to their cytoplasmatic membrane. Gating strategy applied during analysis is presented in Fig 2.

## Results

The percentage of apoptotic cells at diagnosis in leukemic cell population is presented in Fig. 2. No statistically significant difference in percentage of apoptotic cells in different risk groups was observed (p>0,05, Fig. 3). No correlation between the percentage of apoptotic cells in leukemic blasts population and time of remission achievement was noted (r=0,07226, p>0,05, Fig. 4.). In small group of patients who died prior to remission achievement the percentage of apoptotic cells was slightly higher that in the other group, but the difference was not significant (p>0,05, Fig 5).

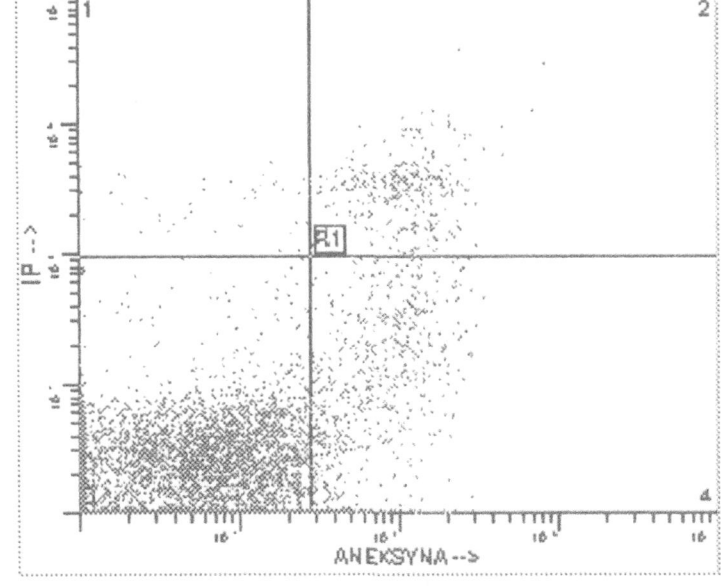

**Fig. 2.** Gating strategy applied for identification of apoptotic cells. R2 – dead and late apoptotic cells acumulating PI and binding Annexin V, R3 – viable Annexin V negative cells excluding PI, R4 – Annexin V positive early apoptotic cells excluding PI.

121

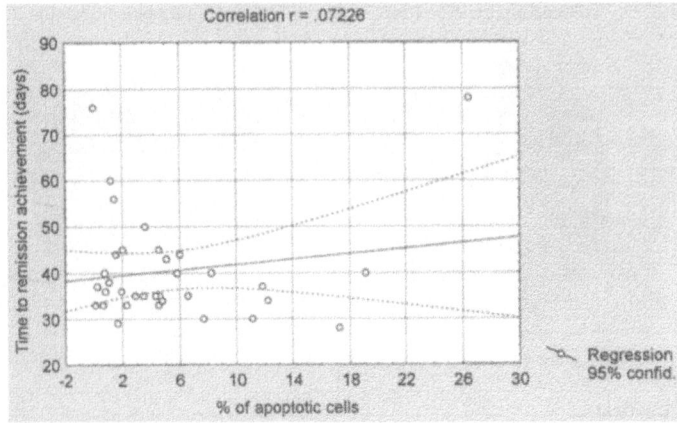

**Fig. 3.** Percentage of apoptotic cells at diagnosis in bone marrow of children with ALL and AML

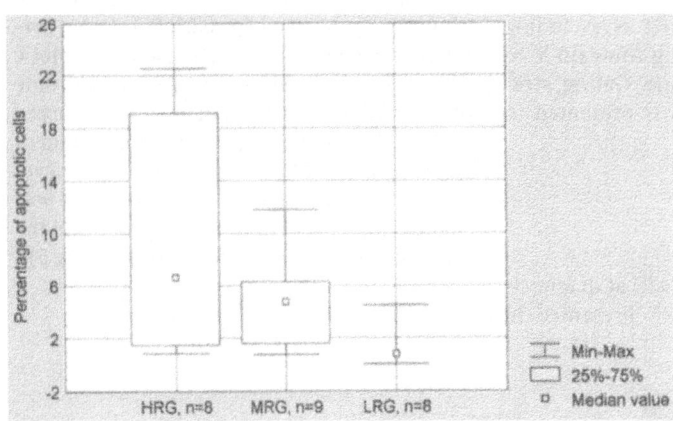

**Fig. 4.** Percentage of apoptotic cells at diagnosis in children with ALL stratified to different risk groups

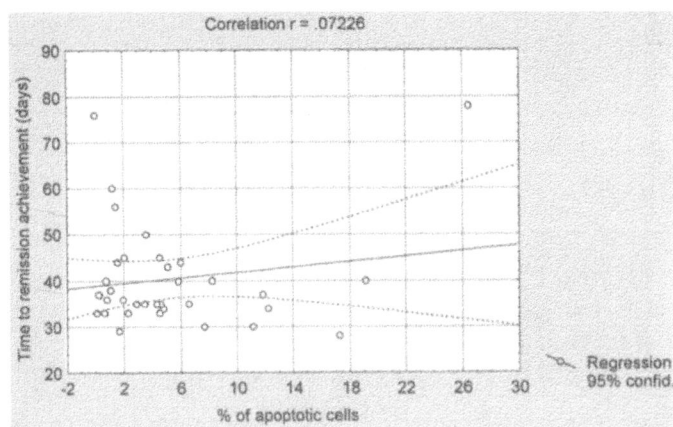

**Fig. 5.** Correlation of apoptosis and time of remission achievement

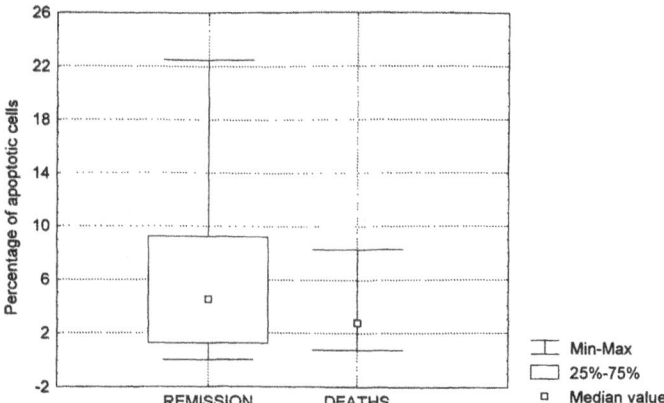

**Fig. 6.** Apoptosis in children who achieved remission or died prior to remission achievement

| | |
|---|---|
| ⊥ | Min-Max |
| ☐ | 25%-75% |
| □ | Median value |

## Discussion

Tissue homeostasis results from fragile balance between cell proliferation and death. Defect occurring in the latter process may lead to uncontrolled cell accumulation – well known feature of cancer. A disturbance of apoptosis is considered one of the most important causes of successful neoplasmatic transformation. The more profound such disturbance is in leukemic cells the worse prognosis and response to therapy could be anticipated. To test this hypothesis we analyzed percentage of cells undergoing spontaneous apoptosis in bone marrow aspirates at the diagnosis and tried to correlated results with risk group stratification and early response to treatment.

For identification of apoptotic cells flow cytometric test with Annexin V and propidium iodide was used. It is very convenient, gives strictly quantitative results easy to compare and allows discriminating of dead cells. The test is based upon early changes of apoptotic cells surface resulting in ability to bind Annexin V. The cells, however, are still capable of excluding PI, what makes their discrimination from dead cells possible [3]. Alternations of apoptotic cell surface resulting from disturbed asymmetry of phospholipids in plasma membrane are early morphological events in apoptotic process, probably leading to enhanced recognition and phagocytosis of such cells [4].

Our results confirmed that leukemic cells generally do not undergo spontaneous apoptosis. Percentage of apoptotic cells at diagnosis in bone marrow never exceeded 10%. Spontaneous apoptosis is similarly low in children belonging to different risk groups and responding differently to initial therapy. Slightly lower level of apoptosis in children who died before remission achievement was not significant. Our initial conclusion is that percentage of spontaneous apoptosis at the beginning of therapy has no predictive value in childhood acute leukemia. In our future studies, we will explore prognostic and clinical significance of leukemic cells ability to undergo apoptosis induced by strong pro-apoptotic substances.

## References

1. Hale AJ, Smith CA, Sutherland LC, Stoneman VEA, Longthorne VL, Culhane AC, Williams GT (1996) Apoptosis. Molecular regulation of cell death. Eur J Biochem 236:1-26
2. Martin SJ, Green DR (1994) Apoptosis as a goal of cancer therapy. Curr Opin Oncol 6:616-621
3. van Engeland M, Nieland LJW, Ramaekers FCS, Schutte B, Reutelingsperger CPM (1998) Annexin V-affinity assay: a review on an apoptosis detection system based on phosphatidylserine exposure. Cytometry 31:1-9
4. Fadok VA, Voelker DR, Campbell PA, Cohen JJ, Bratton DI, Henson PM (1992) Exposure of phosphatidylserine on the surface of apoptotic lymphocytes triggers specific recognition and removal by macrophages. J Immunol 148:2207-2216
5. Cohen JJ (1993) Apoptosis. Immunol Today 14(3):126-130

# Evaluation of Spontaneous and Therapeutically Induced Apoptosis in Childhood Leukemias

I. Malinowska, M. Wasik, A. Stelmaszczyk, E. Górska, M. Steczowicz and R. Rokicka-Milewska

*AIM:* To observe the sequence of spontaneous apoptosis and apoptosis after treatment in acute lymphoblastic leukemia (ALL) in children.

*Methods:* Ten patients (4 girls and 6 boys, aged 2 to 13 years) with ALL were included in the study. Blood was taken aseptically before therapy and after each new drug was administered in induction chemotherapy according to BFM protocol. The aliquoted whole blood was incubated at 37 °C and examined at 0, 6, 24, 48 and 72 hours.

Morphological apoptosis was assessed by light microscopy. Nuclear, membrane and intracellular pH changes typical for apoptosis were assessed by flow cytometry in propidium iodide (PI) assay, annexin-V-FITC assay and in carboxy-SNARF-1-AM assay.

*Results:* Results were expressed as a percentage of apoptotic cells. Blood blasts from ALL patients showed delayed spontaneous apoptosis in comparison to therapeutically induced apoptosis. Immediately after administration of each new drug no apoptotic forms were found in light microscopy or PI and annexin assays. However, they appeared during incubation with peaks at 48 hours. Apoptotic cells were detected by SNARF assay at 0 hours with peak at 24 hours.

*Conclusions:* SNARF assay permitted the detection of early phases of apoptosis not detected by other methods. A good correlation was found between the degree of apoptosis in light microscopy, PI DNA staining and Annexin V–FITC assay in later stages of apoptotosis of leukaemic cells.

## Introduction

Cells from a wide variety of human malignancies show a decreased ability to undergo apoptosis in response to several physiologic stimuli. Many chemotherapeutic agents kill tumour cells by initiating apoptosis. Tumours that demonstrate little or no apoptosis are assumed to be relatively resistant to therapeutic intervention [1]. The aim of our study was to observe the degree and sequence of spontaneous apoptosis (before treatment) and apoptosis after administration of each new drug in acute lymphoblastic leukaemia (ALL) in children.

In ninety–five percent of children with de novo ALL complete remission initially occurs. However there is a relapse in 30% of these patients and they eventually die of the disease.

Apoptosis is a process of cell death characterized by morphological and biochemical changes occurring at different stages. Once triggered, the apoptosis process progresses in different ways depending on cell types and culminates with cell disruption and formation of apoptotic bodies. In the critical stage of apoptosis these cells are phagocyted.

Recently, it has been shown that cells in the initial stages of apoptosis disturb the phospholipid asymmetry of their plasma membrane and expose phospholipid phospatidylserine (PS) which is translocated to the outer

Department of Paediatrics, Haematology and Oncology; Department of Laboratory Diagnostics and Immunology; Medical University of Warsaw, Poland

layer of the membrane, while the cell membrane remains intact [2, 3, 4].

The origin of chromatin condensation is thought to be DNA fragmentation [5]. Usually this fragmentation arises from internucleosomal digestion of genomic DNA by endonucleases. Mammalian cells contain a variety of endonucleases, any of which could be involved in apoptosis, but many cells appear to lack this enzyme. One of these nucleases is deoxyribonuclease II activated by decreased pH [5, 6, 7]. We wanted to find out whether intracellular acidification was associated with induction of apoptosis in ALL blasts.

Flow cytometry assays were used to measure DNA degradation, membrane changes and pH alteration.

This study was the initial part of a project examining the relationship between the degree of spontaneous apoptosis, therapeutically induced apoptosis and results of treatment in terms of remission, survival and death.

## Materials and Methods

### Patients

Ten patients (4 girls and 6 boys, aged 2 to 13 years) with ALL referred to the Department of Paediatrics, Haematology and Oncology were included in the study. Blood was taken aseptically before therapy and after each new drug was administered in induction chemotherapy according to BFM protocol (Prednisone, Vincristin, Daunorubicyn, L-Asparaginase). Investigation in a given patient were continued until the peripheral blasts disappeared.

The aliquoted whole blood was incubated at $37^0$C and examined before therapy and then at intervals of 0, 6, 24, 48 and 72 hours.

### Morphology

Apoptotic morphology of leukaemic cells was assessed by light microscopy. 100 µl of cells at 1 x $10^6$ cells/ml were loaded in a cytospin centrifuge and centrifuged at 350 rpm for 5 min. The cells were fixed with methanol and stai-

ned using the Wright–Giemsa method. Nuclei were scored as apoptotic if chromatin was notably condensed, marginated or divided.

### Cell Cycle Analysis

Cell cycle analysis was performed on cells stained with propidium iodide (PI). The cells were analyzed in a Coulter flow cytometer. The cell suspension was washed and adjusted to a concentration of 1.5 x $10^6$ cell/ml in PBS. The 200xg centrifuged cell pellet was gently resuspended in 1.5 ml hypotonic fluorochrome solution (PI 50 µg/ml in 0.1% sodium citrate plus 0.1% Triton X, Sigma). The tubes were placed in the dark overnight at 40 °C before flow-cytometric analysis. The PI fluorescence of individual nuclei was measured using the Coulter flow cytometer and the data was registered on a logarithmic scale.

### Membrane Changes

Membrane changes were examined using Annexin-V assay. Cells were washed in PBS and 5x $10^5$ of them were resuspended in 100 ul of binding buffer (10 mM Hepes/NaOH, pH 7.4, 140 mM NaCl, 2.5 mM $CaCl_2$). 10 µl of Annexin V and 10 µl of 20 µl/ml of PI were added. Cells were incubated for 10 minutes, washed and analysed in a Coulter flow cytometer. Staining of cells simultaneously with FITC-Annexin V and PI allowed discrimination of intact cells (FITC-PI-), early apoptotic (FITC+PI-) and late apoptotic or necrotic cells (FITC+PI+).

### PH Assessment

Intracellular pH measurement was performed by flow cytometry as described previously (8). 1x106 cells were loaded with 5 uM of the acetoxymethylester derivative of Carboxy SNARF-1 (SNARF-1-AM) in 2 ml of medium at $37^0$C in a $CO_2$ incubator. Intracellular carboxy-SNARF-1 was excited at 488 nm and the emission measured at both 585 and 640 nm. The 585/640 ratio was calculated electronically as an instrument parameter. Intracellular pH was estimated by comparison of the mean ratio values of a sample to a calibration curve of intracellular pH, generated by incubation of carboxy SNARF-1 loaded cells in varied pH buffers, in the presence of proton ionophore nigericin.

To assess intracellular pH the results were displayed on a 2-dimensional dot plot with 585 nm fluorescence on the x-axis and 640 nm fluorescence on the y-axis. Cells on the same line out from the axis posses the same intracellular pH. A shift to the right represents cells with lower intracellular pH while a shift to the left represents cells with higher intracellular pH.

## Results

Apoptotic cell frequencies were expressed as percentages of the total cell number. The spontaneous and therapeutically induced apoptotic responses of ALL cells varied considerably. Preliminary assays demonstrated that the most marked changes in cell cycles and membranes were seen when cells were examined in the first 24 hours of incubation.

### Spontaneous Apoptosis

Morphologically assessed apoptotic cells appeared in the population of ALL blasts within 6 hours of incubation. After 48 hours most cells were not present in incubated blood which suggested that they had disintegrated. Early apoptotic cells appearing as cells with DNA content less than G1 began to appear after 24 hours. The impressive reduction of diploid peaks and an enhancement of hypodiploid peaks were observed during incubation.

The percentage of hypodiploid cells was almost the same as the percentage of apoptotic cells measured by annexin assay in 7 patients. Three patients had no apoptosis in PI assay but 30%–35% of apoptosis in Annexin V assay. In 2 patients there was the same degree of apoptosis in annexin assay, PI assay and morphological assessment. No changes in pH were detected by SNARF assay before treatment.

### Therapeutically Induced Apoptosis

ALL cells after treatment showed widely variable apoptosis. Treatment specific apoptosis was determined by subtracting spontaneous percent apoptosis from treated percent apoptosis. After 24 hours apoptosis varied from 5% to 50% in PI assay. ALL cells from two out of 10 examined patients showed an equal percentage of apoptosis in PI assay, annexin assay and morphological assessment. Blasts from 7 patients showed an equal percentage of apoptosis in PI and Annexin V assays. In 8 examined children blood blasts showed delayed spontaneous apoptosis in comparison to therapeutically induced apoptosis. Immediately after induction chemotherapy no apoptotic forms were found in light microscopy and PI while Annexin V assay showed same apoptotic cells.

In 2 patients SNARF assay showed changes in intracellular pH with peak at 24 hours in ALL cells after treatment with a full dose of Prednisone.

In one child changes were observed towards basic pH with 0.4 pH units above normal and in the other toward acidic pH with 0.6 units below normal.

## Discussion

Apoptosis is a process of cell death characterised by plasma membrane, cytoplasm and nuclear changes [1, 3, 6]. Loss of plasma membrane asymmetry seems to be a universal phenomenon of apoptosis. Thus, all cell types undergoing apoptosis can be quantitated by staining with Annexin V–FITC and PI. Apoptotic cells become Annexin V positive after nuclear condensation has started, but before the cell becomes permeable to PI. This binding assay appears to be sensitive compared with traditional methods like microscopy, DNA electrophoresis and DNA flow cytometry. It correlates with other tests and is easy, fast reliable and reproducible.

In our study the Annexin V binding test allowed for quantitation of cells at the early stages of apoptosis or when apoptosis occurred in the absence of DNA fragmentation.

SNARF assay permitted the detection of pH changes in two examined cells.

It is known that intracellular pH measurements by SNARF assay represent the average intracellular pH of the entire population of cells. Therefore, it is possible that the marginal changes observed in the cell population could result in an underestimation of the subpopulation of acidic or basic cells. Some cells load SNARF inefficiently and SNARF assay is cell line dependent. However, the ALL cells used in our study loaded carboxy SNARF efficiently, making them a good model. Changes in pH were observed in ALL blasts, but were not constant in apoptosis.

Further studies are needed to prove the efficacy of SNARF in research on children with ALL.

## References

1. Thatte U, Dahanukar S (1997) Apoptosis. Clinical relevance and pharmacological manipulation. Drugs 54:511–532
2. Vermes I, Haanen C, Steffens-Nakken H, Reutelingsperger C (1995) A novel assay for apoptosis flow cytometric detection of phosphatidyserine expression on early apoptotic cells using fluorescein labelled Annexin V. J Immunol Meth 184:39–51
3. Koopman G, Reutelingsperger GAM, Kuijten RMJ, Keehnen ST, Pals ST, van Oers MHJ (1994) Annexin V for flow cytometric Detection of Phosphatidylserine Expression on B cells undergoing Aapoptosis. Blood 84:1415–1420
4. Martin SJ, Reutelingsperger CPM, McGahon AJ, Rader JA, van Schie RCAA, LaFace DM, Green DR (1995) Early Redistribution of plasma membrane Phosphatidylserine is a general Feature of apoptosis regardless of the initiating stimulus: inhibition by overexpression of bcl–2 and abl. J Exp Med. 182:1545–1556
5. Nicoletti I, Migliorati G, Pagliacci M., Grignani F, Riccardi C (1991) A rapid and simple method for measuring thymocyte apoptosis by propidium iodide staining and flow cytometry. J Immunol Meth 139:271–279
6. Li J, Eastman A (1995) Apoptosis in an Interleukin–2–dependent Cytotoxic T lymphocyte cell line is associated with intracellular acidification. J Biol Chem 270:3202–3211
7. Barry MA, Reynolds JE, Eastman A (1993) Etoposide–induced apoptosis in human HL-60 cells is associated with intracellular acidification. Cancer Res 53:2349–2357
8. Karwatowska-Prokopczuk E, Nordberg JA, Li HL, Engler RL, Gottlieb RA (1998) Effect of vacuolar proton ATPase on pHi, Ca 2+ and apoptosis in neonatal cardiomyocytes during metabolic inhibition/recovery. Circ Res 82:1139–1144

The study was supported by KBN grant No 4P05E09214

# Involvement of BCL-2 and Bax in the IL-7-Induced Inhibition of Spontaneous Apoptosis in Childhood T-ALL

V. Ruppert, C. Wuchter, B. Dörken, W.-D. Ludwig and L. Karawajew

*Abstract.* Induction of apoptosis by cytokine deprivation and its inhibition by cytokines in growth factor-dependent cell lines has been demonstrated to be under the control of Bcl-2-related proteins. Recently, we have demonstrated that leukemic cells of patients with newly diagnosed T-ALL underwent spontaneous apoptosis upon culturing *in vitro* and that this kind of apoptosis could be effectively inhibited by IL-7. In the present study, we addressed the role of Bcl-2 and Bax proteins, the two major members of the Bcl-2 family, in the regulation of spontaneous and IL-7-modulated apoptosis in T-ALL. To this end, we investigated leukemic blasts from childhood T-ALL patients as to expression levels of Bcl-2 and Bax, which were quantified by flow cytometry in units of molecules of equivalent soluble fluorochrome (MESF) before and after the treatment with IL-7 (100 U/ml, 24h, $37^0$C), and their relative changes were correlated with the extent of apoptosis in leukemic cells *in vitro*. We found that expression changes of Bax, but not Bcl-2, positively correlated with the extent of spontaneous apoptosis (Spearman correlation: p=0.022 and p=0.991, respectively; 20 patients). By contrast, changes of Bax expression levels did not correlate with the inhibition of apoptosis by IL-7 (p=0.47, 30 patients). However, inhibition of spontaneous apoptosis by IL-7 was associated with upregulation of Bcl-2 and, even stronger, with Bcl-2/Bax ratios (linear regression: r=0.51, p=0.004 and r=0.59, p=0.0006, respectively, 30 patients). Therefore, our data suggest a differential involvement of Bcl-2 and Bax in the induction of spontaneous apoptosis and its regulation by IL-7 in T-ALL.

## Introduction

Normal T-lineage development has recently been shown to crucially depend on the so-called common gamma ($\gamma_c$) chain of the IL-2 receptor shared by the receptors to cytokines IL-2, IL-4, IL-7, IL-9, and IL-15 [1]. Most of these cytokines seem, however, to be functionally redundant, since mice deficient in single cytokines revealed unimpaired lymphopoiesis [2, 3]. The only exception is IL-7, which when deficient in mice has been shown to result in a drastically reduced number of thymocytes, though with a normal subset distribution [4, 5].

The analysis of thymocytes from IL-7-deficient mice disclosed their developmental arrest on the triple-negative (TN: CD3-, 4-, 8-) stage [5]. These cells revealed increased rates of spontaneous apoptosis associated with decreased expression levels of anti-apoptotic protein Bcl-2. Treatment of TN-thymocytes with IL-7 resulted in upregulation of Bcl-2 expression and inhibition of apoptosis. Moreover, an overexpression of Bcl-2 in IL-7-deficient mice largely restored the normal T-cell development, thus suggesting that IL-7 might exert its survival function by the upregulation of Bcl-2 [6].

Recently, we investigated the ability of IL-7, IL-4, and IL-2 to modulate spontaneous apoptosis of leukemic blasts from childhood T-ALL patients [7]. T-ALL cells were found to be sensitive to IL-7 in terms of apoptosis inhibition in 56% of cases (32 of 57), whereas almost all T-ALL samples were refractory to IL-4 and IL-2.

In the present study, we addressed the role of Bcl-2 in spontaneous apoptosis and its

Dept. of Hematology, Oncology and Tumor Immunology, Robert-Rössle-Clinic, Charité, Humboldt-University of Berlin, D-13125 Berlin, Germany.

inhibition by IL-7. To this end, Bcl-2 expression levels and their alterations following culturing of leukemic cells in the presence of IL-7 were quantified by flow cytometry in 30 T-ALL samples. Furthermore, expression levels of Bax, the apoptosis-promoting homolog of Bcl-2, were evaluated parallel to Bcl-2 measurements.

## Materials and Methods

### Cell samples

Leukemic blasts from childhood patients with newly diagnosed T-lineage ALL (n=30) were included. The diagnosis was based on bone marrow (BM) aspirates, and the smears were classified as ALL according to the FAB criteria using light microscopy and cytochemistry [8]. Immunophenotyping was carried out on leukemic blasts isolated by standard Ficoll-Hypaque density gradient centrifugation, and cell-surface as well as cytoplasmic antigens were detected using direct or indirect immunofluorescence techniques as described elsewhere [9, 10]. The criteria for marker positivity as well as the subclassification of T-lineage ALL (pro-T-, pre-T-, cortical, and mature T-ALL) were adopted from the guidelines proposed by the 'European Group for the Immunological Characterization of Leukemias' (EGIL) [11]. In the present study, 10 samples were subclassified as pro-T/pre-T-ALL, 16 samples as cortical T-ALL, and 4 samples as mature T-ALL.

### Cell purification and culture

Leukemic cells recovered from fresh patient samples were purified by density gradient centrifugation using Ficoll-Hypaque separation (Pharmacia, Uppsala, Sweden). Viability of cells was always more than 90% as determined by trypan blue or propidium iodide (PI) (Sigma, Deisenhofen, Germany) exclusion. All samples contained more than 90% leukemic cells based on morphological criterias. Leukemic cells were maintained in RPMI 1640 (Biochrom, Berlin, Germany) standard medium containing 2mM L-glutamine, 100 U/ml penicillin, 100 µg/ml streptomycin and supplemented with 10% heat-inactivated fetal calf serum (FCS) (Gibco BRL, Paisley, Scotland).

To assess spontaneous apoptosis, $0.5 \times 10^6$ leukemic cells/well were cultured in 96-well microtiter plates (Nunc, Roskilde, Denmark) in standard medium for 24 hours at 37 °C in a humidified atmosphere of 5% $CO_2$ in air. To investigate cytokine-mediated effects, leukemic cells were cultured for 24 hours in the presence of recombinant human cytokine IL-7 (100 U/ml) (Pharma Biotechnologie Hannover PBH, Hannover, Germany) [12, 13]. Functional assays performed with samples from several patients in the presence and absence of FCS gave similar results.

### Assessment of apoptosis

To determine the extent of apoptosis, cells were stained with FITC-conjugated Annexin V and PI using the Annexin V kit (Immunotech, Marseille, France) as recommended by the manufacturer. Thereafter, samples were analysed by flow cytometry (FACScan, Becton Dickinson, San Jose, CA, USA) for the presence of viable (Annexin V- and PI- negative), early apoptotic (Annexin V-positive, PI-negative), and late apoptotic (Annexin V- and PI-positive) cells. The extent of apoptosis (N%) was quantified as percentage of Annexin V-positive cells. The extent of spontaneous apoptosis was calculated as difference of N% values in leukemic samples following and prior to culture in medium, ($\Delta N^{spont} = N^{medium} - N^{0h}$). The IL-7-specific modulation of apoptosis was calculated as difference between apoptosis extents after culturing in the absence and presence of the cytokine ($\Delta N^{IL-7} = N^{medium} - N^{IL-7}$). All tests were performed in doublets, with mean value of standard deviation (SD) of 2%. The 2.5-fold SD-value (i.e. $\Delta N = 5\%$) was used as a threshold value for cytokine-induced inhibition of apoptosis.

### Assessment of Bcl-2 and Bax expression

To evaluate the expression of the intracellular antigens Bcl-2 and Bax, leukemic cells were fixed and permeabilized using the fixation-permeabilization kit (Fix & Perm; An-der

Grub, Kaumberg, Austria) as recommended by the manufacturer. Bcl-2 antigen was detected by the FITC-conjugated anti-Bcl-2 antibody clone 124 (Dako, Glostrup, Denmark). FITC-conjugated irrelevant mouse antibodies of the appropriate subclasses (Immunotech, Marseille, France) were used as negative controls.

To detect Bax, Bax-specific rabbit polyclonal antibodies raised against synthetic peptide sequences (I-19, Santa Cruz Biotech., CA) and FITC-conjugated goat anti-rabbit serum (Medac, Hamburg, Germany) as a secondary staining reagent were used. As negative controls, cells stained with Bax antibody in the presence of the blocking synthetic peptide (provided by the manufacturer, Santa Cruz) were taken.

Immunofluorescence analysis was performed on a FACScan flow cytometer (Becton Dickinson) using CellQuest software (Becton Dickinson). Since late apoptotic cells lose their membrane integrity and may have a reduced protein content, the expression of antigens only in viable cells have been considered. Viable cells were discriminated from apoptotic cells by criteria of higher forward and lower side scatter intensities [14, 15].

The expression of antigens was quantified by flow cytometry in units of molecules of equivalent soluble fluorochrome (MESF) using calibration beads as fluorescence standards (DAKO FluoroSpheres, DAKO, Glostrup, Denmark). Relative changes of expression (RCE) of Bcl-2 and Bax due to the culturing in standard medium were quantified as the ratio $RCE^{spont} = MESF^{medium}/MESF^{0h}$. IL-7-specific relative changes of expression of Bcl-2 and Bax were calculated from the ratio of antigen expression levels in IL-7-treated and untreated cells, $RCE^{IL-7} = MESF^{IL-7}/MESF^{medium}$.

## Statistical analysis

Evaluations of the association of protein expression levels with extent of spontaneous or IL-7-modulated apoptosis were performed using linear regression or Spearman correlation statistics. Differences were considered to be significant for P values < 0.05.

## Results

### Involvement of Bcl-2 and Bax in spontaneous apoptosis

To investigate an involvement of Bcl-2 and Bax in spontaneous cell death, their intracellular levels were determined parallel to the apoptosis detection in 20 T-ALL samples. The mean extent of spontaneous apoptosis was 24% ± 3%, with values ranging between 5% and 54%. All samples endogeneously expressed Bcl-2 and Bax with mean values of (7.0 ± 1.7) x 10³ MESF and (161 ± 20) x 10³ MESF, respectively (Table 1). In individual samples, the levels of expression were highly variable and failed to correlate with the extent of spontaneous apoptosis (data not shown). However, higher rates of spontaneous apoptosis were correlated with increased expression levels of Bax following culturing of leukemic cells in standard medium when compared with initial Bax levels (p=0.02, Spearman correlation) (Fig. 1). In contrast, neither Bcl-2 levels (Fig. 2) nor Bcl-2/Bax ratios (not shown) were correlated with the spontaneous apoptosis.

**Table 1.** Endogeneous expression levels of Bcl-2 and Bax in leukemic cells from T-ALL patients.

| T-ALL samples (n=20) | Bcl-2 [MESF] [×10⁻³]ᵃ | Bax [MESF] [×10⁻³] |
|---|---|---|
| mean expression | 7.0 ± 1.7 [b] | 161 ± 20 |
| range | 0.5–24.9 | 42–358 |

a Expression levels of Bcl-2 and Bax were quantified as MESF (molecules of equivalent soluble fluorochrome) using calibration standards.
b mean ± SEM

### Involvement of Bcl-2 and Bax in the apoptosis inhibition by IL-7

To investigate an involvement of Bcl-2 and Bax in the IL-7-induced inhibition of spontaneous apoptosis, their expression levels were determined parallel to the assessment of apoptosis following incubation in the absence and presence of IL-7. All T-ALL samples studied (30/30) revealed spontaneous apoptosis, to an extent ranging between 5% and 70% and a mean value of 26% ± 3.4%. IL-7 was

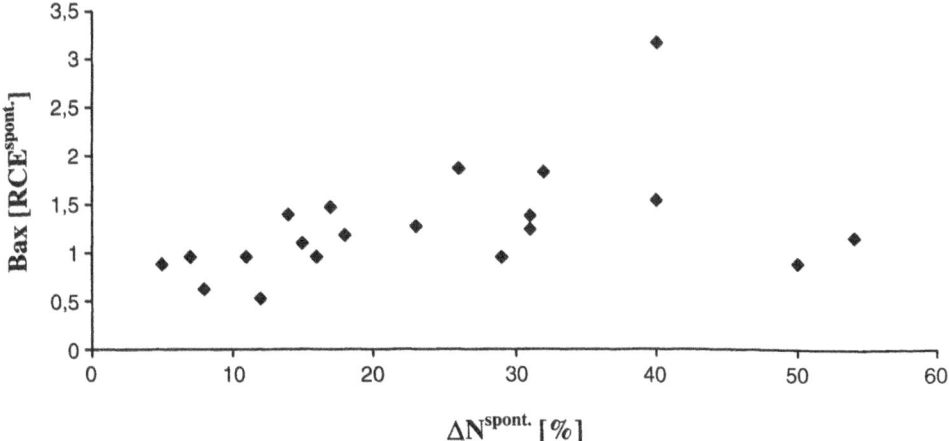

**Fig. 1.** Relative expression changes of Bax, Bax (RCE$^{spont}$), positively correlate with the extent of spontaneous apoptosis (20 T-ALL samples; Spearman correlation: p=0.02).

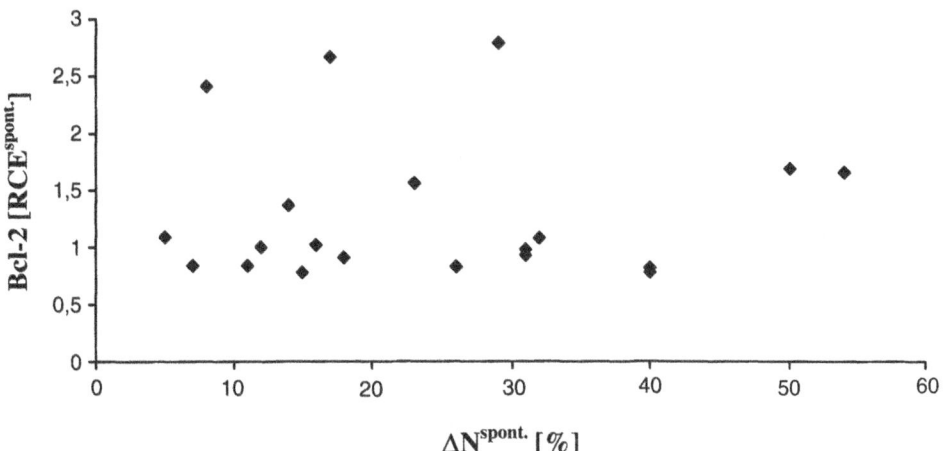

**Fig. 2.** Relative expression changes of Bcl-2, Bcl-2 (RCE$^{spont}$), do not correlate with the extent of spontaneous apoptosis (n=20; n.s.).

able to inhibit apoptosis ($\Delta N^{IL-7} \geq 5\%$) in the majority of the T-ALL cases (57% of all cases, 17 of 30 patients). Bcl-2 expression following treatment with IL-7 increased significantly when compared with untreated samples (Fig. 3). In contrast to Bcl-2, IL-7-induced changes of Bax were variable and did not correlate with the ability of IL-7 to prevent apoptosis in leukemic samples (Fig. 4). Interestingly, examination of Bcl-2/Bax ratios resulted in a better correlation with IL-7 effect than for Bcl-2 levels alone (Fig. 5).

## Discussion

Recently, we demonstrated that leukemic cells of patients with newly diagnosed T-ALL underwent spontaneous apoptosis upon culturing *in vitro* and that this kind of apoptosis could be effectively inhibited by IL-7 [7]. Since proteins of the Bcl-2 family have been implicated in the modulation of apoptosis mediated by cytokines, in the present study we addressed the role of Bcl-2 and Bax proteins, the two major members of the Bcl-2

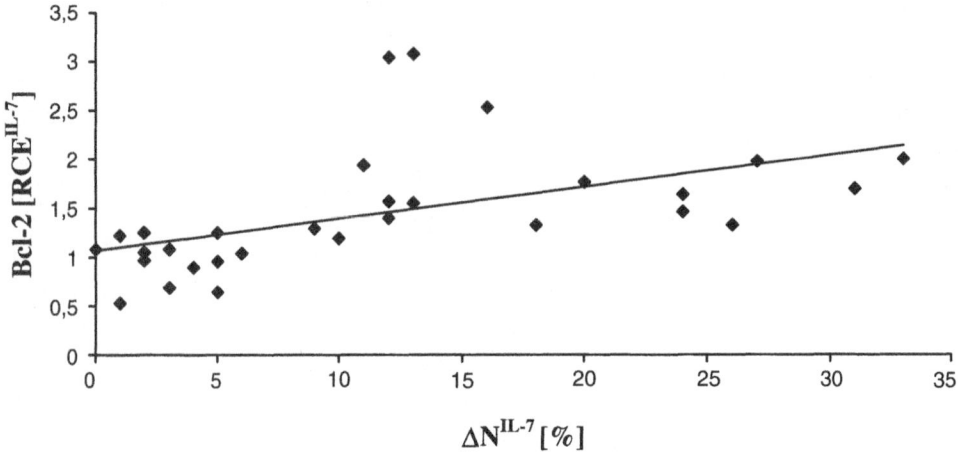

**Fig. 3.** Relative expression changes of Bcl-2 protein are positively correlated with the extent of IL-7-specific apoptosis inhibition (n=30; linear regression: r=0.51, p=0.004).

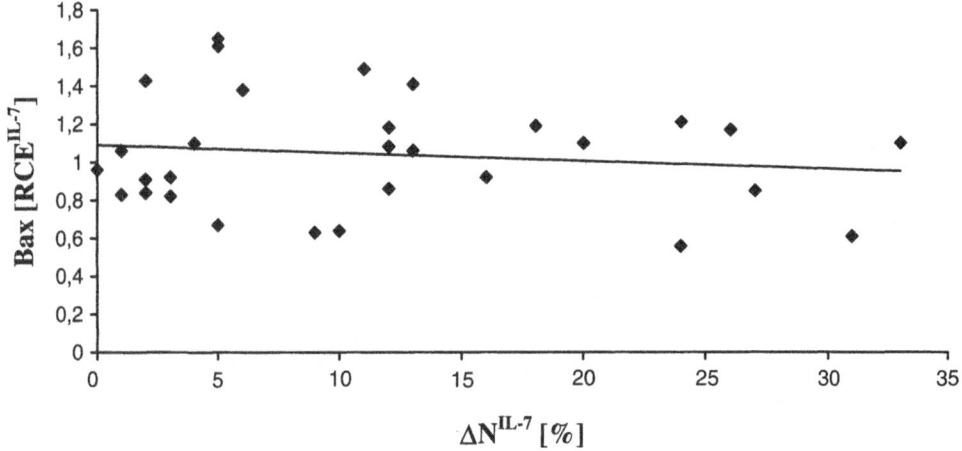

**Fig. 4.** Relative expression changes of Bax protein do not correlate with the extent of IL-7-specific apoptosis inhibition (n=30; linear regression: r=-0.14, n.s.).

family, in the regulation of spontaneous and IL-7-modulated apoptosis in T-ALL. To this end, relative changes of protein expression were examined by flow cytometry and correlated with the extent of apoptosis in leukemic cells *in vitro*. We found that expression changes of Bax, but not Bcl-2, positively correlated with the extent of spontaneous apoptosis. By contrast, changes of Bax expression levels did not correlate with the inhibition of apoptosis by IL-7. However, the IL-7-induced inhibition of apoptosis was associated with an upregula-

tion of Bcl-2 and, even stronger, with Bcl-2/Bax ratios. Therefore, our data suggest a differential involvement of Bcl-2 and Bax in the induction of spontaneous apoptosis and its regulation by IL-7 in T-ALL.

Spontaneous death of haematopoietic malignant cells observed *in vitro* is presumably due to deprivation of humoral and cellular factors capable of protecting these cells from apoptosis *in vivo* [16–19]. A variety of cytokines, such as Flt3-L and SCF in AML, IL-4, IL-10 and IL-13 in B-CLL, have been identi-

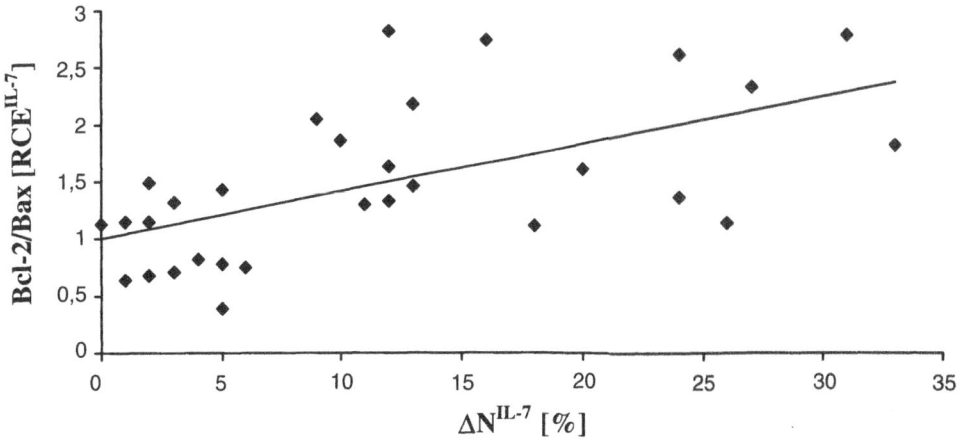

**Fig. 5.** Changes of Bcl-2/Bax ratio by IL-7 revealed a stronger positive correlation with rates of IL-7-induced apoptosis inhibition than Bcl-2 alone (n=30; linear regression: r=0.59, p=0.0006).

fied as anti-apoptotic, survival factors [14, 16, 20–22]. Although molecular pathways of spontaneous apoptosis and its modulation by cytokines remain to be elucidated, there is abundant evidence that Bcl-2 family members are involved in the regulation of these processes. An overexpression of Bcl-2 has been shown to delay a cytokine deprivation-triggered apoptosis in growth factor-dependent cell lines, while an overexpression of Bax was able to induce or enhance spontaneous cell death without additional factors [23–25]. Studies on constitutive expression of Bcl-2 and Bax in freshly isolated leukemic cells revealed correlations between rates of spontaneous apoptosis and expression levels of these proteins in AML, B-lineage ALL and CLL [14, 26–29]. With respect to T-lineage cells and IL-7, a cytokine-induced inhibition of apoptosis and its correlation with increased levels of Bcl-2 was observed in mouse normal pro-T and malignant T-lymphoma cells and in human activated T lymphocytes [6,30-33]. In contrast, no Bax expression changes were found in mouse malignant T-lymphoma cells [33] and human activated T cells [30], although an apoptosis-associated upregulation of Bax and its prevention by IL-7 was reported for pro-T-cells [32].

Our data suggest that Bcl-2, rather than Bax, is involved in the anti-apoptotic signaling by IL-7 in T-ALL. The Bcl-2 dependent function of IL-7 as survival factor in T-ALL exhibits similarity to the function of IL-7 in the early T-cell development. Mice lacking IL-7 or IL-7R alpha genes have been found to be severely deficient in developing thymocytes [4,5]. The analysis of thymocytes from IL-7-deficient mice disclosed their developmental arrest on the triple-negative (TN: CD3-, 4-, 8-) stage [5]. The freshly isolated TN-cells from IL-7-deficient mice exhibited spontaneous apoptosis *in vitro*, which was markedly higher than in normal thymocytes and could be inhibited by the addition of IL-7 [34]. Interestingly, bcl-2-deficient mice also revealed an impaired development of lymphoid lineages [35]. Moreover, bcl-2 overexpression in IL-7-deficient mice largely restored the maturation of thymocytes, suggesting a developmental point in pro-T cells, in which IL-7 exerts an anti-apoptotic function by upregulating or maintaining of Bcl-2 levels [34].

In conclusion, our data demonstrated that changes of Bax but not Bcl-2 expression were associated with the extent of spontaneous cell death in T-ALL. By contrast, IL-7-induced inhibition of apoptosis significantly correlated with expression alterations of Bcl-2, rather than with these of Bax, thus suggesting a differential involvement of Bcl-2 and Bax in the induction and prevention of apoptosis in T-ALL blasts. In an ongoing study we investigate whether T-ALLs differing in their response to IL-7 *in vitro* may reveal specific clinical features and differential response to therapy *in vivo*.

*Acknowledgements.* We are grateful to Karin Ganzel, Mathilde Martin and Karin Liebezeit for valuable technical assistance.
This work was supported in part by the Deutsche Leukämie-Forschungshilfe (grant no. DLFH-98.04) and by the Deutsche Jose Carreras Leukämie-Stiftung (grant no. DJCLS-98/NAT-3).

# References

1. DiSanto JP, Muller W, Guy Grand D, Fischer A, Rajewsky K: Lymphoid development in mice with a targeted deletion of the interleukin 2 receptor gamma chain. Proc Natl Acad Sci U S A 92:377, 1995
2. Schorle H, Holtschke T, Hunig T, Schimpl A, Horak I: Development and function of T cells in mice rendered interleukin-2 deficient by gene targeting. Nature 352:621, 1991
3. Kuhn R, Rajewsky K, Muller W: Generation and analysis of interleukin-4 deficient mice. Science 254:707, 1991
4. Peschon JJ, Morrissey PJ, Grabstein KH, Ramsdell FJ, Maraskovsky E, Gliniak BC, Park LS, Ziegler SF, Williams DE, Ware CB, et al.: Early lymphocyte expansion is severely impaired in interleukin 7 receptor-deficient mice. J Exp Med 180:1955, 1994
5. von Freeden Jeffry U, Vieira P, Lucian LA, McNeil T, Burdach SE, Murray R: Lymphopenia in interleukin (IL)-7 gene-deleted mice identifies IL-7 as a nonredundant cytokine. J Exp Med 181:1519, 1995
6. Akashi K, Kondo M, von Freeden Jeffry U, Murray R, Weissman IL: Bcl-2 rescues T lymphopoiesis in interleukin-7 receptor-deficient mice. Cell 89:1033, 1997
7. Karawajew L, Kösser A, Ruppert V, Martin M, Schrappe M, Dörken B, Ludwig W-D: Capability of IL-7 to prevent in vitro spontaneous apoptosis of T-lineage acute lymphoblastic leukemia (ALL) cells correlates with a cortical/mature phenotype and a good initial in vivo response to chemotherapy. Blood 90:560a, 1997
8. Bennett JM, Catovsky D, Daniel MT, Flandrin G, Galton DA, Gralnick HR, Sultan C: Proposals for the classification of the acute leukaemias. French-American-British (FAB) co-operative group. Br J Haematol 33:451, 1976
9. Ludwig W-D, Rieder H, Bartram C-R, Heinze B, Schwartz S, Gassmann W, Löffler H, Hossfeld D, Heil G, Handt S, Heyll A, Diedrich H, Fischer K, Weiss A, Völkers B, Aydemir Ü, Fonatsch C, Gökbuget N, Thiel E, Hoelzer D: Immunophenotypic and genotypic features, clinical characteristics, and treatment outcome of adult pro-B acute lymphoblastic leukemia: results of the German multicenter trials GMALL 03/87 and 04/89. Blood 92:1898, 1998
10. Creutzig U, Harbott J, Sperling C, Ritter J, Zimmermann M, Löffler H, Riehm H, Schellong G, Ludwig WD: Clinical significance of surface antigen expression in children with acute myeloid leukemia: results of study AML-BFM-87. Blood 86:3097, 1995
11. Béné MC, Castoldi G, Knapp W, Ludwig WD, Matutes E, Orfao A, van't Veer MB: Proposals for the immunological classification of acute leukemias. European Group for the Immunological Characterization of Leukemias (EGIL). Leukemia 9:1783, 1995
12. Vella AT, Dow S, Potter TA, Kappler J, Marrack P: Cytokine-induced survival of activated T cells in vitro and in vivo. Proc Natl Acad Sci U S A 95:3810, 1998
13. Skjonsberg C, Erikstein BK, Smeland EB, Lie SO, Funderud S, Beiske K, Blomhoff HK: Interleukin-7 differentiates a subgroup of acute lymphoblastic leukemias. Blood 77:2445, 1991
14. Lisovsky M, Estrov Z, Zhang X, Consoli U, Sanchez Williams G, Snell V, Munker R, Goodacre A, Savchenko V, Andreeff M: Flt3 ligand stimulates proliferation and inhibits apoptosis of acute myeloid leukemia cells: regulation of Bcl-2 and Bax. Blood 88:3987, 1996
15. Dive C, Gregory CD, Phipps DJ, Evans DL, Milner AE, Wyllie AH: Analysis and discrimination of necrosis and apoptosis (programmed cell death) by multiparameter flow cytometry. Biochim Biophys Acta 1133:275, 1992
16. Campana D, Coustan Smith E, Kumagai MA, Manabe A: Growth requirements of normal and leukemic human B cell progenitors. Leuk Lymphoma 13:359, 1994
17. Moqattash S, Lutton JD: Leukemia cells and the cytokine network. Proc Soc Exp Biol Med 219:8, 1998
18. Lagneaux L, Delforge A, Bron D, De Bruyn C, Stryckmans P: Chronic lymphocytic leukemic B cells but not normal B cells are rescued from apoptosis by contact with normal bone marrow stromal cells. Blood 91:2387, 1998
19. Nishigaki H, Ito C, Manabe A, Kumagai M, Coustan Smith E, Yanishevski Y, Behm FG, Raimondi SC, Pui CH, Campana D: Prevalence and growth characteristics of malignant stem cells in B-lineage acute lymphoblastic leukemia. Blood 89:3735, 1997
20. Hassan HT, Zander A: Stem cell factor as a survival and growth factor in human normal and malignant hematopoiesis. Acta Haematol 95:257, 1996
21. Chaouchi N, Wallon C, Goujard C, Tertian G, Rudent A, Caput D, Ferrera P, Minty A, Vazquez A, Delfraissy JF: Interleukin-13 inhibits interleukin-2-induced proliferation and protects chronic lymphocytic leukemia B cells from in vitro apoptosis. Blood 87:1022, 1996
22. Kitabayashi A, Hirokawa M, Miura AB: The role of interleukin-10 (IL-10) in chronic B-lymphocytic leukemia: IL-10 prevents leukemic cells from apoptotic cell death. Int J Hematol 62:99, 1995
23. Cerezo A, Martinez AC, Gonzalez A, Gomez J, Rebollo A: IL-2 deprivation triggers apoptosis which is mediated by c-Jun N-terminal kinase 1 activation and prevented by Bcl-2. Cell Death Differentiation 6 (1):87, 1999

24. Hockenbery D, Nunez G, Milliman C, Schreiber RD, Korsmeyer SJ: Bcl-2 is an inner mitochondrial membrane protein that blocks programmed cell death. Nature 348:334, 1990

25. Oltvai ZN, Milliman CL, Korsmeyer SJ: Bcl-2 heterodimerizes in vivo with a conserved homolog, Bax, that accelerates programmed cell death. Cell 74:609, 1993

26. Manabe A, Coustan Smith E, Kumagai M, Behm FG, Raimondi SC, Pui CH, Campana D: Interleukin-4 induces programmed cell death (apoptosis) in cases of high-risk acute lymphoblastic leukemia. Blood 83:1731, 1994

27. Kitada S, Andersen J, Akar S, Zapata JM, Takayama S, Krajewski S, Wang HG, Zhang X, Bullrich F, Croce CM, Rai K, Hines J, Reed JC: Expression of apoptosis-regulating proteins in chronic lymphocytic leukemia: correlations with In vitro and In vivo chemoresponses. Blood 91:3379, 1998

28. McConkey DJ, Chandra J, Wright S, Plunkett W, McDonnell TJ, Reed JC, Keating M: Apoptosis sensitivity in chronic lymphocytic leukemia is determined by endogenous endonuclease content and relative expression of BCL-2 and BAX. J Immunol 156:2624, 1996

29. Tangye SG, Raison RL: Human cytokines suppress apoptosis of leukaemic CD5+ B cells and preserve expression of bcl-2. Immunol Cell Biol 75:127, 1997

30. Akbar AN, Borthwick NJ, Wickremasinghe RG, Panayoitidis P, Pilling D, Bofill M, Krajewski S, Reed JC, Salmon M: Interleukin-2 receptor common gamma-chain signaling cytokines regulate activated T cell apoptosis in response to growth factor withdrawal: selective induction of anti-apoptotic (bcl-2, bcl-xL) but not pro-apoptotic (bax, bcl-xS) gene expression. Eur J Immunol 26:294, 1996

31. Kinoshita T, Yokota T, Arai K, Miyajima A: Suppression of apoptotic death in hematopoietic cells by signalling through the IL-3/GM-CSF receptors. EMBO J 14:266, 1995

32. Kim K, Lee CK, Sayers TJ, Muegge K, Durum SK: The trophic action of IL-7 on pro-T cells: inhibition of apoptosis of pro-T1, -T2, and -T3 cells correlates with Bcl-2 and Bax levels and is independent of Fas and p53 pathways. J Immunol 160:5735, 1998

33. Lee SH, Fujita N, Mashima T, Tsuruo T: Interleukin-7 inhibits apoptosis of mouse malignant T-lymphoma cells by both suppressing the CPP32-like protease activation and inducing the Bcl-2 expression. Oncogene 13:2131, 1996

34. von Freeden Jeffry U, Solvason N, Howard M, Murray R: The earliest T lineage-committed cells depend on IL-7 for Bcl-2 expression and normal cell cycle progression. Immunity 7:147, 1997

35. Nakayama K, Nakayama K, Negishi I, Kuida K, Shinkai Y, Louie MC, Fields LE, Lucas PJ, Stewart V, Alt FW, et al.: Disappearance of the lymphoid system in Bcl-2 homozygous mutant chimeric mice. Science 261:1584, 1993

# Analysis of the Apoptotic Signal Transduction Cascade and New Differentially Expressed Genes in Drug Resistant and Sensitive Hematopoetic Cell Lines

G. Beyer-Sehlmeyer, M. Kneba*, W. Hiddemann⁺, B. Wörmann and J. Bertram

*Abstract.* The development of a therapy-induced drug resistance is still one of the most important therapeutic limitations, but the mechanisms involved are largely unknown. In order to study supposed common steps in the development of a resistance against cytotoxic drugs with a quite different mode of action, we established drug resistant (doxorubicin, methotrexate, cisplatinum, vincristine) derivatives of six hematopoetic cell lines (Jurkat, U937, HL60, DoHH-2, K562, ARH77). Gene expression of drug resistant and the respective sensitive parental cell lines was analysed by suppressive subtractive hybridization (SSH). Differential expression of cDNA fragments was confirmed by Northern Blot analysis. As a result of this screening, the following genes showed a higher (at least 2-fold) or exclusive expression in the drug resistant variants: hsp90, serglycin, sorcin, BMPG (bone marrow proteoglycan gene) and PTI-1 (prostate-tumor-inducing gene 1).

Whereas the overexpression of specific drug target proteins (eg. P-glycoprotein, thymidylate synthase or cytosine deaminase) can be regarded as the „proximal" part of the development of a drug resistant phenotype, alterations in the apoptotic signal transduction cascade might be the „distal" mechanism of this process. Therefore, besides looking for the postulated „superimposed" link between these two mechanisms, the expression of proteins involved in the apoptotic signal transduction cascade (FAS, FAS-ligand, bcl-2, bcl-$x_L$, bax, cyt.c, FLICE and others) was investigated. A reduced expression of the pro-apoptotic bax protein (Jurkat MTX$^R$) and an increased expression of anti-apoptotic bcl-2 and bcl -$x_L$ proteins (ARH D60 DxR) was detected by Western Blot analysis.

## Introduction

Cancer patients that initially respond to standard chemotherapeutic agents often relapse, with the selective outgrowth of a tumor cell subpopulation that is resistant to further treatment. Therefore, drug resistance is still a therapeutic challenge. Many reports in the past decade have demonstrated that overexpression of a variety of membrane or intracellular proteins confer drug resistance not only in experimental models but are also of clinical significance, eg. P-glycoprotein overexpression in human AML (Huang et al., 1997; McGuire, 1997; Nooter, 1996; Bellamy, 1996). Cytotoxic drugs used for the treatment of different tumor entities but also restricted to the treatment of patients with hematologic malignancies exhibit quite different modes of action (Kinsella, 1997; Fisher, 1994). However, tumors frequently display resistance not only to the specific drug initially used for treatment, but also to a variety of structurally and functionally unrelated agents.

It is speculated, that drug induced changes in cellular homöostasis can be sensored by a postulated cellular mechanism. If this putative sensor signals a moderate damage caused by any single or combined drug, a repair program is initiated. Besides repair, also cell differentiation or senescence may be initiated to avoid the proliferation of an aberrant cell. If the postulated sensor notices a damage above a certain threshold level, the cellular suicide is

Dept. of Hematology/ Oncology, University Clinics, R. Koch Str. 40, Goettingen,
*2. Med. Clinic Christian-Albrechts Universität Kiel, ⁺ Dept. of Internal Medicine University Hospital Grosshadern, Munich, Germany.

initiated. However, there are no hints of the components and/or the mechanism of such a common cellular damage sensor, although inhibition of drug induced apoptosis by different mechansims itself might be a kind of superimposed drug resistance mechanism (Rowan and Fisher, 1997; Landowski, 1997).

In order to shed some light on this speculative superimposed cellular mechanism we established a variety of resistant sublines of six different hematopoetic cell lines (Jurkat, HL60, U937, ARH77, DoHH-2, K562). Selected drugs leading to more or less different resistance mechanisms were used: doxorubicin, which is mainly related to P-glycoprotein overexpression (Nooter, 1996), methotrexate, which is known to be related to an overexpression of the dihydrofolate reductase (McGuire, 1997), cisplatinum, an alkylating agent resulting in DNA damage (Dassonneville, 1998), 5-fluorouracil, which causes overexpression of the thymidylate synthase (Rustum, 1997), and vincristine, which besides increasing P-glycoprotein expression interacts with components of the cytoskeleton (Jordan, 1998).

Using suppressive subtractive hybridization (SSH), a variety of different combinations of drug resistant cell lines established during this study as well as their sensitive counterparts were compared for genes exclusively or at least overexpressed in the drug resistant cell lines. Recently, a growing family of anti-apoptosis gene products have been shown to modulate drug cytotoxicity via regulation of drug-induced apoptotic cell death (Scaffidi et al., 1998; Rowan and Fisher, 1997). For example, overexpression of Bcl-2 or Bcl-$x_L$ (Miyashita and Reed, 1993; Datta et al., 1995) as well as down-regulation of Bax (Krajewski et al., 1995) have been demonstrated to inhibit apoptosis and reduce the cytotoxic effects of a variety of anticancer drugs exhibiting diverse modes of action. Therefore, besides screening of our established drug resistant hematopoetic cell lines for components of a possible common cellular sensor of drug induced damage, we investigated the expression of different components of the apoptosis signal transduction cascade in these drug resistant and sensitive cell lines.

## Materials and Methods

### Cell culture conditions and selection of drug resistant cells

Cell lines K562 (DSM ACC 10), HL60 (DSM ACC 3), U937 (DSM ACC 5) and DoHH-2 (DSM ACC 83) were obtained from the German collection of microorganisms and cell cultures (DSM), Braunschweig, Germany. ARH77 and the doxorubicin resistant variant ARHD60 Dx$^R$ were a kind gift from Dr. Bellamy, Tucson, USA. The Jurkat cell line was derived from the laboratory cell culture stock. All cells were grown in Click´s-RPMI-1640 medium supplemented with 10% FCS (GibcoBRL, Eggenstein, Germany), 10mM HEPES, 1% L-glutamine (Biowhitaker, Boehringer Ingelheim, Germany) at 37•C in an atmosphere of 5% $CO_2$ in air and 100% humidity.

Methotrexate (MTX), vincristine (Vin), doxorubicin (DX) and 5-fluorouracil (5-FU) were obtained from Lederle (Wolfratshausen, Germany) and cisplatinum (cisPt) from HexalPharm (Holzkirchen, Germany). Doxorubicin was diluted in 0,9% NaCl (w/v), for all other drugs phosphate buffered saline (PBS) was used. Cells were initially exposed to drug concentrations representing the respective $IC_{80}$ value (MTT assay) determined previously. Fresh drugs were added to the medium whenever it was changed (app. two to three times a week). Drug concentration was gradually increased to the respective final concentration. After selection of drug resistant sublines, drugs were added only once a week to maintain the selective pressure. The vincristine resistant variant of K562 was established by subsequent elimination of dead cells using a lymphocyte separation medium (Ficoll, Biochrom, Berlin, Germany) (Bhalla et al., 1994). At weekly intervals the concentration of vincristine was increased, dead cells were removed several times and surviving cells were maintained in Click`s-RPMI-1640 medium as described. Prior to each experiment cells were maintained in a drug-free medium for one week.

**Table 1.** Sensitivity of resistant cell lines to selected cytostatic drugs.*†

| cell line | vincristine | doxorubicin | cisplatinum | methotrexate | 5-fluorouracil |
|---|---|---|---|---|---|
| HL60 MTXR | 0,8 | 0,8 | 1,0 | **1214** | 0,4 |
| HL60 cisPtR | 0,8 | 1,1 | **3,1** | 2,5 | 0,7 |
| ARHD60R | 400 | 43 | 1,5 | 1,3 | 2,3 |
| ARH77 VinR | **1250** | 22 | 1,9 | 1,3 | 3,2 |
| Jurkat MTXR | 0,8 | 1,7 | 0,8 | **14** | 2 |
| Jurkat DXR | 1,3 | **13** | 0,7 | 20 | 3 |
| Jurkat cisPtR | 0,7 | 0,8 | **4** | 0,5 | 2 |
| U937 MTXR | 1,3 | 0,8 | 0,6 | **150** | 1,0 |
| U937 VinR | **960** | 12 | 0,3 | 0,7 | 0,1 |
| DoHH-2 cisPtR | 1,5 | 9,3 | **16** | 2,7 | 1,9 |
| K562 VinR | **83** | 18 | 1,8 | 1,7 | 1,6 |

* data represent the resistance factors (rf) of the drug resistant derivatives: Resistance factors were calculated as ratio of the IC50 value for the drug resistant and the respective parental cell line. IC50 values were determined by MTT assay.
† underlined numbers mark that cytostatic drug used for selection of the corresponding cell line.

## Drug sensitivity assay

For the drug sensitivity assay, cells were harvested and cultured for 24 h in fresh medium, subsequently cells were plated into 96 well microtiter plates (Nunc, Wiesbaden, Germany) at $5 \times 10^4$ cells/ml. Sensitivity of the cell lines to MTX, Dx, Vin and cisPt was determined after 96 hours of drug exposure using a MTT assay (Mosmann, 1983). The $IC_{50}$ represents the drug concentration resulting in 50% growth inhibition and was calculated from linear transformation of the dose response curves. The resistance factors (rf's) were calculated as ratio of the $IC_{50}$ of the drug-resistant cell line and the sensitive parental cell line (Table 1).

## RNA extraction and Northern blot analysis

Total cellular RNA of drug resistant, sensitive or stressed sensitive cells was prepared using standard protocols (Chirgwin et al., 1979). Stress treatment was performed as described elsewhere (Bertram et al., 1998). Total cellular RNA (5 µg/lane) was denatured at 70°C for 20 min in 50% formamide; 6.5% formaldehyde; 1x MOPS buffer (20mM morpholinopropansulfonic acid MOPS, 5mM sodium acetate, 1mM EDTA); 0.7% Na-dodecylsulfate (SDS); 3.3% glycerine; 0.007% bromphenol blue, and 2µg ethidiumbromide and subjected to electrophoresis in MOPS buffer on a 1.5% (w/v) denaturing agarose gel in the presence of 5% (v/v) formaldehyde. RNA was transferred to a nylon membrane (Roche Molecular Biochemicals GmbH, Mannheim, Germany) in 20x SSC (3M NaCl, 0.3M sodium citrate) for app. 8 h according to Chomczysnki (1992) and immobilized by baking the nylon membrane at 120°C for 30 min. Filters were prehybridized in high-SDS buffer (7% SDS; 50% formamide; 5x SSC; 0.2M phosphate buffer; 2% blocking reagent (Roche Molecular Biochemicals GmbH, Mannheim, Germany); 0.01% laurylsarcosine; 50µg/ml salmon sperm DNA) for 20 min at 68°C. Hybridization was carried out at 68°C for 16 hours with digoxigenin-labelled RNA-probes complementary to the respective mRNA target (primer sequences for probe synthesis: rsp, 5′- CAG GAA ACA GCT ATG ACC- 3′; usp, 5′-GTA AAA CGA CGG CCA GTG- 3′; serglycin 5`, 5`- CCT GTT CCA TTT CCG TTA G- 3`; serglycin 3′-T7, 5′- GGC TAA TAC GAC TCA CTA TAG GGA GAC CTG TTC CAT TTC CGT TAG- 3′; sorcin 5′, 5′- CAG GAT GGG CAG ATA GAT G- 3′; sorcin 3′-T7, 5′- GGC TAA TAC GAC TCA CTA TAG GGA GAG GTG ATC TTT CCA TTG GTG C- 3′; bone-marrow-proteoglycan 5′, 5′- GGA TGA GGA GAC ACC AGA G- 3′; bone-marrow-proteoglycan 3′-T7, 5′- GGC TAA TAC GAC TCA CTA TAG GGA GAG AGC AGC CCA GTA CGC AAA G- 3′). RNA-probes were generated by *in vitro* transcription (Megashortscript Kit, ITC Heidelberg, Germany) of PCR products containing a T7-promoter at the 3′-primer. Membranes were washed twice in 2x SSC, 0.1% SDS for 15 min at room temperature, and twice in 0.3x SSC, 0.1% SDS for 15 min at 68 °C. After an incubation in blocking solution (1% blocking reagent reagent (Roche Molecular Biochemicals GmbH, Mannheim, Germany) in maleinic acid buffer (0.1M maleinic acid, 0.15M NaCl, pH 7.5) for 30 min at RT, the nylon membranes were incubated with an alkaline phosphatase (AP) conjugated anti-digoxigenin antibody (1:1000) in 1% blocking solution for 30 min. 2 additional washings of the membranes for 15 min in 0.3% Tween-20 in maleinic acid buffer were followed by a 5 min incubation with the CDP-Star substrate (Roche Molecular Biochemicals GmbH, Mannheim, Germany) diluted 1:5000 in detection buffer (100mM Tris, 100mM NaCl, pH 9.5). Subsequently, the nylon membranes were exposed to X-ray films (Amersham LIFE SCIENCE, Braunschweig, Germany) for 2 to 30 min. The densitometric analysis was carried out using WinCam 2.2 software of ImagePro V (Cybertech, Berlin, Germany). To normalize the densitometric analysis for RNA-loading differences, membranes were hybridized with a human ß-actin probe (Roche Molecular Biochemicals, Germany).

## Suppressive Subtractive Hybridization (SSH)

mRNA was synthesized starting from 100 µg of total RNA of the corresponding cells using the Dynal kit for mRNA synthesis as recommended by the manufacturer (Deutsche Dynal, Hamburg, Germany). SSH was carried out according to the user manual of the Clontech PCR-Select cDNA Subtraction Kit (Clontech, Heidelberg, Germany). According to the user manual the cDNA containing specific overexpressed transcript is called „tester cDNA", and the reference cDNA is called „driver cDNA". The subtracted cDNA was amplified in a Thermal Cycler (MJ-Research, Biozym, Hameln, Germany) for 30 cycles: 94 °C, 60 sec; 60 °C, 45 sec; and 72 °C, 90 sec using KlenTaq polymerase mix and buffer (Clontech. Heidelberg, Germany). The nested PCR was performed using 12 and 16 cycles, respectively (94 °C, 60 sec; 68 °C, 30 sec; and 72 °C, 90 sec). After 12 cycles of nested PCR no products were detectable in an agarose gel. Therefore, an aliquot of the PCR reaction was withdrawn after 12 cycles and additional 4

cycles were run with the remaining reaction mixture. An aliquot of both nested PCR products was ligated into the pCR$^{II}$-vector of TA-Cloning Kit (Clontech, Heidelberg, Germany) and transformed into competent *E. coli* DH5( cells.

For a rapid screening of the obtained clones for putative differentially expressed cDNAs before sequencing, 96 clones were cultured in 100 µl LB-medium supplemented with ampicillin (100 µg/ml) in a 96 well microtiter plate. 1µl of bacterial suspension was denatured in PCR buffer for 10 min at 98 °C. Amplification of cDNA inserts was done using a Thermal-Cycler (MJ Research, Biozym, Hameln, Germany) and the reverse (rsp) and universal sequencing primer (usp) for 35 cycles: 95 °C, 30 sec; 68 °C, 3 min, an additional extension period at 72 °C for 5 min was added. Positive PCR products were ethanol precipitated, dotted onto two nylon membranes (Roche Molecular Biochemicals, Germany) and cross-linked to the membrane by baking at 120 °C for 30 min. Membranes were hybridized with two probes synthesized of total digoxigenin-labelled cDNAs of the sensitive and the resistant cell line, respectively. Labelling of cDNAs of resistant and sensitive cell lines was performed with 1 µg of cDNA prepared according to the protocol of the Gibco/BRL Superscript$^{TM}$ Preamplfication System using 200 µM dATP, 200 µM dCTP, 200 µM dGTP, 100 µM dTTP, 100 µM DIG-11-dUTP, 3 mM MgCl$_2$, Tfl-buffer, 1 µl random hexamer (50ng), and 2 U Klenow-fragment at 37•C for 16 h. Dotted PCR samples that were positive with labelled „tester"-cDNA probe and negative with labelled „driver"-cDNA were further analysed by sequencing on an ABI 373 A sequencer (Applied Biosystems, Weiterstadt, Germany) using ABI-DNA-sequencing kit (genauer Name). The sequences obtained were compared with reported sequences (GenBank) using the BlastN network service (advanced ncbi-blast-search).

## Western Blot analysis

The expression of Bcl-2 , Bax, Bcl-x$_L$, CPP 32, FAS, FAS-ligand, FLICE and p53 were determined by Western Blot analysis as described priviously (Bertram et al., 1996). The following antibodies were used: Bcl-2 (clone 124, DAKO Hamburg, Germany), Bax (Calbiochem Bad Soden/Ts., Germany), Bcl-x$_L$ CPP 32, FAS (clone G254-274), FAS-ligand (clone G247-4), FLICE (clone B9-2), cyt. c (Pharmingen, Hamburg, Germany) and p53 (clone DO-7, DAKO Hamburg, Germany) at a dilution of 1:1000 or 1:2000. Blots were incubated for 1-3 h at room temperature with the respective antibody and then with anti-mouse or anti-rabbit peroxidase-conjugated secondary IgG antibodies. Immune complexes were detected with an enhanced chemiluminescence detection method by immersing the blot for 1-5 min in a 1:1 mixture of chemiluminescence reagents A and B (NEN, Köln, Germany) and then exposing to Amersham ECL films (Amersham, Braunschweig, Germany) for 20 sec to 20 min depending on signal intensity.

## Results

### Characterization of the drug resistance profile of newly established drug resistant hematopoetic cell lines

In order to study potentially new molecular mechanisms of drug resistance development in hematopoetic cell lines a panel of drug-resistant variants of the cell lines HL60, ARH77, U937, Jurkat, DoHH-2, and K562 was established. To determine their relative resistance (rf) to the selected drugs, the ratio of the IC$_{50}$ values of the resistant and the sensitive cell lines was determined in cytotoxicity assays (MTT). The resistance factors of the newly established resistant cell lines to five different drugs are shown in Table 1.

A doxorubicin and vincristine cross-resistance was found for the doxorubicin resistant ARH D60 Dx$^R$ cell line investigated in this study (rf vincristine: 400), as well as for the newly established vincristine resistant (ARH Vin$^R$, rf doxorubicin: 22) variant of ARH77 (Table 1). This cross-resistance to doxorubicin was also found for the established vincristine resistant U937 Vin$^R$ (rf doxorubicin: 12) and K562 Vin$^R$ (rf doxorubicin: 18) cell lines. No cross-resistances to the investigated antimetabolites methotrexate and 5-fluorouracil or the alkylating agent cisplatinum were found in these three vincristine/doxorubicin resistant cell lines.

Unexpected cross-resistances were observed for drug resistant variants of Jurkat, HL60 and DoHH-2 cell lines. Besides a resistance against the drug used for selection of the respective resistant subline, a cross-resistance against drugs exhibiting a different mechanism of cell poisoning was found. The doxorubicin (rf: 13) resistant Jurkat cells are also resistant to methotrexate (rf: 20) but not to vincristine, the cisPt resistant DoHH-2 variant is also resistant to doxorubicin (rf: 9.3) and the cisplatinum resistant HL60 derivative is also resistant to methotrexate (rf 2.5). However, none of the methotrexate resistant sublines showed a significant cross-resistance to 5-fluorouracil, although the resistance factor of the methotrexate resistant variant is rather high (rf up to 1214 for HL60 MTX$^R$). Moreover, methotrexate resistant variants showed no cross-resistance to any of the other drugs tested (Table 1). Therefore, the established panel of drug resistant hematopoetic cell lines offers the possibility to study candidate genes for putative „superimposed" steps in drug resistance development.

### Detection of differentially expressed genes and verification by Northern Blot analysis

In an attempt to investigate new genes that might be involved in drug resistance development in hematopoetic cell lines, the cDNA of HL60 cells was subtracted from the cDNA of the methotrexate resistant HL60 variant by selective subtractive hybridization (SSH). In addition, several drug resistant cell lines as well as their sensitive counterparts were pooled for SSH. After cloning of PCR products derived of the putative differentially expressed cDNA fragments a prescreening (ref. Materials and Methods) was done to minimize the number of positive clones. Candidate cDNA-fragments found by sequencing after the prescreening procedure and identified by a homology search using ncbi advanced BLAST search (2.0) are listed in Table 2. Higher or exclusive expression of the identified candidate genes in the resistant variants was confirmed by Northern Blot analysis.

Further analysis of the candidate genes listed in Tab. 2 revealed a three fold increased expression of thymosin ß4 in the vincristine

**Table 2.** Candidate genes obtained after subtractive suppressive hybridization from cDNAs of resistant and sensitive hematopoetic cell lines. **bold:** differentially expressed genes identified by Northern Blot analysis.

| A | B | C |
|---|---|---|
| **serglycin** | **PTI-1** | **sorcin** |
| **thymosin ß 4** | glycyl-t-RNA-synthetase | **bone- marrow-proteoglycan** |
| MCP 1 | hexokinase 1 | L5 |
| TafII31 | Hsc70 | |
| TCTP | E6-AP-ubiq.-protein-ligase | |
| TCP-1 | | |
| U32 | | |

A: cDNA of HL 60 cells was subtracted from the cDNA of the corresponding methotrexate resistant variant HL 60 MTXR
B: cDNA of Jurkat cells was subtracted from the pooled cDNAs of resistant cell lines Jurkat MTXR/DxR/cisPtR
C: cDNAs of ARH77 and U937 were pooled and subsequently subtracted from pooled resistant sublines ARH77 VinR, ARHD60 DxR, U937 MTXR, U937 VinR and vice versa

resistant U937 cell line in comparison to the sensitive line. However, all other hematopoetic cell lines investigated showed a nearly uniform expression level of thymosin ß4 (data not shown). Only in the doxorubicin resistant colon carcioma cell line LoVo DxR a 4-fold increase of thymosin ß4 was observed in the resistant variant in comparison to the sensitive cell line. High expression levels of serglycin (CD44-ligand) in methotrexate and vincristine resistant U937 cells were confirmed by Northern Blot analysis, while in sensitive U937 cells nearly no serglycin mRNA was detected (Fig. 1). A similar phenomenon was found in vincristine resistant and sensitive ARH77 cells, respectively. However, neither in drug resistant nor in sensitive Jurkat cells serglycin expression was detected.

The calcium binding protein sorcin is expressed in the resistant variants K562 Vin$^R$, ARH77 Vin$^R$ and ARHD60 DX$^R$, while in the sensitive parental cell lines nearly no expression of sorcin was detected (Fig.1). However,

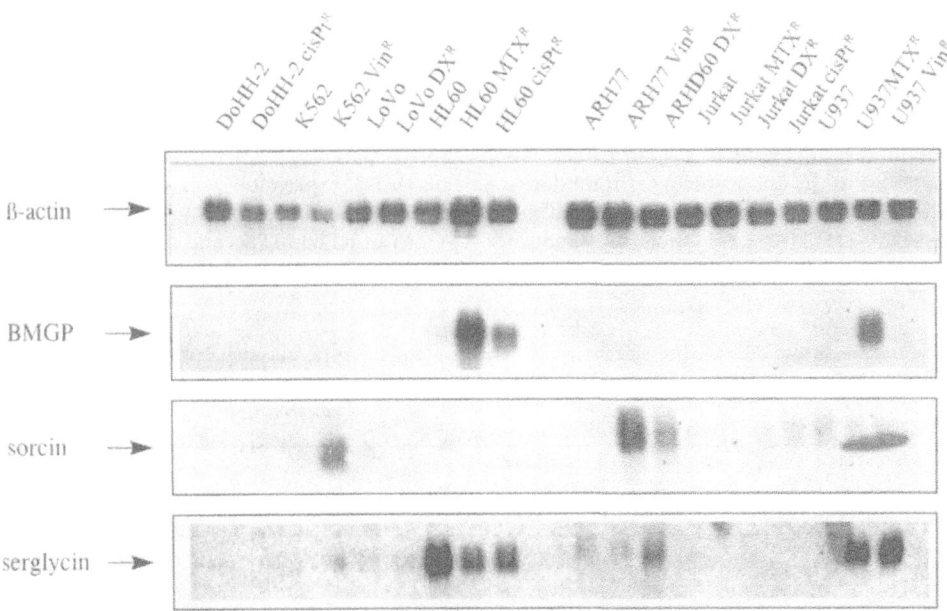

**Fig. 1.** Expression of sorcin, serglycin and bone-marrow-proteoglycan (BMPG) mRNA in different drug resistant and sensitive hematopoetic cell lines as well as in the doxorubicin resistant and sensitive colon cancer cell line LoVo H67P (LoVo and LoVo Dx$^R$, respectively) as determined by Northern Blot analysis. Total RNA was extracted from drug-resistant and -sensitive cell lines and hybridized with the respective DIG-labelled probes as described in Materials and Methods. A ß-actin probe (Roche Molecular Biochemicals, Germany) was used as a standard for RNA load (5µg/lane).

the vincristine resistant variant of U937 as well as the doxorubicin resistant Jurkat clone do not express detectable amounts of sorcin.

While the bone-marrow proteoglycan (BMPG) is expressed in the resistant variants U937 MTX^R, HL60 MTX^R and HL60 cisPt^R (Fig. 1), BMPG expression was detected neither in the other methotrexate or cisplatinum resistant sublines (DoHH-2 cisPt^R, Jurkat cisPt^R or Jurkat MTX^R) nor in any of the six drug sensitive hematopoetic cell lines investigated.

## Expression of proteins of the apoptotic signal transduction cascade

To investigate the possibility of an altered expression of proteins of the cellular apoptotic signal transduction cascade as a potentially common mediator of drug induced resistance, the expression of various known proteins involved in this signal pathway was investigated by Western Blot analysis (Fig. 2, Tab. 3). Bcl-2 expression was increased in doxorubicin resistant ARH plasmocytoma cells, however there was no difference between the sensitive and the vincristine resistant ARH cells. Surprisingly, Bax expression was increased in both resistant ARH cell lines (Fig. 2). The anti-apoptotic Bcl-x$_L$ was decreased in the vincistine resistant variant and increased in the doxorubicin resistant derivative (Fig. 2). On the other hand, cisplatinum resistant DoHH-2 cells showed a reduced expression of the anti-apoptotic proteins Bcl-

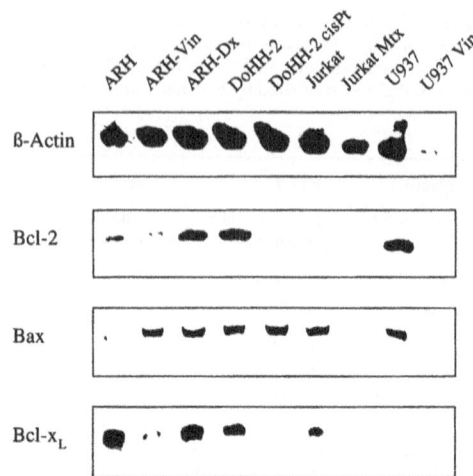

**Fig. 2.** Protein levels of Bcl-2, Bcl-x$_L$ and Bax in drug resistant and sensitive hematopoetic cell lines ARH, DoHH-2, Jurkat and U937 as analysed by Western Blotting. ß-actin was used as control for protein load (20μg/lane). Due to a lower amount of protein for U937 Vin, the data for this couple were derived from a different analysis. For these analyses, 20μg of the cytosolic protein were probed with the respective monoclonal or polyclonal antibody. Further details of the Western Blot procedure and the sources of antibodies are given in Materials and Methods.

2 and Bcl-x$_L$. Bax expression was not changed (Fig. 2) in comparison to the sensitive t(14;18) positive parental B-cell leukemia DoHH-2 cell line. Bcl-2 expression was also reduced in K562 Vin^R, in U937 Vin^R, in U937 MTX^R as well as in HL60 MTX^R and in HL60 cisPt^R in comparison to the respective drug sensitive

**Table 3.** Expression of different proteins involved in the apoptotic signal transduction cascade in drug resistant and sensitive hematopoetic cell lines
For these analyses, 20 μg of the cytosolic protein were probed with the respective monoclonal or polyclonal antibody. For p53 only a weak signal was obtained.

| antibody | | | | cell line | | | |
|---|---|---|---|---|---|---|---|
| | ARH | ARH Vin | ARH D60 | DOHH-2 | DoHH-2 cistPt | Jurkat | Jurkat MTX |
| FAS-lig. | + | + | + | ++ | +++ | ++ | + |
| FAS | + | ++ | ++ | ++ | ++ | +++ | + |
| Bcl-2 | + | + | ++ | +++ | + | + | + |
| Bcl-xL | ++ | + | ++ | ++ | + | ++ | + |
| Bax | + | ++ | ++ | ++ | ++ | ++ | + |
| CPP32 | ++ | ++ | ++ | ++ | ++ | ++ | ++ |
| FLICE | ++ | ++ | ++ | ++ | ++ | ++ | ++ |
| cyt.c | + | + | + | + | + | + | + |

+ low, ++ intermediate, +++ high expression

parental cell lines (data not shown). However, reduction of Bcl-2 expression was less pronounced in U937 MTX$^R$ in comparison to U937 Vin$^R$ and in HL60 cisPt$^R$ in comparison to HL60 MTX$^R$. There was no difference in Bcl-2 expression in the methotrexate resistant and the sensitive parental Jurkat T-cell line, however, Bcl-x$_L$ and Bax expression were reduced (Fig. 2). Expression of FLICE and CPP32 in the sensitive parental and in the resistant sublines of ARH, DoHH-2 and Jurkat, respectively (Table 3) was comparable. Taken together, no common alterations in the expression of proteins of the signal transduction cascade, eg. overexpression of anti-apoptotic proteins and/or reduced expression of pro-apoptotic genes was detected in the investigated drug resistant hematopoetic cell lines in comparison to the sensitive parental lines.

## Discussion

In this study we established hematopoetic cell lines which are resistant to cytotoxic drugs exhibiting rather different mechansims of cell poisoning (Gottesman et al.,1998). It was the aim of the work to compare the expression profile of genes potentially related to the development of these drug resistant phenotypes using suppressive subtractive hybridization. We wanted to look for a potentially common cellular sensor for drug poisoning postulated by us and others (Lit) and to identify parts of the cellular regulatory network sensoring drug induced damage. Based on the „read-out" of this speculative cellular sensor, the cell has to „make a decision" between cell cycle arrest allowing for damage repair, differentiation, senescence or even active regulated cell death called apoptosis (Rowan and Fisher, 1997), thereby protecting the whole organism against a mal-functioning maybe resistant and hyperproliferative cell clone.

Evidence was found for some unexpected cross-resistances (Tab. 1), indicating mechanisms of drug resistance development not only related to well known endpoints of resistance development. These „proximal" resistance mechanisms are for instance the multiple drug resistance phenotype (MDR,

Bellamy, 1996) or overexpression of the target gene of the drug used during selection of the respective resistant cell lines. Using various combinations of „tester" and „driver" cDNAs during SSH we tried to eliminate genes which might be found due to cell line to cell line variations although focus was already put on hematopoetic cell lines. For the elimination of genes which might be related to the resistance development for a single drug only, cDNAs of different resistant sublines (eg. Jurkat MTX$^R$, cisPt$^R$ and Dx$^R$) were pooled. A couple of genes which are up-regulated or exclusively expressed in the resistant derivatives were identified and differential expression was confirmed by Northern Blot analysis (Tab. 2, Fig. 1).

The screening performed during this study revealed candidate genes for a role in drug resistance development (Table 1) which are thymosin ß4 (Paciucci, 1996; Bao, 1998), serglycin (Robinson, 1997), sorcin (Meyers, 1995) and bone-marrow-proteoglycan (Popken-Harris, 1998). Nevertheless, these candidate genes are not uniformly upregulated in all drug resistant hematopoetic cell lines investigated (ref. Results). Although six different hematopoetic cell lines were selected for resistant subclones raised against four different drugs with rather different modes of action and known resistance mechanisms, and although a strategy of suppressive subtractive hybridization was used were different combinations of drug resistant and sensitive cell lines in different „tester" and „driver" combinations were used, no candidate gene was detected which was uniformly upregulated or even exclusively expressed in the drug resistant variants. Taken together, so far no hints were found for a common cellular sensor of drug induced damage.

Although the identified genes upregulated in drug resistant hematopoetic cell lines do not support a common cellular drug induced response, some of the genes are involved in the interaction of the cell with its environment: serglycin (a CD 44 ligand), bone-marrow-proteoglycan, CAPL (S100A4) and maybe also thymosin ß4 and sorcin (Robinson, 1997; Popken-Harris, 1998; Paciucci, 1996; Bao, 1998; Meyers, 1995). Therefore it is tempting to speculate, that at least one aspect of cellular drug resistance development is a dysregulated communication between the resistant cell and its environment (Rabbani, 1998; Braun, 1997). This might be due to the upregulation of proteins interacting with the extracellular matrix, eg. metalloproteinases. A recent paper reports on selection for drug resistance resulting in a co-selection of resistance to FAS-mediated apoptosis (Landowski et al., 1997). In this context it might be interesting, that drug resistant Jurkat cell lines established during this study exhibited an increased synthesis of metalloproteinases (Bertram et al., unpublished results). On the other hand, these drug resistant Jurkat cell lines showed a decreased expression of the FAS/APO-1 receptor (Bertram et al., unpublished results) which might be due to a metalloproteinase catalyzed shedding of the external domain of the receptor resulting in an impaired response of the drug resistant Jurkat cells to apoptotic stimuli via the FAS/APO-1 receptor. It is well known that shedding of the FAS-ligand is involved in an altered responsiveness of metalloproteinase overexpressing cell lines to apoptotic stimuli (Kayagaki, 1995; Schneider; 1998; Tanaka, 1998).

The analysis of various proteins involved in apoptotic signal transduction in the drug resistant hematopoetic cell lines however did not reveal a uniforme alteration in the expression of anti-apoptotic proteins (eg. upregulation) or pro-apoptotic proteins (downregulation). Whereas Bcl-2 is upregulated in the doxorubicin resistant ARH cell line (Fig. 2), it is downregulated in cisplatinum resistant DoHH-2 cells as well as in K562 Vin$^R$, in U937 Vin$^R$, in U937 MTX$^R$ as well as in HL60 MTX$^R$ and in HL60 cisPt$^R$ in comparison to the respective drug sensitive parental cell line (data not shown). Therefore it might be speculated that a Bcl-2 dependent apoptotic signaling is involved in doxorubicin mediated cell poisoning, whereas a less Bcl-2 dependent pathway might be involved in vincristine, methotrexate or cisplatinum dependent cytotoxic effects. These findings are in agreement with a recent paper by Scaffidi et al. (1998), showing evidence for two CD95 (APO-1/FAS) signaling pathways with a different involvement of the mitochondrial, Bcl-2 responsive part of apoptotic signaling.

Dowregulation of the anti-apoptotic Bcl-x$_L$ was found in vincristine resistant ARH cells and in the cisplatinum resistant DoHH-2 cells, whereas an increased expression as for Bcl-2 was observed in the doxorubicin resistant ARH cells. The pro-apoptotic Bax was decreased in methotrexate resistant Jurkat cells, however it was increased in vincristine and doxorubicin resistant ARH cells. One possible explanation for the upregulation of Bcl-2 and Bcl-x$_L$ expression in doxorubicin but not in vincristine resistant ARH cells might be due to the different level of resistance of the two cell lines (Tab. 1). Whereas the vincristine resistant ARH cell line is highly resistant to vincristine (rf: 1250) it has a significantly lower resistance towards doxorubicin (rf: 22) in comparison to the doxorubicin resistant ARH variant (rf doxorubicin: 43). This difference may be reflected by the above mentioned two CD95 signaling pathways and the respective involvement of Bcl-2. However, the dowregulation of Bcl-2 or Bcl- x$_L$ in the other resistant cell lines shown in Fig. 2 is hardly to explain, as well as it is the upregulation of the pro-apoptotic bax in some resistant cell lines. At least it can be concluded that even though drug resistance in part may be due to some „distal" regulators involved in apoptotic cell death (Huang et al., 1997), no uniforme changes in anti-apoptosis gene products were found in the cell lines established and investigated in this study. However, besides changes in the expression level of proteins involved in the apoptotic signal transduction cascade, protein modifications such as phosphorylation/dephosphorylation or others as well as alterations in downstream pathways might be involved in the cellular response to drug induced apoptosis. Therefore a functional analysis of the induction of apoptosis in drug resistant and sensitive cells is necessary. Work is in progress to deciffer the possible impact of some selected of the candidate genes (Tab. 2) overexpressed in the drug resistant hematopoetic variants establishing stable transfectants for hsp 90ß and serglycin.

*Acknowledgements.* These studies were supported by DFG grant SFB 500.

# References

Bao L, Loda M, Janmey PA, Stewart R, Anand-Apte B, Zetter BR (1996) Thymosin ß15: a novel regulator of tumor cell motility upregulated in metastatic prostate cancer. Nat Med 1:1322-1328

Bellamy WT (1996) P-glycoproteins and multidrug resistance. Annu Rev Pharmacol Toxicol 36:161-183

Bellamy WT (1996) Development of of an orthotropic SCID mouse-human tumot xenograft model displaying the multidrug-resistant phenotype. Cancer Chemother Pharmacol 37: 305-316

Bertram J, Palfner K, Hiddemann W, Kneba M (1996) Increase of P-glycoprotein-mediated drug resistance by hsp 90ß. Anti-Cancer Drugs 7:838-845

Bertram J, Palfner K, Hiddemann W, Kneba M (1998) Overexpression of ribosomal proteins L4 and L5 and the putative alternative elongation factor PTI-1 in the doxorubicin resistant human colon cancer line LOVoDx$^R$. Eur J Cancer 34: 731-736

Bhalla K, Huang Y, Tang C, Self S, Ray S, Mahoney ME, Ponnathpur V, Tourkina E, Ibrado AM, Bullock G, Willingham MC (1994) Characterization of a human myeloid leukemia cell line highly resistant to taxol. Leukemia 8: 465-475

Braun DP, Preissler HD (1997) Cytolytic activity of peripheral blood blast cells from patients with acute myeloid leukemia. Leuk. Lymphoma 27: 459-467

Chirgwin JM, Przybyla AE, MacDonald RJ, Rutter WJ (1979) Isolation of biologically active ribonucleic acid from sources enriched in ribonulease. Biochemistry 18: 5294-5299

Chomczynski P (1992) One-hour downward alkaline capillary transfer for blotting of DNA and RNA. Anal Biochem 201: 134-139

Dassonneville L, Bailly C (1998) Chromosome translocations and leukemias induced by inhibitors of topoisomerase II anticarcinogenis drugs. Bull Cancer 85: 254-261

Datta R, Manome Y, Taneja N, Boise LH, Weichselbaum R, Thompson CB, Slapak CA, Kufe D (1995) Overexpression of Bcl-x$_L$ by cytotoxic drug exposure confers resistance to ionizing radiation-induced internucleosomal DNA fragmentation. Cell Growth Diff 6:363-370

Fisher DE (1994) Apoptosis in cancer therapy: crossing the threshold. Cell 78: 539-542

Gottesman MM, Cardarelli C, Goldenberg S, Licht T, Pastan I (1998) Selection and maintenance of multidrug resistant cells. Methods Enzymol 292:248-258

Gottlicher M, Heck S, Herrlich P (1998) Transcriptional cross-talk, the second mode of steroid hormone receptor action. J Mol Med 76: 489-489

Jordan A, Hadfield JA, Lawrence NJ, McGown AT (1998) Tubulin as a target for anticancer drugs: agents which interact with the mitotic spindle. Med Res Rev 18: 259-296

Kayagaki N, Kawasaki A, Ebata T, Ohmoto H, Ikeda S, Inoue S, Yoshino K, Okumura K, Yagita H (1995) Metalloproteinase-mediated release of human FAS ligand. J Exp Med 182: 1777-1783

Kinsella AR, Smith D, Pickard M (1997) Resistance to chemotherapeutic antimetabolites: a function of salvage pathway involvement and cellular response to DNA damage. Br J Cancer 75:935-945

Krajewski S, Blomqvist C, Franssila K, Krajewska M, Wasenius VM, Niskanen E, Nordling S, Reed JC (1995) Reduced expression of pro-apoptotic BAX is associated with poor response rates to combination chemotherapy and shorter survival in women with metastatic breast adenocarcinoma. Cancer Res 55: 4471-4478

Landowski TH, Gleason-Guzman MC, Dalton WS (1997) Selection for drug resistance results in resistance to FAS-mediated apoptosis. Blood 89: 1854-1861

McGuire JJ, Magee KJ, Russell CA, Canestrari JM (1997) Thymidylate synthase as a target for growth inhibition in methotrexate-sensitive and -resistant human head and neck cancer and leukemia cell lines. Oncol Res 9: 139-147

Meyers MB, Zamparelli C, Verzili C, Dicker AP, Blanck TJJ, Chiancone E (1995) Calcium-dependent translocation of sorcin to membranes: functional relevance in contractile tissue. FEBS Letters 357: 230-234

Miyashita T, Reed JC (1993) BCL-2 oncoprotein blocks chemotherapy-induced apoptosis in human leukemia cell line. Blood 81:151-157

Mosmann T (1983) Rapid colorimetric assay for cellular growth and survival: Application to proliferation and cytotoxicity assays. J. Immunol. Methods 65: 55-61

Nooter K, Stoter G (1996) Molecular mechanisms of multidrug resistance in cancer chemotherapy. Pathol Res Pract 192: 768-780

Paciucci R, Berrozpe G, Tora M, Navarro E, Garcia-de-Herreros A, Real FX (1996) Isolation of tissue-type plasminogen activator, cathepsin H, and non-specific cross-reacting antigen from SK-PC-1 pancreas cancer using subtractive hybridization. FEBS Lett 385: 72-76

Popken-Harris P, Checkel J, Loegering D, Madden B, Springett M, Kephart G, Gleich GJ (1998) Regulation and processing of a precursor form of eosinophil granule major basic protein (ProMBP) in differentiating eosinophils. Blood 92: 623-631

Rabbani SA, Xing RH (1998) Role of urokinase (uPA) and ist receptor (uPAR) in invasion and metastasis of hormone-dependent malignancies. Int J Oncol 12: 911-920

Robinson L, Panayiotakis A, Papas TS, Kola I, Seth A (1997) ETS target genes: identification of egr1 as a target by RNA differential display and whole genome PCR techniques. Proc Natl Acad Sci USA 94:7170-7175

Rowan S, Fisher DE (1997) Mechanisms of apoptotic cell death. Leukemia 11: 457-465

Rustum YM, Harstrick A, Cao S, Vanhoefer U, Yin MB, Wilke H, Seeber S (1997) Thymidylate synthase inhibitors in cancer therapy: direct and indirect inhibitors. J Clin Oncol 15: 389-400

Scaffidi C, Fulda S, Srinivasan A, Friesen C, Li F, Tomaselli KJ, Debatin KM, Krammer PH, Peter ME (1998) Two CD95 (APO-1/FAS) signaling pathways. EMBO J 17:1675-1687

Schneider P, Holler N, Bodmer JL, Hahne M, Frei K, Fontana A, Tschopp J (1998) Conversion of membrane-bound FAS (CD 95) ligand to ist soluble form is associated with downregulation of its proapoptotic activity and loss of liver toxicity. J Exp Med 187: 1205-1213

Tanaka M, Itai T, Adachi M, Nagata S (1998) Downregulation of FAS ligand by shedding. Nat Medicine 4: 31-36

# Transforming Activity of Flt3 in 32D Cells

M. Mizuki, W. Grüning, R. Schmidt, S. Serve, R. Fenski, K. Kratz-Albers, T. Büchner, J. Kienast, W. E. Berdel and H. Serve

## Introduction

The type III receptor tyrosine kinase Flt3 (Matthews et al., 1991) and its ligand FL (Hannum et al., 1994) play an important role in survival and self renewal of early multipotent hematopoietic progenitors, of monocytic precursors and in early lymphoid development (Lyman and Jacobsen, 1998).

Incubation of leukemic blasts with FL results in enhanced DNA synthesis in some, but not all cases of AML and in a reduced rate of spontaneous apoptosis of AML blasts. Interestingly, the proliferative response to FL is not necessarily predicted by surface expression of the receptor (Stacchini et al., 1996).

Since the description of Flt3 expression on leukemic blasts (Drexler, 1996) speculation arose that it might play a role in malignant transformation of hematopoietic progenitors. Reports about a proliferative and antiapoptoic response to FL supported that hypothesis (Drexler, 1996; Lisovsky et al., 1996). We have reported previously that Flt3 receptor of two third AML patients shows ligand dependent phosphorylation and 10% AML patients show ligand-independent autophosphorylation of Flt3 receptor. The mechanism of the observed activation remains unknown. Internal tandem repeat (ITR) mutations involving exon 11 of Flt3, which cause an insertion of several amino acids in the juxtamembrane region of the protein and are detectable in about 20% of AML samples, have been suggested as a mechanism of Flt3 activation (Kiyoi et al., 1998). However, we have shown that ITR mutations do not correlate with Flt3 autophosphorylation (Fenski et al., submitted for publication). An activating point mutation in

the kinase domain of two other receptor tyrosine kinases has been linked to neoplastic diseases. Substitution of Asp 814 by Valin (Furitsu et al., 1993) in the structurally and functionally closely related protein c-kit (Qiu et al., 1988) has been associated with systemic mastocytosis (Longley et al., 1996). A similar mutation(Met 918 Thr) in the protooncogene ret is found in germ line of families with multiple endocrine neoplasin type 2b and as a somatic mutation in about 30–40% of sporadic cases with medullary thyroid carcinoma (reviewed in Kolibaba and Druker, 1997). In order to analyse the consequences of constitutive activation of Flt3 in myeloid cells, we introduced the wildtype receptor into 32D cells, a murine IL-3-dependent hematopoietic cell line without endogenous Flt3 expression. Furthermore, we constructed a mutation of Flt3, substituting Asp 838 with Valin, (Flt3$^{D838V}$), which we also transfected into these cells. This mutation is homologous to the activating mutation found in c-kit in neoplastic mast cell disorders. Here, we show that Flt3 signalling can mediate proliferation and survival of 32D cells, and that the D838V mutation confers ligand independent proliferation of these cells. We also demonstrate possible signalling pathways and in-vivo effects of Flt3 activation in 32Dcl3 cells.

## Materials and Methods

### cDNA Constructs and Expression Systems

The cDNA of murine Flt3 was kindly provided by Dr. Ihor Lemischka (Princeton, NJ, USA). The complete coding sequence was

University of Münster, Department of Hematology/Oncology, Albert-Schweitzer-Straße 33, 48129 Münster, Germany subcloned into the retroviral vector pGD at the Bcl I site under the control of the long terminal repeat of the myeloproliferative sarcoma virus (MPSV). After site-directed mutagenesis of Flt3, integrity of the complete Flt3 coding region was confirmed by sequence analysis. Hybrid receptor containing the extracellular domain of mouse c-kit and the transmembrane and intracellular domains of human Flt3 was constructed by PCR-based methods and the construct was cloned into pcDNA3.1 (Clontech). For transfection, 10 µg plasmid DNA of either plasmid was linearized by HindIII digestion and added to the cell suspensions. Samples were electroporated with a Gene Pulser (Biorad) in 0,4 cm cuvettes at 300 V and 960 µF and were selected with 0,6 mg/ml G418. 14 days later the Geniticin resistant cells were purified twice with a magnetic cell sorting (MACS)-column (Miltenyi Biotec) using rat anti-mouse-Flt3 monoclonal antibody and goat anti-rat-ferrobeads according to the manufacturer's instructions. COS-1 cells were transiently transfected by the DHEA-method.

### Proliferation and Apoptosis Assays

Proliferation was measured by $^3$H thymidine incorporation into cells, which had been arrested in $G_0/G_1$ prior to the assay. Apoptis was induced by growth factor and serum deprivation of the cells for the indicated times combined with ionising irradation when indicated. For this purpose, cells were γ-irradiated with 10 Gy and FL or IL-3 was added as indicated. Inhibition of cytokine activities was done by 15 min-preincubation with 100 nM wortmannin (Sigma) and/or 40 µM PD98059. Apoptosis assay was done with the Annexin-V assay kit (Genzyme). Annexin-V$^-$ Propidium Ionide$^-$ cells were counted as viable cells.

### Immunoprecipitation, Western blot and MAPK Assays

After starving from cytokines cells were lysed 50 mM HEPES pH 7.4, 10% Glycerol, 150 mM NaCl, 1% Triton x-100, 1 mM EDTA, 1 mM EGTA, 50 µM ZnCl, 25 mM NaF, proteinase

inhibitors, 1 µM pepstain and 1 mM sodium orthovanadate) and immunoprecipitation was performed with the indicated antibodies. MAPK activity was measured by adding MBP as a substrate and GGG[$^{32}$P]-ATP. The kinase reaction was allowed to proceed für 20 min at 30°C. Reactions were spotted onto phosphocellulose paper, washed extensively with 0.85% phosphoric acid and incorporated radioactivity was determined. For western blot analysis, immunoprecipitates were separated by SDS-PAGE (7%), blotted onto PVDF membrane and immunoblots were performed using the indicated antibodies and ECL (Amersham) as a detection system.

### In vivo Tumorigenicity

C3H/HeJ-mice were injected with 1x10$^6$ cells of 32Dcl3/Flt3 or 32Dcl3/Flt3$^{D838V}$. Control mice received 32Dcl3/vector. The animals were observed on a daily basis. Moribund animals were sacrificed and bone marrow samples were smeared onto glass slides and stained with May-Grünwald Giemsa stain.

## Results

In order to analyse the effects of activating mutations of Flt3, we stably transfected Flt3 and Flt3$^{D838V}$ into 32D cells (Fig. 1). Similar levels of surface expression could be reached for both protein isoforms. 32Dcl3/Flt3 cells responded to addition of FL by increased $^3$H thymidine incorporation, whereas 32Dcl3/vector were not influenced by addition of FL. In contrast to these two cell lines, 32Dcl3/Flt3$^{D838V}$ cells proliferate without exogenously added growth factors, and exogenously added FL does not influence DNA synthesis in these cells (Fig. 2). 32Dcl3/Flt3$^{D838}$ continued to grow for several weeks without exogenously added growth factors (data not shown). Thus, Flt3$^{D838V}$ expression causes factor-independent growth of 32Dcl3 cells.

32Dcl3 cells are IL-3 dependent cell lines, and IL-3 deprivation induces apoptosis on these cells. When depleted from IL-3 and serum, 90% of 32Dcl3 cells die by 40h (Fig. 3A). Ionising irradiation induces more rapid death in 32Dcl3 cells, and after 16 h over 90%

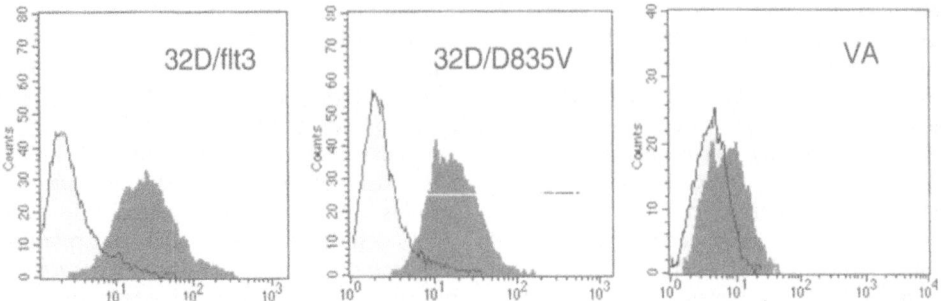

**Fig. 1.** Expression of Flt3 isoforms in transfected 32Dcl3 cells. 32D cells transfected with the indicated cDNA constructs were stained with PE-conjugated anti-Flt3 (dark grey) or control (light grey) antibody and analysed by flow cytometry.

of cells are apoptotic (Fig. 3B). FL rescues 32Dcl3/Flt3 cells dose dependently in both conditions. Notably, 32Dcl3/Flt3$^{D838V}$ cells could not survive as 32Dcl3/Flt3 supplemented with Flt3-ligand.

Having shown, that Flt3 induces proliferation and survival in 32D-cells, we were interested in elucidating the signalling events involved. We first analysed the signalling pathways activated by Flt3. In an immunocomplex kinase assay, Flt3-ligand induced MAPK activity in Flt3-transfected cells approximately 10 times over basal activity (Fig. 4). The MEK1 inhibitor PD98059 inhibits this rise in activity by 85%. We also analysed the association of Flt3 with p85$^{PI3K}$, a first step

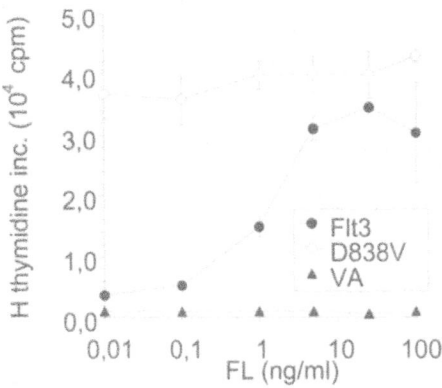

**Fig. 2.** Proliferation of Flt3 transfected cells in the presence of FL. 10$^4$ serum-starved cells transfected as indicated were incubated with increasing concentrations of FL for 40 h. For the last 16 h of the incubation period 1 μCi $^3$H thymidine was added. Cells were lysed and thymidine incorporation was measured by liquid scintillation counting.

in PI3K activation by receptor tyrosine kinases. We could not find significant association of p85 with murine Flt3 (data not shown). Since we were concerned about the sensitivity of the immunocomplex formation with the antibody we used, we constructed a hybrid molecule of the extracellular domain of c-kit containing the epitope binding to a monoclonal c-kit antibody (ACK2) fused with the transmembrane and intracellular domains of human Flt3. We then compared the amount of p85 bound to roughly equal amounts of c-kit and this hybrid molecule. No p85 could be found to be associated with the immunoprecipitated intracellular domain of Flt3 under conditions, which easily demonstrated association of c-kit and p85 (Fig. 5). Thus, no direct association of Flt3 with p85 could be demonstrated. We then were interested in the functional significance of Flt3-dependent signalling pathways for Flt3-mediated functions. The PI3K inhibitor wortmannin had minor effects on FL-mediated survival, whereas the MEK1 inhibitor PD98059, blocking the MAPK erk-1, inhibited FL-mediated survival quite effectively. Combination of both inhibitors completely blocked survival effect of Flt3 (Fig. 6). Finally, we injected 32D cells expressing the two isoforms of Flt3 into syngeneic, immunocompetent mice. Mice injected with 32Dcl3/vector cells did not show any disease during 4 months observation after injection. In contrast, mice injected with 32Dcl3/Flt3 or 32Dcl3/Flt3$^{D838V}$ suffered from subcutaneous tumors and bone marrow infiltration with myeloid cells of blast morphology starting at 4 weeks after injection.

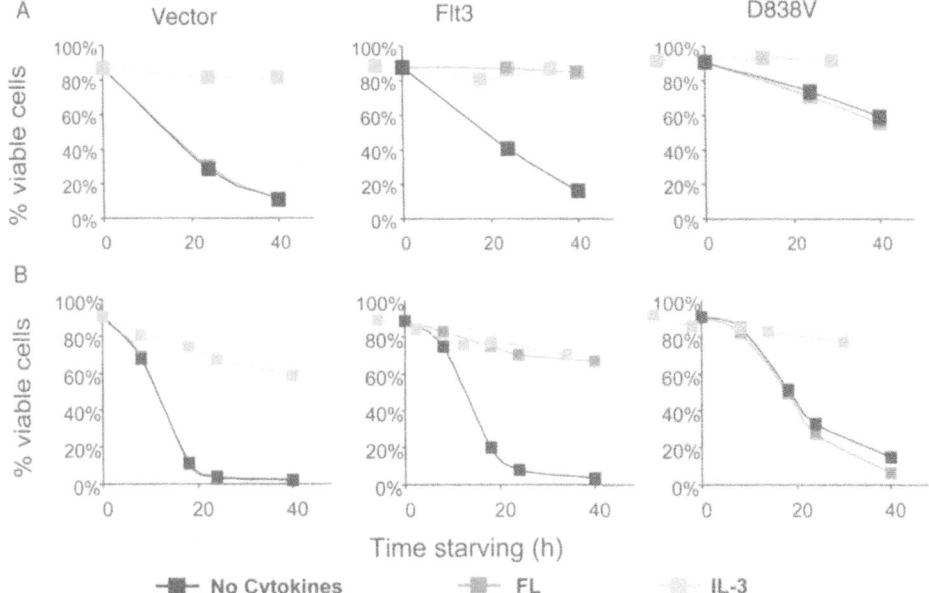

**Fig. 3.** Flt3-mediated rescue of 32D cells from apoptosis. Apoptosis was induced in 32Dcl3 cells by A) cytokine depletion or B) cytokine depletion and ionising irradiation. In order to rescue cells from death, IL-3 and FL were added as indicated at time 0. The y axis shows the percentage of cells staining negative for Anexin-V and propidium iodide.

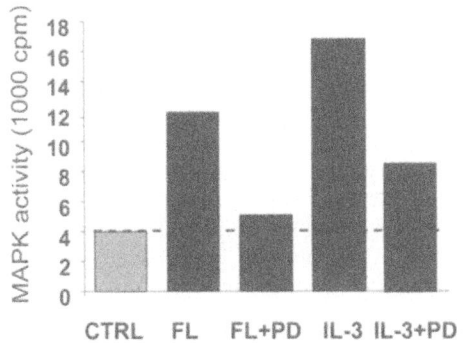

**Fig. 4.** MAP kinase activation by Flt3
32Dcl3/Flt3 cells were starved for 12 hours, stimulated with/without cytokines for 10 minutes, lysed and immunocomplex kinase assays for Erk-1 and Erk-2 were performed. FL; 100 ng/ml, IL-3; 10 ng/ml, PD; 40 μg/ml

## Discussion

In this report, we show that Flt3 mediates proliferation and survival of 32Dcl3 cells, substituting for IL-3. A point mutation in Flt3 kinase domain confers ligand independent proliferation. As determined by analysis with chemical inhibitors, Flt3 signal is mediated by MAPK- and PI3K-dependent pathways. Finally, we determine the significance of Flt3 for in vivo leukemogenesis.

**Fig. 5.** Weak association of p85PI3K protein with Flt3.
A hybrid molecule of mouse c-kit (extracellular) and isoforms of human flt3 (transmembrane and intracellular) as indicated were expressed in COS-1 cells. Immunoprecipitates with ACK-2, recognizing an extracellular epitope on c-kit, were blotted with antibodies against phosphotyrosine (PY) and p85$^{PI3K}$ (p85). Note the lack of association of p85 to the intracellular domain of Flt3, in contrast to c-kit. The ligand-independent autophosphorylation of D838V and the lack of autophosphorylation of D811N (homologous to W$^{42}$ of Kit, constitutive negative mutant) are also indicated.

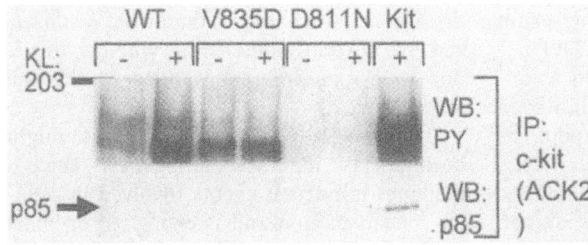

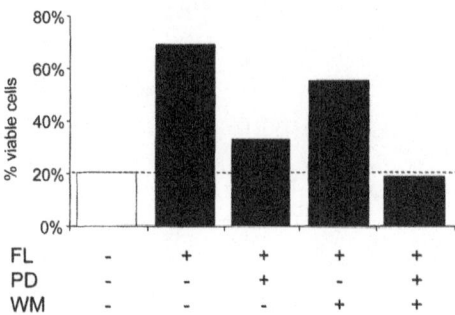

FL   -   +   +   +   +
PD   -   -   +   -   +
WM   -   -   -   +   +

**Fig. 6.** Inhibition of Flt3-mediated survival by PI3K and MAP kinase inhibitors.
Induction of apoptosis was done by irradiation as shown in Fig. 3B. PI3K inhibitor, wortmannin (WM; 100 nM) and MAP kinase inhibitor, PD98059 (PD; 40 µM) were preincubated for 15 min before the addition of FL as indicated. Viability was evaluated 16 hours after irradiation.

We introduced a mutation D838V into the Flt3 cDNA which we reasoned to be activating, since a homologous mutation has been described in c-kit. This c-kit mutation activates proliferation of mouse and human mast cell lines (Furitsu et al., 1993), induces differentiation and tumorigenicity in primary mast cells (Hashimoto et al., 1996) and adult mouse bone marrow (Kitayama et al., 1996) and is associated with neoplastic mast cell disease in humans (Longley et al., 1996). The mechanism of activation of this type of mutation described here is still an unsolved matter. Recently it was shown, that substitution of the homologous Asp at position 814 in c-kit by Tyr causes enhanced degradation of SHP-1, a tyrosine specific protein phosphatase, and a change in the substrate specifity of c-kit (Piao et al., 1996). A similar mechanism could be operative in the described mutation in Flt3.

We could demonstrate, that Flt3 receptor expression endows FL dependent proliferation and survival on 32Dcl3 cells. This survival effect is observed both in cytokine/serum depletion and ionising irradiation. Flt3$^{D838V}$ induced factor independent growth as a constitutive active mutant. Interestingly however, Flt3$^{D838V}$ could rescue cells from apoptosis less effectively than ligand-activated wtFlt3. This difference could be due to qualitative differences of the wtFlt3 and Flt3$^{D838V}$ signal. So, Flt3$^{D838V}$ might serve as a tool for future

studies to dissect the proliferative and antiapoptotic signaling pathways of Flt3. Flt3 is reported to mediate survival in primitive hematopoietic stem cell and fresh AML blasts in serum-free culture (Lisovsky et al., 1996). However, the signal transduction pathway of Flt3 leading to cell survival has not been examined. In this report, we show that Flt3 activates the MAP kinase pathway and that this pathway is important for Flt3-mediated survival. Although activation of ras, an upstream regulator of MAP kinase activity, has been reported to be involved in survival mediated by the GM-CSF-receptor (Kinoshita et al., 1995) as well as by bcr-abl (Cortez et al., 1996), ras can also activate PI3K, an enzyme implicated as a key protein for antiapoptotic signals (Campbell et al., 1998). Moreover, it has been reported, that the MEK-1 inhibitor PD98059 can not inhibit the survival effect of GM-CSF (Scheid and Duronio, 1998). On the other hand, there is emerging evidence suggesting that the MAP kinase pathway is involved in inhibition of apoptosis mediated by many other cytokines (Jarpe et al., 1998). Our results support these findings. However, the major pathway implicated in cytokin-mediated survival involves the lipid kinase PI3K, which generates small second messenger molecules activating the serine/threonine-kinase Akt. The proapoptotic protein Bad is phosphorylated by Akt and is thus inactivated, which results in cell survival. Our studies involving the PI3K inhibitor wortmannin showed only minor importance of this pathway for Flt3-mediated survival.

We show for the first time, that wildtype and constitutively active Flt3 greatly enhances the malignant potential of 32D cells. It has been reported previously, that c-kit expression on 32Dcl3 cells enhances their leukemogenic potential (Hu et al., 1995). However, in the study reported on c-kit, the lag period until the animals developed a leukemic disease was much longer, than what we observed. We currently determine, whether this is due to clonal differences between the cell lines used.

Thus, we provide evidence, that Flt3 might be important for AML pathogenesis, since it mediates important events involved in cellular transformation and is expressed on most AML samples. In the future, studies examining Flt3-dependent signalling events might reveal important targets for oncogene-specific therapies.

# References

Campbell SL, Khosravi-Far R, Rossman KL, Clark GJ, Der CJ (1998) Increasing complexity of Ras signaling. Oncogene 17: 1395-1413

Cortez D, Stoica G, Pierce JH, Pendergast AM (1996) The BCR-ABL tyrosine kinase inhibits apoptosis by activating a Ras-dependent signaling pathway. Oncogene 13: 2589-2594

Drexler HG (1996) Expression of FLT3 receptor and response to FLT3 ligand by leukemic cells. Leukemia 10: 588-599

Furitsu T, Tsujimura T, Tono T, Ikeda H, Kitayama H, Koshimizu U, Sugahara H, Butterfield JH, Ashman LK, Kanayama Y et al. (1993) Identification of mutations in the coding sequence of the proto-oncogene c-kit in a human mast cell leukemia cell line causing ligand- independent activation of c-kit product. J Clin Invest 92: 1736-1744

Hannum C, Culpepper J, Campbell D, McClanahan T, Zurawski S, Bazan JF, Kastelein R, Hudak S, Wagner J, Mattson J et al. (1994) Ligand for FLT3/FLK2 receptor tyrosine kinase regulates growth of haematopoietic stem cells and is encoded by variant RNAs. Nature 368: 643-648

Hashimoto K, Tsujimura T, Moriyama Y, Yamatodani A, Kimura M, Tohya K, Morimoto M, Kitayama H, Kanakura Y, Kitamura Y (1996) Transforming and differentiation-inducing potential of constitutively activated c-kit mutant genes in the IC-2 murine interleukin-3-dependent mast cell line. Am J Pathol 148: 189-200

Hu Q, Trevisan M, Xu Y, Dong W, Berger SA, Lyman SD, Minden MD (1995) c-KIT expression enhances the leukemogenic potential of 32D cells. J Clin Invest 95: 2530-2538

Jarpe MB, Widmann C, Knall C, Schlesinger TK, Gibson S, Yujiri T, Fanger GR, Gelfand EW, Johnson GL (1998) Anti-apoptotic versus pro-apoptotic signal transduction: checkpoints and stop signs along the road to death. Oncogene 17: 1475-1482

Kinoshita T, Yokota T, Arai K, Miyajima A (1995) Suppression of apoptotic death in hematopoietic cells by signalling through the IL-3/GM-CSF receptors. Embo J 14: 266-275

Kitayama H, Tsujimura T, Matsumura I, Oritani K, Ikeda H, Ishikawa J, Okabe M, Suzuki M, Yamamura K, Matsuzawa Y, Kitamura Y, Kanakura Y (1996) Neoplastic transformation of normal hematopoietic cells by constitutively activating mutations of c-kit receptor tyrosine kinase. Blood 88: 995-1004

Kiyoi H, Towatari M, Yokota S, Hamaguchi M, Ohno R, Saito H, Naoe T (1998) Internal tandem duplication of the FLT3 gene is a novel modality of elongation mutation which causes constitutive activation of the product. Leukemia 12: 1333-1337

Kolibaba KS, Druker BJ (1997) Protein tyrosine kinases and cancer. Biochim Biophys Acta 1333: F217-248

Lisovsky M, Estrov Z, Zhang X, Consoli U, Sanchez-Williams G, Snell V, Munker R, Goodacre A, Savchenko V, Andreeff M (1996) Flt3 ligand stimulates proliferation and inhibits apoptosis of acute myeloid leukemia cells: regulation of Bcl-2 and Bax. Blood 88: 3987-3997

Longley BJ, Tyrrell L, Lu SZ, Ma YS, Langley K, Ding TG, Duffy T, Jacobs P, Tang LH, Modlin I (1996) Somatic c-KIT activating mutation in urticaria pigmentosa and aggressive mastocytosis: establishment of clonality in a human mast cell neoplasm. Nat Genet 12: 312-314

Lyman SD, Jacobsen SE (1998) c-kit ligand and Flt3 ligand: stem/progenitor cell factors with overlapping yet distinct activities. Blood 91: 1101-1134

Matthews W, Jordan CT, Wiegand GW, Pardoll D, Lemischka IR (1991) A receptor tyrosine kinase specific to hematopoietic stem and progenitor cell-enriched populations. Cell 65: 1143-1152

Piao X, Paulson R, van der Geer P, Pawson T, Bernstein A (1996) Oncogenic mutation in the Kit receptor tyrosine kinase alters substrate specificity and induces degradation of the protein tyrosine phosphatase SHP-1. Proc Natl Acad Sci U S A 93: 14665-14669

Qiu FH, Ray P, Brown K, Barker PE, Jhanwar S, Ruddle FH, Besmer P (1988) Primary structure of c-kit: relationship with the CSF-1/PDGF receptor kinase family-oncogenic activation of v-kit involves deletion of extracellular domain and C terminus. Embo J 7: 1003-1011

Scheid MP, Duronio V (1998) Dissociation of cytokine-induced phosphorylation of Bad and activation of PKB/akt: involvement of MEK upstream of Bad phosphorylation. Proc Natl Acad Sci USA 95: 7439-7444

Stacchini A, Fubini L, Severino A, Sanavio F, Aglietta M, Piacibello W (1996) Expression of type III receptor tyrosine kinases FLT3 and KIT and responses to their ligands by acute myeloid leukemia blasts. Leukemia 10: 1584-1591

# Evidence of Angiogenesis in Acute Myeloid Leukemia

T. Padro[1], S. Ruiz[1], R. H. Bürger[2], M. Steins[1], R. Bieker[1], J. Kienast[1], T. Büchner[1], W. Böcker[2], W.E. Berdel[1] and R.M. Mesters[1]

*Abstract.* Angiogenesis plays a key role in the growth of solid tumors and in the development of metastases. An increased angiogenesis in bone marrow has been reported in children with acute lymphoblastic leukemia (*Am J Pathol 150: 815-821, 1997*). The purpose of the present study was to assess angiogenesis in bone marrow biopsies from 47 patients with newly diagnosed, untreated acute myeloid leukemia (AML). Control specimens (n=20) were obtained from patients with neoplasic disorders without bone marrow involvement. The FAB distribution of the AML cases was as follows: 7 M1, 21 M2, 1 M3, 7 M4, 7 M5, 2 M6 and 2 AMLs without defined subtype. The endothelial cells of microvessels were highlighted by immunohistochemical staining for thrombomodulin (TM) and von Willebrand factor (vWF). The 3 areas with the highest microvessel density in representative sections of each bone marrow core biopsy specimen were selected and the microvessels scored in x500 fields by two observers using light microscopy. A significant correlation was found between microvessel counts in bone marrow sections stained by vWF and TM antibodies ( r = 0.828; $p <$ 0.001). Using TM staining, AML marrows had (median [interquartile range]) 25.5 [22.1-29.3] microvessels / field while normal marrows had 13.2 [11.4-14.8] microvessels / field. Using vWF staining of the same specimens, AML marrows had 22.9 [16.1-26.2] microvessels / field while normal marrows had 9.8 [7.7-10.5] microvessels / field. The differences between the number of vessels / field in AML and controls were statistically significant for both TM ($p =$ 0.0003) and vWF ($p =$ 0.001) staining.

When analyzed by FAB category, there was no difference in the average number of microvessels / field between the different subgroups of AML. In summary, we demonstrated that bone marrow in AML is associated with increased microvessel density. These findings suggest that antiangiogenic therapy might constitute a novel strategy for the treatment of acute myeloid leukemia.

## Introduction

Formation of new blood vessels (angiogenesis) is an absolute requirement for the viability and growth of solid tumors [1,2]. This neovascularization is mediated by angiogenic molecules released by tumor cells themselves and by accessory host cells such as macrophages, mast cells and lymphocytes. In turn, the newly formed endothelial cells of the tumor can stimulate tumor growth in a paracrine fashion [3-5]. Furthermore, angiogenesis is important for the development of a malignant phenotype [6-7], and numerous studies have demonstrated that the vascular density of a tumor directly correlates with metastasis and patient outcome [8-17].

In contrast to solid tumors, few data are available regarding angiogenesis in hematologic malignancies. In multiple myeloma, bone marrow neovascularization correlates with disease activity [18-19], and in B-cell non-Hodgkin's lymphomas a correlation of the degree of angiogenesis with the stage of the lymphoma was reported [20]. Recently, an increased microvessel density has been demonstrated in the bone marrow of children

From the [1]Department of Medicine / Hematology and Oncology and the [2] Gerhard-Domagk Institute of Pathology, University of Münster, Germany.

with acute lymphoblastic leukemia (ALL) [21].

Until now, information concerning bone marrow neovascularization in acute myeloid leukemia (AML) has been limited to two recent abstract reports with conflicting results [22,23]. The present study was undertaken to investigate the extent of angiogenesis in the bone marrow of adult patients with newly diagnosed, untreated AML.

## Materials and Methods

### Materials

Bone marrow specimens from 47 adult patients with newly diagnosed, untreated AML were studied. Diagnosis and classification of AML according to the criteria of the French-American-British (FAB) Cooperative Group [24] were confirmed by centralized review of bone marrow morphology, cytochemistry and immunophenotyping within the AML Cooperative Group (AMLCG) [25]. Patient characteristics including AML FAB-subtypes are depicted in Table 1. A bone marrow core biopsy (iliac crest) for histological diagnosis was obtained from all patients at presentation. To establish controls, we studied bone marrow biopsies obtained at diagnosis, i.e. before any chemo- / radiotherapeutic treatment from 20 adult patients with various diseases but normal bone marrow morphology. In case of non-Hodgkin's lymphomas, Hodgkin's disease and solid tumors, the bone marrow was histologically not involved by the underlying disease (Table 1). After every core biopsy, a bone marrow aspiration was obtained through a separate puncture for cytological analyses.

### Immunohistochemical staining

Bone marrow specimens were fixed in paraformaldehyde, embedded in paraffin and decalcified with EDTA. 4-µm-thick serial sections of each sample were processed for immunohistochemical identification of microvascular endothelial cells with anti-human von Willebrand factor (vWF monoclonal antibody [MoAb], clone F8/86, Dako,

**Table 1.** Patient characteristics

| AML patients | n = 47 |
|---|---|
| Age (years)* | 60 [18–84] |
| Sex (males / females) | 25 / 22 |
| FAB distribution § | 7 M1, 21 M2, 1 M3, 7 M4, 7 M5, 2 M6, 2 AML without defined subtype |
| Percentage of leukemic blasts* (bone marrow) | 80% [30–99] |
| Controls | n = 20 |
| Age (years)* | 60 [17 - 82] |
| Sex (males / females) | 13 / 7 |
| Disease | 1 Hodgkin's disease, 6 non-Hodgkin's lymphomas, 2 solid tumors, 11 non-malignant disorders |

\* median [range]
§ French-American-British classification for AML [24]

Glostrup, Denmark; working dilution 1:25) and anti-human thrombomodulin antibodies (TM MoAb, clone 1009, Dako; working dilution 1:50). Anti-vWF antibodies are commonly used for highlighting endothelial cells [26,27], although on paraffin sections anti-CD31 antibodies have been suggested as first option on the basis of sensitivity / specificity [27,28]. However, immunohistochemistry employing anti-CD31 (clone JC/70A, Dako) as well as anti-CD34 antibodies (clone QBEND 10, Immunotech, Marseille, France) was not further pursued because of the frequently observable strong staining of leukemic blasts in our study (data not shown). Since TM is constitutively expressed in high density by a restricted number of cells, including endothelial and mesothelial cells [29], we used TM as an endothelial marker. Applying anti-TM antibodies we observed low background staining and a highly specific and intense labeling of endothelial cells. Controls for immunostaining using non-immune mouse IgG (20µg/ml; Sigma Chemical Co, St Louis, MO) in substitution for the specific first antibodies were consistently negative (data not shown).

Immunohistochemical localization was performed by the alkaline phosphatase/antialkaline phosphatase double bridge technique (Dako-APAAP Kit; Dako). Before staining, tissue sections were deparaffinized in xylene, rehydrated in a graded ethanol series and permeabilized by treatment with 0.23% (w/v) pepsin (Sigma Chemical Co) for 6 minutes at

37°C. The primary antibodies were applied overnight at 4°C. Subsequent steps were performed according to the manufacturer's instructions. The fast red substrate (Dako) supplemented with 0.1% (w/v) levamisole was employed for revelation of phosphatase activity (30 min at room temperature). Sections were counterstained with 0.1% (w/v) erythrocin solution.

## Microvessel counting

The degree of angiogenesis was determined by the microvessel density in defined areas of bone marrow sections according to the method of Weidner et al. [8] and an international consensus report [27]. Microvessel counting was simultaneously assessed by two independent experienced investigators using light microscopy. The investigators were not aware of the diagnosis and clinical characteristics of the patient before performing the microvessel counting. The entire bone marrow section was systematically scanned, i.e. field per field, at x100 magnification in order to find the areas showing the most intense vascularization. The magnification was then changed to x250, or to x500, and the investigators were allowed to reposition the slide until the highest number of microvessels were within the x500 field. This area was defined as a hot-spot after achievement of a consensus between both investigators, thus reducing the interobserver error of microvessel counting [30,31]. These vascular hot-spots were only suitable for analysis provided they were within cellular areas of the marrow, since the non-cellular areas (bone lamellae, fat and connective tissue areas, necrotic foci) are devoid of microvessels and hamper comparison between sections [18]. Areas of vascularization adjacent to bone or dense connective tissue were also excluded, because vascularization is not representative of neoangiogenesis in these areas. In each hot-spot, both investigators performed individual microvessel counting in a x500 field (0.126 mm$^2$ field area). In a slight modification of the method described by Weidner *et al.* [8], any red staining endothelial cell or endothelial cell cluster, with or without a lumen, that was clearly separated from adjacent microvessels, blasts and other bone marrow cells, was considered as a single, countable microvessel. Besides the endothelial cells, megakaryocytes were also strongly stained with anti-vWF and at lower intensity with anti-TM antibodies. However, these were easily recognized by their characteristic size and morphology. Other TM- or vWF-positive staining cells were rarely found in the bone marrow samples and were also easily differentiated from endothelial cell positivity on the basis of morphological differences. In each biopsy sample, microvessels were counted at least in three independent hot-spots per section (range 3-5) and in two to three sections stained with vWF as well as TM antibodies. The microvessel density of a bone marrow specimen was calculated as the mean value of all independent readings and recorded as the number of microvessels per x500 field.

## Quantification of leukemic blast infiltration and criteria for response to chemotherapy.

Quantitative analysis of leukemic blast infiltration was performed in bone marrow aspirates by routine cytological analysis as described by the FAB Cooperative Group [24]. A complete remission was defined as a bone marrow with normal hematopoiesis of all cell lines, less than 5% blast cells, and a peripheral blood count with at least 1,500 neutrophils / µL and 100,000 platelets / µL [32].

## Statistics

Data are presented as individual data plots or as medians, interquartile ranges (low quartile – high quartile [LQ-HQ]). Differences in microvessel density between AML and control groups were analyzed by the Mann-Whitney rank sum test for independent groups. Statistical significance of overall differences between more than two groups was analyzed by the Kruskal-Wallis one-way analysis of variance. Correlation between variables was assessed by the Pearson's coefficient (r). Two-sided p values of 0.05 or less were considered significant.

## Results

At presentation, areas with intense neovascularization (hot-spots) were widely distributed in cellular regions of the bone marrow from AML patients. Endothelial cell sprouts and microvessels without visible lumina prevailed in these samples, contrasting with the bigger and well shaped microvessels in the controls (data not shown). When counting the number of vessels in these hot-spots (area of 0.125 mm$^2$), the bone marrow microvessel density was significantly increased in AML patients compared with controls: median [LQ-HQ] values for TM as well as vWF staining were 25.5 [22.1-29.3] and 22.9 [16.1-26.2] microvessels / x500 field in AML *versus* 13.2 [11.4-14.8] and 9.8 [7.7-10.5] microvessels / x500 field in the controls (TM: $p= 0.0003$; vWF: $p= 0.001$; Fig. 1).

The pattern of angiogenesis in the bone marrow specimens was consistently similar when sections were stained with anti-TM or anti-vWF antibodies. Indeed, there was a strong correlation between microvessel counts in adjacent marrow sections stained with these endothelial cell markers (r = 0.828, $p< 0.0001$; Fig 2).

Microvessel counts were not related to age or sex of the patients in the AML and in the control group (AML patients: <60 *vs* ≥60 years, 22.9 *vs* 25.5; males *vs* females, 23.8 *vs* 23.4; control patients: <60 *vs* ≥60 years, 9.5 *vs*

**Table 2.** Bone marrow microvessel density according to the AML subtype

| AML subtype (FAB – classification) | | Microvessel counts* (x500 field) |
|---|---|---|
| M1 | (n= 7) | 21.8 [10.8-24.8] |
| M2 | (n=21) | 22.3 [20.7-26.3] |
| M3 | (n= 1) | 13.9 |
| M4 | (n= 7) | 23.0 [20.8-24.0] |
| M5 | (n= 7) | 24.6 [17.8-30.1] |
| M6 | (n= 4) | 33.1 [27.9-38.2] |
| Not defined | (n= 2) | 31.7 [30.3-31.3] |

* Values represent medians and interquartile ranges. No significant differences between the groups were observed by Kruskal-Wallis analysis.

10.1; males *vs* females, 10.1 *vs* 9.1). Furthermore, statistical analysis did not reveal any significant differences in microvessel density between the AML FAB-subtypes (Kruskal-Wallis test: $p= 0.109$; Table 2).

Bone marrow in the AML patients studied was usually highly infiltrated by blast cells. The median [LQ-HQ] percentage of blasts was 80% [50-90]. However, microvessel density in the biopsies of AML patients did not correlate with the percentage of blasts found in the marrow aspirates (r= -0.161, $p= 0.212$).

## Discussion

The present investigation has unequivocally demonstrated a significant increase of bone

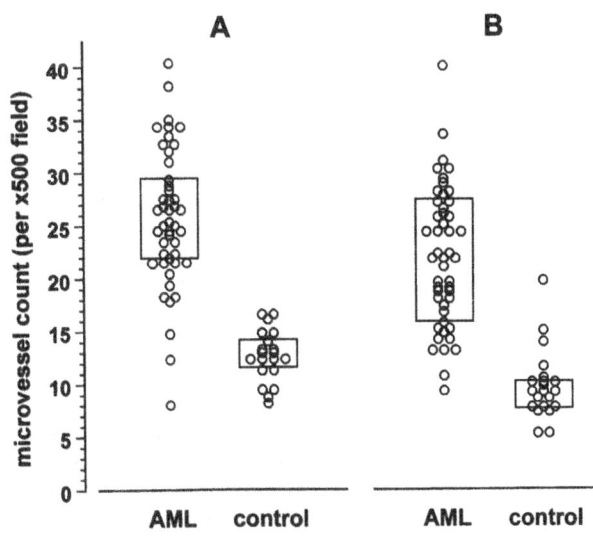

**Fig. 1.** Microvessel density in the bone marrow from 47 AML patients at presentation and 20 controls. Microvessel quantification was performed in adjacent sections of each bone marrow biopsy stained in parallel for TM (A) and vWF (B) as described in Materials and Methods. Data are presented as individual values (open circles) and interquartile ranges (boxes). The difference in microvessel counts between the two groups was statistically significant ( $p= 0.0003$ for TM and $p= 0.001$ for vWF; Mann-Whitney rank sum test for independent groups).

155

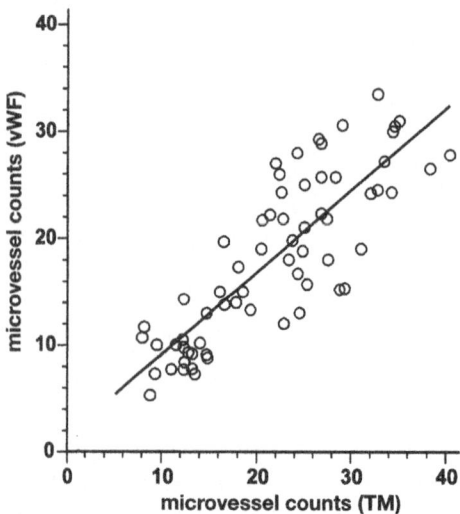

**Fig. 2.** Relationship between microvessel counts per x500 field in adjacent sections of the bone marrow stained for TM or vWF. For each sample (47 patients with AML and 20 controls), microvessel density measured by vWF staining was plotted against the microvessel density obtained with TM staining. Significance of the regression analysis was calculated by the Pearson test (r= 0.828, p< 0.001).

marrow microvessel density in patients with newly diagnosed, untreated AML compared with controls. Indeed, the bone marrow of 75% of the patients with AML showed a two- to three- fold higher microvessel count than the median of the control group. This finding suggests that bone marrow angiogenesis might play an important role in the pathogenesis of AML.

Our results are in line with the reports of increased bone marrow microvessel density in pediatric patients with ALL [21] and in adult patients with multiple myeloma [18] compared with control subjects. Moreover, more intense vascularization has been described in B-cell non Hodgkin's lymphoma compared with benign lymphadenopathies [20], and in colorectal cancers compared with adjacent unaffected mucosa [33].

In contrast to anti-vWF antibodies, immunostaining with anti-TM antibodies has not been described for quantification of angiogenesis up to now. Our study shows a strong correlation between microvessel counts obtained by anti-vWF and anti-TM antibo-

dies, two highly specific endothelial cell markers. This underscores the validity of our findings. Furthermore, staining with the anti-TM antibody displayed a slightly better sensitivity and a higher reproducibility for quantifying angiogenesis. Other groups have also reported that vWF, although highly specific for the vasculature, was partly absent in the capillary endothelium of tumor tissues [33,34]. This and the higher focal background frequently observed with the vWF antibody (probably due to plasma vWF) may explain the lower microvessel counts found in bone marrow sections stained with this endothelial marker. We therefore suggest TM staining as a reliable tool for quantification of angiogenesis in paraffin embedded AML bone marrow samples. Immunohistochemistry with anti-CD31 and anti-CD34 antibodies is not useful, because of the frequently observable strong staining of myeloid leukemic blasts.

The degree of angiogenesis found in our study with a median of 190 vessels / mm$^2$ for AML patients and 89 vessels / mm$^2$ for controls is in accordance with a recent report in multiple myeloma patients (mean: 294 / mm$^2$ vs 93 / mm$^2$ in the controls) [35]. However, these counts were approximately two- to three-fold higher than those obtained in pediatric ALL patients [21]. The reasons for this apparent discrepancy may be differences in age (adults vs children), different sensitivities of the antibodies or the magnification at which microvessel counting was performed. Indeed, a two-fold higher microvessel density has been reported when the magnification was increased from x200 to x400 in CD31 stained breast cancer sections, provided microvessel density was expressed in microvessels / mm$^2$ [30].

Of course it cannot be excluded that the marked increase in microvessel counts in the bone marrow of AML patients is related to reactivation of dormant marrow sinusoids that do not react with the anti-vWF antibody due to low level vWF expression. This nonreactivity to the vWF antigen has been reported in normal hepatic sinusoids [36-40]. These hepatic sinusoids become reactive to the vWF antibody in certain disorders of the liver, including chronic hepatitis, alcohol liver disease, and nodular regeneration [36-40]. However, such a phenomenon has not been described for the TM antigen. Furthermore, the highly variable morphology of the microvessels with arborizing branching, the presence of endothelial sprouts without discernible lumina, the presence of hot-spots and the high microvessel density all suggest a truly neoangiogenic phenomenon. This pattern of angiogenesis is in accordance with the observations reported in pediatric patients with ALL [21].

The mechanisms by which AML blasts induce angiogenesis, however, remain to be elucidated. Among the large number of identified angiogenic factors produced by tumor cells themselves and by accessory host cells, attention has recently focused on members of the fibroblast growth factor (FGF) and vascular endothelial growth factor (VEGF) families as the most common angiogenic factors in tumors [41-43]. These cytokines stimulate migration and proliferation of endothelial cells. Indeed, VEGF expression by leukemic blasts has recently been demonstrated in AML patients [44]. An excess of urokinase plasminogen activator (UPA), a key enzyme for regulation of pericellular proteolysis and degradation of matrix proteins [45], has been found in the bone marrow of AML patients [46]. Furthermore, increased urinary basic FGF levels were reported in children with ALL [21]. Together, these data support the hypothesis of an important role of angiogenesis in acute leukemias.

The lack of correlation between microvessel density and the bone marrow blast count at diagnosis may be due to the low variation of the percentage of blast infiltration in our study population (median: 80; HQ-LQ: 50-90) or interindividual differences in expression of pro- and antiangiogenic factors by leukemic blasts. This observation is in line with the findings in multiple myeloma, in which the degree of bone marrow angiogenesis did not correlate with the percentage of plasma cell infiltration [18].

In summary, we have demonstrated that acute myeloid leukemia is associated with increased bone marrow microvessel density. These findings suggest that antiangiogenic therapy could constitute a novel strategy for the treatment of AML.

# References

1. Gimbrone M, Leapman S, Cotran R, Folkman J (1972) Tumor dormancy in vivo by prevention of neovascularization. J Exp Med 136:261-276
2. Folkman J, Watson K, Ingber D, Hanahan D (1989) Induction of angiogenesis during the transition from hyperplasia to neoplasia. Nature 339:58-61
3. Nicosia RF, Tchao R, Leighton J (1986) Interaction between newly formed endothelial channels and carcinoma cells in plasma clot culture. Clin Exp Metastasis 4:91-104
4. Hamada J, Cavanaugh PG, Lotan O, Nicholson G (1992) Separable growth and migration factors for large-cell lymphoma cells secreted by microvascular endothelial cells derived from target organs for metastasis. Br J Cancer 66:349-354
5. Rak JW, Filmus J, Kerbel RS (1996) Reciprocal paracrine interactions between tumor cells and endothelial cells: the angiogenesis progression hypothesis. Eur J Cancer 32:2438-2450
6. Hanahan D, Folkman J (1996) Patterns and emerging mechanisms of the angiogenic switch during tumorigenesis. Cell 86:353-364
7. Skobe M, Rockwell P, Goldstein N, Vosseler S, Fusenig NE (1997) Halting angiogenesis suppresses carcinoma cell invasion. Nature Medicine 3:1222-1227
8. Weidner N, Semple JP, Welch WR, Folkman J (1991) Tumor angiogenesis and metastasis-correlation in invasive breast carcinoma. N Eng J Med 324:1-8
9. Gasparini G, Weidner N, Maluta S, Pozza F, Boracchi P, Mezzetti M, Testolin A, Bevilacqua P (1993) Intratumoral microvessel density and p53 protein: correlation with metastasis in head -and - neck squamous cell carcinoma. Int J Cancer 55:738-744
10. Weidner N, Carroll PR, Flax J, Blumenfeld W, Folkman J (1993) Tumor angiogenesis correlates with metastasis in invasive prostate carcinoma. Am J Pathol 143:401-409
11. Yamazaki K, Abe S, Takeka H, Sukoh N, Watanabe N, Ogura S, Nakajima I, Isobe H, Inoue K, Kawakami Y (1994) Tumor angiogenesis in human lung adenocarcinoma. Cancer 74: 2245-2250
12. Ellis LM, Fidler IJ (1995) Angiogenesis and breast cancer metastasis. Lancet 346:388-390
13. Gasparini G, Harris AL (1995) Clinical importance of the determination of tumor angiogenesis in breast carcinoma: much more than a new prognostic tool. J Clin Oncol 13:765-782
14. Maeda K, Chung YS, Takasuka S, Ogawa Y (1995) Tumor angiogenesis as a predictor of recurrence in gastric carcinoma. J Clin Oncol 13:477-481
15. Wiggins DL, Granai CO, Steinhoff MM, Calabresi P (1995) Tumor angiogenesis as a prognostic factor in cervical carcinoma. Gynecol Oncol 56:353-356
16. Fontanini G, Lucchi M, Vignati S, Mussi A, Ciardiello F, De Laurentiis M, de Placido S, Basolo F, Angeletti CA, Bevilacqua G (1997) Angiogenesis as a prognostic indicator of survival in non-small cell lung carcinoma. A prospective study. J Natl Cancer Inst 89:881-886
17. Fernández AceLucchi M, Vignati S, Mussi A, Ciardiello F, De Laurentiis M, de Placido S, Basolo F, Angeletti CA, Bevilacqua G (1997) Angiogenesis as a prognostic indicator of survival in non-small cell

lu18. Vacca A, Ribatti D, Roncali L, Ranieri G, Serio G, Silvestris F, Dammacco F (1994) Bone marrow angiogenesis and progression in multiple myeloma. Br J Haematol 87:503-508

19. Vacca A, Ribatti D, Presta M, Minischetti M, Iurlaro M, Ria R, Albini A, Bussolino F, Dammacco F (1999) Bone marrow neovascularization, plasma cell angiogenic potential, and matrix metalloproteinase-2 secretion parallel progression of human multiple myeloma. Blood 93:3064-3073

20. Ribatti D, Vacca A, Nico B, Fanelli M, Roncali L, Dammacco F (1996) Angiogenesis spectrum in the stroma of B-cell non Hodgkin's lymphomas. An immunohistochemical and structural study. Eur J Haematol 56:45-53

21. Perez-Atayde AR, Sallan SE, Tedrow U, Connors S, Allred E, Folkman J (1997) Spectrum of tumor angiogenesis in the bone marrow of children with acute lymphoblastic leukemia. Am J Pathol 150:815-821

22. Shami PJ, Hussong JW, Rodgers GM (1998) Evidence of increased angiogenesis in the bone marrow of patients with acute nonlymphocytic leukemia. Blood 92(suppl 1):512a, (abstr)

23. Aguayo A, Kantarjian H, Talpaz M, Estey E, Koller C, Estrov Z, O'Brien S, Keating M, Barlogie B, Albitar M (1998) Increased angiogenesis in chronic myeloid leukemia and myelodysplastic syndromes. Blood 92(suppl 1):607a, (abstr)

24. Bennett JM, Catovsky D, Daniel MT, Flandrin G, Galton DAG, Gralnick HR, Sultan C (1985) Proposed revised criteria for the classification of acute myeloid leukemia: A report of the French-American-British Cooperative Group. Ann Intern Med 103:620-625

25. Büchner T, Hiddemann W, Wörmann B, Löffler H, Gassmann W, Haferlach T, Fonatsch C, Haase D, Schoch C, Hossfeld D, Lengfelder E, Aul C, Heyll A, Maschmeyer G, Ludwig WD, Sauerland MC, Heinecke A (1999) Double induction strategy for acute myeloid leukemia: the effect of high-dose cytarabine with mitoxantrone instead of standard-dose cytarabine with daunorubicin and 6-thioguanine: a randomized trial by the german AML cooperative group. Blood 93:4116-4124

26. Mukai K, Rosai J, Burgdorf WHC (1980) Localisation of FVIII-R ag in vascular endothelial cells using an immunoperoxidase method. Am J Surg Pathol 4:273-276

27. Vermeulen PB, Gasparini G, Fox SB, Toi M, Martin L, McCulloch P, Pezzella F, Viale G, Weidner AL, Harris AL, Dirix LY (1996) Quantification of angiogenesis in solid tumors: an international consensus on the methodology and criteria of evaluation. Eur J Cancer 32A:2474-2484

28. Miettinen M, Lindenmayer AE, Chaubal A (1994) Endothelial cell markers CD31, CD34 and BNH9 antibody to H- and Y-antigens - evaluation of their specificity and sensitivity in the diagnosis of vascular tumors and comparison with von Willebrand factor. Mod Pathol 1:82-90

29. Mayurama I, Bell C, Majerus P (1985) Thrombomodulin is found on endothelium of arteries, veins, capillaries, and lymphatics and on syncytiotrophoblasts of human placenta. J Cell Biol 101:363-371

30. Vermeulen PB, Libura M, Libura J, O'Neill PJ, van Dam P, van Mark E, van Oosteron AT, Dirix LY (1997) Influence of investigator experience and microscopic field size on microvessel density in node-negative breast carcinoma. Breast Cancer Res Treat 42:165-172

31. Hansen S, Grabau DA, Rose C, Bak M, Sorensen FB (1998) Angiogenesis in breast cancer: a comparative study of the observer variability of methods for determining microvessel density. Lab Invest 78:1563-1573

32. Cheson BC, Cassileth PA, Head DR, Schiffer CA, Bennett JM, Bloomfield CD, Brunning R, Gale RP, Grever MR, Keating MJ, Sawitsky A, Stass S, Weinstein H, Woods WG (1990) Report of the national cancer institute-sponsored workshop on definitions of diagnosis and response in acute myeloid leukemia. J Clin Oncol 8:813-819

33. Vermeulen PB, Verhoven D, Fierens H, Hubens G, Goovaerts G, Van Marck E, De Bruijn EA, Van Oosterom AT, Dirix LY (1995) Microvessel quantification in primary colorectal carcinoma: an immunohistochemical study. Br J Cancer 71:340-343

34. Stephenson TJ, Mills PM (1985) Monoclonal antibodies to blood group isoantigens: an alternative marker to factor VIII related antigen for benign and malignant vascular endothelial cells. J Pathol 147:139-148

35. Rajkumar SV, Fonseca R, Witzig TE, Gertz MA, Greipp PR (1999) Bone marrow angiogenesis in patients achieving complete response after stem cell transplantation for multiple myeloma. Leukemia 13:469-472

36. Bhunchet E, Fujieda K (1993) Capillarization and venularization of hepatic sinusoids in porcine serum-induced rat liver fibrosis: a mechanism to maintain liver blood flow. Hepatology 18:1450-1458

37. Martinez-Hernandez A, Martinez J (1991) The role of capillarization in hepatic failure: studies in carbon tetrachloride-induced cirrhosis. Hepatology 14:864-874

38. Dubuisson L, Boussarie L, Bedin CA, Balabaud C, Bioulac-Sage P (1995) Transformation of sinusoids into capillaries in a rat model of selenium-induced nodular regenerative hyperplasia: an immunolight and immunoelectron microscopic study. Hepatology 21:805-814

39. García-Monz, Boussarie L, Bedin CA, Balabaud C, Bioulac-Sage P (1995) Transformation of sinusoids into capillaries in a rat model of selenium-induced nodular regenerative hyperplasia: an immunolight and immunoelectron microscopic study. Hepatology40. Urashima S, Tsutsumi M, Nakase K, Wang JS, Takada A (1993) Studies on capillarization of the hepatic sinusoids in alcoholic liver disease. Alcohol Alcohol Suppl 1B:77-84

41. Fernig DG, Gallaher JT (1994) Fibroblast growth factors and their receptors: an information network controlling tissue growth, morphogenesis and repair. Prog Growth Factor Res 5:353-377

42. Dvorak HF, Brown LF, Detmar M, Dvorak AM (1995) Vascular permeability factor / vascular endothelial growth factor, microvascular hyperpermeability, and angiogenesis. Am J Pathol 146:1029-1039

43. Claffey KP, Robinson GS (1996) Regulation of VEGF / VPF expression in tumor cells: consequences for tumor growth and metastasis. Cancer Metastasis Rev 15:165-176

44. Fiedler W, Graeven U, Ergün S, Verago S, Kilic N, Stockschläder M, Hossfeld DK (1997) Vascular endothelial growth factor, a possible paracrine growth factor in human acute myeloid leukemia. Blood 89:1870-1875

45. Senger DR (1996) Molecular frame for angiogenesis: a complex web of interactions between extravasated plasma proteins and endothelial cell proteins induced by angiogenic cytokines. Am J Pathol 149:1-7

46. McWilliam N, Robbie L, Booth N, Bennet B (1998) Plasminogen activator in acute myeloid leukemic marrows: u-PA in contrast to t-PA in normal marrows. Br J Haematol 101:626-631

# Significance of AC133 and CD34 Expression on Acute Myeloid Leukemia Cells

P.A. Horn, H. Tesch, P. Staib, C. Schoch*, D. Kube, V. Diehl and D. Voliotis

*Abstract.* AC133 is a novel monoclonal antibody that recognizes a CD34bright subset of human progenitor cells (Yin et al., 1997). Very little data exists so far on expression of AC133 on leukemic blasts. This seems important, however to evaluate its usefulness in immunophenotyping of leukemias and to be able to adress the question whether it may be used for purging purposes in autologous bone marrow transplants for these patients. The aim of this study was therefore to investigate the expression of the AC133 antigen on blast cells of acute myeloid leukemias. 43 cases of AML were examined for expression of AC133, CD34 and other cell surface and cytoplasmatic markers using multicolour flow cytometry in addition to the routinely performed morphological, cytochemical and cytogenetic analysis. 32/43 (74%) AML samples were positive for AC133. AC133 was often but not always associated with CD34 expression. Interestingly, five out of eleven AML that were negative for AC133 showed expression of CD34. In our analysis AC133 expression was found on all FAB subtypes examined except FAB M3 (with only two samples examined). Chromosomal aberrations were found with a similar frequency in both AC133 dim and bright AMLs (58%) and with a slightly lower frequency in AC133 negative AMLs (55%). There was no detectable correlation to cytogenetic abnormalities associated with a more favourable prognosis (e.g. t(8;21), inv(16), t(16;16)) or unfavourable prognosis (e.g. -7, del(7q), del(5q)). Neither the number of leukocytes nor LDH levels were significantly different in AC133 positive and negative AML.

Complete remission rates did not significantly differ in AC133 positive and negative AMLs, although there was a trend towards better outcome in AC133negative AMLs. Further analysis of CD34pos/AC133neg AMLs has to be performed to clarify whether there exists a leukemia-free subset of AC133pos normal hematopoetic stem cells which could serve as a source for autologous stem cell preparation in combination with high dose chemotherapy in these patients who would obviously not benefit from a CD34 based selection.

## Introduction

The AC133 antigen is a glycosylated protein with a molecular weight of 120 kD. The molecular cloning of a cDNA encoding this antigen was reported by Miraglia et al. [1]. The AC133 polypeptide has a predicted size of 97 kD and contains five-transmembrane (5-TM) domains with an extracellular N-terminus and a cytoplasmic C-terminus. Whereas the expression of tetraspan (4-TM) and 7-TM molecules is well documented on mature and immature hematopoietic cells and leukocytes, this 5-TM type of structure containing two large extracellular loops is unique and does not share sequence homology with any known multi-TM family members.

AC133 antigen is selectively expressed on CD34bright hematopoietic stem and progenitor cells derived from human fetal liver and bone marrow, and blood. It is not detectable on other blood cells, cultured human umbili-

Clinic I for Internal Medicine, University of Cologne, Cologne, Germany and
*Department of Internal Medicine III, Ludwig-Maximilians-University, Munich, Germany

cal vein endothelial cells (HUVECs), or fibroblast cell lines by standard flow cytometric procedures. All of the noncommitted CD34+ cell population, as well as the majority of CD34+ cells committed to the granulocytic/monocytic pathway, are stained with the AC133 antibody. AC133-selected cells engraft successfully in a fetal sheep transplantation model, and human cells harvested from chimeric fetal sheep bone marrow have been shown to successfully engraft secondary recipients, providing evidence for the long-term repopulating potential of AC133+ cells.

Very little data exists so far on expression of AC133 on leukemic blasts. This seems important, however, in order to evaluate its usefulness in immunophenotyping of leukemias, to asses its clinical and prognostic significance and to be able to adress the question whether it may be used for purging purposes in autologous bone marrow transplants for AML patients.

## Materials and Methods

### Patients

Bone marrow aspirates performed at initial diagnosis or relapse from 43 patients with AML were examined for expression of AC133. Patients were admitted to the Clinic I for Internal Medicine at the University of Cologne (Koeln, Germany). Diagnosis and classification of AML was based on light microscopy of Pappenheim-stained slides, and on cytochemical reaction with periodic acid shiff (PAS), myeloperoxidase, and esterase. Slides were reviewed by two independent hematologists according to the criteria of the French-American-British (FAB) classification [2]. Demographic data and pertinent medical history were also collected.

### Treatment schedule and definition of response

Patients with de-novo AML received the sequence TAD-HAM as double-induction therapy consisting of cytosine arabinoside (Ara-C) 100 mg/m2 continuous i.v. days 1-2, then 100 mg/m2 twice daily i.v. days 3-8 combined with daunorubicin 60 mg/m2 i.v. days

3-5 and thioguanine 100 mg/m2 twice daily p.o. days 3-9 followed by Ara-C 3 g/m2 twice daily i.v. over three hours days 21-23 combined with mitoxantrone 10 mg/m2 i.v. days 23-25.

Patients with relapsed or secondary AML were treated according to the Ida-FLAG protocol consisting of idarubicin 8 mg/m2 i.v. days 1, 3, 5 combined with fludarabine 25 mg/m2 i.v. days 1-5 followed four hours later by Ara-C 1 g/m2 twice daily i.v. days 1-5, and filgastrim 400 µg/m2 continuous infusion from day 0 until recovery of leukocytes > 1.000/µl.

Complete remission (CR) was defined as a normocellular bone marrow containing < 5% blasts and a peripheral blood count with > 2.500/µl leucocytes and > 100.000/µl platelets.

## Immunofluorescent staining and flowcytometric analsyis

Mononuclear cells from heparinized fresh bone marrow aspirates (BM) were isolated using Ficoll-Hypaque [3] (Pharmacia LKB, Uppsala, Sweden), washed twice in either RPMI 1640 (PAA, Linz, Austria) or phosphate buffered saline (PBS) and resuspended in PBS at a concentration of approximately 2 ( 107 cells/ml. In some cases, frozen cells isolated previously from patients with AML were quickly thawed at 37¡ C, washed twice, and resuspended in PBS at approximately 2 ( 107 cells/ml.

Cells were incubated at approximately 5 ( 105 per test with the corresponding MoAbs for 15 min for direct staining of membrane antigens with FITC or PE conjugated monoclonal antibodies (MoAb),. After staining cells were washed with PBS. Flowcytometric data was obtained on a FACSCalibur(tm) (Becton Dickinson) equipped with Cell Quest Software (Becton Dickinson).

A gate was set on blast cells primarily according to FSC/SSC characteristics. This cell population was then confirmed to be myeloid blasts by determination of the expression profile of surface antigens in combination with FSC/SSC characteristics of these cells. For determination of AC133 expression the commercially available AC133 antibody from Miltenyi Biotec (Bergisch-

Gladbach, Germany) was employed. A gate was set on the blast population according to the above mentioned criteria and staining with CD34-FITC/AC133-PE was used to determine the expression of the corresponding two progenitor cell antigens. Propidium iodide (PI) was added freshly to gate out dead cells by PI staining in a FL2/FL3 dot plot.

Leukemias were considered positive for an antigen according to the guidelines of the European Group for the Immunological Characterization of Leukemias (EGIL) [4] by expression of membrane antigens on more than 20% of blasts and/or intracytoplasmatic antigens on more than 10% of blasts. An isotype matched control antibody was used for the definition of the negative cell population. Similar to the procedure stated by Miraglia et al. [1] AC133dim was defined by a mean relative fluorescence intensity of the gated blast population in the second decade of relative fluorescence intensity and AC133bright by a mean relative fluorescence intensity above the second decade of relative fluorescence intensity.

To compare the brightness of AC133-staining to the brightness of a CD34-staining, a CD34-PE antibody (Becton Dickinson) was used.

### In vitro culture and cytogenetics

Chromosome analyses were performed on metaphases from short term (24h, 48h) cultures of bone marrow cells. Methods of cell cultivation, of chromosome preparation and staining are described elsewhere [5]. A modified GAG-banding technique [6] was used to classify the chromosomes according to the ISCN [7].

## Results

### Patient characteristics

Fourty-three patients with AML were studied. Demographic and clinical data are shown in Table 1. Patient ages ranged from 24 to 69 years (median = 51). 29 patients (67%) were male, and 14 (33%) were female. Bone marrow (BM) cells were collected at initial pre-

sentation of the disease for 37 patients and during relapse for 6 patients. Median white blood cell (WBC) count was 56062/(l (range: 570-246000/(l) and median lactate dehydrogenase (LDH) was 733 U/ml (range: 130-3607 U/ml). The distribution according to the French-American-British (FAB) criteria [2 and 8] was: M1 (n=5), M2 (n=13), M3 (n=2), M4 (n=9), M4eo (n=4), M5 (n=6), M6 (n=1). The FAB classification of one patient was unavailable. There were two cases of secondary AML following Myelodysplastic syndrome (MDS).

### AC133 expression

We investigated the expression of AC133 antigen on blast cells of 43 cases of acute myeloid leukemias. 32/43 (74%) AMLs were positive for AC133. Twelve out of 32 expressed bright levels and 20 expressed dim levels of AC133. In most double-positive leukemias the fluorescence signal for CD34 was brighter than for AC133. All AC133bright leukemias expressed CD34, whereas 14 of the AC133dim leukemias were positive and six were negative for CD34. Interestingly, five out of eleven AMLs that were negative for AC133 showed expression of CD34. Our data show that AC133 expression was often but not always associated with CD34 expression.

### AC133 expression and FAB subtype

In our analysis AC133 expression was found on all FAB subtypes except FAB M3 (only two samples). It was always present in FAB M1 (5/5 cases examined) and in most cases of FAB M2 (11/13). Both FAB M3 leukemias stained negative for AC133, but one was positive for CD34. In FAB M4, M4eo, and M5 AC133 is expressed in approximately 78% of cases (12/19). One M6 leukemia expressed bright levels of AC133 and both secondary leukemias (following MDS) were positive for AC133.

### AC133 expression and karyotype

Chromosomal aberrations were found with the same frequency in both AC133 dim and

**Table 1.** Distribution of AC133 and CD34 expression, morphological classification and cytogenetics in AML patients.

| # | AC133 | CD34 | sex | age | FAB | karyotype |
|---|-------|------|-----|-----|-----|-----------|
| 1 | bright | pos | F | 59 | M1 | 48,XX,+13,+20 |
| 2 | bright | pos | F | 28 | M1 | 46,XX |
| 3 | bright | pos | M | 38 | M1 | 46,XY |
| 4 | bright | pos | M | 39 | M2 | 46,XY |
| 5 | bright | pos | M | 51 | M2 | 46,XY,der(18),t(1;18)(q11;p11) |
| 6 | bright | pos | M | 69 | M4 | 47,XY,ins(1;?)(p35;??),+8,del(9)(q22),del(20)(q11) |
| 7 | bright | pos | M | 52 | M4 | 46,XY |
| 8 | bright | pos | M | 61 | M4eo | 47,XY,+8,inv(16)(p13q22) |
| 9 | bright | pos | F | 32 | M5 | 46,X,t(X;5)(q22;p15),t(5;13)(q35;q14) |
| 10 | bright | pos | M | 61 | M6 | 44,XY,dic(5;16)(q13;q22),-7,-20,-18,+2xmar |
| 11 | bright | pos | M | 63 | NA | 48,XY,+8,+21 |
| 12 | bright | pos | F | 68 | secondary | 46,XX |
| 13 | dim | pos | M | 34 | M1 | 46,XY,t(8;21)(q22;q22),del(9)(q22) |
| 14 | dim | pos | F | 41 | M2 | 47,XX,+8 |
| 15 | dim | pos | M | 67 | M2 | 46,XY |
| 16 | dim | pos | M | 29 | M2 | 45,X,-Y,t(8;21)(q22;q22),del(9)(q22) |
| 17 | dim | pos | F | 53 | M2 | 47,XX,del(5)(q15q33),+11,del(17)(q23) |
| 18 | dim | pos | F | 37 | M2 | 46,XX,t(11;19)(p11.2;q13.1) |
| 19 | dim | pos | F | 45 | M2 | 46,XX,t(8;21)(q22;q22) |
| 20 | dim | pos | M | 52 | M2 | 46,XY |
| 21 | dim | pos | M | 43 | M2 | 46,XY |
| 22 | dim | pos | M | 56 | M4 | NA |
| 23 | dim | pos | M | 27 | M4eo | 46,XY,t(16;16)(p13;q22) |
| 24 | dim | pos | M | 24 | M4eo | 46,XY,inv(16)(p13q22) |
| 25 | dim | pos | F | 50 | M4eo | 46,XX,inv(16)(p13q22),+22 |
| 26 | dim | pos | M | 51 | secondary | 47,XY,del(7)(q22),add(17)(p11),+mar |
| 27 | dim | neg | M | 31 | M1 | 46,XY |
| 28 | dim | neg | M | 53 | M2 | 46,XY |
| 29 | dim | neg | M | 62 | M4 | 46,XX |
| 30 | dim | neg | M | 62 | M4 | 46,XY |
| 31 | dim | neg | M | 63 | M5 | 46,XY |
| 32 | dim | neg | F | 35 | M5 | 47,XY,+8,t(9;11)(p22;q23) |
| 33 | neg | pos | F | 60 | M2 | 45,X,-X,t(8;21) |
| 34 | neg | pos | M | 38 | M3 | 46,XX,+8,t(15;17)(q22;q21) |
| 35 | neg | pos | M | 44 | M4 | 47,XY,+10 |
| 36 | neg | pos | F | 48 | M5 | 46,XY,i(7)(q10) |
| 37 | neg | pos | F | 51 | M5 | 46,XX |
| 38 | neg | neg | M | 62 | M2 | 46,XY |
| 39 | neg | neg | F | 57 | M3 | 46,XX,add(7)(q22),t(15;17)(q22;q21) |
| 40 | neg | neg | M | 61 | M4 | 46,XY |
| 41 | neg | neg | M | 62 | M4 | 46,XX,add(16)(p13.3) |
| 42 | neg | neg | M | 51 | M4 | 46,XY |
| 43 | neg | neg | M | 47 | M5 | 46,XY |

bright AMLs (58%). The frequency was slightly lower in AC133 negative AMLs (55%). All AML patients were subgrouped into risk groups according to their karyotype with t(8;21), inv(16)/t(16;16), and t(15;17) being considered as a good prognostic group, -5/5q-, -7/7q-, inv(3)/t(3;3), t (9;22), t(6;9), 17p-anomalies, 11q23-anomalies and complex chromosomal aberrations (three or more numeric or structural changes) as a poor prognostic group. All other karyotypes including normal ones were considered intermediate risk [similar to 9]. No clear correlation between AC133 expression and karyotype based prognosis group was evident.

Chromosomal aberrations were found with a significantly higher frequency in CD34positive than in CD34negative AMLs (70% vs. 25%). This result is consistent with the findings of Fruchart et al. [10].

### AC133 expression and clinical presentation / outcome

The peripheral leukocyte count (WBC) is known to be a prognostic factor in AML [11 and 12]. Serum lactate dehydrogenase (LDH) levels >400 IU/I is significantly related to an adverse clinical outcome and has been shown to significantly influence disease-free survival, and therefore thought to be a main prognostic factor in AML of the elderly [13 and 14].

There was no significant correlation between the number of leukocytes and lactate dehydrogenase (LDH) levels as clinical prognostic markers and AC133 expression.

26 patients receiving TAD/HAM induction therapy could be evaluated for treatment outcome. 19 of these (73%) reached complete remission (CR). Complete remission did not significantly differ in AC133 positive and negative AMLs, although there was a trend towards better outcome in AC133negative AMLs.

### Discussion

Yin et al. [15] reported the production of AC133, a monoclonal antibody (MoAb) that binds to a novel cell surface antigen present on a CD34bright subset of human hematopoetic stem cells (HSCs) and Miraglia et al. [1] described expression of the AC133 antigen on subsets of CD34+ leukemias.

It was also reported that only myelomonocytic acute leukemia (FAB M4 or M5) expressed bright levels of AC133 [1]. We have previously shown that also other FAB subtypes frequently express bright levels [16]. Still AC133 expression might prove useful in subtyping AMLs.

Only long term follow-up of patients in terms of disease free survival and overall survival of patients classified according to AC133 expression will show, whether its expression is actually related to clinical outcome.

Most patients with AML will obtain a CR after induction chemotherapy but eventually the majority relapses and dies of disease progression [17]. Treatment intensification with autologous bone marrow transplantation (ABMT) may offer a means of improving disease-free survival in relapsed patients [18].

Contamination of the remission marrow with occult malignant cells has been shown to contribute to relapse post transplantation [19], resulting in intense research efforts in finding ways to purge residual tumor cells from remission bone marrows prior to ABMT [20-22]. Our data show that a considerable part of the CD34+ leukemias are AC133- suggesting that isolation of AC133+ HSCs may be a useful purging alternative in these patients, who would obviously not benefit from a CD34 based selection. However, it has to be elucidated, whether the AC133+ cells in these patients are indeed tumor free.

In summary, membrane expression of AC133 in combination with other antigens might facilitate the immunologic characterization of acute myeloid leukemias. It was found in approximately 75% of AML samples and there are indications that it may correlate to clinical outcome. Further investigations are required to evaluate its potential for purging of residual tumor cells in remission marrows in ABMT.

*Acknowledgement.* The authors thank Ms. H. Schultes and Ms. M. Zibulla for excellent technical assistance. Part of this work was supported by a grant from the BMBF, project 12 (01KS9052) and by a grant from the Deutsche Forschungsgemeinschaft (SFB 502).

### References

1. Miraglia, S., Godfrey, W., Yin, A.H., Atkins, K., Warnke, R., Holden, J.T., Bray, R.A., Waller, E.K., Buck, D.W. (1997) A novel five-transmembrane hematopoietic stem cell antigen: isolation, characterization, and molecular cloning. Blood, 90, 5013-5021
2. Bennett, J., Catovsky, D., Daniel, M.-T., Flandrin, G., Galton, D.A.G., Gralnick, H.R., Sultan, C. (1985) Proposed revised criteria for the classification of acute myeloid leukemia. Annals of Internal Medicine, 103, 620-625
3. Boyum, A. (1968) Separation of leukocytes from blood and bone marrow. Scand J of Clin Lab Invest Suppl, 97, 7
4. Bene, M.C., Castoldi, G., Knapp, W., Ludwig, W.D., Matutes, E., Orfao, A., van't Veer, M.B. (1995) Proposals for the immunological classification of acute leukemias. European Group for the Immunological Characterization of Leukemias (EGIL). Leukemia, 9, 1783-1786
5. Stollmann B., Fonatsch Ch. and Havers W. (1985) Persistent Epstein-Barr virus infection associated with monosomy 7 or chromosome 3 abnormality

in childhood myeloproliferative disorders. British Journal of Haematology 60, 183-196

6. Fonatsch Ch., Schaadt M., Kirchner H., Diehl V. (1980) A possible correlation between the degree of karyotype aberrations and the rate of sister chromatid exchanges in lymphoma lines. International Journal of Cancer 26, 749-756

7. ISCN 1995, Guidelines for Cancer Cytogenetics, Supplement to: An International System for Human Cytogenetic Nomenclature (1995) Ed.: F. Mitelman, Publisher: S. Karger.

8. Bennett, J., Catovsky, D., Daniel, M.-T., Flandrin, G., Galton, D.A.G., Gralnick, H.R., Sultan, C. (1976) Proposals for the classification of acute leukemias. A report of the French-American-British Cooperative Group. Br J Haematol, 33, 451-458

9. Mrozek, K., Heinonen, K., de la Chapelle, A., Bloomfield, C.D. (1997) Clinical significance of cytogenetics in acute myeloid leukemia. Semin Oncol, 24, 17-31

10. Fruchart, C., Lenormand, B., Bastard, C., Boulet, D., Lesesve, J.F., Callat, M.P., Stamatoullas, A., Monconduit, M., Tilly, H. (1996) Correlation between CD34 expression and chromosomal abnormalities but not clinical outcome in acute myeloid leukemia. Am J Hematol, 53, 175-180

11. Rigolin GM, Fagioli F, Spanedda R, Scapoli G, Lanza F, Cuneo A, Tomasi P, Castoldi G (1994) Study of prognosis in acute myeloid leukemias (AML) by cluster analysis. Haematologica 79(3): 233-240

12. van der Weide M, Langenhuijsen MM, Huijgens PC, Imandt LM, de Waal FC, Mol JJ, van Rhenen DJ, Kester DA (1987) Relation between leukaemic cell count and degree of maturation in acute myeloid leukaemia. Eur J Cancer Clin Oncol 23(8):1125-1129

13. Ferrara F, Mirto S (1996) Serum LDH value as a predictor of clinical outcome in acute myelogenous leukaemia of the elderly. Br J Haematol 92(3): 627-631

14. Buchner T, Heinecke A (1996) The role of prognostic factors in acute myeloid leukemia. Leukemia Suppl 1: S28-29

15. Yin, A.H., Miraglia, S., Zanjani, E.D., Almeida-Porada, G., Ogawa, M., Leary, A.G., Olweus, J., Kearney, J., Buck, D.W. (1997) AC133, a novel marker for human hematopoietic stem and progenitor cells. Blood, 90, 5002-5012

16. Horn, P.A., Tesch, H., Staib, P., Kube, D., Diehl, V., Voliotis, D., Schoch, C. (1999) Expression of AC133, a novel hematopoetic precursor antigen, on acute myeloid leukemia cells. Blood (letter), 93, 1435-1437

17. Rees, J.K., Gray, R.G., Swirsky, D., Hayhoe, F.G.J. (1986) Principal results of the medical research council's 8th acute myeloid leukemia trial. Lancet, 2, 1236-1241

18. McMillan A.K., Goldstone, A.H., Linch, D.C., et al. (1990) High-dose chemotherapy and autologous bone marrow transplantation in acute myeloid leukemia. Blood, 76, 480-488

19. Brenner, M.K., Rill, D.R., Moen, R.C., et al. (1993) Gene-marking to trace origin of relapse after autologous bone marrow transplantation. Lancet, 341, 85-86

20. Ball, E.D., Mills, L.E., Cornwell, G.G. et al. (1990) Autologous bone marrow transplantation for acute myeloid leukemia using monoclonal antibody-purged bone marrow. Blood, 75, 1199-1206

21. Nimgaonkar, M., Kemp, A., Lancia, J., Ball, E.D. (1996) A combination of CD34 selection and complement-mediated immunopurging (anti CD15 monoclonal antibody) eliminates tumor cells while sparing normal progenitor cells. J Hemato-ther, 5, 39-48

22. Robertson, M.J., Soiffer, R.J., Freedman, A.S. et al. (1992) Human bone marrow depleted of CD33-positive cells mediates delayed but durable reconstitution of hematopoiesis: clinical trial of MY9 monoclonal antibody-purged autografts for the treatment of acute myeloid leukemia. Blood, 79, 2229-2236

# Heterogeneity in the Stem Cell Compartment of Newly Diagnosed Acute Myeloid Leukemia Analyzed by 4-Colour Immunofluorescence

O. ALBRECHT, M. ZÜHLSDORF, G. BAERSCH, J. VORMOOR and T. BÜCHNER

*Abstract.* Leukemic and normal karyotypes have been found in the CD34+CD38-cells in acute myeloid leukemia (AML) irrespective of the CD34 and CD38 expression of the AML. Little is known about the substructure of this CD34+CD38- compartment [3]. We here describe phenotypic subpopulations within the scarce CD34+CD38- cells and differences between this stem cell-like compartment of AML and the bulk of mature leukemic cells.

In 10 cases of AML, the bulk of leukemic blasts was charakterized by 3-colour immunofluorescence and the CD34+CD38- cells were examined by 4-colour analysis. Up to 3 million cells were acquired in a life storage gate. CD33 or HLA-DR versus CD117 (c-kit) were measured in this compartment.

6 of 10 AML were CD34+ in the main population. The CD34+CD38- region appeared to be empty in 9 of 10 cases. However, overacquisition revealed CD34+CD38- cells in 8 of these 9 cases. Different subpopulations were observed. A CD117 lo and HLA-DR lo/- or CD33lo/- population shared by 9 cases was compatible with normal hemopoietic stem cells. 8 of 9 cases showed leukemic subpopulations defined by different marker combinations. In conclusion, overacquisition and 4-colour analysis detected leukemic cells in a compartment where 3- colour immunofluorescence mostly showed no blasts. These results bear on attempts to isolate leukemic or normal stem cells and on the use of anti CD33 monoclonal antibodies

## Materials & Methods

Bone marrow aspirates were obtained from 10 pts. with previously untreated AML. The phenotype of the bulk leukemic population was analysed by 3-colour immunofluores-cence with 20 marker combinations [1,2] . Ammonium chloride lysed cells were stained for CD117 (PE-labelled), CD34 (APC), CD38 (FITC) and HLA-DR (PerCP) or CD33 (PerCP). Up to 3 million cells were acquired and the CD34+CD38- cells collected in a life storage gate . 4-colour analysis was performed on a FACS-Calibur (Becton-Dickinson). Populations were evaluated in Paint-A-Gate 3.0.

## Results

10 Samples of patients with AML were analysed. Patient data are listed in Table 1. All mature blasts of the bulk population were CD38+. In six cases they were also CD34+. In 8 of 9 cases the CD34+CD38- compartment seemed to be empty in the routine3-colour analysis (Figure 1 A), whereas CD34+CD38-cells were well detectable by overaquisition (Figure 1B) . Figure 1 shows the setting of a life storage gate . Populations were coloured in FSC/SSC.

**Table 1.** Basic data of 10 samples from patients with AML. The expression of CD 34 and CD 38 of the bulk population of mature leukemic blasts is indicated.

| Pat # | Age | Gender | FAB | Mature blasts CD34 | CD38 |
|---|---|---|---|---|---|
| 1 | 71 | M | M0 | (+) | + |
| 2 | 44 | M | M1 | + | + |
| 3 | 77 | M | M1 | - | + |
| 4 | 66 | F | M2 | - | + |
| 5 | 43 | F | M3 | - | + |
| 6 | 61 | F | M4 | + | + |
| 7 | 29 | M | M4Eo | + | + |
| 8 | 70 | M | M4Eo | + | + |
| 9 | 63 | M | M5a | - | + |
| 10 | 67 | M | M6 | (+) | + |

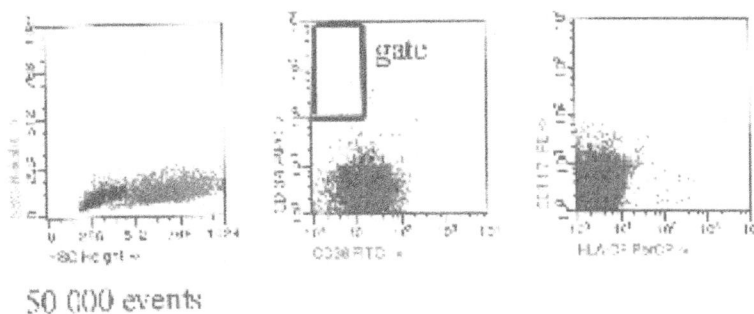

**Fig. 1.** Setting of the live-storage-gate.

50 000 events

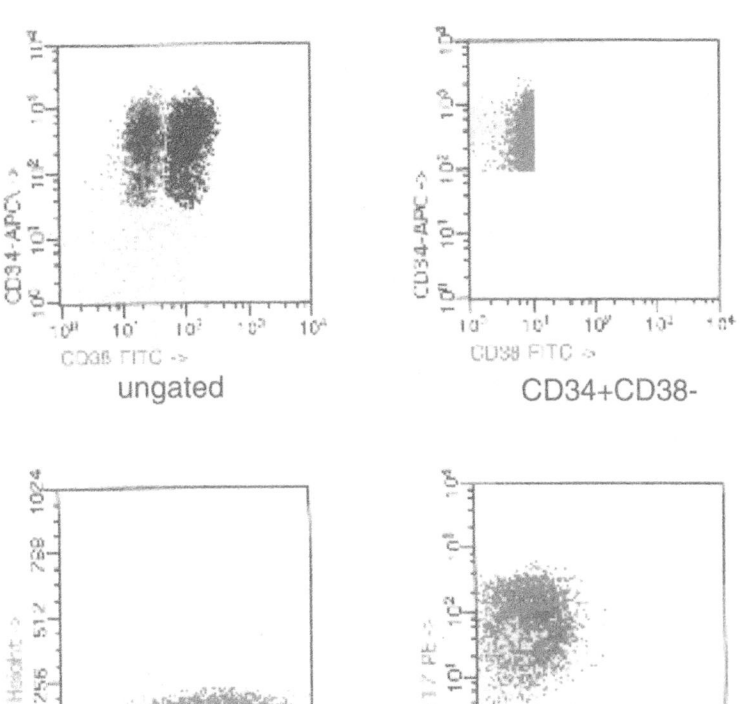

ungated

CD34+CD38-

**Fig. 2.** Example for the evaluation of HLA-DR and CD-117 expression within the CD34+cd38- compartment.

CD34+CD38-

CD34+CD38-

In Figure 2 examples are shown for the evaluation of HLA-DR and CD117 expression within the CD34⁺CD38⁻ compartment . The mature blasts were CD117+ and HLA-DR+ as well as CD34+CD38+ in this case.

Table 2 summarizes the subpopulations within the CD34⁺CD38⁻ cells for each case . The antigen expression in the stem cell compartment was heterogenic. Also the number of events within the storage gate varied between 0 and 154 000, with a mean of 3 000. Five samples ranged from 1000 to 10 000.

## Discussion and Conclusion

Leukemic cells are organized in a hierarchy of proliferation and differentiation similar to

167

**Table 2.** Subpopulations of the CD34+CD38- compartment

| Pat # | CD33lo or HLA-DR lo CD117 lo | other |
|-------|------------------------------|-------|
| 1 | Empty | HLA-DR+CD117+ |
| 2 | 25% | HLA-DR+CD117+ |
| 3 | 24%* | CD33+cd117+/- |
| 4 | 21% | HLA-DR+CD117- |
| 5 | 10% | HLA-DRloCD117+ |
| 6 | 2,4% | HLA-DR+CD117+ |
| 7 | 5,1% | HLA-DR-CD117+ |
| 8 | 1% | HLA-DR-CD117+ |
| 9 | 2,6%* | CD33+CD117+ |
| 10 | 0,3%* | CD33+CD117+ |
| | | HLA-DR+CD117+ |

*CD33loCD117lo #8: 154 000 cells in CD34+CD38-

normal hematopoetic cells [Bornet 1997, Nat.Med. 730-737]. CD34$^+$CD38$^-$ cell are detectable also in leukemic bone marrow. Other have shown leukemic Karyotypes in these cells [7].

We detected CD34$^+$CD38$^-$ cells by overacquisition and 4-colour imunoflorescence in AML samples negative for this compartment in routine analysis. 4-colour analysis reveals further subpopulations in the stem cell compartment of newly diagnosed AML. Leukemic cells display a heterogeneous phenotype within the stem cell compartment. Candidate normal immature cells can be detected at variable low frequencies. These results bear on attempts to immunologically separate normal and leukemic cells and on immunological therapies for AML such as the case of anti CD33 antibodies.. These preliminary data's suggest the coexistence of normal and leukemic stem cells in the CD34$^+$CD38$^-$ compartment. Further analyses will comprise a genotypic characterization of the subpopulations within this compartment.

## References

1. Terstappen LW, Konemann S, Safford M, Loken MR, Zurlutter K, Büchner T, Hiddemann W, Wörmann B: Flow cytometric characterization of acute myeloid leukemia. Part 1. Significance of light scattering properties. Leukemia 5:315-21,1991
2. Wörmann B, Safford M, Könemann S, Büchner T, Hiddemann W, Terstappen LW: Detection of aberrant antigen expression in acute myeloid leukemia by multiparameter flow cytometry. Recent Results Cancer Res 131:185.96,1993
3. Macedo A, OrfaoA, Ciudad J. Gonzalez M, Vidriales B, Lopez Berges MC, Martinez A, Landolfi C, Canizo C, San Miguel JF: Phenotopic analysis of CD34 subpopulations in normal human bone marrow and its application for the detection of minimal residual disease. Leukemia 9:1896-901, 1995
4. Haase D, Feuring Buske M, Schäfer C, Schoch C, Troff C, Gahn B, Hiddemann W, Wörmann B: Cytogenic analysis of CD 34$^+$ subpopulations in AML and MDS characterizes by the expression of CD38 and CD117. Leukemia 11: 674-9, 1997

# Validation of the IPSS and Other Scoring Systems in Patients with Primary MDS

C. Aul, U. Germing, C. Strupp, A. Giagounidis and G. Meckenstock

The International Prognostic Scoring System (IPSS) was proposed to improve risk evaluation in MDS. The IPSS is based on bone marrow blast count, number of peripheral cytopenias and cytogenetic findings. The Düsseldorf score does not include cytogenetics, but uses LDH levels as prognostic parameter. The Spanish-score includes bone marrow blast count, number of peripheral cytopenias and age, the Bournemouthscore includes bone marrow blast count and number of peripheral cytopenias.

In order to evaluate the prognostic impact of the different scores we compared the results of the scores using data of 328 patients with primary MDS and successful chromosomal studies.

The frequency of chromosomal risk groups as defined by the IPSS was as follows: (n = 328) low-risk 236 (72%), intermediate-risk 50 (15%) and high-risk 42 (13%).

The following table shows the results of the scoring systems concerning median survival and risk of AML at 2 and 5 years after diagnosis. Patients who received chemotherapy were excluded from the analysis. It also shows the proportion of patients allocated to different risk groups.

Considering morphological subtypes the IPSS was able to define risk groups only in RARS and RA. The Bournemouth and Spanish scores were not able to define risk groups in any FAB-Subtype group. The Düsseldorf score was able to separate CMML, RAEB and RAEB-T into risk groups with significantly different outcome.

The IPSS was able to separate the large group of intermediate-risk patients into 2 categories. The Spanish score was able to identify more low-risk patients. The Düsseldorf score identified more patients with high-risk MDS.

In conclusion all scores had high prognostic impact. If cytogenetic data are available, the IPSS should be used. If cytogenetic data are missing, the other scores are equally suited to provide risk stratification for MDS patients.

**Table 1**

| Score | Risk group | Pts (%) | Sur | AML (2yr) | AML (5yr) |
|---|---|---|---|---|---|
| IPSS | low | 36 | 108 | 10% | 10% |
| Düsseldorf | low | 23 | 108 | 10% | 10% |
| Spanish | low | 47 | 107 | 10% | 13% |
| Bournemouth | low | 30 | 104 | 11% | 13% |
| IPSS | inter I | 27 | 48 | 15% | 20% |
| | Inter I | 22 | 23 | 22% | 47% |
| Düsseldorf | intermediate | 55 | 48 | 13% | 20% |
| Spanish | intermediate | 39 | 31 | 23% | 42% |
| Bournemouth | intermediate | 55 | 36 | 24% | 49% |
| IPSS | high | 14 | 7 | 72% | 80% |
| Düsseldorf | high | 22 | 8 | 65% | 78% |
| Spanish | high | 14 | 12 | 46% | 66% |
| Bournemouth | high | 15 | 9 | 62% | 84% |

Heinrich-Heine-University of Düsseldorf, Germany

| IPSS | 0 | 0,5 | 1 | 1,5 | 2 |
|---|---|---|---|---|---|
| Number of cytopenias | 0/1 | 2/3 | | | |
| Karyotyp | good | interm. | poor | | |
| Med.blasts (%) | <5% | 5–10% | | 11–20% | >20% |

| | |
|---|---|
| Low: 0 | |
| Intermediate I | 0,5–1 |
| Intermediate II | 1,5–2 |
| High | >2,5 |

Karyotypes:  good risk: normal, 5q-, 20q-, -Y
Intermediate-risk: all other aberrations
High-risk: aberrations of chromosome 7, aberrations of ≥2 chrom.

| Bournemouth-Score | | Spanish-Score | | Düsseldorf-Score | |
|---|---|---|---|---|---|
| Hb <10 | 1 | age >60 | 1 | med.blasts >5% | 1 |
| Neutrophils <2500 | 1 | med.blasts 5–10% | 1 | Hb <9 | 1 |
| Platelets <100000 | 1 | med.blasts >10% | 1 | Platelets <100000 | 1 |
| | | Platelets <50000 | 2 | | |

| | | | | |
|---|---|---|---|---|
| low-risk | 1 | | 0–1 | 0 |
| intermediate-risk | 2–3 | | 2–3 | 1–2 |
| high-risk | 4 | | 4–5 | 3–4 |

**Definitions of Scoring-Systems**

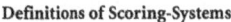

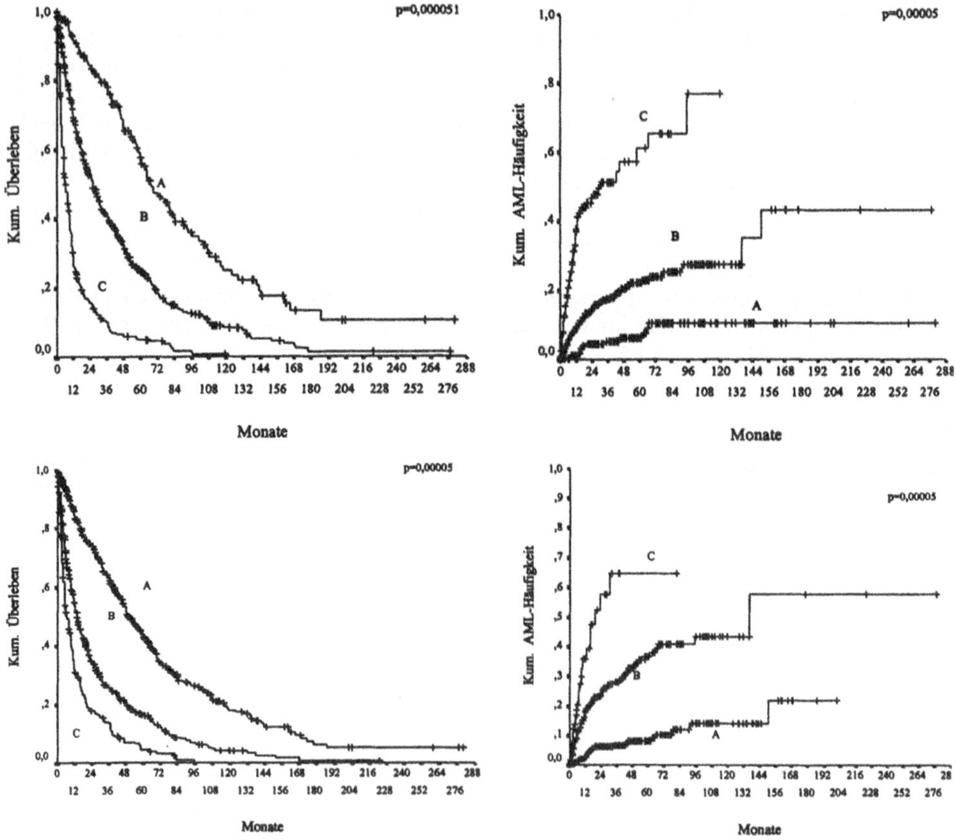

**Fig. 1.** Düsseldorf-Score: Survival and AML-Transformation

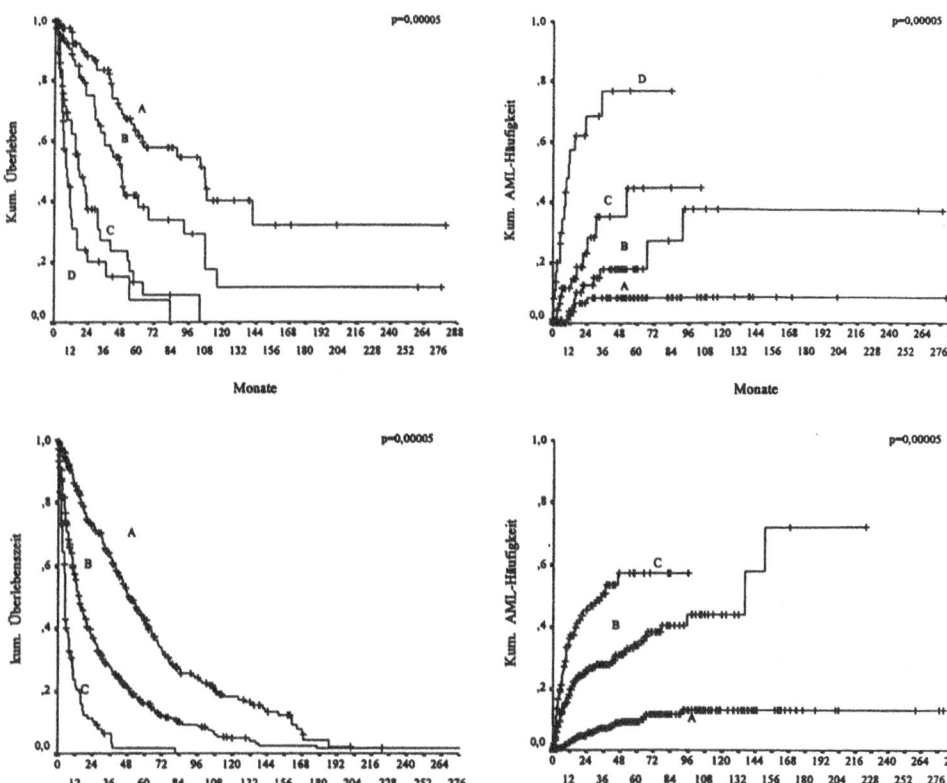

**Fig. 2.** IPSS-Score: Survival and AML-Transformation

## References

Aul C, Gattermann N, Heyll A et al. (1992) Primary myelodysplastic syndromes: analysis of prognostic factors in 235 patients and proposals for an improved scoring system. Leukemia 6, 52

Sanz GJ, Sanz MA, Vallespi T et al. (1989) Two regression models and a scoring system for predicting survival and planning treatment in myelodysplastic syndromes: a multivariate analysis of prognostic factors in 370 patients. Blood 74, 395

Mufti GJ, Stevens JR, Oscier DG et al. (1985) Myelodysplastic syndromes: a scoring system with prognostic significance. Br J Hematol 59, 425

Greenberg P, Cox C, LeBeau MM, Fenaux P, Morel P, Sanz G et al. (1997) International scoring system for evaluating prognosis in myelodysplastic syndromes. Blood 89, 2079

# Although Patients with AML and Complex Aberrant Karyotype Can be Subdivided Into Different Subtypes by Cytogenetics, Prognosis is Equally Poor

C. Schoch[1], M. Klaus[1], S. Bursch[1], T. Büchner[2], H. Löffler[3], T. Haferlach[1] and W. Hiddemann[1]

## Introduction

Complex karyotype abnormalities occur in about 10 to 15% of patients with acute myeloid leukemia (AML). An analysis of 90 patients with complex chromosome aberrations (defined as 3 or more numerical and/or structural chromosome aberrations) treated according to the protocols of the AMLCG study group showed a dismal outcome in 45 patients < 60 years (CR rate 47%, overall survival (OS) rate at 3 years 12%) as well as in 45 patients ≥ 60 years (CR rate 44%, OS rate at 3 years 6%) [1]. In order to analyze the karyotype aberrations in this subgroup of patients in more detail, we performed dual color fluorescence in situ hybridization (FISH) in 50 cases in addition to conventional chromosome analysis. As conventional chromosome analysis by G-Banding often shows rearrangements of chromosomes 5, 7 and 17 in patients with complex aberrant karyotype we used loci specific probes for EGR1 (5q31), D7S522 (7q31) and p53 (17p13) to answer the question whether these loci are deleted in all patients who show rearrangements in these regions by G-banding and whether patients without rearrangements of chromosome 5, 7 or 17 in conventional cytogenetics show deletions by FISH.

## Material and Methods

Fifty patients with acute myeloid leukemia and complex karyotype (3 or more chromosome aberrations) were selected. Fluores-

cence in situ hybridization (FISH) was performed on bone marrow cells prepared as for conventional cytogenetics according to the protocol of the manufacturer.

The following probes were used:
– locus specific probes: EGR1 (5q31) combined with D5S721 (5p15.2), D7S522 (7q31) combined with CEP7 (centromer of chromosome 7) and p53 (17p13) in every patient (probes were directly labeled with spectrum orange or spectrum green, VYSIS).
– whole chromosome paints (WCP) for chromosomes 5, 7 and 17, whenever conventional cytogenetics suggested rearrangements or loss of these chromosomes, further chromosome paints were used in individual patients to clarify complex rearrangements (probes were labeled with biotin, digoxigenin, spectrum orange or spectrum green, Oncor, AGS, VYSIS).

## Results

As reported in the literature the chromosomes most often involved in structural and numerical chromosome aberrations were chromosomes 5, 7 and 17 (Fig. 1 and 2). Loss of genetic material due to terminal or interstitial deletions or unbalanced translocations was more frequent than gain of chromosomal material. Structural aberrations occurred more often than gains and losses of whole chromosomes. Besides 5q, 7q and 17p the following regions were frequently involved in rearrangements: 11p, 11q, 12p and 18q.

[1] Department of Internal Medicine III, University Hospital Grosshadern, Ludwig-Maximilians-University, Munich, Germany
[2] Department of Hematology and Oncology, University of Münster, Germany
[3] St. Peter, Germany

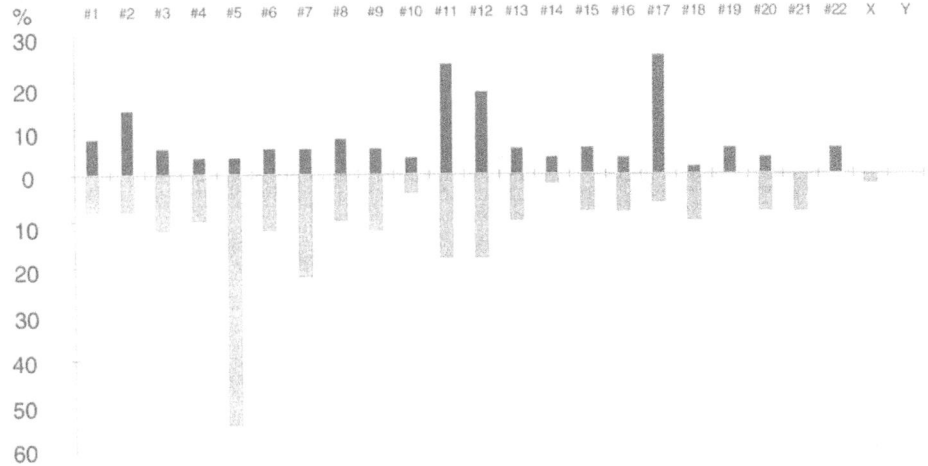

**Fig. 1.** This diagram shows the frequency of the involvement of the different chromosomes in structural aberrations in 50 patients with AML and complex aberrant karyotype. Involvement of the short arm of each chromosome (p) are indicated in columns to the top, involvement of the long arm of each chromosome are shown in the columns to the bottom

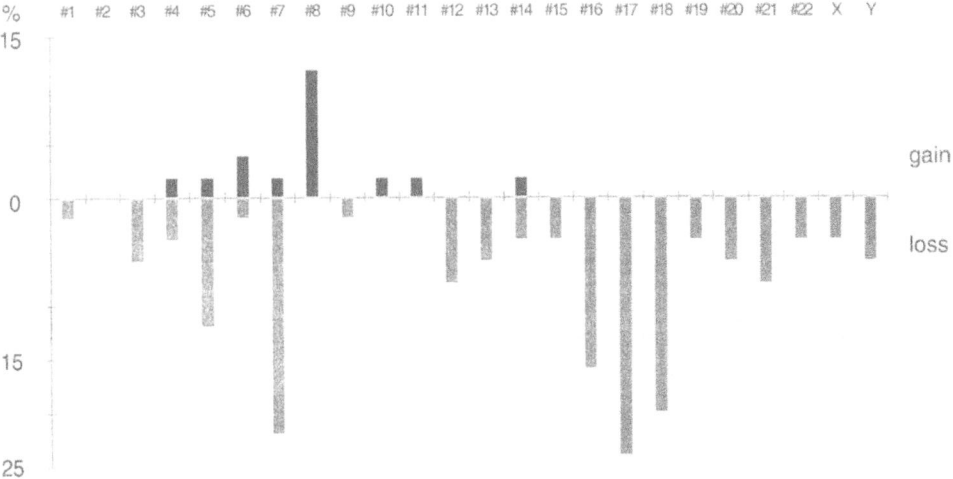

**Fig. 2.** This diagram shows the frequency of the involvement of the different chromosomes in numerical abnormalities in 50 patients with AML and complex aberrant karyotype. The gain of a chromosome is indicated in columns to the top, a loss is shown in the columns to the bottom

FISH with probes for the EGR1-locus (5q31), the D7S522-locus (7q31) and the p53 gene (17p13) revealed a deletion of all three loci in 12 patients, while 27 cases showed a deletion of one to two of these loci.

In all but two cases showing a rearrangement of chromosome 5 in G-banding a 5q31 deletion was found by FISH. In one case each

a 7q31 and a p53 deletion was observed with FISH, despite two normal appearing chromosomes 7 and 17 in G-banding, respectively.

We identified a subgroup of 11 patients showing neither a deletion of 5q31 nor of 7q31 or p53 (Fig. 3). Seven of these patients did not show rearrangements of chromosomes 5, 7 and 17 by G-banding, while in 4 cases

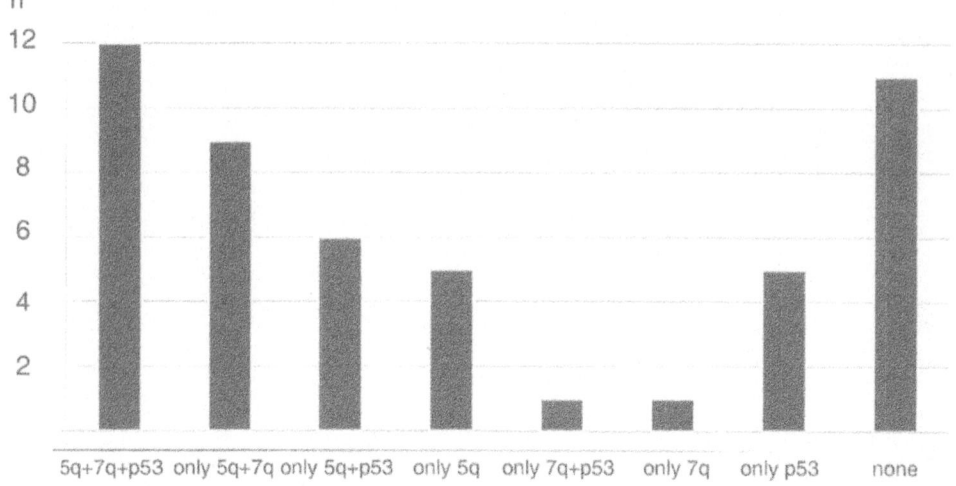

**Fig. 3.** The incidence of the deletion of 5q31, 7q31 and p53 in different combinations is indicated in columns giving the number of patients in each category

balanced translocations involving chromosomes 5 or 7 were observed by FISH with whole chromosome paints.

The incidence of the different deletions was comparable in patients with de novo AML (n=32), secondary AML (n=13) and relapsed AML (n=5).

## Discussion

Among various pretreatment determinants cytogenetics are considered to be the most important independent prognostic parameter [2,3]. For clinical purposes karyotype analysis allows to discriminate between three major prognostic groups. A favorable outcome under currently used treatment regimens was observed in several studies in patients with t[8;21], inv(16) or t(15;17) [4-10] Chromosome aberrations with an unfavorable clinical course are -5/5q-, -7/7q-, inv(3)/t(3;3) and complex aberrant karyotype [4,6,7,9,11-13]. The definition of karyotypes that are associated with an intermediate prognosis is still on debate. Patients with a normal karyotype and rare chromosome aberrations and therefore unknown prognostic impact are assigned to this category in most studies.

A huge amount of data has been collected on the molecular pathogenesis of AML with balanced translocations such as

t(8;21)(q22;q22), t(15;17)(q22;q12) or inv(16)(p13q22), but very little is known about the chromosome abnormalities in detail observed in complex aberrant karyotypes. From the clinical point of view our data and data from the literature show low CR rates and short survival times for patients with complex karyotype aberrations and/or abnormalities of chromosomes 5 and/or 7 [4,6,7,11]. But these aberrations are frequently associated and complex karyotypes often include -5/5q- and -7/7q- abnormalities. Therefore, we asked the question, whether the deletion of distinct gene loci or the complexity of karyotype aberration is associated with poor prognosis. We had identified a group of patients by conventional cytogenetics who showed a complex aberrant karyotype as defined by three or more chromosome abnormalities without rearrangements of chromosomes 5, 7 or 17. Our FISH data show, that even with FISH only in 1 patient each a deletion of 7q31 and p53 was detected in this group of patients. In four patients showing 5q or 7q rearrangements in conventional cytogenetics FISH confirmed balanced translocations without deletion of material of chromosomes 5 and 7. As the clinical outcome of patients with complex aberrant karyotype without 5q31, 7q31 or p53 deletions was as poor as for patients with one to three of these loci deleted, the complexity of the karyotype itself seems to be relevant for prognosis. This hypothesis is further supported by data from Ravandi et al. who reported that patients suffering from AML, MDS RAEB or RAEB-T with simple -5/-7 abnormalities experienced a significantly better outcome than patients with -5/-7 and complex aberrant karyotype abnormalities [14]. In two earlier studies a rather good prognosis for patients with isolated 7q-or -7 was observed as well [7,15]. Data by Pedersen-Bjergaard at al. support this finding as well by demonstrating that the number of chromosome aberrations was an independent prognostic factor for patients with secondary myelodysplastic syndrome [16].

## References

1. Schoch C, Haferlach T, Haase D, Fonatsch Ch, Schlegelberger B, Sauerland MC, Löffler, H, Staib, P, Wörmann B, Büchner Th, Hiddemann W for the German AML Cooperative Group (1997) Complex chromosome aberrations in patients with de novo AML are associated with a very poor prognosis despite intensive treatment: A study of 90 patients Blood 90,Suppl. 1: 62a, abstr.
2. Bloomfield CD, Herzig GP, Caligiuri MA (1997) Introduction: acute leukemia: recent advances. Semin Oncol 24:1-2
3. Mrozek K, Heinonen K, de la Chapelle A, Bloomfield CD (1997) Clinical significance of cytogenetics in acute myeloid leukemia. Semin Oncol 24:17-31
4. Haferlach T. (1996) More individual markers are necessary for patients with acute myeloid leukemia (AML). Does cytomorphology or cytogenetics define the biological entity? Leukemia 10 Suppl 3:S5-S9
5. Dastugue N, Payen C, Lafage Pochitaloff M, Bernard P, Leroux D, Huguet Rigal F, Stoppa AM, Marit G, Molina L, Michallet M, Maraninchi D, Attal M, Reiffers J (1995) Prognostic significance of karyotype in de novo adult acute myeloid leukemia. The BGMT group. Leukemia 9:1491-1498
6. Berger R, Bernheim A, Ochoa Noguera ME, Daniel MT, Valensi F, Sigaux F, Flandrin G, Boiron M. (1987) Prognostic significance of chromosomal abnormalities in acute nonlymphocytic leukemia: a study of 343 patients. Cancer Genet Cytogenet 28:293-299
7. Fenaux P, Preudhomme C, Lai JL, Morel P, Beuscart R, Bauters F. (1989) Cytogenetics and their prognostic value in de novo acute myeloid leukaemia: a report on 283 cases. Br J Haematol 73:61-67
8. Keating M, Cork A, Broach Y, Smith T, Walters RS, McCredie KB, Trujillo J, Freireich EJ (1987) Toward a clinically relevant cytogenetic classification of acute myelogenius leukemia. Leuk Res 11:119-133
9. Hiddemann W, Fonatsch C, Wörmann B, Heinecke A, Sauerland M-C, Scharnhorst S, Büchner T (1995) Cytogenetic subgroups of AML and outcome from high dose versus conventional dose ARA-C as part of double induction. Blood 86: 267a abstr.
10. Warrell RP, Jr (1998) Clinical an molecular aspects of retinoid therapy for acute promyelocytic leukemia. Int J Cancer 70:496-497
11. Yunis JJ, Brunning RD, Howe RB, Lobell M (1984) High-resolution chromosomes as an independent prognostic indicator in adult acute nonlymphocytic leukemia. N Engl J Med 311:812-818
12. Fonatsch C, Gudat H, Lengfelder E, Wandt H, Silling-Engelhardt G, Ludwig W-D, Thiel E, Freund M, Bodenstein H, Schwieder G, Grüneisen A, Aul C, Schnittger S, Rieder H, Haase D, Hild F (1994) Correlation of cytogenetic findings with clinical features in 18 patients with inv(3)(q21q26) ot t(3;3)(q21;q26). Leukemia 8:1318-1326
13. Grimwade D, Walker H, Oliver F, Wheatley K, Harrison C, Harrison G, Rees J, Hann I, Stevens RF, Burnett AK, Goldstone A, on behalf of the Medical Research Council Adult and Children's Leukemia Working Party (1998) The importance of diagnostic cytogenetics on outcome in AML: Analysis of 1,612 patients entered into the MRC AML 10 trial. Blood 92:2322-2333
14. Ravandi F, Keating M, Pierce S, Estey E (1997) Identification of a relatively favorable group within AML/MDS patients with chromosome 5 and/or 7 abnormalities. Blood 90:64a, abstr.
15. Swansbury GJ, Lawler SD, Alimena G, Arthur D, Berger R, Van den Berghe H, Bloomfield CD, de la Chapelle A, Dewald GW, Garson OM, Hagemeijer A, Kaneko Y, Mitelman F, Rowley JD, Sakurai M (1994) Long-term survival in acute myelogenous leukemia: a second follow-up of the Fourth International Workshop on Chromosomes in Leukemia. Cancer Genet Cytogenet 73:1-7
16. Pedersen-Bjergaard J, Philip P, Larsen SO, Jensen G, Byrsting K (1990) Chromosome aberrations and prognostic factors in therapy-related myelodysplasia and acute nonlymphocytic leukemia. Blood 76:1083-1091

# Recent Antileukemic Strategies

# Pharmacokinetics of Idarubicin: Intracellular Events and Extracellular Concentrations

F. GIESELER, M. CLARK, K. STIEBELING, M. PUSCHMANN and S. VALSAMAS

*Abstract.* Although anthracyclines have been used for decades, the pharmacokinetic requirements for optimal therapeutic efficacy (effect versus side effect) are still unclear. Obviously, a high plasma peak that occurs after bolus injection is responsible for delayed cardiotoxicity, which is one of the most serious side effects. Idarubicin is the only anthracycline that can be applied orally, which results in an altered pharmacokinetic with a long terminal half time and a low plasma peak. It is still an open question, how intercellular effects, namely the DNA binding of idarubicin and cytotoxicity, are influenced by a prolongation of application time. We performed in vitro experiments with the human promyelocytic HL-60 leukemia cell line and ex vivo experiments with AML blast cells from patients. The cytotoxicity of idarubicin is in direct and linear correlation with the amount of idarubicin bound to the DNA. However, the extracellular concentrations that are necessary to achieve the maximum DNA binding are well above the levels that are accomplished during therapy. Although a number of clinical studies have shown the efficacy of idarubicin given orally in AML therapy, the significance of the plasma peak has not yet been disclosed. The prolongation of application time in vitro for more than 90 minutes did not have a notable effect upon the induction of cell death in vitro. These experiments have been performed with the HL-60 cell line and must be put into proper perspective: AML blast cells from patients exhibit a variance of three log steps of idarubicin concentration to achieve the IC50 or the IC90.

## Introduction

One of the most serious side effects in the treatment with anthracyclines is delayed cardiotoxicity that develops after repetitive applications of anthracyclines and increases with the given cumulative dose [1]. It has been proposed that the cardiotoxicity is linked to the liberation of free oxygen radicals by the anthrachinon ring system in the presence of magnesium and iron ions [2-4]. As the glutathion system for the detoxification of oxygen radicals is lower in myocardial cells than in other cells of the body, they might be especially sensitive.

Anthracyclines are metabolized by the aldoketoreductase to an alcohol-derivative (idarubicinol). Idarubicinol, in contrast to the metabolites of other anthracyclines, is as active as idarubicin [5]. In addition, idarubicin is the only anthracycline which can be given orally due to its acid stability [6]. After oral application, a high plasma peak is avoided and, due to a more complete metabolization, the area under the time curve of both idarubicin and idarubicinol is higher than after intravenous application [6]. A high plasma peak that occurs after bolus injection of anthracyclines results in a fast increase of oxygen radicals in myocardial cells and should, therefore, be avoided. On the other hand, it is still not clear how important the plasma peak is for the induction of apoptosis in malignant cells, which is the desired effect of treatment.

In this paper, we present a number of experiments that address these questions. First we describe the in vitro conditions which are optimal for apoptosis induction

Klinik für Allgemeine Innere Medizin, Schwerpunkt Hämatologie / Onkologie, Christian-Albrechts-Universität, Kiel, Germany

and then compare it with the pharmacokinetic in vivo after different application forms of idarubicin.

## Material and Methods

### Nuclear uptake of idarubicin and idarubicinol in HL-60-cells

The human promyelocytic leukemia HL-60 cell line has been obtained from ATCC, Bethesda, MD, USA. For fluorimetric determination of drug uptake, 4 x 10⁶ cells were washed and re-suspended in HBSS (Gibco BRL, Paisley, Scotland) plus 2.5 µg/ml verapamil (Knoll, Germany) and incubated for 1 hour at 37°C. An equal volume of HBSS containing twice the desired drug-dosage was added and the samples incubated at 37 °C. The cells were then centrifuged and the pellet re-suspended in either 4 ml lysis buffer (0.3 M sucrose, 0.05 mM EGTA pH 8.0, 60 mM KCl, 15 mM NaCl, 15 mM HEPES pH 7.5 (all from Roth, Karlsruhe, Germany), 150 µM spermine, 50 µM spermidine) containing 20 µl triton X-100 (Sigma Chemie, Deisenhofen, Germany) for nuclear isolation or 400 µl HCl/isopropanol for whole cell lysis. The whole cells in HCl/isopropanol were vortexed and diluted with H₂O to 2 ml. The cells in lysis buffer were mixed and left on ice for 15 minutes before centrifuging. The nuclei (pellet) were then vortexed with 400 µl HCl/isopropanol. Quantification of anthracyclines was done with a Perkin Elmer fluorescence spectrometer with an excitation at 480 nm and an emission maximum at 560-590 nm. A linear relation between fluorescence (AU) and the amount of drugs (anthracyclines from Pharmacia GmbH Erlangen Germany; etoposide from Bristol Meyers Squibb, Munich, Germany), has been found with the following correlations: daunorubicin (µg/ml) = 2.31 x AU - 28.44 (R = 0.99), idarubicin (µg/ml) = 0.95 x AU - 16.19 (R = 0.99), idarubicinol (µg/ml) = 0.68 x AU - 12.65 (R = 0.99).

### DNA binding of anthracyclines

1 x 10⁶ cells/ml were incubated at 37°C for 30 minutes in RPMI (Sigma Chemie, Deisenh-

ofen, Germany) plus 2.5 mg/ml verapamil and subsequently for an additional 30 minutes with 1 mg/ml of the fluorescent AT-binder Hoechst dye 33342 (Hoechst GmbH, Bad Soden, Germany). The total emission of 2 x 10⁴ cells per sample was subsequently measured using a Pasec II flow cytometer equipped with a mercury lamp, excitation from 300 to 600 nm, and a 435 nm excitation filter. The fluorescence of this probe serves as 100 % control. Drugs were added and the cell suspension was again measured as before. DNA binding of drugs was expressed as percent quenching of Hoechst dye fluorescence in the control sample. It has been described, that the quenching of Hoechst dye fluorescence is due to the resonance energy transfer between the two molecules and is directly related to the amount of drug bound to the DNA .

### Patient characteristics

We examined 78 samples from patients with newly diagnosed AML before chemotherapy. The patients characteristics were as follows: 43 female, 35 male; youngest patient 16 years, oldest patient 83 years, median age 60 years. The viability of the cells was > 95%, the blasts were enriched by a two-step lymphocult-gradient following standard procedures (Sigma Chemie, Deisenhofen, Germany). The percentage of blast cells per sample  was > 80% as controlled by light-microscopy of a cytocentrifuge-preparation.

### Determination of cell death

We used the »Alamar Blue« assay (Alamar, Sacramento, CA, USA) which has been described in detail, and trypan blue (Sigma Chemie, Deisenhofen, Germany) exclusion.

## Results

Cell death was determined 72 hours after incubation begin with idarubicin. Depending upon the incubation time and the concentration of idarubicin, we found different amounts of DNA bound idarubicin as measured by the quenching of Hoechst dye 33342. A direct and linear correlation between the

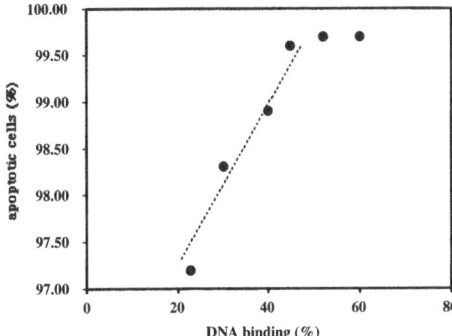

**Fig. 1.** Correlation between the DNA binding of idarubicin and apoptosis in HL-60 cells

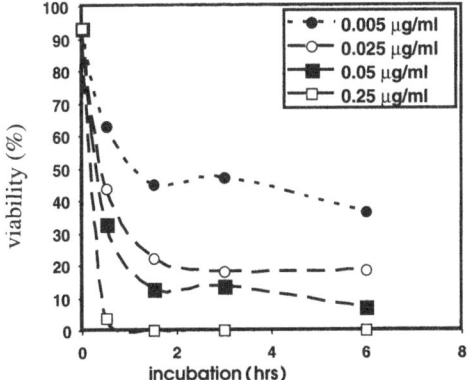

**Fig. 2.** Viability of HL-60 after various incubation times and clinically relevant concentrations of idarubicin

DNA binding and the resulting cell death could be established. With ca. 60 % of Hoechst dye quenching, saturation could be monitored with 100 % cell death. The extracellular concentration of idarubicin that was necessary to achieve this saturation could be determined as 1.5 µg/ml as displayed in table 1. 20 minutes of incubation were necessary at this concentration. Prolongation of the incubation time up to 90 minutes resulted in higher cytotoxicity as shown in Figure 2. The amount of cell death was dependent upon the concentration used, but a prolongation of the incubation time over 90 minutes did not increase cytotoxicity. The concentrations of idarubicin that were used in the experiments shown in Figure 2 cover the plasma peak concentration and the terminal half time concentration. The cells that have been used for these experiments were human promyelocytic HL-60 leukemia cells. These cells are relatively sensitive to anthracyclines. Interestingly, the sensitivity of AML blasts from patients is extremely variable as can be concluded from figure 3. The cells have been continuously incubated in idarubicin for 72 hours and the probability of achieving the IC50 or the IC90 is displayed.

## Discussion

The inhibition of the religation step of topoisomerase II by idarubicin results in DNA double strand breaks. These lesions are diffi-

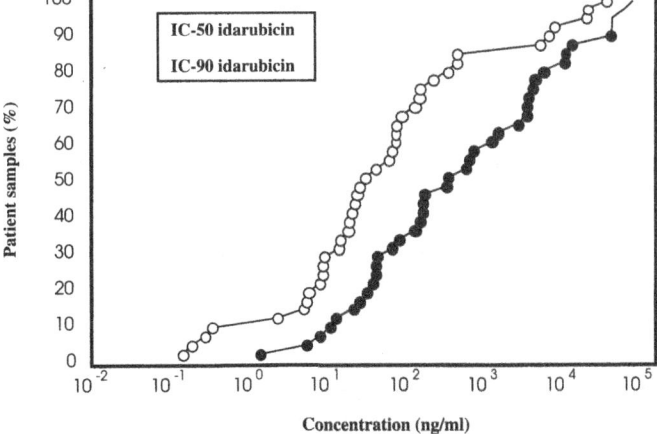

**Fig. 3.** Probability to achieve the IC 90 or IC 50 with idarubicin (AML-blast cells from patients before therapy)

**Table 1.** Intracellular pharmacokinetics of idarubicin in human leukemia cells (HL-60)

| | |
|---|---|
| saturation nucleus | 15.0 min |
| saturation DNA binding* | 20.0 min |
| concentration for DNA saturation** | 1.5 µg/ml |

mean of three independent experiments, SD = 15%
* time to saturation (extracellular conc. 5 µg/ml)
** extracellular concentration for maximal DNA-binding (µg/ml)

cult to repair due to the covalently bound topoisomerase and the loss of the enzyme's function that is important for DNA repair [7-9]. Consistent with this model of action, we found a linear and direct correlation of the DNA binding of idarubicin and the resulting cell death (Fig. 1). For these experiments we used the quenching of H33342-dye to measure the amount of idarubicin bound to the DNA. This method allows relative determination; the absolute quantity of idarubicin can only be estimated: as the maximal intercalation of anthracyclines is 1 molecule per 10 basepairs, the maximum number of anthracycline molecules in a human cell with $3 \times 10^9$ basepairs is $3 \times 10^8$. With the help of Loschmidt's number (1 Mol = $6.02 \times 10^{23}$ molecules), the maximal concentration of anthracyclines at the DNA can be calculated as 0.5 nM / $10^6$ cells.

It is shown in table 1 that the extracellular concentration necessary for the saturation of DNA with idarubicin is 1.5 µg / ml (=2.8 µMol). The incubation time to reach a plateau of maximal DNA binding is at least 20 minutes (table 1). As we found a direct correlation between the DNA binding and apoptosis, these conditions (1.5 µg / ml for 20 minutes) can be defined as the optimum from our in vitro studies. These conditions can never be achieved in therapy. The pharmacokinetic data after bolus infusion of idarubicin 13 mg / $m^2$ are as follows:
– plasma peak level is appr. 200 ng/ml (= 37 µMol)
– terminal half time 72 hours
– plasma concentration during terminal half time 2 ng/ml (370 nMol)
With oral application of idarubicin, the plasma peak is avoided.

As elucidated in the introduction, it does not seem rationale to raise the plasma peak due to the anticipated cardiotoxicity. The question is, whether longer incubation times might be a way to increase the rate of apoptosis-induction without the necessity of a high plasma peak. To address this question, we performed a number of experiments with different incubation times of idarubicin and several clinically relevant concentrations that cover the plasma peak concentration and the concentration during the terminal half time. In figure 2 it is shown that the final level of cell death is dependent upon the utilized concentration even with longer application times. A plateau is reached after 90 minutes of incubation in every set of experiments. The concentrations that were used in these experiments cover the clinically relevant ranges from 5 ng/ml (terminal half time) to 250 ng/ml (plasma peak).

The cells which have been used in these experiments are HL-60 cells, and the sensitivity of this cell-line might not be comparable to patient AML-cells. In order to look for the sensitivity of patient cells to idarubicin, we examined 78 samples of patients with freshly diagnosed AML prior to chemotherapy. The cells have been incubated for 72 hours in idarubicin and the probability of achieving the IC50 or the IC90 is displayed in figure 3. Indeed, the sensitivity of HL-60 cells cannot be compared with AML blasts from patients as the sensitivity of AML blasts is extremely variable and covers more than three log steps of idarubicin concentration.

Can these in vitro experiments be compared to the clinical situation? One of the problems is that the tumor cells we want to reach with therapy are not located in the blood but in other compartments such as the bone marrow or solid tumors. The plasma pharmacokinetic is not necessarily the same as the pharmacokinetic within these compartments. We have shown that a prolongation of the application time to 90 minutes increases the rate of apoptosis. The optimal concentration for maximal DNA binding of idarubicin can not be reached in the clinical situation, but the prolongation of the infusion time to 90 minutes should increase the cellular effect. However, the importance of the plasma peak for cytotoxicity has not yet been completely revealed.

# References

1. Goebel M, Kaplan E (1992)Anthracycline-induced cardiotoxicity-a review. Onkologie 15:198-204.
2. Hershko C, Link G, Tzahor M, Pinson A (1993)The role of iron and iron chelators in anthracycline cardiotoxicity. Leuk Lymphoma 11:207-14.
3. Minotti G, Cairo G, Monti E (1999)Role of iron in anthracycline cardiotoxicity: new tunes for an old song? Faseb J 13:199-212.
4. Hochster H, Wasserheit C, Speyer J (1995)Cardiotoxicity and cardioprotection during chemotherapy. Curr Opin Oncol 7:304-9.
5. Kuffel MJ, Reid JM, Ames MM (1992)Anthracyclines and their C-13 alcohol metabolites: growth inhibition and DNA damage following incubation with human tumor cells in culture. Cancer Chemother Pharmacol 30:51-7.
6. Goebel M (1993)Oral idarubicin—an anthracycline derivative with unique properties. Ann Hematol 66:33-43.
7. Downes CS, Johnson RT (1988)DNA topoisomerases and DNA repair. Bioessays 8:179-84.
8. Larsen AK, Gobert C, Gilbert C, Markovits J, Bojanowski K, Skladanowski A (1998)DNA topoisomerases as repair enzymes: mechanism(s) of action and regulation by p53. Acta Biochim Pol 45:535-44.
9. Nelson WG, Kastan MB (1994)DNA strand breaks: the DNA template alterations that trigger p53-dependent DNA damage response pathways. Mol Cell Biol 14:1815-23.

# Oral Idarubicin in Maintenance Therapy of Acute Myeloid Leukemia

M. Musso, F. Porretto, A. Crescimanno, F. Bondì, V. Polizzi, R. Scalone, M. Tolomeo and G. Mariani

## Summary

More than half of all acute myeloid leukaemia (AML) patients are over 60 years. The disease free survival (DFS) and overall survival (OS) rate of these patients is poor. These unsatisfactory results are associated with adverse cytogenetic characteristics, prior myelodsplasia, adverse phenotypic features, MDR and BCL2 overexpression. Furthermore a large fraction of patients achieving CR early relapses. This is due to two factors: acquired tumor cell drug resistance and tumor re-growth. Maintenance therapy could provide a means to keep leukemic growth under control. We enrolled 31 elderly previous responder patients to standard induction therapy to receive maintenance oral IDA 3mg/m$^2$ daily d 1-14 at a 2 weeks interval for a total of 12 cycles or until disease progression. We also evaluated the cell cycle and apoptosis in leukemic cells from PR patients after IDA administration, and as a control from HL60 cell line exposed to IDA and idarubicinol in vitro. DNA analysis showed an increase of G2/M cell frequencies and evidence of apoptosis (sub G1 peak). In CR patients the median DFS and OS was 8 months and 12.5 months respectively. In PR patient the median OS was 9 months. In contrast comparing these results with an historical control group we observe a lower median cumulative OS (3 vs 11 months) and in CR patients a DFS and OS of 4 and 7 months. The treatment was well tolerated. Low haematological and extrahaematological toxicity were observed. In conclusion, long-term low doses of oral IDA would appear valuable as a maintenance regimen for elderly AML patients.

## Introduction

Acute Myeloid Leukemia (AML) occurs at all ages, however more than half of the patients with AML are over 60 years old [1-2] Despite the increase of AML with age the optimum regimen for elderly patients remains still undefined; in fact the modern therapeutic approaches offer little benefit to these patients. More than 65% of adults who are less than 60 years old achieve complete remission (CR) and survival rates of 35% are commonly obtained, while only 50% of older patients obtain a CR with chemotherapy and only 10% of them have a disease free survival beyond 4 years after diagnosis [3]. The reason for these unsatisfactory results is related to the underlying biology of AML in older patients, adverse cytogenetic characteristics, a prior myelodysplasia, phenotypic features, and MDR1 overexpression, BCL-2 positivity [4-5-6-7 ].

These considerations represent the rationale for offering new therapeutic approaches to older patients with AML. The choice of treatment for elderly patients depends on the balancing of the toxicity and the quality of their life. Increased related treatment toxicity complicates chemotherapy, so most studies about AML in the elderly suggest a less intensive induction therapy to reduce toxicity [8]. However a large fraction of AML patients who achieve CR relapse; this progression of the disease depends on two factors: tumour cell drug resistance and tumour regrowth [9]. Shiller et Al. reported a longer leukemia-free survival in patients treated with high dose ARA-C and autologous stem cell transplantation than in those treated with the standard dose [10].

Chair of Haematology and Stem cell Transplant Unit University of Palermo.

Maintenance treatment could play role in AML elderly patients if we consider that they often cannot be treated with an intensive first line therapy. The choice of post-induction therapy should consider on the one hand the control of leukemia regrowth and on the other the quality of life.

Recently Lowemberg B et al reported in previously untreated AML elderly patients that low dose ARA-C in maintenance may prolong DFS but doesn't improve survival. [11]

Idarubicin (IDA), which can be administered orally is an active anthracycline in AML. Its metabolite idarubicinol (idaol) is also active and it is formed in much larger amount after oral administration. Patients over 60 years old seem to have an impaired idaol elimination so that exposure to it could be prolonged unlike to younger patients treated with the same dosage [12].

Oral IDA could play a role in maintenance treatment of elderly patients at low dose and for long term therapy. We suggest that continuous exposure to IDA and idarubicinol could be efficient in the disease's control through its effects on low rate proliferation residual leukemic cells, inducing an apoptotic cell death, and what is more minor dependence of IDA/Idaol on MDR1.

Therefore we have evaluated the feasibility of oral administration of Idarubicin at the dose of 3 mg/m$^2$/day for a fortnight every 4 weeks for a total of 12 cycles or until disease progression, in responsive older AML patients, in complete or partial remission after standard induction therapy with ARA-C+VP16+IDA/Mitox. In addition we have studied in vitro and in vivo the apoptosis responses to this therapeutic agent in myeloid cells collected from patients in partial remission and in leukemic cell lines (HL60).

The aims of our study were: a) to evaluate the feasibility and tolerability of oral IDA administration; b) to evaluate the impact of this maintenance treatment on DFS and OS; c) to evaluate in vitro the apoptotic effect of this agent

## Materials and Methods

### Patients' Characteristics

31 myeloid leukaemia elderly patients, 13 of them with secondary AML to myelodisplastic syndrome, with a median age of 69 years (range 60-83), M/F ratio 22/9, responsive to first line treatment, 10 in CR and 21 in PR, were enrolled (Table 1).

Inclusion criteria were: age $\geq$ 60 years, diagnosis of AML in complete or partial remission after induction therapy, no eligibility or refused autologous stem cell transplantation, normal hepatic and renal function tests, cardiac fraction of ejection $\geq$ 50%. After informed consent was requested.

Induction and consolidation treatment consisted of ARA-C 100 mg/m$^2$ × 5 days - VP16 100 mg/m$^2$ × 3 days and IDA or Mitox at dosage of 8 mg/m$^2$ and 12 mg/m$^2$ respectively for 3 days; response to therapy was assessed according to the Cancer and Leukaemia B Group Criteria [13].

The maintenance treatment consisted of oral IDA 3 mg/m$^2$/day a fortnight every 4 weeks for total 12 cycles or until disease progression occurred.

Fresh and frozen cell samples were obtained from all elderly pts included in this study at 3 different times: before beginning IDA

**Table 1.** Clinical characteristics of elderly patients treated with maintenance oral Idarubicin

|  | CR | PR |
| --- | --- | --- |
| Pts n° | 10 | 21 |
| Median Age | 68 | 72 |
| Range | 60-78 | 60-83 |
| Sex M/F | 7/3 | 15/6 |
| FAB M$_0$ | 1 | 2 |
| M$_1$ | 1 | 3 |
| M$_2$ | 5 | 9 |
| M$_4$ | 3 | 6 |
| M$_5$ | 0 | 1 |
| Secondary | 6 | 7 |
| Hepatomegaly | 3 | 7 |
| Median LDH U/l | 441 | 402 |
| Range | 195-1493 | 275-1238 |
| Unfavourable Karyotype | 2 | 6 |
| Favourable | 2 | 4 |

administration, during treatment at 7th day and at 14th day for the studies in vivo. These samples were Ficoll purified and contained about $1 \times 10^7$ cells each, a part of the cells were used for cytogenetic analysis.

Ficoll separated cells were suspended at a concentration of $2 \times 10^6$/ml in minimal essential medium (MEM) supplemented with 20% FCS and cultured for 24–48 hours in plastic flasks at 37°C in a humidified atmosphere containing 5% $CO2$, with IDA at the dosage of 0,001 µgr/ml and or with Idaol at the dosage of 0,0012 µgr/ml corresponding to the concentration of 1 ng/ml in vivo.

They were assayed for cell-cycle and apoptosis at 24–48 hours post treatment.

These cells were incubated with PI for DNA stain for 30 minutes and analysed by cytometric assay with the FACScan.

10.000–50.000 cells of each sample were analysed; cell frequencies in cell-cycle phases are expressed as a percentage of the number within the complete cell-cycle.

Apoptosis cell frequencies are expressed as a percentage of the total cell number.

Cells with sub-G1 DNA content were scored as apoptotic according to previous studies [6].

Drugs effects on apoptosis and necrosis were determined also morphologically by fluorescent microscopy after labeling with Acridine Orange and Ethidium bromide as described by Duke and Choen [14]

Surface markers were analysed by flow cytometry as previously described with antibodies of the following features: CD13, CD14, CD15, CD33, CD34, while BCL-2 expression was analysed using the antihuman BCL-2 clone antiserum (DAKO) after permeabilization by Permeaphix (Ortho). The staining was considered positive when 20% of the cells or more in the control were stained.

Overall and Disease free survival were calculated from the date of starting induction therapy until the date of death, whatever the reason, and the date of relapse respectively.

Actuarial curves were computed according the Kaplan-Meier tecnique, we compared survival among the different groups using the log-rank test. [15]

## Results

In CR patients only mild to moderate haematological toxicity was registered.

No transfusion requirement occurred in CR patients while in PR patients a median of 2 units of RBC and 12 Units of PLT were transfused. No major bleeding or documented infection was noted.

Easily controlled mild nausea and vomiting occurred in 3 PR patients (Table 2–3).

Clinical results are shown in Fig1-2. In patients in CR a median of DFS and OS was 8 and 12.5 months respectively and the median OS in those in PR was 9 months. In contrast if we compare these results with another historical group of similar patients for disease state who didn't receive maintenance therapy we observe a lower cumulative median OS (3 vs 11 months) and a DFS and OS, in CR patients of 4 and 7 months respectively (Fig:

**Table 2.** Haematological toxicity and transfusion requirements of elderly patients treated with maintenance oral Idarubicin

| | CR | | PR | |
| | n°Pz | WHO | n°Pz | WHO |
|---|---|---|---|---|
| ANC | 3/10 | 1-2 | 12/21 | 1-3 |
| Hb | 4/10 | 1-2 | 17/21 | 2-4 |
| PLT | 2/10 | 2-3 | 17/21 | 1-4 |
| Rbc units Median (range) | — | | 2 (0-6) | |
| Plt units Median (range) | — | | 8 (0-32) | |

**Table 3.** Extrahaematological toxicity in elderly patients treated with maintenance oral Idarubicin

| | CR | | PR | |
| | Pts n° | WHO | Pts n° | WHO |
|---|---|---|---|---|
| Alopecia | 10 | 0 | 21 | 0 |
| Cardiac | 10 | 0 | 21 | 0 |
| Hepatic | 10 | 0 | 21 | 0 |
| Nausea Vomiting | 3 | 1 | 8 | 1-2 |
| Diarrhoea | 10 | 0 | 1 | 1 |

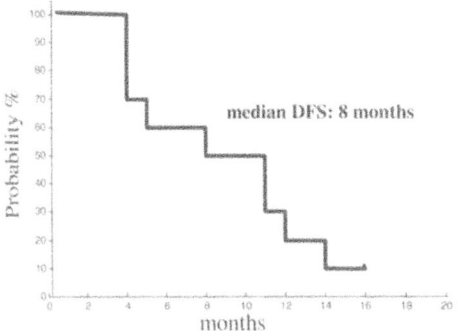

**Fig. 1.** Klapan-Meier cumulative Disease Free Survival of CR elderly patients treated with maintenance oral Idarubicin

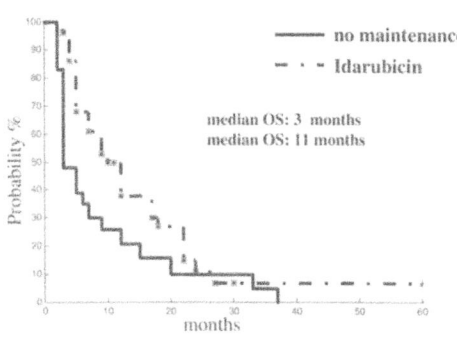

**Fig. 4.** Klapan-Meier cumulative OS of elderly patients responders (CR+PR) to first line therapy: comparation of patients treated with maintenance oral Idarubicin with a non maintained historical control group.

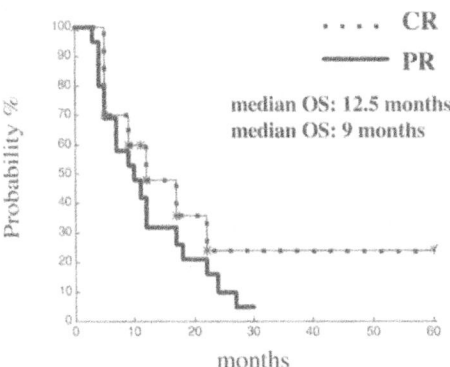

**Fig. 2.** Klapan-Meier cumulative Overall Survival of elderly patients treated with maintenance oral Idarubicin

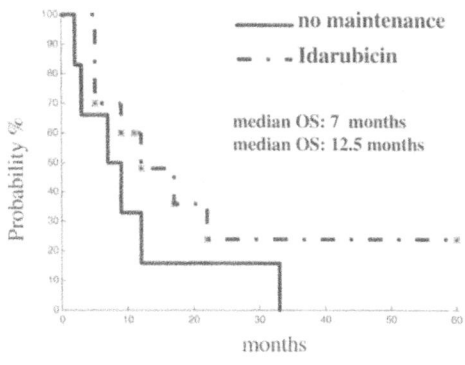

**Fig. 5.** Klapan-Meier cumulative OS of elderly patients achieved CR after first line therapy: comparation of patients treated with maintenance oral Idarubicin with a non maintained historical control group.

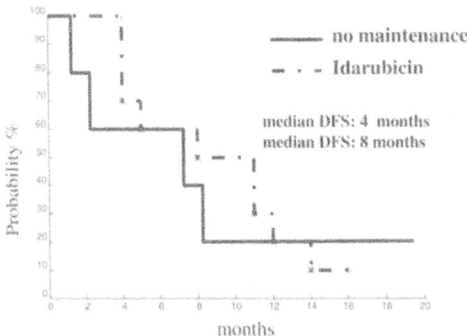

**Fig. 3.** Klapan-Meier cumulative DFS of elderly patients achieved CR after first line therapy: Comparation of patients treated with maintenance oral Idarubicin with a non maintained historical control group.

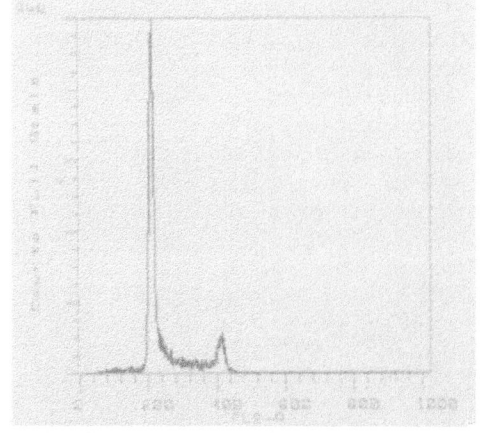

**Fig. 6.** DNA analysis of HL60 cells after 24 hours coulture (control) showing a G2+M cell frequencies of 5.5%

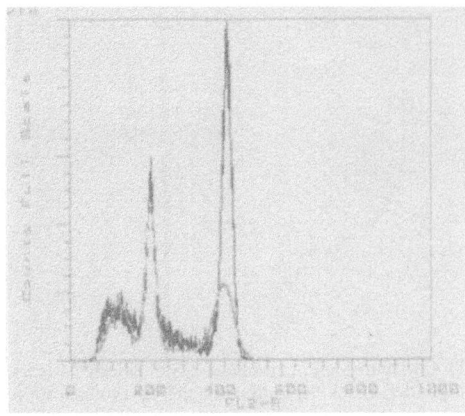

**Fig. 7.** DNA analysis of HL60 cells after 24 hours exposure to IDA/IDAol showing a sub G1 of 13.4 and an increase of G2+M cell frequencies of 48%

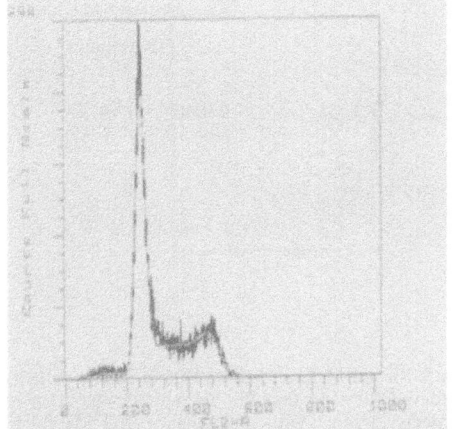

**Fig. 8.** DNA analysis at day 0 of leukemia cells showing G2+M cell frequencies of 8.5%

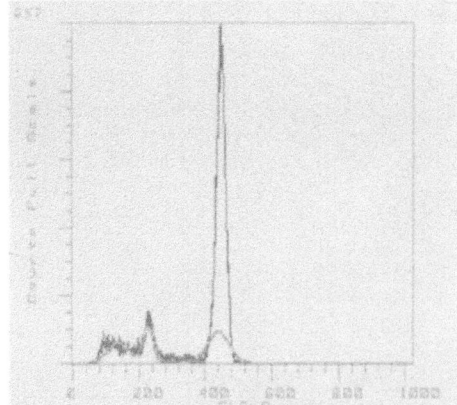

**Fig. 9.** DNA analysis at day 7 from starting Ida treatment of leukemia cells showing an increase of G2+M cell frequencies of 42% and a sub G1 peak of 17.8

**Table 4.** Clinical characteristics of elderly control patients

|  | CR | PR |
| --- | --- | --- |
| Pts n° | 10 | 19 |
| Median Age | 63 | 72 |
| Range | 61-72 | 62-77 |
| Sex M/F | 8/2 | 10/9 |
| FAB $M_0$ | 1 | 1 |
| $M_1$ | 2 | 3 |
| $M_2$ | 4 | 8 |
| $M_4$ | 2 | 4 |
| $M_5$ | 1 | 1 |
| $M_6$ | 0 | 2 |
| Secondary | 3 | 8 |
| Hepatomegaly | 2 | 11 |
| Median LDH U/l | 421 | 492 |
| Range | 195-1023 | 295-1438 |
| Unfavourable | 3 | 4 |
| Karyotype Favourable | 2 | 3 |

3–5, Table 3). DNA analysis shows a sub-G1 peak both in vivo and in vitro samples (only in patients in PR), moreover we observed an increase in G2+M cell frequencies (Fig. 6–9, Table 4). The apoptotic morphology assay confirmed these results (Fig. 10). In all patients in PR the leukemic cells were BCL-2 positive and no change of BCL-2 expression emerged during treatment (data not shown).

**Table 5.** IDA and IDAol induced apoptosis in patient leukemic cells and leukemic cell line

|  | HL60 Control 24h | 48h | PR pts Basal | day 7 |
| --- | --- | --- | --- | --- |
| Sub G1* | 1.05% | 13.4% | 26.2% | 0.8% | 17.8% |
| G2+M* | 9% | 28.8% | 48% | 9.9% | 42% |
| Morphology° | 2% | 8% | 30% | 3% | 18% |

## Discussion

Old age is a major adverse prognostic factor in AML patients both considering achievement of CR and OS , because these patients have frequently a poor performance status and other biological features such as high WBC and the presence of unfavourable cytogenetic features [16].

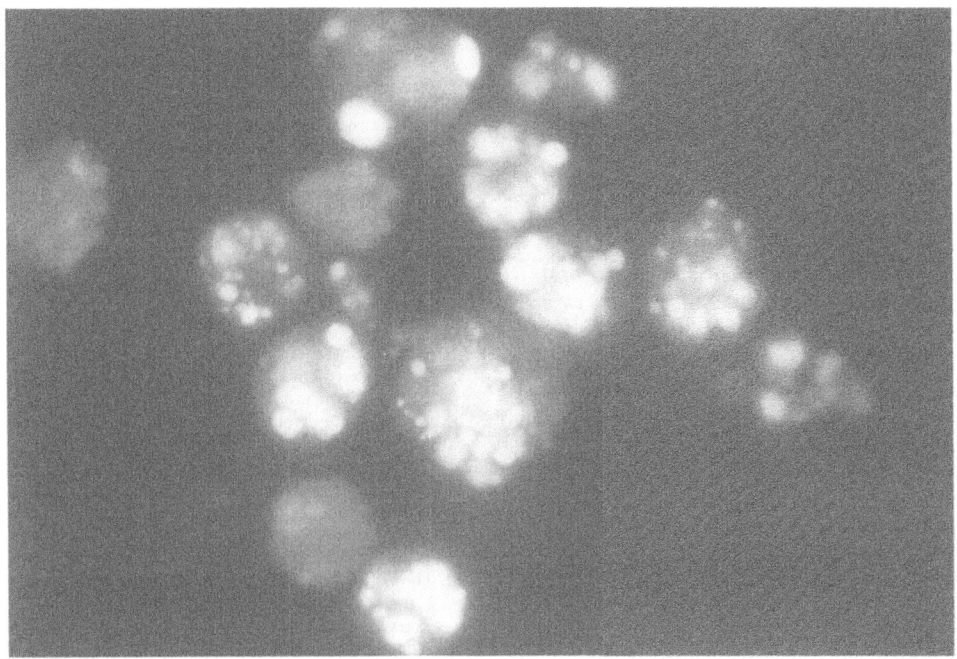

**Fig. 10.** Morphological features of HL60 cells after Ida and Idaol in vitro treatment. Live cells are stained in green, apoptotic cells are stained in orange. By Duke and Choen method.

In fact only 10% of patients will survive free of leukemia beyond 4 years after diagnosis. The choice of treatment for elderly patients depends on the balancing between toxicity and the quality of life. Many studies about AML in the patients over 60 suggest less intensive induction therapy to reduce toxicity. What is more a large percentage of patients who achieve a CR, relapse. One possible explanation is that the post-remission treatment is inadequate. Maintenance treatment could play a role in these patients who often cannot be treated with an intensive first-line therapy. In fact the post-induction therapy by continuous administration of a low dose of IDA in the long term warrants a control of the residual leukemic cells, (inducing apoptotic cell death). Recently studies in cytometric assays report a variable response to treatment-induced apoptotic AML cells after exposure to several drugs (ARA-C, DNR).

In a previous study we demonstrated only in those samples exposed to IDA and IDAol at the same time an increase in apoptosis in the leukemic cells after IDA and IDAol in vitro and in vivo exposure, moreover we have observed an increase in G2+M cell frequencies. On the other hand ARA-C gives similar results, while only an increase in G2+M cell frequencies is reported after DNR exposure [9].

Regarding the BCL-2 positive cells and the prospective apoptosis correlation, we found overexpression in many AML cells of patients in PR, yet these were correlated to treatment-induced apoptosis frequencies. Furthermore only cells from PR patients showed high BCL-2 positive cells, suggesting that tumour drug resistance were in this case more frequent.

The results of this study prove our preliminary observations and seem to confirm the hypothesis that long term exposure to low dose of IDA induces increase of apoptosis in leukemic cells.

Our clinical results showed a very low haematological and extrahaematological toxicity, and a good compliance with this treatment. The results of the study reported here indicate a good OS and DFS. If we compare these results with those obtained in a group of patients who didn't receive maintenance treatment, we can observe that the OS rate at 18 months for patients treated with IDA is almost three-fold that of patients without maintenance (35% v 12% p:0.04).

The DFS rate at 18 months was 20% for IDA treated patients while no patient is alive in the non treated group.

We find these results interesting even if it was not a randomised study and moreover was a small series.

In conclusion sequential cycles of oral IDA show clinically antileukemic activity in maintenance therapy and could be applied to older patients with disregard for toxicity and in an outpatient context, however more extensive and randomised trials are needed to evaluate the real impact on DFS and OS.

## References

1. Brinker H (1985): Estimate of overall treatment results in acute non lymphocytic leukemia based on age-specific rates of incidence and of complete remission.. Cancer Treatment Reports, :69: 5-11,.
2. Cartwright RA & Staines A (1992): Acute leukemias. Epidemiology of Haematological Disease. In:. AT Fleming (eds),. Bailliere's Clinical Haematology vol: 5, pp:1 - 26,
3. Lowenberg B (1996): Acute myelogeneus Leukaemia and Myelodysplasia In AT Fleming (eds) Bailliere's Clinical Haematology, vol.9,pp 147-159.
4. Keating MJ, McCredie KB, Benjamin RS, Bodey GP, Zander A, Smith TJ & FrereichEJ (1981): Treatment of patients over 50 years of age with myelogenous leukemia with a combination of rubidazone and cytosine arabnoside, vincristine and prednisolone (ROAP). Blood, 58: 584-591.
5. Swirsky DM, De Bastos M, Parish SE, Rees JKH & Hayhoe FGJ (1987): Features affecting outcome during remission induction of acute myeloid leukemia in 619 adult patients. British Journal of Haematology, 64: 435-453.
6. Campos L, Roualt JP, Oriol P, Roubi N, Vasselon C, Archimbaud E, Magaud JP,Guyotat D (1993): High expression of BCL-2 protein in acute myelogeneous leukemia cells is associated with poor response to chemotherapy. Blood, Vol.81, n°11: 3091-3096.
7. Liu Yin JA (1993): Acute myeloid leukemia in elderly: biology and treatment. British Journal of Haematology , vol.8: 361-366.
8. Baudard M, Marie JP, Cadiou M, Viguié V & Zittoun R (1994): Acute myelogenous leukemia in the elderly: retrospective study of 235 consecutive patients. British Journal of Hematology, 86: 82-91.
9. Banker DE, Groudine M, Norwood T & Appelbaum FR (1997): Measurement of spontaneous and therapeutic agent-induced apoptosis. Blood, vol. 89, n°1: 243-255,.
10. Shiller JC (1996): Post-remission therapy of acute myeloid leukemia in older adults. Leukemia, 10, suppl.1, S18-S20,.
11. Lowemberg B. (1998): Mitoxantrone versus daunorubicin in induction consolidation chemotherap. The value of low dose Cytarabine for maintenance of remission, and an assessment of prognostic factors in acute myeloid leukemia in the elderly: final report of the Leukemia Cooperative Group of the European Organization for the Research and Treatment of Cancer and the Dutch-Belgian Hemato-Oncology Cooperative Hovon Group randomized phase III study AML-9. Journal Clinical Oncology, 16,3, 872-881
12. Leoni F, Ciolli S, Pascarella A, Caporale R, Salti F, Cervi L & Rossi Ferrini P (1995): Attenuated-dose idarubicin in acute myeloid leukemia in the elderly: pharmacokinetic study and clinical results. British Journal of Haematology, 90: 169-174.
13. Ellison RR, Holland JF, Weil M, Jacquillat C, Boiron M, Bernard J, Sawitsky A , Rosner F, Gussof B, Silver RT, Karanas A, Cuttner J, Spurr CL, Hayes DM, Blom J, Leone LA, Haurani F, Kyle R, Hutchinson JL, Forcier RJ, Moon JH (1968): Arabinosyl citosine: a useful agent in the treatment of acute leukemia in adults. Blood 32:507,.
14. Duke RC, Choen JJ (1992): Morphological and biochemical assay of apoptosis in: Coligan JE, Kruis Beack AM (eds) Current Protocols in Immunology. NY: J Willey and Sons pp:3171-6
15. Kaplan, E. L. & Meier, P. (1958): Nonparametric estimation from incomplete observations. Journal of the American Statistical Association,53: 457-481.
16. Johnson RE, Ryder WDJ, Liu Yin JA(1995): Validation of a model to predict survival in elderly patients with acute myeloid leukemia. British Journal of Haematology , 90: 954-956.

# Phase I Study of Liposomal Daunorubicin (DaunoXome) in Relapsed and Refractory Acute Myeloid Leukemia

C. Lerchenmüller, W.E. Berdel and T. Büchner

*Abstract.* Daunorubicin (DNR) is one of the most important cytotoxic agents in the treatment of acute myeloid leukemia (AML). Its use is usually limited by drug-induced cardiotoxicity depending on the cumulative dose administered. Liposomal encapsulation of DNR (DaunoXome®, DNX) seems to reduce the risk of this severe and sometimes fatal side effect. To investigate the toxicity of DNX in a heavily pretreated patient population, we currently conduct a phase I study including patients (pts) older than 60 years with relapsed or refractory AML. DNX is used at doses of 40, 60, 75, 90 and 100 mg/m2 biweekly. Until now, 13 pts have been treated: median age 69 years (range, 63-77), median number of prior regimen 1,4 (range, 0-2), median cumulative doses of DNR 553.5 mg (range, 0-880), mitoxantrone 16.2 mg (range, 0-60) and idarubicin 33.8 mg (range, 0-80). A total of 47 courses of DNX were administered (3 pts at 40 mg/m2 with a total of 13 courses, 5 at 60 mg/m2 with a total of 20 courses, 4 at 75 mg/m2 with a total of 12 courses and 1 at 90 mg/m2 with a total of 2 courses). Mean cumulative dose of DNX administered was 386,3 mg (range, 120-1200). Hematologic and non-hematologic toxicities were monitored by clinical, laboratory and cardiologic examination (including radionuclide ventriculography and echocardiography) and by a questionaire which was repeatedly filled in by the pts. Grade 1 and 2 elevations of liver enzymes were seen in 2 pts. A 20 % decline in left ventricular ejection fraction (LVEF) without clinical signs and symptoms of heart failure was noticed after a cumulative DNX dose of 480 mg in 2 patients, one with a history of two myocardial infarctions and the other with arterial hypertension. Even at the highest cumulative doses of DNX, no further decline in LVEF was noticed (LVEF prior to DNX: median 53 % (range, 34-67), after last course: median 52,7 % (range, 46-60). Vomiting, alopecia and mucositis were absent. All patients had significant myelosuppression requiring transfusion support. During treatment, 3 pts showed a reduction of leukemic blasts in bone marrow of > 25 %, 8 pts had to be excluded due to AML progression and 2 pts died due to disease-related complications. We conclude from these preliminary data, that DNX might offer a less toxic alternative to DNR and other anthracyclines. We will give a dose recommendation for the palliative treatment of relapsed and refractory AML as soon as our phase I study is finished. A phase II study will then be initiated.

## Introduction

Daunorubicin (DNR) is an integral part of most AML treatment strategies. In the majority of chemotherapy regimens, DNR has been used in concentrations of between 30 and 60 mg/m2 on three consecutive days [1, 2, 3]. Due to the toxic side effects of the drug, dose escalation of DNR has never been systematically investigated in prospective randomized trials, whereas studies using high cumulative doses of DNR have occasionally been published [4]. During the last few years, one phase III study and several phase I/II studies have been published, investigating toxicity and clinical efficacy of a liposomal formulation of DNR (DNX) in a variety of different entities [5, 6, 7]. In these and other

---

Dept. of Internal Medicine, University of Münster, Germany.

studies it could be shown, that DaunoXome® (DNX) has a moderate toxicity profile and could be given in high cumulative doses without significant cardiotoxicity.

DNX is characterised by so-called unilamellar vesicles consisting of phospholipids and cholesterol which enclose an aqueous core containing daunorubicin (DNR). These phospholipids have a diameter of between 40 and 80 nanometers and show a neutral surface charge [8]. The particular chemical composition of the vesicle membrane and its physical features are responsible for the remarkable stability of the liposomes in vivo [9]. While in circulation, the DNX formulation protects the entrapped DNR from chemical and enzymatic degradation, minimizes protein binding, and generally decreases uptake by normal tissue [8]. Further experimental data have shown, that DNR distribution in vivo is altered through the entrappment within liposomes, and that the maximum concentration of the available drug in tumors exceeds that of the free drug, suggesting a preferential accumulation of DNX within tumor tissue [10].

Due to the favourable toxicity data of DNX, and the ability to administer both higher single and cumulative doses of the drug, we intended to investigate this new formulation of DNR in elderly patients with AML, who have already been pretreated with different intercalating drugs during their first-line and salvage treatment. The intention of treatment was palliation and therapy was administered in an outpatient setting.

## Patients and Protocol

In 1998, we started a clinical phase I trial, investigating DNX in elderly patients with relapsed or refractory AML, who were not eligible for intensive treatment strategies due to the clinical course of their leukemia or concomitant disease. Patients were older than 60 years of age and have already been treated within study protocols of the AML Cooperative Group, containing the intercalating drugs daunorubicin, mitoxantrone, and idarubicin. Before entering the study, patients had to undergo a cardiac examination, including electrocardiography, echocardiography and also radionuclide ventriculography. Patients with congestive heart failure showing clinical symptoms according to NYHA grade 3 or higher, or concomitant disease of the lung, liver, kidneys, infectious diseases, or any other clinical condition prohibiting treatment with cytotoxic agents, were excluded from study and treated by supportive care only. Patient characteristics are shown in Table 1.

Study patients were assigned to one of the cohorts and were treated with the corresponding DNX dose in two week intervals (Table 2). After two DNX courses, bone marrow of the patients was examined, and study treatment was continued if leukemic blasts were reduced by more than 25 % compared with the initial blast count („responder"). If complete remission was to be achieved, DNX treatment has to be given for another two courses and then stopped until relapse occured. Patients were excluded from further study treatment in case of persistent or progressive leukemia or the appearance of a dose-limiting toxicity (DLT). If 4 patients have been treated within a cohort without showing a DLT, and at least two of these patients have received 3 or more courses of treatment, the following patients have been assigned to the next cohort. Dose-limiting toxicities were defined as follows: (1) Appearance of grade 4 hematotoxicity in combination with a single grade 3 organ toxicity after two consecutive DNX

**Table 1.** Patient Characteristics

| Patients (n) | 13 |
|---|---|
| Median Age (years) | 69 |
| Range (years) | 63 – 77 |
| Sex (m/f) (n) | 5 / 8 |
| AML type (de novo / prior MDS) (n) | 11 / 2 |
| Relapsed / Refractory AML (n) | 11 / 2 |
| Adverse karyotype at study entry (n) | 5 |

**Table 2.** Study cohorts

| Cohort | DNX (mg/m2) | Treatment interval (wk) |
|---|---|---|
| 1 | 40 | 2 |
| 2 | 60 | 2 |
| 3 | 75 | 2 |
| 4 | 90 | 2 |
| 5 | 100 | 2 |

**Table 3.** Cumulative Doses of Prior Intercalating Drugs

| Drugs | Mean dosage (mg) | Range (mg) |
|---|---|---|
| Daunorubicin | 553.5 | 0 – 880 |
| Mitoxantrone | 16.2 | 0 – 60 |
| Idarubicine | 33.8 | 0 – 80 |

**Table 4.** Number of Treatment Courses and Cumulative DNX doses

| Cohort No. | DNX dose (mg/m$^2$) | Patients (n) | Courses (n) | Maximal DNX doses adminstered (mg/m$^2$) |
|---|---|---|---|---|
| 1 | 40 | 3 | 13 | 650 |
| 2 | 60 | 5 | 20 | 1200 |
| 3 | 75 | 4 | 12 | 840 |
| 4 | 90 | 1 | 2 | 180 |
| Total | | 13 | 47 | |

courses, (2) grade 4 organ toxicity, (3) persistent thrombocytopenia of < 50.000/µl on day 29 of a DNX course, and (4) persistent neutropenia of < 1.000/µl ond day 22 (toxicity grading according to the CTC criteria). Most patients have been pretreated with high cumulative doses of different intercalating drugs (Table 3). Therefore, study patients had to undergo close cardiac monitoring with radionuclide ventriculography and echocardiography in monthy intervals. Left ventricular ejection fraction and shortening fractions were measured and compared to baseline values prior to treatment start.

## Results

The majority of study patients showed a pancytopenia at the time of treatment start, with median values for neutrophils of 400/µl (range, 60–6000/µl), hemoglobin of 9.8 g/dl (range, 7.7–11.5 g/dl), and platelets of 27.000/µl (range, 14.000 – 96.000/µl). The median bone marrow blast count was 70 % (range, 20 – 90 %). At study entry, all patients were transfusion-dependent for either red blood cells or platelets or both.

So far, 13 patients have been included in the study. Meanwhile, cohort 4 has been opened with one patient being treated at a dose of 90 mg/m2. Unfortunately, he died shortly after the second course of treatment and was therefore not evaluable for response and toxi-

city. In Table 4, number of courses and cumulative DNX doses administered are depicted.

Until now, 7/13 study patients did receive a bone marrow examination after the 2$^{nd}$ course of treatment. 3/7 patients showed a reduction of 30, 76 and 40 % of their inital bone marrow blast count and were therfore classified as responders. Responding patients were treated with cumulative doses of 650, 240 and 525 mg/m$^2$, respectively. 2 of the responding patients were eventually excluded from further study treatment due to progressive disease and died shortly thereafter. One of the responding patients ist still under treatment. Repeated bone marrow examinations of the responders showed hypoplastic marrows with residual leukemic blast populations. In one of the cases, further treatment was postponed due to severly hypoplastic bone marrow. This patient showed no regeneration of normal hematopoiesis but proliferation of leukemic blasts and was therefore excluded from the study after having received 4 courses of DNX. Bone marrow examination of the 4 non-responding patients showed an unaltered leukemic infiltration. 3 of the 4 patients developed progressive disease soon therafter, and one patients received further 6 treatment courses until progression occured.

**Table 5.** Early Deaths of Study Patients

| Patient No. | Courses (n) | Death due to | Neutropenia Grad IV | | Thrombocytopenia Grad IV | |
|---|---|---|---|---|---|---|
| | | | Study entry | time of death | Study entry | time of death |
| 1 | 2 | Infection | + | + | + | + |
| 2 | 1 | Hemorrhage | + | + | + | + |
| 3 | 1 | Infection | - | ? | - | ? |
| 4 | 2 | Infection | + | + | + | + |
| 5 | 1 | Infection | + | + | + | + |
| 6 | 1 | Infection | + | + | + | + |

Unfortunately, but not surprisingly, the early death rate was rather high. 6/13 patients died either between the 1st and 2nd or shortly after the 2nd DNX course (Table 5). 5 patients suffered from neutropenic infections, 3 of these patients also showed clinical evidence of a rapidly progressive leukemia. All patients dying from infectious complications have already shown severe neutropenia at study entry. One patient died from cerebral hemorrhage due to severe thrombocytopenia, which was also present before study entry.

Analysis of cardiac toxicity was restricted to patients who received 3 or more treatment courses. Decline of left ventricular ejection fraction was detected in 2 patients, showing a decrease of 22.3 and 20.7 % from baseline values after two treatment courses. Neither of the 2 patients showed clinical signs or symptoms of congestive heart failure. One of the patients had a history of coronary heart disease with 2 myocardial infarctions, and prior anti-leukemic treatment was therefore restricted to amsacrine- and mitoxantrone-containing regimens. The other patient had a history of arterial hypertension and had received prior treatment with daunorubicin and idarubicin at cumulative doses of 390 mg/m2 and 40 mg/m2, respectively. No deterioration of cardiac function was detectable in the remaining patients (n = 5).

Nonhematologic toxicity was assessed by regular clinical and weekly laboratory examinations. Apart from these examinations, EORTC-QLQ 30-questionaires were filled in by patients in monthly intervals. No toxicities exceeding CTC grade 2 were found. General toxicities like fatigue, nausea and weight loss

**Table 6.** Non-hematological toxicity

| Toxicity | Patients (n) | Patients (%) |
|---|---|---|
| Fatigue | 6 | 46 |
| Nausea | 5 | 38 |
| Weight loss | 4 | 31 |
| Fever | 4 | 31 |
| Hospital Admission | 4 | 31 |
| i.v. Antibiotics | 3 | 23 |
| Elevation of liver enzymes | 2 | 15 |
| Neuropathy | 2 | 15 |
| Diarrhea | 1 | 8 |
| Alopecia | 0 | 0 |
| Mucositis | 0 | 0 |

were found in up to 50 % of patients. Hospital admission was necessary in one third of the patients under treatment, for either infections or neurologic deterioration. Slight elevations of liver enzymes were seen in two patients, whereas alopecia and mucositis were not detected in any of the study participants (Table 6).

## Discussion

Although the number of patients included in this study is still low, and the data which can be presented at the moment are preliminar, at least a few conclusions can be drawn which have to be confirmed in the ensuing phase II study. DNX is very well tolerated in these heavily pretreated patient population and can be easily adminstered in an outpatient setting. Due to the fact, that typical anthracycline-associated toxicities like mucositis and alopecia are absent, DNX treatment is suitable as a palliative therapy and the risk of mucositis-associated infectious complications in neutropenic patients might be decreased.

According to the dismal prognosis of the study patients, early death within the first month of treatment start was not surprising but was expected to occur in some of the patients due to AML-related complications. Neither of the deaths was related to treatment, although in one patient who suffered from infection, a treatment-associated neutropenia could not be evaluated due to her sudden death.

3 of 13 patients are responders to study treatment in terms of significant reduction of the leukemic infiltration in the bone marrow. Neither of these 3 patients has actually achieved a complete or even partial response. Therefore, at least in this prognostically dismal patient population and with the dosages used so far, DNX has low therapeutic efficacy as single agent. It remains to be seen whether higher doses of DNX can improve therapeutic efficacy and might overcome multidrug resistance, which is a frequent finding in these patients [11, 12]. Encouraging results of phase I/II studies have been published by several groups, investigating high doses of DNX in the treatment of relapsed or refractory acute myeloid leukemia [13, 14]. In these studies,

DNX was used at doses of up to 250 mg/m2 x 1 day or 150 mg/m2 x 3 days. In this context, it is interesting to investigate, whether the use of the liposomal formulation of daunorubicin might help to circumvent multidrug resistance in AML. In a phase I/II trial published in 1993 [15], the authors investigated cyclosporin A as a modulator of multidrug resistance in a progrostically poor patient population with AML. It was demonstrated, that hyperbilirubinemia was a predictor of response when patients were treated with high doses of cyclosporine A. It was suggested, that in addition to modulation of pgp-function in leukemic blasts, the delayed hepatic clearance of daunorubicin due to inhibition of pgp-mediated biliary excretion and the significantly enhanced daunorubicin levels in plasma might explain the increased cytotoxic effect. In a recently published study [16], it was reported that pgp-positive leukemic blasts from patients with acute leukemia who were clinically daunorubicin-resistant, were still sensitive to daunorubicin in-vitro, provided that they encounter daunorubicin concentrations and exposure times which might be achieved by liposomal rather than by free daunorubicin in-vivo.

It may be said, that the available data pointing to the pharmacologic characteristics of liposomal daunorubicin, the possible advantages in overcoming multidrug resistance, the favourable toxicity profile, and the opportunity to pursue dose-intensification strategies, makes further investigation of the drug both interesting and worthwhile.

# References

1. Yates J, Glidewell O, Wiernik P et al. (1982). Cytosine Arabinoside With Daunorubicin or Adriamycin for Therapy of Acute Myelocytic Leukemia: A CALGB Study. Blood 60: 454-462.
2. Büchner T, Urbanitz D, Hiddemann W et al. (1985). Intensified Induction and Consolidation With or Without Maintenance Chemotherapy for Acute Myeloid Leukemia (AML): Two Multicenter Studies of the German AML Cooperative Group. J Clin Oncol 3: 1583-1589.
3. Mayer RJ, Davis RB, Schiffer CA et al. (1994). Intensive Postremission Chemotherapy in Adults With Acute Myeloid Leukemia. N Engl J Med 331: 896-903.
4. Usui N, Dobashi N, Kobayashi T et al. (1998). Role of Daunorubicin in the Induction Therapy for Adult Acute Myeloid Leukemia. J Clin Oncol 16: 2086-2092.
5. Gill PS, Espina BM, Muggia F et al. (1995). Phase I/II Clinical and Pharmacokinetic Evaluation of Liposomal Daunorubicin. J Clin Oncol 13: 996-1003.
6. Gill PS, Wernz J, Scadden DT et al. (1996). Randomized Phase III Trial of Liposomal Daunorubicin Versus Doxorubicin, Bleomycin, and Vincristin in AIDS-Related Kaposi's Sarcoma. J Clin Oncol 14: 2453-2364.
7. Richardson DS, Kelsey SM, Johnson SA et al. (1997). Early Evaluation of Liposomal Daunorubicin (DaunoXome®, NeXstar) in the Treatment of Relapsed and Refractory Lymphoma. Invest New Drugs 15: 247-253.
8. Forssen EA, Ross ME (1994). DaunoXome® Treatment of Solid Tumours: Preclinical and Clinical Investigations. J Lip Res 4 (1): 481-512.
9. Forssen EA, Coulter DM, Proffit RT (1992). Selective In Vivo Localization of Daunorubicin Small Unilamellar Vesicles in Solid Tumours. Cancer Res 52: 3255-3261.
10. Forssen EA, Malé-Brune R, Adler-Moore JP, Lee MJA, Schmidt PG, Krasieva TB, Shimizu S, Tromberg BJ (1996). Fluorescence Imaging Studies for the Disposition of Daunorubicin Liposomes (DaunoXome®) within Tumor Tissue. Cancer Res 56: 2066-2075.
11. Guerci A, Merlin JL, Missoum N, et al. (1995). Predictive Value for Treatment Outcome in Acute Myeloid Leukemia of Cellular Daunorubicin Accumulation and P-Glycoprotein Expression Simultaneously Determined by Flow Cytometry. Blood 85: 2147-2153.
12. Leith CP, Kopecky KJ, Godwin J, et al. (1997). Acute Myeloid Leukemia in the Elderly: Assessment of Multidrug Resistance (MDR1) and Cytogenetics Distinguishes Biologic Subgroups With Remarkably Distinct Responses to Standard Chemotherapy. A Southwest Oncology Group Study. Blood 89: 3323-3329.
13. Cortes J, Kantarjian H, O'Brien S, et al. (1998). Phase I Study of Liposomal Daunorubicin (LD) in Refractory or Relapsed Acute Myeloid Leukemia (AML) or Blast Phase Chronic Myelogenous Leukemia (CML-BP). ASH-Meeting 1998, Miami (abstr 957).
14. Cripe L, Kneebone P, Roberts L, et al. (1998). A Phase I Trial of Liposomal Daunorubicin (DaunoXome) Administered With High-Dose Cytarabine (HiDAC) to Patients With Relapsed Acute Leukemia. ASH-Meeting 1998, Miami (abstr. 955).
15. List AF, Spier C, Greer J, et al. (1993). Phase I/II Trial of Cyclosporine A as a Chemotherapy-Resistance Modifier in Acute Leukemia. J Clin Oncol 11: 1652-1659.
16. Verdonck LF, Lokhorst HM, Roovers DJ, et al. (1998). Multidrug-Resistant Acute Leukemia Cells are Responsive to Prolonged Exposure of Daunorubicin: Implications for Liposome-Encapsulated Daunorubicin. Leukemia Res 22: 249-256.

# Multi Centre Study of a Combination of Fludarabine Phosphate, Cytosine Arabinoside and Granulocyte Colony Stimulating Factor (FLAG) in Relapsed and Refractory Acute Myeloid Leukaemia and in De Novo RAEB-t

S. Proctor, on behalf of the UK FLAG Collaborative Group

## Introduction

The purpose of the present study was to evaluate the use of the FLAG regimen (fludarabine phosphate in combination with cytosine arabinoside and granulocyte colony stimulating factor (GCSF) in patients with poor risk myeloid malignancy. The rationale for this combination is based on the synergy between fludarabine phosphate and cytosine arabinoside; the cytotoxic activity of cytosine arabinoside is dependent on its intracellular conversion to its active metabolite the 5'-triphosphate (ara-CTP). The intracellular accumulation of ara-CTP is a multistep process, of which phosporylation of ara-C to its monophosphate by deoxycytidine kinase (Cyd kinase) is the rate-limiting event. Fludarabine phosphate increases the activity of this critical enzyme leading to a higher rate of ara-CTP accumulation intracellularly (Gandhi [1]).

The rationale behind the addition of GCSF prior to administration of fludarabine phosphate and cytosine arabinoside is to increase the number of cells in the cell cycle which are vulnerable to cytosine arabinoside (Tafuri [2] and Gandh [3]). Following the initial reports in 1994 by Estey [4] and Visan [5], the present multicentre study began to evaluate prospectively the reponse to FLAG in patients with RAEB-t and refractory and relapsed acute myeloid leukaemia (AML).

## Patients and Methods

### Patients

There were 19 U.K. centres involved in this study. At the inception of the study, it was decided that patients were to be divided into three groups for analysis of treatment results.

*Group A.* Patients with AML who had responded to first line chemotherapy and relapsed more than 6 months from the end of treatment.

*Group B.* Patients with AML who had responded to first line chemotherapy and relapsed within 6 months of stopping treatment or were resistant to first line chemotherapy.

*Group C.* Patients with de novo advanced myelodysplastic syndrome sub-type RAEB-t (refractory anaemia with excess blasts in transformation).

Members of the UK Collaborative Group are:

Mr J Brookes, Schering Health Care Ltd, Burgess Hill; Dr P Carey, Sunderland Royal Hospital, Sunderland; Dr P Chu, Royal Liverpool and Broadgreen University Hospital NHS Trust, Liverpool; Dr M Deane, Norfolk and Norwich Hospitals NHS Trust, Norwich; Dr A Duncombe, Royal South Hants Hospital, Southampton; Dr P Ganly, Western General Hospital, Edinburgh; Dr D Gillett, Pembury Hospital, Tunbridge Wells; Dr M Hutchinson, Leicester Royal Infirmary, Leicester; Dr G Jackson, Royal Victoria Infirmary, Newcastle upon Tyne; Dr S A Johnson, Taunton and Somerset Hospital, Taunton; Dr E Kanfer, Hammersmith Hospital, London; Dr T J Littlewood, John Radcliffe Hospital, Oxford; Dr N P Lucie, Western Infirmary, Glasgow; Dr M J Mackie, Western General Hospital, Edinburgh; Dr R Marcus, Addenbrooke_s Hospital, Cambridge; Dr A Mehta, Royal Free Hospital, London; Dr D Oscier, Royal Bournemouth Hospital, Bournemouth; Dr S Schey, Guy_s Hospital, London; Dr G Scott, Bristol Royal Infirmary, Bristol; Dr A Smith, Royal South Hants Hospital, Southampton; Dr G Smith, Royal United Hospital, Bath; Dr G M Smith, Leeds General Infirmary, Leeds; Dr P Taylor, Royal Victoria Infirmary, Newcastle upon Tyne; Dr S M Tollerfield, Schering Health Care Ltd, Burgess Hill; Dr G E Turner, Norfolk and Norwich Hospitals NHS Trust, Norwich; Dr M P Wilson, Schering Health Care Ltd, Burgess Hill.

## Objectives

The primary objective of the study was to evaluate the complete response rate to the FLAG regimen as remission induction treatment. Secondary objectives were to assess the survival time and to investigate the safety and tolerability of the FLAG regimen.

## Eligibility

Patients had to be aged 18–75 years with a WHO performance status of 0-2. Specific exclusion criteria included de novo AML, previous chemotherapy for RAEB-t, chronic myeloid leukaemia in blast transformation, clinically significant impairmet of renal or liver function and a prior bone marrow or peripheral blood stem cell (PBSC) transplant.

## Treatment

Patients received induction therapy consisting of intravenous infusions of fludarabine phosphate given daily for five days (days 1–5) as a 30 minute intravenous infusion of 30 mg/m$^2$ 4 hours prior to each daily infusion of cytosine arabinoside. Cytosine arabinoside, at a dose of 2 g/m$^2$, was given daily for five days (days 1–5) as a 4 hour intravenous infusion. GCSF, at a dose of 30 million units, was given daily for seven days (day-1 through to day 6) by subcutaneous injection beginning 24 hours prior to the first administration of fludarabine phosphate.

Patients were assessed by bone marrow aspirate for remission status once neutrophil recovery was achieved, this being defined as an absolute neutrophil count of greater than or equal to 1 x 10$^9$/l for three days. The use of GCSF as a supportive agent in the event of unsatisfactory neutrophil recovery post chemotherapy was allowed. After complete remission was achieved with patients having received one or two courses, up to two cycles of consolidation chemotherapy consisting of a four day course of FLAG (fludarabine and ara-C given for 4 days instead of 5) were recommended.

If complete remission was not achieved patients received a second cycle of induction chemotherapy at the clinician's discretion. Patients who did not achieve a complete remission after two cycles of induction chemotherapy were withdrawn. Cytogenetic assessment was recommended in all patients. This was to be performed locally on a bone marrow aspirate, if possible, and the presence of a normal karyotype or any abnormal clone recorded.

## Response to Treatment

A response to treatment was classified as complete remission if there were less than 5% myeloblasts in the bone marrow associated with evidence of trilineage regeneration and an absence of unequivocal leukaemic features. Survival data were analysed by the Kaplan-Meier method.

## Results

89 patients were entered from the 19 centres (range 1–11), of whom 83 were eligible for the trial (21 – Group A, 44 – Group B and 18 – Group C). Reasons for exclusion were: untreated de-novo AML (3), non Hodgkin's lymphoma (1), RAEB (1) and failed second line chemotherapy (1).

### Patient Details and Response to Treatment

The median age of the eligible patients was 49 years (range 18–75); 25 patients were aged > 60 years. There were 42 male patients, 41 females. One patient died before study treatment, having given consent. Further details of the patients and the response to therapy, by disease group, are shown in Table 1. CR rates were 81% in Group A patients, 30% in Group B and 56% in Group C.

### Cytogenetic Analysis

The protocol specified that all patients should have cytogenetic analysis attempted at trial entry; in 20 patients this was not done. It is noteworthy that of those with a successful analysis, only 5 had »favourable« karyotypers:

**Table 1.** Patient details/results

| | Number of Patients | Median Age (years) | CR (%) | 5 month survival (%) |
|---|---|---|---|---|
| Group A (late first relapse AML) | 21 | 48 | 81 | 81 |
| Group B (primary refractory, early first relapse AML) | 44 | 47 | 30 | 34 |
| Group C (de novo RAEB-t) | 18 | 60 | 56 | 78 |

1 t(15;17); in inversion (16) and 3 patients with t(8;21). By contrast 18 patients had the karyotype typical of »secondary« leukaemias with abnormalities including monosomy 7 and trisomy 8 and a further 21 patients had some other cytogenetic abnormality. Nineteen patients had no abnormality detected.

## Toxicity

A total of 133 courses of FLAG were assessed for toxicity (WHO grading). Haematological toxicity is summarised in Table 2. Grade 4 neutropenia ($< 0.5$ x $10^9$/L) occurred in all courses; for each course patients spent a median of 24 days in hospital and were given a median of 7 platelet transfusions. One patient died before treatment commenced after giving consent; two patients were withdrawn from the study due to a rapid rise in white cell count whilst on GCSF, and a further patient was withdrawn following development of venoocculsive disease. There were 13 deaths on treatment: 2 from haemorrhage, 2 from disease progression and 9 from infection including (3 proven fungial infections). After

achieving remission, 12 patients proceeded to transplantation, 8 allogeneic (including 3 MUDs) of whom 5 survive (4 in CR). 4 patients were able to undergo autologous transplantation (3 survine in CR and 1 has relapsed). 37 patients have died since completing the study, mainly due to disease progression (28). Other causes of death included transplant toxicity post allotransplant (3), infection (5) and haemorrhage (1).

## Discussion

The outlook for patients who relapse following primary chemotherapy for AML is poor, and results of treatment outcome can be difficult to find. A recent report (Burnet [6]) showed that in the follow up study of patients entered in the MRC 10 trial, the two year survival in relapsed adults was less than 20% (see Table 3).

A total of 83 eligible patients entered the present study, of whom 82 received treatment. The results in this cohort of patients show promise. The regimen was well tolerated and the CR rates are shown (by group) in Table 1. These results are comparable with previous studies of response to FLAG in patients with poor prognosis myeloid malignancy (Table 4). CR rates in relapsed AML are particularly encouraging although, as expected, a lower CR rate was observed in patients with refractory disease or early relapse (Group B).

Following study chemotherapy with FLAG, further treatment was at the discretion of the physician. In twelve patients, FLAG therapy was followed by transplantation (5 sibling allografts, 3 MUDs and 4 autologous transplants). The overall survival of the group is shown in Figure 1.

**Table 2.** FLAG Therapy in Poor Risk Myeloid Malignancy

| Toxicity-Haematological | |
|---|---|
| Courses assessed | 133 |
| GD IV neutropenia | All courses |
| Days in hospital/course | Median 24 |
| Platelet transfusions/course | Median 7 |

* 2 patients withdrew due to significant increase in WCC
* 1 patient withdrew due to veno-occlusive disease

**Table 3.** AML Relapse Pattern post MRC 10

165 relapses – 139 adults (> 15 years)

| | Previous Auto | No Auto |
|---|---|---|
| 2nd remission achieved | | |
| aged < 35 years | 56% | 48% |
| aged > 35 years | 26% | 62% |
| Two year survival | | |
| aged < 35 years | 7% | 16% |
| aged > 35 years | 17% | 12% |

**Table 4.** Response rate of FLAG therapy in poor risk myeloid malignancy

| Paper | FLAG Regimen | Number of Patients | Age (median range) | Compete Response Rate | Median Survival |
|---|---|---|---|---|---|
| Estey [4] (1994) | Standard | 112 | 63 (range not available) | 63% | 38 weeks |
| Visani [6] (1994) | Standard | 28 | 50 (16–72) | 58% | 24 weeks |
| Huhmann [7] (1996) | Fludarabine 25 mg | 22 | 46 (24–63) | 50% | 13 months |
| Nokes [8] (1997) | Variable doses of cytosine arabinoside | 32 | 60 (14–75) | 80% | Not available |
| Montillo [9] (1998) | Standard | 38 | 41 (11–70) | 55% | 9 months |

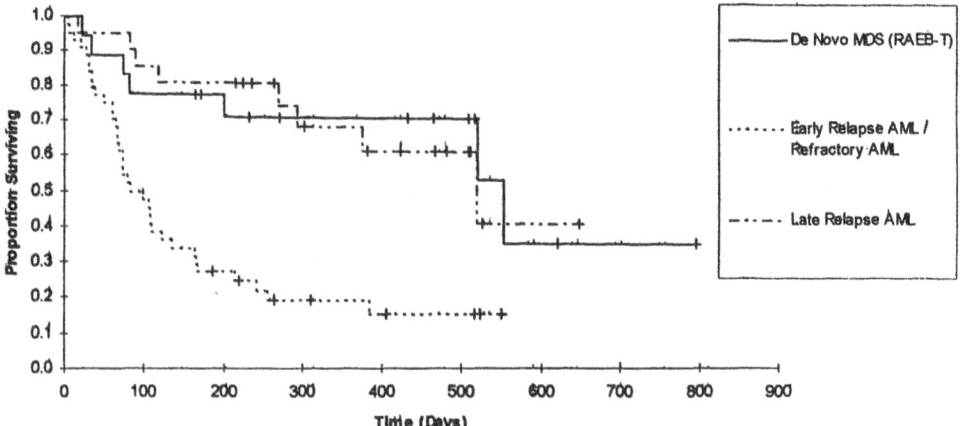

**Fig. 1**

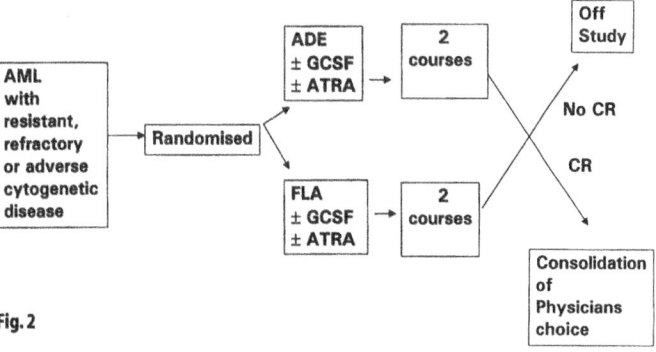

**Fig. 2**

Follow up on the study is short at present and a further assessment of the results will be necessary at a later date.

## Conclusion

We consider that our results confirm the promising results of earlier studies on the impact of treatment with FLAG combination chemotherapy in patients with poor prognosis myeloid malignancy (Table 4). We consider that the newly opened MRC AML HR study (see fig. 2), which is a randomised trial comparing ADE versus FLA chemotherapy in a similar group of patients to those in the present study, merits consideration by doctors treating this group of patients with difficult diseases.

# References

1. Gandhi V, Plunkett W (1988) Modulation of arabinosyl nucleoside metabolism by arabinosylnucleotides in human leukemia cells. Cancer Res 48: 329–334
2. Tafuri A, Andreeff M (1990) Kinetic Rationale for Cytokine-Induced Recruitment of Myeloblastic Leukaemia Followed by Cycle-Specific Chemotherapy In Vitro. Leukemia 4: No 12, 826–834
3. Gandhi V, Estey E, Keating MJ, Plunkett W (1993) Fludarabine Potentiates Metabolism of Cytarabine in Patients With Acute Myelogenous Leukemia During Therapy. Journal of Clinical Oncology 11: No 1, 116–124
4. Estey E, Thall P, Andreeff M, Beran M, Kantarjian H, O_Brien S, Escudier S, Robertson LE, Koller C, Kornblau S, Pierce S, Freireich EJ, Deisseroth A, Keating M (1994) Use of Granulocyte Colony-Stimulating Factor Before, During, and After Fludarabine Plus Cytarabine Induction Therapy of Newly Diagnosed Acute Myelogenous Leukemia or Myelodysplastic Syndromes: Comparison With Fludarabine Plus Cytarabine Without Granulocyte Colony-Stimulating Factor. Journal of Clinical Oncology 12: No 4, 671–678
5. Visani G, Tosi P, Zinzani PL, Manfroi S, Ottaviani E, Testoni N, Clavio M, Cenacchi A, Gamberi B, Carrera P, Gobbi M, and Tura S (1994) FLAG (Fludarabine + High-Dose Cytarabine + G-CSF): An Effective and Tolerable Protocol for the Treatment of `Poor Risk_ Acute Myeloid Leukemias. Leukemia 8: No 11, 1842–1846
6. Burnett AK, Goldstone AH, Stevens RMF, Hann IM, Rees JKH, Gray RG, Wheatley K (1998) Randomised comparison of addition of autologous bone-marrow transplantation to intensive chemotherapy for acute myeloid leukaemia in first remission: results of MRC AML 10 trial. Lancet 351: 700 –708
7. Huhmann IM, Watzke HH, Geissler K, Gisslinger J, Jäger U, Knöbl P, Pabinger I, Korninger L, Mannhalter C, Mitterbauer G, Schwarzinger I, Kalhs P, Haas OA, Lechner K (1996) FLAG (fludarabine, cytosine arabinoside, G-CSF) for refractory and relapsed acute myeloid leukemia. Ann Hematol 73: 265–271
8. Nokes TJC, Johnson S, Harvey D, Goldstone AH (1997) FLAG is a Useful Regimen for Poor Prognosis Adult Myeloid Leukaemias and Myelodysplastic Syndromes. Leukemia and Lymphoma 27: 93–101
9. Montillo M, Mirto S, Petti MC, Latagliata R, Magrin S, Pinto A, Zagonel V, Mele G, Tedeschi A, Ferrara F (1998) Fludarabine, Cytarabine and G-CSF (FLAG) for the Treatment of Poor Risk Acute Myeloid Leukemia. American Journal of Haematology 58: 105–109

# Modulation of AraC by Fludarabine: Results of Salvage Therapy by AMLCG

W. Kern[1], A. Matylis[2], T. Grüneisen[3], C. Huber[4], A. Grote-Metke[5], B. Wörmann[6], T. Büchner[7], J. Ohnesorge[1], W.D. Ludwig[2] and W. Hiddemann[1] for the German AML Cooperative Group

*Abstract.* Fludarabine was shown to increase the intracellular formation of AraCTP during treatment with AraC both in vitro and in vivo and had significant activity in patients with advanced acute myeloid leukemia (AML) when used in combination with AraC in phase II studies. However, the efficacy of fludarabin as chemo-modulatior of the AraC metabolism has not yet been assessed in phase III studies. Based on the S-HAI salvage regimen comprizing high-dose AraC q 12 hours on days 1, 2, 8, and 9 and idarubicin on days 3, 4, 10, and 11, the German AML Cooperative Group initiated a prospective randomized comparison between fludarabine q 12 hours on days 1, 2, 8, and 9 in addition to S-HAI as compared with S-HAI alone. Of 91 patients having entered the ongoing study 66 are fully evaluable at the present time (median age 54 years, range 20-75). Twenty-five patients had refractory disease or early relapses, 39 patients had relapses after a preceding CR of more than six months duration and one patient had a second relapse. Thirty patients achieved a remission (CR, 45%; PR, 3%) while the non-response rate was 32% and 20% suffered from early death. The application of fludarabine resulted in a longer duration of neutropenia (38 versus 32 days). Severe non-hematologic toxicity (WHO III°/IV°) consisted mainly of nausea/vomiting (26% versus 13%), diarrhea (23% versus 10%), mucositis (14% versus 19%), and bleeding (11% versus 0%) and infectious complications included pneumonia (57% versus 39%), FUO (60% versus 45%), and bacteremia (49% versus 16%). The sequential test has not yet decided for either superiority of fludarabine or equality of both study arms.

## Introduction

Cytosine arabinoside (AraC) is the most active single agent in the treatment of adults with acute myeloid leukemia (AML) and provides the basis for most currently used regimens [26]. A substantial improvement of the antileukemic efficacy of the drug has been achieved both in patients receiving first line combination regimens and in cases undergoing salvage therapy by applying higher than conventional doses of AraC [10,32,38]. In attempts to further increase the activity of AraC-containing regimens, fludarabine has been added as a chemo-modulator to augment the intracellular levels of AraC triphosphate (AraCTP) which is the main cytotoxic metabolite of AraC. Pharmacokinetic investigations revealed that, following intracellular phosphorylation of fludarabine, the resulting triphosphate acts as an inhibitor of ribonucleotide reductase, which catalyzes the de novo synthesis of deoxynucleotides. As a consequence, the intracellular levels of these compounds are depleted leading to a diminished inhibition of deoxycytidine kinase. Scince this enzyme catalyses the initial and rate-limiting step in the synthesis of AraCTP, i.e. the phosphorylation of AraC to its mono-

[1] University Hospital Großhadern, Department of Medicine III, Ludwig-Maximilians-University, München;
[2] Robert-Rössle-Klinik, Charité, Humboldt-University, Berlin;
[3] Krankenhaus Neukölln, Berlin;
[4] Department of Medicine III, Johannes-Gutenberg-University, Mainz;
[5] Evangelisches Krankenhaus, Hamm;
[6] Department of Hematology and Oncology, Georg-August-University, Göttingen;
[7] Department of Hematology and Oncology, Westfälische-Wilhelms-University, Münster; Germany.

phosphate, an overall increase in intracellular levels of AraCTP results, which fas been demonstrated in AML blasts both ex vivo and in vivo [22,23]. In several phase II studies applying the fludarabine/AraC regimen [20,46] or combinations of both drugs with G-CSF [21,29,40,41,49] and anthracyclins [17,42] a significant antileukemic efficacy was demonstrated in patients with high-risk AML. CR rates of up to 74% have been achieved with these combinations, although most studies included a small number of patients only. However, the use of fludarabine as a chemomodulator of the AraC metabolism has not yet been proven in a randomized phase III trial. Therefore, the current study addressed the question of improving the activity of a high-dose AraC based regimen by fludarabine on the basis of a prospective randomized comparison of applying fludarabine in addition to the sequential high-dose AraC and idarubicine (S-HAI) regimen versus S-HAI alone in patients with refractory and relapsed AML.

## Patients and Methods

### Patients

Consecutive patients at ages 18 or older with relapsed and refractory AML who were admitted at the participating centers between april 1996 and february 1999 were eligible for the study. The diagnosis of AML was based on the revised French-American-British (FAB) Group criteria [7]. Refractoriness against standard chemotherapy was defined according to previously established criteria [28]: These included
a) primary resistance against two cycles of induction therapy;
b) first early relapse with a remission duration of less than 6 months;
c) second and subsequent relapse.

Patients with first relapses after six months remission duration were not considered refractory to standard therapy and were included as relapsed AML.

All patients were recruited from the first line trials of the German AML Cooperative Group and had thus received a standardized first line treatment. In patients less than 60 years of age first line therapy consisted in double induction therapy with the sequential application of the nine-day-regimen of thioguanine, AraC, daunorubicin (TAD-9) followed by high-dose AraC and mitoxantrone (HAM). Older patients all received one course of TAD-9 and were treated by a HAM course only upon inadequate response to TAD-9. Patients of all ages who achieved a complete remission (CR) subsequently received TAD-9 for consolidation and monthly maintenance therapy for three years [14,15].

Patients with a preceding allogeneic bone marrow transplantation were excluded from the study. Further exclusion criteria comprized coronary heart disease; heart failure; cardiomyopathy; severe arterial hypertension; abnormal liver function tests (aspartate aminotransferase [AST], alanine aminotransferase [ALT], or alkaline phosphatase [AP] more than three times the upper normal limits; total bilirubin > 2.0 mg/dl); impaired renal function (serum creatinine > 2.0 mg/dl); severe infections; or pregnancy.

### Antileukemic Therapy

Patients meeting the entry criteria were enrolled into the current study and were treated by S-HAI [34] comprizing AraC every 12 hours by a 3-hour infusion on days 1, 2, 8, and 9 and idarubicine 10 mg/m²/day as a 30-min infusion on days 3, 4, 10, and 11, respectively (Fig. 1). Based on the results of a previous study comparing two dose levels of high-dose AraC [32], patients younger than 60 years with refractory disease, early relapse following a first CR of less than six months, or second and subsequent relapses received AraC at doses of 3.0 g/m² per application while all other patients were treated with 1.0 g/m² AraC per single dose. All patients were randomly assigned to receive fludarabine in addition to S-HAI or S-HAI alone. Patients randomized for fludarabine received the drug at 15 mg/m² as a 30-min infusion four hours prior to each AraC administration, i.e. twice daily on days 1, 2, 8, and 9. To avoid imbalances in the patients´ risk profile randomization was stratified for the following criteria:

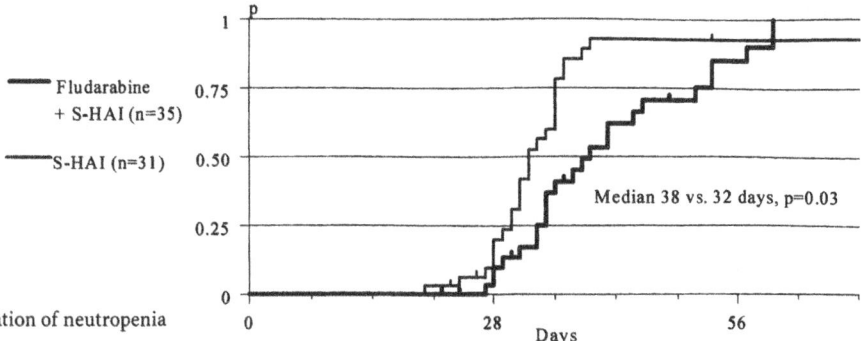

**Fig. 1.** Duration of neutropenia <500/μl

Fludarabine + S-HAI (n=35)

S-HAI (n=31)

Median 38 vs. 32 days, p=0.03

Days

a) primary resistance against two cycles of induction therapy,
b) first early relapse with a remission duration of less than 6 months,
c) first relapse with a remission duration of more than 6 months but less than 18 months,
d) first relapse with a remission duration of more than 18 months,
e) second and subsequent relapse.

Based on prior evaluations of supportive growth-factor administration [43], all patients received G-CSF 5 μg/m² subcutaneously starting on day 14, i.e. two days following the completion of chemotherapy. G-CSF was stopped in case of persistance of more than 5% leukemic blasts on a day 18 bone marrow examination or upon recovery of granulocytes to more than 1500/μl. To prevent high-dose AraC induced photophobia and conjunctivitis all patients received glucocorticoid eye drops every 6 hours starting before the first dose and continuing for 24 hours after the last dose of high-dose AraC. Antimicrobial prophylaxis consisted of co-trimoxazol 960 mg po three times daily, colistine sulphate two million units po four times daily, and amphotericin B suspension 40 mg po six times daily.

**Study Parameters**

Bone marrow examinations were carried out on day 18, i.e. one week after the end of chemotherapy, and upon full recovery of peripheral blood counts. Response to therapy was assessed according to CALGB criteria [54].

CR was defined as a normal cellular bone marrow with normal erythroid and myeloid elements and less than 5% myeloblasts, and with peripheral blood counts of more than 100,000/μl platelets and more than 1,500/μl granulocytes for at least four weeks. Patients with regenerated peripheral blood values but more than 5% and less than 25% myeloblasts were considered to be in partial remission (PR), as were patients fulfilling the bone marrow criteria of CR but without full recovery of peripheral blood platelet and/or white blood cell counts. Patients with persisting leukemic blasts in the bone marrow or blood or with leukemic regrowth within four weeks after initial response were considered as non-responders (NR). Patients dying within six week after the end of antileukemic therapy without evidence of leukemic regrowth were classified as early deaths (ED).

The duration of critical neutropenia was evaluated by the time for granulocyte recovery to more than 500/μl from the onset of S-HAI treatment. The time to CR was measured from the onset of treatment to the date of documented CR and disease free survival from the date of documented CR to relapse or death during remission. Survival and time to treatment failure were measured by the time from the beginning of treatment to death, documentation of persisting leukemia, or relapse, respectively.

Toxicity was evaluated according to the World Health Organization (WHO) grading system [53]. Infectious complications were classified according to the Consensus Report of the Immunocompromised Host Society as reported previously [33].

## Statistics

The primary end point of the present study was the impact of the addition of fludarabine to S-HAI on the time to treatment failure as compared to a randomly assigned control group receiving S-HAI alone. The comparison of both study arms was designed to test whether S-HAI + fludarabine could decrease the one-year treatment failure rate of 75% expected for S-HAI by 15%. On this basis a one-sided sequential test with a working significance level of 0.05 was applied [51]. This procedure allowed to detect the assumed superiority of S-HAI + fludarabine over S-HAI with a probability of 90%. The test statistics were calculated after entry of every evaluable patient.

Secondary end points were the rates of CR, NR, and ED, the disease free and overall survival as well as the incidence of hematologic and non-hematologic side effects. Numerical values were compared by the Fisher´s-exact-test. Response to antileukemic therapy was compared by an ordinal $\chi^2$-test. Remission duration and survival was calculated according to Kaplan Meier estimates. Comparisons were carried out using the log-rank test.

## Study Conduct

Prior to therapy all patients gave their informed consent for participation in the current evaluation after having been advised about the purpose and investigational nature of the study as well as of potential risks. The study design adhered to the declaration of Helsinki and was approved by the ethics committees of the participating institutions prior to its initiation.

## Results

### Patient Characteristics

Ninety-one patients were entered into the ongoing study from 24 centers in Germany, 66 of whom were fully evaluable at the time of analyses. Thirty-five patients were randomized to fludarabine in addition to S-HAI while 31 patients were randomized to S-HAI alone.

The patients´ ages ranged from 20 to 75 years (median 54 years) and did not differ between the respective groups (table 1). All patients had received prior chemotherapy for their disease as indicated above. Overall, 10 (15%) patients had primary refractory disease and 15 (23%) had early relapses after a first CR of less than six months duration. In 24 (36%) and 15 (23%) cases the relapses occured after a CR of more than six but less than 18 months and of more than 18 months duration, respectively; 2 (3%) patients suffered from second or subsequent relapses (Table 1). The comparison of the profile of disease status revealed a similarity for the two study groups. AML subtypes were predominantly M1, M2, M4, and M5. All 66 patients received one course of S-HAI therapy only.

**Table 1.** Patient characteristics

|  | Fludarabine (n=35) | Control (n=31) |
|---|---|---|
| Sex (male/female) | 19/16 | 17/14 |
| Age |  |  |
|   Median/Range (years) | 50/20-75 | 56/24-73 |
|   <60 years | 22 | 19 |
|   >60 years | 13 | 12 |
| FAB-Subtype |  |  |
|   M0 | 1 | 5 |
|   M1 | 13 | 1 |
|   M2 | 11 | 12 |
|   M3 | 1 | - |
|   M4 | 4 | 7 |
|   M5 | 3 | 5 |
|   M6 | - | 1 |
|   n.d. | 2 | - |
| Disease Status |  |  |
|   Refractory AML | 5 | 5 |
|   Duration of CR1 <6 months | 9 | 6 |
|   Duration of CR1 ≥6 <18 months | 13 | 11 |
|   Duration of CR1 ≥18 months | 6 | 9 |
|   ≥2nd relapse | 2 | - |
| Karyotype at diagnosis |  |  |
|   Favorable | 4 | 1 |
|   Normal / intermediate | 19 | 18 |
|   Unfavorable | 3 | 3 |
|   n.d. | 9 | 9 |
| Karyotype at relapse |  |  |
|   Favorable | 4 | - |
|   Normal / intermediate | 10 | 18 |
|   Unfavorable | 5 | 5 |
|   n.d. | 16 | 8 |

## Antileukemic Activity

A bone marrow examination on day 18 was evaluable in 48 cases, in 46 (96%) of whom an adequate reduction of leukemic blasts to less than 5% was achieved. Overall, 30 (45%) and 2 (3%) of the 186 evaluable patients achieved a CR and a PR, respectively, while 21 (32%) cases were NR. Thirteen (20%) patients suffered from ED (Table 2). The sequential analyses of the log-rank test has not yet decided to stop patient recruitment, i.e. it has not yet decided either for superiority of the fluarabine arm or for equal efficacy of both arms. The recruitment of patients is still ongoing.

**Table 2.** Antileukemic efficacy of S-HAI ± Fludarabine

|  | n (%; 95% confidence interval) |
|---|---|
| Complete remission | 30 (45%; 33%-59%) |
| Partial remission | 2 (3%; 0%-11%) |
| Non-response | 21 (32%; 21%-44%) |
| Early death | 13 (20%; 11%-31%) |

## Hematologic Side Effects

The additional administration of fludarabine resulted in a longer recovery time of granulocytes to more than 500/µl, which amounted to a median of 38 vs. 32 days (p=0.03; Table 3). In patients achieving a CR the time till CR was longer in patients receiving fludarabine (median, 62 vs. 49 days; p=0.07).

## Non-hematologic Side Effects

The non-hematologic side effects that were encountered during S-HAI therapy are summarized in Table 3. Overall, the most frequent side effects were nausea/vomiting, diarrhea, mucositis, elevation of bilirubin levels, and bleeding with no significant differences in toxicity according to WHO grade III/IV. Nausea/vomiting (p<0.01), diarrhea (p<0.01), and CNS toxicity (p<0.05) according to WHO grade I/II/III/IV occured more frequently during fludarabine plus S-HAI. There were no major differences in the freuquency and the severity of the remaining toxicities.

**Table 3.** Non-hematologic toxicity

| Toxicity (WHO grade) | Fludarabine n=35 I°/II° | Fludarabine n=35 III°/IV° | Control n=31 I°/II° | Control n=31 III°/IV° |
|---|---|---|---|---|
| Nausea/Vomiting* | 40 % | 26 % | 10 % | 13 % |
| Diarrhea* | 40 % | 23 % | 19 % | 10 % |
| Mucositis | 29 % | 14 % | 16 % | 19 % |
| Bilirubin | 34 % | 11 % | 35 % | 6 % |
| Bleeding | 23 % | 11 % | 26 % | 0 % |
| Cardiac (function) | 0 % | 6 % | 0 % | 0 % |
| Creatinine | 31 % | 0 % | 29 % | 3 % |
| AST/ALT | 14 % | 3 % | 32 % | 0 % |
| AP | 17 % | 0 % | 16 % | 3 % |
| Cardiac (rhythm) | 14 % | 0 % | 6 % | 3 % |
| CNS** | 11 % | 3 % | 0 % | 0 % |
| Skin | 9 % | 0 % | 6 % | 0 % |
| Allergy | 3 % | 0 % | 0 % | 0 % |
| Pericarditis | 3 % | 0 % | 0 % | 0 % |

*p<0.01 **p<0.05

## Infectious Complications

The infectious complications encountered were predominantly fever of unknown origin (FUO, 53%), pneumonia (48%), and bacteremia (33%). Bacteremias were more frequently detected in patients receiving fludarabine plus S-HAI (49% vs. 16%, p<0.01). There were no signifficant differences in the frequency of other documented infections or FUO (Table 4). However, there were slightly more episodes of pneumonia in patients receiving fludarabine plus S-HAI. Only minor differences occured in the frequency of FUO, sepsis syndrome, septic shock, perianal infections, catheter-related infections, and other infections.

**Table 4.** Infectious episodes

|  | Fludarabine n=35 | Control n=31 |
|---|---|---|
| FUO | 60 % | 45 % |
| Pneumonia | 57 % | 39 % |
| Bacteremia* | 49 % | 16 % |
| Septic syndrome | 14 % | 6 % |
| Septic shock | 17 % | 3 % |
| Catheter-related infections | 11 % | 13 % |
| Abdominal infections | 20 % | 10 % |
| Perianale infections | 6 % | 6 % |
| Other infections** | 11 % | 32 % |

*p<0.01 **p<0.05

## Discussion

Improvements of the antileukemic efficacy of combination chemotherapies have been achieved in recent years by adding new effective drugs to AraC-based regimens [4,6,8,9, 11,37,44,45,50,52] and by applying AraC at intermediate and high doses instead of conventional doses [10,12,16,27,32,38,39,47]. However, especially in patients with refractory disease and relapsed AML the results of second-line therapies remain unsatisfactory and warrant the evaluation of new drugs and innovative therapeutic concepts [19]. Fludarabine was shown to significantly increase the intracellular levels of AraCTP in leukemic blasts treated with AraC and thereby serves a new treatment modality to be used as a chemo-modulator in patients with AML [22,23]. The current study addresses for the first time the question of an increase in the antileukemic efficacy of a high-dose AraC based regimen by the addition of fludarabine as a chemo-modulator in way of a prospective randomized comparison of fludarabine plus S-HAI versus S-HAI alone in patients with refractory and relapsed AML. Overall, 45% and 3% of the patients achieved a CR and a PR, respectively, while 32% were NR and 20% suffered from ED. These results are within the range of the previously reported S-HAM regimen [31-33,35] and compare favorably with other intermediate-dose and high-dose AraC based salvage regimens [1,3,5,24,40,48,49]. Since the recruitment of patients into the ongoing study has not yet been stopped, this report focusses on the comparison of the toxicities observed during both treatment arms.

The non-hematologic side effects that were encountered sigificantly more frequent following fludarabin plus S-HAI were nausea/ vomiting, diarrhea, and CNS toxicity. At least in part this was expected, since higher doses of AraC are known to more profoundly damage mucosal membranes and lead to an increased frequency and severity of both stomatitis and diarrhea [13,32]. Furthermore, results of previous trilas which clearly demonstrated a dependance of CNS toxicity on higher doses of AraC [25,30,32] are in accordance to the current data.

As reported in preceding studies on higher doses of AraC [18,36], the more intensive regimen of the current trial, i.e. the S-HAI plus fludarabine combination, resulted in more infectious episodes, mainly bacteremia (49% vs. 16%) and pneumonia (57% vs. 39%). Obviously, this is related to the higher degree of mucosal damage [13,32] and may be due to a longer period of severe neutropenia (38 vs. 32 days, p=0.03). However, these results have to be confirmed in a larger number of patients, since an incidence of 16% for bacteremias might be an underestimate of the true frequency, which was higher in prior studies using high-dose AraC-based salvage regimens [27,31-33]. In contrast to previous reports on patients receiving fludarabine mainly for chronic lymphocytic leukemia [2], however, infections due to impaired lymphocyte function, i.e. viral infections, listeriosis, and pneumocystosis, were not observed more frequently in patients receiving fludarabine plus S-HAI.

In conclusion, these preliminary data on a prospective randomized evaluation of the addition of fludarabine as chemo-modulator to a high-dose AraC-based salvage regimen in patients with refractory and relapsed AML indicate that the resulting infectious complications might be more frequent in the fludarabine arm, probably due to an increased hematologic toxicity and maybe also due to a higher rate of mucosal damage. There is no evidence of an increase in infectious epizodes due to a specific decrease of the number and the function of T-lymphocytes. In improvement of the antileukemic efficacy of the S-HAI regimen by fludarabine, however, remains to be established yet and the analysis of further patients is needed to adequately address this question.

## References

1. Amadori S, Meloni G, Petti MC, Papa G, Miniero R, Mandelli F. (1989) Phase II trial of intermediate dose ARA-C (IDAC) with sequential mitoxantrone (MITOX) in acute myelogenous leukemia. Leukemia 3: 112-114.
2. Anaissie EJ, Kontoyiannis DP, O'Brien S, Kantarjian H, Robertson L, Lerner S, Keating MJ. (1998) Infections in patients with chronic lymphocytic leukemia treated with fludarabine. Ann Intern Med 129: 559-566.
3. Archimbaud E, Fenaux P, Reiffers J, Cordonnier C, Leblond V, Travade P, Troussard X, Tilly H, Auzan-

neau G, Marie JP, et al. (1993) Granulocyte-macrophage colony-stimulating factor in association to timed-sequential chemotherapy with mitoxantrone, etoposide, and cytarabine for refractory acute myelogenous leukemia. Leukemia 7: 372-377.

4. Archimbaud E, Leblond V, Michallet M, Cordonnier C, Fenaux P, Travade P, Dreyfus F, Jaubert J, Devaux Y, Fiere D. (1991) Intensive sequential chemotherapy with mitoxantrone and continuous infusion etoposide and cytarabine for previously treated acute myelogenous leukemia. Blood 77: 1894-1900.

5. Archimbaud E, Thomas X, Leblond V, Michallet M, Fenaux P, Cordonnier C, Dreyfus F, Troussard X, Jaubert J, Travade P, et al. (1995) Timed sequential chemotherapy for previously treated patients with acute myeloid leukemia: long-term follow-up of the etoposide, mitoxantrone, and cytarabine-86 trial [see comments]. J Clin Oncol 13: 11-18.

6. Arlin Z, Case DC, Jr., Moore J, Wiernik P, Feldman E, Saletan S, Desai P, Sia L, Cartwright K. (1990) Randomized multicenter trial of cytosine arabinoside with mitoxantrone or daunorubicin in previously untreated adult patients with acute non-lymphocytic leukemia (ANLL). Lederle Cooperative Group. Leukemia 4: 177-183.

7. Bennett JM, Catovsky D, Daniel MT, Flandrin G, Galton DA, Gralnick HR, Sultan C. (1985) Proposed revised criteria for the classification of acute myeloid leukemia. A report of the French-American-British Cooperative Group. Ann Intern Med 103: 620-625.

8. Berman E, Wiernik P, Vogler R, Velez Garcia E, Bartolucci A, Whaley FS. (1997) Long-term follow-up of three randomized trials comparing idarubicin and daunorubicin as induction therapies for patients with untreated acute myeloid leukemia. Cancer 80: 2181-2185.

9. Bishop JF, Lowenthal RM, Joshua D, Matthews JP, Todd D, Cobcroft R, Whiteside MG, Kronenberg H, Ma D, Dodds A, et al. (1990) Etoposide in acute nonlymphocytic leukemia. Australian Leukemia Study Group. Blood 75: 27-32.

10. Bishop JF, Matthews JP, Young GA, Szer J, Gillett A, Joshua D, Bradstock K, Enno A, Wolf MM, Fox R, et al. (1996) A randomized study of high-dose cytarabine in induction in acute myeloid leukemia. Blood 87: 1710-1717.

11. Bjorkholm M, Liliemark J, Gahrton G, Grimfors G, Gruber A, Hast R, Juliusson G, Jarnmark M, Killander A, Kimby E, et al. (1995) Mitoxantrone, etoposide and ara-C vs doxorubicin-DNA, ara-C, thioguanine, vincristine and prednisolone in the treatment of patients with acute myelocytic leukaemia. A randomized comparison. Eur J Haematol 55: 19-23.

12. Bloomfield CD, Lawrence D, Byrd JC, Carroll A, Pettenati MJ, Tantravahi R, Patil SR, Davey FR, Berg DT, Schiffer CA, Arthur DC, Mayer RJ. (1998) Frequency of prolonged remission duration after high-dose cytarabine intensification in acute myeloid leukemia varies by cytogenetic subtype. Cancer Res 58: 4173-4179.

13. Bow EJ, Loewen R, Cheang MS, Schacter B. (1995) Invasive fungal disease in adults undergoing remission-induction therapy for acute myeloid leukemia: the pathogenetic role of the antileukemic regimen. Clin Infect Dis 21: 361-369.

14. Buchner T, Hiddemann W, Wormann B, Loffler H, Maschmeyer G, Hossfeld D, Ludwig WD, Nowrousian M, Aul C, Schaefer UW, Sauerland C, Heinecke A. (1992) Longterm effects of prolonged maintenance and of very early intensification chemotherapy in AML: data from AMLCG. Leukemia 6 Suppl 2: 68-71.

15. Buchner T, Urbanitz D, Hiddemann W, Ruhl H, Ludwig WD, Fischer J, Aul HC, Vaupel HA, Kuse R, Zeile G, Nowrousian MR, Konig HJ, Walter M, Wendt FC, Sodomann H, Hossfeld DK, von Paleske A, Loffler H, Gassmann W, Hellriegel KP, Fulle HH, Lunscken C, Emmerich B, Pralle H, Pees HW, Pfreundschuh M, Bartels H, Koeppen KM, Schwerdtfeger R, Donhuijsen-Ant R, Mainzer K, Bonfert B, Koppler H, Zurborn KH, Ranft K, Thiel E, Heinecke A. (1985) Intensified induction and consolidation with or without maintenance chemotherapy for acute myeloid leukemia (AML): two multicenter studies of the German AML Cooperative Group. J Clin Oncol 3: 1583-1589.

16. Cassileth PA, Andersen JW, Bennett JM, Harrington DP, Hines JD, Lazarus HM, Mazza JJ, McGlave PP, O'Connell MJ, Paietta E, et al. (1992) Escalating the intensity of post-remission therapy improves the outcome in acute myeloid leukemia: the ECOG experience. The Eastern Cooperative Oncology Group. Leukemia 6 Suppl 2: 116-119.

17. Clavio M, Carrara P, Miglino M, Pierri I, Canepa L, Balleari E, Gatti AM, Cerri R, Celesti L, Vallebella E, Sessarego M, Patrone F, Ghio R, Damasio E, Gobbi M. (1996) High efficacy of fludarabine-containing therapy (FLAG-FLANG) in poor risk acute myeloid leukemia. Haematologica 81: 513-520.

18. Cohen J, Donnelly J, Worsley A, Catovsky D, Goldman J, Galton D. (1983) Septicaemia caused by viridans streptococci in neutropenic patients with leukaemia. Lancet 2: 1452-4

19. Estey E. (1996) Treatment of refractory AML. Leukemia 10: 932-936.

20. Estey E, Plunkett W, Gandhi V, Rios MB, Kantarjian H, Keating MJ. (1993) Fludarabine and arabinosylcytosine therapy of refractory and relapsed acute myelogenous leukemia. Leuk Lymphoma 9: 343-350.

21. Estey E, Thall P, Andreeff M, Beran M, Kantarjian H, O'Brien S, Escudier S, Robertson LE, Koller C, Kornblau S, et al. (1994) Use of granulocyte colony-stimulating factor before, during, and after fludarabine plus cytarabine induction therapy of newly diagnosed acute myelogenous leukemia or myelodysplastic syndromes: comparison with fludarabine plus cytarabine without granulocyte colony-stimulating factor. J Clin Oncol 12: 671-678.

22. Gandhi V, Estey E, Keating MJ, Plunkett W. (1993) Fludarabine potentiates metabolism of cytarabine in patients with acute myelogenous leukemia during therapy. J Clin Oncol 11: 116-124.

23. Gandhi V, Estey E, Keating MJ, Plunkett W. (1993) Biochemical modulation of arabinosylcytosine for therapy of leukemias. Leuk Lymphoma 10 Suppl: 109-114.

24. Harousseau J, Reiffers J, Hurteloup P, et al. (1989) Treatment of relapsed acute myeloid leukemia

with idarubicin and intermediate-dose cytarabine. Journal of Clinical Oncology 7: 45-9

25. Herzig R, Hines J, Herzig G, Wolff S, Cassileth P, Lazarus H, Adelstein D, Brown R, Coccia P, Strandjord S, Mazza J, Fay J, Phillips G. (1987) Cerebellar toxicity with high-dose cytosine arabinoside. Journal of Clinical Oncology 5: 927-32

26. Hiddemann W. (1991) Cytosine arabinoside in the treatment of acute myeloid leukemia: the role and place of high-dose regimens. Ann Hematol 62: 119-128.

27. Hiddemann W, Kreutzmann H, Straif K, Ludwig WD, Mertelsmann R, Donhuijsen Ant R, Lengfelder E, Arlin Z, Buchner T. (1987) High-dose cytosine arabinoside and mitoxantrone: a highly effective regimen in refractory acute myeloid leukemia. Blood 69: 744-749.

28. Hiddemann W, Martin WR, Sauerland CM, Heinecke A, Buchner T. (1990) Definition of refractoriness against conventional chemotherapy in acute myeloid leukemia: a proposal based on the results of retreatment by thioguanine, cytosine arabinoside, and daunorubicin (TAD 9) in 150 patients with relapse after standardized first line therapy. Leukemia 4: 184-188.

29. Huhmann IM, Watzke HH, Geissler K, Gisslinger H, Jager U, Knobl P, Pabinger I, Korninger L, Mannhalter C, Mitterbauer G, Schwarzinger I, Kalhs P, Haas OA, Lechner K. (1996) FLAG (fludarabine, cytosine arabinoside, G-CSF) for refractory and relapsed acute myeloid leukemia. Ann Hematol 73: 265-271.

30. Jolson H, Bosco L, Bufton M, Gerstman B, Rinsler S, Williams E, Flynn B, Simmons W, Stadel B, Faich G, Peck C. (1992) Clustering of adverse drug effects: Analysis of risk factors for cerebellar toxicity with high-dose cytarabine. Journal of the National Cancer Institute 84: 500-5

31. Kern W, Aul C, Maschmeyer G, Kuse R, Kerkhoff A, Grote-Metke A, Eimermacher H, Kubica U, Wormann B, Buchner T, Hiddemann W, for the German AML Cooperative Group. (1998) Granulocyte colony-stimulating factor shortens critical neutropenia and prolongs disease free survival after sequential high-dose cytosine arabinoside and mitoxantrone (S-HAM) salvage therapy for refractory and relapsed acute myeloid leukemia. Ann Hematol 77: 115-122.

32. Kern W, Aul C, Maschmeyer G, Schönrock-Nabulsi R, Ludwig WD, Bartholomaus A, Bettelheim P, Wormann B, Buchner T, Hiddemann W, for the German AML Cooperative Group. (1998) Superiority of high-dose over intermediate-dose cytosine arabinoside in the treatment of patients with high-risk acute myeloid leukemia: results of a age-adjusted prospective randomized comparison. Leukemia 12: 1049-1055.

33. Kern W, Behre G, Rudolf T, Kerkhoff A, Grote-Metke A, Eimermacher H, Kubica U, Wormann B, Buchner T, Hiddemann W, for the German AML Cooperative Group. (1998) Failure of fluconazole prophylaxis to reduce mortality and the requirement of systemic amphotericin B therapy during treatment for refractory acute myeloid leukemia: results of a prospective randomized phase III study. Cancer 83: 291-301.

34. Kern W, Matylis A, Gruneisen T, Huber C, Grote-Metke A, Wormann B, Buchner T, Ohnesorge J, Ludwig WD, Hiddemann W, for the German AML Cooperative Group. (1999) Modulation of arac by fludarabine: results of salvage therapy by AMLCG. Ann Hematol 78: S5

35. Kern W, Schleyer E, Unterhalt M, Wormann B, Buchner T, Hiddemann W. (1997) High antileukemic activity of sequential high dose cytosine arabinoside and mitoxantrone in patients with refractory acute leukemias. Results of a clinical phase II study. Cancer 79: 59-68.

36. Lazarus HM, Vogler WR, Burns CP, Winton EF. (1989) High-dose cytosine arabinoside and daunorubicin as primary therapy in elderly patients with acute myelogenous leukemia. A phase I-II study of the Southeastern Cancer Study Group. Cancer 63: 1055-1059.

37. Lowenberg B, Suciu S, Archimbaud E, Haak H, Stryckmans P, de Cataldo R, Dekker AW, Berneman ZN, Thyss A, van der Lelie J, Sonneveld P, Visani G, Fillet G, Hayat M, Hagemeijer A, Solbu G, Zittoun R. (1998) Mitoxantrone versus daunorubicin in induction-consolidation chemotherapy—the value of low-dose cytarabine for maintenance of remission, and an assessment of prognostic factors in acute myeloid leukemia in the elderly: final report. European Organization for the Research and Treatment of Cancer and the Dutch-Belgian Hemato-Oncology Cooperative Hovon Group. J Clin Oncol 16: 872-881.

38. Mayer RJ, Davis RB, Schiffer CA, Berg DT, Powell BL, Schulman P, Omura GA, Moore JO, McIntyre OR, Frei E. (1994) Intensive postremission chemotherapy in adults with acute myeloid leukemia. Cancer and Leukemia Group B. N Engl J Med 331: 896-903.

39. Mitus AJ, Miller KB, Schenkein DP, Ryan HF, Parsons SK, Wheeler C, Antin JH. (1995) Improved survival for patients with acute myelogenous leukemia [see comments]. J Clin Oncol 13: 560-569.

40. Montillo M, Mirto S, Petti MC, Latagliata R, Magrin S, Pinto A, Zagonel V, Mele G, Tedeschi A, Ferrara F. (1998) Fludarabine, cytarabine, and G-CSF (FLAG) for the treatment of poor risk acute myeloid leukemia. Am J Hematol 58: 105-109.

41. Nokes TJ, Johnson S, Harvey D, Goldstone AH. (1997) FLAG is a useful regimen for poor prognosis adult myeloid leukaemias and myelodysplastic syndromes. Leuk Lymphoma 27: 93-101.

42. Parker JE, Pagliuca A, Mijovic A, Cullis JO, Czepulkowski B, Rassam SM, Samaratunga IR, Grace R, Gover PA, Mufti GJ. (1997) Fludarabine, cytarabine, G-CSF and idarubicin (FLAG-IDA) for the treatment of poor-risk myelodysplastic syndromes and acute myeloid leukaemia. Br J Haematol 99: 939-944.

43. Patt YZ, Peters RE, Chuang VP, Wallace S, Mavligit G. (1983) Effective retreatment of patients with colorectal cancer and liver metastases. Am J Med 75: 237-240.

44. Pavlovsky S, Gonzalez Llaven J, Garcia Martinez MA, Sobrevilla P, Eppinger Helft M, Marin A, Lopez Hernandez M, Fernandez I, Rubio ME, Ibarra S, et al. (1994) A randomized study of mitoxantrone plus cytarabine versus daunomycin plus cytarabine in the treatment of previously untrea-

ted adult patients with acute nonlymphocytic leukemia. Ann Hematol 69: 11-15.

45. Reiffers J, Huguet F, Stoppa AM, Molina L, Marit G, Attal M, Gastaut JA, Michallet M, Lepeu G, Broustet A, Pris J, Maraninchi D, Hollard D, Faberes C, Mercier M, Hurteloup P, Danel P, Tellier Z, Berthaud P. (1996) A prospective randomized trial of idarubicin vs daunorubicin in combination chemotherapy for acute myelogenous leukemia of the age group 55 to 75. Leukemia 10: 389-395.

46. Russo D, Candoni A, Grattoni R, Bertone A, Zaja F. (1998) Fludarabine and cytosine-arabinoside for poor-risk acute myeloid leukemia [letter]. Haematologica 83: 281-282.

47. Schiller G, Gajewski J, Territo M, Nimer S, Lee M, Belin T, Champlin R. (1992) Long-term outcome of high-dose cytarabine-based consolidation chemotherapy for adults with acute myelogenous leukemia. Blood 80: 2977-2982.

48. Spadea A, Petti MC, Fazi P, Vegna ML, Arcese W, Avvisati G, Aloe Spiriti MA, Latagliata R, Meloni G, Testi AM, et al. (1993) Mitoxantrone, etoposide and intermediate-dose Ara-C (MEC): an effective regimen for poor risk acute myeloid leukemia. Leukemia 7: 549-552.

49. Visani G, Tosi P, Zinzani PL, Manfroi S, Ottaviani E, Testoni N, Clavio M, Cenacchi A, Gamberi B, Carrara P, et al. (1994) FLAG (fludarabine + high-dose cytarabine + G-CSF): an effective and tolerable protocol for the treatment of 'poor risk' acute myeloid leukemias. Leukemia 8: 1842-1846.

50. Vogler WR, Velez Garcia E, Weiner RS, Flaum MA, Bartolucci AA, Omura GA, Gerber MC, Banks PL. (1992) A phase III trial comparing idarubicin and daunorubicin in combination with cytarabine in acute myelogenous leukemia: a Southeastern Cancer Study Group Study. J Clin Oncol 10: 1103-1111.

51. Whitehead J. AnonymousNew York: Ellis Horwood, (1992) The design and analysis of sequential clinical trials (second edition).

52. Wiernik PH, Banks PL, Case DC, Jr., Arlin ZA, Periman PO, Todd MB, Ritch PS, Enck RE, Weitberg AB. (1992) Cytarabine plus idarubicin or daunorubicin as induction and consolidation therapy for previously untreated adult patients with acute myeloid leukemia. Blood 79: 313-319.

53. World Health Oraganization. AnonymousA handbook for reporting results of cancer treatment. Geneva: WHO publications, (1979)

54. Yates J, Glidewell O, Wiernik P, Cooper MR, Steinberg D, Dosik H, Levy R, Hoagland C, Henry P, Gottlieb A, Cornell C, Berenberg J, Hutchison JL, Raich P, Nissen N, Ellison RR, Frelick R, James GW, Falkson G, Silver RT, Haurani F, Green M, Henderson E, Leone L, Holland JF. (1982) Cytosine arabinoside with daunorubicin or adriamycin for therapy of acute myelocytic leukemia: a CALGB study. Blood 60: 454-462.

# Colony Stimulating Factors in Myelodysplastic Syndromes

G. VERHOEF

*Abstract.* The potential for recombinant growth factors to augment hematopoiesis has been extensively investigated with a wide range of clinical benefit. Among more than 18 trials using varied routes and schedules of erythropoietin, a rise in hemoglobin or reduction in transfusion requirement was reported in 16 % of patients. Most responding patients had an erythropoietin level less than 200 U/l, were not transfusion dependent, and had FAB types other than RARS. Recombinant myeloid growth factors (G-CSF, GM-CSF) restore granulocyte production in 75-90 % of neutropenic patients without a consistent change in red cell transfusion requirements or platelet production. Only one randomized trial, using GM-CSF for 90 days, reported on a significantly reduction in infections without adversely affecting disease progression. Because of the excessive cost of these cytokines and the necessity for continuous administration, there use has been relegated to the management of neutropenic patients with intercurrent infection. Cytokines such as IL-3 have shown limited benefit in MDS. Most encouraging results have been reported with combined administration of G-CSF and erythropoietin. 40-50 % of patients experienced a 50 % reduction in red blood cell transfusion needs. Erythropoietic responses occurred primarily in patients with an inappropriately low erythropoietin level, higher basal reticulocyte count, low leukemic burden and a normal karyotype. Combination of differentiating agents (ATRA, tocopherol) and growth factors gives similar results. Other cytokines, such as thrombopoietin to augment platelet levels, are under investigation. We recently performed a randomized study of G-CSF applied during and after AML-type chemotherapy in 62 patients with bad risk MDS with a CR rate of 73 % in the G-CSF arm and 52 % in the control group. The median overall survival was 16 months for the G-CSF group and 9 months for the control arm. However, these differences were not statistically different, possible because of the low numbers of patients. G-CSF certainly plays an important role in the mobilization of peripheral stem cells in MDS.

## Introduction

The myelodysplastic syndromes (MDS) comprise a heterogeneous group of clonal bone marrow failure syndromes, characterized by different levels of uncoupling of proliferative and differentiative responses of haematopoietic stem cells, leading to progressive cytopenias, qualitative abnormalities in erythroid, granulocytic and megakaryocytic series, and increased transformation into acute leukemia.

The overall incidence rates are estimated to be around 3 to 5 /100.000/year, but in the age group over 70 years the incidence may rise as high as 15/100.000/year [1]. Whether the incidence of MDS is rising - possibly in relation to environmental factors - is a matter of much debate. Undoubtedly the diagnostic possibilities and the investigative efforts have increased, but a true, steady increase can probably not be denied [2].

Department of Haematology, University Hospital Leuven, Herestraat 49, B-3000, Leuven, Belgium.

## Prognosis

The biologic and clinical course of MDS can roughly be divided in 3 patterns, corresponding to three major risk groups i.e. low, intermediate and high risk.

Some MDS-patients, mostly elderly, have a rather stable, indolent course over many years. Additional chromosomal abnormalities rarely occur and most of these patients will die of incidental causes. Other patients will initially show a stable disease, but will then undergo an abrupt transition from MDS to acute leukaemia, which is frequently associated with additional cytogenetic abnormalities or new oncogene activations/mutations. The third category of patients display a gradual, relentless increase in bone marrow blasts, leading to early death from acute leukaemia for most, from pancytopenic complications for some.

Since its introduction in 1982 the French-American-British-classification (FAB) of MDS-subtypes [3] based on the percentage of blood and bone marrow blasts, the percentage of ringed sideroblasts, monocytes and presence or absence of Auer-rods, has been extensively applied to subtype MDS. Although it has been proven to be a valid tool in clinical practice, the classification has several shortcomings concerning its use in evaluating clinical outcome for MDS patients. Firstly, the FAB proposal completely relies on the bone marrow and peripheral blood blast counts while many studies have suggested the prognostic importance of other morphological, clinical and biological variables (degree, number and type of cytopenias, bone marrow biopsy findings, LDH value, bone marrow culture studies and cytogenetics). Secondly, for the RAEB and the CMML subtypes a wide range of bone marrow blasts is used, respectively 5 to 20 % and 1 to 20 %. Thirdly, there are significant differences in clinical outcome among patients belonging to the same FAB-subtype [4]. These problems have led to the development of numerous additional classification systems but their clinical usage is still debated.

To improve the prognostic utility of these systems, an international workshop combined data of MDS patients of seven previously reported studies and analyzed these data centrally. Significant variables for survival and AML evolution were bone marrow blast count, number of cytopenia and cytogenetic abnormalities. In addition, a more refined cytogenetic classification was developed with prognostic significance. Age and gender were also prognostic parameters for survival but not for AML evolution. Combining these variables in a multivariate analysis resulted in the design of the International Prognostic Scoring System (IPSS) [5].

Although the IPSS seems to be an effective method for predicting survival or AML evolution in MDS patients, further studies are necessary to proof its validity in the design and the analysis of therapeutic trials. In view of this, the IPSS has certain limitations: the choice of therapy can not exclusively be based on prognosis but will also depend on the age and the performance status of the patient, since curative treatment modalities for MDS are aggressive. Secondly, it is not clear whether the IPSS predicts for the response to treatment, although in previous studies the percentage of bone marrow blasts and the karyotype were two important factors« affecting relapse rate and disease-free survival after different therapy strategies in MDS patients. Third limitation of the IPSS is the inclusion of karyotype as a prognostic factor. Cytogenetic results are sometimes not available at the time of diagnosis due to problems inherent to the technique.

## Treatment

Therapeutic strategies in MDS have historically been inspired by either »missionary« approaches i.e. converting malignant cells into normal behavior, or by »crusader« tactics i.e. destroying non compliant elements at the expense of innocent bystanders. Transplantation of haematopoietic stem cells has thereby proven to be the only truly curative treatment option, at least for younger patients. Whether any of the new cytokine combinations or differentiation inducers will improve at least the quality, possibly also the quantity of life of MDS patients, remains to be proven.

A variety of treatment approaches have been used in MDS. Due to the advanced age of these patients and their relatively poor responses to chemotherapy, supportive therapy with antibiotics and/or transfusions of blood cell products has remained the main therapeutic option. This article will focuse on the role of haematopoietic growth factors in MDS.

## Haematopoietic growth factors

In theory, the haematopoietic growth factors could exert their action in various ways: decreasing the morbidity and mortality associated with prolonged anaemia, neutropenia and/or thrombocytopenia by stimulation of the proliferation and maturation of residual normal or leukaemic haematopoietic cells into respectively red cells, granulocytes and/or thrombocytes; they could enhance the impaired functional capacities of granulocytes [6] and may synchronize the leukaemic cells, thereby increasing the effectivity of S-phase-specific agents; they may shorten the aplastic phase after intensive chemotherapy.

## Erythropoietin in MDS

Thirty one separate trials, involving 520 MDS patients, have been reported (Table 1) [for review, see reference 7]. An increase in hemoglobin level was noticed in 20%, and a reduction of RBC transfusion requirements in 24% of patients. There was considerable variation in rHuEPO dosing, ranging from as low as 30 U/kg three times weekly, up to 100.000 U two times weekly. Erythroid response, if seen, will usually occur within the first 8 weeks of rHuEPO treatment. The current practice of rHuEPO administration is three times per week, subcutaneously, with a starting dose of 150 U/kg, with escalation up to 300 U/kg in patients not initially responding after 4 to 8 weeks of rHuEPO treatment. As expected from the known in vitro actions of erythropoietin, there was virtually no effect on neutrophils and only occasional improvements in platelet counts.

A recently published meta-analysis of 205 patients from 17 studies identified factors associated with response to erythropoietin therapy [8]. These factors included no transfusion need (44% versus 10%), endogenous serum erythropoietin level below 200 U/L, and absence of ringed sideroblasts (21% versus 7.5%). This meta-analysis could identify a group of patients (i.e. patients without transfusion need and MDS other than RARS) with a response rate of $50%, irrespective of their serum level of erythropoietin. At the other extreme, no response was seen in patients with RARS and serum erythropoietin levels $200 U/l.

## Granulocyte (G-CSF) and Granulocyte-macrophage colony stimulating factor (GM-CSF) in MDS

G-CSF has been administered by both intraveneous infusion and subcutaneous injection. Pooled data from five trials that have previously been summarized [9] have shown increased neutrophils in 90% of MDS patients and minimal effect on anaemia and thrombocytopenia (Table 1), although there have been rare reports of MDS patients who showed trilineage haematologic responses to G-CSF [10]. There was no correlation between the subtype of MDS and response rate. Toxicity during G-CSF therapy was minimal, although sharp decline in platelet counts after starting G-CSF therapy can create serious bleeding problems in the first weeks of therapy. The best dose of G-CSF to be used in MDS is still a matter of debate. A practical approach would be to start with 1 μg/kg/d and to adjust the G-CSF dose to obtain neutrophils around 2500/μL.

Several investigators have reported the results of phase I/II therapeutic trials with GM-CSF [9, 11, 12]. These trials have utilized different drug preparations, dosages and schedules of administration of GM-CSF for varied intervals. The combined data from these studies, including 263 MDS patients, showed that GM-CSF was effective in increasing neutrophil counts in 76% of the patients (Table 1). In addition to the increase of neutrophils, further cell lineages were stimulated, including eosinophils, monocytes, and lymphocytes. The counts generally returned to baseline levels upon discontinuation of the cytokine. The responses in other cell lineages such as platelets and hemoglobin were limited to only a fraction of the patients (2-5%). Adverse effects of GM-CSF which occur in

**Table 1.** Response rates to colony-stimulating factors in patients with myelodysplastic syndromes[§]

| | No. of patients | Increase in neutrophils (%)* | Increase in hemoglobin (%)* | Increase in platelets (%)* | Increase in blasts (%) |
|---|---|---|---|---|---|
| G-CSF | 73 | 66 (90%) | 6 (8%) | 4 (5%) | 3 (4%) |
| GM-CSF | 263 | 199 (76%) | 4 (2%) | 14 (5%) | 32 (12%) |
| IL-3 | 135 | 49 (36%) | 6 (4%) | 29 (21%) | 11 (8%) |
| IL-6 | 22 | 0 (0%) | 0 (0%) | 8 (36%) | 2 (9%) |
| Epo | 520 | 0 (0%) | 133 (25%) | 8 (1%) | 4 (0.7%) |
| IL-3 + GM-CSF | 9 | 7 (77%) | 0 (0%) | 3 (33%) | 1 (11%) |
| Epo + G-CSF | 71 | 62 (87%) | 18 (25%) | 1 (1%) | 6 (8%) |
| Epo + GM-CSF | 24 | 19 (79%) | 8 (33%) | 3 (12%) | 2 (8%) |
| Epo + IL-3 | 23 | 16 (70%) | 4 (17%) | 5 (21%) | 0 (0%) |
| Epo + G-CSF + ATRA + $\alpha$-tocopherol | 10 | 9 (90%) | 4 (40%) | 2 (20%) | NS |

[§] data based on references quoted in the text
*Response criteria included an increase in neutrophils (doubling with a minimum of $0.5 \times 10^9$/L, or platelets (doubling with a minimum of $50 \times 10^9$/L, a rise in hemoglobin by 2 g/dl, or reduction in transfusion requirements by 50%; NS, not stated.

25% of patients at "conventional dose" (60-250 µg/m²), include fever, bone pain, local erythema, phlebitis, decrease in platelet counts, fluid overload, and, rarely an adult respiratory distress syndrome. An interesting approach for long-term GM-CSF therapy seems the administration of "very low dose" of GM-CSF (0.25-0.5 µg/kg), since recent studies suggest that it might be possible to divorce the toxic effects of GM-CSF from the therapeutic benefits [12].

Two central questions in the use of G-CSF and GM-CSF are whether they produce survival benefit or significant decrease in morbidity from infection, and whether the use of these growth factors causes increased rate of progression to leukaemia. A significant proportion of patients with RAEB and RAEBt receiving GM-CSF (and to a lesser extent G-CSF) do develop transient increases in blast cell counts while undergoing therapy that revert to pretreatment levels when therapy is withdrawn. In contrast, several reports have documented the induction of leukaemic transformation by GM-CSF in CMML [13, 14]. Preliminary results of a randomized, controlled clinical trial comparing GM-CSF for 90 days versus observation, did not show differences in transformation to RAEBt/ANLL in the different treatment arms [15]. As expected, there was a significant increase in WBC in the treatment arm which was associated with fewer major infections during the 90 day treatment period. A multicenter study comparing G-CSF and observation did not show significant differences in the rate of progression to ANLL between treated and untreated patiens [16]. However, there was a shorter median survival in the G-CSF treated group of patients with RAEB. Death was due to non-leukaemic, disease-related causes. Decreased survival in treated RAEB patients was probably due to the increased number of high-risk patients included in the G-CSF treated arm and the unusually long survival of RAEB patients in the control arm. Infection rates in the two groups have not yet been reported. No survival benefit has yet been demonstrated for growth factor therapy in MDS. While prophylactic administration of G-CSF or GM-CSF cannot be recommended, treatment with febrile neutropenia might benefit from G-CSF in combination with antibiotics.

Combined therapy with low-dose Ara-C and GM-CSF or G-CSF, respectively, has not proven to be superior to therapy with low-dose Ara-C alone, with regard to survival, or toxicity, and resulted in CR rate of 15% to 20% and a PR rate of 20% [17, 18].

## Interleukin-3 (IL-3) in MDS

One long-term and seven short-term studies have reported the effects of IL-3 therapy in 135 MDS patients (Table 1) [19-22]. There is an overall response rate for neutrophils of approximately 36% , increase in hemoglobin level of 4%, platelets 21%, and a 8% increase in bone marrow blasts. Trilineage response was only seldom seen. These data indicate that IL-3 must be combined with other haematopoietic growth factors to achieve substantial improvement in MDS cytopenias. Adverse effects of IL-3 were significant, especially at higher doses, and consisted of eosinophilia, fever, bone pain, myalgias and headache, necessitating discontinuation of IL-3 in several patients.

## Interleukin-6 (IL-6) in MDS

One short-term study has reported the effects of IL-6 in 22 low-risk MDS patients with < 5% bone marrow blasts and < 100.000/μL platelets (Table 1) [23]. Eight patients experienced at least a transient improvement in platelet counts. Two of three patients who received maintenance therapy with IL-6 had a persistent increase in platelet counts, during 3 and 12 months of IL-6 therapy, respectively. Moderate to severe toxicity with constitutional symptoms occurred without leukocyte improvement, and worsening anemia developed, but without a significant effect on transfusion requirements.

## Combination of cytokines in MDS

The infrequent multilineage responses with recombinant human growth factors have led to studies involving combinations of growth factors, either simultaneously or sequentially, in order to target proliferation and differentiation of both early and late stages of haematopoietic progenitor cells. However, combination of growth factors, especially that act early in haematopoiesis, must be balanced against potential risk of increased rate of progression to acute leukaemia, and side effects of combinations of growth factors may be additive.

Preliminary trials with the combination of erythropoietin and G-CSF or GM-CSF, respectively, have yield impressive results with erythroid responses of 42% compared to 20-25% with erythropoietin alone [24-26]. Additional studies, however, could not support these synergistic effects of combination therapy, and resulted in erythroid responses comparable to erythropoietin alone (Table 1) [27-29]. Dose schedule, timing and duration of the growth factors and difference in the study population may, at least partly, explain these conflicting results.

Recently, data have been published from a randomized phase II study of 71 MDS patients with anemia, receiving G-CSF and erythropoietin [30]. Patients were randomized to treatment starting with G-CSF for 4 weeks followed by the combination for 12 weeks, or starting with erythropoietin for 8 weeks followed by the combination for 10 weeks. The overall response rate to G-CSF and erythropoietin was 38 % and was identical in the two treatment groups indicating that an initial treatment with G-CSF was not necessary for a response to the combination. Patients, receiving long-term maintenance treatment, showed a median duration of response of 24 months.

A prognostic scoring system has been proposed to predict responses when using the combination of G-CSF and erythropoietin [31]. The score based on the serum epo level (<100, 100-500 or > 500 U/l) and RBC transfusion need (<2 or ≥2 units per month) divided patients into three groups: one group with a high probability of erythroid responses (74 %), one intermediate group (23 %) and one group with poor responses to treatment (7 %). This predictive scoring system could be used in decisions regarding use of these cytokines for treating the anaemia of MDS patients.

Treatment with IL-3 and erythropoietin has so far been disappointing [32, 33]. A worrisome finding was the development of thrombocytopenia in 50% of the patients, probably related to the induction of tumor necrosis factor α (TNF-α), a rather potent inhibitor of megakaryopoiesis.

The combination of ATRA with G-CSF, erythropoietin and tocopherol resulted in increased neutrophils in 90%, an erythroid response in 40%, and increased thrombocytes in 30% of the patients, respectively [34]. The induction of TNFα might be responsible for treatment failure.

Sequential therapy with interleukin-3 followed by GM-CSF gave improved absolute neutrophil count in 77% and improved platelets in 33% [35]. However, toxicity was unacceptable.

Administration of growth factors in MDS rarely induces polyclonal haematopoiesis as evaluated by repeated cytogenetic investigations and analysis of restriction fragment length polymorphisms [9, 36].

### Thrombopoietin (TPO)

Recombinant TPO or the mpl-ligand has recently become available for clinical testing. TPO stimulates MDS granulocyte-macrophage and erythroid progenitor cells in vitro [37]. No clinical data of TPO in MDS are at present available.

### Intensive AML-type chemotherapy with CSF

Using varying combinations of AML-type chemotherapy in MDS it has been shown that complete remissions can be reached. However on average, CR rates are lower than in AML treated with more or less identical protocols. A longer duration of the pancytopenic period resulting in a high hypoplastic death rate is one of the explanation for the lower CR rate. Resistance to chemotherapy has also been argued to be responsible for treatment failure in MDS. Haemopoietic growth factors administered simultaneously with chemotherapy and after stopping treatment might prime the malignant cells to make them more susceptible for cell killing, and might shorten the pancytopenic period. Recently, we investigated in a randomized study the application of G-CSF during and after chemotherapy in patients with bad risk MDS [38]. CR rate in

the G-CSF arm was 73 % and 52 % in the control group (not yet statistically significant). The median overall survival in the G-CSF arm was longer (16 months versus 9 months) and also the duration of neutropenia was significantly shorter in the G-CSF arm. However, this did not result in less infectious complications, less antibiotic use or shorter hospitalization. In contrast, a recently published randomized study comparing aggressive chemotherapy with or without G-CSF support (starting after stopping chemotherapy) for high-risk MDS showed a lower incidence of infections, shorter duration of neutropenia and significantly better responses (CR and PR). However, chemotherapy and G-CSF did not prolong either CR duration or survival. The growth factor support, however, increased the number of allo-transplantable cases by inducing higher remission rates and improving clinical conditions [39].

### Autologous stem cell mobilization with G-CSF and transplantation in MDS

A pilot study demonstrated the feasibility of peripheral blood progenitor cell harvest and transplantation (PBPCT) in selected patients with high risk myelodysplasia after mobilization with G-CSF. Consistent with the rapid haematopoietic recovery after infusion (median time to ANC > 0.5 x $10^9$/l: 14 days, range: 10-18; and platelets > 20 x $10^9$/l: 41 days, range: 8-144 in 4 patients), requirements for supportive care were restricted [40]. Repopulation data after at least 100 days follow-up were compared for 10 patients receiving ABMT versus 7 patients after PBPCT after identical induction therapy. The mean number of CFU-GM (x $10^4$/kg) reinfused in the ABMT group was 5.2 versus 68.5 in the PBPC group. After BM reinfusion, leucocytes $ 0.5 and 1.0 x $10^9$/l were reached after a median of respectively 34.5 and 39.5 days, versus 11 and 13 days in the PBPCT group. In 5/10 ABMT patients, platelet counts > 20 x $10^9$/l were reached after a median of 80 days. In 5/7 PBPCT patients, platelets were > 20 x $10^9$/l after a median of 17.5 days. Five of 10 ABMT recipients were still transfusion dependent 100 days after reinfusion, in contrast to 1/7 recipients of PBPC. Immediate transplant-related mortality (< 100 days) was 0/10 in ABMT versus 1/7 after PBPCT. These data indicate that PBPC transplantation is feasible in selected MDS patients and leads to more rapid and complete repopulation when compared to ABMT. Further study will be necessary to determine whether this approach has any value. A major concern remains the possible contamination of autologous stem cells by clonal malignant cells. Polyclonal, putative benign, CD34+ stem cells have been demonstrated in PBPC harvests after chemotherapy with G-CSF support of female patients by techniques based on X-chromosome inactivation patterns (PCR-analysis with the HUMARA-probe) [41-42]. Further identification and purification of polyclonal stem cells in patients with myelodysplastic syndromes will help to explore this approach further.

# References

1. Aul C, Schneider W (1989a) The role of low dose cytosine arabinoside and aggressive chemotherapy in advanced myelodysplastic syndrome. Cancer 64: 1812-1818.
2. Reizenstein P, Dabrowski L (1991) Increasing prevalence of the myelodysplastic syndromes: an international Delphi study. Anticancer Research 11:1069-1070.
3. Bennett JM, Catovski D, Daniel MT et al (1982) Proposals for the classification of the myelodysplastic syndromes. Br J Haematol 51: 189-199.
4. Verhoef GEG, Pittaluga S, De Wolf-Peeters C, Boogaerts M (1995) FAB classification of myelodysplastic syndromes: merits and controversies. Ann Hematol 71: 3-11.
5. Greenberg P, Coc C, LeBeau M, et al. (1998) International Scoring System for evaluating prognosis in myelodysplastic syndromes. Blood 89:2079-2092
6. Verhoef G & Boogaerts M (1991) In vivo administration of granulocyte-macrophage colony stimulating factor enhances neutrophil function in patients with myelodysplastic syndromes. Br J Haematol 79: 177-184.
7. Verhoef G & Boogaerts M (1995) Recombinant human erythropoietin in the treatment of the myelodysplastic syndromes. In Smythe JF, Boogaerts M, Ehmer B (eds) RhErythropoietin in Cancer Supportive Treatment. New York, Marcel Dekker, Inc.
8. Hellström-Lindberg E (1995) Efficacy of erythropoietin in the myelodysplastic syndromes: a meta-analysis of 205 patients from 17 studies. Br J Haematol 89: 67-71.
9. Ganser A & Hoelzer D (1992) Treatment of myelodysplastic syndromes with hematopoietic growth factors. In Koeffler HP (ed) Hematology/Oncology Clinics of North America, pp 633-653. Philadelphia: WB Saunders Company.
10. Chiba S, Inamori K, Mitani K, Hirai H, Yazaki Y (1994) Marked and reproducible increase in trilineage blood cell counts by administration of granulocyte colony-stimulating factor in a patient with refractory anemia with excess blasts in transformation. Br J Haematol 86:665-667.
11. Kaczmarski RS, Pozniak A, Lakhani A, Harvey E, Mufti GJ (1993) A pilot study of low-dose recombinant human granulocyte-macrophage colony-stimulating factor in chronic neutropenia. Br J Haematol 84: 338-340.
12. Rose C, Wattel E, Bastion Y, Berger E et al (1994) Treatment with very low-dose GM-CSF in myelodysplastic syndromes with neutropenia. A report on 28 cases. Leukemia 8: 1458-1462.
13. Ganser A, Völkers B, Greher J et al (1989) Recombinant human granulocyte-macrophage colony stimulating factor in patients with myelodysplastic syndromes-a phase I/II trial. Blood 73: 31-37.
14. Rosenfeld CS, Sulecki M, Evans C, Shadduck RK (1991) Comparison of intravenous versus subcutaneous recombinant human granulocyte-macrophage colony-stimulating factor in patients with primary myelodysplasia. Exp Hematol 19: 273-277.
15. Schuster MW, Thompson JA, Larson R et al (1990) Randomized trial of subcutaneous granulocyte-macrophage colony-stimulating factor versus observation in patients with myelodysplastic syndrome. Int J Canc Res Clin Oncol 116 (suppl II): 1079.
16. Greenberg P, Taylor K, Larson R et al (1993) Phase III randomized multicenter trial of G-CSF vs. Observation for myelodysplastic syndromes. Blood 82 (suppl 1): 196a.
17. Im T, Yamane T, Mugitani A et al (1994) Treatment with cytosine arabinoside and granulocyte colony-stimulating factor in patients with myelodysplastic syndrome and its leukemic phase. Int J Hematol 60: 215-223.
18. Gerhartz HH, Marcus R, Delmer A et al (1994) A randomized phase II study of low-dose cytosine arabinoside (LD-AraC) plus granulocyte-macrophage colony stimulating factor (rhGM-CSF) in myelodysplastic syndromes with a high risk of developing leukemia. Leukemia 8: 16-23.
19. Kurzrock R, Talpaz M, Estrov Z et al (1991) Phase I study of recombinant human interleukin-3 in patients with bone marrow failure. J Clin Oncol 9: 1241-1250.
   of myelodysplastic syndromes. Eur J Haematol 54: 39-45.
20. Willemze R, Fenaux P, Gerhartz H et al (1992) A randomized phase I/II multicenter study (EORTC 06891) of rh-IL-3 in patients with myelodysplastic syndromes at relatively low risk of developing leukemia (MDS-LR). Blood 80 (suppl): 86a.
21. Ganser A, Ottmann OG, Seipelt G et al (1993) Effect of long-term treatment with recombinant interleukin-3 in patients with myelodysplastic syndromes. Leukemia 7: 696-701.
22. Legare RD & Gilliland DG (1995) Myelodysplastic syndrome. In Bernstein ID (ed) Current Opinion in Hematology, pp 283-292. Philadelphia: Current Science.

23. Gordon MS, Nemunaitis J, Hoffman R et al (1995) A phase I trial of recombinant human interleukin-6 in patients with myelodysplastic syndromes and thrombocytopenia. Blood 85: 3066-3076.

24. Hansen PB, Johnson HE, Hippe E et al (1993) Recombinant human granulocyte-macrophage colony-stimulating factor plus recombinant human erythropoietin may improve anemia in selected patients with myelodysplastic syndromes (1993) Am J Hematol 44: 229-236.

25. Hellström-Lindberg E, Birgegård G, Carlsson M et al (1993) A combination of granulocyte colony-stimulating factor and erythropoietin may synergistically improve the anaemia in patients with myelodysplastic syndromes. Leuk Lymph 11: 221-228.

26. Negrin RS, Stein R, Vardiman J et al (1993) Treatment of the anemia of myelodysplastic syndromes using recombinant human granulocyte colony-stimulating factor in combination with erythropoietin. Blood 82: 737-743.

27. Imamura M, Kobayashi M, Kobayashi S et al (1994) Failure of combination therapy with recombinant granulocyte colony-stimulating factor and erythropoietin in myelodysplastic syndromes. Ann Hematol 68: 163-166.

28. Musto P, Falcone A, Carotenuto M et al (1994) Granulocyte colony stimulating factor and erythropoietin for the anemia of myelodysplastic syndromes: A real improvement with respect to erythropoietin alone? [letter] Blood 84: 1687-1688.

29. Runde V, Aul C, Ebert A et al (1995) Sequential administration of recombinant human granulocyte-macrophage colony-stimulating factor and human erythropoietin for the treatment of myelodysplastic syndromes. Eur J Haematol, 54: 39-45

30. Hellström et al (1998) Treatment of anemia in myelodysplastic syndromes with granulocyte colony stimulating factor plus erythropoietin: results from a randomized phase II study and long-term follow-up of 71 patients. Blood 92: 68-75

31. Hellström et al (1997) Erythroid response to treatment with G-CSF plus erythropoietin for the anaemia of patients with myelodysplastic syndromes: proposal for a predictive model. Br J Haematol, 99: 344-351

32. Verhoef G, Demuynck H, Zachée P et al (1993) Treatment of myelodysplastic syndromes with the combination of interleukin-3 and erythropoietin. Blood 82 (suppl): 377a.

33. List AL, Noyes W, Power J et al. (1999) Limited erythropoietic response to combined treatment with recombinant human interleukin 3 and erythropoietin in myelodysplastic syndromes. Leuk-Res, 23: 77-83.

34. Maurer AB, Ganser A, Seipelt G et al (1995) Changes in erythroid progenitor cell and accessory cell compartments in patients with myelodysplastic syndromes during treatment with all-*trans* retinoid acid and haemopoietic growth factors. Br J Haematol 89: 449-456.

35. Nand S, Sosman J, Godwin JE, Fisher RI (1994) A phase I/II study of sequential interleukin-3 and granulocyte-macrophage colony-stimulating factor in myelodysplastic syndromes. Blood 83: 357-360.

36. Verhoef G, van den Berghe H, Boogaerts M (1992) Cytogenetic effects of cells derived from patients with myelodysplastic syndromes during treatment of hematopoietic growth factors. Leukemia 6: 766-770.

37. Ferrajoli et al.(1998). Thrombopoietin stimulates myelodysplastic syndrome granulocyte-macrophage and erythropoid progenitor proliferation. Leuk-Lymphoma, 30: 279-292

38. Ossenkoppele G, van der Holt B, Verhoef G. et al. A randomized study of granulocyte-colony stimulating factor applied during and after chemotherapy in patients with bad risk myelodysplastic syndromes. Submitted.

39. Bernasconi et al. (1998). Randomized clinical study comparing aggressive chemotherapy with or without G-CSF support for high-risk myelodysplastic syndromes or secondary leukemia evolving from MDS. Br J Haematol, 102: 678-683

40. Demuynck H, Delforge M, Verhoef GEG et al (1996) Feasibility of peripheral blood progenitor cell harvest and transplantation in patients with poor-risk myelodysplastic syndromes. Br J Haematol, 92: 351-359

41. Delforge M, Van Duppen V, Demuynck H, Verhoef GEG, Vandenberghe P, Zachée P, Boogaerts MA (1995) Polyclonal primitive haematopoietic progenitors can be demonstrated in mobilized PBPC collections of patients with myelodysplastic syndromes. Blood, 86: 3660-3667

42. Delforge M, Demuynck H., Verhoef G (1998) et al (1999) Patients with high-risk myelodysplastic syndrome can have polyclonal or clonal haemopoiesis in complete haematological remission. Br J Haematol, 102: 486-495

# Modulation of Ara-C Toxification by Fludarabine and Hydroxyurea in Leukemic Blasts

M.AHLMANN, K. LÜMKEMANN, C.LANVERS, A.FREUND, C.RÖSSIG and J.BOOS

*Introduction.* Arabinosyl-cytosine (ara-C) is one of the most effective drugs in the treatment of childhood acute leukemia. Deficiency of desoxycytidine-kinase (dCK), the rate limiting enzyme in the phosphorylation of cellular ara-C to the active metabolite arabinosyl-cytosine-triphosphate (ara-CTP), is considered to be an important mechanism of ara-C resistance. Ribonucleotide reductase inhibitors such as fludarabine (F-ara) and hydroxyurea (HU) are known to potentiate ara-CTP by increasing dCK activity.

*Purpose.* We wished to determine the effect of the ribonucleotide reductase inhibitors, F-ara and HU, on ara-CTP formation in blast cells from children with acute leukemia, in order to test the potential effect of these modifying strategies for pediatric leukemia.

*Methods:* Blast cells from 19 patients with acute leukemia (AML:9, T-ALL:4, non-T-ALL:4, relapsed ALL:2, classification by immunphenotyping) were isolated by Ficoll-Hypaque gradient centrifugation. After preincubation for 4h with 5µM F-ara or 0,5mM HU blast cells were incubated for 1h with 10µM ara-C. Intracellular formation of ara-CTP was measured by high-performance liquid chromatography (HPLC) and compared to ara-CTP levels reached in non-pretreated control blast cells (ara-C 10µM for 1h only).

*Results.* The ara-CTP enhancement by pretreatment with ribonucleotide reductase inhibitors differed significantly among the individual groups. In blast cells of lymphoblastic leukemia, T-ALL and non-T-ALL, no ara-C modulatory effect was observed. In myeloge-nous blasts preincubation with F-ara and HU increased ara-CTP levels by 100 resp 50%.

*Conclusion.* F-ara tended to increase ara-CTP more efficiently than HU, nevertheless the difference was not significant. Thus, HU should be further tested as an alternative modifier of ara-C in the treatment of AML for children and adults.

## Introduction

The pyrimidine analogue arabinosyl-cytosine (ara-C) plays a central role in the treatment of childhood acute leukemia. The ability to accumulate and retain the active metabolite arabinosyl-cytosine-triphosphate (ara-CTP) correlates with cytotoxicity and clinical outcome [1-6]. Rate limiting in the ara-C toxification pathway is the first phosphorylation step catalyzed by the deoxycytidinkinase (dCK), which is partly regulated by deoxycytidine triphospate (dCTP) feedback inhibition. Development of ara-C resistance is a major cause of treatment failure and can partly be traced back to deficiency of the dCK [7]. Ribonucleotide reductase inhibitors like fludarabine (F-ara) [8-12] and hydroxyurea (HU) [13-17] deplete intracellular dCTP pools thus increasing activity of dCK and enhancing intracellular ara-CTP levels. Therefore, ribonucleotide reductase inhibitors might help to overcome ara-C resistance.

The combination of F-ara and ara-C is already clinically applied in the treatment of relapsed acute myelogenous leukemia of adults and children [11,17,18]. However, the combination of HU, a comparatively low

Dept. of Pediatric Oncology, University of Münster, Albert Schweitzer Straße 33, 48129 Münster, Germany

cytotoxic agent, and ara-C is hardly used in AML therapy today, although the ability of HU to enhance intracellular ara-CTP has been shown in some solid tumors and leukemias in the 1980s [14-17]. In the light of this we tried to compare the effect of pretreatment with F-ara and HU on ara-CTP levels in different subtypes of childhood acute leukemia.

## Methods

### Drugs

Ara-C, F-ara, HU, natural nucleotides and ara-CTP were obtained from Sigma Chemical Co (Deisenhofen, Germany). All chemicals were of the highest purity available.

Ara-C and HU stock solution were prepared in sterile water, F-ara was dissolved in ethanol at final concentrations which did not effect cell growth. Incubation experiments were carried out at therapeutically relevant concentrations.

Stock solutions were stored at –20°C.

### Patients

Blood samples or bone marrow aspirates of pediatric patients were obtained prior to drug administration after informed consent. So far, blasts of 19 children have been examined. According to immunephenotyping, 9 patients had AML, 4 T-ALL , 4 non-T-ALL and 2 relapsed acute leukemia.

### Separation of blast cells

Peripheral blood or bone marrow aspirates were immediatley placed on ice, diluted with 15 ml RPMI 1640 medium (GIBCO Laboratories, Eggenstein Germany) and isolated by Ficoll-Hypaque centrifugation (Lymphoprep™, Nycomed Norway).

Mononuclear cells at the interface were harvested, washed three times with 50 ml medium and centrifugated at 400g (10 min/4°C).

The total number of blasts was counted and then resuspended in RPMI-1640 with 10% heat-inactivated fetal calf serum (GIBCO) for incubation experiments.

### Cellular pharmacology

Concordant with Plunkett et al. 1993 [9] blast cells were preincubated with F-ara 5µM respectively HU 500µM for 4h, washed twice and resuspended in ara-C containing medium and incubated in a shaking water bath at 37°C for 1h. Incubation time and final ara-C concentration were in the linear range of ara-CTP accumulation.

Ara-CTP was separated from other nucleotide triphosphates by an isocrated ion pair high performance liquid chromatography (HPLC) method using a reversed phase C18 column (Nova Pak, Waters-FRG) and 0.09 M phosphate puffer (pH6, tetrahydrofuran 0.35%, tetrabutyl ammonium hydrogen sulfate 0.01M) and measured with UV detection at 270nm against anthranilic acid as internal standard. The limit of detection was 25ng/ml ara-CTP. Ara-CTP levels were expressed as picogram (pg) ara-CTP per $10^7$ cells [20].

### Statistical analysis

Intracellular ara-CTP concentrations with and without preincubation were compared using the Rank-Sum test.

## Results

### Accumulation of ara-CTP in different subtypes of leukemia

Enhancement of intracellular ara-CTP levels by ribonucleotide reductase inhibitors, F-ara and HU, differed clearly between different types of acute leukemia (Fig.1, 2).

In myelogenous blasts preincubation with F-ara and HU exhibited increased ara-CTP accumulation compared to non-pretreated controls, whereas in T-ALL pretreatment did not exert any effect. In non-T-ALL treatment with ribonucleotide reductase inhibitors showed variable results in ara-CTP enhancement. In 3 out of 4 patients no significant augmentation of ara-CTP metabolism was reached, whereas the cellular ara-CTP levels of 1 patient showed a 4 fold increase after preincubation with F-ara and a 2 fold increase after preincubation with HU. In

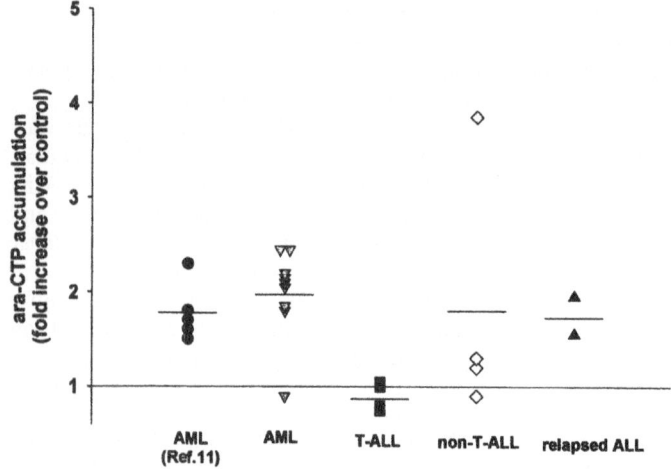

**Fig. 1.** Effect of preincubation with F-ara on ara-CTP accumulation in different acute leukemia subtypes as compared to non-pretreated controls.

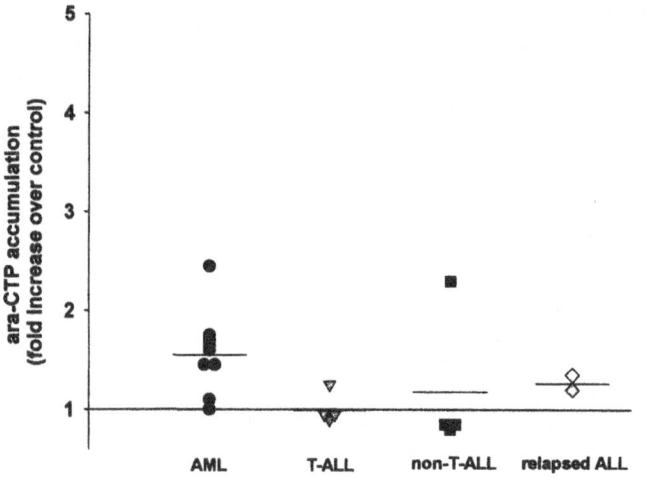

**Fig. 2.** Effect of preincubation with HU on ara-CTP accumulation in different leukemia subtypes as compared to non-pretreated controls

blasts of relapsed ALL pretreatment with F-ara resulted in 1.9 respectively 1.5 fold increase of ara-CTP levels, whereas pretreatment with HU resulted in 1.3 respectively 1.2 fold ara-CTP levels.

## Comparison of ara-C modulatory efficacy of F-ara and HU in AML blasts

In myelogenous blasts preincubation with HU showed 1.5 fold ara-CTP accumulation (range:0.88-2.41) compared to blasts treated with ara-C alone. Preincubation with F-ara increased ara-CTP levels about 2.0 times

(range:0.96-2.43). These results are in accordance with Gandhi et al., who determined a 1.7 fold increase of ara-CTP accumulation in blasts of adults with relapsed acute myelogenous leukemia after F-ara infusion and ex vivo treatment with ara-C. In comparison to HU F-ara tends to be more effective, but the difference was not statistically significant (p=0.062) (Fig.3).

## Discussion

The level of ara-CTP reached under antileukemic treatment is of prognostic significance

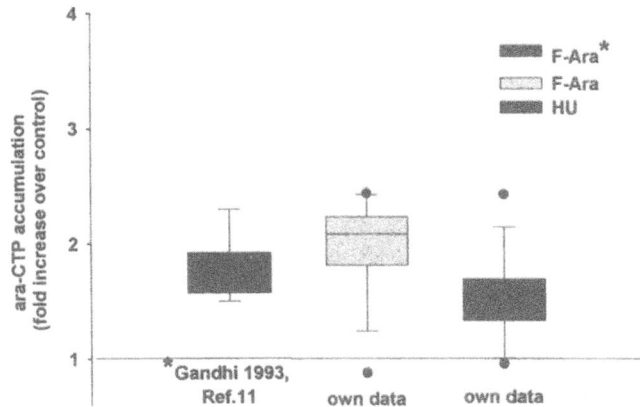

**Fig. 3.** Comparison of ara-CTP levels after preincubation with F-ara and HU in myelogenous blasts

[1, 6]. Strategies to increase therapeutic efficacy and to overcome ara-C resistance focussed on the enhancement of intracellular ara-CTP levels by pretreatment with ribonucleotide reductase inhibitors [8,13].

The combination of F-ara and ara-C is already successfully applied in the treatment of both adult and childhood relapsed acute leukemia in clinical studies. Avramis et al. found in children with relapsed acute leukemia 5 fold levels of intracellular ara-CTP after *in vivo* infusion of fludarabine and *ex vivo* treatment of separated blasts with ara-C [19]. Though HU has also been shown to increase ara-CTP levels and though it shows a favorable toxicity profile it is hardly used in combination with ara-C in clinical studies today.

In our experiments on T-ALL blasts pretreatment with HU and F-ara did not influence ara-CTP levels. However, in myelogenous blasts we found a 1.5 fold increase of ara-CTP (range:0.88-2.41) by pretreatment with HU and a 2-fold increase by pretreatment with F-Ara compared to treatment with ara-C alone. Concordant with our results Gandhi et al.[11] observed a 1.7 fold increase of ara-CTP accumulation in blasts of adults with relapsed acute myelogenous leukemia after F-ara infusion and *ex vivo* treatment with ara-C.

In conclusion, pretreatment with F-ara and HU increases ara-CTP levels in blast cells of children with acute myelogenous leukemia. Comparing the efficacy of F-ara and HU on the ara-C toxification, we observed no statistically significant difference between F-ara and HU. Therefore, HU should be further tested for its potential role as an ara-C modifier in AML in children and adults.

*Acknowledgments.* This work was supported by the Federal Department of Research and Technology (#01EC9401).

## References

1. Rustum YM (1978) Metabolism and intracellular retention of 1-ß-D-arabinofuranosylcytosine as predictors of response of animal tumors. Cancer Res 38: 543-549
2. Kufe D, Spriggs D, Egan EM, Munroe D (1984) Relationship among ara-CTP pools, formation of (ara-C) DNA, and cytotoxicity of human leukemic cells. Blood 64: 54-58
3. Shewach DS, Plunkett W (1982) Correlation of cytotoxicity with total intracellular exposure to 9-ß-D-arabinofuranosyladenine 5´-triphosphate. Cancer Res. 42: 3637-3641
4. Plunkett W, Iacoboni S, Estey EH, Danhauser L, Liliemark JO, Keating MJ (1985) Pharmacologically directed ara-C therapy for refractory leukemia. Sem Oncol 12 (suppl): 20-30
5. Estey E, Plunkett W, Dixon DO, Keating M, Mc Credie K, Freireich EJ (1987) Variables predicting response to high dose cytosine arabinoside therapy with refractory acute leukemia. Leukemia 1: 580-583
6. Boos J, Hohenlöchter B, Schulze Westhoff P, Schiller M, Zimmermann M, Creutzig U, Ritter J, Jürgens H (1996) Intracellular retention of cytosine arabinoside triphosphate in blast cells from children with acute myelogenous and lymphoblastic leukemia. Med Ped Oncol 26: 397-404
7. Zühlsdorf M, Vormoor J, Boos J (1997) Cytosine Arabinoside in Childhood Leukemia. Int J Pediatr Hematol/Oncol 4:565-581
8. Gandhi V, Plunkett W (1988) Modulation of arabinosylnucleoside metabolism by arabinosylnucleotides in human leukemia cells Cancer Res 48: 329-334

9. Plunkett W, et al. (1993) Fludarabin: Pharmacocinetics, mechanism of action, and rationales for combination therapies. Sem Oncol 20 (Suppl.7): 2-12

10. Gandhi V, Nowak B, JKeating MJ, PlunkettW (1989) Modulation of arabinosylcytosine metabolism by arabinosyl-2-fluoroadenine in lymphocytes from patients with chronic lymphocytic leukemia: Implication for combination therapy. Blood 74: 2070-2075

11. Gandhi V, Kemena A, Keating MJ, Plunkett W (1992) Fludarabin infusion potentiates arabinosylcytosine metabolism in lymphocytic leukemia. Cancer Res 52: 897-903

12. Gandhi V, Estey E, Keating MJ, Plunkett W (1993) Fludarabin potentiates metabolism of cytarabine in patients with acute myelogenous leukemia. J Clin Oncol 11: 116-124

13. Donehower RC (1992) An overview of the clinical experience with hydroxyurea. Sem Oncol 19: 11-19

14. Plagemann PGW, Marz R, Wohlhueter RM (1978) Transport and metabolism of 1-ß-D-arabinofuranosylcytosine into cultured Novikoff rat hepatoma cells, relationship to phosphorylation, regulation of triphosphate synthesis. Cancer Res 38: 978-989

15. Walsh CT, Craig RW, Agarwal RP (1980) Increased activation of 1-ß-D-arabinofuranosylcytosine by hydroxyurea in L1210 cells. Cancer Res 40: 3286-3292

16. Steife JA, Mendelsohn J, Howell SB (1981) Modulation of cytosine arabinoside triphosphate (ara-CTP) and trinucleotide pools in a human acute leukemia cell line (HL-60) by thymidine (dThd) and hydroxyurea (HU). Proc AM Assoc Cancer Res 22: 213

17. Rauscher III F, Cadman E (1983) Hydroxyurea and effect of 1-ß-D-arabinofuranosylcytosine metabolism and cytotoxicity. Cancer Res 43: 2688-2693

18. Fleischhack et al. (1998) IDA-FLAG (idarubicin, fludarabin, cytarabin, G-CSF), an effective remission-induction therapy for poor-prognosis AML of childhood prior to allogenic or autologous bone marrow transplantation: experiences of a phase II trial. BR J Haematol., 102(3): 647-655

19. Avramis VI, et al (1998) Pharmacokinetic and pharmacodynamic studies of fludarabine and cytosine arabinoside administrated as loading boluses followed by continuous infusions after a phase I/II study in pediatric patients with relapsed leukemias. The Children´s Cancer Group. Clin Cancer Res 4(1): 45-52

20. Boos J (1991) A simple isocratic high performance liquid chromatographic determination of 1-ß-D-arabinofuranosylcytosine 5´-triphosphate for intracellular drug monitoring and in vitro incubation assays. Pharm Biom Anal 9: 47-52

# Drug Monitoring of Doxorubicin in Children

S. Flege, G. Hempel, P. Schulze-Westhoff, N. Laubrock and J. Boos

## Introduction

Anthracyclines show activity against both haematological malignancies and solid tumours. Doxorubicin is an important part of many treatment protocols for children with leukemia. A very serious side effect of anthracyclines is myocardial degeneration causing congestive heart failure. Apart from the cumulative dose the peak plasma levels seem to be an independent risk factor. In the literature fractional dosing and prolongation of infusion times have been suggested to reduce the risk of congestive heart failure [1,4]. This admits the presumption that high peak plasma levels are responsible for the cardiotoxicity by short infusions full dose. Therefore, a drug monitoring program has been established to measure the peak plasma levels of children receiving doxorubicin in different treatment protocols. Plenty of preanalytical problems had to be solved before.

## Methods

A simple and sensitive method using capillary electrophoresis with laser-induced fluorescence detection has been developed. This method requires only very small sample volumes which allows doxorubicin monitoring from capillary blood. A plasma volume of only 10 µl is sufficient to determine the peak plasma levels [3].

## Patients

During the period of january to december 1998 58 patients between 1.5 and 22.9 years receiving doxorubicin were monitored in informed consent. Doxorubicin was administered with a perfusor. Capillary blood was taken at the end of the infusion between the perfusor alarm and the beginning of the rinse.

Until now 220 samples of 58 patients with 9 different diagnosis and 12 different treatment schedules have been collected and measured. A detailed analysis has been done for the two frequent schedules: ALL-BFM 95, Eicess 92 and 98, respectively.

## Results

### Stability problems

Initially, experiments were carried out to reduce the preanalytical mistakes during sample collection and preparation. Collecting capillary blood and immediate centrifugation at 4°C for 5 minutes is a convenient and reproducible procedure. Subsequently, the samples have to be frozen by at least –20°C. A temperature of –80°C is necessary if the storage will take more than four weeks. The instability of the drug at room temperature and the parallel increase of doxorubicinol in whole blood are two reasons for this rapid preparation to produce reliable measurements for the parent compound (Fig.1).

WWU Münster - Klinik und Poliklinik für Kinderheilkunde – Pädiatrische Hämatologie und Onkologie – Albert-Schweitzer Str. 33, 48129 Münster – Germany

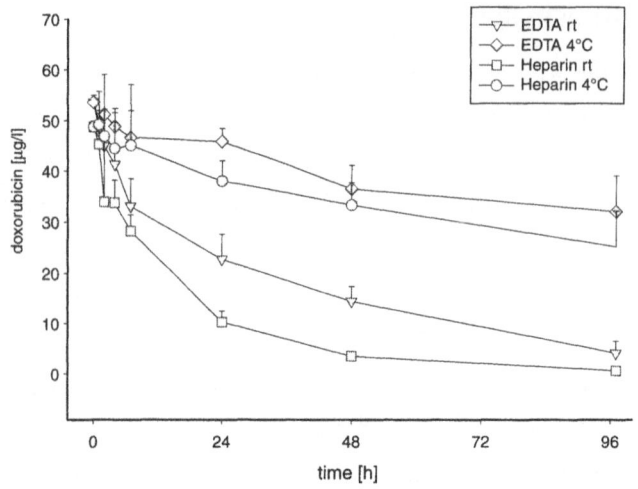

**Fig. 1.** Stability of doxorubicin at room temperature and at 4°C in heparin- and EDTA-plasma

## Simulations

Because of the short half-life of doxorubicin a peak plasma level has to be taken at steady state but before the end of the infusion. Therefore, the optimal time to take the sample is between the perfusor alarm and the start of the rinse. One main preanalytical mistake of the measurements is the balance of doxorubicin in the perfusor syringe which will be given in dash to attach the rinse. The results are artificial high peak plasma levels (Fig. 2).

The peak plasma levels of doxorubicin infusions will be reduced massively by prolonging the infusion time. Figure 3 shows the measurements in comparison to simulations

based on literature values [2]. Prolonging the infusion time to 1 hour (mean $C_{max}$ 555 µg/l) in comparison to bolus (mean $C_{max}$ 3550 µg/l) results in a reduction of the peak plasma levels to about one seventh. Further, the simulation shows that prolonging the infusion time for more than 4 hours no worth mentioning alterations of the maximal concentration of doxorubicin are detectable (Fig.3).

## Clinical observations

61 samples of 20 patients (9 boys and 11 girls) are derived from patients with ALL treated with 30 mg/m2 as a 1 or 2h-infusion. Alto-

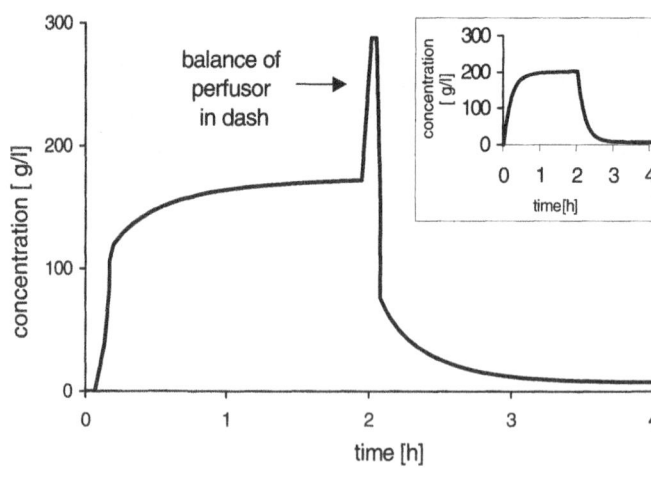

**Fig. 2.** Simulations of 2 hour doxorubicin infusions ( dose: 30 mg/m2) with and without correct handling at the end of infusion

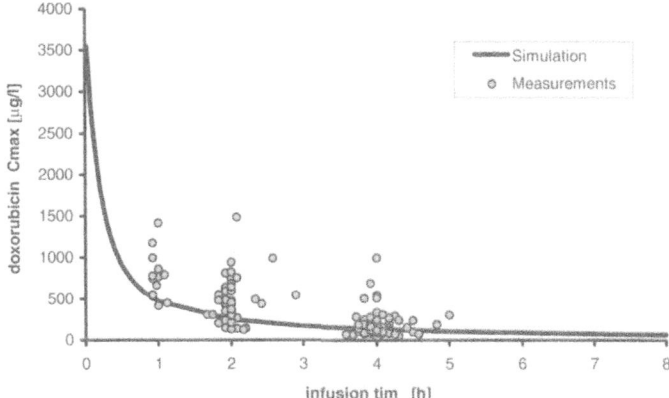

**Fig. 3.** Simulation of the peak plasma levels and measurements at different infusion times

gether doxorubicin has been given weekly for one month. The mean $C_{max}$ for these patients was 555 ± 293 µg/l for a 1h-infusion and 294 ± 115 µg/l for a 2h-infusion, respectively (mean ± SD). The peak plasma levels are not significantly different between boys and girls.

The values of the ALL patients are not directly comparable due to modest variations in the real infusion times. Consequently the concentrations were corrected with factors derived from a pharmacokinetic model [2]. The fourth figure describes the high intra- (7 boys, dark grey and 7 girls, light grey bars) and interindividual variability (boys, first and girls, second white bar as well as both together, scattered bar, mean ± SD). The interindividual variability was calculated from the first measurement in each patient. All 14 patients have at least 3 samples from maximal 4 doxorubicin administrations.

**Table 1.** Comparison of the peak plasma levels of boys and girls

|  |  | mean [µg/l] | standard deviance [µg/l] | median [µg/l] |
|---|---|---|---|---|
| boys | 1h | 553 | 260 | 497 |
| n=9 | 2h | 281 | 116 | 284 |
| girls | 1h | 557 | 335 | 443 |
| n=11 | 2h | 306 | 116 | 290 |
| altogether | 1h | 555 | 293 | 470 |
| n=20 | 2h | 294 | 115 | 287 |

## Conclusions

Capillary electrophoresis with laser-induced fluorescence detection requires small sample volumes to quantify doxorubicin. Therefore, capillary blood sampling is sufficient. One

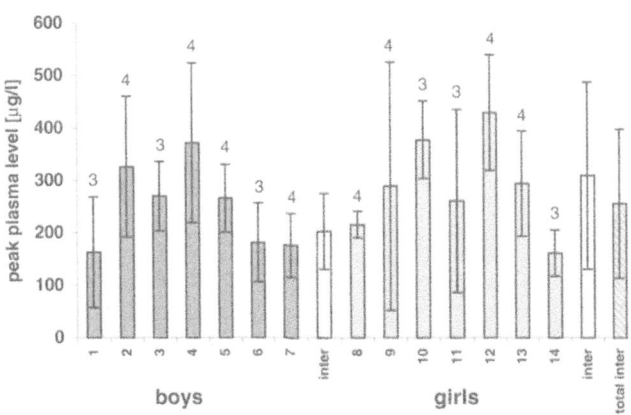

**Fig. 4.** Intra- and interindividual variability of boys and girls in ALL-BFM 95 protocol

further advantage in sampling capillary blood is the good compliance of children to this method.

The optimal time to collect the peak plasma levels has been standardised to the end of infusion between the perfusor alarm and the start of the rinse. No differences between blood sampling into heparinised or EDTA-tubes have been found. An important problem is the short half-life and the instability of doxorubicin (temperature, light) in whole blood after withdrawal. To get veritable measurements rapid preparation and swift cooling is necessary.

In comparison to the literature data from adults the data show similar interindividual fluctuations. There are only few data in the literature estimating the intraindividual variability.

As expected, the consequence of lower dosages and prolonged infusion times are lower peak plasma levels.

With reference to the literature [5] girls have a higher risk to develop a cardiomyopathie as boys. Up to now, the peak plasma levels showed no significant difference between gender. Likewise, great intraindividual fluctuations demonstrated that individual dose adaptation is not feasible.

Supported by the Federal Department of Research and Technology (#1EC9401)

## References

1. Bielack SS et al. (1996) Impact of Scheduling on Toxicity and Clinical Efficacy of Doxorubicin: What Do We Know in the Mid-Nineties?. Eur J Cancer, Vol.32A, No.10, pp 1652-1660
2. Eksborg S et al. (1985) Pharmacokinetic Study of IV Infusions of Adriamycin. Eur J Clin Pharmacol 28: pp 205-212
3. Hempel G et al. (1998) Therapeutic drug monitoring of doxorubicin in paediatric oncology using capillary electrophoresis. Electrophoresis 19: pp 2939-2943
4. Hortobágyi GN (1997) Anthracyclines in the Treatment of Cancer - An Overview. Drugs 54, Suppl. 4: pp 1-7
5. Silber JH et al. (1993) Increased Risc of Cardiac Dysfunction After Anthracyclines in Girls. Medical and Pediatric Oncology 21: pp 477-479

# Pharmacokinetics of Daunorubicin Entrapped in Liposomes or Erythrocytes – Phase II Study in Refractory Acute Leukemias

V. G. Savchenko, E. N. Parovitchnikova, A. A. Skorokhod, T. Z. Garmaeva, V. G. Isaev, A. V. Pivnik, V. M. Vetvitsky and F. I. Attaulakhanov

## Introduction

Anthracyclines are basic cytostatic drugs for the treatment of acute leukemias. Pharmacokinetics of these drugs determins their efficacy. Peak concentration (PC) correlates with response rate, for example in acute myeloid leukemia (AML) [1]. Area under the curve (AUC) parameters of daunorubicin are not optimal due to very fast phase of distribution and slow phase of elimination of the anthracycline. The usage of drug carriers - liposomes and erythrocytes - provides a new tool for overcoming these negative points. It was already proved that liposomal daunorubicin creates very high PC and large AUC [2]. It's also supposed that liposomal formulation of daunorubicin can overcome P-glycoprotein related resistance of leukemic cells [3]. Erythrocytes as carriers of anthracyclines (doxorubicin) were already tested in a small cohort of lymphoma patients, and it was shown that this drug formulation did not create high PC but enlarge AUC [4].

The other side of the efficacy of the anthracyclines is their toxicity, especially cardiotoxicity. It's mostly related to the high peak concentration of the drug leading to the formation of free radicals leading to the damage of cardiomyocytes [5]. It could be avoided by selective accumulation of liposomal daunorubicin in the tumor cells, and more than twice less concentration in myocardiocytes [6,7].

Taking all above mentioned points in consideration the phase II study on comparison of pharmacokinetics, toxicity and tolerability of free, lyposomal (DaunoXome, DX) and erythrocytes entrapped (DEE) daunorubicin in 7+3 like courses for refractory acute leukemias was initiated in our center. It was additionally planned to investigate the pharmacokinetics of 5 day DaunoXome combined with ATRA for relapsed acute promyelocytic leukemias.

## Materials and methods

Since May 1998 till January 1999 3 patients with relapsed and resistant AML were treated with DX, 5 patients (2-ALL,3-AML) with DEE, 2 patients with relapsed APL - with 5-days monotherapy with DX. The pharmacokinetics data on 3 patients with *de novo* AML treated with free daunorubicin (45 mg/m2) served as a control.

DX in 7+3 course was infused at the dose of 100 mg per day (for each patient it constituted _ 50 mg/m2) for three days with ARA-C 100 mg/m2 bid 1-7 days. DEE were prepared by 1 hour (t=37⁰C) incubation of donor or auto erythrocytes with Daunorubicin (45 mg/m2) deluted in 100 ml of saline and infused on the third day of the 7+3 course. 5 days therapy with DX for APL cases was conducted at the dose of 60 mg/m2 per day in combination with ATRA 45 mg/m2.

The samples for drug concentration measurement were collected at the folowing time points: 1, 15, 30 min, 1, 6, 24 hours after infusion of daunorubicin on days 1-3 and following 4-7 days of 7+3 course at the time of anthracyclines infusion. In APL patients the concentration of daunorubicin after DX infusions was also measured in bone marrow (BM) aspirate (day 2 of the course, 4 hours after infusion) and spinal fluid (lumbar pun-

National Research Center for Hematology, Moscow, Russia

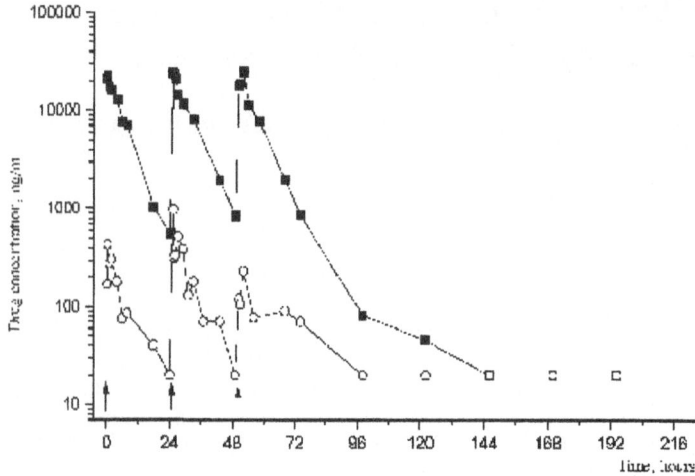

**Fig. 1.** Cumulative plasma concentration curves of free (open circles) and liposomal (black squares) daunorubicin in 7+3 courses. Arrows point the moments of anthracyclines infusions.

cture on day 3 of the course, 4 hours after infusion).

The daunorubicin concentration was measured by spectrofluorometric method in chlorophorm's extracts of plasma, whole blood, bone marrow and spinal fluid [8].

## Results and discussion

Totally there were made 66 sample measurements for 9 infusions in the patients of control group, 66 – for 12 infusions in DX 7+3 group, 72 - in 10 infusions of 5-days DX, 50 - 5 infusions of DEE.

Pharmacokinetics parameters of free and entapped in erythrocytes or liposomes Daunorubicin are shown in Table 1.

DX demonstrated statistically higher peak concentrations at 15 and 30 min time points and AUC parameters (p<0,001) due to slow clearance and prolonged sirculation. No diffe-

rence was noted at time point 1 min after infusion due to wide range of obtained concentration parameters. It's worth of note that there was no accumulation of daunorubicin concentration within three days of DX infusions in 7+3 course (Fig.1). The Figure 1 also demonstrates the difference between the cummulative curves of 3 DX patients and 3 control group patients at start point of 15 min after infusion It's clearly seen that concentration of free daunorubicin is almost 2 logs less than of liposomal form (p<0,001).

Despite higher concentration and prolonged circulation of the drug, DX was better tolerated, less nausea, vomiting were noted comparing with previous free daunorubicin infusions in the same patients. The duration of critical neutropenia (L<1*10⁹/l) after DX containing course was 16 days. In 1 of 2 resistant AML cases (M6, M4) and in 1 relapsed APL CR was attained. High and stable peak consentrations together with prolonged expo-

**Table 1.** Pharmacokinetic parameters of free and encapsulated in erythrocytes and liposomes Daunorubicin

| Form of the drug (number of infusions/patients) | Time of circula-tion, h | T1/2, h ($\alpha$-fast phase) | T 1/2, h ($\beta$-slow phase) | AUC, ng h/ml | Clea-rance ml/min | PC at 1 min ng/ml | PC at 15 min, ng/ml | PC at 30 min, ng/ml |
|---|---|---|---|---|---|---|---|---|
| Free (n=9/3) | 24 | 0,13 | 5, 4 | 6 540 | 245.9 | 19100± 11700 | 665 | 340 |
| DEE (n=6/5) | 92 | 1.4 | 14.3 | 14 556 | 80.8 | 9000± 7400 | 1 410 | 940 |
| DX (n=9/3) | 78 | 4.7 | 16.1 | 205127 | 12.3 | 26 080± 4900 | 21000 | 22700 |

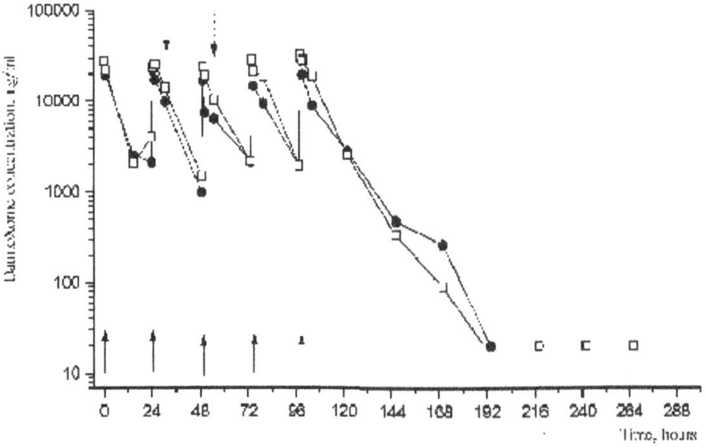

**Fig. 2.** Plasma (open squares) and blood (black circles) concentration of DanuoXome in 5-days course for relapsed APL. Solid arrows point the moments of DX infusions, dotten arrows - time of bone marrow and spinal punctures.

sure of the drug plus possibility to overcome P-glycoprotein resistance create a clear evidence of DX benefits over free daunorubicin. All these suggestions should be proved by following investigations and randomized comparison in *de novo* AML patients.

Peak consentration immediately after infusion (1 min) of DEE did not differ statistically from the free daunorubicin's one, though it seemed to be somewhat less. At 15 and 30 min time points the concentration exceeded the control more than twice. AUC of DEE is 2 times larger than AUC of the free drug and there's a statistical difference. No complications while DEE procedure were noted, infusions of erythrocytes carreing daunorubicin were well tolerated and did not cause the prolongation of neutropenia (15 days). One main negative point exists regarding DEE - manipulations with blood demanding extremely accurate fulfilment of all sanitary-epidemiologic rules. It's still experimental way of anthracyclines infusions and, as it obviously increases the time of drug exposure, it may be used instead of continuous i.v. infusion (pharmacokinetics not yet investigated) thus avoiding infusomats and patients' attachment to i.v. lines. It's also may be a choice for the elderly patients or those with compromised cardiac function or can be used in VAD-like courses for multiple myeloma.

Coming back to pharmacokinetics it should be stressed that peak concentration of daunorubicin at the time point immediately after infusion did not differ in three groups

(p>0,05) and is really high for all three formulations of the drug. All differences appeared after time. So free daunorubicin also provides exrtemely high peak concentrations after infusion but having very short (_7min) α-phase of elimination, it demonstrates quick dramatic decreasement of its levels in blood and plasma.

The 5-days DX infusions combined with ATRA were applied in two relapsed APL patients. The concentration curves for 5-days DX in blood and plasma are shown in Fig.2. This data once more proved the absence of accumulation of DX. In both patients the concentration of daunorubicin after DX infusions in bone marrow (BM) aspirate (day 2 of the course) and spinal fluid (lumbar puncture on day 3 of the course) was measured. It appeared that 4 hour after infusion the concentration of the drug in BM was the same as in blood and plasma. No drug was find in spinal fluid. In both cases CR was achieved after the first course and the treatment is continued with the same 5-days DX. DX may be considered to be the drug of choice for relapsed APL patients as in the most of them the total acceptable dose of daunorubicin have been already reached but they still need anthracyclines as the most effective drugs in these leukemias.

## Conclusions

It's too early to evaluate the durable clinical efficacy and delayed toxic effects of both forms of Daunorubicin but sufficient improvement in pharmacokinetics parameters inspire some optimism regarding these approaches. DX may be used in relapsed leukemia patients with exceeding total acceptable dose of anthracyclines and may be recommended as monotherapy combining with ATRA for APL. DEE may replace prolonged anthracyclines infusions for example in patients with defective myocardial function or in VAD-like courses.

# References

1. Preisler H.D, Gesser T., Azarnia N et al (1984) Relationship between plasma adriamycin levels and outcome of remission induction therapy for acute non-lymphocytic leukemia. Cancer Cemother.Parmacol. 12(2) pp 125-30
2. Gill P.S., Espina B.M., Muggia F et al (1995) Phase I/II clinical and pharmacokinetic evaluation of liposomal daunorubicin. J.Clin.Oncol. v 13 pp 996-1003
3. Verdonck L.F., Lokhorst H.M., Roovers D.J. et al (1998) Multi-drug resistant acute leukemia cells are responsive to prolonged esposure of daunorubicin: implications for liposome-encapsulated daunorubicin Leuk.Res. v 22 N3 pp249-256
4. F.Ataullakhanov,V.Isaev, A.Kohno et al (1997) Pharmacokinetics of doxorubicin in patients with lymphoproliferative disorders after infusion of doxorubicin-loaded erythrocytes. In: U.Sprandel and J.L.Way (eds) "Erythrocytes as drug carriers in medcine" Plenium Press pp.137-142
5. Abraham R., Basser R.L., Green M.D. et al (1996) A risk-benefit assessment of anthracycline antibiotics in antineoplastic therapy. Drug.Saf. v 15 (6) pp 406-29
6. Forssen E.A., Male-Brune R., Adler-Moore S.P. et al (1996) Fluorescence imaging studies for the disposition of daunorubicin liposomes (DaunoXome) within tumor tissue. Cancer Res. v 56 (9) pp 2066-75
7. Richardson D.S., Johnson S.A. (1997) Anthracyclines in hematology: preclinical studies, toxicity, and delivery systems. Blood Rev. v11 (4) pp 201-223
8. Ataullakhanov F., Vetvitsky V., Kovaleva V. (1992) Plenum Press v 326 pp 209-213

# Drug Monitoring During Maintenance Therapy In Children with ALL

T. WESSEL, G. HEMPEL and J. BOOS

*Abstract.* The period of remission maintenance therapy is an important, but less investigated part in the treatment of common
acute lymphoblastic leukaemia (ALL) in
children. In this part of treatment in the ALL-
BFM-Trial the patient has to take daily 6-Mer-
captopurine (6-MP) and weekly Methotrexate
(MTX) orally. The aspect to be examined is
the influence of non-compliance on the patient outcome. Case reports and experiences in
other chronic diseases in children let us presume that there is an unknown high part of
non-compliers. Therefore, we have developed
a new non-invasive method to quantify MTX
and 6-MP in urine with capillary electrophoresis (CE) as an additional assessing method
to investigate the degree of non-compliance.
The analytical method has been validated
and first patient measurements revealed a
case of possible non-compliance.

## Introduction

Therapy protocols in the treatment of common acute lymphoblastic leukaemia (ALL)
are commonly divided into the (three) parts:
induction, consolidation and maintenance
therapy. These scheme has often been modified and changed in the last decades, mainly
in the section of induction and consolidation
therapy. Maintenance therapy is an important, but less investigated part in the treatment of common ALL in children [1]. The
period of remission maintenance therapy to
be investigated in the ALL-BFM 94 protocol
is extended for up to 2.5 years after diagnosis. According to the BFM-ALL 94 treatment
protocol, in this outpatient treatment the
patient has to take daily 6-Mercaptopurine
(6-MP, 50 mg/m2 BSA) and weekly Methotrexate (MTX, 20 mg/m2 BSA) orally, depending on WBC.

## Non-compliance

The aspect to pay more attention on is the
influence of possible non-compliance on the
patient outcome. Compliance is defined
according to R.B. Haynes as the ratio between
the really taken to the prescribed dose. A
similar used term is adherence.. O`Hanrahan
and O`Malley define the problem by sug-
gesting it to be "when failure to comply is sufficient to interfere appreciable with achieving
the therapeutic goal" [2]. At present, it is
unknown if a given number of missed tablets
can substantially increase the risk of disease
relapse. As tolerable is commonly accepted a
maximum of 5% of lacking doses until the
degree and extent of non-compliance is more
completely understood and it is possible to
define the threshold of compliance more precisely [3].

Case reports and experience in other chronic diseases in children (e.g., *diabetes mellitus*
[4], *juvenile chronic arthritis* [5]) let us presume that there is an unknown high part of
non-compliers. In these reports the presumed
or investigated medication non-compliance
ranges from 10 up to 42% and first improvements for correction are examined. The range
of estimated non-compliance in the few investigations on children with acute leukaemia
were: 19-42% for urinary assessing, 10-40%

Klinik und Poliklinik für Kinderheilkunde, Pädiatrische Hämatologie/Onkologie, Albert-Schweitzer-Str. 33,
D-48129 Muenster Germany ())

for plasma assessing and 20-30% for inter-view assessing [3].

Until now, there is no sufficient examination about this problem in the area of a multi-center german treatment protocol for acute leukaemia. Therefore, we developed a new and additional non-invasive instrument for direct assessing non-compliance in urine. The method allows simultaneous urine measurements of 6-Mercaptopurine (6-MP), Methotrexate (MTX) and Sulfamethoxazole (SMX). Urine rather than blood was selected because of ease of the collection in children.

### Drug monitoring in urine with CE

Drug monitoring is a rapidly developing area in the clinical laboratory. To be effective, drug monitoring requires the valid acquisition of specimens followed by routine, timely, and reliable determinations of the drug concentrations. The use of CE for clinically relevant assays is attractive since it presents several advantages over contemporary methods.

CE involves a separation of charged molecules in a buffer-filled capillary by the application of a high voltage. The outstanding characteristic of CE is the high separation efficiency which can be achieved. $10^6$ theoretical plates are able to be attained at an applied voltage of 30 kV. This allows an analysis time in the order of a few minutes [6]. The use of CE results in high speed, on-line sample pretreatment if necessary and automatic separation and quantification. These aspects will probably make CE the most attractive technique for routine and emergency analysis of drugs. Furthermore it is possible to perform single-step analyses, with direct injection of body fluids on-column. This is quite often feasible in CE because the open capillary columns are less prone to irreversible modification by sample matrix components than a packed HPLC column and there are few limits on the use of aggressive cleaning steps which can be taken. Urine contains many components, including high concentrations of ions, and pushes the resolving power of CE to the limits. Nevertheless, drug analyses in urine with direct injection has the advantage that the time and effort of extraction procedures are eliminated [7].

A clear relationship between plasma area under the curve (AUC)/ plasma concentration and the 24-h urinary excretion of the unchanged drugs for 6-MP (r = 0.9381, p < 0.01) [8] and for MTX (r = 0.7, p < 0.001; on day 2 and 7) has been published, respectively [9]. Focussing on urine-data, therefore, seems to be easy and representative. As an additional parameter we focus on Sulfamethoxazole (SMX), which is frequently used together with Trimethoprim for P. carinii prophylaxis. An aliquot of 1.5 ml from the 12-h sample is sufficient for the determination of the amount of unchanged drug excreted after dose.

### Experimental

For the detection a Beckman P/ACE 5510 capillary electrophoresis system was used. To avoid the difficulty of peak identification in the direct analysis of urine, a diode-array-detector (DAD) was used. DAD allows a simultaneous detection of Sulfamethoxazole at 254 nm, Methotrexate and 6-Mercaptopurine at 310 nm (absorption maxima: SMX 255 nm, MTX 300 nm, 6-MP 314 nm). The possibility of multi-wavelength scans can be used for peak identification and for the estimation of peak purity.

Untreated fused silica capillaries with an inner diameter of 50 µm and an effective length of 30 cm were used (Beckman). The running buffer contained 60 µM Borate at pH 9.7. The capillary was rinsed between the runs with 100 mM NaOH and the running buffer for 2 minutes. Separation was performed at 400 V/cm (14.8 kV), with a current of 78 µA and a running time of less than 20 minutes. The sample injection was done by pressure (0.5 psi) for 10 seconds.

A sample preparation is not necessary and 25µl of the Internal Standard (I.S.: Methylmercaptopurine, 7.16 mg/ml) have to be added to 1500 µl of the sample. The urine samples were collected over night for 12 h before the next ambulatory examination date. To asses long-term compliance, additional measurements were done of the major toxic metabolites of 6-MP and MTX (E-6-TGN and E-MTX) in erythrocytes.

## Results and discussion

For quantification 6 different spiked urine-samples in a range of: 7 – 164 µM MTX, 10 – 200 µM 6-MP and 10 – 199 µM SMX were analysed. The calibration graphs were calculated from the corrected peak area-data by the method of weighted last square regression. The data for the quantification of spiked urine-samples are in accordance with the international standards concerning reproducibility and precision. The limits of quantification are 12 µM for MTX, 17 µM for 6-MP and 14 µM for SMX, respectively. The limits of detection are 5 µM for both MTX and SMX and 10 µM for 6-MP, respectively.

Up to now the method has been applied to samples from 11 patients. The data of two of them are demonstrated beneath. Fig. 1 and 2 shows two typical treatment histories of maintenance therapy of two children with ALL. The patient in Fig. 1 shows the clear attempt to reach the given target: <3000/µl leukocytes by dose escalation of MTX and 6-

MP. Striking at the patient in Fig. 1 is the treatment history and, on the other hand, a very high and stabilised WBC. Our urine measurements revealed low MTX, 6-MP and SMX values (absolute: 22 µM, 23 µM, <14 µM; in % of given dose: 10%, 1.2%, 0.6%) which is in accordance to the results of MTX and 6-MP metabolites levels in erythrocytes. In addition, the low E-MTX (3.8 nmol/mmol Hb) and the low E-6TGN (170 nmol/mmol Hb) data, as indicator of long-term compliance, indicates possible non-compliance, too.

In contrast, the patient in Fig.2 has an unconspicuous treatment history and urine levels (absolute: 49 µM MTX, 25 µM 6-MP, 27 µM SMX; in % of given dose: 76%, 5.5%, 1.7%). The patient in Fig.1 was treated with 50 mg MTX/w, 150 mg 6-MP/d and 240 mg SMX (1.4 m$^2$ BSA, intended regimen dose: 28 mg MTX/w, 71 mg 6-MP/d)

The patient in Fig. 2 was treated with 17.5 mg MTX/w, 50 mg 6-MP and 240 mg SMX (1.6 m$^2$ BSA, intended regimen dose:32 mg MTX/w, 80 mg 6-MP/d), respectively.

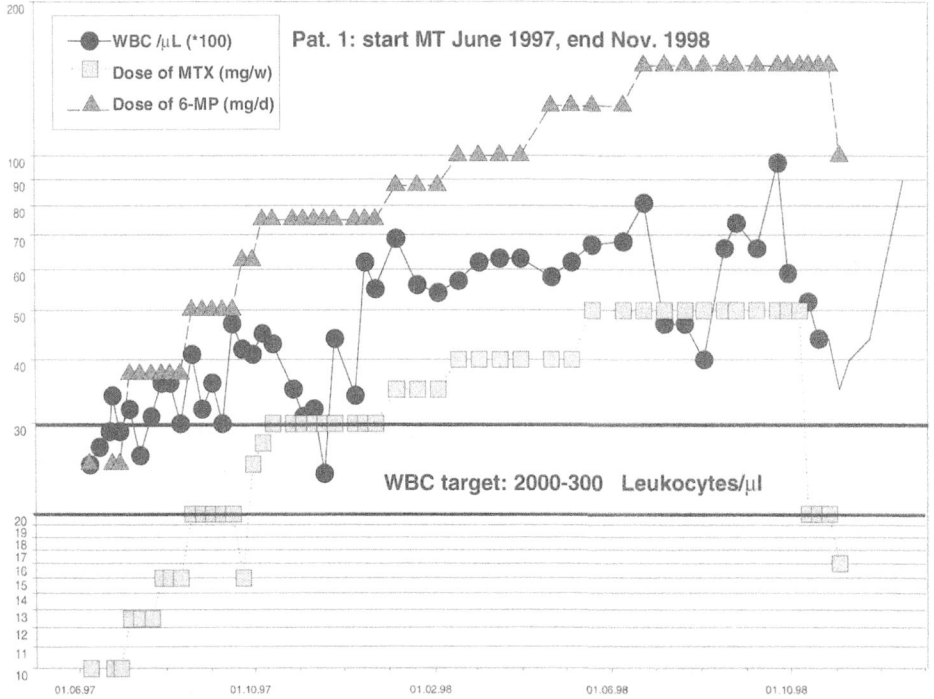

**Fig. 1.** Maintenance therapy treatment history of a patient with ALL suspicious to be non-compliant. Demonstrated are the WBC and the prescribed doses of MTX and 6-MP.

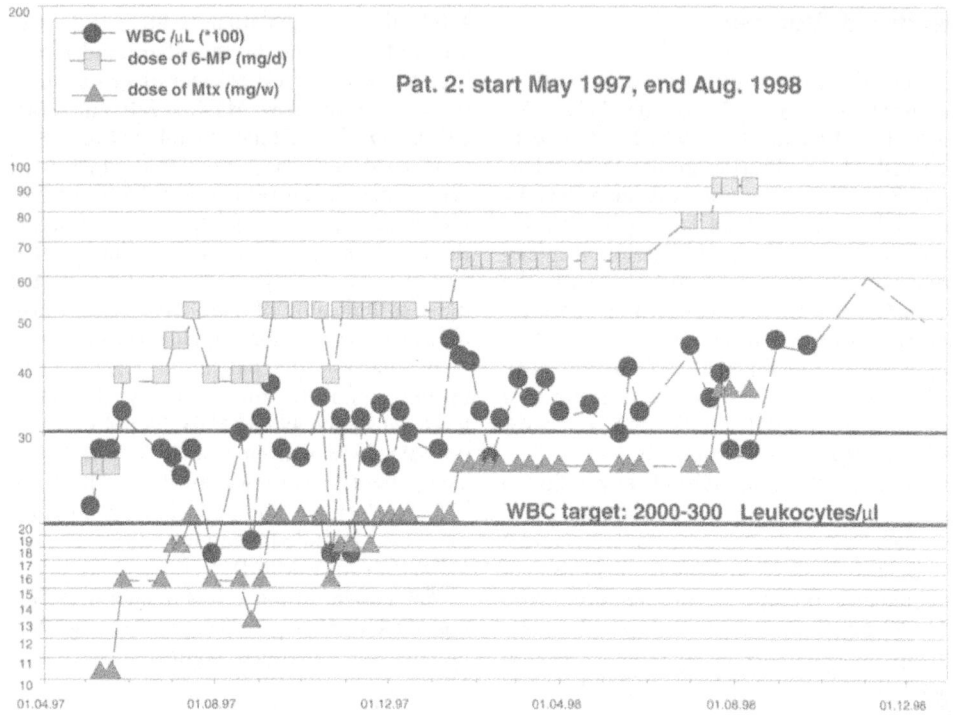

**Fig. 2.** This maintenance therapy treatment history demonstrates an patient to be unconspicuous of non-compliance.

The antimetabolite 6-MP, an analogue of hypoxanthine, is now used in combination with MTX in the treatment of ALL, in rheumatic diseases and in bowel disease, e.g. Morbus Crohn. The bioavailability of 6-MP is poor and highly variable between and within patients when studied on multiple occasion (5-37% in patient with ALL). This is due to the hydrolysis mediated by the enzyme xanthine oxidase which is abundant in the liver. 2-8 % percent of the given dose are excreted as the unchanged drug, mostly by renal excretion within twelve hours [10].

The antifolate MTX is the other important component in the maintenance therapy regimens used in childhood acute lymphoblastic leukaemia. Numerous factors can influence the pharmacokinetics of MTX (including age, renal function and hydration) leading to large interpatient variability [11].

At low dose MTX is excreted predominately unchanged by renal excretion (2-15 mg/kg: 40-50%, 150 mg/kg: 90%). The bioa-

vailability reaches up to 100 % (at 30mg/m2 BSA) [12].

In patient treated for rheumatoid arthritis with low dose MTX (15 mg/m2 BSA) Seideman et al. found that MTX was mainly excreted in urine as intact drug. The median 24 h recovery was 80.5 % following oral administration [13].

Macdougall et al. detected 6-MP in 81% of first morning urine samples, indicating compliance with medication the preceding evening. But she recommends to consider that the absence of 6-MP in the urine samples does not necessarily indicate poor compliance because of the variability in 6-MP excretion and unpredictable night voiding in children. The average for the oral dose excreted unchanged was 5.6% ± 3.3% (6-MP dose: 73.6 ± 16.7 mg) [14]. The significance of drug compliance as a variable factor in the long-term prognosis is receiving increasing attention and the monitoring of blood or urine levels has been advocated [3]. Therefore we developed and validated a robust, non-invasive and simple method for the simultaneous detection of Methotrexate, 6-Mercaptopurine and Sulfamethoxazole in urine. Urine can be given directly to the capillary without preparation by pressure injection. A linear correlation in the range of 20–200 μM between the concentration and peak area for each substance was found. Separation is performed within 20 minutes. The problem of the variability in 6-MP and MTX excretion will be reduced by repeated measurements of the same patient over time. To assess long-term compliance in children with repeatedly negative samples, we cooperate with Mr. Schmiegelow`s laboratory in Copenhagen. They measured the erythrocyte concentration of MTX polyglutamates and 6-thioguanine nucleotides (E-6-TGN and E-MTX) mentioned above, the respective major cytotoxic metabolites of 6-MP and MTX. During maintenance therapy, E-MTX and E-6-TGN accumulate intracellularly, also in erythrocytes, and this can be used as an indicator of long-term compliance [15].

The CE method described here can be used as an additional assessing method to detect possible short-term non-compliance and to control sufficient medication in the maintenance therapy of children with acute leukaemia's. Currently we are testing this method in clinical practice together with other methods for assessing non-compliance like electronic monitoring devices (MEMS®) [16], interviews and diaries.

The authors wish to thank Mr. K. Schmiegelow, Copenhagen for measuring the erythrocyte-metabolites and for classifying the results.

This work was funded by the Bundesministerium für Forschung und Technologie (#1EC94041).

## References

1. Hoelzer D, Seipelt G (1998) Leukämietherapie. Uni-med Verlag, Bremen
2. O'Hanrahan M, O'Malley K (1981) Compliance with drug treatment. British Medical Journal, 283:298-300
3. Davies-HA et al. (1995) Compliance with oral chemotherapy in childhood lymphoblastic leukaemia. Cancer Treatment Reviews, 21:93-103
4. Blanz B (1994) Die psychischen Folgen chronischer Krankheiten im Kindes- und Jugendalter. In Petermann F (ed) Chronische Krankheiten bei Kindern und Jugendlichen. Quintessenz, Berlin, pp 11-28
5. Wiedebusch S (1994) Langzeitcompliance im Kindesalter - am Beispiel der juvenilen chronischen Arthritis. In Petermann F (ed) Chronische Krankheiten bei Kindern und Jugendlichen. Quintessenz, Berlin, pp 37-46
6. Jenkins MA, Guerin MD (1996) Capillary electrophoresis as a clinical tool. Journal of Chromatography B, 682:23-34
7. Lloyd DK (1996) Capillary electrophoretic analyses of drugs in body fluids: sample pre-treatment and methods for direct injection of biofluids. Journal of Chromatography A, 735:29-42
8. Skoglund-AK et al. (1994) Plasma and urine levels of MTX and 7-OH-MTX in children with ALL during maintenance therapy with weekly oral MTX. Medical and Pediatric Oncology, 22:187-93
9. Endresen-L et al. (1990) Pharmacokinetics of oral 6-MP: Relationship between plasma levels and urine excretion of parent drug. Therapeutic Drug Monitoring, 12:227-34
10. Schäfer-Korting M (1993) Mercaptopurin. In Hartke H, Mutschler E (Eds) DAB 10 Kommentar. Wissenschaftliche Verlagsgesellschaft, Stuttgart, M 45, p 4
11. Masson E, Zamboni WC (1997) Pharmacokinetic optimisation of cancer chemotherapy. Clinical Pharmacokinetics, 32 (4): 324-343
12. Schäfer-Korting M: Methotrexat. In Hartke H, Mutschler E (Eds), DAB 10 Kommentar, Wissenschaftliche Verlagsgesellschaft, Stuttgart, M 56, pp 4-7
13. Seideman P, Beck O, Eksborg S, Wennberg M (1993) The pharmacokinetics of methotrexate and 7-hydroxy metabolite in patients with rheumatoid arthritis. British Journal of Clinical Pharmacology, 35:409-412
14. Macdougall LG, McElligott SE, Ross E, Greeff MC, Poole JE (1992) Pattern of 6-Mercaptopurine urinary excretion in children with Acute Lymphoblastic Leukemia: Urinary assays as a measure of drug compliance. Therapeutic Drug Monitoring, 14:371-375
15. Schmiegelow K, Schrøder H, Schmiegelow M (1994) Methotrexate and 6-mercaptopurine maintenance therapy for childhood acute lymphoblastic leukemia: dose adjustments by white cell counts or pharmacokinetic parameters? Cancer Chemotherapy and Pharmacology, 34:209-215
16. Lau RCW et al. (1998) Electronic measurements of compliance with 6-MP in pediatric patients with ALL. Medical and Pediatric Oncology, 30:85-90

# Modulation of Glucocorticoid Resistance in Childhood Acute Lymphoblastic Leukemia; Preliminary Results

E.G. Haarman[1], G.J.L. Kaspers[1], R. Pieters[2], M.M.A. Rottier[1] and A.J.P. Veerman[1]

*Abstract.* Glucocorticoid (GC) resistance is a major adverse prognostic factor in childhood acute lymphoblastic leukemia (ALL). Cell line studies have elucidated several mechanisms of GC resistance and corresponding possibilities to modulate or circumvent this phenomenon. In the present study we evaluated whether in vitro GC resistance, as determined by the MTT assay, could be modulated by meta-iodobenzylguanidine (MIBG; increases receptor/hormone binding), 5-aza-2'-deoxy-cytidine (5-AZA; decreases DNA-methylation), buthionine sulfoximine (BSO; reduces glutathione-levels), ethacrynic acid (ETH; inhibits glutathione-S-transferase) and 3-aminobenzamide (3-AB; inhibits poly-(ADP)-ribose-polymerase). All modulators showed dose dependent antileukemic activity in vitro when tested as single agents at 6 concentrations in 12 patients. Next, eighteen ALL samples taken at initial diagnosis (iALL) and 1 taken at relapse (rALL) were incubated with two concentrations of the modulators and two concentrations of dexamethasone (DXM) both separately and in combination during 4 days in triplicate. We determined the additive leukemic cell kill (extra cell kill after co-incubation compared to that induced by DXM alone) and the extent of synergism (leukemic cell kill after co-incubation with correction for the cell kill by the modulator and DXM alone). MIBG, 5-AZA and 3-AB respectively showed a dose-dependent additive leukemic cell kill in 12 out of 19 samples (up to 49% extra cell kill; in 3 samples (up to 49%) synergism), in 13 out of 16 samples (up to 37% extra cell kill; in 1 sample (up to 27%) synergism) and in 4 out of 11 samples (up to 56% extra cell kill; in 1 sample (up to 11%) synergism). All samples in which we found synergism were intermediately or highly resistant to glucocorticoids. BSO and ETH did not induce any significant additive leukemic cell kill. In conclusion, both MIBG and 5-AZA induced additive cell kill after co-incubation in the majority of patient samples and in a small sub-group synergism was found, predominantly induced by MIBG. (Supported by the Dutch Cancer Society, VU 97-1564.)

## Introduction

Glucocorticoid (GC) resistance, when assessed clinically or in vitro, is a major adverse prognostic factor in childhood acute lymphoblastic leukemia (ALL) [11, 12, 16, 22]. Moreover acute myeloid leukemia patients and patients suffering from relapsed ALL, subgroups with a relatively poor prognosis [9], are at least 75 fold more resistant in vitro to prednisolone and dexamethasone [8, 15].

As GC resistance has a major impact on the success of chemotherapy, it is of clinical importance to identify possibilities to modulate or circumvent this type of drug resistance. Cell line studies have elucidated several mechanisms of GC resistance and corresponding strategies for modulation.

MIBG is an analogue of the neurotransmitter norepinephrine and is used in its radio-iodinated form as radiopharmaceutical in the diagnosis and treatment of neuroectodermal tumors [4, 6]. MIBG is also a selective inhibitor of mono-ADP-ribosylation [26]. Treatment of the L1210 cells with MIBG

---

[1] Department of Pediatric Hematology/Oncology, University Hospital Vrije Universiteit, De Boelelaan 1117, 1081 HV, Amsterdam, The Netherlands.
[2] Dept. of Pediatric Hematology/Oncology, Sophia Children Hospital, Dr. Molewaterplein 60, 3015 GJ Rotterdam, The Netherlands.

increased the total number of GC-binding sites, enhanced the affinity of the receptor to DXM and restored glucocorticoid sensitivity [25].

Gasson et al. described a thymic lymphoma cell line in which DNA methylation was associated with the acquisition of glucocorticoid resistance [3]. Hypomethylation induced by 5-azacytidine (an analogue of 5-aza-2'-deoxycytidine) restored glucocorticoid sensitivity. 5-aza-2'-deoxycytidine (5-AZA) may also induce differentiation of leukemic cells and has been reported to down-regulate c-myc expression (an anti-apoptotic oncoprotein) [18], which adds to the potential value of this drug.

Glutathione (GSH) and glutathione-S-transferases have also been implicated in glucocorticoid resistance. In one study raised GSH levels were correlated with in vitro drug resistance against prednisolone, among other drugs, in ALL cases [17]. Hall et al. reported a significantly worse prognosis in case of GST mu positivity [5]. It is of particular interest that the levels of these compounds can be modulated [20]. Ethacrynic acid (ETH) inhibits GST by blocking the substrate binding site. Buthionine sulfoximine (BSO) depletes GSH levels by the specific inhibition of gamma-glutamyl-cysteine synthetase; a key enzyme in the GSH synthesis.

Studies on cell lines have demonstrated the role of DNA repair in glucocorticoid-induced cell lysis, mainly by showing that inhibition of poly(ADP-ribose) polymerase (PARP) assisted DNA repair potentiated the glucocorticoid-induced cell lysis of lymphoid cells [28]. This suggests that 3-AB, an inhibitor of PARP, may be of value in potentiating glucocorticoid induced cell lysis in patient samples.

In this study we tested whether in vitro glucocorticoid resistance as determined by the MTT assay could be modulated in pediatric ALL samples using MIBG, 5-AZA, BSO, ETH and 3-AB.

## Materials and methods

### Leukemic samples

Fresh leukemic samples were obtained from bone marrow or peripheral blood taken for routine diagnostic procedures from 30 iALL patients and 1 rALL patient. Twelve samples were used to determine the in vitro cytotoxicity of each modulator separately, 19 samples (including the rALL sample) were used to determine the in vitro modulating effects of the compounds tested. Mononuclear cells were isolated by Ficoll density gradient centrifugation (Ficoll Paque, density 1.077g/ml; Pharmacia, Sweden) for 15 minutes (room temperature, 1000g). Next cells were washed twice in RPMI 1640 (Dutch modification, Gibco, Uxbridge, UK) with 10 minute periods of centrifugation at 300g and resuspended in cell culture medium containing supplements as previously described [21]. Cytospins were prepared by centrifugating 50 µl aliquots of 2 x 10^6 cells/ml leukemic cell suspension for 7 minutes at 50g. Cytospins were air dried, fixed for 3 minutes in methanol and stained with May-Grünwald-Giemsa. We counted 200 cells using a light microscope to determine the proportion of malignant cells of each sample. All samples contained >80% blasts at the start of cell culture.

### Preparation of drug solutions

We prepared 96-well microculture plates containing 20 µl aliquots of drug solution and stored them at –80ºC. First we tested the in vitro cytotoxicity of each modulator separately in order to determine the concentrations inducing a median cell kill of approximately 10-20%; concentrations potent enough to have biological effects and influence cell survival, but not inducing cell kill to such an extent that modulating effects cannot be determined. The following final concentrations were tested: 5-AZA 2.44, 9.77, 39, 156, 625, 2500 µg/ml; BSO and 3-AB 1.95, 7.8, 31, 125, 500, 2000 µg/ml; ETH 0.031, 0.125, 0.5, 2, 8, 32 µg/ml and MIBG 1.25, 2.5, 5, 10, 20, 40 µg/ml. Next 96-well microculture plates were prepared containing 20 µl aliquots of the selected concentrations of the modulators and two concentrations of DXM (0.012 and 0.75 µg/ml; concentrations known to induce a limited amount of cell kill in sensitive and resistant leukemic cells after 4 days culturing respectively) both in combination and separately in triplicate.

## In vitro leukemic cell kill

In vitro drug cytotoxicity was determined using the MTT assay. The assay conditions were essentially the same as previously described [21]. Briefly, aliquots of 80 µl cell suspension were added to 96-well microculture plates containing 20 µl aliquots of drug solutions. Leukemic cells were incubated at 37°C during 4 days. Eight wells with cells in medium without drugs were used to determine the control cell survival. May-Grünwald-Giemsa stained cytospins of control cells showed that all samples contained ≥70% blasts after 4 days culturing, which is required for reliable test-results [10]. Next, we added 10 µl of 5 mg/ml MTT (Sigma) to each well. The microculture plates were shaken gently for 1 minute and incubated for 6 hours. The yellow tetrazolium salt MTT is reduced to dark colored formazan by viable cells only. Formazan crystals were dissolved in 100 µl acidified isopropanol. The optical density (OD) was measured at 565 nm with an EL-312 microplate reader (Biotek Instruments Inc., Winooski, USA). The OD is linearly related to the number of viable cells. After correction for the optical density of the culture medium, leukemic cell survival (LCS) was calculated as follows:

$$LCS = (OD_{\text{drug-exposed well}}) / (\text{mean } OD_{\text{control wells}}) \times 100\%.$$

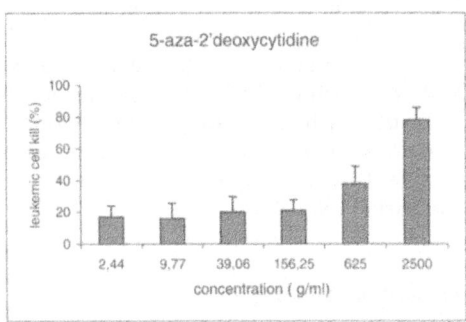

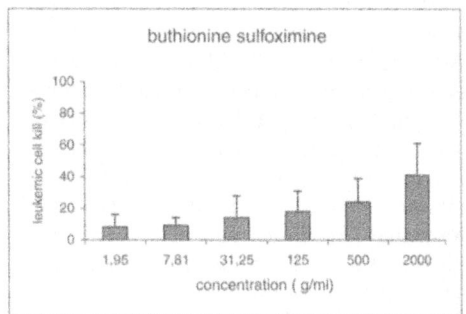

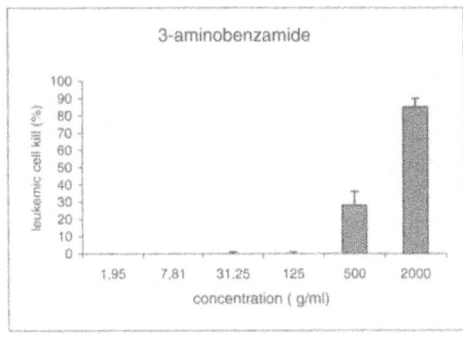

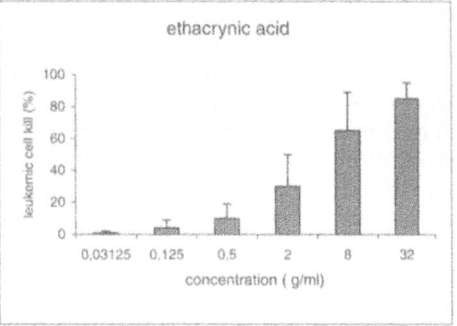

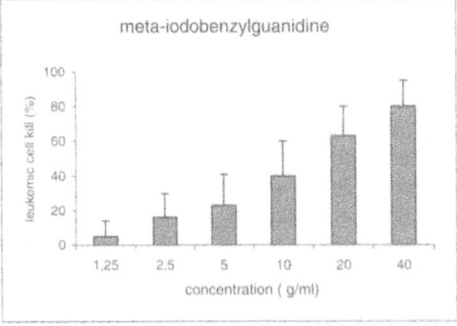

**Fig. 1.** In vitro cytotoxicity of the modulators tested. Bars represent median % LCK, vertical lines represent 75th percentiles. Two concentrations were selected for the modulation study: 5-aza 2.4 µg/ml and 39 µg/ml, BSO 1.95 µg/ml and 31 µg/ml, 3-AB 250 µg/ml and 500 µg/ml, ETH 0.5 µg/ml and 1.0 µg/ml and MIBG 2.5 µg/ml and 5 µg/ml.

By comparing leukemic cell kill (LCK=100-LCS) in wells containing DXM with LCK in wells containing the modulator and wells containing both DXM and the modulator, we were able to calculate any additive leukemic cell kill or synergism. The extent of additive leukemic cell kill was defined as the extra cell kill after co-incubation compared to that induced by DXM alone (=$LCK_{DXM+modulator}$ - $LCK_{DXM}$). ($LCK_{DXM+modulator}$ - $LCK_{DXM}<0$). The extra cell kill after co-incubation with correction for the cell kill by the modulators and DXM alone was defined as the extent of synergism. Example: for DXM LCK=30%, for the modulator LCK=20% and after co-incubation LCK= 60%. Based on the LCK induced by the single agents we would expect to find a LCK of 44% (DXM kills 30% of the blasts, of the remaining 70% the modulator kills 20%; 56% of the cells survive theoretically). After co-incubation a LCK of 60% was observed, thus 60-44=16% synergism. In each patient sample 4 combinations of DXM and the modulators were tested (2 concentrations DXM, 2 concentrations modulator. We defined that the modulator induced leukemic cell kill additi-

vely or synergistically respectively in a specific sample, if in at least 3 combinations additive leukemic cell kill or synergism was found.

## Results

### In vitro antileukemic activity

The antileukemic activity of each modulator separately was tested in 12 iALL samples. A dose-dependent leukemic cell kill was observed for all modulators. Median leukemic cell kill increased gradually for MIBG from 5% at 1.25 µg/ml MIBG to 80% at 40 µg/ml, for 5-AZA from 18% at 2.44 µg/ml to 78% at 2500 µg/ml, for BSO from 7% at 1.95 µg/ml to 42% at 2000 µg/ml, for ETH from 1% at 0.031 µg/ml to 83% at 32 µg/ml and for 3-AB from 0% at 1.95 µg/ml to 82% at 2000 µg/ml (Fig.1). For the modulation studies we used he following concentrations: 5-AZA 2.4 µg/ml and 39 µg/ml, BSO 1.95 µg/ml and 31 µg/ml, ETH 0.5 µg/ml and 1 µg/ml, 3-AB 250 µg/ml and 500 µg/ml and MIBG 2.5 µg/ml and 5 µg/ml.

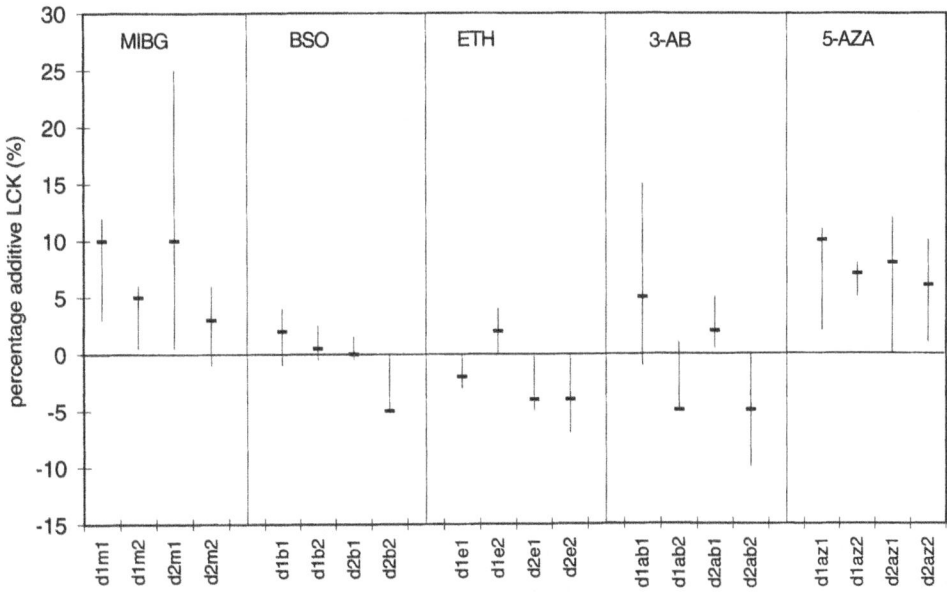

**Fig. 2.** Median additional cell kill after co-incubation for each drug combination. Vertical lines represent the 25th and 75th percentiles; d=DXM, m=MIBG, b=BSO, e=ETH, ab=3-AB, az=5-AZA, 1=high concentration, 2=low concentration.

### Additive leukemic cell kill

MIBG, 5-AZA and 3-AB showed a dose-dependent additive leukemic cell kill in 12 out of 19 samples (up to 49%), 13 out of 16 samples (up to 37%) and 4 out of 11 samples (up to 56%). ETH and BSO did not induce significant additive leukemic cell kill. The median additive leukemic cell kill after co-incubation for each drug combination is summarized in Fig. 2.

### Synergism

In 5 patients synergism was observed (Table 1). MIBG and DXM induced LCK synergistically in 4/19 samples (up to 49%), 5-AZA in 1/16 (up to 27%) and 3-AB in 1/11 samples (up to 11%). The extent of synergism was higher at higher concentrations of the modulators. All samples in which we observed synergism, were intermediately or highly resistant in vitro to glucocorticoids as indicated in Table 1.

**Table 1.** Modulation observed in patient samples. Indicated are [1]the expected leukemic cell kill (based on the leukemic cell kill by the modulator and DXM as single agents; see materials and methods), [2]the observed leukemic cell kill after co-incubation and [3]the extent of synergism (=observed LCK – expected LCK). Indicated is if the sample is resistant (R), intermediately resistant (I) or sensitive (S) to glucocorticoid induced cell kill (MTT assay).

| | [1]expected | $MIBG_{high}$ [2]observed | [3]synergism | [1]expected | $MIBG_{low}$ [2]observed | [3]synergism | Glucocorticoid resistance |
|---|---|---|---|---|---|---|---|
| 9130 | | | | | | | R |
| $DXM_{high}$ | 39 | 41 | 2 | 25 | 23 | -2 | |
| $DXM_{low}$ | 38 | 48 | 10 | 24 | 25 | 1 | |
| 9134 | | | | | | | I |
| $DXM_{high}$ | 85 | 88 | 3 | 80 | 86 | 6 | |
| $DXM_{low}$ | 50 | 66 | 16 | 31 | 48 | 17 | |
| 9139 | | | | | | | R |
| $DXM_{high}$ | 0 | 49 | 49 | 0 | 33 | 33 | |
| $DXM_{low}$ | 2 | 11 | 9 | 2 | 0 | -2 | |
| 9312 | | | | | | | R |
| $DXM_{high}$ | 55 | 70 | 15 | 47 | 52 | 5 | |
| $DXM_{low}$ | 31 | 40 | 9 | 20 | 24 | 4 | |

| | [1]expected | $AZA_{high}$ [2]observed | [3]synergism | [1]expected | $AZA_{low}$ [2]observed | [3]synergism | |
|---|---|---|---|---|---|---|---|
| 9139 | | | | | | | R |
| $DXM_{high}$ | 10 | 37 | 27 | 0 | 13 | 13 | |
| $DXM_{low}$ | 12 | 18 | 3 | 2 | 8 | 6 | |

| | [1]expected | $3Ab_{high}$ [2]observed | [3]synergism | [1]expected | $3Ab_{low}$ [2]observed | [3]synergism | |
|---|---|---|---|---|---|---|---|
| 9127 | | | | | | | I |
| $DXM_{high}$ | 79 | 82 | 3 | 77 | 79 | 2 | |
| $DXM_{low}$ | 39 | 50 | 11 | 35 | 35 | 0 | |

## Discussion

Glucocorticoid resistance is a major adverse prognostic factor in childhood ALL [11, 12, 16, 22]. Cell line studies have elucidated several mechanisms of and corresponding possibilities for modulating GC resistance. However studies on patient samples, apart from one study performed within our laboratory by Klumper et al., have not yet been performed [14]. In the present study we tested the in vitro modulating effects of MIBG, 5-AZA, BSO, ETH and 3-AB in childhood ALL samples.

Each modulator as a single agent induced in vitro cytotoxicity dose dependently. Previously it has been demonstrated that MIBG displayed cytotoxic properties in a large panel of histogenetically different cell lines, including a L1210 leukemia cell line [24]. Also 5-aza and BSO are known to induce leukemic cell kill, both in vivo and in vitro [1, 18, 23]. Initial studies conducted by Nagourney et al. with ETH showed that 1 µg/ml was toxic to a substantial number of adult leukemic specimens in vitro[19]. In the present study we also found that ETH was cytotoxic to pediatric leukemic blasts. 3-AB displayed cytotoxic properties only at the highest concentrations.

After co-incubation of DXM with ETH or BSO, no additive leukemic cell kill or synergism was observed. Recent studies performed within our laboratory showed that expression levels of GSTα, µ and π class were not correlated with in vitro glucocorticoid resistance [2]. In addition no correlation was found between GSH expression levels and in vitro GC resistance [13]. Based on these results it seems less likely that GSH and GSTs are involved in GC resistance in childhood ALL.

MIBG induced additive leukemic cell kill in 12/19 patients, and in 4/19 patients synergism was observed. These results are in agreement with data previously reported by Klumper et al., who showed that MIBG and prednisolone induced cytotoxicity synergistically in 3/13 samples and further support the previously proposed hypothesis that increased ADP-ribosylation inhibits GC receptor activity [7, 14, 25, 27]. This modulatory effect may be of clinical relevance as all samples in which we found modulation were intermediately or highly resistant to GC induced cell kill.

3-AB induced additive leukemic cell kill in 4/11 patients and in 1 patient modulation was observed to a limited extent (up to 11%). These results are suggestive that DNA damage is a terminal, rather than a causative step in glucocorticoid induced apoptosis in childhood ALL. In other words, DNA fragmentation may be an apoptotic phenomenon occurring at a moment when cell death is already inevitable, whereas other (earlier) processes, like mitochondrial depolarization, determine whether the leukemic cell dies. Inhibition of DNA repair may therefore not result in potentiation of apoptosis inducing agents like glucocorticoids.

5-aza-2'-deoxycytidine not only induced leukemic cell death as a single agent, but also induced additive leukemic cell kill after co-incubation with DXM in 13/16 samples (up to 37%). However synergism was only observed in 1 sample. Therefore it seems less likely that DNA methylation is involved in the development of GC resistance in childhood ALL.

In summary, though all of the modulators were cytotoxic to leukemic cells as single agents, only MIBG and 5-AZA induced additive leukemic cell kill in a majority of patients after co-incubation with DXM. Synergism was observed in a small subgroup of patients (all intermediately or highly resistant to GC induced cell kill), predominantly induced by MIBG. These results do not provide evidence that regulation of intracellular redox state, DNA-methylation or DNA-repair are major mechanisms involved in GC resistance in childhood ALL. ADP ribosylation however, may be involved as a negative regulator of GC receptor activity. Further studies have to point out whether treatment of pediatric leukemic cells with MIBG is associated with alterations in GR status. In addition, we will test the modulators in rALL and AML samples, subgroups known to be highly resistant to GC induced cell kill. Finally, we will test whether pre-exposure of leukemic cells to the modulators influences DXM cytotoxicity differentially compared to the co-incubation described in present study.

*Acknowledgements.* This work is supported by The Dutch Cancer Society (grant VU 97-1564)

# References

1. Curtis JE, Hedley DW, Minden MD, McCulloch EA (1999) Antileukemic effects of buthionine sulfoximine (BSO) (NSC326231) in vivo. Ann Haematol 78 (Suppl II): 36 (abstract)

2. Den Boer ML, Pieters R, Kazemier KM, Janka-Schaub GE, Henze G, Creutzig U, Kaspers GJL, Kearns PR, Hall AG, Pearson ADJ, Veerman AJP (1999) Different expression of glutathione S-transferase alpha, mu and pi in childhood acute lymphoblastic and myeloid leukemia. Br J Haem 104: 321–327

3. Gasson JC, Ryden T, Bourgeois S (1983) Role of de novo DNA methylation in the glucocorticoid resistance of a T lymphoid cell line. Nature 302: 621–623

4. Gelfand MJ (1993) Metaiodobenzylguanidine in children. Sem Nucl Med 23: 231–241

5. Hall AG, Autzen P, Cattan AR, Malcolm AJ, Cole M, Kernahan J, Reid MM (1994) Expression of mu class glutathione S-transferases correlates with event-free survival in childhood acute lymphoblastic leukemia. Cancer Res 54: 5251–5254

6. Hoefnagel CA (1994) Metaiodobenzylguanidine and somatostatin in oncology: role in the management of neural crest tumors. Eur J Nucl Med 21: 561–581

7. Johnson GS, Ralhan R (1986) Glucocorticoid agonists as well as antagonists are effective inducers of mouse mammary tumor virus RNA in mouse mammary tumor cells treated with inhibitors of ADP-ribosylation. J Cell Physiol 129: 36–42

8. Kaspers GJ, Kardos G, Pieters R, Van Zantwijk CH, Klumper E, Hählen K, de Waal FC, Van Wering ER, Veerman AJP (1994) Different cellular drug resistance profiles in childhood lymphoblastic and non-lymphoblastic leukemia: a preliminary report. Leukemia 8:1224–1229

9. Kaspers GJL, Pieters R, Klumper E, De Waal FC, Veerman AJP (1994) Glucocorticoid resistance in childhood leukemia-A review. Leuk Lymphoma 13: 187–201

10. Kaspers GJ, Veerman AJP, Pieters R, Broekema GJ, Huismans DR, Kazemier KM, Loonen AH, Rottier MA, Van Zantwijk CH, Hählen K, Van Wering ER (1994) Mononuclear cells contaminating acute lymphoblastic leukaemic samples tested for cellular drug resistance using the methyl-thiazol-tetrazolium assay. British Journal of Cancer. 70:1047–52

11. Kaspers GJL, Veerman AJP, Pieters R, van Zantwijk CH, Smets LA, Van Wering ER, Van Der Does-Van Den Berg A (1997) In vitro cellular drug resistance and prognosis in newly diagnosed childhood acute lymphoblastic leukemia. Blood 90: 2723–2729

12. Kaspers GJL, Pieters R, Van Zantwijk CH, Van Wering ER, Van Der Does-Van Den Berg A, Veerman AJP (1998) Prednisolone resistance in childhood acute lymphoblastic leukemia – vitro-vivo correlations and cross resistance to other drugs. Blood 92: 259–266

13. Kearns PR, Pieters R, Rottier MMA, Veerman AJP, Hall AG, Pearson ADJ (1997) Glutathione and drug resistance in childhood acute lymphoblastic leukemia. Med Ped Oncol 29: 391 (abstract)

14. Klumper E, Pieters R, Kaspers GJL, Huismans DR, Henze G, Veerman AJP (1995) Modulation of resistance to prednisolone in childhood acute lymphoblastic leukemia by meta-iodobenzylguanidine (MIBG). Leukemia 9: 538 (abstract)

15. Klumper E, Pieters R, Veerman AJP,. Huismans DR, Loonen AH, Hahlen K, Kaspers GJL, van Wering ER, Hartmann R, Henze G (1995) In vitro cellular drug resistance in children with relapsed/refractory acute lymphoblastic leukemia. Blood 86: 3861–3868

16. Mastrangelo R, Riccardi R, Corbo S, Marchetti P, Iacobelli S (1984) Prediction of clinical response to glucocorticoids in children with acute lymphoblastic leukemia. Eur Paediatr Haematol Oncol 1: 33–36

17. Maung ZT, Hogarth L, Reid MM, Proctor SJ, Hamilton PJ, Hall AG (1994) Raised intracellular glutathione levels correlate with in vitro resistance to cytotoxic drugs in leukaemic cells from patients with acute lymphoblastic leukemia. Leukemia 8: 1487–1491

18. Momparler RL, Dore BT, Momparler LF (1990) Effect of 5-aza-2'-deoxycytidine and retinoic acid on differentiation and c-myc expression in HL-60 myeloid leukemic cells. Cancer Lett 54: 21–28

19. Nagourney RA, Messenger JC, Kern DH, Weisenthal LM (1990) Enhancement of anthracycline and alkylator cytotoxicity by ethacrynic acid in primary cultures of human tissues. Cancer Chemotherapy & Pharmacology 26: 318–322

20. O'Dwyer PJ, Hammilton TC, Yao K-s, Twe KD, Ozols RF (1995) Modulation of glutathione and related enzymes in reversal of resistance to anticancer agents. Hematol/Oncol Clin North Am 9: 383–396

21. Pieters R, Loonen AH, Huismans DR, Broekema GJ, Dirven MWJ, Heyenbrok MW, Hählen K, Veerman AJP (1990) In vitro drug sensitivity of cells from children with leukemia using the MTT assay with improved culture conditions. Blood 76: 2327–2336

22. Riehm H, Reiter A, Schrappe M, Berthold F, Dopfer R, Gerein V, Ludwig R, Ritter J, Stollmann B, Henze G (1986) Die Corticoisteroid-Abhängige Dezimierung der Leukämiezellzahl im Blut als Prognosefaktor bei der Akuten Lymphoblastischen Leukaämie im Kinderalter (Therapiestudie ALL-BFM 83). Klin Pädiatr 199: 151–160

23. Rivard GE, Momparler RL, Demers J, Benoit P, Raymond R, Lin K, Momparler LF (1981) Phase I study on 5-aza-2'-deoxycytidine in children with acute leukemia. Leukemia Research 5: 453–462

24. Smets LA, Bout B, Wisse J (1988) Cytotoxic and antitumor effects of the norepinephrine analogue meta-iodo-benzylguanidine (MIBG). Cancer Chemotherapy & Pharmacology 21: 9–13

25. Smets LA, Metwally E, Knol E, Martens M (1988) Potentiation of glucocorticoid induced cell lysis in refractory and resistant leukemia cells by inhibitors of ADP-ribosylation. Leuk Res 12: 737–747

26. Smets LA, Loesberg C, Janssen M, Van Rooij H (1990) Intracellular inhibition of mono (ADP)-ribosylation by metaiodobenzyl-guanidine: specificity, intracellular concentration and effects on glucocorticoid-mediated cell lysis. Biochim Biophys Acta 1054: 49–55

27. Smith AC, Harmon JM (1987) Structural organization of the human glucocorticoid receptor determined by one- and two-dimensional gel electrophoresis of proteolytic receptor fragments. Biochemistry 26: 646–652

28. Wielckens K, Delfs T (1986) Glucocorticoid-induced cell death and poly-[adenosine diphosphate (ADP)-ribosyl]-ation: Increased toxicity of dexamethasone on mouse S49.1 lymphoma cells with the poly (ADP-ribosyl)-ation inhibitor benzamide. Endocrinology 119: 2383–2392

# In-Vitro Cellular Drug Resistance in Acute Non-Lymhoblastic Leukemia: Comparisons Between Adults and Children

T.G.K.J. de Haas[1], Ch.M. Zwaan[1], M.J. Wondergem[1], R. Pieters[4], G.J.L. Kaspers[1], A.H. Loonen[1], M.M.A. Rottier[1], R. Wünsche[1], U. Creutzig[2], S. Bartl[3], K. Hählen[4], H.J. Broxterman[5], G.J. Ossenkoppele[6] and A.J.P. Veerman[1]

## Introduction

Children with acute non-lymphoblastic leukemia (ANLL) experience a better clinical outcome than adults with ANLL. For younger adults (arbitrarily defined as age <60 years of age) complete remission (CR) rates are usually about 70-80% with a long term disease free survival (DFS) of 25-50% in patients achieving CR [1,2]. Elderly patients with ANLL (age at diagnosis ≥60 years of age) experience a poor clinical outcome: CR rates are <50% and long term DFS for those achieving CR is only 5-15% [1,3,4]. For pediatric ANLL the best results published so far are from the MRC group in their trial MRC AML 10, which led to a CR rate of 92% and to a 5 year DFS of 54% [5].

Generally, differences in clinical outcome can be caused by pharmacokinetic factors (determining the drug-exposure of the malignant cells), cellular drug resistance and the regrowth potential of residual malignant cells [6]. From the literature it is known that the dismal prognosis of elderly ANLL patients is caused by several factors influencing intrinsic drug-resistance and by less tolerance to cytostatic treatment [7]. It is also suggested that adult ANLL patients <60 years of age are more intrinsically resistant to chemotherapy in comparison with children.

To analyze whether cellular drug resistance contributes to the poorer prognosis in adult ANLL we compared adult and childhood ANLL samples taken at initial diagnosis with regards to in-vitro drug resistance as determined with the MTT-assay.

## Materials and methods

### Patients and patient samples

We tested samples from 127 children (age <18 years) and 123 adults (age ≥18 years) with untreated ANLL, of whom either bone marrow or peripheral blood, taken at initial diagnosis, was sent to the research laboratory of pediatric hematology/oncology at the University Hospital Vrije Universiteit in Amsterdam. Children were treated according to BFM-like protocols and adults according to HOVON-protocols. The MTT assay was successful in 94 pediatric and 93 adult samples. Cells of pediatric ANLL with a successful MTT assay were obtained from the following institutions: BFM AML Study Group (n=67), Sophia Children's Hospital, Rotterdam (n=10) and the University Hospital Vrije Universiteit in Amsterdam (n=17). Cells from adult patients with a successful MTT assay were obtained from the Department of Hematology, University Hospital Vrije Universiteit, Amsterdam.

Patient characteristics for the children and adults are shown in Table 1. No significant differences occurred between children and adults considering white blood cell count (WBC; p=0.26), FAB classification (p=0.77) or sex (p=0.82).

The adult ANLL group was further divided in 2 groups of patients according to age (n=4 age unknown): those aged ≥18 yr and <60 yr (n=60, median age 44 yr), and those who were ≥60 yr (elderly ANLL; n=29, median age 67 yr). Sex distribution, WBC and FAB classifica-

Department of Pediatric Haematology/Oncology[1], Dept. of Hematology[6], Dept. of Medical Oncology[5], University Hospital Vrije Universiteit, De Boelelaan 1117, POB 7057, 1007 MB Amsterdam, The Netherlands
BFM AML Study Group[2], Münster, Germany
Children's University Hospital, Hamburg[3], Germany
Sophia Children's Hospital/University Hospital Rotterdam[4], Rotterdam, The Netherlands

**Table 1.** Characteristics of patients with ANLL, successfully tested for cellular drug resistance

| | Children (n=94) | Adults (n=93) | p[(1)] | **Adults** (<60 yr., n=60) | Elderly (≥60yr., n=29) | p[(2)] |
|---|---|---|---|---|---|---|
| **Age** (yrs) (median and range) | 8.1 (0.1-17.2) | 49 (18-89) | | 44 (18-59) | 67 (60-89) | |
| **WBC** 10⁹/l | 24.0 (0.7-416) | 37.2 (1.7-341) | 0.26 | 36.0 (1.7-306) | 46.0 (1.7-341) | 0.28 |
| **Male;female** | 50 / 44 | 52 / 41 | 0.82 | 34 / 26 | 16 /13 | 0.9 |
| **FAB** | | | | | | |
| M0 | 2 | 4 | | 2 | 2 | |
| M1 | 12 | 8 | | 3 | 4 | |
| M2 | 23 | 21 | | 12 | 7 | |
| M3 | 3 | 5 | | 4 | 1 | |
| M4 | 14 | 20 | 0.77 | 10 | 9 | 0.013 |
| M4 Eo | 12 | 8 | | 8 | 0 | |
| M5 | 13 | 20 | | 17 | 3 | |
| M6 | 1 | 1 | | 1 | 0 | |
| M7 | 4 | 2 | | 2 | 0 | |
| MDS | 4 | 1 | | 1 | 0 | |
| Unknown | 6 | 3 | | 0 | 3 | |

[1)] Mann-Whitney U test, differences between childhood and adult ANLL.
[2)] Mann-Whitney U test, differences between adult (<60 yr) and elderly (≥ 60yr) ANLL.

tion are given in Table 1. Sex distribution (p=0.9) and WBC (p=0.28) do not differ significantly, however, FAB classification in elderly ANLL differs significantly from adult ANLL (p=0.013), showing less FAB M5 and no FAB M4Eo cases in elderly ANLL. When comparing childhood ANLL either with adult <60yr or elderly (≥60 yr) patients with regards to FAB-classification, WBC and sex distribution no significant differences were found.

## MTT-assay

In vitro drug resistance of leukemia samples was assessed using a 4 day cell culture assay based on the principle that living cells are able to reduce 3-(4,5-dimethylthiazol-2,5-diphenyl) tetrazolium bromide (MTT) to a colored formazan product, which can be determined spectrophotometrically at 562 nm, as described earlier [8]. Data from bone marrow (BM) and peripheral blood (PB) samples were evaluated together, as were data from fresh and cryopreserved samples, as this does not influence the results of in-vitro drug-resistance testing [9,10]. Twelve drugs were tested, each at 6 different concentrations

and in duplicate in 96-well microculture plates. The following drugs were tested (minimal and maximal concentration): Cytarabine (Ara-C; 0.002-2.5 mg/ml), Daunorubicin (DNR; 0.002-2 µg/ml), Idarubicin (Ida; 0.002-2 µg/ml), Doxorubicin (Dox; 0.008-8 µg/ml), Amsacrin (Amsa; 0.006-20 µg/ml), Mitoxantrone (Mitox; 0.001-1 µg/ml), Etoposide (VP16; 0.05-50 µg/ml), Vincristine (VCR; 0.05-50 µg/ml), Prednisolone (Pred; 0.008-250 µg/ml), L-Asparaginase (L-ASP; 0.003-10 IU/ml), 6-Thioguanine (6-TG; 1.56-50 µg/ml), 4 hydroperoxy ifosfamide (0.1-100 µg/ml) and Busulfan (Bus; 1.23-300 µg/ml). The optical density (OD) is linearly related to the cellnumber [9]. Six wells contained cells with culture medium but no drugs, to determine the control cell survival. Six wells with culture medium only were used to blank the spectrophotometer. Leukemia cell-survival was calculated at each drug concentration by the equation: LCS = (OD treated well/mean OD control wells) x 100% after correction for the background OD. Samples were considered evaluable only if the control wells contained ≥70% malignant cells after 4 days of culture when the MTT is added [11]. This was determined by morphology (May-Grünwald-Giemsa staining). Also, the mean control OD after correction for the background at day 4 must exceed 0.05 arbitrary units. The LC50 value was used as a measure of resistance, which is the drug concentration needed to kill 50% of the leukemia cells.

## P-glycoprotein activity

From elderly ANLL patients the P-glycoprotein (P-gp) activity was determined by Broxterman et al. (Dept. of Medical Oncology, University Hospital Vrije Universiteit, Amsterdam) by means of a functional assay; i.e. the modulation of rhodamine 123 accumulation by PSC833, as described in detail in a recent study [12]. Results were expressed as the ratio between the rhodamine accumulation with and without PSC833 ('RHO-ratio'). Parts of the results have been published already but without focus on elderly ANLL specifically [12].

## Statistics

Differences in the distribution of LC50 values were analyzed using the Mann-Whitney U test for unpaired samples. Correlations were calculated using the Spearman's Rank Correlation Coefficient (rho). P-values of £ 0.05 were considered statistically significant (2-tailed test).

## Results

### Cellular drug resistance testing

From all samples sent to our laboratory 74% of 127 childhood ANLL-samples and 76% of 123 adult ANLL samples could be tested successfully with the MTT-assay. Excluding those samples with a percentage of malignant cells below 70 at day 0 (n=15 children and n=9 adults), the technical success rate of the MTT-assay was 84% in childhood ANLL and 82% in adult ANLL samples. Reasons for technical failure of the MTT assay were as follows:
- in childhood ANLL: blasts day 4 <70% (n=11), OD below 0.05 (n=2), other (n=5)
- in adult ANLL: blasts day 4 <70% (n=10), OD below 0.05 (n=8), infection (n=1), other (n=2).

No statistically significant differences in in-vitro drug resistance were detected between childhood and adult ANLL samples (Table 2). When comparing the childhood ANLL samples with the samples from adults <60 yr a significant difference for DNR was detected (p=0.041). However, this difference is only small; cells from adults are median 1.2 fold more resistant (Fig. 1). When comparing cells from children with elderly ANLL or when comparing cells from adults <60 yr with elderly ANLL again no significant differences in in-vitro drug resistance were detected.

**Table 2.** Median LC50 values in untreated and pediatric ANLL-samples

| Drugs | Median and range LC50 adults (µg/ml) | N | Median and range LC50 children (µg/ml) | N | RR [1] | p-value [2] |
|---|---|---|---|---|---|---|
| Ara-C | 0.38 (0.03->2.5) | 91 | 0.46 (0.01->2.5) | 87 | 0.8 | 0.46 |
| DNR | 0.27 (0.04->2.0) | 85 | 0.22 (0.002 - 1.32) | 83 | 1.2 | 0.06 |
| Ida | 0.10 (0.02-0.38) | 15 | 0.17 (0.01-1.12) | 62 | 0.6 | 0.27 |
| Dox | 0.54 (0.14-5.80) | 24 | 0.48 (0.01-1.71) | 63 | 1.1 | 0.23 |
| Mitox | 0.17 (0.008->1.0) | 29 | 0.09 (<0.001->1.0) | 78 | 2.0 | 0.12 |
| Amsa | 0.54 (0.03-5.31) | 28 | 0.59 (0.03-3.43) | 66 | 0.9 | 0.83 |
| VP16 | 7.47 (0.6->50) | 28 | 6.36 (0.11->50) | 84 | 1.2 | 0.73 |
| 6-TG | 8.4 (1.77->50) | 24 | 5.9 (<1.56-50) | 85 | 1.4 | 0.16 |
| VCR | 7.17 (<0.05->50) | 18 | 3.13 (<0.05->50) | 87 | 2.3 | 0.88 |
| L-ASP [3] | 1.33 (<0.003->10.0) | 16 | 1.02 (<0.003->10) | 73 | 1.3 | 0.24 |
| Pred | >250 (9.1->250) | 26 | >250 (0.4->250) | 91 | 1.0 | 0.29 |
| Bus | 37.3 (10.1-288) | 28 | 33.3 (5.5-204) | 67 | 1.1 | 0.52 |
| Ifos | 12.84 (4.9-19.4) | 9 | 12.15 (2.2-44.7) | 68 | 1.1 | 0.84 |

[1] RR = resistance ratio: ratio between median LC50 adults divided by median LC50 children
[2] Mann-Whitney U test (2-tailed)
[3] L-Asparaginase: in IU/ml

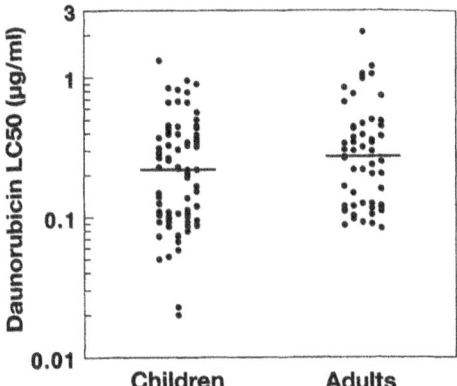

**Fig. 1.** In-vitro DNR resistance (µg/ml) in childhood (n=83) versus adult ANLL <60 years of age (n=60) at initial diagnosis. The dots represent the individual DNR LC50 values, the horizontal lines the median LC50 value for each group. The median LC50 value between children and adults (<60 yr) differs significantly (1.2 fold, p=0.041). DNR LC50 values >2 µg/ml are depicted as 2.1 µg/ml.

## P-gp activity

In a part of the elderly ANLL samples (n=19) the rhodamine accumulation with and without PSC833 (RHO) was also determined and could be compared to the in-vitro DNR resistance in this group. The RHO-ratio ranged from 0.97-4.16, median 1.14. Higher RHO-ratios (=higher P-gp activity) were associated

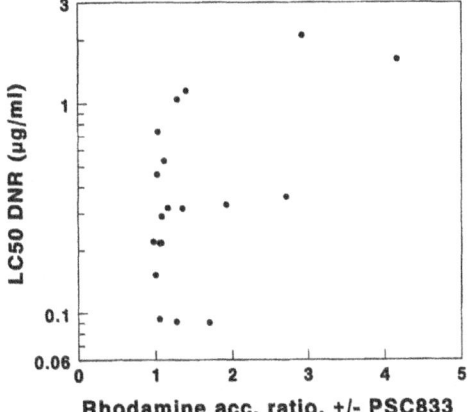

**Fig. 2.** Relationship between P-gp activity as determined by rhodamine 123 accumulation with and without PSC833 and depicted as a ratio (RHO-ratio) versus in-vitro daunorubicin resistance (µg/ml) in elderly (≥ 60 yr) ANLL only. Rho=0.66, p=0.002.

with relatively DNR resistant cells (rho=0.66; p=0.002; Figure 2).

## Discussion

From clinical trials in ANLL it is clear that increasing age is an adverse prognostic factor. Our hypothesis that enhanced cellular drug resistance with increasing age could explain this could not be clearly demonstrated in this study. Although adults <60 years of age were statistically significant more in-vitro resistant to DNR in comparison with pediatric ANLL the clinical impact is probably limited as the difference was only 1.2 fold. When comparing adult ANLL as a total group with pediatric ANLL borderline significance for DNR was found, but again the difference in median LC50 was only very small (resistance ratio 1.2, p=0.06). In a previous study we compared pediatric ANLL with pediatric acute lymphoblastic leukemia (ALL) and showed pediatric ANLL to be 1.7 fold more in-vitro DNR resistant (p<0.001) [13]. Therefore ANLL is relatively DNR resistant in all age groups when compared with pediatric ALL.

Apart from cellular drug-resistance several other explanations for the difference in prognosis between childhood and adult ANLL exist. Of those patients achieving CR in adult ANLL almost half relapse in the first year after treatment [14]. In pediatric ANLL the relapse rate is lower: Stevens et al. reported a relapse rate of 26 and 11% in the first and second year respectively [5]. Therefore the regrowth potential of residual malignant cells [6] may play an important role in the different prognosis of pediatric and adult ANLL. Also, pharmacokinetic differences between children and adults, especially elderly patients, may exist. Moreover, due to poor performance status it is estimated that about 25-50% of elderly patients can not tolerate intensive chemotherapy, and are therefore either not offered induction chemotherapy or are treated with a palliative regimen only [15,16]. If treated with aggressive chemotherapy the rate of toxic and infectious complications is much higher [17].

We could not demonstrate clear differences in in-vitro drug resistance between childhood and adult ANLL, and suggest the following explanations. The MTT-assay may not be able to detect small, but resistant, subpopulations of cells, which may cause relapse. Also, we may have tested selected patient groups. Apart from age at least 2 other prognostic factors have emerged. A high WBC is associated with a poor prognosis, but in our study children and adults did not differ significantly in WBC. Secondly, both poor and good cytogenetic risk-groups are defined [18,19], but we lack data from cytogenetic analysis in our patients. Therefore we cannot rule out the possibility of overrepresentation of good risk cytogenetics in our elderly or poor risk cytogenetics in the pediatric patients, possibly influencing cellular drug resistance. When considering FAB-classification only the SWOG reported a significantly better prognosis according to FAB-type in adult ANLL, with FAB M2, M3 and M4 being favorable, probably corresponding with the good cytogenetic riskgroups [20]. In childhood ANLL the BFM reported a favorable prognosis in M1/M2 with Auer rods, M3 and M4 [21]. The FAB-type distribution between children and adults <60 yr is almost equal, only FAB M3 is more frequently diagnosed in adults [1,5,21]. In elderly ANLL a higher percentage of FAB M1 and M2 is found in comparison with children and adults [3,7]. This is in accordance with our data, where we find a relatively low percentage of FAB M4 and M5 in elderly patients with an increased frequency of FAB M0, M1 and M2. Therefore there seems to be no selection in our patient cohort according to FAB-types.

In the elderly patients it is assumed that MDR1-overexpression, leading to extrusion of the so-called natural product drugs out of the cell by P-gp, is a major cause of primary drug-resistance. For example Leith et al. described that the absence or presence of MDR1 overexpression, trilineage dysplasia and cytogenetic subgroup changes CR rates in elderly ANLL from 0 to 81 %, thus influencing intrinsic drug resistance [7]. Other studies confirm the relevance of MDR1 overexpression in adult ANLL [22-25]. The MDR1 over-expression frequency ranges from 15% in childhood ANLL up to 70% in elderly ANLL [7,26]. In our study we could not demonstrate enhanced in-vitro resistance to anthracyclines or other natural product drugs in relation to age. Broxterman et al. recently

described that there is no correlation between P-gp activity or P-gp level (MRK16 protein detection by FACS analysis) and in-vitro DNR resistance as determined by the MTT-assay in a combined group of adult (<60 yr) and elderly (≥ 60 yr) ANLL patients [12]. The ANLL patients studied by Broxterman partially overlap with the patients described in our study presented here. Focusing on the elderly patients exclusively, however, we did find a significant correlation between P-gp activity and in-vitro DNR resistance. In the study of Norgaard et al. significant correlations between MDR1 gene expression and in-vitro drug resistance to DNR, Dox and VP16 in adult ANLL were found, which was not restricted to elderly patients only [27]. In pediatric ANLL the role of P-gp is very limited [13,26]. Therefore, in pediatric ANLL DNR-resistance may be related to other factors, such as the expression of other resistance associated proteins, for instance LRP overexpression [13], as is also described in adult ANLL [28,29].

The prognostic value of the MTT assay in childhood and adult ANLL has been described earlier by our group in 2 pilot-studies by Klumper et al. [9,30]. In adult ANLL CR rate could be predicted by in-vitro DNR resistance, whereas survival was determined by in-vitro cytarabine resistance [9]. In pediatric ANLL in-vitro cytarabine resistance was able to predict CR rate. Also relapsed childhood ANLL was 3-fold more cytarabine resistant than the untreated ANLL group [30]. Other studies confirm the prognostic value of cellular drug resistance in childhood ANLL, as is recently reviewed by Kaspers et al [31].

In conclusion: we did not observe clear differences in in-vitro drug resistance between pediatric and adult ANLL that explain the poorer prognosis within the latter group. Other causes to explain their unfavorable prognosis may play a major role. In elderly ANLL we did find a correlation between P-gp activity and in-vitro DNR resistance. The prognostic value of cellular drug resistance in both pediatric and adult ANLL has been described in pilot studies but needs confirmation in larger series of patients.

# References

1. Bennett JM, Young ML, Andersen JW, Cassileth PA, Tallman MS, Paietta E, Wiernik PH, Rowe JM (1997) Long term survival in acute myeloid leukemia. The Eastern Cooperative Oncology Group Experience. Cancer 80: 2205-2209
2. Hann IM, Stevens RF, Goldstone AH, Rees JKH, Wheatley K, Gray RG, Burnett AK on behalf of the Adult and Childhood Leukaemia Working Parties of the Medical Research Council (1998) Randomized comparison of DAT versus ADE as induction chemotherapy in children and younger adults with acute myeloid leukemia. Results of the Medical Research Council's 10th AML Trial. Blood 89: 2311-2318
3. Löwenberg B, Suciu S, Archimbaud B, Haak H, Stryckmans P, De Cataldo R, Dekker AW, Berneman ZN, Thyss A, Van der Lelie J, Sonneveld P, Visani G, Fillet G, Hayat M, Hagemeijer A, Solbu G, Zittoun R (1998) Mitoxantrone versus daunorubicin in induction-consolodation chemotherapy – the value of low-dose cytarabine for maintenance of remission, and an assessement of prognostic factors in acute myeloid leukemia in the elderly: final report of the Leukemia Cooperative Group of the European Organization for the Research and Treatment of Cancer and the Dutch-Belgian Hemato-Oncology Cooperative Hovon Group Randomized Phase III Study AML 9. J Clin Oncol 16: 872-881
4. Feldman EJ, Seiter K, Damon L, Linker C, Rugo H, Ries C, Case DC Jr, Beer M, Ahmed T (1997) A randomized trial of high- versus standard-dose mitoxantrone with cytarabine in elderly patients with acute myeloid leukemia. Leukemia 11:485-489
5. Stevens RF, Hann IM, Wheatley K, Gray RG on behalf of the MRC Childhood Leukemia Working Party (1998) Marked improvements in outcome with chemotherapy alone in paediatric acute myeloid leukemia: results of the United Kingdom Medical Research Council's 10th AML trial. Br J Haematol 101: 130-140
6. Preisler HD, Gopal V (1994) Regrowth resistance in leukemia and lymphoma: the need for a new system to classify treatment failure and for new approaches to treatment. Leuk Res 18: 149-160
7. Leith CP, Kopecky KJ, Godwin J, McConnell T, Slovak ML, Chen I-M, Head DR, Appelbaum FR, Willman CL (1997) Acute myeloid leukemia in the elderly: assessment of multidrug resistance (MDR1) and cytogenetic distinguishes biologic subgroups with remarkably distinct responses to standard chemotherapy. A Southwest Oncology Group Study. Blood 89: 3323-3329
8. Pieters R, Loonen AH, Huismans DR, Broekema GJ, Dirven MWJ, Heyenbrok MW, Hählen K, Veerman AJP (1990) In vitro drug sensitivity of cells from children with leukemia using the MTT assay with improved culture conditions. Blood 76: 2327-2336
9. Klumper E, Ossenkoppele GJ, Pieters R, Huismans DR, Loonen AH, Rottier A, Westra G, Veerman AJP (1996) In vitro resistance to cytosine arabinoside, not to daunorubicin, is associated with the risk of relapse in de novo acute myeloid leukemia. Br J Haematol 93: 903-910
10. Pieters R, Huismans DR, Leyva A, Veerman AJP (1989) Comparison of a rapid automated tetrazolium based (MTT) assay with a dye exclusion assay for chemosensitivity testing in childhood leukemia. Br J Cancer 64: 217-220
11. Kaspers GJL, Veerman AJP, Pieters R, Broekema GJ, Huismans DR, Kazemier KM, Loonen AH, Rottier MMA, Van Zantwijk CH, Hählen K, Van Wering ER (1994) Mononuclear cells contaminating acute lymphoblastic leukaemic samples tested for cellular drug resistance using the methyl-thiazol-tetrazolium assay. Br J Cancer 70: 1047-1052
12. Broxterman HJ, Sonneveld P, Pieters R, Lankelma J, Eekman CA, Loonen AH, Schoester M, Ossenkoppele GJ, Löwenberg B, Pinedo HM, Schuurhuis GJ (1999) Do P-glycoprotein and major vault protein (MVP/LRP) expression correlate with in vitro daunorubicin resistance in acute myeloid leukemia. Leukemia 13: 258-265
13. Den Boer ML, Pieters R, Kazemier KM, Rottier MMA, Zwaan CM, Kaspers GJL, Janka-Schaub G, Henze G, Creutzig U, Scheper RJ, Veerman AJP (1998) Relationship between major vault protein/lung resistance protein, multidrug resistance associated protein, P-glycoprotein expression and drug resistance in childhood leukemia. Blood 91: 2092-2098
14. Estey E, deLima M, Strom S, Pierce S, Freireich EJ, Keating MJ (1997) Long-term follow-up of patients with newly diagnosed acute myeloid leukeima treated at the University of Texas M.D. Anderson Cancer Center. Cancer 80: 2176-2180
15. Rowe J. Prognostic factors in AML: a statement of issues (1997) In: New treatment considerations for AML: the clinician's challenge. Proceedings of the 39th Annual Meeting of the American Society of Hematology, pre-congress symposium, December 5, 1997: 6-7
16. Stasi R, Venditti A, Del Poeta G, Aronica G, Dentamaro T, Cecconi M, Stipa E, Scimo MT, Masi M, Amadori S (1996) Intensive treatment of patients over 60 years of age and older with de novo acute myeloid leukemia. Analysis of prognostic factors. Cancer 77: 2476
17. Stasi R, Del Poeta G, Venditti A, Masi M, Stipa E, Cox MC, Amadori S (1998) Prognostic value of cytogenetics and multidrug resistance (MDR1) in elderly patients with acute myeloid leukemia. Blood 92: 695-696
18. Dastugue N, Payen C, Lafage-Pochitaloff M, Bernard P, Lerous D, Huguet-Rigal F, Stoppa A-M, Marit G, Molina L, Michallet M, Maraninchi D, Attal M, Reiffers J (1995) Prognostic significance of karyotype in de novo adult acute myeloid leukemia. Leukemia 9: 1491-1498
19. Bloomfield CD, Shuma C, Regal L, Philip PB, Hossfeld DK, Hagemeijer AM, Garson OM, Peterson BA, Sakurai M, Alimena G, Berger R, Rowley JD, Ruutu T, Mitelman F, Dewald GW, Swansbury J (1997) Long term survival of patients with acute myeloid leukemia. A third follow-up of the fourth international workshop on chromosomes in leukemia. Cancer 80: 2191-2198
20. Appelbaum FR, Kopecky KJ (1997) Long-term survival after chemotherapy for acute myeloid leukemia. Cancer 80: 2199-2204

21. Creutzig U, Harbott J, Sperling C, Ritter J, Zimmermann M, Löffler H, Riehm H, Schellong G, Ludwig W (1995) Clinical significance of surface antigen expression in children with acute myeloid leukemia: results of study AML-BFM 87. Blood 86: 3097-3108

22. Wood P, Burgess R, MacGregor A, Liu Yin JA (1994) P-glycoprotein expression on acute myeloid leukaemia blast cells at diagnosis predicts response to chemotherapy and survival. Br J Haematol 87: 509-514

23. Guerci A, Merlin JL, Missoum N, Feldmann L, Marchal S, Witz F, Rose C, Guerci O (1995) Predictive value for treatment outcome in acute myeloid leukemia of cellular daunorubicin accumulation and P-glycoprotein expression simultaneously determined by flow cytometry. Blood 85: 2147-2153

24. Zöchbauer S, Gsur A, Brunner R, Kyrle PA, Lechner K, Pirker R (1994) P-glycoprotein expression as unfavorable prognostic factor in acute myeloid leukemia. Leukemia 8: 974-977

25. Van den Heuvel-Eibrink MM, Ven der Holt B, Te Boekhorst PAW, Pieters R, Schoester M, Löwenberg B, Sonneveld P (1997) MDR1 expression is an independent prognostic factor for response and survival in de novo acute myeloid leukemia. Br J Haematol 99: 76-83

26. Sievers EL, Smith FO, Woods WG, Lee JW, Bleyer WA, Willman CL, Bernstein ID (1995) Cell surface expression of the multidrug resistance P-glycoprotein (P-170) as detected by monoclonal antibody MRK-16 in pediatric acute myeloid leukemia fails to define a poor prognostic group: a report from the Childrens Cancer Group. Leukemia 9: 2042-2048

27. Norgaard JM, Bukh A, Langkjer ST, Clausen N, Palshof T, Hokland P (1998) MDR1 gene expression and drug resistance of AML cells. Br J Haematol 100: 534-540

28. List AF, Spier CS, Grogan GM, Johnson C, Roe DJ, Greer JP, Wolff SN, Broxterman HJ, Scheffer GL, Scheper RJ, Dalton WS (1996) Overexpression of the major vault transporter protein lung-resistance protein predicts treatment outcome in acute myeloid leukemia. Blood 87: 2464-2469

29. Borg AG, Burgess R, Green LM, Scheper RJ, Liu Yin JA (1998) Overexpression of lung-resistance protein and increased P-glycoprotein function in acute myeloid leukemia cells predict a poor response to chemotherapy and reduced patient survival. Br J Haematol 103: 1083-1091

30. Klumper E, Pieters R, Kaspers GJL, Huismans DR, Loonen AH, Rottier MMA, Van Wering ER, Van der Does-Van den Berg A, Hählen K, Creutzig U, Veerman AJP (1995) In vitro chemosensitivity assessed with the MTT-assay in childhood acute non-lymphoblastic leukemia. Leukemia 9: 1864-1869

31. Kaspers GJL, Zwaan ChM, Veerman AJP, Rots MG, Pieters R, Bucksy P, Domula M, Goebel U, Graf N, Havers W, Jorch N, Kabisch K, Spaar H-J, Ritter J, Creutzig U (1999) Cellular drug resistance in acute myeloid leukemia: literature review and preliminary analysis of on ongoing collaborative study. Klin Padiatr: in press

# Prognostic Relevance of In-Vitro Drug Sensitivity Testing in Adult AML

P. Staib, T. Schinköthe, S. Wiedenmann, T. Dimski, C. Schoch*, D. Voliotis, P.A. Horn, H. Tesch, B. Lathan and V. Diehl

*Abstract.* The prognostic accuracy of *in-vitro* drug sensitivity tests such as the differential staining cytotoxicity (DISC) assay must be assessed by correlation with response rates and also patient survival. We prospectively investigated the prognostic relevance of the DISC assay in adult patients (pts) with AML by using a new evaluation system called chemosensitivity index $C_i$.

*Patients and Methods.* Pts with de-novo AML were treated according to the TAD-HAM regimen and pts with relapsed or secondary AML according to the Ida-FLAG regimen. DISC assay was performed as described previously. Dose-response curves for each clinically used drug were calculated by logarithm and linear regression, then the area under the curve (AUC) as an exact measure for the *in-vitro* dose-response relation was transformed into an index called chemosensitivity index $C_i$. The cut off point between resistance and sensitivity was adjusted at 0,5 for each drug by the AUC data of a subgroup of clinically resistant patients: $C_i \leq 0,5$ predicts resistance, $C_i > 0,5$ sensitivity to the particular drug.

*Results.* 115 pts were evaluable; 91 received TAD-HAM and 24 Ida-FLAG for induction therapy. 75 pts (65%) achieved CR and 25 (22%) reduction of BM blasts <10%, in both groups the maximum $C_i$ ($C_i$-max) was >0,5 for at least one drug clinically used (TP=true positive correlation). 12 pts (10%) were non-responders and identified with $C_i$-max $\leq 0,5$ of all drugs given for therapy (TN=true negative). 3 pts with Ci-max >0,5 did not reach CR (FP=false positive correlation). TP=100, TN=12, FP=3,

($\chi^2$: p<0,001). Overall predictive accuracy was 97%. Pts with $C_i$-max >0,5 lived significantly longer with 26 months (median) than pts with $C_i$-max $\leq 0,5$ who lived 2 months (logrank, p<0,001). Karyotypes were available in 95 pts as follows: 29 unfavourable, 53 normal and 13 favourable. The rate of 64% (7/11) of unfavourable karyotypes among non-responders was substantially higher as compared with 26% (22/84) in the responder group.

*Conclusions.* The DISC assay evaluated by the $C_i$ provides accurate prediction of clinical response and also survival in pts with AML. Cytogenetics, one of the strongest known prognostic parameters in AML, may still not precisely predict individual prognosis. Further studies are needed to proof the $C_i$ as a possible independent prognostic factor in AML, which may serve for risk-adapted therapy strategies.

## Introduction

*In-vitro* drug sensitivity tests were developed in order to predict individual treatment outcome in various neoplastic diseases. Since the early 1980s a variety of short-term tests, e.g. the colorimetric methyl-thiazol-tetrazolium (MTT) assay or the differential staining cytotoxicity (DISC) assay, have been invented to study *in-vitro* cellular drug resistance [1-2,4-8]. The DISC assay and the MTT assay, having shown comparable results with stem cell or colony assays [3], were identified as the short term *in-vitro* drug sensitivity tests of choice in acute leukemias [1-2,4-7,9-12]. We adapted

---

Clinic I for Internal Medicine, University of Cologne, Germany.
*Clinic III for Internal Medicine Großhadern, University of Munich, Germany.

the DISC assay which allows direct evaluation of the cells tested by light microscopy [1-2].

Since the individual prognosis in acute myeloid leukemia may still not be determined by known prognostic factors such as age or karyotype, the *in-vitro* chemosensitivty profile may help to predict individual treatment outcome more precisely [5-6,11,13-16].

For *in-vitro* assays, defining a cut off point between sensitive and resistant is difficult as the results will usually make up a continuum from very sensitive through very resistant [11,14]. This may compromise the accuracy of an *in-vitro* assay, especially if preset cut off points such as a certain percentage of tumor cell survival (TCS) or various levels of inhibitory concentrations ($IC_{50}$, $IC_{90}$) are used for the evaluation of test results [11,14]. We, therefore, developed an evaluation system for the interpretation of DISC assay results that takes the complete dose-response relation into account [16].

The accuracy of an *in-vitro* assay and its evaluation system should be assessed not only by correlation of assay results with response rates but also with survival [11,14]. We, therefore, conducted a prospective study to correlate response to therapy and overall survival with DISC-assay results in adult patients with AML applying this new evaluation methodology, that we called „chemosensitivity index $C_i$".

## Materials and Methods

### Patients and Treatment

At our institution patients with de-novo AML were included into the German prospective randomized multicenter trial of the AML-Cooperative Group (AMLCG-'92 trial) [17]. Induction therapy consisted of the TAD-HAM double induction regimen containing thioguanine, Ara-C, daunorubicin - high dose Ara-C, mitoxantrone. Patients suffering from relapsed AML or AML with a history of pre-existing myelodysplastic syndrorme (MDS-AML) were treated with the Ida-FLAG regimen consisting of idarubicin, fludarabine, Ara-C and G-CSF [18].

### DISC assay

The DISC-assay was performed according to the methods described by Weisenthal et al. with minor modifications [1-2,9]. Briefly, bone marrow or peripheral blood specimens from each patient with AML were collected into heparin prior to the administration of chemotherapy. Leukemic blast cells were isolated by Ficoll density gradient centrifugation, washed and suspended in RPMI 1640 culture medium supplemented with fetal calf serum (FCS). Drugs were tested at five concentrations in triplicate [19]. All drugs used for treatment in the TAD-HAM or the Ida-FLAG regimen were routinely tested: thioguanine, Ara-C, daunorubicin, mitoxantrone, idarubicin and fludarabine [17-18]. The middle test concentration of each drug was chosen within the range of clinically relevant steady state plasma levels [19]. Drug (20 µl) was added to 90,000 cells in 180 µl medium; phosphate-buffered saline (PBS) in medium served as a control. After 94 hours of incubation (37°C, humidified 5% $CO_2$), 50,000 fixed duck erythrocytes (DRBCs) were added to each tube in 10 µl PBS containing 2% fast-green and 1% nigrosin. The cells were transferred to collagen surfaced microscope slides by cytocentrifugation, air-dried and counter-stained with May-Grünwald-Giemsa stain. Subsequent evaluation of slides by light microscopy facilitated the determination of drug efficacy at each concentration compared with controls. Assay results are expressed as percent tumor cell survival (% TCS).

### New Evaluation System: Chemosensitivity Index Ci

TCS-data were transformed into the following mathematical equation by logarithm and linear regression for description of the dose response curve:

$$TCS(conc) = e^{-\,dist\,+\,rise*conc}$$

(conc = drug test concentration; e = Euler number; TCS = percent tumor cell survival; dist = y-intercept; rise = gradient)

The dose-response curve allowed the determination of the area under the curve (AUC),

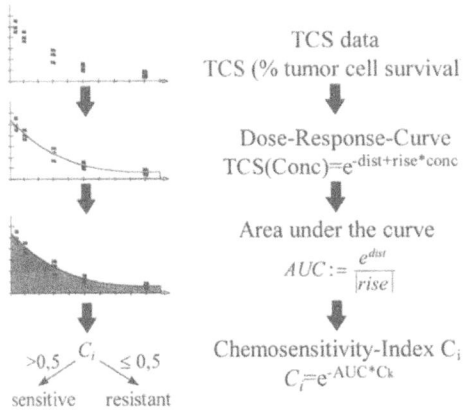

TCS data
TCS (% tumor cell survival)

$\downarrow$

Dose-Response-Curve
$TCS(Conc) = e^{-dist + rise \cdot conc}$

$\downarrow$

Area under the curve
$$AUC := \frac{e^{dist}}{|rise|}$$

$\downarrow$

Chemosensitivity-Index $C_i$
$C_i = e^{-AUC \cdot C_k}$

>0,5 $\swarrow$ $C_i$ $\searrow$ ≤ 0,5
sensitive    resistant

**Fig. 1.** Illustration of data processing for the chemosensitivity index $C_i$; (conc = drug test concentration; e = Euler number; TCS = percent tumor cell survival; dist = y-intercept; rise = gradient; $C_k$ = drug specific constant)

which is an exact measure of the complete dose-response relation. In order to compare the various drugs tested the AUC was transformed into an index ranging from 0 to 1. We called this index „chemosensitivity index $C_i$". The cut off point between resistance and sensitivity was adjusted at 0,5 for each drug by the AUC data of clinically resistant patients, since in these patients obviously all cytotoxic agents given for treatment are ineffective. If the $C_i$ is ≤ 0,5 resistance to the particular drug is predicted, and if the $C_i$ is > 0,5 sensitivity to the drug is postulated. The whole data processing is illustrated in Figure 1.

## Clinical Correlation

The highest scoring $C_i$ of those drugs clinically used was called $C_i$-max. The $C_i$-max was correlated with clinical outcome after induction chemotherapy in terms of complete

remission (CR), reduction of bone marrow blasts less than 10%, refractory disease and also, most importantly, overall survival.

Overall survival curves were estimated according to the method described by Kaplan and Meier. Differences in survival between patients with $C_i$-max ≤ or > 0,5 were assessed by the logrank test.

## Results

A total of 115 patients with AML were eligible for evaluation of DISC assay results and clinical outcome after chemotherapy. Of these 115 evaluable patients, 71 were male and 44 female. Median age was 50 years, range 18-75 years. The DISC assay was performed in 103 patients at the first diagnosis of AML and in 12 patients at relapse of the disease. 97 patients had de-novo AML, 14 patients suffered from secondary AML and 4 from biphenotypic acute leukemia. FAB subtypes of the de-novo AML cases were as follows: 4 M0, 11 M1, 36 M2, 6 M3, 22 M4, 14 M5, 3 M6, 1 M7. 91 patients received the TAD-HAM regimen and 24 patients the Ida-FLAG regimen for induction therapy. Ida-FLAG was used for high-risk AML such as relapsed, secondary AML or AML with trilineage dysplasia.

After induction therapy 75 patients (65%) reached a complete remission and 25 patients (22%) an effective reduction of bone marrow blasts below 10%, whereas 15 patients (13%) had refractory disease. The correlation between the $C_i$-max of only those drugs clinically used and the three response categories is shown in table 1. All the 100 patients in the responder group were found with a $C_i$-max value > 0,5 of at least one drug given for therapy, and 12 of 15 non-responders showed $C_i$-max values below 0,5 (see Table 1). Only three patients with $C_i$-max > 0,5 did not reach

**Table 1.** Correlation between $C_i$-max and clinical outcome.

| Treatment outcome | $C_i$-max > 0,5 | $C_i$-max ≤ 0,5 | p-value |
|---|---|---|---|
| CR, BM-Blasts < 10% | 100 (87%) (true positive, TP) | 0 (false negative, FN) | $\chi^2$: p<0,001 |
| Non-response | 3 (2,6%) (false positive, FP) | 12 (10,4%) (true negative, TN) | |

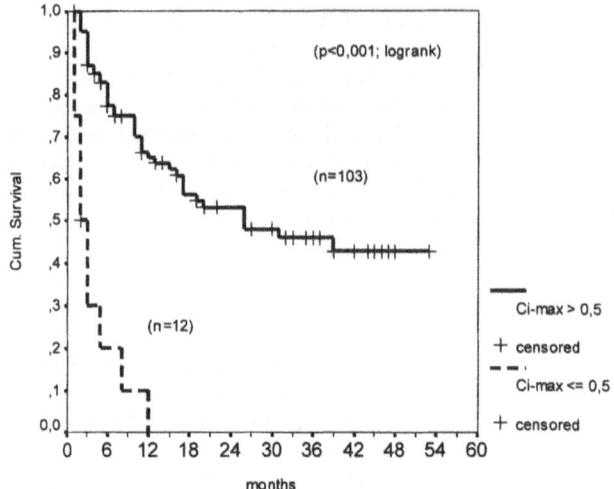

Fig. 2. Overall survival of AML patients dependent on $C_i$-max $> 0,5$ or $\leq 0,5$.

CR or effective blast reduction in the bone marrow. Thus, the vast majority of non-responders (12/15) was precisely identified from the total group of patients. No significant difference of $C_i$-max values was found for the two responder-groups. The overall predictive accuracy was 97,4%, and the correlation of $C_i$-max with immediate treatment outcome was highly significant in the chi-square test.

Correlation of $C_i$-max with overall survival is shown in Figure 2. Median survival of patients with $C_i$-max $> 0,5$ was 26 months (775 days) compared to less than two months (57 days) in patients with $C_i$-max $\leq 0,5$. The difference in overall survival between the two groups was statistically highly significant ($p<0,001$; logrank).

Cytogenetic analysis was available in 95 patients. Unfavourable chromosomal abnormalities were found in 29 (30%) patients, favourable abnormalities in 13 (14%) patients

**Table 2.** Frequencies of cytogenetic subgroups in relation to clinical outcome. Favourable: t(15;17), t(8;21), inv16. Unfavourable: complex ($\geq 3$) abnormalities, deletions of chromosome 5 or 7. Intermediate: other abnormalities, normal karyotype.

| Karyotype | Non-Responders (n=11/15) | Responders (n=84/100) |
|---|---|---|
| Favourable | 0 | 13 (16%) |
| Intermediate | 4 (36%) | 49 (58%) |
| Unfavourable | 7 (64%) | 22 (26%) |
| n.d. | 4 | 16 |

and a normal or intermediate risk karyotype in 53 (56%) patients. The rate of 64% (7/11) of unfavourable karyotypes among non-responders was substantially higher compared with 26% (22/84) in the responder group. There were no favourable karyotypes found among the non-responders. (see Table 2)

## Discussion

*In-vitro* chemosensitivity assays have been developed with the ultimate aim of predicting clinical drug resistance and to tailor chemotherapy in individual patients with resistant disease or poor prognosis [1-14,15-16,19-22]. For the assessment of the accuracy of an *in-vitro* chemosensitivity assay it is necessary to compare the test results not only with short term outcome in terms of complete remission or persistent disease, but also with patient survival [11,14]. This clinical correlation is usually obtained by categorising into sensitive or resistant both test results and patient response and comparing the two. The definition of patient response is usually easy (response = CR or PR) whilst test results are not so easily categorized as the test results will usually make up a continuum from very sensitive through very resistant [11,14]. Defining a cut off point between sensitive and resistant in vitro can in many cases only be done by comparison with the clinical data. In many studies the percentage of surviving tumor cells (e.g. 30%) at a particular drug concentration or the inhibitory drug concentration to achieve a certain percentage of killed tumor cells (e.g. $IC_{50}$ or $IC_{90}$) were used for cut off points [1-2,4-7,10,12,15]. In contrast to these conventional, rigid cut off point systems the newly developed chemosensitivity index $C_i$ takes the total dose response relation into account by using the AUC [16].

The application of the $C_i$ methodology for analysing DISC-assay results in this series of AML patients demonstrated a correct prediction of clinical response to induction chemotherapy in almost all patients with a positive predictive accuracy of 97% (100/103). It is also important to notice that 12 of 15 patients with primary resistant disease were precisely identified as non-responders within a few days. Thus, the negative predictive accuracy of 100% (TN/TN+FN = 12/12) together with the overall predictive accuracy of 97,4% are promising results of the $C_i$ methodology for analysing DISC-assay results. The most important fact we found is, however, that patients with a $C_i$-max over 0,5 lived significantly longer than patients with a $C_i$-max below 0,5. Nevertheless, as the the three missed non-responders demonstrate, no *in-vitro* test can hope to mimic the *in-vivo* complexities of drug delivery, metabolism and excretion that a perfect predictive accuracy results.

The majority (64%) of the non-responders had prognostic unfavourable cytogenetic abnormalities. However, the rate of 26% of unfavourable karyotypes in the responder-group implies that the karyotype - although one of the strongest known prognostic factors - is not the only determinant of the biology in AML.

Our data confirm that the DISC-assay is one of the most suitable *in-vitro* drug sensitivity test for acute myeloid leukemias. By application of the chemosensitivity index $C_i$ evaluation methodology the DISC-assay provides a valuable tool for the prediction of individual treatment outcome in adult AML in terms of clinical response and also overall survival. In childhood ALL *in-vitro* drug sensitivity test results were shown to be one of the strongest independent prognostic factors [21-22]. For AML this still remains an open question, but our data encourage further prospective evaluation to find out whether the $C_i$ is an independent new prognostic factor in AML and whether it may serve for the stratification of treatment in clinical trials. Prospective clinical trials where patients are randomised to receive best available therapy or assay directed therapy or, alternatively, treatment is stratified according to risk groups identified by assay results are definitely justified [13,20]. For childhood ALL such a strategy has already been adapted, since within the German childhood ALL BFM study protocol treatment is partly stratified according to drug resistance assay results [22].

*Acknowledgements.* This work was partly supported by the Deutsche Krebshilfe e.V. Bonn, Germany, and partly by the Frauke-Weiskam-Stiftung, Stifterverband für die deutsche Wissenschaft e.V., Essen, Germany.

# References

1. Weisenthal LM, Dill PL, Kurnick NB and Lippman ME (1983) Comparison of dye exclusion assays with a clonogenic assay in the determination of drug-induced cytotoxicity. Cancer Res 43:258-264
2. Weisenthal LM, Marsden JA, Dill PL and Macaluso CK (1983) A novel dye exclusion test for testing *in-vitro* chemosensitivity of human tumors. Cancer Res 43:749-757
3. Delmer A, Marie JP, Thevenin D, Cadiou M, Viguie F and Zittoun R (1989) Multivariate analysis of prognostic factors in acute myeloid leukemia: value of clonogenic leukemic cell properties. J Clin Onc 7:738-746
4. Kirkpatrick DL, Duke M, Goh TS (1990) Chemosensitivity testing of fresh human leukemia cells using both a dye exclusion assay and a tetrazolium dye (MTT) assay. Leukemia Res 14:459-466
5. Klumper E, Ossenkoppele GJ, Pieters R, Huismans DR, Loonen AH, Rottier A, Westra G and Veerman AJP (1996) In vitro resistance to cytosine arabinoside, not to daunorubicin, is associated with the risk of relapse in de novo acute myeloid leukaemia. Br J Haematol 93:903-910
6. Pieters R, Huismans DR, Loonen AH, Hählen K, van der Does-van den Berg A, van Wering ER and Veerman AJP (1991) Relation of cellular drug resistance to long-term clinical outcome in childhood acute lymphoblastic leukaemia. Lancet 338:399-403
7. Sargent JM, Taylor CG (1989) Appraisal of the MTT assay as a rapid test of chemosensitivity in acute myeloid leukaemia. Br J Cancer 60:206-210
8. Bird MC, Godwin VAJ, Antrobus JH, Bosanquet AG (1987) Comparison of *in-vitro* drug sensitivity by the differential staining cytotoxicity (DISC) assay and colony-forming assays. Br J Cancer 55:429-431

9. Bird MC, Bosanquet AG, Forskitt S, Gilby ED (1986) Semi-micro adaption of a 4-day differential staining cytotoxicity (DISC) assay for determining the *in-vitro* chemosensitivity of haematological malignancies. Leuk Res 10:445-449

10. Bosanquet AG (1993) The DISC assay - 10 years and 2000 tests further on. In: Kaspers GJL, Pieters R, Twentyman PR, Weisenthal LM & Veerman AJP (eds) Drug Resistance in Leukemia and Lymphoma. The Clinical Value of Laboratory Studies. Harwood, London, pp 373-384

11. Bosanquet AG (1991) Correlations between therapeutic response of leukaemias and *in-vitro* drug sensitivity assay. Lancet 337:711-714

12. Kaspers GJL, Pieters R, Van Zantwijk CH, De Laat PAJM, De Waal FC, Van Wering ER and Veerman AJP (1991) *In-vitro* drug sensitivity of normal peripheral blood lymphocytes and childhood leukaemic cells from bone marrow and peripheral blood. Br J Cancer 64:469-474

13. Bosanquet AG (1993) *In-vitro* drug sensitivity testing for the individual patient: an ideal adjunct to current methods of treatment choice. Clin Oncol 5:195-197

14. Bosanquet AG (1994) Short-term *in-vitro* drug sensitivity tests for cancer chemotherapy. A summary of correlations ot test result with both patient response and survival. Forum Trends Exp. Clin. Med. 4:179-189

15. Lathan B, von Tettau M, Verpoort K, Diehl V (1990) Pretherapeutic drug testing in acute leukemias for prediction of individual prognosis. In: Büchner T, Schellong G, Hiddemann W, Ritter J (eds) Haematology and Blood Transfusion. Vol. 33. Acute Leukemias II. Springer Verlag, Berlin, Heidelberg, pp 295-298

16. Staib P., Lathan B., Michel K., Janz E., Schinköthe T. and Diehl V (1998) Predictive value of prethera-peutic *in-vitro* chemosensitiviti testing in adult AML. Haematology and Blood Transfusion 39: 509-519

17. Büchner T, Hiddemann W, Wörmann B, Löffler H, Gassmann W, Haferlach T, Heyll A, Aul C, Lengfelder E, Maschmeyer G, Ludwig WD, Sauerland MC and Heinecke A (1996) Intensive consolidation versus prolonged maintenance following intensive induction and conventional consolidation in primary AML: a study by AMLCG. Blood 88 (No 10): 214a (suppl. 1)

18. Wickramanayke PD, Steinmetz HT, Katay I, Glasmacher A, Staib P and Diehl V (1995) Phase II trial of idarubicine, fludarabine, Ara-C and filgrastim (G-CSF) (Ida-FLAG) for the treatment of poor prognosis acute myeloid leukemia (AML). Blood 86 (No 10): 755a (suppl. 1)

19. Tidefelt U, Sundman-Engberg B, Rhedin AS, Paul C (1989) In vitro drug testing in patients with acute leukemia with incubations mimicking in vitro intracellular drug concentrations. Eur J Haematol 43:374-384

20. Veerman AJP and Pieters R (1990) Drug sensitivity assays in leukemia and lymphoma. Br J Haematol 74:381-384

21. Kaspers GJL, Veerman AJP, Pieters R, Van Zantwijk CH, Smets LA, Van Wering ER, Van Der Does-Van Den Berg A (1997) In-vitro cellular drug resistance and prognosis in newly diagnosed childhood acute lymphoblastic leukemia. Blood 90 (No7):2723-2729

22. Kaspers GJL, Pieters R, Van Zantwijk CH, Van Wering ER, Van Der Does-Van Den Berg A and Veerman AJP (1998) Prednisolone resistance in childhood acute lymphoblastic leukemia: vitro-vivo correlations and cross-resistance to other drugs. Blood 92 (No 1):259-266

# Antileukemic Effects of Buthionine Sulfoximine (BSO) (NSC 326231) in Vivo: A Pilot Study in Acute Myeloblastic Leukemia

J. Curtis, D.W. Hedley, M.D. Minden, M.A. Moore and E.A. McCulloch

*Abstract.* In this pilot study we have tested the in vivo effects of the potent glutathione (GSH)-depleting agent buthionine sulfoximine (BSO) on the peripheral blood blast cells of 6 patients with acute myeloblastic leukemia (AML) in relapse. The clinical trial was designed to extend the observation that in the presence of BSO the cells of some blast populations are depleted of GSH and undergo apoptosis. Each patient received a continuous intravenous infusion of BSO over 72 hours. A loading dose of 3 Gm/m$^2$ body surface area (BSA) was given over 30 minutes followed by a continuous infusion at a rate of 0.75 Gm/m$^2$ BSA/hour. Blood was drawn before the start of BSO, at 24, 48 and 72 hours and later times after BSO to determine clonogenic cell recovery (CCR) and to measure by flow cytometry intracellular GSH and reactive oxygen intermediates (ROI). In vitro BSO dose responses were determined by exposing AML blast cells to a range of doses of BSO for 48 hours in suspension culture; cells were then washed, counted and an aliquot plated in methylcellulose to enable calculation of CCR. BSO levels were measured every 12 hours during the infusion of BSO. The AML continuous cell line OCI/AML-5 was used to determine the effect of BSO on resistance to cytosine arabinoside (ARA-C) in culture. For 5 patients CCR in vivo was measured serially; CCR for two patients decreased to <20% of control, for two patients to <70% and for one patient there was no change. Serial intracellular GSH values were available for 4 of these patients with reductions ranging from 32 to 45% of control. Plasma BSO levels showed patient to patient heterogeneity. Clinical status and blood counts remained stable during BSO; no significant toxicity was observed. The ARA-C resistance of OCI/AML-5 cells was reduced in the presence of BSO.

The studies demonstrate the in vivo cytotoxic effect of BSO on the blast cells of AML patients and suggest that the effect is mediated through GSH depletion. Higher doses of BSO and/or longer durations of infusion might be associated with larger effects on blast cells and have greater therapeutic potential. The adjuvant role of BSO with chemotherapeutic agents such as ARA-C may lead to new therapeutic options for patients with AML.

## Introduction

The outcomes of patients with acute myeloblastic leukemia have improved in recent years [1-4]. Despite better results with remission induction treatment and bone marrow transplantation, most patients continue to die leukemia-related deaths. In this paper we present the results of a pilot study that demonstrates that the potent glutathione (GSH)-depleting agent, buthionine sulfoximine (BSO), is cytotoxic to AML blast cells in vivo. The trial based on pre-clinical investigations in our laboratory [5,6] was designed as the initial step in the development of a new treatment strategy for AML.

Recently it has been appreciated that oxidative mechanisms may be important in the effective chemotherapy of AML and in the cytotoxicity of cytosine arabinoside (ARA-C)(5,7). When AML blast cells were exposed to ARA-C in culture, multi-parameter flow

Department of Medical Oncology and Hematology, Princess Margaret Hospital and Division of Cellular and Molecular Biology, Ontario Cancer Institute, Toronto, Canada

cytometry revealed the following sequence of events. Initially, there was a transient increase in both GSH and reactive oxygen intermediates (ROI), second, a dramatic fall in GSH levels and a further increase in ROI and, finally, cell death by apoptosis (5). Exposure of AML blast cells to BSO in cell culture was associated with a dose-dependent reduction in clonogenic cell recovery (CCR). Flow cytometry demonstrated that the mechanism of apoptosis with BSO exposure was similar to that seen with ARA-C, depletion of GSH and increase in ROI (6). GSH deficiency can be readily induced in cells with BSO, a selective inhibitor of γ-glutamylcysteine synthetase, the enzyme controlling the rate-limiting step in GSH synthesis (8,9). Phase I studies in patients with solid tumours have confirmed that BSO is relatively non-toxic in very large doses for human cells and that its administration is associated with substantial reductions in levels of cellular (GSH) (10-12). GSH-mediated detoxification of common cytotoxic drugs such as alkylating agents, anthracyclines and platinum compounds has been suggested as a mechanism of chemotherapy resistance (13-15). In vivo GSH depletion by BSO would be thus anticipated to enhance the anti-tumour effects of these drugs as well as ARA-C, one of the most useful drugs in the treatment of AML.

In the study described below patients with AML in relapse were given infusions of BSO. Using cell culture methods and flow cytometry, an in vivo decrease both in the CCR of blast cells and the depletion of GSH in blast cell populations has been demonstrated.

## Materials and Methods

### Patient Selection

The patients entered on this study had a diagnosis of AML established according to the criteria of the FAB classification [16]. The clinical features of the patients are summarized in Table 1. All patients were in relapse after one or more courses of intensive remission induction therapy; patients had neither chemotherapy nor radiation treatment in the two weeks before commencing BSO. Study patients were considered in "stable" relapse and unlikely to require chemotherapy in the next two weeks. All patients had circulating peripheral blood blast cells. Patients had normal renal function as indicated by normal serum creatinine, adequate liver function with hepatic enzymes less than 1.5 times normal and all had a central venous catheter in place. Patients gave written informed consent according to institutional guidelines before entry on the BSO pilot study.

**Table 1.** Patients – Clinical Characteristics

| UPN | AGE/ SEX | FAB CLASS | Peripheral Blood[a] TOTAL WBC | ABS BLASTS | CLINICAL STATUS |
|-----|----------|-----------|-------------------------------|------------|-----------------|
| 1432 | 38/M | M5B | 13.6 | 5.6 | Ca thyroid treated with $I^{131}$; prior MDS; primary non-responder to DNR and HDara-c and etoposide and topotecan remission inductions |
| 1350 | 73/M | M1 | 28.5 | 16.2 | prior MDS-no treatment; CR with DNR, Hdara-c, ATRA; duration 6 months |
| 1326 | 53M | M4 | 21.1 | 13.9 | CR with DNR and HDara-c; remission 9 months; no response CYCLO and etoposide |
| 1330 | 68M | M0 | 2.6 | 1.9 | CR with DNR,HDara-c,ATRA; duration 2months |
| 1440 | 43M | M4E | 4.8 | 3.9 | Primary non-responder;DNR and Hdara-c and etoposide and topotecan remission inductions |
| 1410 | 35M | M1 | 10.2 | 6.0 | Primary non-responder DNR, ara-c; then MITOX and HDara-c |

MDS – myelodysplastic syndrome; DNR – daunorubicin; HDara-c – high-dose cytosine arabinoside; CR- complete remission; ATRA- all-trans retinoic acid; MITOX – mitoxantrone [a] $\times 10^9$ per litre

## Treatment Plan

Prior to starting BSO patients were admitted to the inpatient leukemia service at the Princess Margaret Hospital, Toronto, and remained in hospital for 24 hours after completion of the BSO infusion. BSO (NSC 326231) was given by continuous intravenous infusion over 72 hours. Initially a loading dose of 3 gm per $m^2$ body surface area (BSA) was administered over 30 minutes followed by a continuous infusion at the rate of 0.75 gm per $m^2$ BSA per hour. All patients received the same dose and schedule of BSO as in this trial only one dose and schedule was tested. BSO was supplied by the Division of Cancer Treatment, Diagnosis and Centers, National Cancer Institute, Bethesda, MD.

After completion of the BSO infusion patients were followed for up to two weeks. If their clinical condition indicated, patients were given additional treatment with chemotherapy at the discretion of their attending physician. Toxicity was graded using the Expanded Common Toxicity Criteria of the National Cancer Institute of Canada Clinical Trials Group.

## Laboratory Studies

BSO DOSE RESPONSE IN VITRO. Peripheral blood cells were obtained prior to starting the BSO infusion for measurement of BSO dose response in culture. Purified preparations of blast cells were prepared by a two-step Ficoll-Hypaque procedure as previously described [17-19]. Blast cells were then cultured one to 3 days before addition of BSO in α-minimal essential medium (α-MEM) supplemented with 10% fetal calf serum (FCS) and c-kit ligand (KL) obtained from the supernatant of c-kit transfected CHO cells (Genetics Institute, Cambridge, MA). Aliquots of cells were cultured with and without a range of doses of BSO (L-buthionine sulfoximine, Sigma, St Louis, MO) for 48 hours in suspension culture containing α-MEM medium, 10% each of FCS, KL and 5637CM (prepared from the bladder cancer cell line 5637 and used as source of G-CSF and GM-CSF)[20]. For the clonogenic assay cells were plated in quadruplicate in α-MEM medium containing 0.8%

methylcellulose, 10% FCS, KL and 5637CM for 5 to 7 days in 96-microwell plates (Linbro, Flow Laboratories, McLean, VA) for 5 to 7 days at $37^0C$ in a moist atmosphere containing 5% $CO_2$. Colonies containing >20 cells were counted using an inverted microscope giving the plating efficiency in methylcellulose [18]. The colony counts were used to calculate clonogenic cell recovery (CCR) and prepare the dose response curves as previously described [19,21].

## Clonogenic Cell Recovery in Vivo

For this purpose peripheral blood was drawn from the patient and plated as quickly as possible. The blast cell containing population was separated by a single Ficoll-Hypaque procedure, the mononuclear fraction was washed, counted and aliquots plated in methylcellulose in quadruplicate in microwell plates with growth factors as described above. Colonies were counted between 5 and 7 days. In vivo CCR was expressed as a percentage of the number of colonies per $10^4$ cells plated compared with the number of colonies before BSO.

## ARA-C Dose Response Curves

The continuous AML cell line OCI/AML-5 was used study the effect of BSO on ARA-C sensitivity (21). Cells were exposed to a range of doses of ARA-C for 48 hours in suspension culture either with or without a single dose of BSO. The dose of BSO chosen was one that in preliminary tests was found to be non-toxic for OCI/AML-5 cells. After suspension culture, the cells were washed, counted and an aliquot by volume plated in methylcellulose with 10% FCS and 5637CM as described above. OCI/AML-5 cells for optimal growth require GM-CSF provided by 5637CM. After 5 days in culture, colonies were counted and dose response curves to ARA-C were constructed [22].

## Flowcytometry

Reduced GSH was measured using the sulphydryl probe monobromobimane (MBBr) at a final concentration of 50 mm for 5 minutes [6,23]. This compound binds avidly to glutathione, yielding a brightly fluorescent conjugate. When applied to AML samples, approximately 80% of the fluorescence is derived from the binding of MBBr to GSH, with the remainder coming from the other low molecular weight thiols, particularly cysteine. A dual-labeling technique was used to measure reactive oxygen intermediates (ROI) and GSH simultaneously. ROI were measured by using dihydrorhodamine 123 (Molecular Probes, Eugene, OR) by methods previously described [5].

### L-Buthionine (SR)-Sulfoximine Plasma Levels

Blood samples for BSO determinations were drawn every 12 hours during the BSO infusion. Samples were centrifuged and the plasma immediately stored at $-20^0C$ until required for analysis. Plasma samples were extracted and analyzed by HPLC using a modified procedure of Koyama et al [24].

## Results

The patients at the time of entry into the study and the start of the BSO infusion were all in relapse but were asymptomatic and clinically stable (Table 1).. Patient UPN 1432 had treatment with $I^{131}$ for carcinoma of the thyroid 10 years previously and was considered to have secondary AML. Patients 1432 and 1350 had documented myelodysplasia before the onset of AML; the other patients had de novo AML. The total leukocyte count, absolute neutrophils, platelets, hemoglobin, serum creatinine and liver function tests remained constant during and immediately after BSO.

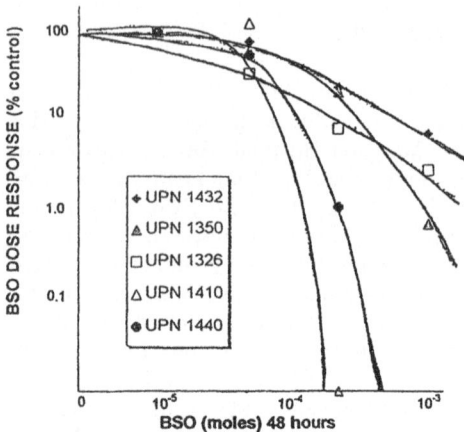

**Fig. 1.** BSO dose responses of peripheral blast cells of patients with AML who subsequently received intravenous infusions of BSO. Cells were exposed to BSO in suspension culture for 48 hours and then plated in methylcellulose to measure CCR. Marked heterogeneity in sensitivity to BSO in culture was observed.

For one patient (UPN 1440) there was a steady increase in the absolute blast cell count during and after BSO; for the others the blast cell counts remained within a narrow range. Serious toxicity to BSO was not encountered in any patients in this pilot study. The severest toxicity was grade 2 nausea and vomiting (NCIC criteria) in patients 1440 and 1350 (Table 2).

The BSO dose response curves of the blast cells of 5 patients demonstrated marked heterogeneity (Figure 1); the peripheral blood

**Table 2.** In Vivo Effects of BSO on Blasts of Six Patients Receiving a Continuous Infusion of BSO

| UPN | Maximum Reduction During BSO | | ADVERSE EFFECTS |
| | CLONOGENIC CELL RECOVERY[a] | INTRACELLULAR GSH[a] | |
| --- | --- | --- | --- |
| 1432 | 70 | 45 | NONE |
| 1350 | <20 | 38 | HEADACHES; VOMITING X2 |
| 1326 | 69 | NOT DONE | NONE |
| 1330 | NOT DONE | NOT DONE | MILD NAUSEA DAYS 2 AND 3 |
| 1440 | <20 | 38 | NAUSEA; VOMITING NEEDED ANTI-EMETICS |
| 1410 | 84 | 32 | NONE |

[a] maximum reduction during BSO infusion expressed as percent of value before starting infusion

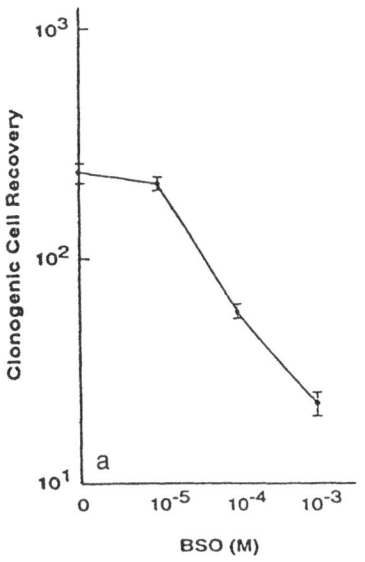

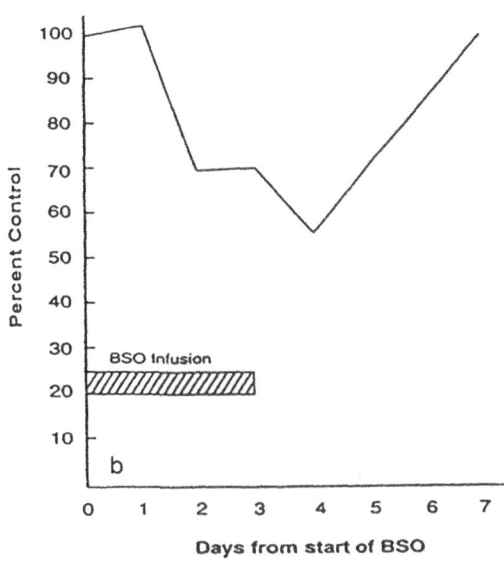

**Fig. 2.** BSO associated changes in CCR as measured in vitro (panel A) and in vivo (panel B) for patient UPN 1432. The responses in vivo and in vitro were typical of the results obtained for the blast cells of patients treated with BSO in this study.

blast cells of one patient (UPN 1330) did not grow in cell culture. The in vitro dose response to BSO for patient UPN 1432 (Figure 2A) and the in vivo CCR for the cells of the same patient (Figure 2B) are illustrative of the effects of BSO on leukemic cell growth. CCR in vivo during the BSO infusion was obtained for 5 of the patients (Table 2). For two patients in vivo CCR was reduced during the BSO infusion to less than 20% of the value immediately before BSO. The CCR in vivo for the blasts of another two patients was reduced to less than 70% of control; for one patient the reduction was less than 20%. Decrease in CCR was limited to the time of BSO infusion as in vivo CCR recovered promptly to control (pre-treatment) levels with completion of the BSO infusion.

Intracellular GSH in the blast cells of 4 patients was determined serially during the BSO infusions (Figure 3). The reductions of GSH ranged from 32 to 45% of control or pretreatment GSH concentrations. As with the changes in in vivo CCR, the reductions in GSH were transient and confined to the period of BSO infusion. The method used for measuring GSH does not distinguish binding of the stain (MMBr) to cysteine and may have

resulted in underestimating GSH depletion (23). In this small study we could not demonstrate a correlation between the decrease in in vivo CCR and blast cell intracellular GSH depletion. Similarly no correspondence of

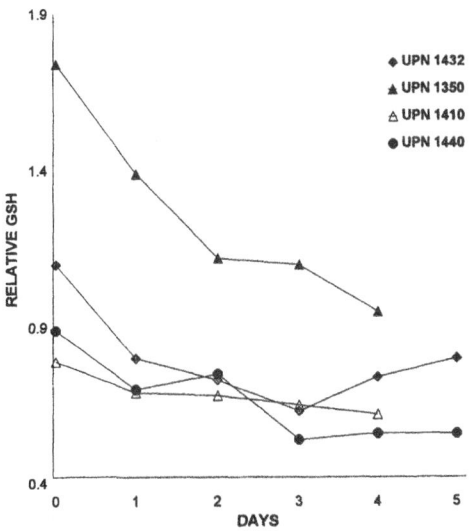

**Fig. 3.** GSH concentrations in the blast cells of 4 patients were measured serially during BSO infusion. Marked heterogeneity in GSH depletion was observed.

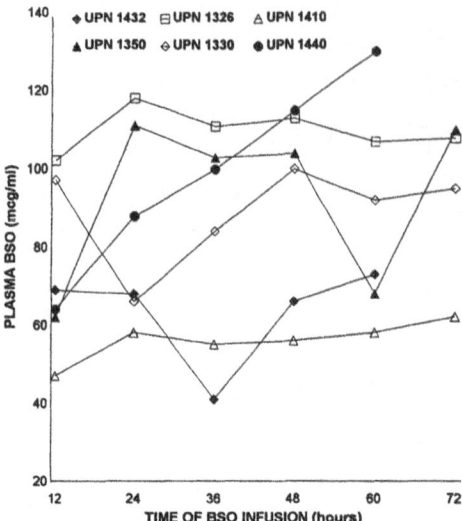

**Fig. 4.** Plasma levels of BSO in patients during BSO infusion. Considerable heterogeneity was found between patients. In patient UPN 1440 plasma BSO levels rose steadily during the BSO infusion. For this patient no decrease in CCR or GSH was identified; in contrast with the other patients the peripheral blood blast count increased during the BSO infusion.

BSO sensitivity in vitro with in vivo CCR reduction or GSH depletion was observed. In contrast to our previous study (5), an increase in ROI was not observed in blast cells exposed to BSO in vitro and despite the evidence of GSH depletion increase in ROI was not found after in vivo administration of BSO.

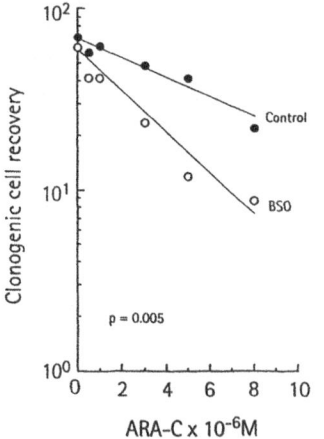

**Fig. 5.** The sensitivity to ARA-C of the continuous AML cell line OCI/AML-5 was significantly increased in the presence of BSO.

The plasma levels of BSO showed variation from patient to patient and for 5 of the patients the BSO levels were relatively constant during the BSO infusion (Figure 4). For one patient (UPN 1440) there was a steady rise in BSO plasma concentrations during the infusion. This patient was metabolically stable during the BSO infusion but unlike the other patients there was a rise in the absolute blast cell count during the time of the BSO infusion.

Cells from the ARA-C resistant continuous cell line OCI/AML-5 were used to test the effect of BSO on ARA-C resistance (Figure 5). For this purpose a dose of BSO was chosen that in preliminary experiments was found not to have a cytotoxic effect on the growth of OCI/AML-5 cells [25]. In the presence of BSO there was a significant decrease in the resistance of the cells to ARA-C.

## Discussion

In this study GSH depletion in vivo and reduction in CCR in vivo were found for the blast cells of some patients. The observations confirm and validate the pre-clinical studies as the in vivo effects of BSO on AML blasts parallel those found in vitro, a cytotoxic effect on blast cells associated with GSH depletion [5]. Further, BSO in the dose and schedule employed was well tolerated by all the patients in the study. In the current pilot study the supply of BSO permitted the testing of only one dose and schedule of BSO. A higher dose of BSO might induce greater GSH depletion although the maximum decrease in experimental systems of GSH by BSO has been to 20% of normal cellular concentrations of GSH [7]. A reduction in GSH to this level has been associated with mitochondrial damage and may be sufficient to enhance apoptosis [26]. As the reductions in in vivo CCR and GSH were limited to the time of BSO administration, longer durations of BSO infusions might have more lasting cytotoxic effect on AML blast cell populations. This has been the experience when non-chemotherapeutic agents such as all-trans retinoic acid (ATRA) and arsenic trioxide have been used to treat the t(15;17) variant of AML [27,28]. Our results indicate the need for additional clinical trials using higher doses and longer times of infusion to assess adequately the activity of BSO in AML.

The responses of AML blast cell progenitors both in vitro and in vivo are heterogeneous. With blast populations ranging from very sensitive to highly resistant to BSO, significant anti-leukemic activity may easily be missed in studies with very small numbers of patients. If a GSH-depleting agent is effective in the treatment of AML, it would only be expected to benefit a small fraction of the patient population with AML. This again supports the need for more extensive testing of BSO in AML.

Finally, BSO in a very small non-toxic dose was found in cell culture to reduce the resistance of the continuous AML cell line, OCI/AML-5 to ARA-C. The cytotoxic activity of ARA-C may be mediated in part through the generation of ROI [6] and could be potentially enhanced in vivo in the presence of BSO. The role of BSO as a biological response modifier for other cytotoxic drugs including the anthracyclines and platinum compounds, both of which have significant activity in AML, has not yet been explored. While BSO alone may provide effective treatment for a small group of patients, BSO as an adjuvant to chemotherapy may have greater applicability in the treatment of AML.

# References

1. Mayer RJ, Davis RB, Schiffer CA, Berg BL, Schulman P, Omura GA, Moore JO, McIntyre OR. Frei 3rd E. Intensive postremission chemotherapy in adults with acute myeloid leukemia. N Engl J Med 1994, 31:896-903.
2. Bishop JF, Mathews JP, Young GA, Szar J, Gillet A, Joshua D, Bradstock K, Enno A, Wolf MM, Fox R, Cobcroft R, Herrmann R, Van Der Weyden M, Lowenthal RM, Page F, Garson OM, Juneja S. A randomized study of high-dose cytarabine in induction in acute myeloid leukemia. Blood 1996, 87:1710-7.
3. Mitus AJ, Miller RB, Schenkein DP, Ryan HF, Parsons SK, Wheeeler C, Antin JH. Improved survival for patients with acute myelogenous leukemia. J Clin Oncol 1995, 13:560-9.
4. Cassileth PA, Harrington DP, Appelbaum FR, Hillard M, Lazarus MD, Rowe JM, Paietta E, Willman C, Hurd DD, Bennett JM, Blume KG, Head DR, Wiernik PH. Chemotherapy compared with autologous or allogeneic bone marrow transplantation in the management of acute myeloid leukemia in first remission. N Engl J Med 1998, 339:1649-56.
5. Hedley DW, McCulloch EA. Generation of reactive oxygen intermediates after treatment of blasts of acute myeloblastic leukemia with cytosine arabinoside: role of bcl-2. Leukemia 1996, 10:1143-49.
6. Hedley DW, McCulloch EA, Minden MD, Chow S, Curtis JE. Antileukemic action of buthionine sulfoximine: evidence for an intrinsic death mechanism based on oxidative stress. Leukemia 1998, 12:1545-52.
7. Hu Z-B, Minden MD, McCulloch EA. Direct evidence for the participation of bcl-2 in the regulation by retinoic acid of the cytosine arabinoside sensitivity of leukemic stem cells. Leukemia 1995, 9:1667-73.
8. Meister A. Glutathione deficiency produced by inhibition of its synthesis, and its reversal; applications in research and therapy. Pharmac Ther 1991, 51:155-194.
9. Tew KD. Glutathione-associated enzymes in anticancer drug resistance. Cancer Res 1994, 54:4313-20.
10. O'Dwyer PJ, Hamilton TC, Young RC, LaCreta FP, Carp N, Tew KD, Padavic K, Comis RL, Ozols RF. Depletion of glutathione in normal and malignant human cells in vivo by buthionine sulfoximine: clinical and biochemical results. J Natl Cancer Inst 1992, 84:264-67.
11. Bailey HH, Mulcahy RT, Tutsch KD, Arzoomanian RZ, Alberti D, Tombes MB, Wilding G, Pomplun M, Spriggs DR. Phase I clinical trial of intravenous L-buthionine sulfoximine and melphalan: an attempt at modulation of glurathione. J Clin Oncol 1994, 12:194-204.
12. O'Dwyer PJ, Hamilton TC, LaCreta FP, Gallo JM, Kilpatrick D, Halbherr T, Brennan J, Bookman MA, Hoffman J, Young RC, Comis RL, Ozols RF. Phase I trial of buthionine sulfoximine in combination with melphalan in patients with cancer. J Clin Oncol 1996,14:249-56.
13. Siemann DW, Beyers KL. In vivo therapeutic potential of combination thiol depletion and alkylating chemotherapy. Br J Haematol 1993, 68:1071-79.
14. Zaman GJR, Lankelma J, van Tellingen O, Beijnen J, Dekker H, Paulusma C, Oude Elferink RPJ, Baas F, Borst. Role of glutathione in the export of compounds from cells by the multidrug-resistance-associated protein. Proc Natl Acad Sci USA 1995, 92:6790-4.
15. Goddard P, Valenti M, Kelland LR. The role of glutathione (GSH) in determining sensitivity to platinum drugs in vivo in platinum-sensitive and –resistant leukaemia and plasmacytoma and human ovarian carcinoma xenografts. Anticancer Res 1994, 14:1065-70.
16. Bain BJ. Leukaemia Diagnosis 2nd ed. Oxford, UK, Blackwell Science 1999.
17. Minden MD, Buick RN, McCulloch EA. Separation of blast cell and T-lymphocyte progenitors in the blood of patients with acute myeloblastic leukemia. Blood 1979, 54:186-95.
18. Buick RN, Till JE, McCulloch EA. Colony assay for proliferating blast cells circulating in myeloblastic leukemia. Lancet 1977, 1:862-3.
19. Nara N, McCulloch EA. The proliferation in suspension of the progenitors of the blast cells in acute myeloblastic leukemia. Blood 1985, 65:1484-93.

20. Hoang T, McCulloch EA. Production of leukemic blast cell growth factor by a human bladder carcinoma cell line. Blood 1985, 66:745-51.

21. Curtis JE, Minden MD, Minkin S, and McCulloch EA. A Comparison of the Sensitivities of AML Blast Stem Cells to Idarubicin and Daunorubicin. Leukemia. 1995, 9: 396-404.

22. Curtis JE, Minkin S, Minden MD and McCulloch EA. A Role for Paclitaxel in the Combination Chemotherapy of Acute Myeloblastic Leukemia: Preclinical Cell Culture Studies. 1996, Br J Haematol, 95: 354-363.

23. Chow S, Hedley DW. Flow cytometric measurement of glutathione in clinical samples. Cytometry 1995, 21:68-71.

24. Koyama H, Sugioka N, Hirata I, Ohta T, Kishimoto H. Determination of L-buthionin (SR)-sulfoximine, gamma-glutamylcysteine synthetase inhibitor in rat plasma with HPLC after prelabeling with dansyl chloride. J Chromatogr Sci 1996;34:326-9.

25. Curtis JE. Unpublished observations.

26. Meister A. Glutathione, ascorbate, and cellular protection. Cancer Res (suppl) 1994, 1969s-1975s.

# Dendritic Cells Generated out of Blasts from Patients with Acute Leukemia

T. Köhler, R. Plettig, W. Wetzstein, G. Ehninger and M. Bornhäuser

*Abstract.* We investigated the ability of both acute myelogenous and lymphoblastic (ALL) cells to differentiate into dendritic cells (DC) in vitro. Cytokine supplemented suspension cultures of leukemic blasts in 30 patients with AML and 3 patients with BCR/ABL positive ALL were performed. Mononuclear cells out of peripheral blood or bone marrow containing between 60 and 90% leukemic blasts were cultured for 8 days using granulocyte-macrophage colony-stimulating factor, tumor necrosis factor-$\alpha$ and Flt-3 ligand and interleukin-4. The content of CD1a+/CD14- cells after 8 days of culture varied between 1 and 2 % in ALL and between 2 and 28 % in AML samples. In 4 informative AML patients CD1a+/CD14- cells were sorted by fluorescence activated cell sorting (FACS). Cytogenetic and PCR analysis showed known primary chromosomal aberrations (monosomy 7 and inversion 16) in the sorted fractions, respectively. In the ALL patients the sorted CD1+/CD14- fractions were BCR/ABL negative when analyzed with fluorescence in-situ hybridization indicating their non-leukemic origin. BCR/ABL positive lymphoblasts could not be transformed into cells with a early dendritic phenotype with the cytokines used in our experiments. In contrast, a significant number of dendritic cells can be generated out of leukemic blasts in 78% of AML patients. There seemed to be a trend towards a higher remission rate in patients with > 1.0 % CD1a+/14- cells after culture. Leukemic DC might be useful for autologous and allogeneic immunotherapy in selected patients.

## Introduction

Long-term remission can only be achieved in a small number of patients with acute myelogenous leukemia [1]. Besides allogeneic blood stem cell transplantation, autologous immunotherapy might be a way to optimize the treatment outcome especially in older patients. Dendritic cells carrying and presenting leukemic antigens are supposed to be helpful in targeting residual leukemic stem cells. Since the development of leukemic progeny resembles the normal hematopoiesis, the in-vitro generation of leukemic dendritic cells seems possible with similar cytokine combinations [2,3]. Those dendritic cells might elicit potent antileukemic T cell responses with more specificity and might be useful for in vivo vaccination strategies.

Efforts to generate dendritic cells with a leukemic genotype in serum-free cultures have been successful in acute (AML) and chronic myelogenous leukemia (CML)[4,5]. Dendritic cells (DC) presenting leukemic antigens seem to be potent effectors for induction of cytotoxic T cell responses in-vivo or in-vitro [6]. Only recently two groups have suggested that DC with the leukemic genotype or leukemia specific antigen markers can be grown in vitro out of AML cells [7,8]. Those DC were able to induce specific cytotoxicity of autologous T cells against leukemic targets cells.

Although this seems to be a promising approach to immunotherapy of AML, both groups reported cases where no DC could be cultured at all. Some AML cells behave different in cytokine driven cultures and leukemic stem cells can not be differentiated into DC.

Universitätsklinikum Carl Gustav Carus, Med. Klinik I, Dresden, Germany.

Patients with BCR/ABL positive acute lymphoblastic leukemia (ALL) have a poor prognosis even after allogeneic blood stem cell transplantation and do not respond to infusion of donor leukocytes in most cases. This seems to be either due to a resistance against the induction of apoptosis or the insufficient presentation of leukemic antigens and costimulatory signals.

We performed experiments using mononuclear cells of ninety-five patients with AML and 3 patients with BCR/ABL positive ALL. In most cases we compared the leukemic cells originating from peripheral blood and bone marrow. These cells were cultured in serum-free medium with addition of different cytokines. The aim of the study was to find the culture conditions with relevant in vitro growth of DC in most patients. The leukemic origin of those DC was tested by Fluorescence in situ Hybridization or PCR analysis, when chromosomal aberrations were known. The in vitro data were correlated with the myelogenous and lymphoblastic origin, the FAB subtypes and the response to induction chemotherapy.

## Materials and Methods

### Patient samples

Blood or bone marrow from 30 AML patients and 3 patients with Ph positive ALL was collected after informed consent at the time of sample collection. The clinical study including the drawing of all diagnostic and research samples had been approved by institutional ethical board. The cells were diluted with PBS DULBECCO'S w/o Magnesium and Calcium, pH 7.2 (Gibco, Paisley, Scotland). Density gradient centrifugation was performed as follows:

Blood was centrifuged with Immuflot (Immucor GmbH, Rödermark, Germany) at 800 g for 20 minutes, mononuclear cells were collected and washed twice with PBS, supplemented with 0.5 % Human Serum Albumin (HSA 5%, Immuno GmbH, Heidelberg, Germany).

Pellets were resuspended in 5 ml of X-VIVO 20 (Bio-Whittaker, Walkersville, Maryland). Cells were counted automatically by Technicon H 3 RTC™ (Bayer Diagnostics GmbH, München, Germany).

### Generation of DC from AML and ALL cells.

Mononuclear cells, containing AML-blasts, were cultured at 1 x 10$^6$ cells/ml in 25 cm$^2$ flasks containing 10 ml serum-free medium (X-VIVO 20, Bio-Whittaker) at 37°C and 5% $CO_2$ for eight days. Four growth factor cocktails containing GM-CSF (Amgen, Munich, Germany), TNF-α, Flt-3l, SCF, TGF-ß (R&D, Wiesbaden, Germany), IL-4, and IL-13 like seen in Table 1.

### Phenotypic analysis of cells by flow cytometry

Flow cytometric analysis of all samples before and after expansion was performed with FACS SCAN (Becton Dickinson, San Jose, USA) using the standard software LYSIS II. Double color staining and analysis were performed for all samples using the following antibodies: anti-CD1a-PE, anti-CD14-FITC, anti-CD80-FITC, anti-CD83-FITC, anti-CD86-FITC (Pharmingen), anti-CD11c-FITC, anti-HLA-DR-FITC (Serotec), anti Dendritic cells (X-11), anti-CD64-FITC, anti-CD38-FITC (Coulter-Immunotech Diagnostics, Miami, USA) and anti-CD34-PE (HPCA-2), a class III CD34 antibody (Becton Dickinson, San Jose,

**Table 1. Growth factor cocktails.** The culture was supplemented by GM-CSF, TNF-α and Flt-3l on principle. To obtain better yields an addition of the other cytokines was tested.

| | GM-CSF [U/ml] | TNF-α [U/ml] | Flt-3l [ng/ml] | IL-4 [U/ml] | IL-13 [ng/ml] | TGF-ß [ng/ml] | SCF [U/ml] |
|---|---|---|---|---|---|---|---|
| Cocktail DC 1 | 1000 | 60 | 100 | - | - | - | - |
| Cocktail DC 2 | 1000 | 60 | 100 | 1000 | - | - | - |
| Cocktail DC 3 | 1000 | 60 | 100 | 1000 | 10 | - | - |
| Cocktail DC 4 | 1000 | 100 | 100 | - | - | 0.25 | 50 |

USA). Double staining of CD1a and CD14, CD80, CD83, CD86, CD11c, CD64, or HLA-DR was performed to quantitate the DC phenotype. A "dendritic cell" antibody X-11 was tested before and after the cell culture period.

To test for vitality propidiumiodide (PI) staining was performed in all experiments. Annexin (R&D, Wiesbaden, Germany) was used to determine the percentage of apoptotic cells. PI-/Annexin+ events defined early apoptosis whereas PI+/Annexin+ signals were counted as late apoptosis. PI+/Annexin- cells are necrotic cells.

## Dendritic cell purification after in vitro culture

Cell sorting of DC was performed after the culture period. Two selection methods were used:

In 4 cases DC were separated with the help of a FACS VANTAGE (Becton Dickinson, San Jose, USA). All cells were labeled with a double color staining, using anti-CD14-FITC and anti-CD 1a-PE. Unspecific staining was removed, using the correction with the isotype controls IgG1-FITC/IgG1-PE and the compensation with CD14-FITC/IgG1-PE as well as CD1a-PE/IgG1-FITC. Sorted dendritic cells, that are CD1a+/CD14- were collected in a tube prefilled with PBS and 1% HSA.

Alternatively, DC were enriched using the MACS system according to the manufacturers instructions. Briefly, cells were washed and resuspended in PBS, 0.5% bovine serum albumin and 5 mmol/l EDTA. Cells were first incubated with CD1a antibody (mouse antihuman CD1a, Pharmingen) in the presence of human IgG as blocking reagent. After one cell wash, another incubation step with 100μl CD14 microbeads per $10^8$ cells followed. Labeled cells were loaded onto a column installed in a magnetic field. Trapped cells were removed and the CD14 negative fraction was used for further staining. These cells were incubated with 100μl rat anti mouse IgG1 microbeads per $10^8$ cells. Labeled cells were loaded onto another column installed in a magnetic field. Trapped cells were eluted after removal of the column.

## Genetic analysis of cells by fluorescence in situ hybridization (FISH) and polymerase chain reaction (PCR).

To prove the clonal origin of the sorted DC FISH for monosomy 7 was performed in 3 cases. Cells were sorted on slides. A commercial SO CEP 7 (α satellite) DNA probe was used together with a centromer specific probe for chromosome 11 as a control (Vysis, Stuttgart, Germany). In the samples from ALL patients interphase FISH for the BCR/ABL rearrangement was performed using a LSI bcr-abl dual color DNA probe (Vysis). The probes were used according to manufacturer's instructions. At least 300 interphase nucleii were examined in each experiment.

In 2 patients a sensitive nested RT-PCR for the fusion transcript CBFß-MYH1/inversion 16 was performed in the sorted CD1a+/14- cells as described before [9].

## Induction therapy

The patients characteristics are summarized in Table1. AML patients less than 60 years included in a multicenter trial received induction therapy with ara-C 8 x 100 mg/m², etoposide 5 x 100 mg/m² and mitoxantrone 5 x 10 mg/m². On day 28 ara-C 5 x 2000 mg/m² and amsacrine 5 x 100 mg/m² was infused (MAMAC). Patients older than 65 years were treated with 2 x 45 mg/m² daunorubicine and 7 x 100 mg/m² ara-C. Complete remission was defined as less than 5 % atypical blasts in a bone marrow aspirate when the platelet count was above 100 x 10⁹/l. Partial remission was defined as > 5-30% residual blasts.

## Results

### Cytokine combinations

The cytokine combinations tested are summarized in Table 1. The percentage of CD1a+/14- cells as well as the expression of costimulatory molecule CD80 was highest with cocktail 4 containing SCF, TGF-ß, TNF-alpha, GM-CSF and Flt3-ligand. (Fig. 1)

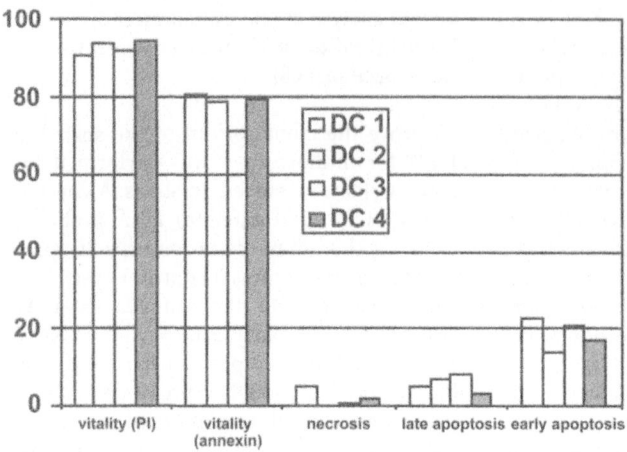

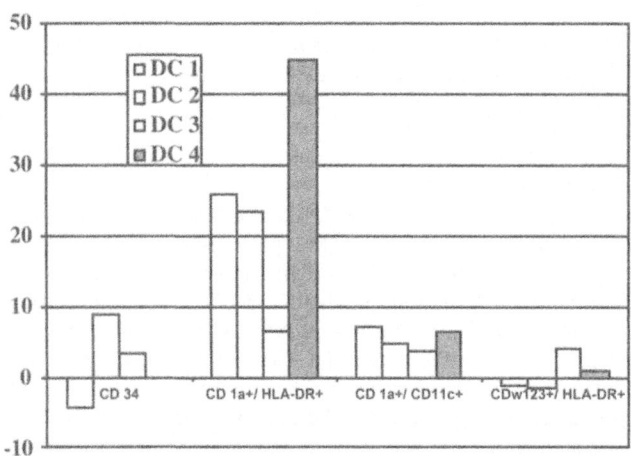

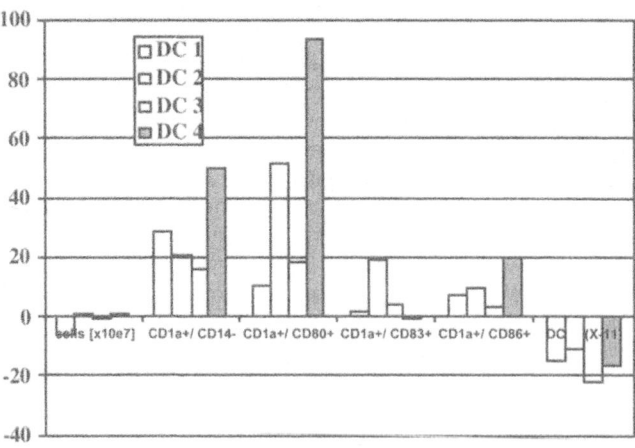

**Fig. 1.** Results of cultures with four different growth factor cocktails. The cytokines of the cocktails are provided in Table 1. The bars represented the percentage of the respective cell type after culture in percent.

## Phenotype analysis

The mean number of viable cells tested by propidium iodide staining and apoptosis data are provided in Table 2. DC could be obtained in 78 % of AML patients.

There was a significant increase of CD1a+/14- cells compared to the initial sample in some cases. The same was true for class II (DR) and the costimulatory CD80 and CD86 molecule.

The ALL samples contained somewhat less DC after culture compared to AML patients. The results of pre-and postculture analyses are depicted in Figure 2.

## Detection of clonal aberrations in sorted CD1a+/14- cells

In 3 patients with monosomy 7 FISH analysis confirmed the progeny of the leukemic DC. The same was possible in 2 patients with inversion 16 by PCR. In all ALL patients the sorted fractions were negative for the BCR/ABL transcript although BM analysis had shown 60-70% positive metaphases when PB or BM had been drawn.

## Clinical data

Out of 20 patients with > 1.0 % CD1a+/14- cells postculture 11/12 evaluable patients have

**Table 2.** Results of phenotypic analysis before and after 8 days of culture. The median and range (in brackets) for 30 AML (left) and 3 Ph+ ALL (right) samples are provided.

|  | AML | | ALL | |
|---|---|---|---|---|
|  | pre culture | post culture | pre culture | post culture |
| total nucleated cells [107] | 1 | 1.65 (0.04 - 3.39) | 1 | 1.0 (0.91 - 1.6) |
| vitality (PI) [%] | 98.5 (53 -99.9) | 91.7 (54.4 - 98.2) | 99.9 | 88.5 (79.2 - 93.1) |
| vitality (annexin) [%] | 88.0 (50.8 - 96.7) | 75.9 (37.7 - 92.2) | 89.9 | 71.4 (52.0 - 85.3) |
| necrosis [%] | 0.1 (0 - 9) | 0.7 (0 - 14.2) | 0 | 2.5 (0.3 - 6.3) |
| late apoptosis [%] | 1.2 (0 - 38) | 6.5 (0.6 - 31.4) | 0.2 | 9.0 (6.6 - 14.5) |
| early apoptosis [%] | 10.6 (1.2 - 94.3) | 12.6 (6.1 - 54.2) | 10 | 22 (5.7 - 33.5) |
| CD 34 [%] | 21.1 (0 - 88.5) | 10.2 (0 - 66.3) | 5.5 | 0.3 (0.1 - 18.7) |
| CD 1a+/ CD 14- [%] | 0.0 (0 - 0.2) | 2.65 (0 - 24.8) | 0 | 1.2 (0.7 - 3.8) |
| CD 1a+/ CD 80+ [%] | 0.05 (0 - 0.3) | 1.32 (0 - 5.8) | 0 | 1.4 (0.9 - 3.8) |
| CD 1a+/ CD 83+ [%] | 0.0 (0 - 0.2) | 0.21 (0 - 2.1) | 0 | 0.0 (0 - 0.6) |
| CD 1a+/ CD 86+ [%] | 0.06 (0 - 0.9) | 0.66 (0 - 4.1) | 0 | 1.2 (0.6 - 10.6) |
| CD 1a+/ HLA-DR+ [%] | 0.0 (0 - 0.4) | 1.90 (0 - 16.8) | 0 | 2.2 (0.9 - 9.5) |
| CD 1a+/ CD 11c+ [%] | 0.0 (0 - 0.2) | 1.06 (0 - 7.6) | 0 | 0.8 (0.2 - 1.2) |
| CD 1a+/ CD 64+ [%] | 0.0 (0 - 0.2) | 0.29 (0 - 2.6) | 0 | 1.1 (0.4 - 3.0) |
| CDw123/ HLA-DR+ [%] | 14.1 (0.2 - 55.4) | 6.73 (0.8 - 18.9) | 7.3 | 6.6 (6.4 - 17.6) |
| DC (X-11) [%] | 7.58 (0 - 63.3) | 2.26 (0 - 18.2) | 10.9 | 1.1 (0.4 - 1.6) |

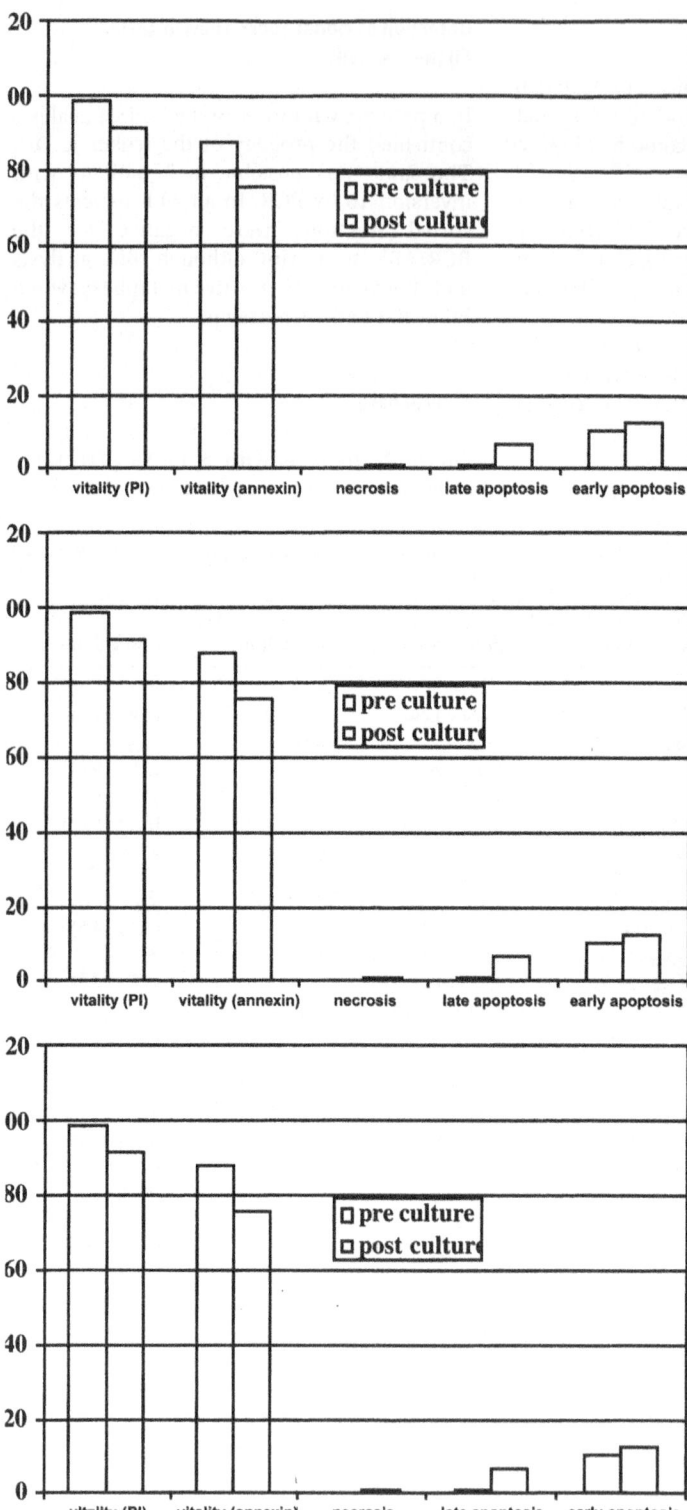

**Fig. 2.** Results of pre- and post culture analysis of 30 cultures with AML blasts.

achieved complete Remission. In 6 patients with primary refractory disease no DC could be generated in vitro.

## Discussion

Successful immunotherapy for acute leukemia is an attractive goal for immunological and clinical research in the near future. Since it has been difficult to isolate specific antigens in different AML and ALL patients [10,11] the generation of DC with leukemic genotype which might act as professional antigen presenting cells seems attractive. Different groups have shown that CML cells can be cultured with cytokines, which are known to promote DC growth [3,6]. Those DC are Philadelphia chromosome positive and seem to elicit significant T cell responses against CML targets. Immunotherapeutic trials are underway to test for the clinical usefulness of these DC.

Two recent reports have shown that the same might become possible for patients with AML. Although the success of DC cultures was varying form patient to patient, there seem to be some patients whose leukemic cells are able to differentiate along the dendritic differentiation pathway. Using different flow cytometric analysis, those authors have found a far higher percentage of so called' DC. This might be either due to different culture conditions or the small number of patients investigated. Beyond these limitations, we believe the use of these DC for autologous immunotherapy might be hampered by several circumstances.

First patients with AML undergo multiple cycles of chemotherapy with immunosuppressive drugs and therefor cytotoxic T cells might be difficult to obtain. On the other hand, our clinical data show, that high-risk patients even generate no DC in-vitro. So we believe the potential to generate a significant amount of DC in-vitro might correspond to good clinical responses. This hypothesis is underlined by the observation that no Ph+ DC could be obtained in ALL patients. One might argue that lymphoblastic B cells need different cytokines for dendritic differentiation. Nevertheless, DC have been derived from CD10 positive B cell precursors in healthy individuals.

The sorted fractions of AML patients have provided evidence for the differentiation of leukemic stem cells into DC with different maturation grades. FISH analysis of unselected cultures performed by other groups might be clouded by the mixture of different cells in the samples [8].

The clinical use of immunotherapy in AML patients is difficult because they suffer from profound lymphopenia and autologous T cells are difficult to harvest during initial presentation or remission. Therefor the priming of allogeneic T cells might be a potential alternative. Besides leukemic DC, peptides derived and eluted from blasts by high performance liquid chromatography can be used together wit allogeneic DC to prime specific responses [12]. These experiments are somehow complicated and large amounts of leukemic blasts have to be available to elute enough peptides. Lysates of leukemic blasts have to be explored in this context for the induction of specific responses and feasibility in vivo.

An another drawback of immunotherapy in AML is the known downregulation of costimulatory signals also seen in our experiments. This might be overcome by some extent by differential cell cultures in vitro or by transfection of blasts with the genes for CD80 or CD86. First encouraging results have been documented with this approach [13].

Our data give further insights into the biology of acute myeloid leukemia which hierarchy resembles normal hematopoiesis. Whether the lack of leukemic DC after culture in some patients can be seen as an independent negative prognostic factor has to be studied with a longer follow-up. Ph + ALL blasts behave differently and show no significant growth of dendritic cells. This might be one reason for the poor outcome of these patients even after allogeneic stem cell transplantation. Clinical studies using leukemic DC as adjuvant immunotherapy for maintenance therapy are warranted.

*Acknowledgments.* The authors thank M. Ritter for PCR analysis, B. Mohr for the cytogenetical analysis, U. Oelschlägel and C. Brendel for the cell sorting.

# References

1. Anderlini P, Luna M, Kantarjian HM, et al (1996) Causes of initial remission induction failure in patients with acute myeloid leukemia and myelodysplastic syndromes. Leukemia 10:600-608
2. Ye Z, Gee AP, Bowers WE, Lamb LS, Turner MW, Henslee Downey PJ (1996) In vitro expansion and characterization of dendritic cells derived from human bone marrow CD34+ cells. Bone Marrow Transplant 18:997-1008
3. Eibl B, Ebner S, Duba C, et al (1997) Dendritic cells generated from blood precursors of chronic myelogenous leukemia patients carry the Philadelphia translocation and can induce a CML-specific primary cytotoxic T- cell response. Genes Chromosomes Cancer 20:215-223
4. Fearnley DB, McLellan AD, Mannering SI, Hock BD, Hart DN (1997) Isolation of human blood dendritic cells using the CMRF-44 monoclonal antibody: implications for studies on antigen- presenting cell function and immunotherapy. Blood 89:3708-3716
5. Choudhury A, Toubert A, Sutaria S, Charron D, Champlin RE, Claxton DF (1998) Human leukemia-derived dendritic cells: ex-vivo development of specific antileukemic cytotoxicity. Crit Rev Immunol 18:121-131
6. Choudhury A, Gajewski JL, Liang JC, et al (1997) Use of leukemic dendritic cells for the generation of antileukemic cellular cytotoxicity against Philadelphia chromosome-positive chronic myelogenous leukemia. Blood 89:1133-1142
7. Robinson SP, English N, Jaju R, Kearney L, Knight SC, Reid CD (1998) The in-vitro generation of dendritic cells from blast cells in acute leukaemia. Br J Haematol 103:763-771
8. Choudhury A, Liang JC, Thomas EK, et al (1999) Dendritic cells derived in vitro from acute myelogenous leukemia cells stimulate autologous, antileukemic T cell responses. Blood 93:780-786
9. Ritter M, Thiede C, Schäkel U, et al (1997) Underestimation of inversion (16) in acute myeloid leukaemia using standard cytogenetics as compared with polymerase chain reaction: results of a prospective investigation. Br J Haematol 98:969-972
10. Colovai AI, Suciu Foca N, Baiulescu GE, Harris PE (1994) HLA class I self peptides isolated from a T-cell leukemia reveal the allele-specific motif of HLA-B38. Tissue Antigens 44:65-72
11. Dolstra H, Fredrix H, Maas F, et al (1999) A human minor histocompatibility antigen specific for B cell acute lymphoblastic leukemia. J Exp Med 189:301-308
12. Ostankovitch M, Buzyn A, Bonhomme D, et al (1998) Antileukemic HLA-restricted T-cell clones generated with naturally processed peptides eluted from acute myeloblastic leukemia blasts. Blood 92:19-24
13. Mutis T, Schrama E, Melief CJM, Goulmy E (1998) CD80-transfected acute myeloid leukemia cells induce primary allogeneic T-cell responses dircetd at patient specific minor histocompatibility antigens and leukema-associated antigens. Blood 92:1677-1684

# Generation of Leukemia-Derived Dendritic Cells from Patients with AML

A. Berer[1], F. Keil[2], O. Haas[3], K. Lechner[1], K. Geissler[1] and L. Öhler[1]

*Abstract.* Although AML cells are highly sensitive to cytotoxic agents the majority of AML patients relaps after conventional chemotherapy due to the persistence of minimal residual disease. Leukemia cell derived dendritic cells (DCs) generated by in vitro differentiation of AML cells may be useful for anti-leukemia vaccination strategies.

We cultured in FCS-free media PBMC from 15 newly diagnosed AML patients with WBC counts ranging from 17,500 to 260,000/ml supplemented with different cytokine combinations (SCF, GM-CSF, IL-4, TNFα). Cultured cells were analyzed by flow cytometry with respect to DC-associated surface-molecules (CD1a, CD83, CD40, CD80, CD86, HLA-DR) when they showed significant DC-morphology in culture (14 cases). A surface molecule expression was defined as positive when more than 20% of cells stained with the indicated antibody (mAb). Prior to culture, PBMC stained positive (>20%) with mAb against HLA-DR in 11 patients, CD40 in 3 patients, CD86 in 3 patients and CD1a in 1 patient, whereas CD80 and CD83 expression was not detected. After cultivation, neo-expression/up-regulation of CD1a antigen was found in 8 samples, CD83 in 2, CD40 in 14, CD80 in 7, and CD86 in 9 patients. Each of the AML samples, in which DC morphology could be induced upon cultivation, showed up-regulation of at least 2 DC-associated molecules. In 6 from 14 samples tested, a marked increase of the T cell stimulatory capacity could be demonstrated in the allogeneic mixed lymphocyte reaction (10 to 400 fold). The leukemic origin of these DCs was demonstrated by fluorescence in situ hybridization in a patient with translocation t(15;17). Our results suggest that cells with the morphological, phenotypical and functional characteristics of DCs can be induced in vitro from PBMC of patients with newly diagnosed AML using appropriate culture conditions.

## Introduction

Acute myeloid leukemia (AML) is a clonal disorder of immature hematopoietic cells [1]. Despite considerable progress in treatment most patients will die from relapsing disease within the following five years after diagnosis. Therefore, new treatment strategies seems clearly warranted. It is generally believed that the immune system plays a critical role not only in the acquisition of malignant diseases but also to reject both microscopic and established tumor cells [2]. Failure of the immune system to eliminate tumor cells may be, among others, due to an insufficient presentation of tumor antigens. Dendritic cells (DCs) are bone marrow derived leukocytes with a unique capacity to initiate primary immune responses [3,4]. In the past few years culture techniques were developed which made DCs from individual patients easily available in large quantities [5]. This led to new concepts for the development of immune-based therapies [6]. Studies from leukemic cell lines and freshly isolated leukemic blast cells have shown, that these cells can be induced to differentiate along one or several pathways [7]. Thus, differentiation of AML cells towards highly immunostimulatory DCs should theo-

Department of Internal Medicine I, Division of Hematology[1] and the Bone Marrow Transplantation Unit[2], University of Vienna, A-1090 Vienna, Austria, and the St. Anna Children Hospital[3], Kinderspitalgasse 14, A-1090 Vienna, Austria

retically be possible. Choudhury et al have very recently reported the in vitro generation of leukemia specific cytotoxic T cells by using autologous AML-derived DCs [8]. However, the presented data showed a shift of only a small sub-population of AML cells towards the DC-lineage. This is also reflected by the data of the allogeneic MLR, which show rather poor T cell stimulatory capacity in most cases. Here we demonstrate, that culture condition needed for optimal induction of DC differentiation vary from different AML samples.

## Materials and Methods

### Patients

Blood samples for this study were collected from 15 patients with AML prior to induction chemotherapy after obtaining informed consent. Diagnosis was made on the basis of the French-American-British (FAB) classification. Median leukocyte count was L (range 17,500–260,000) (see Table 1).

### Media and Reagents

As a culture media RPMI 1640 supplemented with 2 mM L-glutamine, 100 U/mL penicillin, 100 mg/mL sptreptomycin and 10% fetal calf serum (FCS) or 1% human serum was used. The synthetic culture medium X-VIVO 20 was obtained from BioWhittaker (Walkersville, Maryland). Recombinant human (rh) GM-CSF was a kind gift from Novartis (Basel, Switzerland), rhIL-4 was kindly provided by Schering-Plough Corp. (Kenilworth, NJ) and TNFα was purchased from PBH (Pharma Biotechnologie Hannover, Germany).

### Antibodies

The fluorescein-labeled antibodies specific for CD1a (clone HI149), CD40 (clone 5C3), HLA-DQ (clone TÜ169), CD80 (clone BB1) and the phycoerythrin-labeled antibodies against CD86 (clone IT2.2) and HLA-DR (clone TÜ36) were obtained from PharMingen (San Diego, CA). Fluorescein-conjugated

antibodies against CD83 (clone HB15A), CD14 (clone RMO52), CD11b (clone BEAR1), and the isotype controls IgG1-FITC (clone 679.1Mc7) and IgG1-PE (clone 679.1Mc7) were purchased from Immunotech (Marseille, France). The fluorescein-labeled antibody specific for CD54 (clone RR1/1) was from Bender MedSystems (Vienna, Austria).

### Cultivation of Cells

Cells were cultured at a density of $5 \times 10^5$ cells/mL in standard culture flasks (Costar, Cambridge, MA) at 37°C in a humidified $CO_2$ containing atmosphere. For induction of cell differentiation RPMI 1640 plus 1% human serum supplemented with GM-CSF (1000 U/mL, IL-4 (500 U/mL), and TNFα (1000 U/mL) or GM-CSF (1000 U/mL), TNFα (1000 U/mL), SCF (20 ng/mL), and TGFb (0,5 ng/ml) was used. As a second medium, X-VIVO 20 supplemented with GM-CSF, IL-4, and TNFα or GM-CSF, TNFα, SCF, and TGFb was used. Cells were harvested between days four and twenty-one when they showed significant DC morphology. Culture medium was exchanged according to the in vitro behavior (i.e. proliferation) or otherwise every four days of culture.

### Morphological cell analyses

Freshly isolated cells and cells cultured for four to twenty-one days were evaluated for development of DC morphology on an inverted microscope (Olympus IMT-2, Tokyo, Japan). Harvested cells were centrifuged onto microscope slides (Cytospin-2, Shandon Southern Products, Astmoor, UK), stained with May-Grünwald-Giemsa solution and analyzed by light microscopy.

### Proliferation assay (MLR)

A constant number of $10^5$ allogeneic highly purified T cells were incubated with graded numbers of irradiated (3,000 rad, $^{137}Cs$ source) AML cells prior to culture or AML cells that were cultured for four to twenty-one days. Experiments were performed in 96-well culture plated in RPMI 1640 supplemented with 10% human serum. Proliferation of T cells was monitored by measuring [methyl-³H]-thymidine uptake (Amersham, Buckinghamshire, UK) incorporation on day 4 of culture. Cells were harvested 18h later and radioactivity was determined on microplate scintillation counter (Packard, Topcount Instrument Cop., Meriden, CT).

### Fluorescence in situ hybridization

For detection of translocation t(15;17) in a patient with AML M3, a mixture of digoxigenin-labeled DNA probes specific for the 17q12 chromosome breakpoint, and biotin-labeled DNA probes specific for the 15q22 chromosome breakpoint were used according to manufacture instructions (ONCOR, Inc, Gaithersburg, MD).

### Results

### Culture conditions, morphological changes and growth characteristics

PBMCs from 15 patients with de novo AML of FAB types M0 to M5 were cultured to generate DCs (Table 1). There is a great heterogeneity in AMLs, reaching from very immature blasts cells which seem more related to CD34+ progenitor cells, to cells from AML M5 sharing many features with normal peripheral

blood monocytes. Therefore, we have chosen two different cytokine combinations for DC generation, containing GM-CSF plus IL-4 plus TNFα, and GM-CSF plus TNFα plus SCF plus TGFb, respectively, and used two different culture media. In all but one patient sample (pat.15) morphological features of DCs could be induced upon cultivation (Figure 1, pat. 7). However, a marked variability in the behavior of cultured AML-PBMCs was observed. Viability of cells and proliferation was usually but not always higher in medium containing 1% human serum when compared to X-VIVO 20 (data not shown). Moreover, optimal induction of cell differentiation did not correlate with FAB subtype and the cytokine cocktail used. Time of harvest depended on the appearance of cells with a typical DC morphology and reached from day 6 to day 21.

### Phenotypic changes

As mentioned above, we could not identify a single culture condition for optimal induction of cell differentiation. Figure 2 shows antigen expression pattern of cells from an AML M0 (pat.1) before and after cultivation in RPMI 1640 plus 1% human serum containing GM-CSF, TNFα, SCF, and TGFb. Interestingly, viability of cells rapidly decreased in both cultures containing GM-CSF, IL-4 and TNFα and no viable cells could be harvested, whereas clear neo-expression of the costimulatory molecules CD40, CD80, and CD86 was

**Table 1.** Clinical Characteristics and Cytogenetics of AML Patients

|    | FAB-type | Age/sex | WBC     | %blasts/mono | karyotype              |
|----|----------|---------|---------|--------------|------------------------|
| 1  | M0       | 51/f    | 18,040  | 83/0         | 46XX                   |
| 2  | M1       | 79/m    | 101,000 | 86/1         | del(11)(p15)           |
| 3  | M1       | 41/f    | 37,450  | 61/7         | 46XX                   |
| 4  | M3       | 33/m    | 103,000 | 91/2         | t(15;17)               |
| 5  | M4       | 54/f    | 27,420  | 29/28        | 46XX                   |
| 6  | M4       | 72/f    | 17,500  | 34/22        | 46XX                   |
| 7  | M4       | 78/m    | 260,000 | 40/26        | 46XY                   |
| 8  | M5       | 22/f    | 100,300 | 67/19        | t(9;11),t(1;10)        |
| 9  | M5       | 28/m    | 78,000  | 76/15        | t(Y;1),t(1;12)t(1;16)  |
| 10 | M5       | 31/m    | 71,000  | 51/17        | inv(16)                |
| 11 | M5       | 32/f    | 140,000 | 11/67        | 46XX                   |
| 12 | M5       | 41/m    | 128,100 | 12/72        | 46XY                   |
| 13 | M5       | 68/m    | 86,830  | 34/31        | 46XY                   |
| 14 | M5       | 78/f    | 41,700  | 2/56         | 46XX                   |
| 15 | M1       | 70/f    | 105,000 | 65/14        | 46XX                   |

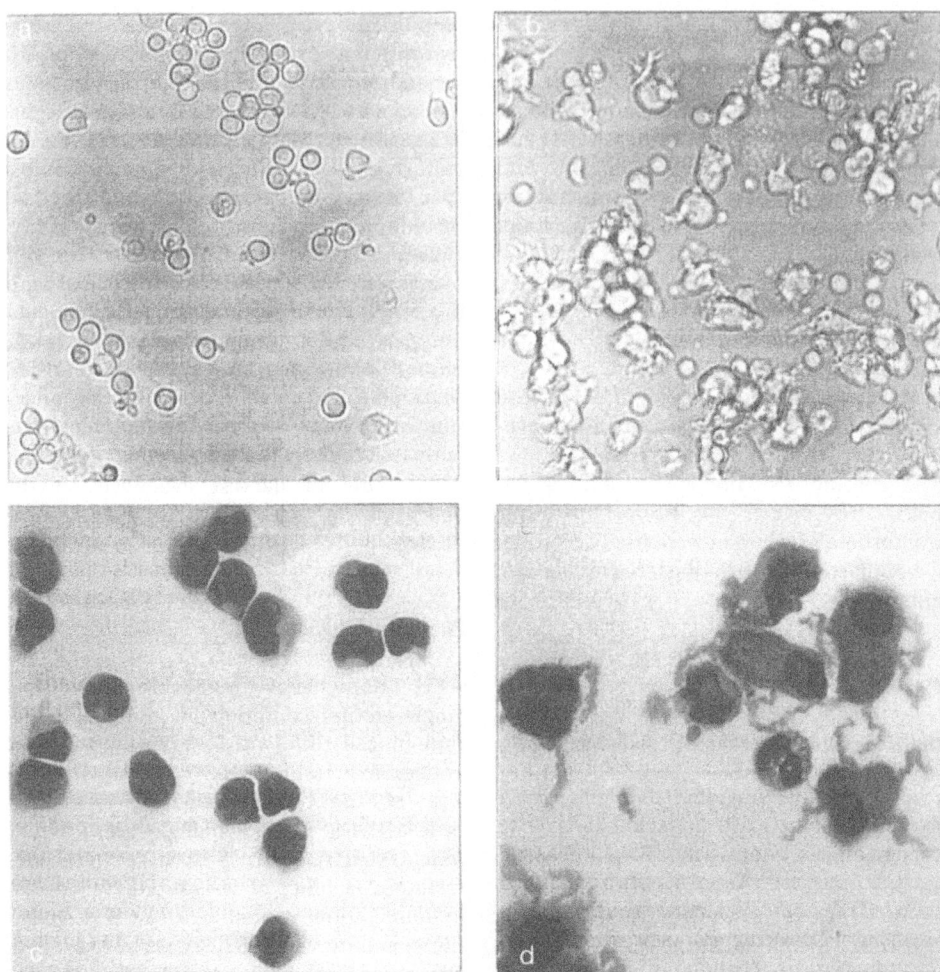

**Fig. 1.** Appearance of cells in liquid culture and cytospin preparations (AML FAB M4 / patient 7). Characteristic phase contrast morphology of freshly isolated AML cells showing a homogeneous population of equally sized, round cells (A), and after 6d of culture in RPMI+1% human serum containing GM-CSF + IL-4 + TNFα, imposing with widespread cytoplasmic projections (B). May-Grünwald-Giemsa stained cytospin preparations of freshly isolated (C) and cultured cells are shown of the same patient (D).

observed in both culture media containing GM-CSF, TNFα, SCF, and TGFb.

Figure 3 shows an overlay histogram of AML cells (FAB M4, pat. 7) prior and post cultivation. In contrast to patient 1, better results were obtained in both media containing GM-CSF, IL-4 and TNFα. Consistent with the observed increase of cell size and development of long cytoplasmic projections, upregulation/neoexpression of DC-related surface molecules CD1a, CD83, CD54, CD40, CD80, and CD86 occurred upon cultivation.

Table 2 gives an overview of the expression pattern of AML cells before and after culture. Prior to culture, >20% of cells stained with mAb against HLA-DR in 11 patients, CD40 in 3 patients, CD86 in 3 patients and CD1a in 1 patient, whereas CD80 and CD83 expression was not detected. After cultivation, neo-expression/ up-regulation of CD1a antigen was found in 8 samples, CD40 in 14, CD80 in 7, CD83 in 2 and CD86 in 9 patients. Each of the AML samples, in which DC morphology could be induced upon cultivation, showed

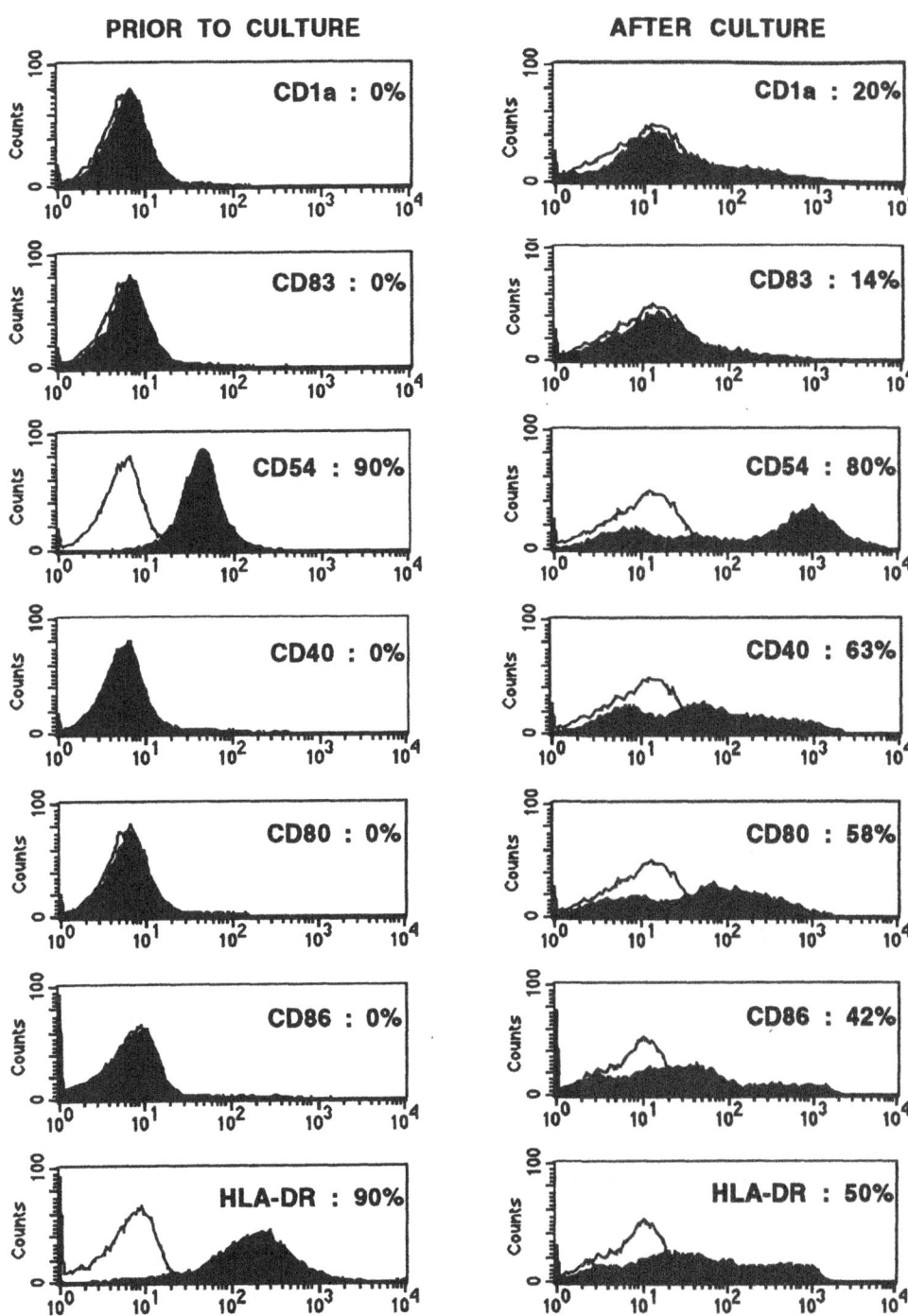

**Fig. 2.** Expression pattern of AML-PBMCs (AML M0, pat. 1) prior and post cultivation in RPMI1640 + 1% human serum containing GM-CSF + SCF + TNFα + TGFb. The left column represents cells prior to culture upon staining with the indicated mAbs (black profiles), white profiles indicate staining with non-binding control mAb. The right column represent expression pattern of cells after cultivation.

**Table 2.** Expression Pattern of AML Cells Before and After Culture

| Pat. | FAB | Cult. | HLA-DR | CD1a | CD80 | CD86 | CD40 | CD83 | MLR |
|------|-----|-------|--------|------|------|------|------|------|-----|
| 1 | M0 | 2 | +/+ | -/+ | -/+ | -/+ | -/+ | -/- | + |
| 2 | M1 | 1 | -/+ | -/- | -/- | -/- | -/+ | -/- | - |
| 3 | M1 | 1 | -/+ | -/- | -/- | -/- | -/+ | -/- | - |
| 4 | M3 | 1 | -/+ | -/+ | -/+ | -/+ | +/+ | -/- | + |
| 5 | M4 | 1 | +/+ | -/- | -/+ | -/- | -/+ | -/- | - |
| 6 | M4 | 3 | +/+ | -/+ | -/+ | +/+ | +/+ | -/- | + |
| 7 | M4 | 1 | +/+ | -/+ | -/+ | -/+ | -/+ | -/- | + |
| 8 | M5 | 2 | +/+ | -/+ | -/- | -/+ | +/+ | -/+ | + |
| 9 | M5 | 1 | +/+ | -/- | -/- | -/- | -/+ | -/- | - |
| 10 | M5 | 1 | +/+ | -/+ | -/- | -/+ | -/+ | -/- | - |
| 11 | M5 | 3 | +/+ | -/- | -/+ | -/+ | -/+ | -/- | - |
| 12 | M5 | 2 | +/+ | -/- | -/- | +/- | -/+ | -/- | - |
| 13 | M5 | 3 | +/+ | -/+ | -/+ | -/+ | -/+ | -/- | - |
| 14 | M5 | 1 | +/+ | +/+ | -/+ | +/+ | -/+ | -/+ | + |

Surface molecules: + means ≥ 20% positive cells
MLR: T cell stimulation of 800 ld-DCs is ≥ 12.500 uncultivated AML cells
Culture:  1: RPMI+1% huSerum / GM-CSF+IL-4+TNFα, 2: RPMI+1% huSerum / GM-CSF+TNFα+SCF+TGFβ
3: X-VIVO20 / GM-CSF+IL-4+TNFα

up-regulation of at least 2 DC-associated molecules.

## Functional changes

Potent induction of primary MLR responses is a characteristic functional feature of DCs. We, therefore, compared the allostimulatory capacity of freshly isolated AML-PBMC with AML cells which were cultured with different cytokine combinations. Together with the observed morphological and phenotypic changes, the ability of AML cells to induce a potent stimulation of allogeneic T cells markedly increased upon cultivation. The criteria for an optimal MLR response was defined as an equal or superior T cell stimulatory capacity of 800 cultivated cells compared with 12.500 AML cells prior to culture. Figure 4A shows the potent induction of MLR of cultured AML cells from patient 1 even at very low stimulator cell counts. Consistent with the observed neo-expression of the co-stimulatory molecules CD40, CD80, and CD86 the allogeneic T cell stimulation of AML cells from patient 7 markedly increased upon cultivation in media containing GM-CSF plus IL-4 and TNFα. As can also be seen in Table 2, the ability of cultured cells to induce a potent MLR correlated with the acquisition of DC-related molecules, most strikingly with the up-regulation of co-stimulatory molecules.

## FISH-analysis of leukemia derived DCs

The results of the experiments described above show that, by using appropriate culture conditions, a substantial number of AMLs can be driven in vitro to acquire the morphological, phenotypic, and functional features of DCs. In order to proof that they were of leukemic origin, we highly enriched by FACS sorting CD1a+ cells from a culture of a patient with known translocation t(15;17). By using interphase FISH we were able to detect t(15;17) in 67% of CD1a+ cells. This result confirms that DCs of leukemic origin can be obtained in vitro from AML cells.

## Discussion

T cell-mediated immunity seems to play a critical role in the acquisition and rejection of malignant diseases [2,9]. Especially in minimal residual disease (MRD) in patients with leukemia, experimental as well as clinical data indicate an important role of cellular immunity [10,11]. Patients with AML who receive bone marrow transplants from syngeneic

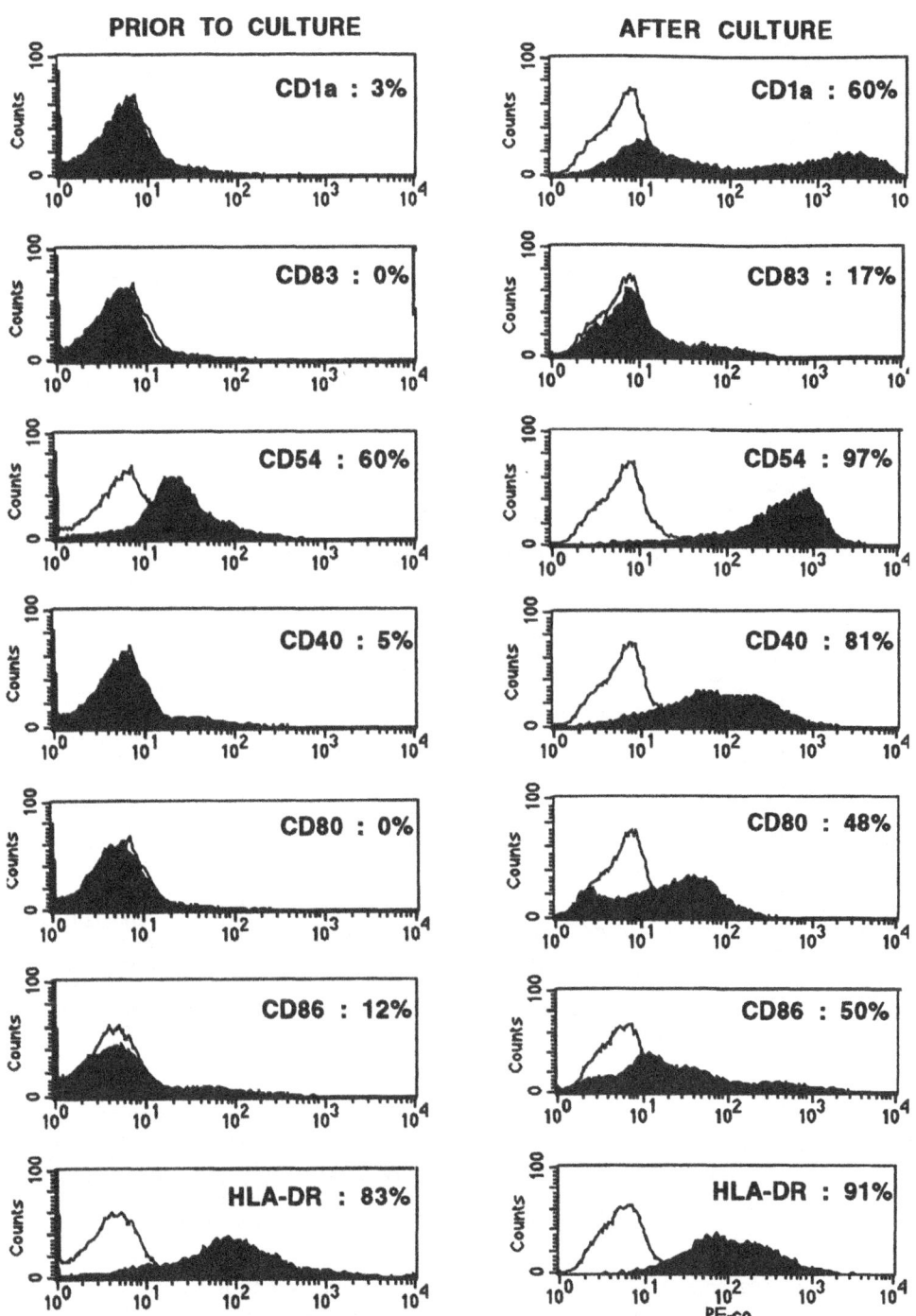

**Fig. 3.** Overlay histograms of AML-PBMCs (AML M4, pat. 7) prior and post cultivation. PBMC were cultured for 6 days in RPMI1640 + 1% human serum containing GM-CSF + IL-4 + TNFα. The left column represents cells prior to culture upon staining with the indicated mAbs (black profiles), white profiles indicate staining with non-binding control mAb. The right column represent expression pattern of cells after cultivation.

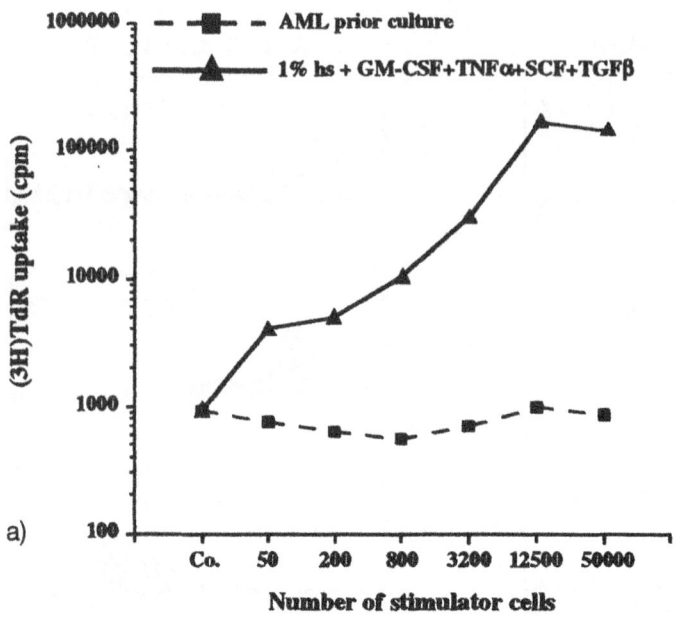

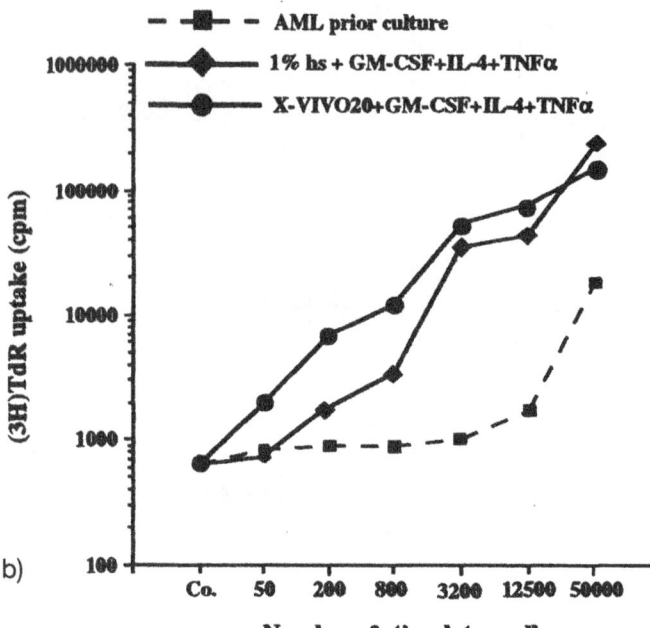

**Fig. 4.** T cell stimulatory capacity of AML-derived DCs. $10^5$ allogeneic highly purified T cells were incubated with graded numbers of irradiated, either freshly isolated AML-PBMCs or cells cultured with GM-CSF + SCF + TNFα + TGFb. (Fig. 4A, pat. 1) or GM-CSF + IL-4 + TNFα (Fig. 4B, pat. 7). Proliferation of T cells was monitored by adding ($^3$H)-thymidine on day 4 of culture followed by measuring incorporated radioactivity 18 hours later.

donors and recipients of T cell depleted transplants are at much higher risk of relapse compared with patients, who receive unmanipulated transplants from allogeneic donors. Intensive chemotherapy or autologous bone marrow transplantation can induce remission in most patients with AML. Due to underlying minimal residual disease (MRD) or presence of malignant cells in the marrow graft relapse of disease will occur in the majority of the patients. The use of adoptive immunotherapy may offer a key to eliminate MRD.

With the new ability of effectively generating dendritic cells from normal hematopoietic cells including monocytes and CD34$^+$ progenitor cells, immunotherapy became an interesting approach in the treatment of malignant diseases. Several studies proved the feasibility of inducing a cytotoxic T cells response against tumor cells by using peptide pulsed DCs, both in vitro and in vivo [12,13]. Because of the wide spectrum of chromosomal abnormalities that underlie AMLs [14,15] and, therefore, a variety of potential tumor antigens, a concept of inducing features of DCs in the tumor cells itself might be of principle advantage. These malignant DCs may induce anti-leukemic reactivity in autologous T cells without the necessity of additional exogenous antigens. In this study we show that acute myeloid leukemia cells can differentiate in vitro to cells with the characteristic morphological, phenotypic, and functional properties of DCs. The results of the FISH analysis confirms the leukemic origin of AML-derived DCs.

The use of fetal calf serum (FCS) in the generation of DCs might present problems to the clinical use of these cells. We present data that effective generation of DCs is also possible with cultures containing human serum or in serum-free media. There exists a great variability of AML cells with regard to morphology, phenotype, and in vitro behaviour. Thus, blast cells of AML M1 seem to be more closely related to immature progenitor cells whereas cells of AML M5 share many features with normal peripheral blood monocytes. As shown in Table 2, the culture requirements for optimal induction of DC differentiation varied between different AMLs. However, we could not assign a certain cytokine combination to a certain AML subtype.

In conclusion, this study shows that functional leukemia derived-DCs can be generated from patients with AML by using appropriate culture conditions. These DCs may be used as a cellular vaccine to induce anti-tumor immunity for AML patients in remission after chemotherapy.

# References

1. Bonnet D, Dick JE. Human acute myeloid leukemia is organized as a hierarchy that originates from a primitive hematopoietic cell. Nature Med 3: 730, 1997
2. Hellström I, Hellström KE. T cell immunity to tumor antigens. Crit Rev Immunol 18:1, 1998
3. Cella M, Sallusto F, Lanzavecchia A. Origin, maturation and antigen-presenting function of dendritic cells. Curr Opin Immunol 9: 10, 1997
4. Steinman RM. The dendritic cell system and its role in immunogenicity. Annu Rev Immunol 9: 271, 1991
5. Pickl WF, Majdic O, Kohl P, Stöckl J, Riedl E, Scheinecker C, Bello-Fernandez C, Knapp W. Molecular and functional characteristics of dendritic cells generated from highly purified CD14$^+$ peripheral blood monocytes. J Immunol 157: 3850, 1996
6. Danussi-Joannopoulos K, Weinstein HJ, Nickerson PW, Strom TB, Burakoff SJ, Croop JM, Arceci RJ. Irradiated B7-1 transduced primary acute myelogenous leukemia (AML) cells can be used as therapeutic vaccine in murine AML. Blood 87: 2938, 1996
7. Choudhury A, Gajewski JL, Liang JC, Popat U, Claxton DF, Kliche KO, Andreeff M, Champlin RE. Use of leukemic dendritic cells for generation of anti-leukemic cellular cytotoxicity against Philadelphia chromosome-positive chronic myelogenous leukemia. Blood 89: 1133, 1997
8. Choudhury A, Liang JC, Thomas EK, Flores-Romp L, Xie QS, Agusala K, Sutaria S, Sinha I, Champlin RE, Claxton DF. Dendritic Cells Derived In Vitro From Acute Myelogenous Leukemia Cells Stimulate Autologous, Antileukemic T Cell Response. Blood 93: 780, 1999
9. Sherman LA, Theobald M, Morgan D, Hernandez J, Bacik I, Yewdell J, Bennink J, Biggs J. Strategies for tumor elimination by cytotoxic T lymphocytes. Crit Rev Immunol 18:47, 1998
10. Kolb HJ, Schattenberg A, Goldman JM, Hertenstein B, Jacobson N, Arcese W, Ljungman P, Ferrant A, Verdonck L, Niederwieser D, Van Rhee F, Mittermueller J, De Witte T, Holler E, Ansari H. Graft-versus-leukemia effect of donor lymphocyte transfusions in marrow grafted patients. Blood 86: 2041, 1995
11. Giralt S, Hester J, Hun J, Hirsh-Ginsberg C, Rondon G, Seong D, Lee M, Gajewski J, Van Besien K, Khouri I, Mehra R, Prezepiorka D, Korbling M, Talpaz M, Kantarjian HM, Fischer G, Deisseroth A, Champlin R. CD8-depleted donor lymphocyte infusions as treatment for relapsed chronic myelogenous leukemia after allogeneic bone marrow transplantation. Blood 86: 4337, 1995
12. Celluzzi CM, Mayordomo JI, Storkus WJ, Lotze MT, Falo LDJr. Peptide-pulsed dendritic cells induce antigen-specific CTL-mediated protective immunity. J Exp Med 183: 283, 1996
13. Molldrem J, Dermime S, Parker K, Jiang YZ, Mavroudis D, Hensel N, Fukushima P, Barret AJ. Targeted T-cell therapy for human leukemia: Cytotoxic T lymphocytes specific for a peptide derived from proteinase 3 preferentially lyse human myeloid leukemia cells. Blood 88:2450, 1996
14. Bloomfield CD, de la Chapelle A. Chromosome abnormalities in acute nonlymphocytic leukemia: clinical and biological significance. Semin Oncol 14: 372, 1987
15. Rabbitts TH. Chromosomal translocations in human cancer. Nature 372: 143

# Dendritic Cells from AML Patients in Complete Remission are Capable to Present Antigen to Autologous T Lymphocytes

D.K. Schui, L. Singh, A. Krapohl, B. Schneider, D. Hoelzer and E. Weidmann

Abstract. Evidence for immunogenicity of AML blasts is supported by graft versus leukemia reaction, the effect of donor lymphocyte transfusion and *in vitro* studies with cytotoxic T cells. Because of the potency of dendritic cells (DC) to present antigens, it seems feasible to study, whether functional DC can be generated in AML patients with the perspective of future vaccination strategies. Therefore, peripheral blood was obtained from 19 patients in complete remission of AML and 13 healthy controls (HC). DC were established from monocytes by culturing in the presence of GM-CSF and IL-4 for 8 days. To collect mature DC GM-CSF and TNF-α were added to cultures until day 12. At days 8 and 12 cell numbers were counted and expression of surface markers typical for DC was analyzed by flowcytometry. The ability of established DC to present antigens was tested using tetanus toxoid (TT) as a recall antigen. Furthermore day 8 DC were incubated with lysates of leukemic blasts and cocultured with autologous lymphocytes. Cytotoxicity against autologous blast cells was measured by a PKH67 assay. The numbers of DC were significantly lower in AML patients >2 months after chemotherapy as compared to HC (p=0,04) or AML patients during hematopoietic regeneration following chemotherapy (p=0,01). There was no statistical difference in expression of surface markers by DC from AML patients and HC. CD83, the most specific marker for DC, was comparable in both groups (day 8: HC 11-62%, AML 10-67% p=0,07; day 12: HC 42-91%, AML 23-78% p=0,08). TT was presented efficiently to autologous lymphocytes by DC from HC and AML patients. At an effector:target-ratio of

20:1 lymphocytes from one patient stimulated with DC pulsed with blast lysates killed 20,3% of autologous blasts compared to 13,6% lysis by effector cells from HC. Cloning of these T cells is currently in progress. In conclusion dendritic cells can be efficiently generated in AML patients especially during hematopoietic regeneration following chemotherapy. Preliminary results indicate the activation of autologous T cells after stimulation by DC pulsed with blast lysates.

Supported by Deutsche Krebshilfe (10-0930-Be 2).

## Introduction

Dendritic cells are strong antigen-presenting cells capable of inducing primary T cell responses [1]. Specific T cell responses have been demonstrated in different tumors [2] including acute leukemias [3, 4].

Although complete remission can be obtained in the majority of AML patients, most of them relapse. Therefore it seems feasible to search for immunotherapeutical approaches to maintain complete remission.

Evidence for the immunogenicity of leukemic blast cells is supported by graft versus leukemia reaction [5] and *in vitro* generation of T cells with cytotoxic activity against AML blasts. In melanoma patients several investigators have demonstrated induction of cytotoxic T-cell responses using DC pulsed with peptides derived from different melanoma associated antigens e. g. gp100 [6]. So far specific AML related antigens have not been identified. However, in scope of the possibility

---

Department of Medicine III, Hematology/Oncology, J. W. Goethe University, Frankfurt, Germany.

to use DC pulsed with tumor cell lysates [7, 8] or gene-modified DC [9, 10] it seems feasible to investigate whether DC can induce specific antileukemic T cell responses.

The aim of the present study was to analyze the phenotype and function of DC established in complete remission of AML patients with the future perspective of immunotherapeutical approaches to prevent relapse.

## Material and Methods

### Generation of dendritic cells

DC were established from 40mL heparinized peripheral blood of 19 AML patients and 13 healthy controls as previously described with minor modifications [11]. Mononuclear cells were isolated by Ficoll-Hypaque (Biochrom, Berlin, FRG)sedimentation and monocytes were separated by adherence to plastic. Adherent cells were cultured in RPMI 1640 (GIBCO, , FRG) 1% autologous serum supplemented with 1000 IU/mL GM-CSF and 1000 IU/mL IL-4 for 8 days. For functional tests DC of day 8 were used. To analyze mature DC cells were cultured for another 3-4 days with 1000 IU/mL GM-CSF and 100 IU/mL TNF-a (Biochrom, Berlin, FRG). On day 8 and 12 cell numbers were counted and expression of surface markers CD1a, CD54, CD58, CD83 (Immunotech, Hamburg, FRG), HLA-DR (Becton Dickinson, Heidelberg, FRG), CD80 and CD86 (Pharmingen, Hamburg, FRG) was studied by flowcytometry on a FACScan‰ (Becton Dickinson, Heidelberg, FRG).

### Presentation of tetanus toxoid

DC from day 8 were incubated with 50mg/mL tetanus toxoid, kindly provided by Dr. Hungerer (Chiron Behring, Marburg, FRG), for four hours at 37∞ C. Cells were washed and irradiated with 30 Gy. Subsequently declining numbers of DC ($10^4$-$10^1$) were incubated with $10^5$ autologous lymphocytes for three days. Finally 1mCi/well $^3$H-Thymidine (Amersham Buchler, Braunschweig, FRG) was added and after 18 hours the incorporation was measured on a β-counter (Canberra Packard, Neu-Isenburg, FRG).

### Stimulation of lymphocytes with autologous blast cell lysates

DC from day 8 were incubated with blast cell lysates prepared by repeated cycles of freezing in liquid nitrogene and thawing at 37°C. Three days later autologous lymphocytes were added and until the fifth day of coculture medium was supplemented with 1000 IU/mL Interleukin-2. After two weeks of coculture stimulated lymphocytes were used as effector cells in a cytotoxicity assay.

### Cytotoxicity assay

Autologous and allogeneic blast cells from AML patients were used as target cells. These were labeled with PKH67 according to the instructions of the manufacturer (Sigma, Deisenhofen, FRG). Briefly, 2x106 blast cells were labeled with $2x10^{-7}$ M PKH67 dye, washed three times and used as target cells. DC stimulated lymphocytes were incubated with labeled target cells in effector:target-ratios 20:1, 10:1, 5:1 and 1:1. IL-2 stimulated lymphocytes from healthy donors were used as control for the susceptibility of blast cells to lysis. After three hours the killing of target cells was analyzed by flowcytometry using propidiumiodide to indicate dead cells. Results are expressed as percent lysis of target cells after substraction of spontanous lysis.

## Results

The yield of DC on day 8 was comparable between AML patients in complete remission and healthy controls (Table 1). However, when the patients were subdivided in those during regeneration of hematopoiesis and those analyzed two months or later after finishing of treatment the number of DC from patients of the latter group was significantly lower compared to the regenerating population of patients (p=0,01) or healthy donors (p=0,04).

Analysis of cell surface molecules on day 8 DC of AML patients in complete remission and healthy individuals showed no statistical difference regarding CD83, the most specific marker for DC, CD1a, CD54, CD58, CD80 and

**Table 1.** Establishment of DC from healthy donors, AML patients >2months following chemotherapy and AML patients during hematopoietic regeneration. There was no significant correlation between the monocyte count in the starting cell population and yield of DC on day 8. The No. of DC on day 8 as well as the expression of HLA-DR was significantly (p<0.05) lower in AML patients >2 months after chemotherapy as compared to healthy donors and AML patients during hematopoietic regeneration. There were no significant differences in expression of CD83 and CD1a between the 3 groups.

| | healthy donors Median (range) | AML patients >2 months after chemo-therapy Median (range) | AML patients during hematopoietic regeneration Median (range) |
|---|---|---|---|
| No. | 13 | 11 | 8 |
| monocytes [µL] | 370 (288-493) | 387 (101-732) | 747 (191-3069) |
| No. of DC day 8 [*10$^6$] | 1,0 (0,3-2,7) | 0,4 (0,1-1,2) | 1,05 (0,2-2,1) |
| CD83 day 8 [%] | 50 (10-70) | 17 (10-67) | 18 (5-53) |
| HLA-DR day 8 [%] | 95 (87-100) | 77 (33-98) | 99 (92-99) |
| CD1a day 8 [%] | 85 (28-99) | 60 (25-98) | 74 (13-99) |

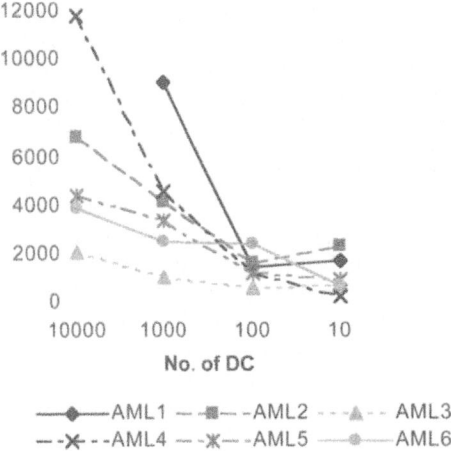

**Fig. 1.** Stimulation of T-cells with tetanus toxoid processed by autologous dendritic cells in AML patients

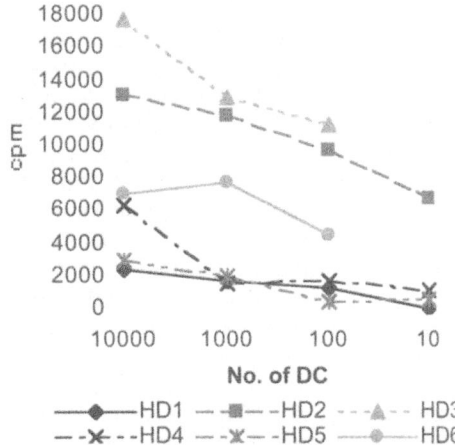

**Fig. 2.** Stimulation of T-cells with tetanus toxoid processed by autologous dendritic cells in healthy controls

CD86. AML patients two months or longer after chemotherapy showed a slightly reduced expression of HLA-DR (Table 1). In a smaller amount of patients the expression of cell surface markers was analyzed on day 12, additionally. Besides a higher expression of CD58 in AML patients there were no significant differences in expression of DC associated surface molecules between AML patients in CR and healthy controls (data not shown).

Efficient antigen presentation to autologous lymphocytes by DC from six AML patients (4/6 during hematopoietic regeneration) and six healthy individuals was demonstrated using tetanus toxoid as recall antigen (Figure 1, 2). There was no significant difference between both groups.

The stimulation of lymphocytes with blast lysates by DC was analyzed in an autologous system in one patient. After two weeks of coculture stimulated lymphocytes killed 20,3% of autologous blast cells at an effector:target-ratio of 20:1 compared to 13,6% lysis by effector cells of healthy controls (Figure 3). Using allogeneic blasts as targets DC stimulated lymphocytes lysed 26,2% whereas HC effector cells killed 41,8% (Figure 4). These results may suggests a specific effect of DC stimulated lymphocytes against autologous blast cells.

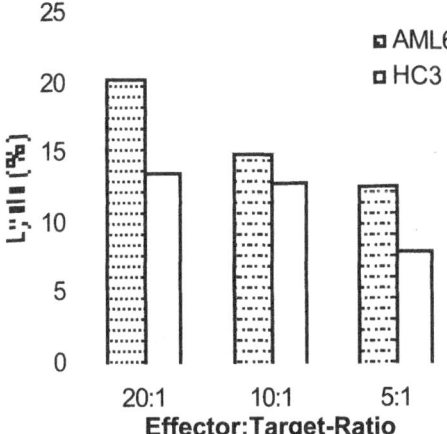

**Fig. 3.** Lysis of autologous blast cells by lymphocytes stimulated with dendritic cells pulsed with blast cell lysates. AML= patient with acute myelogenous leukemia, HC= healthy control

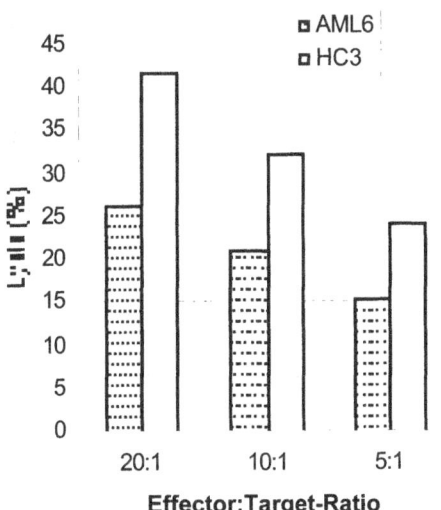

**Fig. 4.** Lysis of allogeneic blast cells by lymphocytes stimulated with dendritic cells pulsed with blast cell lysates. AML= patient with acute myelogenous leukemia, HC= healthy control

## Discussion

Dendritic cells have been suggested to be capable of presenting tumor associated or tumor specific antigens to T lymphocytes. Several investigators have demonstrated the effective presentation of bcr-abl as a specific antigen to T cells by DC differentiated from leukemic precursors from chronic myeloid leukemia, thereby inducing a cytotoxic T cell response against leukemic cells [12-14].

To date no AML specific antigens have been identified. Nevertheless DC may have a potential for immunotherapy approaches in AML e. g. by pulsing DC with tumor cell lysates [7, 8] or transfecting DC with tumor cell cDNA libraries [15], which have been suggested for other tumor entities and may offer senseful strategies also in AML. A possible role of DC in the efficacy of donor lymphocyte transfusions has been suggested by Kolb&Holler [16]. Moreover, DC are supposed to be key effectors regarding the induction of tolerance in donor host chimeras [17] and may therefore have a major impact on treatment strategies using so called stem cell minitransplantation [18].

In conclusion, from our results functional DC can be efficiently generated from peripheral blood of AML patients especially during hematopoietic regeneration following chemotherapy. The higher yield of DC in regenerating patients may be an effect of endogenous release of monocyte promoting growth factors or elevated generation of DC precursors in regenerating bone marrow. Whether the lower counts of DC in patients two months or longer after treatment is of any clinical relevance remains unclear. One could speculate that reduced numbers of DC causes a lack in T cell stimulation may be resulting in higher amounts of infectious diseases or leukemia relapses due to diminished immune response against residual blast populations. Supporting this hypothesis several investigators demonstrated a better outcome in patients with different solid tumors if there are higher amounts of DC in the tumor [reviewed by 19]. Preliminary results from one patient indicate the possible specific activation of autologous T lymphocytes by stimulation with DC pulsed with blast cell lysates. These results have to be confirmed by analysis of more patients. However, for the potential use of DC in vaccination strategies to prevent relapse it may be appropriate to state that functional DC are easily to obtain in sufficient numbers during regeneration of hematopoiesis after chemotherapy of AML.

# References

1. Austyn JM (1998) Dendritic cells. Curr opin Hematol 5:3-15
2. Weidmann E, Trucco M, Whiteside TL (1994) Relevance of the T cell receptor for immunotherapy of cancer. Cancer Immunol Immunother 39:1-14
3. Ostankovitch M, Buzyn A, Bonhomme D, Connan F, Bouscary D, Heshmati F, Dreyfus F, Choppin J, Guillet JG (1998) Antileukemic HLA-restricted T-cell clones generated with naturally processed peptides eluted from acute myeloblastic leukemia blasts. Blood 92:19-24
4. Jahn B, Bergmann L, Weidmann E, Brieger J, Fenchel K, Schwulera U, Hoelzer D, Mitrou PS (1995) Bone marrow-derived T-cell clones obtained from untreated acute myelocytic leukemia exhibit blast directed autologous cytotoxicity. Leukemia Res 19:73-82
5. Kolb HJ, Schattenberg A, Goldman JM, Hertenstein B, Jacobsen N, Arcese W, Ljungman P, Ferrant A, Verdonck L, Niederwieser D, van Rhee F, Mittermueller J, de Witte T, Holler E & Ansari H (1995) Graft-versus-leukemia effect of donor lymphocyte transfusions in marrow grafted patients. Blood 86:2041-2050
6. Tsai V, Southwood S, Sidney J, Sakaguchi K, Kawakami Y, Appella E, Sette A, Celis E (1997) Identification of subdominant CTL epitopes of the gp100 melanoma-associatedtumor antigen by primary in vitro immunization with peptide-pulsed dendritic cells. J Immunol 158:1796-1802
7. Tjoa B, Erickson S, Barren III R, Ragde H, Kenny G, Boynton A, Murphy G (1995) In vitro propagated dendritic cells from prostate cancer patients as a component of prostate cancer immunotherapy. Prostate 27:63-69
8. Nestle FO, Alijagic S, Gilliet M, Sun Y, Grabbe S, Dummer R, Burg G, Schadendorf D 1998) Vaccination of melanoma patients with peptide- or tumor lysate-pulsed dendritic cells. Nature Med 4:328-332
9. McArthur JG & Mulligan RC (1998) Induction of protective anti-tumor immunity by gene-modified dendritic cells. J Immunother 21:41-47.
10. Szabolcs P, Gallardo HF, Ciocon DH, Sadelain M, Young JW (1997) Retrovirally transduced human dendritic cells express a normal phenotype and potent T-cell stimulatory capacity. Blood 90:2160-2167
11. Romani N, Reider D, Heuer M, Ebner S, Kämpgen E, Eibl B, Niederwieser D, Schuler G (1996) Generation of mature dendritic cells from human blood. An improved method with special regard to clinical applicability. J Immunol Meth 196:137-151
12. Eibl B, Ebner S, Duba C, Bock G, Romani N, Erdel M, Gachter A, Niederwieser D, Schuler, G (1997) Dendritic cells generated from blood precursors of chronic myelogenous leukemia patients carry the Philadelphia translocation and can induce a CML-specific primary T-cell response. Genes, Chromosomes & Cancer 20: 215-223.
13. Choudhury A, Gajewski JL, Liang JC, Popat U, Claxton DF, Kliche KO, Andreef M & Champlin RE (1997) Use of leukemic dendritic cells for the generation of antileukemic cellular cytotoxicity against philadelphia chromosome-positive chronic myelogenous leukemia. Blood 89:1133-1142
14. Lim SH & Coleman S (1997) Chronic myeloid leukemia as an immunological target. Am J Hematol 54:61- 67
15. Nair SK, Boczkowski D, Morse M, Cumming RI, Lyerly HK, Gilboa E. (1998) Induction of primary carcinoembryonic antigen (CEA)-specific cytotoxic T-lymphocytes in vitro using human dendritic cells transfected with RNA. Nat Biotechnol 16:364-369
16. Kolb, H.J. & Holler E. (1997) Adoptive immunotherapy with donor lymphocyte transfusions. Curr Opin Oncol 9:139-145
17. Lu L, Rudert W, Quain S, McCaslin D, Fu F, Rao AS, Trucco M, Fung JJ, Starzl TE, Thomson AW (1995) Growth of donor-derived dendritic cells from the bone marrow of murine liver allograft recipients in response to granulocyte/macrophage colony-stimulating factor. J Exp Med 182:379-87
18. Storb R, Yu C, Deeg HJ, Georges G, Kiem HP, McSweeney PA, Nash RA, Sandmaier BM, Sullivan KM, Wagner JL, Walters MC (1998) Current and future preparative regimens for bone marrow transplantation in thalassemia. Ann N Y Acad Sci 850:276-287
19. Troy AJ & Hart DNJ (1997) Dendritic cells and cancer: progress toward a new cellular therapy. J Hematother 6:523-533

# Antibody Response to Neuraminidase of the Influenza Virus in Children with Acute Lymphoblastic Leukaemia Vaccinated against Influenza after Chemotherapy

R. Rokicka-Milewska[1], L. B. Brydak[2], M. Machala[2] and T. Jackowska[1]

## Introduction

Influenza is one of the most common respiratory diseases. It may be very serious and can result in high morbidity and increased mortality, mainly due to severe complications. Most of them occur in patients with underlying medical conditions, including chronic disorders of the pulmonary or cardiovascular system, metabolic diseases like diabetes, renal dysfunction, haemoglobinopathies and immunosuppression [1, 2]. Patients subjected to chemotherapy also belong to the high-risk group and they should be vaccinated against influenza every year.

The aim of this study was to assess the humoral immune response of the influenza virus to neuraminidase in children with acute lymphoblastic leukaemia immunised against influenza after chemotherapy treatment.

## Material and methods

The study group consisted of 22 patients (age 7-16 years) in complete remission of acute lymphoblastic leukaemia, vaccinated in the epidemic seasons 1993/94 and then in 1996/97. They were treated according BFM protocols. In 10 of them chemotherapy was completed before 1991 (A) and in 12 children chemotherapy was completed after 1991 (B). The second group consisted of 20 patients immunised against influenza for the first time in the season 1996/97 and similarly divided into groups A (n=10) and B (n=10). All patients received one 0.5ml dose of subunit vaccine ('Flushield', Wyeth – 1993/94, 'Influvac', Solvay Duphar – 1996/97) containing 15 μg haemagglutinin of each of the following strains: A/Texas/ 36/91 (H1N1), A/Beijing/32/92 (H3N2) and B/Panama/45/90 in the season 1993/94; A/Singapore/6/86 (H1N1), A/Wuhan/359/95 (H3N2) and B/Beijing/184/93 in the epidemic season 1996/97. Antineuraminidase (NI) antibody titres were determined by the neuraminidase inhibition test in sera samples collected before immunisation and then after 3 weeks and after 6 months. The neuraminidase inhibition test was carried out according to Aymard-Henry`s method (modification of A. Douglas) with fetuin as a substrate [3, 4]. The same procedures were carried out in healthy non-vaccinated children.

## Results

After vaccination NI antibody levels significantly increased when compared with the values recorded before vaccination. In group A patients vaccinated in the epidemic seasons 1993/94 and then in 1996/97 mean fold increase indexes – MFIs (increase of mean titres of antibodies in pre- and postvaccination sera) determined three weeks after vaccination were between 10.5 and 19.5 in season 1993/94 and between 11.2 and 18.9 in season 1996/97. In group B patients MFI values were more diverse and ranged from 10.8 to 56.5 and from 3.8 to 9.2 respectively (Table 1). In the case of patients vaccinated for the first time in the epidemic season 1996/97 MFI indexes were between 5.1 and 6.5 in group A and between 4.7 to 11.6 in group B (Table 2).

Six months after immunisation a further slight increase of NI antibody titres was

[1] Dept. of Paediatric Haematology and Oncology, Medical School Warsaw,
[2] National Influenza Centre WHO, Nat. Inst. of Hygiene, Warsaw, Poland

**Table 1.** Antineuraminidase antibody kinetics in children with acute lymphoblastic leukaemia vaccinated against influenza in Poland in the epidemic seasons 1993/94 and 1996/97

| Epidemic season | Antigen | Group | | Geometric mean titres of antineuraminidase antibodies | | | Mean fold increase | |
|---|---|---|---|---|---|---|---|---|
| | | | | before vaccination | 3 weeks after vaccination | 6 months | 3 weeks after vaccination | 6 months |
| 1993/94 | | A | vaccinated | 2.9 | 42.9 | 149.3 | 14.8 | 51.5 |
| | A/Texas/36/91 | | control | 2.1 | 2.7 | 4.0 | 1.3 | 1.9 |
| | (H1N1) | B | vaccinated | 3.5 | 37.8 | 67.3 | 10.8 | 19.2 |
| | | | control | 3.0 | 2.9 | 3.8 | 1.0 | 1.2 |
| | | A | vaccinated | 4.6 | 89.9 | 59.3 | 19.5 | 12.9 |
| | A/Beijing/32/92 | | control | 4.0 | 16.2 | 2.0 | 4.1 | < 1.0 |
| | (H3N2) | B | vaccinated | 2.2 | 119.9 | 56.6 | 54.5 | 25.7 |
| | | | control | 3.8 | 13.1 | 1.8 | 3.4 | < 1.0 |
| | | A | vaccinated | 7.1 | 74.6 | 24.1 | 10.5 | 3.4 |
| | B/Panama/45/90 | | control | 1.6 | 14.1 | 0 | 8.8 | < 1.0 |
| | | B | vaccinated | 1.5 | 84.8 | 49.5 | 56.5 | 33.0 |
| | | | control | 2.1 | 15.0 | 0 | 7.1 | < 1.0 |
| 1996/97 | | A | vaccinated | 1.6 | 30.3 | 42.2 | 18.9 | 26.4 |
| | A/Singapore/6/86 | | control | 1.3 | 3.2 | 5.8 | 2.4 | 4.4 |
| | (H1N1) | B | vaccinated | 15.0 | 58.1 | 47.6 | 3.8 | 3.2 |
| | | | control | 1.2 | 3.2 | 6.3 | 2.7 | 5.3 |
| | | A | vaccinated | 2.0 | 32.5 | 65.0 | 16.3 | 32.5 |
| | A/Wuhan/359/95 | | control | 0 | 4.0 | 10.7 | 4.0 | 10.7 |
| | (H3N2) | B | vaccinated | 4.1 | 37.8 | 63.5 | 9.2 | 15.5 |
| | | | control | 1.2 | 4.6 | 8.7 | 3.8 | 7.3 |
| | | A | vaccinated | 5.4 | 60.6 | 105.6 | 11.2 | 19.6 |
| | B/Beijing/184/93 | | control | 0 | 6.3 | 14.1 | 6.3 | 14.1 |
| | | B | vaccinated | 7.6 | 59.9 | 89.8 | 7.9 | 11.9 |
| | | | control | 1.2 | 6.8 | 14.1 | 5.7 | 11.8 |

A - chemotherapy completed before 1991 (n=10)
B - chemotherapy completed after 1991 (n=12)


**Table 2.** Antineuraminidase antibody kinetics in children with acute lymphoblastic leukaemia vaccinated against influenza for the first time in the epidemic season 1996/97

| Epidemic season | Antigen | Group | | Geometric mean titres of antineuraminidase antibodies | | | Mean fold increase | |
|---|---|---|---|---|---|---|---|---|
| | | | | before vaccination | 3 weeks after vaccination | 6 months | 3 weeks after vaccination | 6 months |
| 1996/97 | | A | vaccinated | 3.2 | 16.2 | 52.8 | 5.1 | 16.5 |
| | A/Singapore/6/86 | | control | 1.3 | 3.2 | 5.8 | 2.4 | 4.4 |
| | (H1N1) | B | vaccinated | 3.2 | 16.2 | 69.6 | 5.1 | 21.8 |
| | | | control | 1.2 | 3.2 | 6.3 | 2.7 | 5.3 |
| | | A | vaccinated | 5.0 | 32.5 | 65.0 | 6.5 | 13.0 |
| | A/Wuhan/359/95 | | control | 0 | 4.0 | 10.7 | 4.0 | 10.7 |
| | (H3N2) | B | vaccinated | 3.2 | 37.3 | 65.0 | 11.6 | 20.3 |
| | | | control | 1.2 | 4.6 | 8.7 | 3.8 | 7.3 |
| | | A | vaccinated | 4.0 | 23.0 | 75.0 | 5.8 | 18.8 |
| | B/Beijing/184/93 | | control | 0 | 6.3 | 14.1 | 6.3 | 14.1 |
| | | B | vaccinated | 7.9 | 37.3 | 69.6 | 4.7 | 8.8 |
| | | | control | 1.2 | 6.8 | 14.1 | 5.7 | 11.8 |

A - chemotherapy completed before 1991 (n=10)
B - chemotherapy completed after 1991 (n=10)

observed in most cases. Differences were recorded in the season 1993/94 in groups A and B where mean fold increases of NI antibody levels for neuraminidase N2 and NB were from 1.5 to 3.1 times lower than those noted 3 weeks after vaccination (Table 1).

The vaccines used in this study were well tolerated and did not cause any serious adverse reactions in the vaccinated patients.

## Discussion

The percentage of immunised patients for whom annual vaccination against influenza is recommended by WHO and the Advisory Committee on Immunisation Practices is still low and amounts to less than 20% [5]. Knowledge about the severity of influenza infections and their complications is still insufficient. Many people are not convinced about the efficacy of influenza vaccines; they expect the vaccines to protect them against all respiratory infections, although it is known that these can be caused by over 100 other respiratory viruses, as well as by bacteria's.

In the case of patients with proliferative diseases, altered humoral and cellular immunity has been noted [6-10]. Influenza vaccines stimulate B lymphocytes via T cells. Chemotherapy may weaken immunological response to viral infections in this group. Therefore, influenza vaccinations for patients such as these should have special priority, although the expected efficacy of immunisation can be less than in healthy persons. Influenza vaccines induce the production of antibodies against two surface influenza glycoproteins, i.e. haemagglutinin and neuraminidase. The role of antineuraminidase antibodies in immunity against influenza is considered to be less significant in comparison with the antihemagglutinin antibodies. Immunity against influenza is connected with neutralising HI antibodies, which in titres of $\geq 1:40$ are considered to have a protective effect. Nevertheless, although NI antibodies do not prevent the infection, they contribute to a milder course of the disease [11]. They inhibit the release of progeny viruses from the infected cells or aggregate virions reducing the number of infectious units [12]. In contrast to established levels of HI antibodies, there are no determined levels of NI antibodies considered to have a beneficial effect on immunity against influenza infections. Serological response after influenza vaccination is assessed by the haemagglutinin inhibition test or ELISA tests, whereas response to neuraminidase is not well characterised [13]. It is worth adding that humoral response to neuraminidase is poorer when compared with response to haemagglutinin. This is due to the intravirionic antigenic competition between these two antigens [14]. Nevertheless, it can be supposed that, in the present study, high antineuraminidase antibody levels recorded after influenza vaccination provided some protection in children with acute lymphoblastic leukaemia. No influenza infections were observed in the vaccinated patients, and NI antibody levels remained high even 6 months after immunisation.

An immunological response to the influenza vaccine and its protective effect depends on the antigenic correlation between the strains in the vaccine and currently circulating viruses, earlier exposures to the influenza virus, age of the vaccinated subjects and their medical condition [1, 15, 16]. However, in the present study the time that elapsed after the completion of chemotherapy treatment did not influence antibody response to neuraminidase antigens.

## Conclusions

NI antibodies do not give protection against influenza infection but they contribute to a milder course of the disease, while antihaemagglutinin antibodies protect patients against the infection. Results of this study confirm the immunogenicity of influenza vaccines, which induce the production of antihaemagglutinin antibodies (data presented earlier), as well as antineuraminidase antibodies in high titres, regardless of the time that has elapsed after chemotherapy treatment.

## References

1. Brydak LB (1998) Influenza and its prophylaxis. Springer PWN, Warsaw

2. Centers for Disease Control and Prevention (1998) Prevention and control of influenza: recommendations of the Advisory Committee on Immunization Practices (ACIP). MMWR 47 (No. RR-6): 5
3. Aymard-Henry M, Coleman MT, Dowdle WR, Laver WG, Schild GC, Webster RG (1973) Influenza virus neuraminidase and neuraminidase-inhibition test procedures. Bull WHO 48, 199
4. Douglas AR (1993) Assay of neuraminidase (NA) activity and neuraminidase inhibition test. Report of the WHO International Collaborative Center for Reference and Research on the Influenza Virus at Mill Hill. NIMR. London
5. Hall CB (1987) Influenza: A Shot or Not? Pediatrics 79 (4): 564-566
6. Kempe A, Hall CB, MacDonald NE, Foye HR, Woodin KA, Cohen HJ, Lewis ED, Gullace M, Gala CL (1989) Influenza in children with cancer. The Journal of Pediatrics 115 (1): 33-39
7. Ridgway D, Wolfe LJ (1993) Active immunization of Children with Leukemia and Other Malignancies. Leukemia and Lymphoma 9: 177-192
8. Smithson WA, Siem RA, Ritts RE, Gilchrist GS, Burgert EO, Ilstrup DM, Smith TF (1978) Response to influenza virus vaccine in children receiving chemotherapy for malignancy. The Journal of Pediatrics 93: 632-634
9. Steinherz PG, Brown AE, Gross PA, Braun D, Ghavimi F, Wollner N, Rosen G, Armstrong D, Miller DR (1980) Influenza Immunization of Children with Neoplastic Diseases. Cancer 45 (4): 750-756
10. Sumaya CV, Williams TE (1982) Persistance of Antibody After the Administration of Influenza Vaccine to Children with Cancer. Pediatrics 69(2): 226-229
11. Rott R, Becht H, Orlich M (1974) The significance of influenza virus neuraminidase in immunity. J Gen Virol 22: 35-41
12. Couch R, Kasel J, Gerin J, Schulman J, Kilbourne E (1974) Induction of partial immunity to influenza by a neuraminidase-specific influenza A virus vaccine in humans. J Infect Dis 129: 4110
13. Johansson BE, Matthews JT, Kilbourne ED (1998) Supplementation of conventional influenza A vaccine with purified viral neuraminidase results in a balanced and broadened immune response. Vaccine 16 (9/10): 1009-1015
14. Johansson B, Moran T, Kilbourne E (1987) Antigen-presenting B cells and helper T cells cooperatively mediate intravirionic antigenic competition between influenza A virus surface glycoproteins. Proc Natl Acad Sci USA 84:6869
15. Brydak LB, Rokicka-Milewska R, Jackowska T, Rudnicka H, Regnery H, Cox N (1997) Kinetics of humoral response in children with acute lymphoblastic leukemia immunized with influenza vaccine in 1993 in Poland. Leukemia Lymphoma 26: 163-169
16. Brydak LB, Rokicka-Milewska R, Machala M, et al. Immunogenicity of subunit trivalent influenza vaccine in children with acute lymphoblastic leukemia. Pediatr Infect Dis J 1998; 17: 125-129

# Expansion and Fibronectin-Enhanced Retroviral Transduction of Primary Human T Lymphocytes for Adoptive Immunotherapy

M. Stockschläder, S. Exner, O. Schmah and J. Finke

*Abstract.* Human lymphocytes remain one of the most promising target cells for gene therapy. Gene modified lymphocytes have been successfully used to treat ADA-deficient patients and to control GvHD after allogeneic bone marrow transplantation. Since activation and proliferation of T cells is necessary for efficient retrovirus-mediated gene transfer and subsequent selection of transduced cells, mononuclear cells (MNC) from steady-state and G-CSF stimulated peripheral blood were activated by short exposure to the mitogen phytohemagglutinin (PHA) and/or the anti-CD3 antibody OKT3 in the presence of different concentrations of recombinant interleukin-2 (Il-2). Using OKT3 (10 or 30 ng/ml) and Il-2 (100 U/ml), T cells expanded efficiently during a 14-day culture period. Cell expansion was similar under serum-free conditions. The immunophenotypic profile over time showed a marked increase in CD8$^+$ cells leading to a reversed CD4/CD8 ratio of 1:2 and a slight increase in CD56$^+$ cells. Supernatant-based centrifugational transduction of primary human T lymphocytes was compared with supernatant transduction on the extracellular matrix protein fibronectin. Transduction with cell-free retrovirus-containing supernatant in tissue culture flasks coated with human plasma fibronectin led to significantly higher transduction efficiencies (20.0±7.5%) than centrifugational transduction in uncoated culture flasks (13.6±5.1%)(p=0.041). To both rapidly characterize transduced cells and to isolate these from residual nontransduced but biologically equivalent cells, an amphotropic Mo-MuLV based retroviral vector containing the intracytoplasmatically-truncated human low-affinity nerve growth factor receptor (ΔLNGFR) cDNA as a marker gene was used. FACS sorting of T cells after transduction resulted in > 90 % LNGFR$^+$ cells and was much faster than enrichment of transduced cells through growth in G418-selection medium. These results show that supernatant-based retroviral gene transfer into primary human T lymphocytes can be enhanced by extracellular matrix proteins such as fibronectin approaching levels of transduction that can otherwise only be achieved by cocultivation of virus-producing cells with target cells. Ectopic expression of a cell surface protein can be used to rapidly and conveniently quantitate transduction efficiency through FACS analysis and to efficiently enrich transduced cells through FACS sorting.

## Introduction

The transfer of immune cells with antitumor activity into cancer patients is the principle of adoptive immunotherapy. Various immune cells (lymphokine-activated killer cells [LAK], natural killer cells [NK], tumor-infiltrating lymphocytes [TIL], *in vitro* sensitized [IVS] lymphocytes, cytotoxic T lymphocytes [CTL]) have proven valuable for this purpose. Autologous and allogeneic human lymphocytes have been cultured *ex vivo* in an attempt at expanding their numbers, augmenting their antitumor function, or improving gene transfer for further use in therapeutic protocols for adoptive immunotherapy. Administration of donor leukocyte infusions or donor lymphocytes to induce a graft-versus-leukemia (GvL) effect has pro-

Department of Hematology and Oncology, University Hospital of the Albert-Ludwigs-Universität Freiburg

duced hematologic, cytogenetic, and molecular remissions in approximately 80% of patients with chronic myelogenous leukemia (CML) relapsing after allogeneic bone marrow transplantation (BMT)[1,2]. However, associated graft-versus-host disease (GvHD) has resulted in significant morbidity and mortality which may be overcome through transduction of infused T cells with a „suicide gene" [3-5]. To obtain sufficient numbers of gene-modified T cells, blood-derived mononuclear cell (MNC) cultures can be used by inducing nonspecific T cell proliferation through activation signals which lead to continuous expression of the Il-2 receptor as well as continuous Il-2 production [6].

Retroviral vector mediated gene transfer is currently used in many gene marking and gene therapy protocols for advanced cancer, HIV infection [7-9], and the treatment of inherited and acquired diseases [10-13]. Genetically modified peripheral blood lymphocytes have been used to treat adenosine deaminase (ADA) deficient patients [14-21] and patients developing graft-versus-host disease (GvHD) after allogeneic bone marrow transplantation [3,22]. Because efficient and stable gene delivery is central to all lymphocyte-based gene therapy, the primary limitation of using retroviral vectors for genetic modification of T lymphocytes has been the inefficiency of gene transfer by standard supernatant transduction ranging from 0.1–10 % [15,17,20,23-25]. To overcome this problem, different improved supernatant-based transduction protocols have been proposed [26,27] thus avoiding cocultivation of primary cells with the retrovirus packaging cell line [3,17,24] which for various safety reasons is not desirable for clinical use.

Recently, it has been shown that supernatant-based retroviral transduction of hematopoietic stem cells can be enhanced through colocalization of retrovirus particles and target cells on specific domains of fibronectin. Since activated T cells express very late antigen (VLA)-4 and VLA-5 [28-32], integrins known to interact with fibronectin [31,33], we examined whether fibronectin would also increase gene transfer into human T cells.

In this study, we have compared several methods for blood-derived MNC activation and subsequent proliferation of T cells. Furthermore, we demonstrate efficient transduction of primary human T cells with cell-free supernatant containing a retroviral vector on fibronectin-coated surfaces. Through ectopic expression of a cell surface protein (ΔLNGFR), transduced T cells cells could be rapidly and accurately identified through FACS analysis and were efficiently enriched through FACS sorting.

## Materials and Methods

### Primary cells and cell lines

After informed consent, mononuclear cells (MNC) were isolated from peripheral blood, bone marrow, or (rhGCSF-mobilized) leukapheresis products by centrifugation on a Ficoll-gradient (density 1077g/l, Pharmacia, Freiburg, Germany) for 20 min at 20°C and washed twice with phophate-buffered saline (PBS, Gibco, Eggenstein, Germany) prior to use. For the cell expansion studies, MNC (1 x $10^6$ cells/ml) were activated with soluble CD3-Mab (OKT-3: 10, 30, and 100 ng/ml; Cilag, Neuss, Germany), and/or phytohemagglutinin (PHA: 10 and 50 µg/ml; Sigma, Deisenhofen, Germany) and recombinant human interleukin-2 (Il-2; 25, 100, and 1000 U/ml; Proleukin, Chiron, Ratingen, Germany) and incubated in RPMI 1640 (Seromed, Biochrom, Berlin, Germany) supplemented with 10 % [vol/vol] heat-inactivated fetal calf serum (Hyclone Europe, Erembodegem, Belgium), 50 µM 2-mercaptoethanol, 2 mM glutamine, 1 mM sodium pyruvate, and 1 % penicillin-streptomycin (Gibco). Cells were cultured in 12-well plates (flat bottom multiwell tissue culture plate; Falcon 3043; 2 x $10^6$ cells/well) and fed 4, 7, and 10 days after culture initiation. For retroviral transduction, MNC (2 x $10^6$ cells/ml) were activated three to four days in tissue culture flasks (Falcon, Becton Dickinson, Heidelberg, Germany) with OKT-3 (10–30 ng/ml) and Il-2 (100 U/ml). Long-term cultures were set up in T-75 flasks (Falcon, Becton Dickinson, Heidelberg, Germany) at 2 x $10^6$ cells/ml. Expanding cells were split every two to three days with 50% of the medium being replaced with fresh medium supplemented with 100 U of rh Il-2/ml. For expansion in serum-free media, cells were cultured in CellGro SCG medium (Cellgenix, Freiburg, Germany) or X-VIVO-15 medium (Biowhittaker-Serva, Germany) ± 5 % human AB-serum. On day 0, PBMNC (1 x 10⁶ cells/ml; 5 ml) were seeded in T25-flasks with 30 ng/ml OKT3 and 100 U/ml rhIl-2. Cells were counted on days 3,5,7,10,12, and 14 and fed according to the following guidelines: 1) if the cell concentration was < 1.5 x 10⁶ cells/ml, cells were centrifuged and half the medium was replaced by fresh medium + Il-2; 2) if the cell concentration was > 1.5 x 10⁶ cells/ml, cell concentration was adjusted to 1.0 x 10⁶ cells/ml with half-medium change. The amount of medium was kept constant at 5 ml during expansion.

The amphotropic packaging cell line HSRBM-01 containing split helper genome sequences [34,35] was established by Boehringer Mannheim GmbH (Penzberg, Germany) releasing high-titer (1 x 10⁶ cfu/ml) replication-deficient retroviral vector (LXSN-based construct [36]]. The retrovirus vectors containing the cDNA of an intracytoplasmatically truncated version of the human low-affinity nerve growth factor receptor (ΔLNGFR) have been described [37]. In addition to ΔLNGFR, one vector contained the cDNA of the neomycin phosphotransferase gene (neoᴿ) and in the other vector the neoᴿ gene was replaced by the viral Herpes-simplex thymidine kinase gene (Fig. 1). Packaging cell lines producing replication-deficient retroviral vectors were kept in Dulbecco's modified Eagle's medium (DMEM, Gibco) supplemented with 10% heat-inactivated fetal calf serum (FCS, HyClone) and 1 mM sodium pyruvate.

HeLa cells were kept in Dulbecco's modified Eagle's medium (DMEM) supplemented with 10% heat-inactivated FCS and sodium pyruvate. Jurkat cells, a human T cell line, were cultured in RPMI (Seromed) supplemented with 10% heat-inactivated FCS (HyClone), 1mM sodium pyruvate, and 2 mM glutamine (Gibco). All cells were kept at 37°C in a humidified atmosphere of 5% CO₂ in air.

### Transduction protocol

After three days of stimulation with OKT-3 and Il-2, cultured cells were transduced on the fourth day with retroviral vectors at an MOI of 1 in the presence of 4 µg/ml polybrene (Sigma Aldrich, Deisenhofen, Germany) or protamine sulfate (Sigma Aldrich) and Il-2 (100 U/ml) according to the following protocols:

1. resuspension of T cells in retrovirus-containing supernatant supplemented with 100 U/ml Il-2 for 24 hours;
2. resuspension of T cells in retrovirus-containing supernatant supplemented with 100 U/ml Il-2 and subsequent centrifugation in 6-well plates for 1–2 hours at different centrifugational forces (1 x 10⁶ cells/ml; 4 ml/well; temperature was kept at 32°C during centrifugation);
3. resuspension of T cells in retrovirus-containing supernatant supplemented with 100 U/ml Il-2 and incubation in fi-

**Fig. 1.** ΔLNGFR retroviral vectors based on LXSN (Miller and Rosman, 1989). (A) Retroviral vector containing an intracytoplasmatically truncated version of the human low-affinity nerve growth factor receptor cDNA (ΔLNGFR; C. Bordignon, Milano, Italy) and the neomycin phosphotransferase cDNA (NEO) from Transposon Tn5. (B) Retroviral vector containing the ΔLNGFR cDNA and the Herpes-simplex thymidine kinase cDNA; SV indicates the SV40 early promoter.

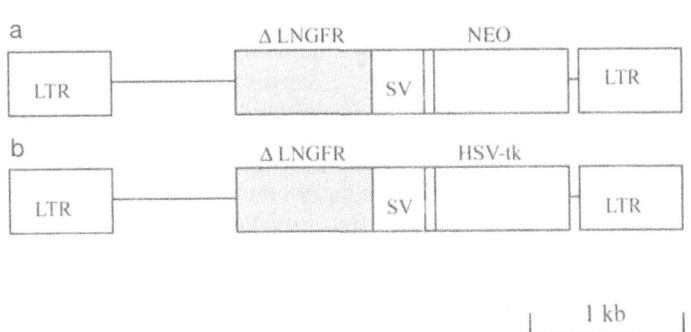

bronectin-coated tissue culture plates (human plasma fibronectin, Biocoat; Falcon, Heidelberg) for 24 hours;

4. cocultivation of T cells with the irradiated virus-producing cell line in RPMI supplemented with 10 % FCS and 100 U/ml Il-2 for 24 hours. Aliquots of cryopreserved supernatant were used in most experiments.

## Flow cytometry

FACS analysis was performed on a FACScan flow cytometer (Beckton Dickinson, San Jose; USA). Data were analyzed using Lysis II software (Beckton Dickinson). The following MAbs and polyclonal antibodies were purchased as phycoerythrin or fluorescein isothiocyanate conjugates: CD3, CD4, CD8, CD16, CD56, HLA-DR, CD25, CD134 (Ox40) CD45RO, CD45RA, CD95, goat anti-mouse from Becton Dickinson (Heidelberg, Germany), goat anti-mouse IgG1-antibody from Dako (Glostrup, Denmark), mouse immunoglobulin G isotype control from Serotec (Oxford, England). Antibodies were used at saturating concentrations in accordance with the manufacturer's instructions. During acquisition, a gate was set on the lymphocyte population so that at least 10000 events were analyzed in every experiment.

## Analysis of gene transfer efficiency, retrovirus titer, and FACS sorting

Gene transfer efficiency was measured by flow cytometry using a monoclonal unconjugated anti-LNGFR-antibody (Boehringer Mannheim GmbH, Penzberg, Germany). Cells were washed twice in PBS (Gibco) and stained with a PE-coupled anti-IgG$_1$-antibody (Dako).

Viral titers were estimated by the infection of HeLa cells with serial tenfold dilutions of virus-containing supernatant and subsequent G418 selection for neo$^R$ containing vectors. Vectors not containig neo$^R$ were titered through FACS analysis. For determination of the titer by FACS analysis, HeLa cells were plated the day before infection (0.5 x 10$^6$ cells/6-cm tissue culture dish; 4 ml). One

replicate dish was obtained at the time of infection to measure the exact target cell number. To avoid the measurement of false-positive cells through flow cytometry after retroviral transfer of cell surface markers [38], cells were harvested 72 hours after infection, counted, and stained with the anti-LNGFR antibody and analyzed by FACS analysis. The concentration of infectious particles was calculated as follows: (% of LNGFR-positive cells/100) x (target cell number at the time of infection) x (1000/viral supernatant used in µl) = (% of LNGFR-positive cells) x (target cell number at the time of infection) x (10/viral supernatant used in µl). The target cell number and and the amount of viral supernatant used for this calculation were chosen so that FACS analysis yielded between 2 % and 50 % positive cells [39].

Transduced T-lymphocytes were enriched for transgene expression through a high-speed sorter (MoFlo; Cytomation Inc., Fort Collins, Colorado, USA). A 488 nm argon ion laser and a 530/40 band pass filter were used. Cells were sorted at a total event rate of 20000 cells/sec. Approximately, 1 x 10$^7$ cells were resuspended in 750 µl PBS and incubated with murine monoclonal anti-ΔLNGFR Ab for 20 min at 20°C in 15-ml tubes. After washing in PBS, phycoerythrin-labeled goat anti-mouse antibody was added and the suspension again incubated for 20 min at 20°C. Cells were resuspended in one ml of PBS and kept on ice for sorting.

## Statistical analysis

The means of transduction efficiencies were compared by an unpaired two-sided student t test.

## Results

### T cell expansion and immunophenotypic characterization

Mononuclear cells from peripheral blood and leukapheresis products were seeded on day-1 at a cell density of 0.5 x 10$^6$/ml and stimulated with different agents in various combinations at different concentrations (OKT3 10, 30, and

100 ng/ml; Il-2 25, 100, and 1000 U/ml; PHA10 and 50 µg/ml) to define optimal conditions for T-cell activation and short-term (14 days) proliferation. Proliferation of the cells during a 14-day culture period under the different conditions was expressed as percentage in relation to the combination leading to the highest proliferation as determined by cell number. As can be seen in Table 1 and 2, peripheral blood and leukapheresis-derived T-cells grew best when stimulated with 10 ng/ml OKT-3 and 1000 U/ml Il-2. At a lower Il-2 concentration (100 U/ml), growth was similar at day 7, and only slightly reduced at day 14. This was true for OKT3 at either 10 or 30 ng/ml. In comparison to cells grown in RPMI + 10 % FCS, similar (CellGro, X-VIVO-15) or slightly better (X-VIVO-15 or CellGro + 5 % human AB-serum) growth kinetics were found when T-cells were grown in serum-free medium (Fig. 2).

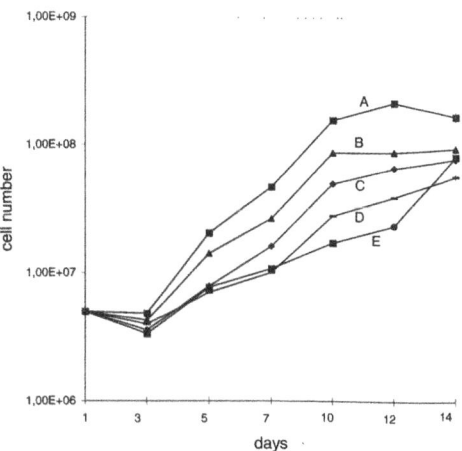

**Fig. 2.** T-cell expansion during a 14-day culture period. MNC were stimulated with 30 ng/ml OKT3 and grown in 100 U/ml recombinant human Il-2 (Proleukin). The absolute cell number on day-0 is 5 x 10^6 cells/ml. Depicted is the cell expansion (logarithmic scale). A: X-VIVO-15 + 5 % AB-serum; B: CellGro + 5 % AB-serum; C: RPMI + 10 % FCS; D: X-VIVO-15 alone; E: CellGro alone; N=3.

**Table 1.** Expansion of peripheral blood derived T lymphocytes under different conditions (N=5). Mononuclear cells from peripheral blood were seeded on day-1 at a cell density of 0.5 x 10^6/ml and stimulated with OKT3, PHA, and Il-2 in various combinations at different concentrations (OKT3 10, 30, and 100 ng/ml; Il-2 25, 100, and 1000 U/ml; PHA10 and 50 µg/ml). Proliferation of the cells during a 14-day culture period (day7 and day 14) under the different conditions was expressed as percentage in relation to the combination leading to the highest proliferation as determined by cell number (10 ng/ml OKT-3 and 1000 U/ml Il-2).

| Stimulation | day 7 | day 14 |
|---|---|---|
| Okt3 10ng/ml + IL-2 1000U/ml | 100±1,1 | 100±3,0 |
| no stimulation | 10,9 ± 0,3 | 0,8 ± 0,3 |
| IL-2 25U/ml | 19,7 ± 0,4 | 7,8 ± 1,5 |
| IL-2 100U/ml | 19,8 ± 0,5 | 7,8 ± 0,8 |
| IL-2 1000U/ml | 20,1 ± 5,7 | 7,6 ± 1,9 |
| Okt3 10ng/ml + IL-2 25U/ml | 94,5 ± 2,0 | 46,4 ± 30,7 |
| Okt3 10ng/ml + IL-2 100U/ml | 114,1 ± 1,8 | 86,7 ± 29,4 |
| Okt3 30ng/ml + IL-2 25U/ml | 81,7 ± 1,4 | 27,6 ± 6,9 |
| Okt3 30ng/ml + IL-2 100U/ml | 101,9 ± 1,3 | 81,6 ± 15,1 |
| Okt3 30ng/ml + IL-2 1000U/ml | 85,7 ± 1,6 | 78,3 ± 12,2 |
| Okt3 100ng/ml + IL-2 25U/ml | 62,1 ± 0,4 | 25,2 ± 9,0 |
| Okt3 100ng/ml + IL-2 100U/ml | 58,0 ± 2,3 | 69,1 ± 11,0 |
| Okt3 100ng/ml + IL-2 1000U/ml | 67,4 ± 0,8 | 68,0 ± 6,1 |
| PHA 10µg/ml + IL-2 25U/ml | 65,1 ± 0,4 | 19,4 ± 3,9 |
| PHA 10µg/ml + IL-2 100U/ml | 79,2 ± 0,6 | 62,1 ± 15,3 |
| PHA 10µg/ml + IL-2 1000U/ml | 79,2 ± 1,4 | 74,5 ± 11,0 |
| PHA 50µg/ml + IL-2 25U/ml | 53,2 ± 1,2 | 14,2 ± 3,5 |
| PHA 50µg/ml + IL-2 100U/ml | 59,1 ± 0,8 | 38,6 ± 2,0 |
| PHA 50µg/ml + IL-2 1000U/ml | 65,0 ± 0,5 | 58,9 ± 17,0 |
| Okt3 10ng/ml + PHA 10µg/ml + IL-2 25U/ml | 48,5 ± 0,6 | 10,5 ± 4,1 |

**Table 2.** Expansion of leukapheresis derived T lymphocytes under different conditions (N≥7). Mononuclear cells from G-CSF stimulated peripheral blood were seeded on day-1 at a cell density of 0.5 x 106/ml and stimulated with OKT3, PHA, and Il-2 in various combinations at different concentrations (OKT3 10, 30, and 100 ng/ml; Il-2 25, 100, and 1000 U/ml; PHA10 and 50 µg/ml). Proliferation of the cells during a 14-day culture period (day7 and day14) under the different conditions was expressed as percentage in relation to the combination leading to the highest proliferation as determined by cell number (10 ng/ml OKT-3 and 1000 U/ml Il-2).

| Stimulation | day 7 | day 14 |
|---|---|---|
| Okt3 10ng/ml + IL-2 1000U/ml | 100 ± 28,1 | 100 ± 42,2 |
| no stimulation | 5,3 ± 4,5 | 0,3 ± 0,3 |
| IL-2 25U/ml | 9,5 ± 6,9 | 4,9 ± 5,1 |
| IL-2 100U/ml | 8,5 ± 7,7 | 4,1 ± 0,6 |
| IL-2 1000U/ml | 10,9 ± 7,7 | 4,2 ± 0,6 |
| Okt3 10ng/ml + IL-2 25U/ml | 54,1 ± 36,3 | 20,7 ± 22,5 |
| Okt3 10ng/ml + IL-2 100U/ml | 98,1 ± 21,9 | 68,5 ± 26,2 |
| Okt3 30ng/ml + IL-2 25U/ml | 50,2 ± 28,3 | 21,3 ± 25,0 |
| Okt3 30ng/ml + IL-2 100U/ml | 90,6 ± 19,3 | 69,8 ± 32,3 |
| Okt3 30ng/ml + IL-2 1000U/ml | 74,5 ± 22,3 | 93,0 ± 48,1 |
| Okt3 100ng/ml + IL-2 25U/ml | 37,6 ± 31,2 | 33,8 ± 24,8 |
| Okt3 100ng/ml + IL-2 100U/ml | 70,7 ± 22,6 | 64,2 ± 41,0 |
| Okt3 100ng/ml + IL-2 1000U/ml | 58,2 ± 4,5 | 73,6 ± 0,3 |
| PHA 10µg/ml + IL-2 25U/ml | 33,3 ± 14,3 | 11,1 ± 9,0 |
| PHA 10µg/ml + IL-2 100U/ml | 31,4 ± 15,7 | 15,3 ± 0,1 |
| PHA 10µg/ml + IL-2 1000U/ml | 26,9 ± 14,0 | 24,0 ± 2,8 |
| PHA 50µg/ml + IL-2 25U/ml | 22,6 ± 8,6 | 6,7 ± 4,4 |
| PHA 50µg/ml + IL-2 100U/ml | 22,8 ± 10,6 | 8,2 ± 0,8 |
| PHA 50µg/ml + IL-2 1000U/ml | 22,4 ± 7,5 | 12,7 ± 1,0 |
| Okt3 10ng/ml + PHA 10µg/ml + IL-2 25U/ml | 38,3 ± 7,2 | 19,5 ± 13,2 |

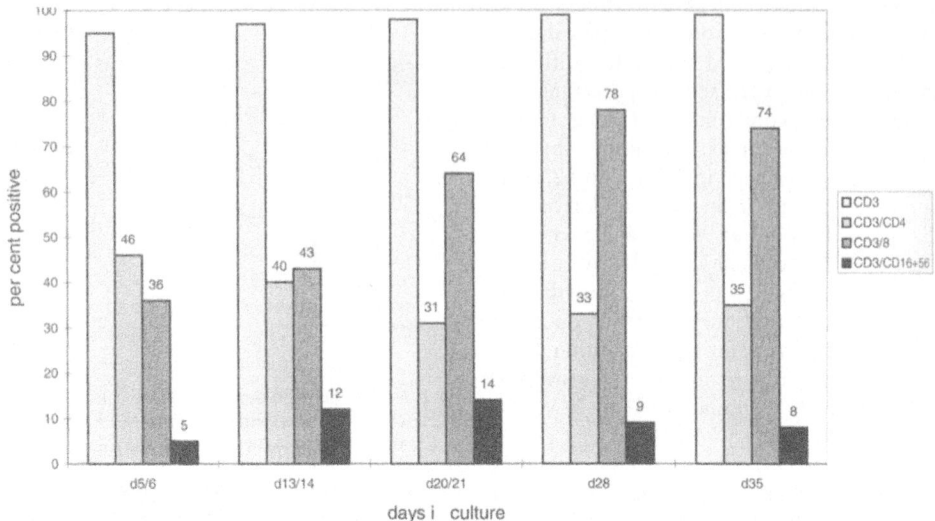

**Fig. 3.** Immunophenotype of cultured T lymphocytes during a 5-week culture period (N=3). Per cent of cells expressing the CD3, CD3/CD4, CD3/CD8, and CD16+56 antigens (means).

Flow cytometric analysis showed that reproducibly more than 90 % and more than 95 % of the cells were CD3$^+$ three to four and five days after activation, respectively. During a 5-week culture period, the majority of the cells (≥ 95 %) remained CD3$^+$ (Fig. 3). Regarding the percentage of CD4$^+$ and CD8$^+$ cells, there was a marked decrease in CD4/CD8-ratio leading to a reversed ratio of 1:2 compared with fresh PBMNC (Fig. 3). The percentage of CD56$^+$ cells increased slightly during the culture period (Fig. 3). The relative number of

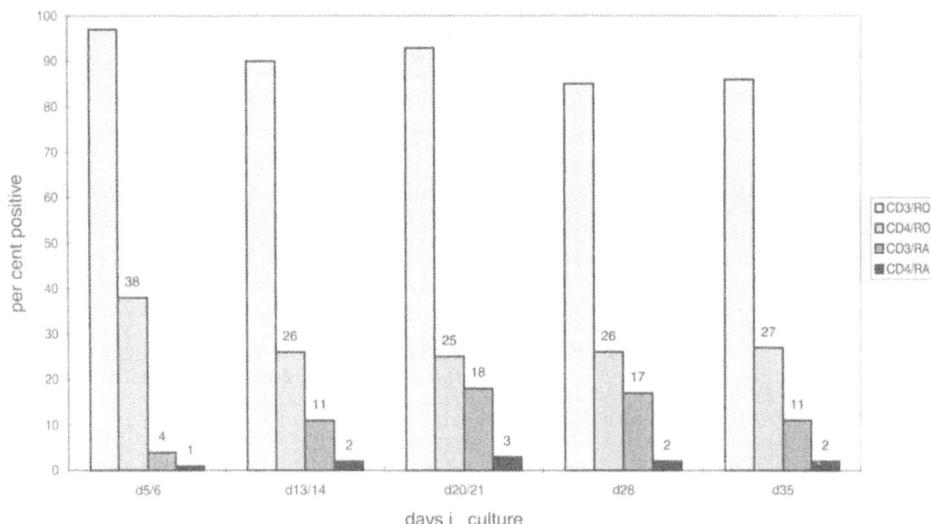

**Fig. 4.** Immunophenotype of cultured T lymphocytes during a 5-week culture period (N=3). Per cent of cells expressing the CD3/CD45RO, CD4/CD45RO, CD3/CD45RA and CD4/CD45RA antigens (means).

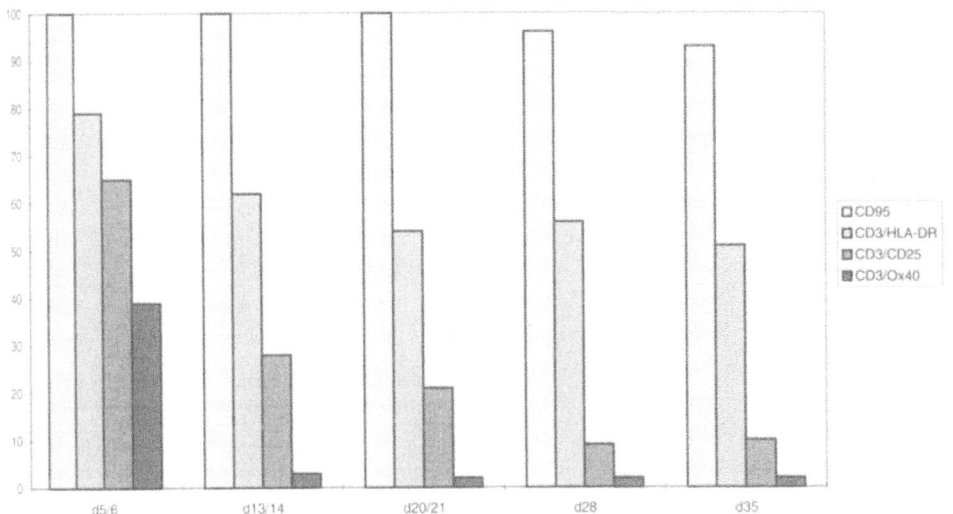

**Fig. 5.** Immunophenotype of cultured T lymphocytes during a 5-week culture period (N=3). Per cent of cells expressing the CD3/CD134 (Ox40), CD3/CD25 (Il-2R), CD3/CD95 (Fas), and CD3/HLA-DR antigens (means)

naive (CD3⁺CD45RA⁺) and memory (CD3⁺CD45RO⁺) T-cells did not significantly change during the culture period (Fig. 4). Almost all T lymphocytes (≥ 93 %) continued to express the FAS-antigen (CD95) whereas other activation markers such as HLA-DR, Il-2R (CD25), and the Ox40-antigen (CD134; mainly expressed on CD4⁺ cells) steadily decreased over the 35-day culture period with different kinetics (Ox40 > CD25 > HLA-DR)(Fig. 5).

When cells were grown in serum-free Cell-Gro medium supplemented with 5 % human AB-serum, there was a marked increase in the percentage of CD56⁺ cells (20.3 ± 0.9 %) at the end of the culture period. After expansion of cells in X-VIVO ± 5 % human AB-serum, a CD4/CD8 ratio of approximately 1 was observed (44.1 ± 8.1 % CD4⁺ cells and 57.9 ± 2.6 % CD8⁺ cells, respectively).

viral supernatant, an almost linear correlation was found between the amount of supernatant and the percentage of transduced ΔLNGFR-expressing cells as determined by flow cytometry (Fig. 6). Using less than 1 μl supernatant, the percentage of transduced cells was below the threshold of detection by FACS analysis. Using more than 100 μl supernatant, there was no correlation between the amount of supernatant and the percentage of transduced cells (Fig. 6; inserts). The titer was calculated from the target cell number, the amount of supernatant, and the percentage of transduced HeLa cells (Materials and Methods). Parallel determination of the titer through FACS analysis and the conventional method of counting the number of G418-resistant colonies after serial dilution showed an excellent correlation.

## Rapid determination of retroviral titer by FACS analysis

Retroviral vectors not containing the neomycin phosphotransferase gene as selectable marker were titered on HeLa cells by a newly established method through FACS analysis. Using 10–100 μl fresh or cryopreserved retro-

## Transduction of the Jurkat cell line

Jurkat cells were transduced through centrifugation in retrovirus containing supernatant in the presence of different concentrations of polybrene (4, 8, and 12 μg/ml) or protamine sulfate (4, 8, and 12 μg/ml). Transduction efficiency ranged from 32.9±14.7 % (polybrene

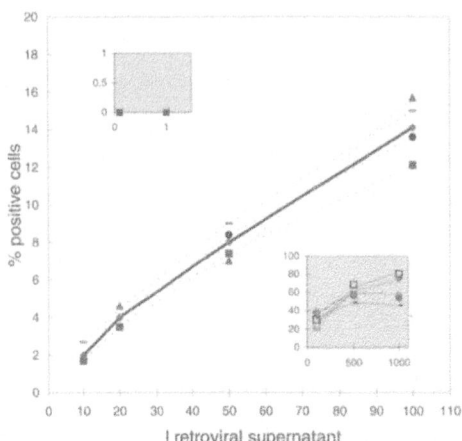

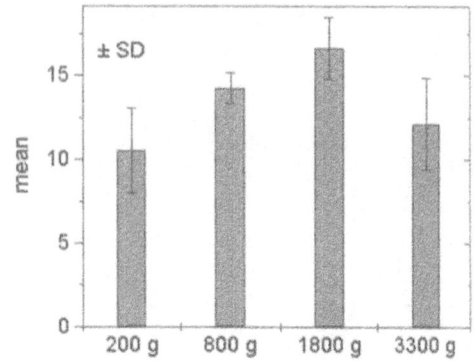

**Fig. 7.** Transduction efficiency of primary T cells after supernatant-based centrifugational transduction at different centrifugational forces (200, 800, 1800, and 3300 g). Per cent of ΔLNGFR-positive cells. Centrifugational transduction of primary T-cells as well as ΔLNGFR expression were donor-dependent and ranged from 4 % to 23 %. Transduction efficiency: 200g: 10.5±5.1%, 800g: 14.3±4.8%, 1800 g: 16.7±3.2%, and 3300 g: 12.1±7.3% of ΔLNGFR-positive cells, respectively.

**Fig. 6.** Titration of ΔLNGFR-vectors on HeLa cells through FACS analysis. For determination of the titer by FACS analysis, HeLa cells were plated the day before infection (0.5 x 10⁶ cells/6-cm tissue culture dish; 4 ml). One replicate dish was obtained at the time of infection to measure the exact target cell number. Cells were harvested 72 hours after infection with 10, 20, 50, and 100 μl filtered supernatant, counted, and stained with the anti-LNGFR antibody and analyzed by FACS analysis. The concentration of infectious particles was calculated as follows: (% of LNGFR-positive cells) x (target cell number at the time of infection) x (10/viral supernatant used in μl). The target cell number and and the amount of viral supernatant used for this calculation were chosen so that FACS analysis yielded between 2 % and 50 % positive cells. Inserts: Using less than 1 μl supernatant, the percentage of transduced cells was below the threshold of detection by FACS analysis (upper left). Using more than 100 μl supernatant, there was no correlation between the amount of supernatant and the percentage of transduced cells (lower right).

### Transduction of primary human T lymphocytes

Centrifugational transduction of primary T-cells as well as ΔLNGFR expression were donor-dependent and ranged from 4 % to 23 %. As shown in Fig. 7, there was an increase in the transduction efficiency depending on the centrifugational force (200g: 10.5±5.1%, 800g: 14.3±4.8%, and 1800 g: 16.7±3.2%, respectively). Recovery of cells after centrifugation (200, 800, and 1800 g) ranged from 75–81 %. A further increase in centrifugation force (3300 g), however, resulted in a lower transduction efficiency (12.1±7.3%) and significant cell damage. Centrifugational transduction led to significantly higher infection rates than standard retroviral supernatant transduction (usually less than 10%).

There was no difference in the transduction efficiency at 1800 g between freshly isolated (13.5±5.2%), cryopreserved (16.3±1.2%), bone marrow-derived (14.0±3.5%), leukapheresis-derived (13.7±5.3%), patient (13.8±4.6%), or healthy donor cells (14.0±5.9%)(Fig. 8).

12 μg/ml) to 64.8±9.1 % (protamine sulfate 12 μg/ml). A polybrene concentration > 8 μg/ml appeared to be toxic to the cell line with a significant reduction in transduction efficiency (polybrene 4 vs 12 μg/ml: 46.8± 17 % and 32.9±14.7 %, respectively; t-test p=0.012) whereas a higher protamine sulfate concentration led to an increased transduction efficiency (protamine sulfate 4 vs 12 μg/ml: 56±6.2 % and 64.8±9.1 %, respectively).

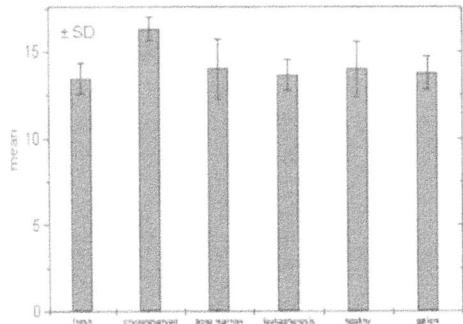

**Fig. 8.** Transduction efficiency of primary T cells from freshly isolated (13.5±5.2%), cryopreserved (16.3±1.2%), bone marrow-derived (14.0±3.5%), leukapheresis-derived (13.7±5.3%), patient (13.8±4.6%), or healthy donor (14.0±5.9%) cells after supernatant-based centrifugational transduction at a centrifugational force of 1800 g. Per cent of ΔLNGFR-positive cells

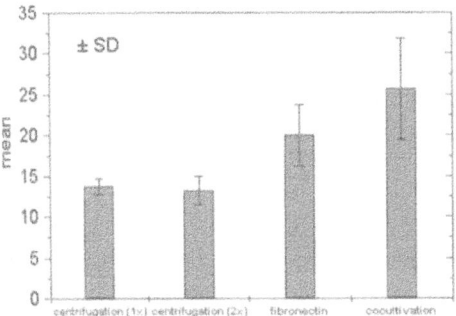

**Fig. 9.** Transduction efficiency of primary T cells after one (day 4) or two (day 4 and 5) rounds of supernatant-based centrifugational transduction (13.8±5.2% and 13.3±4.8%, respectively) vs transduction through cocultivation of target cells with virus-producing packaging cells (25.7±10.7 %) vs supernatant-based transduction in fibronectin-coated tissue culture plates (20.0±7.5 %). Per cent of ΔLNGFR-positive cells.

### Fibronectin increases gene transfer into primary human T cells

Supernatant-based centrifugational transduction of T lymphocytes (one round of centrifugation on day 4 vs two rounds of centrifugation on days 4 and 5; mean transduction efficiency ± SD: 13.8±5.2 % and 13.3±4.8 %, respectively) was compared with transduction through cocultivation of the packaging cells (25.7±10.7 %) and with supernatant transduction on fibronectin coated tissue culture dishes (20.0±7.5 %). As shown in Figure

9, cocultivation and fibronectin-based supernatant transduction led to significantly higher transduction efficiencies than centrifugational transduction (t test p=0.0019 and p=0.041, respectively).

### Efficient enrichment of transduced cells through ectopic cell surface expression of ΔLNGFR or selection in G418-containing medium

To determine the G418 sensitivity of non-transduced cells, T cells were incubated in G418 at different concentrations (0.2, 0.4, 0.6, 0.8, 1.0, and 1.2 mg/ml). As depicted in Figure 10, non-transduced T cells could be reproducibly eliminated by G418 at all tested concentrations. Depending on the G418 concentration, non-transduced cells survived between 10 (1.2 mg/ml) and 23 (0.2 mg/ml) days. FACS analysis of transduced cells which were grown in medium without G418 showed that gene expression of primary T-lymphocytes remained stable during the 5-week culture period (12-16% ΔLNGFR expressing cells) (Fig. 11). When transduced cells were grown under selection pressure (0.4 mg/ml active G418) almost 90 % of the T-lymphocytes became ΔLNGFR-positive within 20 days. Growth in selection medium for a longer period of time was necessary for lower G418 concentrations and led to an enrichment of only 78% ΔLNGFR-positive after 30 days (Fig. 11).

Enrichment for transduced cells through one round of FACS sorting was rapid (less than 2 hours) and highly efficient (93.1±1.3% ΔLNGFR-positive cells).

### Discussion

In this report, we have compared different conditions for expansion of blood-derived mononuclear cells by using various modes of T cell activation. Furthermore, we present both a strategy and a protocol for reproducibly achieving improved gene transfer efficiencies in primary human T lymphocytes.

Our results show that activation with the monoclonal anti-CD3 antibody OKT3 approved for clinical use was at least as efficient as activation with phytohemagglutinin

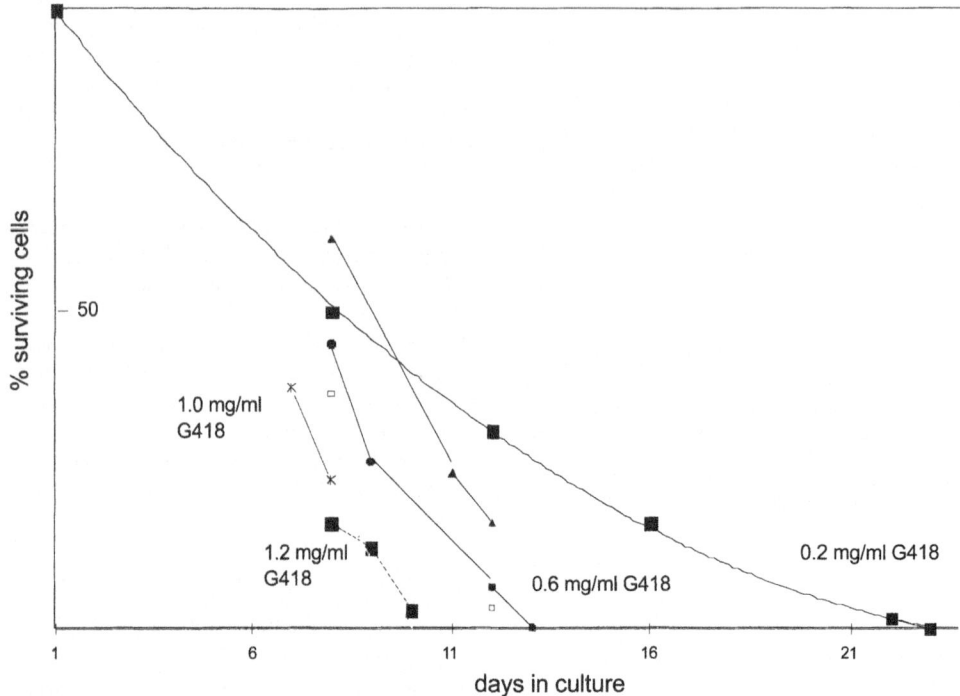

**Fig. 10.** Growth of non-transduced primary human T cells in medium containing G418 at different concentrations (0.2, 0.4, 0.6, 0.8, 1.0, and 1.2 mg/ml)(N=4). Per cent of surviving cells (day 1 = 100 %).

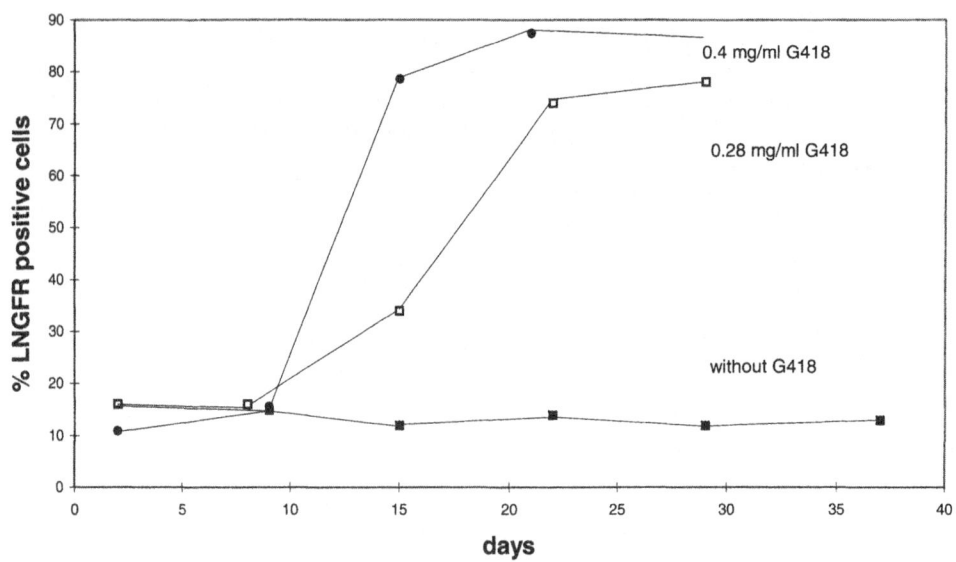

**Fig. 11.** Growth of transduced primary human T cells in medium without and with G418. Per cent of ΔLNGFR-positive cells. When transduced cells were grown in 0.4 mg/ml G418 almost 90 % of the T-lymphocytes became ΔLNGFR-positive within 20 days. Growth in selection medium for a longer period of time was necessary at 0.28 mg/ml G418 and led to an enrichment of only 78% ΔLNGFR-positive after 30 days. FACS analysis of transduced cells which were grown in medium without G418 showed that gene expression of primary T-lymphocytes remained stable during the 5-week culture period (12-16% ΔLNGFR expressing cells).

(PHA). Anti-CD3 activation of T cells induces the expression of the high-affinity Il-2 receptor and at low Il-2 concentrations promotes growth of antigen-specific T cells displaying HLA-restricted killing while reducing the growth of NK-like LAK cells lacking the high-affinity IL-2 heterodimer receptor and T-cell receptors [6,40-42]. As shown previously [43], proliferation of anti-CD3 activated PBMNC gave rise to phenotypically heterogenous cell populations with a reversed ratio of CD4[+] and CD8[+] cells and an increased number of CD56[+] cells compared to freshly isolated, unstimulated PBMNC. As both CD8[+] and CD56[+] cells express cytotoxic activities, increasing their relative and absolute cell numbers in the expanded cultures might play a significant role in improving antitumor activity *in vivo*. Earlier studies in a mouse model have demonstrated that *ex vivo* Il-2 expanded T cells were capable of significant *in vivo* alloreactivity [44]. However, an increase in the number of cultured T cells administered or the introduction of a short resting culture period prior to infusion was necessary in order to achieve *in vivo* alloreactivity identical to the alloreactivity observed with fresh T cells [45]. Whether the recently observed increased and prolonged proliferation of polyclonal T cells through immobilized anti-CD3 and anti-CD28 antibodies leads to a preferential expansion and transduction of TH1 cells warrants further study [46,47]. As a further step towards increased saftey (transmission of viruses, immunogenicity of xenogeneic proteins [48]) for clinical application, the use of serum-free media is desirable. Using two different serum-free media, we show that in the presence of low contrations of human AB-serum expansion of primary T cells was similar to the results obtained with media containing fetal calf serum. The effect of the selected growth medium on the distribution of immunophenotypically defined subsets of the expanded cells at the end of the culture period, however, should be closely monitored.

Currently, retroviral vectors have several advantages as a gene delivery system. Retroviral vectors have been shown to stably transduce animal and human hematopoietic cells and appear safe as long as they are devoid of replication-competent virus [10]. In addition, retroviral vectors are the best characterized gene delivery system and have been used in a number of preclinical and clinicall studies. Genetically modified lymphocytes have been used to treat adenosine deaminase (ADA) deficient patients [14-21,24,49] and patients developing graft-versus-host disease (GvHD) after allogeneic bone marrow transplantation [3,22]. The success and wide applicability of the use of gene-modified lymphocytes is limited, however, by the usually only low transduction efficiency of human T lymphocytes by standard supernatant transduction protocols ranging from 0.1 - 10 % [15,17,20,23-25]. To overcome this problem, different improved supernatant-based transduction protocols have been proposed thus avoiding cocultivation of primary cells with the retrovirus packaging cell line [3,17,20,24,50] which for various safety reasons is not desirable for clinical use. Use of optimized transduction protocols combining centrifugation of the lymphocytes at the inception of transduction with phosphate depletion, low-temperature incubation, and the use of the cell line PG13 [51,52], a packaging cell line which produces vector virions pseudotyped with the gibbon ape leukemia virus envelope, has resulted in high-efficiency retroviral-mediated gene transfer into human and nonhuman primate peripheral blood lymphocytes [26,27,39,48,53]. The two parameters which increased the gene transfer efficiency the most in the present study were the use of a centrifugation step confirming earlier results and fibronectin. We found an increase in transduction efficiency depending on the centrifugational force which was limited by cell viability at the highest speed centrifugation. Interestingly, multiple rounds of transduction did not improve gene transfer efficiency.

Since infection efficiency of T lymphocytes with amphotropic retroviral vectors has been shown to be cell cycle dependent [54] and most cells require attachment to a substrate to enter the cell cycle, the question arose whether extracellular matrix proteins such as fibronectin would improve gene transfer efficiency. A link between adhesion and growth has been shown in T cells where costimulation of the T-cell receptor and the ß$_2$-integrin receptor lymphocyte function antigen-I (LFA-1) caused a synergistic enhancement of T-cell proliferation [55,56]. The extracellular matrix protein fibronectin (FN) contains several functional sites with cell binding properties. The alternatively-spliced type III connecting segment (IIICS) region of FN contains two cell binding sites. The major site, CS-1, located within the first 25 amino acids of IIICS and the COOH-terminal of the heparin-binding domain (HBD) are recognized by very late antigen-4 (VLA-4)[57,58]. The central cell-binding domain (CBD) which includes the minimal essential sequence, RGD(S), is recognized by VLA-5. In the CD4 subset of T cells, the interaction of $\alpha_4\beta_1$ (VLA-4) and $\alpha_5\beta_1$ (VLA-5) integrins with fibronectin [31,33,59] facilitates CD3-mediated cell growth [31,32,60-63]. Furthermore, it has been shown that supernatant-based retroviral transduction of hematopoietic stem cells can be enhanced through colocalization of retrovirus particles and target cells on specific domains of fibronectin [33,37,64]. It remains to be determined whether the observed enhanced retroviral transduction of primary human T cells on fibronectin in our study was only due to the „colocalization effect" mediated by fibronectin or whether fibronectin-facilitated activation and proliferation of T cells expressing VLA-4 and VLA-5 [28-32] contributed to the increased gene transfer into human T cells. Since transduction on fibronectin did not require centrifugation of cells, was reproducible and almost as efficient as cocultivation, the availibility of recombinant human fibronectin fragments will facilitate its use for clinical application in gene therapy protocols.

For many years, the standard approach of measuring gene transfer efficiency in hematopoietic cells has been the determination of the number of cells that had been transduced with vector-encoded genes conferring cellular resistance to drugs such as neomycin, hygromycin, or methotrexate [21,65]. However, this method is limited by prolonged *in vitro* selection and non-specific toxicity of the selection drugs to primary cells. Other methods to determine the number of transduced cells include PCR or *in vitro, ex vivo,* or *in situ* staining with substrates for the bacterial ß-galactosidase (ßgal), the human placental alkaline phosphatase (AP), or green fluorescent protein (GFP)[66,67]. An alternative strategy has relied on the expression of transgene encoded cell surface antigens such as human CD24 [68], its murine homologue heat-stable antigen [HSA][69,70], murine CD2 [71], mutated murine prion protein [mPrP][72], human CD4z [73], and the multidrug resistance gene *mdr-1* [74-76].

The more recently described intracytoplasmatically truncated version of the LNGFR (ΔLNGFR)[20,27,77,78] offers several advantages. Because of its human origin and the intracytoplasmatic truncation, it should neither be immunogenic nor mediate signal transduction. Our results show that quantitative determination of the transduction efficiency of T cells by FACS is fast (within 48 hours)[3,20,37,79]. Furthermore, vectors containing the ΔLNGFR cDNA could be used for the rapid determination of viral titers. This might be of special benefit for vectors containing no other selectable marker gene. Titering of the vector particles was fast and correlated well with the conventional titer assay.

For the clinical application of „suicidegene" modified lymphocytes in allogeneic bone marrow transplantation an absolute prerequisite is that all transfused lymphocytes carry and express the transgene. For this purpose, an enrichment step is necessary after transduction. Most protocols have relied on growth of transduced cells in selection medium containing the aminoglycoside analogue G418. In the present study, we could show that non-transduced T cells were susceptible to G418 at all used concentrations, but eliminated with different kinetics. Previously, it has been shown that although viable nontransduced cells persisted after 1 week of G418 (300 and 600 µg/ml) selection, these cells were not capable of subsequently responding to Il-2 [24]. Selection of transduced cell in G418 resulted in a highly enriched population expressing ΔLNGFR (> 80%) after two weeks. Previously, it has been shown that one week of selection at G418 concentrations greater than 500 µg/ml always resulted in cells inhibited by GCV [24]. Clinical studies have demonstrated that *ex vivo* retroviral-mediated into ADA-deficient PHA-Il-2 stimulated lymphocytes can not only reconstitute enzyme function but also allow the development *in vivo* of a functional immune repertoire with the reconstitution of specific immune functions such as proliferative response to alloantigens, tetanus toxoid, and viral antigens [18]. Other studies with neo<sup>R</sup>-transduced tumor-infiltrating lymphocytes (TIL) have suggested that the transduced populations were representative of the total TIL population in terms of the T-cell receptor repertoire as well as mRNA cytokine pattern [80] and that the phenotype and cytotoxicity profile of the gene-transduced TIL was similar to those of naive TIL [25]. These various studies therefore suggest that, after *ex vivo* gene transfer and culture in G418 and Il-2, transduced human T lymphocytes will maintain *in vivo* specific immune functions such as alloreactivity and GvL effects [81].

Another strategy to enrich transduced cells relies on the ectopic expression of cell surface markers wich permits selection of transduced cells using flow cytometry [68,69]. Evidence that selection of transduced cells leads to an almost pure population of cells expressing the transgene after transplantation has been published [3,68]. Using FACS sorting, we were able to enrich ΔLNGFR expressing cells to a purity of greater than 91 % within a few hours.

In a recently published clinical study on the utility of gene-modified donor lymphocyte transfusions, it has been demonstrated that there was no linear correlation between the number of infused transduced lymphocytes and persitence of detection. Rather, the intensity of antigen response and proliferation of transfuesd cells seemed to affect the levels of detection [3]. Furthermore, *in vivo* data in humans suggest that expression in lymphocytes of the ADA gene under the control of the LTR is durable (> 6 months)[15]. When examining ΔLNGFR expression in primary T-lymphocytes, we found no loss of expression up to 38 days after transduction without selective pressure. The recent finding that proviral gene regulation is downmodulated in the absence of T-cell signaling events has important implications for clinical strategies using retrovirus-modified T cells [82]. It can be envisioned that reinfused „suicide-gene" modified T cells causing severe GvHD after allogeneic bone marrow transplantation

upregulate transgene expression upon stimulation. This will contribute to the selectivity of the approach since GvHD-causing T cells will show increased HSV-tk gene expression and thus GCV sensitivity. Furthermore, stimulation and subsequent proliferation of transduced T cells has been shown to be crucial for the cell replication-dependent activity of HSV-tk [83].

In summary, the use of the ΔLNGFR vector system described in this report allowed the development of an fibronectin-based efficient and clinically applicable procedure for transducing primary human T cells. Because of the the low background, the vector system permitted the accurate quantification of gene transfer efficiency and the enrichment of transduced cells through FACS sorting.

# References

1. Kolb HJ, Schattenberg A, Goldman JM, et al: Graft-versus-leukemia effect of donor lymphocyte transfusions in marrow grafted patients. European Group for Blood and Marrow Transplantation Working Party Chronic Leukemia [see comments]. Blood 86:2041, 1995
2. Mackinnon S, Papadopoulos EB, Carabasi MH, Reich L, Collins NH, O'Reilly RJ: Adoptive immunotherapy using donor leukocytes following bone marrow transplantation for chronic myeloid leukemia: is T cell dose important in determining biological response? Bone Marrow Transplant 15:591, 1995
3. Bonini C, Ferrari G, Verzeletti S, et al: HSV-TK gene transfer into donor lymphocytes for control of allogeneic graft-versus-leukemia. Science 276:1719, 1997
4. Cohen J, Boyer O, Salomon B, et al: Prevention of graft-versus-host-disease in mice using a suicide gene expressed in T lymphocytes. Blood 89:4645, 1997
5. Link CJ, Jr., Burt RK, Traynor AE, et al: Adoptive immunotherapy for leukemia: donor lymphocytes transduced with the herpes simplex thymidine kinase gene for remission induction. HGTRI 0103. Hum Gene Ther 9:115, 1998
6. Siegel J, Sharon M, Smith P: The Il-2 receptor chain (p70) role in mediating signals for LAK, NK, and proliferative activities. Science 238:75, 1987
7. Ranga U, Woffendin C, Verma S, et al: Enhanced T cell engraftment after retroviral delivery of an antiviral gene in HIV-infected individuals. Proc Natl Acad Sci U S A 95:1201, 1998
8. Caruso M, Bank A: Efficient retroviral gene transfer of a Tat-regulated herpes simplex virus thymidine kinase gene for HIV gene therapy. Virus Res 52:133, 1997
9. Manca F, Fenoglio D, Franchin E, et al: Anti-HIV genetic treatment of antigen-specific human CD4 lymphocytes for adoptive immunotherapy of

opportunistic infections in AIDS. Gene Ther 4:1216, 1997

10. Miller AD: Human gene therapy comes of age. Nature 357:455, 1992

11. Anderson WF: Human gene therapy. Science 256:808, 1992

12. Gilboa E, Eglitis M, Kantoff P, Anderson WF: Transfer and expression of cloned genes using retroviral vectors. Biotechniques 7:1986

13. Karlsson S: Treatment of genetic defects in hematopoietic cell function by gene transfer. Blood 78:1991

14. Blaese R, Culver K, Anderson F, et al: Treatment of severe combined immunodeficiency disease (SCID) due to adenosine deaminase deficiency with autologous lymphocytes transduced with a human ADA gene. Hum Gene Ther 4:521, 1993

15. Blaese RM, Culver KW, Miller AD, et al: T lymphocyte-directed gene therapy for ADA- SCID: initial trial results after 4 years. Science 270:475, 1995

16. Blaese RM: Development of gene therapy for immunodeficiency: adenosine deaminase deficiency. [Review] [27 refs]. Pediatr Res 33:S49, 1993

17. Bordignon C, Notarangelo L, Nobili N, et al: Gene therapy in peripheral blood lymphocytes and bone marrow for ADA- immunodeficient patients. Science 270:470, 1995

18. Ferrari G, Rossini S, Nobili N, et al: Transfer of the ADA gene into human ADA-deficient T lymphocytes reconstitutes specific immune functions. Blood 80:1120, 1992

19. Gervaix A, Li X, Kraus G, Wong-Staal F: Multigene antiviral vectors inhibit diverse human immunodeficiency virus type 1 clades. J Virol 71:3048, 1997

20. Mavilio F, Ferrari G, Rossini S, et al: Peripheral blood lymphocytes as target cells of retroviral vector-mediated gene transfer. Blood 83:1988, 1994

21. Bayever E: Gene transfer into hematopoietic cells. Blood 75:1587, 1990

22. Munshi N, Govindarajan R, Drake R, et al: Thymidine kinase (TK) gene-transduced human lymphocytes can be highly purified, remain functional, and are killed efficiently with ganciclovir. Blood 89:1334, 1997

23. Braun SE, Pan D, Aronovich EL, Jonsson JJ, McIvor RS, Whitley CB: Preclinical studies of lymphocyte gene therapy for mild Hunter syndrome (mucopolysaccharidosis type II). Hum Gene Ther 7:283, 1996

24. Tiberghien P, Reynolds CW, Keller J, et al: Ganciclovir treatment of herpes simplex thymidine kinase-transduced primary T lymphocytes: an approach for specific in vivo donor T-cell depletion after bone marrow transplantation? Blood 84:1333, 1994

25. Culver K, Cornetta K, Morgan R, et al: Lymphocytes as cellular vehicles for gene therapy in mouse and man. Proc Natl Acad Sci U S A 88:3155, 1991

26. Bunnell BA, Muul LM, Donahue RE, Blaese RM, Morgan RA: High-efficiency retroviral-mediated gene transfer into human and nonhuman primate peripheral blood lymphocytes. Proc Natl Acad Sci U S A 92:7739, 1995

27. Rudoll T, Phillips K, Lee SW, et al: High-efficiency retroviral vector mediated gene transfer into human peripheral blood CD4+ T lymphocytes. Gene Ther 3:695, 1996

28. Yabkowitz R, Dixit V, Guo N, Roberts D, Shimizu Y: Activated T cell adhesion to thrombopondin is mediated by the alpha 4 beta 1 (VLA-4) and alpha 5 beta 1 (VLA-5) integrins. J Immunol 151:149, 1993

29. Pallis M, Robins A, Powell RA: Peripheral blood lymphocyte binding to a soluble FITC-fibronectin conjugate. Cytometry 28:157, 1997

30. Wayner E, Garcia-Pardo A, Humphries M, McDonald J, Carter W: Identification and characterization of the T lymphocyte adhesion receptor for an alternative cell attachment domain (CS-1) in plasma fibronectin. J Cell Biol 109:1321, 1989

31. Takada Y, Huang C, Hemler M: Fibronectin receptor structures within the VLA family of heterodimers. Nature 326:607, 1987

32. Matsuyama T, Yamada A, Kay J, et al: Activation of CD4 cells by fibronectin and anti-CD3 antibody. J Exp Med 170:1133, 1989abstract

33. Hanenberg H, Xiao L, Diloo D, Hashino K, Kato I, Williams D: Colocalization of retrovirus and target cells on specific fibronectin fragments increases genetic transduction of mammalian cells. Nat Med 2:876, 1996

34. Markowitz D, Goff S, Bank A: A safe packaging line for gene transfer: separating viral genes on two different plasmids. J Virol 62:1120, 1988

35. Markowitz D, Goff S, Bank A: Construction and use of a safe and efficient amphotropic packaging cell line. Virology 167:400, 1988

36. Miller AD, Rosman GJ: Improved retroviral vectors for gene transfer and expression. Biotechniques 7:980, 1998

37. Fehse B, Uhde A, Fehse N, et al: Selective immunoaffinity-based enrichment of CD34+ cells transduced with retroviral vectors containing an intracytoplasmatically truncated version of the human low-affinity nerve growth factor receptor gene. Hum Gene Ther 8:1815, 1997

38. Comoli P, Diloo D, Hutchings M, Hofmann T, Heslop H: Measuring gene-transfer efficiency. Nat Med 2:1280, 1996

39. Gallardo HF, Tan C, Ory D, Sadelain M: Recombinant retroviruses pseudotyped with the vesicular stomatitis virus G glycoprotein mediate both stable gene transfer and pseudotransduction in human peripheral blood lymphocytes. Blood 90:952, 1997

40. Garbrecht F, Russo C, Weksler M: Long-term growth of human T cell lines and clones on anti-CD3 antibody-treated tissue culture plates. J Immunol Methods 107:137, 1988

41. Ueda M, Joshi I, Dan M: Preclinical studies for adoptive immunotherapy in bone marrow transplantation. Generation of anti-CD3 activated cytotoxic T cells from normal donors and autologous bone marrow transplant candidates. Transplantation 56:351, 1993

42. Masucci G, Svensson A, Hansson M, et al: Efficient harvest of in vivo Il-2 activated CD3+ lymphocytes for adoptive immunotherapy by selective leukapheresis (lymphocytapheresis). J Hematother 6:253, 1997

43. Morecki S, Gelfand Y, Levi S, et al: Activated long-term peripheral blood cultures as preparation for adoptive alloreactive cell therapy in cancer patients. J Hematotherapy 6:115, 1997

44. Vella AT, Dow S, Potter TA, Kappler J, Marrack P: Cytokine-induced survival of activated T cells in vitro and in vivo. Proc Natl Acad Sci U S A 95:3810, 1998

45. Contassot E, Murphy W, Angonin R, et al: In vivo alloreactive potential of ex vivo-expanded primary T lymphocytes. Transplantation 65:1365, 1998

46. Pollok KE, Hanenberg H, Noblitt TW, et al: High-efficiency gene transfer into normal and adenosine deaminase-deficient T lymphocytes is mediated by transduction on recombinant fibronectin fragments. J Virol 72:4882, 1998

47. Levine BL, Bernstein WB, Connors M, et al: Effects of CD28 costimulation on long-term proliferation of CD4+ T cells in the absence of exogenous feeder cells. J Immunol 159:5921, 1997

48. Bunnell BA, Metzger M, Byrne E, Morgan RA, Donahue RE: Efficient in vivo marking of primary CD4+ T lymphocytes in nonhuman primates using a gibbon ape leukemia virus-derived retroviral vector. Blood 89:1987, 1997

49. Onodera M, Ariga T, Kawamura N, et al: Successful peripheral T-lymphocyte-directed gene transfer for a patient with severe combined immune deficiency caused by adenosine deaminase deficiency. Blood 91:30, 1998

50. Altenschmidt U, Klundt E, Groner B: Adoptive transfer of in vitro-targeted, activated T lymphocytes results in total tumor regression. J Immunol 159:5509, 1997

51. Miller D: Construction ans properties of retrovirus packaging cells based on gibbon ape leukemia virus. J Virol 65:2220, 1991abstract

52. Onodera M, Nelson DM, Yachie A, et al: Development of improved adenosine deaminase retroviral vectors. J Virol 72:1769, 1998

53. Matsuoka H, Miyake K, Shimada T: Improved methods of HIV vector mediated gene transfer. Int J Hematol 67:267, 1998

54. Springett GM, Moen RC, Anderson S, Blaese RM, Anderson WF: Infection efficiency of T lymphocytes with amphotropic retroviral vectors is cell cycle dependent. J Virol 63:3865, 1989

55. de Fourgerolles A, Qin X, Springer T: Characterization of the function of intracellular adhesion molecule (ICAM)-3 and comparison with ICAM-1 and ICAM-2 in immune responses. J Exp Med 179:619, 1994

56. Bachmann M, McKall-Faienza K, Schmits R, et al: Distinct roles for LFA-1 and CD28 during activation of naive T cells: adhesion versus costimulation. Immunity 7:549, 1997

57. Pierschbacher M, Hayman E, Ruoslathi E: Location of the cell-attachment site in fibronectin with monoclonal antibodies and proteolytic fragments of the molecule. Cell 26:259, 1981

58. Humphries M, Akiyama S, Komoriya A, Olden K, Yamada K: Identification of an alternatively spliced site in human plasma fibronectin that mediates cell type-specific adhesion. J Cell Biol 103:2637, 1986

59. Fehse B, Schade U, Li Z, et al: Highly-efficient gene transfer with retroviral vectors into human T lymphocytes on fibronectin. Br J Haematol 102:566, 1998

60. Shimizu Y, van Seventer G, Horgan K, Shaws S: Costimulation of proliferative responses of resting CD4+ T cells by the interaction of VLA-4 and VLA-5 with fibronectin or VLA-6 with laminin. J Immunol 145:59, 1990

61. Davis L, Oppenheimer-Marks N, Bednarczyk J, McIntyre B, Lipsky P: Fibronectin promotes proliferation of naive and memory T cells by signalling through both the VLA-4 and VLA-5 integrin molecules. J Immunol 145:785, 1990

62. Finkelstein LD, Reynolds PJ, Hunt SW, Shimizu Y: Structural requirements for beta1 integrin-mediated tyrosine phosphorylation in human T cells. J Immunol 159:5355, 1997

63. Salomon D, Mojcik C, Chang A, et al: Constitutive activation of integrin alpha4beta1 defines a unique stage of human thymocyte development. J Exp Med 179:1573, 1994

64. Moritz T, Dutt P, Xiao X, et al: Fibronectin improves transduction of reconstituting hematopoietic stem cells by retroviral vectors: evidence of direct viral binding to chymotryptic carboxy-terminal fragments. Blood 88:855, 1996

65. Bayever E, Haines K, Duprey S, Rappaport E, Douglas SD, Surrey S: Protection of uninfected human bone marrow cells in long-term culture from G418 toxicity after retroviral-mediated transfer of the NEOr gene. Exp Cell Res 179:168, 1988

66. Persons DA, Allay JA, Allay ER, et al: Retroviral-mediated transfer of the green fluorescent protein gene into murine hematopoietic cells facilitates scoring and selection of transduced progenitors in vitro and identification of genetically modified cells in vivo. Blood 90:1777, 1997

67. Ramiro A, de Yebenes V, Trigueros C, Carrasco Y, Toribio M: Enhanced green fluorescent protein as an efficient reporter gene for retroviral transduction of human multipotent lymphoid precursors. Hum Gene Ther 9:1103, 1998

68. Pawliuk R, Kay R, Lansdorp P, Humphries RK: Selection of retrovirally transduced hematopoietic cells using CD24 as a marker of gene transfer. Blood 84:2868, 1994

69. Conneally E, Bardy P, Eaves CJ, et al: Rapid and efficient selection of human hematopoietic cells expressing murine heat-stable antigen as an indicator of retroviral-mediated gene transfer. Blood 87:456, 1996

70. Medin JA, Migita M, Pawliuk R, et al: A bicistronic therapeutic retroviral vector enables sorting of transduced CD34+ cells and corrects the enzyme deficiency in cells from Gaucher patients. Blood 87:1754, 1996

71. Champseix C, Marechal V, Khazaal I, et al: A cell surface marker gene transferred with a retroviral vector into CD34+ cord blood cells is expressed by their T-cell progeny in the SCID-hu thymus. Blood 88:107, 1996

72. Tumas DB, Spangrude GJ, Brooks DM, Williams CD, Chesebro B: High-frequency cell surface expression of a foreign protein in murine hemato-

poietic stem cells using a new retroviral vector. Blood 87:509, 1996

73. Tran A, Zhang D, Byrn R, Roberts M: Chimeric zeta-receptors directed human natural killer effector function to permit killing of NK-resistant tumor cells and HIV-infected T lymphocytes. J Immunol 159:1000, 1995

74. Choi K, Frommel TO, Stern RK, et al: Multidrug resistance after retroviral transfer of the human MDR1 gene correlates with P-glycoprotein density in the plasma membrane and is not affected by cytotoxic selection. Proc Natl Acad Sci U S A 88:7386, 1991

75. Ward M, Richardson C, Pioli P, et al: Transfer and expression of the human multiple drug resistance gene in human CD34+ cells. Blood 84:1408, 1994

76. Richardson C, Bank A: Preselection of transduced murine hematopoietic stem cell populations leads to increased long-term stability and expression of the human multiple drug resistance gene. Blood 86:2579, 1995

77. Machl AW, Planitzer SA, Kubbies M: 1-NGFR receptor is a new flow cytometric tool for rapid cell cycle-correlated gene therapy complementation studies in viable cells. Cytometry 29:371, 1997

78. Gallardo HF, Tan C, Sadelain M: The internal ribosomal entry site of the encephalomyocarditis virus enables reliable coexpression of two transgenes in human primary T lymphocytes. Gene Ther 4:1115, 1997

79. Phillips K, Gentry T, McCowage G, Gilboa E, Smith C: Cell-surface markers for assessing gene transfer into human haematopoietic cells. Nat Med 2:1154, 1996

80. Fukayama M, Kanno T, Brody SL, Kirby M, Crystal RG: Respiratory tract gene transfer. Transplantation of genetically modified T-lymphocytes directly to the respiratory epithelial surface. J Biol Chem 266:18339, 1991

81. Contassot E, Ferrand C, Certoux JM, et al: Retrovirus-mediated transfer of the herpes simplex type I thymidine kinase gene in alloreactive T lymphocytes. Hum Gene Ther 9:73, 1998

82. Quinn E, Lum L, Trevor K: T cell activation modulates retrovirus-mediated gene expression. Hum Gene Ther 9:1457, 1998

83. Cheng Y, Huang E, Lin J et al.: Unique spectrum of activity of 9[(1,3-dihydroxy-2-propoxy)methy]-guanine against herpesviruses in vitro and its mode of action against herpes simplex virus type 1. Proc Natl Acad Sci USA 80:2767, 1983

**Recent Strategies Against
Opportunistic Infections**

# Early Empiric Antifungal Treatment of Infections in Neutropenic Patients with Hematological Malignancies Comparing Fluconazole with Amphotericin B and 5-Flucytosine

G. Silling, W. Fegeler, N. Roos, M. Essink and T. Büchner

## Introduction

Intensification of chemotherapy in patients with hematological malignancies has improved prognosis with regard to the underlying disease. Despite advances in supportive care and antibiotic therapy, prolonged periods of neutropenia constitute the most important risk factor for opportunistic infections, especially for those of fungal origin [1–4]. Granulocyte counts of less than $0,1 \times 10^9$ /l and duration of more than one week predispose about 85% of the patients to infectious complications [5,6]. Because of the high mortality, empiric strategies have been introduced [7–11]. Results of the first German multicenter study of the Paul-Ehrlich-Society [7], showed that infections during the early phase of neutropenia were predominantly caused by gram-positive pathogens. In contrast the longer the neutropenic period the higher was the incidence of fungal infections. This correlated with the result, that after nonresponse to the first line empiric antibiotic therapy the response rate improved more by adding amphotericin B than by change of the antibiotic regimen. In addition, especially patients suffering from pneumonia – half of those caused by fungi – had a worse outcome. So it appears reasonable to not only apply empiric antibiotic therapy but also empiric antifungal treatment at an early stage. So we conducted a prospective randomized study to compare the toxicity and efficacy of fluconazole and amphotericinB/5-flucytosine in neutropenic patients and stratified patients according to fever of unknown origin (FUO) or documented or highly suspected fungal infection.

## Patients and treatment regimen

Patients qualified for this study if prolonged neutropenia that means about more than one week had to be expected. They were included when first fever of > 38.5°C occured and neutrophils were <1000/µl. In case of fever of unknown origin and nonresponse to a combination of antibiotics, a beta-lactam and an aminoglycoside, for at least 72 hours, the antibiotic treatment was changed and the antifungal regimen – fluconazole (FCA) or amphotericin B/5-flucytosine (ABF) was randomly assigned (Fig. 1). If patients had pulmonary infiltrates or other evidence of fungal infection they received their antifungal regimen upfront with the antibiotic combination. After one week of antifungal treatment there was a second evaluation. If patients did not respond to FCA a crossover was planned and under the suspicion of resistant fungi, for example candida krusei, resistant candida glabrata or aspergillus they received ABF. In case of nonresponse to ABF physicans were freee to choose any other agent or to continue ABF bescause a better alternative agent was lacking. In order to take no risk change of the antifungal regimen was allowed earlier if signs of progressive infection occured.

## Dose

Amphotericin B was administered at a dose of 0.5. mg/kg (0.1 + 0.4) on day 1 and 0.75 mg/kg/day (max 50 mg) on days 2–7; after day 7 it was given every other day except for those patients who had evidence of aspergillosis. These patients received a daily dose of 1.0 mg/kg. 5-FC was administered at a daily dose 150 mg/kg/day devided into 4 equal doses on days 1–14 and was adjusted when

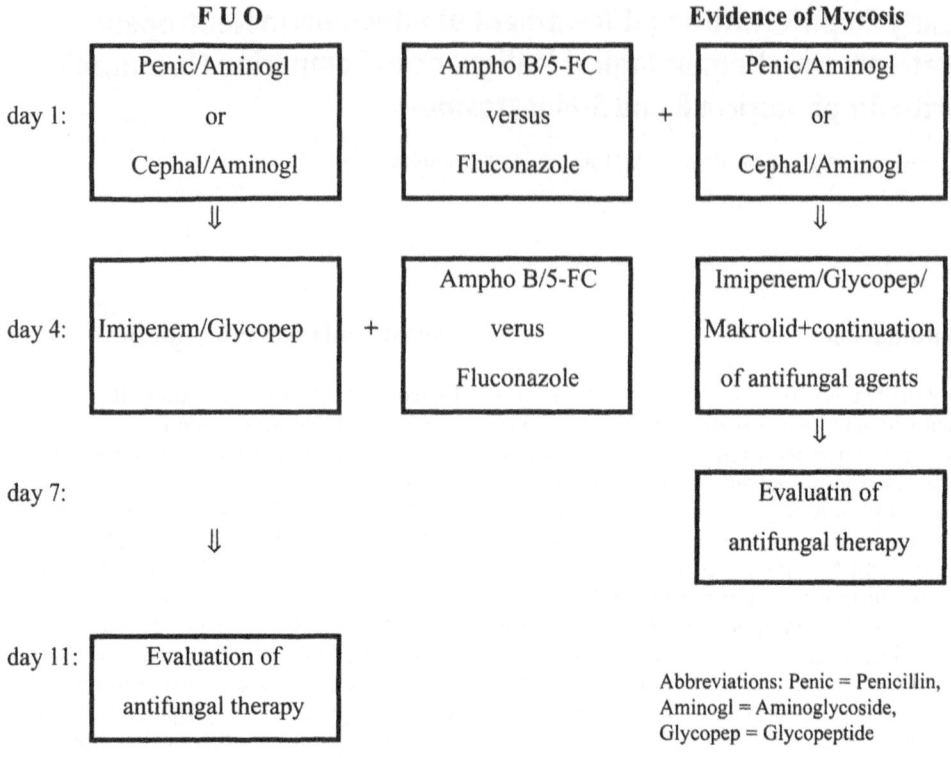

|  | **F U O** | | **Evidence of Mycosis** |
|---|---|---|---|

day 1:

| Penic/Aminogl or Cephal/Aminogl | | Ampho B/5-FC versus Fluconazole | + | Penic/Aminogl or Cephal/Aminogl |

⇓ ⇓

day 4:

| Imipenem/Glycopep | + | Ampho B/5-FC verus Fluconazole | | Imipenem/Glycopep/ Makrolid+continuation of antifungal agents |

⇓

day 7:
⇓

Evaluatin of
antifungal therapy

day 11:

Evaluation of
antifungal therapy

Abbreviations: Penic = Penicillin,
Aminogl = Aminoglycoside,
Glycopep = Glycopeptide

**Fig. 1.** Treatment regimen

creatinine level rose. By administering the parenteral form of 5-FC patients got a high concentration of sodium – about 6–8 grams per day dependant on their dose. So we applied no additional sodium load to prevent or mitigate nephrotoxicity.

Concomitant use of paracetamol, pethidine or corticosteroids were allowed, but it was recommended to avoid steroids.

On day 1 patients received a loading dose of 11.4 mg/kg (max 800 mg) of fluconazole and 5.7 mg/kg/day (max 400 mg) on the following days.

## Results

Of the 98 randomized patients, 47 received ABF and 51 FCA. All randomized patients were evaluated. The study population consisted of 57 males and 41 females, aged 16 to 76 years (mean: 46.1 years). 51 patients were treated with FCA (26 males, 25 females), and

47 were treated with ABF (31 males and 16 females). The demographic data and risk factors were well balanced in both groups (Table 1). More than 80% of the patients suffered from acute leukemia, and 24/74 patients with acute myeloid leukemia as 5/9 with acute lymphoid leukemia suffered from resistant or relapsed leukemia. One of the two patients with myelodysplastic syndromes had refractory anemia with excess of blasts and the other one had transformation to acute leukemia. Additionally 6/8 patients with non-Hodgkin's lymphoma had high grade lymphoma and all of these as the two patients with Hodgkin's lymphoma had relapsed or chemoresistant disease. Since these patients had a worse prognosis intensified regimens of chemotherapy associated with prolonged periods of neutropenia were used. Consequently this was a population of very high risk patients. Again, there was homogeneity with regard to the distribution of de novo, relapsed and refractory diseases.

**Table 1.** Patients' Characteristics

|  | Fluconazole | Ampho B + 5-FC |
|---|---|---|
| *n =* | 51 | 47 |
| *gender* | | |
| male | 26 (51%) | 31 (66%) |
| female | 25 (49%) | 16 (34%) |
| *age* | | |
|  | 47,8 | 44,2 |
|  | (16–76 years) | (17–70 years) |
| *underlying disease* | | |
| ALL | 4 | 5 |
| de novo | 2 | 2 |
| relapse | 2 | 3 |
| AML | 40 | 34 |
| de novo | 25 | 25 |
| relapse/resistent | 15 | 9 |
| MDS | 1 | 1 |
| NHL | 5 | 3 |
| HD (relapse) | 1 | 1 |
| CLL | 0 | 2 |
| CML blast crisis | 0 | 1 |

Abbreviations: All = acute lymphoblastic leukemia, AML = acute myeloid leukemia, MDS = myelo-dysplastic syndrome, NHL = non-Hodgkin's lymphoma, HD = Hodgkin's disease, CLL = chronic lymphocytic leukemia, CML = chronic myeloid leukemia

## Fever

Fever often is the only symptom of infection in neutropenic patients and in this study it was the reason for inclusion and therefore the best criterion to evaluate response. Defervescence occured in 28/51 FCA and 37/47 ABF patients. Another 16/22 FCA responded after switching to ABF. So the overall response was 44/51 in the FCA arm and 37/47 in the ABF arm (Table 2). Die difference in response rates was statistically not signifikant by use of the one-sided Farrington-Manning test.

Response after 7 days of antifungal treatmant – the timepoint of first evaluation – was achieved in 23 FCA and in 26 ABF

**Table 2.** Response of Fever

|  | FCA | ABF | |
|---|---|---|---|
| n = 98 | 51 | 47 | |
| defervescence | 28 (55%) | 37 (79%) | p< 0,05 |
| after change to ABF | 16 | | |
| overall response | 44 (86%) | 37 (79%) | n.s. |
| within 7 days | 23 (45%) | 26 (55%) | n.s. |
| while neutropenic | 22 (43%) | 29 (62%) | n.s. |

patients. So the difference in response of fever between both treatment regimens can be accounted for the fact that ABF patients were maintained on their assigned treatment longer than FCA patients.

Twenty-two FCA and 29 ABF patients responded when they were still neutropenic. This shows that defervescence was not mainly a consequence of neutrophil recovery. So on the basis of an intention-to-treat-analysis, both antifungal treatment regimens seem to be equally effective in neutropenic patients.

Overall, defervescence was achieved in 81 patients. Time to response was 5.7 days (median: 4) in the FCA and 6.9 days (median: 6) in the ABF group, and was thus similar in both groups for patients who did not switch to a different treatment arm (65 patients). In those who did not respond within 7 days and consequently received ABF afterwards, time to defervescence was 15.6 days (median: 11). One may speculate whether this is due to initial waisting of time by using not the optimal agents, or the illness was more severe and needed longer to improve.

As we changed the antibiotic regimen for FUO patients and added the antifungal agents one may argue that the response was due to the change of the antibiotic regimen and ask whether it is necessary to add the antifungals already on day 4. The concept of early antifungal therapy was confirmed by the data of the PEG II Study [12]. Here patients not responding to the initial antibiotic therapy were randomized to receive a glycopeptide and a carbapeneme alone, with fluconazole or with amphotericin B and 5-flucytosine and received response rates of 55.6%, 62.5% and 77.8% respectively. The results showed a significant difference in favour of an antifungal treatment despite having any evidence of mycosis whereas the difference between adding FCA or ABF did not reach statistical significance.

These results are very similar to internationally reported data, regardless of whether patients were neutropenic or nonneutropenic, suffered from proven or suspected candidiasis, or were treated as part of an empiric strategy (Table 3), e.g. Anaissie [13] included patients undergoing bone marrow transplantation as well as patients suffering from acute leukemia, solid tumors or other diseases who were treated because of proven or suspected candidiasis. Despite the heterogeneity response rates to FCA and AB were similar, 64% and 66% respectively, as were response rates at 48 hours or 5 days or median time to response, 5 days in each group.

Rex [14] reported about nonneutropenic suffering from candidemia and with the highest response rates 70% for FCA and 79% for AB patients, whereas Kujath [15] treated surgical patients with systemic mycosis and reaches response rates of 60% and 70% respectively

**Table 3.** Studies comparing fluconazole and amphotericin B + 5-flucytosine

| Author | Indication | FCA | AB ± FC |
|--------|-----------|-----|---------|
| Anaissie '96 | Candidiasis | 64 % | 66 % |
| Kujath '93 | System. Mycosis | 60 % | 70 % |
| Rex '94 | Candidemia | 70 % | 79 % |
| Viscoli '96 | Empiric Therapy | 75 % | 66 % |
| Malik '98 | Empiric Therapy | 56 % | 46 % |
| Silling (in press) | Empiric Therapy | 55 % | 79 % |

Studies with an empirical design were published by Viscoli (16) and Malik (17). Nearly half of the neutropenic patient population studied by Viscoli had undergone bone marrow transplantation and/or suffered from acute leukemia. Consequently the median age was low, 27 for FCA and 24 years for AB treated patients. As response rates showed a non signifikant preponde-rance for FCA (75% vs 66%) this was a consequence of a higher rate of discontinuation of AB therapy due to a higher rate of life threatening toxicity.

Malik [17] found lower response rates (56% FCA and 46% AB) and a high incidence of pneumonia in 32 of 100 patients associated with low response rates of 19 % not differentiated with regard to the antifungal treatment. In addition he found a high associated mortality (25% FCA and 31% AB). In contrast to this results Abele-Horn [18] examined patients of an intensive care unit, where one third of the patients developed pneumonia, either, but response rates to candida pneumonia were 73% for FCA and 67% for ABF. So neutropenia or a higher rate of aspergillosis may be responsible for the worse outcome of the empirically treated patients of Malik [17].

## Pneumonia

As already shown by Maschmeyer [7] or Malik [17] patients of our study had a high incidence of pneumonia either, 21/51 in the FCA arm and 25/47 in the ABF arm. Resolution of infiltrates was seen in 20/25 ABF and only 5/21 FCA patients. Again we have to consider that infiltrates often requires longer treatment than one week and we do not know how many patients would have responded, if FCA had been continued. On the other hand 5 patients had radiological signs of aspergillosis as perivascular necrosis, peripheral triangular pulmonary infarctions, halo or air crescent sign in the high-resolution computed tomography. Because of the resistance pattern of fluconazole to aspergillosis all five profited from amphotericin B therapy. On the whole 10 of 15 initially not responding patients showed regression of pulmonary infiltrates when switched to ABF, especially all patients with evidence of aspergillosis.

## Mycosis

Results are presented according to proven and highly suspected fungal infection. Since proven fungal infections were defined by autopsy or biopsy it was difficult to establish a diagnosis in thrombocytopenic patients, because of the high risk of bleeding associated with taking biopsies. So the diagnosis of proven fungal infection could only be confirmed at autopsy in all but one patient. Proven mycosis occured in 4 FCA and 2 ABF patients. Consequently the antimicrobial regimen had failed in all but one. This patient had proven aspergillosis and respnded after switching to ABF.

Fungal infections were regarded as highly suspected, if they showed typical radiological signs of aspergillosis in the high-resolution computed tomography as described above. Seven FCA and 9 ABF patients had highly suspected mycosis, 4 and 5 respectively had evidence of aspergillosis. None of these patients responded to FCA, however, response was achieved after they switched to ABF; so no one died because of delayed adequate treatment. 4/5 of the ABF patients responded as well. Of note, the incidence of aspergillosis

| | FCA Response | | | ABF Response | |
|---|---|---|---|---|---|
| | | FCA | Crossover | | |
| Proven mycosis | 4 | 0 | 1 | 2 | 0 |
| Candida | 2 | 0 | 0 | 1 | 0 |
| Aspergillus | 2 | 0 | 1 | 1 | 0 |
| Suspected mycosis | 7 | 1 | 5 | 9 | 7 |
| Candida | 3 | 1 | 1 | 4 | 3 |
| Aspergillus | 4 | 0 | 4 | 5 | 4 |

**Table 4.** Response of Fungal Infections

did not increase in the FCA group. On the whole 8 of 9 patients with highly suspected aspergillosis responded, so a high response rate could be achieved and may be due to the early antifungal intervention.

In order to get informations about the spectrum of candida species we also looked at surveillance cultures. It is important ro recognize a shift in favour of candida glabrata, regarding the whole number of isolates as well as a preponderance in the FCA group though it did not reach statistical significance. This cannot be explained by former use of fluconazole as fluconazole was not used in our institution for prophylaxis of neutropenic patients. The occurence of candida krusei was not favoured by the use of fluconazole in our group as only three were isolated, two in the FCA and one in the ABF group.

## Outcome

In this high risk group of severely immuno-compromised patients, death occurred in 18 patients, with three patients dying of cerebral hemorrhage or infarction, the other deaths were due to infection (7 FCA and 8 ABF). Of the deaths due to infection, 4 patients in each group died of fungal infection. Aspergillosis was found in 1 FCA and 2 ABF patients. On the whole, there was no significant difference regarding the incidence and cause of the infections leading to death, except for the non-infectious causes all of which occurred in the ABF arm. However, the number is too small to draw further conclusions.

## Side effects

All adverse events were recorded, regardless of their causative relationship to the study drugs. Side effects with an at least suspected relationship to the antifungal drugs were seen in 19.6 % of FCA and 97.6 % of ABF patients. Patients did not get any premedication before receiving the antifungals the first time, but when they developed fever or chills after the infusion of amphotericin B they got a premedication consisting of paracetamol, antihistamines and if necessary pethidine. Corticosteroids were avoided. Symptoms were less severe using a premedication but did not disappear in most patients. None of them suffered from severe side effects leading to death, discontinuation or change of the antifungal agents. In addition two third of the adverse events were classified als mild in FCA patients, whereas ABF patients graded them as mild 36%, moderate 32% or even severe 30%. So they suffered not only more frequently but also from more severe side effects.

## Conclusion

In conclusion, fluconazole and amphotericin B seem to be equally effective in the empiric treatment of fever of unknown origin in neutropenic patients suffering from hematological malignancies. In view of its lower toxicity, fluconazole may be preferable as first line and early empiric antifungal agent, but an empirical treatment should not instill a false sense of security. Diagnostic procedures – especially early detection of aspergillosis by high-resolution computed tomography – have to be done precisely and close-meshed, as fluconazole is not effective in aspergillosis but it does not favour the occurence of aspergillosis. In case of nonresponse, pneumonia or aspergillosis, it may be replaced by amphotericin B and 5-flucytosine.

## References

1. Armstrong D, Young LS, Meyer RD, Blevins AH (1971): Infectious complications of neoplastic disease. Med Clin North AM 55: 729–745

2. Degregorio MW, Lee WMF, Linker CA, et al (1982): Fungal infections in patients with acute leukemia. Am J Med 73: 543–548
3. Robertson MF, Larson RA (1988): Recurrent fungal pneumonias in patients with acute nonlymphocytic leukemia undergoing multiple courses of intensive chemotherapy. Am J Med 84: 233–239
4. Mirsky HS, Cuttner J (1972): Fungal infections in acute leukemia. Cancer 50: 348–352
5. Bodey GP (1986): Infection in cancer patients – a continuing association. Am J Med 81: 11–26
6. Brown AE (1984): Neutropenia, fever, and infection. Am J Med 76; 421–428
7. Maschmeyer G, Link H, Hiddemann W, et al (1994): Empirische antimikro- bielle Therapie bei neutropenischen Patienten, Ergebnisse einer multizentrischen Studie der Arbeitsgruppe Infektionen in der Haematologie der Paul-Ehrlich-Gesellschaft. Med Klin 89 (3): 114–123
8. EORTC International Antimicrobial Therapy Cooperative Group (1989): Empirical antifungal therapy in febrile granulocytopenic patients. Am J Med 86: 668–672
9. Pizzo PA, Robichaud KJ, Gil FA, et al (1982): Empiric antibiotic and antifungal therapy for cancer patients with prolonged fever and granulocytopenia. Am J Med 72: 101–111
10. Sugar AM (1990): Empiric treatment of fungal infections in the neutropenic host. Arch Intern Med 150: 2258–2264
11. Bodey GP (1986): Fungal infections and fever of unknown origin in neutropenic patients. Am J Med 80 (suppl 5C): 112–119
12. Cornely OA, Hiddemann W, Link H, et al. For the Study Grouup of the PEG (1997): Interventioneal antimicrobial therapy in febrile neutropenic patients – Paul-Ehrlich-Society for chemotherapy (PEG) Study II. Ann Hematol 74 (Suppl I): A 51, Abstract 204
13. Anaissie EJ, Darouiche R, Abi-Said D, et al (1996): Management of invasive candidal infections: Results of a prospective, randomized, multicenter study of fluco-nazole versus amphotericin B and review of the literature. Clin Infect Dis 23: 964–972
14. Rex JH, Pfaller MA, Galgiani JN, et al (1997): Development of interpretive breakpoints for antifungal susceptibility testing: Conceptual framework and analysis of in vitro – in vivo correlation data for fluconazole, itraconazole, and candida infections. Clin Infect Dis 24: 235–247
15. Kujath P, Lerch K, Kochendörfer P, Boos C (1993): Comparative study of the efficacy of fluconazole versus amphotericin B/5-flucytosine in surgical patients with systemic mycosis. Infection 21 (6): 376–381
16. Viscoli C, Castagnola E, Vant Lint MT, et al (1996): Fluconazole versus amphotericin B as empirical antifungal therapy of unexplained fever in granulocytopenic cancer patients: a pragmatic, multicentre, prospective and randomised clinical trial. Eur J Cancer 32A (5): 814–820
17. Malik IA, Moid I, Aziz Z, Khan S, Suleman M (1998): A randomized comparison of fluconazole with amphotericin B as ermpiric anti-fungal agents in cancer patients with prolonged fever and neutropenia. Am J Med (105): 479- 483
18. Abele-Horn M, Kopp A, Sternberg U, et al (1996): A randomized study comparing fluconazole with amphotericin B/5-flucytosine for the treatment of systemic candida infections in intensive care patients. Infection 24 (6): 426–432

# The Role of Newer Quinolones in the Management of Infections in Patients with Hematologic Malignancies

K. V. I. ROLSTON

## Introduction

Patients with hematologic malignancies are at substantial risk for developing infections particularly during episodes of profound and persistent neutropenia [1]. Strategies for the management of such patients include:
- infection prevention (prophylaxis)
- empiric therapy of febrile neutropenia
- therapy of specific infections

The newer quinolones play an important role in all of these strategies and are an important component of the therapeutic armamentarium available to clinicians who take care of patients with hematologic malignancies [2]. Most of these strategies are utilized in hospitalized patients. In recent years, risk predic-tion rules have enabled clinicians to reliably identify a ìlow-riskî subset among febrile neutropenic patients. Alternative treatment strategies such as oral, out-patient, antibiotic therapy are being evaluated. The newer quinolones form the backbone of such strategies as well, since they are the only antimicrobial agents with an adequate spectrum, that are available for oral administration. These agents are also useful for the therapy of specific infections caused by common (enteric gram-negative bacilli) or uncommon (mycobacteria, *Legionella* etc.) organisms that are susceptible to them. Newer indications including meningitis, and pediatric usage are also being evaluated, and are summarized in Table 1.

**Table 1.** Indications for Use of Fluoroquinolones in Patients with Hematological Malignancies

| Indication | Comment |
| --- | --- |
| Prophylaxis in high-risk neutropenic patients | Reduction in febrile episodes and gram-negative infections. Can lead to emergence of resistance |
| Empiric therapy in febrile neutropenic patients | Second-line therapy. Mono-therapy not recommended. Use limited to patients not receiving quinolone chemoprophylaxis |
| Step-down or out-patient therapy in "low-risk" neutropenic patients | Appropriate selection of patients, antimicrobial regimen, and close monitoring required. Still subject of investigation |
| Treatment of specific infections | Legionellosis-considered to be agents of choice. Mycobacterial infections – useful against multi-drug resistant isolates and MOTT.* Salmonellosis – including carrier state/suppressive therapy. Newer agents with expanded gram-positive activity and potency useful for treatment of susceptible isolates (eg PNSP)Ü |
| Newer indications (still investigational) | Pediatric usage. Meningitis |

\* MOTT – mycobacteria other than tuberculosis
Ü PNSP – penicillin non-susceptible pneumococci

From the Section of Infectious Diseases, Department of Internal Medical Specialties, The University of Texas M. D. Anderson Cancer Center, 1515 Holcombe Blvd., Houston, Texas 77030

## Infection Prevention

Enteric gram-negative bacilli, particularly *Escherichia coli, Klebsiella* spp., and *Pseudomonas aeruginosa*, are common pathogens in patients with hematologic malignancies [3]. Most of these infections arise from the patients endogenous microflora and are particularly common during episodes of neutropenia. Since infections caused by gram-negative bacilli are associated with considerable morbidity and mortality, one approach in the overall management of patients with hematologic malignancies is to administer antimicrobial chemoprophylaxis during high-risk periods [4]. The effect of the quinolones on the endogenous microflora of humans has been extensively studied. The quinolones exhibit a selective suppressive effect. The aerobic, gram-negative component is most strongly suppressed by agents like ciprofloxacin, ofloxacin, norfloxacin etc. The aerobic gram-positive component of the intestinal microflora is less influenced, and the anaerobic component even less so. Newer fluorquinolones with anaerobic activity (clinafloxacin, trovafloxacin, moxifloxacin) are likely to cause substantial suppression of the anaerobic flora. Administration of quinolones for chemoprophylaxis results in a 4–7 log/g of faeces reduction in the colony counts of enteric gram-negative bacilli within 3–5 days of administration, and upon discontinuation of therapy, a return to baseline values occurs within 7–14 days.

A large number of studies conducted in high-risk, patients with hematologic malignancies have demonstrated that quinolone prophylaxis results in a significant decrease in the frequency of febrile episodes in neutropenic patients, and also in a significant reduction in documented gram-negative infections [5]. There is minimal impact, or occasionally an increase in gram-positive infections, particularly those due to streptococci. However, the overall mortality is not reduced. Combining quinolones with penicillin, rifampin, a macrolide, or vancomycin (a practice which is not recommended) does significantly reduce the development of gram-positive infections as well [6]. Newer, broad-spectrum quinolones might achieve similar results when used as single agents, but clinical data are lacking.

In general chemoprophylaxis with the fluoroquinolones is well tolerated. In particular, myelosuppression does appear to be a concern.

The development of resistant gram-negative bacilli (*E. coli, P. aeruginosa* etc.), is of concern, and has led to some controversy regarding their use as prophylactic agents [7,8]. Current recommendations suggest that quinolone prophylaxis should not be used routinely, but should be limited to high-risk patients who are likely to experience profound neutropenia for more than 10–14 days [9]. In this situation, the benefit of reducing potentially lethal gram-negative infections might justify chemoprophylaxis, despite the risk of the emergence of resistant isolates.

## Empiric Therapy of Febrile Neutropenia

The standard management of patients with hematologic malignancies who develop neutropenic fever is to administer parenteral, broad-spectrum, empiric, antimicrobial therapy in the hospital, to facilitate close observation of the patient [10]. This is usually achieved by using combination regimens, or selected, broad-spectrum drugs as single-agents (monotherapy) Table 2. The role of the fluoroquinolones for empiric therapy has been limited owing to their widespread use as prophylactic agents. However, susceptibility surveillance studies among gram-negative bacilli isolated from cancer patients continue to demonstrate the potent in-vitro activity of these agents, and increasing, but still relatively low levels of fluoroquinolone resistance despite extensive clinical use [11]. Several studies have examined the therapeutic role of the quinolones (particularly ciprofloxacin – which still retains the best gram-negative activity among this class) as empiric therapy in febrile neutropenic patients. With gram-positive organisms now accounting for 50–75 percent of documented bacterial infections and many of these organisms being resistant or only moderately susceptible to agents like ciprofloxacin, ofloxacin, and levofloxacin, quinolone monotherapy using these agents cannot be recommended. Monotherapy might be feasible using newer generation quinolones (trovafloxacin, gatifloxacin, moxiflo-

**Table 2.** Antimicrobial Regimens for Empiric Therapy in Febrile Neutropenic Patients

| Regimens(s) | Examples in Common use |
| --- | --- |
| Combinations | |
| Aminoglycoside + beta-lactam or quinolone | Amikacin + ceftazidime or cefepime |
| | Amikacin + piperacillin – tazobactam or ticarcillin – clavulanate |
| | Amikacin + imipenem or meropenem |
| | Amikacin + ciprofloxacin |
| Vancomycin + beta-lactam or quinolone | Vancomycin + ceftazidime or cefepime |
| | Vancomycin + aztreonam |
| | Vancomycin + piperacillin-tazobactam or ticarcillin – clavulanate |
| | Vancomycin + imipenem or meropenem |
| | Vancomycin + ciprofloxacin |
| Quinolone + beta-lactam (or other agent) | Ciprofloxacin + piperacillin – tazobactam or amoxicillin – clavulanate |
| | Ciprofloxacin + clindamycin |
| Monotherapy | |
| Extended spectrum agents | Ceftazidime, cefepime, imipenem, meropenem |

xicin etc.) which have a broader antimicrobial spectrum, including substantially enhanced activity against gram-positive organisms. Clinical evaluation of these agents, in this setting, is clearly warranted.

Quinolone based combination regimens have been shown to be as effective as other standard regimens, in small, single institution, clinical trials. However, their equivalence to standard regimens has not yet been demonstrated in a large, sufficiently powered, multicenter trial. They should therefore be considered as second-line regimens in febrile neutropenic patients, and local quinolone susceptibility patterns should be taken into consideration at individual institutions. Their use should also be limited to patients who have not received quinolone chemoprophylaxis.

## Alternative Treatment Strategies/Settings

It has long been recognized that the risk for developing infections, complications, and response to therapy differs substantially in different subsets of febrile neutropenic patients. In the past decade or so, with the development of risk-prediction rules and clinical criteria, it has become possible to identify ìlow-riskî febrile neutropenic patients early enough in the course of a febrile episode to consider alternative treatment strategies or settings. These include the following:

- Oral antibiotic therapy in hospitalized patients
- Hospital based parenteral therapy followed by oral therapy upon discharge (sequential or switch therapy)
- Parenteral, sequential, or oral out-patient antibiotic therapy

The development of the newer quinolones, most of which are available for parenteral and oral administration, has been largely responsible for the success of many of these treatment options. Two recently published trials have demonstrated what several smaller previously published trials initially suggested – that oral antibiotics (ciprofloxacin + amoxicillin/clavulanate) are as safe and effective as parenterally administered agents in hospitalized low-risk patients [12,13]. Several other trials have demonstrated that febrile neutropenic patients can initially be stabilized on parenteral antibiotic therapy administered in a closely monitored hospital setting – followed by early discharge on quinolone-based oral regimens once stabilization has been achieved. Several small, single-institutional studies have also demonstrated the safety and efficacy of empiric parenteral or oral antibiotic regimens administered to low-risk patients (both pediatric and adult patients) without the need for hospitalization [14–16]. Key elements for the success of these strategies are:
- selection of appropriate patients

- selection of appropriate antimicrobial regimens
- adequate monitoring to ensure safety
- possession of a team/infrastructure to handle logistic and/or medical problems expeditiously

Although these alternative treatment strategies/settings have not become part of the mainstream of medical practice as yet, increasing numbers of patients are receiving such therapies, and several organizations including the Infectious Diseases Society of America (IDSA), and the National Comprehensive Cancer Network (NCCN) have incorporated these strategies into their guidelines for the management of febrile neutropenic patients [9,17].

## Treatment of Specific Infections

The fluoroquinolones are active against a number of "atypical" or uncommon microorganisms that cause opportunistic infections in immunosuppressed patients, including those with hematologic malignancies. These include Legionella spp., mycobacteria, and various organism that cause gastrointestinal infections. The quinolones are playing an increasingly important role in the treatment of such infections.

## Legionellosis

As a class, the fluoroquinolones possess potent in vitro activity against Legionella pneumophila and other Legionella spp. In the opinion of several leading authorities, the quinolones have now replaced the macrolides as the agents of choice for the treatment of infections caused by Legionella spp. [18]. Although no prospective, controlled human trials for the treatment of Legionellosis exist, ciprofloxacin, ofloxacin, and pefloxacin have all been used successfully for this indication. Parenteral and/or oral therapy with these agents has been reported to be effective in several patients with documented Legionellosis, including patients with severe immunosuppression. Combination therapy appears to offer no advantages over monotherapy using

potent quinolones. Occasional failures have been reported, mostly in patients receiving inadequate doses. Parenteral therapy is preferable in patients who are severely immunosuppressed or severely ill. A switch to oral therapy can be made when such patients are clinically stable and/or are able to tolerate oral therapy. Additionally, the quinolones are the preferred agents for the treatment of Legionella spp. infections in patients receiving immunosuppressive therapy with cyclosporine or tacrolimus because unlike the macrolides and rifampin, they do not alter the metabolism of cyclosporine or tacrolimus.

In summary, the therapy of legionellosis has changed substantially with the quinolones having replaced the macrolides as agents of choice, even though these recommendations are based on accumulated clinical experience, and not on controlled clinical trials.

## Mycobacterial Infections

The quinolones possess in-vitro activity against Mycobacterium tuberculosis and many non-tuberculous mycobacteria including M. avium-complex, M. kansasii, M. fortiutum , and M. leprae. Ofloxacin and ciprofloxacin are not considered first-line antituberculous drugs and are not included in standard therapeutic regimens for the treatment of tuberculosis. However, these agents (and other quinolones) are proving to be extremely useful in the treatment of tuberculosis caused by multi-drug resistant strains [19].

Disseminated infection caused by M. avium-complex is not only common in HIV-infected individuals, but also in patients with hairy-cell leukemia, and other hematological malignancies. Although the ideal therapy for M. avium-complex infection has not yet been developed, the quinolones are considered important components of combination regimens that are used to treat such infections. The development of newer quinolones that have greater in-vitro activity and more favorable pharmacokinetics than currently available agents will undoubtably lead to further investigation into their role in the treatment of M. avium-complex infections.

M. fortuitum and other mycobacterial infections have been successfully treated with quinolone containing regimens. Prolonged therapy using two or three agents with activity against these isolates is recommended because monotherapy is likely to lead to the development of resistance.

## Other Infections/Indications

The quinolones are very active against enteric bacteria including *Salmonella* spp., *Shigella* spp., and *Aeromonas* spp. and are now considered to be agents of choice for the treatment of such infections including the chronic carrier state for Salmonella. They are also very effective for the treatment and/or prophylaxis of travelers diarrhea. Although these infections are uncommon in patients with hematologic malignancies, they can progress rapidly or disseminate when they do occur, and the prompt administration of effective agents can be critical. Additionally, global travel has become increasingly popular and common, even in patients with malignant disorders and the need for providing such patients with agents such as the quinolones while they travel, has become quite pressing.

Gram-positive bacterial infections are far more common than gram-negative bacterial infections in patients with hematologic malignancies [20]. Many of these organisms are resistant or have reduced susceptibility to commonly used therapeutic agents including (occasionally) the glycopeptides. The newer, extended-spectrum quinolones (trovafloxacin, gatifloxacin, moxifloxacin, clinafloxacin) are active against many such organisms including *Corynebacterium jeikeium*, *Listeria monocytogenes*, viridans-streptococci, *Leuconostoc* spp., *Pediococcus* spp., *Lactobacillus* spp., and *Rhodococcus* spp. These agents are also active against penicillin-susceptible, and penicillin-nonsusceptible *Streptococcus pneumoniae*, and are likely to prove useful in the treatment and/or prevention of these infections. The newer quinolones also have good CSF penetration and are being evaluated for newer indications such as meningitis. Accumulated clinical experience with currently available quinolones (ciprofloxacin, ofloxacin, levofloxacin) clearly indicates that these agents are safe to use in the pediatric age group and are not toxic to growing bone and cartilage, as had initially been feared. These agents will soon be approved for pediatric usage, further expanding their clinical utility.

## Summary

The fluoroquinolones play an important and ever increasing role in the overall management of patients with hematologic malignancies. As we approach a new millennium, newer quinolones, with expanded gram-positive, gram-negative, and even anaerobic activity are being developed and evaluated. Many of these newer aspects also have a more favorable pharmacokinetic profile, making oral, once-a-day administration feasible. This ìuser-friendlyî nature of quinolone therapy, and the large number of indications for which they can be used, make it very tempting (and very likely) to overuse them, or to use them inappropriately, thereby encouraging the development of resistance. It is up to us as health care providers, to use these agents responsibly in order to derive maximal therapeutic benefit, both for current and future generations of patients.

## References

1. Rolston KVI, Bodey GP: Infections in patients with cancer. In: Holland JF, Frei E III, Bast RC Jr., Kufe DW, Morton DL, Weichselbaum RR (eds.): Cancer Medicine – 4th Edition. Philadelphia, Pa: Lea and Febiger, 1996, pp 3303–3333.
2. Rolston KVI: Use of the quinolones in immunocompromised patients. In: Andriole VT (ed). The Quinolones, Second Edition. San Diego, Academic Press, 1998, pp 303–326.
3. Rolston KVI, Tarrand JJ. (1999) *Pseudomonas aeruginosa* – Still a frequent pathogen in patients with cancer: 11-year experience from a comprehensive cancer center. Clin Infect Dis 29:463–464.
4. Pizzo Pa. (1989) Considerations for the prevention of infectious complications in patients with cancer. Rev Infect Dis 11(suppl 7):S1551–63.
5. Cruciani M, Rampazzo R, Malena M, et al. (1996) Prophylaxis with fluoroquinolones for bacterial infections in neutropenic patients: a meta-analysis. Clin Infect Dis 23:795–805.
6. Bow E J, Mandell LA, Louie TJ, et al. (1996) Quinolone-based antibacterial chemoprophylaxis in neutropenic patients: effect of augmented gram-positive activity on infectious morbidity. Annals 125:183–190.
7. Kern WV, Androf E, Oethinger M, et al. (1994). Emergence of fluoroquinolone-resistant Escherichia coli at a cancer center. Antimicrob. Agents Chemother. 38, 681–687.

8. Rolston KVI: (1998) Commentary: Chemoprophylaxis and bacterial resistance in neutropenic patients. Infect Dis Clin Pract 7:202–204.
9. Hughes WT, Armstrong D, Bodey GP, et al. (1997) 1997 Guidelines for the use of antimicrobial agents in neutropenic patients with unexplained fever. Clin Infect Dis 25:551–573.
10. Pizzo PA. (1993). Management of fever in patients with cancer and treatment. Induced neutropenia. N. Engl. J. Med. 328:1323–1332.
11. Jacobson K, Rolston K, Elting L, et al. (1999) Susceptibility surveillance among gram-negative bacilli at a cancer center. Chemotherapy 45:325–334.
12. Kern WV, Cometta A, DeBock R, et al. (1999) Oral versus intravenous empirical antimicrobial therapy for fever in patients with granulocytopenia who are receiving cancer chemotherapy. N Engl J Med 341:312–318.
13. Freifeld A, Marchigiani D, Walsh T, et al. (1999) A double-blind comparison of empirical oral and intravenous antibiotic therapy for low-risk febrile patients with neutropenia during cancer chemotherapy. N Engl J Med 341:205–311.
14. Malik IA, Khan WA, Karim M, et al. (1995) Feasibility of outpatient management of fever in cancer patients with low-risk neutropenia: results of a prospective randomized trial. Am J Med 98:224–231.
15. Rubenstein EB, Rolston K, Benjamin RS, et al. (1993) Outpatient treatment of febrile episodes in low-risk neutropenic patients with cancer. Cancer 71: 3640–3646.
16. Rolston K, Rubenstein EB, Elting L, et al. Ambulatory management of febrile episodes in low-risk neutropenic patients. (Abstract 2235) 35th Interscience Conference on Antimicrobial Agents and Chemotherapy. San Francisco, California. September 17–20, 1995.
17. National Comprehensive Cancer Network. (NCCN Leukopenic Sepsis Guidelines Panel Members). (1999) NCCN Practice Guidelines for Fever and Neutropenia. NCCN Proceedings, Oncology 13:197–257
18. Edelstein P. (1998) Antimicrobial chemotherapy for Legionnaires Disease: Time for a change. Ann Intern Med 128:328–330.
19. Iseman, M.D. (1993) Drug therapy: Treatment of multidrug resistant tuberculosis. N Engl J Med 329: 784–791.
20. Koll BS and Brown A E (1993) The changing epidemiology of infections at cancer hospitals. Clin Infect Dis 17: (Suppl. 2):S322–S328.

# Fungal Infections in Paediatric Haematology

I. M. Hann

## Introduction

At long last we are entering a new era wherein we have an array of antifungal agents and the potential for new diagnostic tests in the management of immunocompromised children. The problem with the former is that the therapy has always been relatively unsuccessful and toxic. Diagnostic laboratory tests have been neither specific nor sensitive but new methodology such as PCR looks promising [9] but may still not deal with the often symbiotic or "innocent bystander" aspect of colonisation by the organisms. In the current state of knowledge the mainstays of management are a high level of clinical vigilance (e.g. looking for hepatosplenomegaly as a sign of disseminated candidosis) and radiological scans looking for instance for pulmonary aspergillus and splenic candidiasis.

The problem of diagnosis has led to the use of early empirical therapy for persistently neutropenic patients who do not respond to intravenous broad spectrum antibiotics. In many situations where the patients are at high risk of fungal infection, this approach is just a few days short of prophylactic therapy.

## Prophylaxis

Even the newest of agents are unsuccessful in curing advanced fungal mass lesions such as cerebral or sino/pulmonary aspergillus infections. It is possible that accurate and early diagnosis will obviate the need for prophylaxis, or that new combinations of therapy (e.g.

speculatively liposomal amphotericin and an echinocandin) will cure most or all patients with established fungal infections. At present, it would thus seem most logical to prevent systemic fungal infection and we now have a variety of agents, some of which have been in clinical trials for nearly 20 years e.g. itraconazole and others of which are still at an early stage of development. Two crucial aspects of such therapies in children is that they should be very well tolerated and that they should preferably be orally absorbed. Thus the intravenous formulation of some of the echinocandins is one major drawback and the up to one fifth non-compliance with the newer formulations of itraconazole is another [1, 5]. Itraconazole is also associated with more gastroinestinal disturbances than fluconazole [5].

At the present time, the evidence that itraconazole prevents aspergillus infection more effectively than fluconazole or placebo is not convincing [1, 3, 5, 7] one study [3] actually demonstrating a higher rate of infection with itraconazole prophylaxis that with placebo [3]. Other studies have shown the oppositive but no trial to date has had enough endpoints to be able to elucidate the matter. In future, all trials of prophylaxis must comply with the following.

1. Use the approved guidelines for investigation and definition of fungal infection [4].
2. Target high risk patients e.g. those with acute myeloid leukaemia (AML), mismatched or unrelated bone marrow transplant (BMT) and aplastic anaemia not responding to immunosuppressive therapy.
3. Enter enough patients such that proven systemic fungal infection can be effectively

Paediatric Haematologist, Haematology Department Level 2, Camelia Botnar Laboratories, Great Ormond Street Hospital for Children NHS Trust, London WCIN 3JH

analysed between arms (this will usually mean several hundred patients in each arm at a minimum).

At this point in time, there is some evidence that fluconazole can improve survival after BMT [7] and that both fluconazole and itraconazole can reduce oropharyngeal and probably systemic candidiasis. We do not as yet know whether the current evidence of emergent strains (e.g. Candida Krusei) will increase as a problem and thus there is even more reason to continue clinical trials, and to target prophylaxis at the high risk groups already mentioned. On the balance of evidence and despite its restricted spectrum of activity, fluconazole is the gold standard against which others should be tested. Larger trials are required versus itraconazole, maybe voriconazole, echinocandins and one other innovative approach which is prophylactic intravenous liposomal amphotericin which has a very long half-life in the tissues and could perhaps be examined at a dose of 10 mg/kg once a week. Preliminary reduced-dosage studies with liposomal amphotericin [8] have used doses of 1 mg/kg/day [8] or 2 mg/kg/day three times a week, with significant reduction in fungal colonisation and possible benefits in reducing proven fungal infection.

It must never be forgotten that strict antisepsis when dealing with indwelling catheters is essential in reducing the risk of deep fungal infection, and that high efficiency particulate air filters reduce the risk of infection with organisms like aspergillus in high risk patients. Other preventive measures such as avoidance of high spore counts from building works, peppers and spices, composts heaps and some herbal preparations can also be of value.

## Empirical Therapy

In the early 1990's we were provided with various alternatives to straight forward amphotericin B deoxycholate (ampho B). Intravenous or oral (as appropriate) fluconazole has proven to be very well tolerated and useful if a sensitive candida albicans is proven to be the causative organism, but not as an empiric agent. A number of anecdotal studies with the lipid-associated amphotericin agents (liposomal ambisome, abelcet and amphotericin colloidal dispersion ABCD) were carried out (e.g. [2, 11]) and appeared to show that and of them had less nephroxicity than ampho-B and that some ampho-B failures with deep-seated fungal infections responded; a group that previously had had an extremely poor prognosis. What none of these studies and none of the in vitro or animal data showed was, what was the least toxic agent, which were the more efficacious and for what fungi and what location. We now know that ambisome is the safest agent in randomised studies, but we have very limited data on efficacy.

The first large randomised study in adults and children was an open-label comparison of ampho-B at 1 mg/kg/day compared with ambisome at 1 mg/kg/day and at 3 mg/kg/day [6]. The problem of nephrotoxicity was significantly reduced with the use of ambisome and a more successful outcome for pyrexia of unknown origin with the liposomal product. In addition, we showed that the mean dose of ampho-B which can be delivered is approximately 0,7 mg/kg/day and that more than a third of patients miss days of therapy because of toxicity and that there is a greatly reduced need for premedication with steroids and other drugs for infusion-related reactions. In fact, ambisome can be readilly used on a day case ore home care basis in children with very few problems due to reactions or hypokalaemia.

The next and largest study so far [10] demonstrated the ambisome at 3 mg/kg/day was as effective as ampho-B for empirical antifungal therapy in patients with fever and neutropenia and was associated with fewer breakthrough proven systemic fungal infections, being further evidence that the liposomal product at this dosage is more effective than the achievable doses of ampho-B. They also confirmed that severe infusion related reactions including those associated with hypotension were less common with ambisome and that hypokalaemia and nephrotoxicity was commoner with ampho-B. The use of premedications was necessary in almost all ampho-B patients and can be avoided with the liposomal preparation. This is particularly relevant when we consider the bizarre situation whereby a high proportion of patients receiving ampho-B and the non-liposomal lipid products need the very drugs (steroids) which impair response to fungi.

Sadly there is a paucity of comparative information with regard to the lipid-associated products and we await what will hopefully be very large trials with proven infection end-points from the newer azoles and other agents. The only other randomised trial which was large enough to have any chance of analysing meaningful end-points, i.e. severe toxicity, compared ambisome at 3 mg/kg/day and 5 mg/kg/day with abelect at 5 mg/kg/day in a double-blind trial. Ambisome was proven, at both dosages, to have less nephrotoxicity, fewer discontinuations due to toxicity, fewer infusion-related reactions and reduced need to prevent and treat infusion-related reactions than with abelect. Of interest was the 42% incidence of doubling of creatinine with abelect compared with 14% with ambisome and the need for 35% of patients on abelect to receive steroids in order to be able to use this drug, compared with 15% on ambisome. Hypoxia occurred in 11.5% of patients receiving abelect on day 1, compared with 1.2% with the higher dose of ambisome and zero at the lower ambisome dose. Severe adverse events occurred twice as commonly with abelect and a third of abelect patients had the drug discontinued due to toxicity, compared with only 10–11% on ambisome. Thus, there is no doubt that ambisome is the safest known amphotericin preparation which may be suitable for prophylaxis. However, we need more studies with regard to efficacy, the only convincing available data being that ambisome 3 mg/kg/day prevents emergent proven systemic infection when used empirically.

We are approaching a new and exciting era in antifungal therapy whereby clinicians may be able to diagnose infections at an early and treatable stage and whereby agents are available which are less toxic and may be usable in combination. We must learn from the errors of the past and solve the problem through large co-operative randomised trials with valid and important end-points.

# References

1. Huijgens PC, Simoons-Smit AM, van Loenen AC et al. Fluconazole versus itraconazole for the prevention of fungal infections in haemato-oncology. J Clin Path
2. Leenders ACAP, Daenen S, Jansen RLH et al. (1993) Liposomal amphotericin B compared with amphotericin B deoxycholate in the treatment of documented and suspected neutropenia-associated invasive fungal infections. Br J Haem 98: 711
3. Menichetti F, del Favero A, Martino P et al. (1999) Itraconazole oral solution as prophylaxis for fungal infections in neutropenic patients with haematological malignancies: A randomised placebo-controlled double-blind multicentre trial. Clin Infect Dis 28: 250–255
4. Denning DW, Evans EGV, Kibbler CC et al. (1997) Guidelines for the investigation of invasive fungal infection in haematological malignancy and solid organ transplantation. Europ J Clin Microbiol & Inf Dis 16: 424–434+
5. Morgenstern GR, Prentice AG, Prentice HG et al. (1999) A randomised controlled trial of itraconazole versus fluconazole for the prevention of fungal infections in patients with haemtological malignancies. Br J Haem 105: 901–911
6. Prentice HG, Hann IM, Herbrecht R et al. (1997) A randomised comparison of liposomal versus conventional amphotericin B for the treatment of pyrexia of unknown origin in neutropenic patients. Br J Haem 98: 711
7. Slavin MA, Osborne B, Adams R (1995) Efficacy and safety of fluconazole prophylaxis for fungal infections after marrow transplantation – a prospective randomised, double-blind study. J Inf Dis 171: 1545–1552
8. Tollemar J, Ringden O, Andersson S (1993) Randomised double-blind study of liposomal amphotericin prophylaxis of invasive fungal infection in bone marrow transplant recipients. Bone Marrow Transp 12: 577–582
9. Verwey PE, Donnelly JP, De Pa WBE, Meis JFGM (1996) Prospects for the early diagnosis of invasive aspergillosis in the immunocompromised patient. Rev Med Microbiol 7: 105–113
10. Walsh TJ, Finberg RW, Arndt C et al. (1999) Liposomal amphotericin B for empirical therapy in patients with persistent fever and neutropenia. N Engl J Med 34: 764–771
11. White MH, Kusne S, Wingard JR et al. (1997) Amphotericin B colloidal dispersion versus amphotericin B in the therapy of invasive aspergillosis. Clin Inf Dis 24: 635
12. Wingard JR, White MH, Anaissie EJ et al. (1999) A randomised double-blind comparative safety trial of ambisome and abelect in febrile neutropenic patients. 9th focus on fungal infections, San Diego

# Empirical Antimicrobial Therapy of FUO and Proved Infections in Neutropenic Patients

M. WILHELM[1], W. HIDDEMANN[2], G. MASCHMEYER[3], H. LINK[4], D. BUCHHEIDT[5], B. GLASS[6], O. CORNELY[7], M. HELMERKING[8], D. ADAM[8] and PEG Study Group

## Summary

Infections in neutropenic patients still represent a great challenge since they often lack other signs of infection except fever, and infection rapidly can become fatal if not treated appropriately. Empirical treatment of those patients has already been shown to be very effective with a high overall response rate (RR) of more than 90%. However, patients with pneumonia have a much lower RR and survival when treated with anti-microbial therapy. In addition, a significant proportion of patients, which do not respond to first or second line therapy have persistent fever for many days, which might result in worsening of the general condition and prolongation of chemotherapy treatment. Therefore improvement of sequential treatment strategies is necessary. The PEG study group initiated 3 studies (PEG I-III), in which efficacy of a three step interventional treatment strategy for high-risk neutropenic patients with fever of unknown origin (FUO) and documented infections was investigated. In the PEG II study 767 patients with FUO and <1000 neutrophils/µl following intensive chemotherapy for hematological diseases were included. Overall a high RR (>90%) could be achieved with a stepwise supplementation and modification of treatment. RR to first line therapy with piperacillin plus aminoglycoside or ceftazidim/cefotaxim plus aminoglycoside could not be improved in PEG II compared to the previous PEG I study (RR=65%). However, for non-responders additional antifungal therapy with amphotericin-B (RR=78%) or fluconazol (RR=63%) significantly (p=0,03) improved RR compared to antibacterial therapy alone (RR=56%, 78% vs. 56%, p=0,03); and the time until patients responded to an empirical treatment was shortened. In addition, it was demonstrated, that in comparison to PEG I, empirical amphotericin-B treatment should be additionally given in patients with lung infiltrates (RR=76% vs. 61%). Based on these results the PEG III study was recently initiated with the following objectives: Can the results of the first line therapy be improved by using piperacillin/tazobactam plus aminoglycosides and will the RR persist with monotherapy (carbapenem or cefepime). In addition, since the important role of antifungals in second line treatment was demonstrated: is therapy with amphotericin-B more effective compared to fluconazole?

## Introduction

Infections in neutropenic patients are still an important cause of treatment failure and represent a great challenge since patients often lack other signs of infection except fever [1, 2]. Therefore, it is essential to assume that every patient with fever more than 38,5 degrees Celsius and neutropenia below 1000 per µl is harboring an infection until proven otherwise [3].

Since infection can rapidly become fatal if not treated appropriately, empirical antimicrobial treatment is necessary before the causative microorganism has been identified [4]. Empirical treatment has already been shown to be very effective. In a study published in 1988 a very high overall survival rate of more than 90% in a neutropenic patient population has been described [5].These results in mind, one can ask whether there is still any improvement necessary or even possible. Other studies, however, have identified several risk factors as predictive of poor out-

Wuerzburg[1], Munich[2], Berlin[3], Kaiserslautern[4], Mannheim[5], Kiel[6], Cologne[7], PEG Study Center, Munich[8], Germany

come, resulting in a much lower response rate to antimicrobial therapy in contrast to the Rubin-study [1–3, 6, 7]. These are patients with persistent neutropenia, hematological diseases, active cancer, pneumonia and a low performance status. Patients with any of these high-risk conditions are more likely to have serious complications including death, than were patients without any risk factor [8]. These results emphasize the need of better therapeutic strategies for febrile neutropenia in patients with risk factors especially hematological diseases or documented infections such as pneumonia.

There are additional reasons to try to improve treatment results: Although finally cured from infection, patients not responding to empirical first-line therapy may have persistent fever for many days. This may have severe consequences for those patients: Worsening of general condition, increase of costs, prolongation of treatment interval, and reduction of dose intensity of the following chemotherapy, which may finally decrease treatment results. However, few data are reported on escalating antimicrobial therapy for patients not responding to first line treatment [9]. The study group of the German Paul Ehrlich Society (PEG) is one of the few investigating second- and third-line randomized treatment strategies [10, 11]. Results of the first study of the PEG study group (PEG I) underline the inferior prognosis of patients with pneumonia [11]. In this study patients with fever of unknown origin (FUO) had a response rate (RR) of over 90% compared to patients with pneumonia, whose RR was only 60% and the death rate over 20%. Although the cumulative RR of patients with FUO in this study was over 90% at the end of the study, nearly 20% of the FUO patients had persistent fever for more than 10 days.

This in mind the PEG Study group initiated a second study for patients with FUO and documented infections (PEG II). For this study it was again very important to investigate a sequential treatment strategy to improve not only the RR for first line empirical therapy but also for the non responders.

## Patients and Methods

### Patient eligibility

Patients over 18 years of age with high-grade hematological disorders were eligible for the protocol. Entry criteria were a granulocyte count < 1000/µl and fever ≥ 38.5 degrees Celsius not related to drugs or blood transfusion. Further exclusion criteria were parenteral or oral (except cotrimoxazol) antimicrobial drugs within 7 preceding days and severe impairment of renal or hepatic function as well as pregnancy and HIV infection.

### Study design

PEG I and II Studies were prospective randomized studies, consisting of three-step se-

| Phase I | | |
|---|---|---|
| A | | B |
| Piperacillin | | Ceftazidime or Cefotaxim |
| Aminoglycoside | | Aminoglycoside |
| No response, persistant fever: day 4 - 6 | | |
| Phase II | | |
| C | D | E |
| Imipenem | Imipenem | Imipenem |
| Glycopeptide | Glycopeptide | Glycopeptide |
| | Amphotericin-B/5-FC | Fluconazole |
| No response, persistant fever: day 9 - 11 | | |
| Phase III | | |
| F | | G |
| Piperacillin | | Ciprofloxacin/Ofloxacin |
| Ceftazidime/Cefotaxime | | Aminoglycoside |
| Aminoglycoside | | Amphotericin-B/5-FC |
| Amphotericin-B/5-FC | | |

Fig. 1. PEG II study design for patients with unexplained fever

325

quential antimicrobial treatment regimens, which were adapted to clinical features and previous treatment responses.

In Figure 1 the study design of the PEG II study for patients with FUO is shown. In phase I, patients were randomized between two antibacterial regimens. Non-responders or recurrent fever after 72 to 96 hours were again randomized between change of antibacterials or a combination with antifungal drugs (amphotericin-B or fluconazol). In phase III, all non responders were treated with amphotericin-B but different antibacterial drugs.

If a patient developed lung infiltrates during therapy for FUO, the same regimens will be followed, but randomized between supplementation with amphotericin-B alone or amphotericin-B plus 5-flucytosine (5-FC).

### Response criteria

In the case of FUO, response was defined as defervescence with no requirement for further antimicrobial treatment for at least 7 days after termination of therapy. In documented infections, resolution of the clinical sign and elimination of the causative pathogen was also required.

## Results

### Patients

767 patients were included (Table 1). All patients suffered from a hematological disease and nearly 70% from acute leukemia. Nearly 90% had a neutrophil count below 500/μl. These represented a high risk group according to the risk factors described before.

**Table 1.** Patients characteristics

| Patient entry: 767 patients | | |
|---|---|---|
| Median age: 46 years, range: 18–92 | | |
| – Acute myeloid leukemia: | 416 | (54,2 %) |
| – Acute lymphblastic leukemia: | 105 | (13,7 %) |
| – High grade lymphoma: | 150 | (19,6 %) |
| – Hodgkin`s disease: | 55 | (7,2 %) |
| – Other hematolog disorders: | 41 | (5,3 %) |
| – Neutropenia: | > 100/μl | (45,6 %) |
| | 100–500/μl | (41,3 %) |
| | 501–1000/μl | (5,7 %) |

### Response to first-line therapy

Table 2 shows treatment results of first line empirical therapy. There was no difference between both arms (piperacillin/aminoglycoside or ceftazidim/cefotaxim/aminoglycoside) with a response rate (RR) of 51% and a death rate of about 2% in both. The overall RR might look relatively low, however this analysis shows response according to the randomized therapy. If treatment was modified because of isolation of a causative bacteria or the occurrence of pneumonia, patients were listed in this analysis as non responders. If the patients with modified therapy were also counted among the responders, patients with FUO had a cummulative RR of 65%, patients with bacteriemia or pneumonia of 94% and 79%, respectively. In about 50% of patients with sepsis, treatment was modified according to the isolated species and all patients with pneumonia received additional amphotericin-B.

### Response to second line therapy

Table 3 shows RR of the non responders to first line therapy. Changing antibiotics to imi-

**Table 2.** Response to first-line therapy

| | N | Responder (%) | Non-responder (%) | Death (%) | Response with modification (%) |
|---|---|---|---|---|---|
| A: PEN/AMG | 373 | 51.5 | 46.4 | 2.1 | 63,8 |
| B: CEPH/AMG | 344 | 51.2 | 46.5 | 2.3 | 66.9 |
| Total | 717 | 51.3 | 46.4 | 2.2 | 65.3 |

**Table 3.** Response to second-line therapy

| | N | Responder (%) | Non-responder (%) | Death (%) | Response with modification (%) |
|---|---|---|---|---|---|
| C: IMI/GLP | 54 | 55.6 | 44.4 | 0 | 64,8 |
| D: IMI/GLP/AM-B | 45 | 77.8 | 20.0 | 2.2 | – |
| E: IMI/GLP/FLUC | 56 | 62.5 | 35.7 | 1.8 | 71.4 |
| | | **C vs. D: p = 0.033** | | **C vs. E: p = 0.561** | |

**Table 4.** Response of patients with lung infiltrates

| | N | Responder (%) | Non-responder (%) | Death (%) |
|---|---|---|---|---|
| A – C + Ampho-B/5-FC | 61 | 72.1 | 10 | 18 |
| A – C + Ampho-B | 25 | 88.0 | 0 | 12 |
| Total | 86 | 76.7 | 7 | 16.3 |

penem plus teicoplanin or vancomycin resulted in a RR of 56% of this patient group, the addition of anti-fungal drugs could increase RR further up to 78% in the amphotericin-B group and 63% for fluconazole treated patients. The difference between the antibacterials alone and additional amphotericin-B was statistically significant (p=0,033), the difference between antibacterials alone and additional fluconazole, not. The difference between amphotericin-B and fluconazol was not significant either.

## Response of patients with pneumonia

All patients, who developed pneumonia after randomization for FUO, received additional amphotericin-B and were randomized for addition of 5-FC or not. Overall RR for these patients was between 72% and 88%, respectively (Table 4). There was no statistically significant difference between amphotericin-B with or without addition of 5-FC.

## Overall response

Table 5 shows the overall response to therapy. At the end of the study nearly 100% of patients with FUO were cured with one or more phases of treatment. Although lower, patients with documented infections also had an improved RR compared to the previous PEG I study. However, patients with pneumonia still had the lowest RR (76%) and highest death rate of all patients.

**Table 5.** Overall response of a sequential antimicrobial therapy (PEG II study)

| | N | Responder (%) | Non-responder (%) | Death (%) | Response with modification (%) |
|---|---|---|---|---|---|
| FUO | 434 | 92.9 | 5.5 | 1.6 | 97.7 |
| Bact/Fungemia | 96 | 44.8 | 48.9 | 6.3 | 93.8 |
| Lung infiltrates | 90 | – | 73.3 | 16.7 | 75.6 |
| Other | 87 | 26.4 | 65.6 | 8.0 | 89.7 |
| Total | 707 | 66.1 | 27.4 | 5.0 | 93.4 |

## Discussion

At the end of PEG II study a high overall RR for all patient subpopulations could be achieved with the described sequential treatment strategy.

For first line treatment we found no difference between the two investigated antibacterial regimens. The RR of FUO patients at this stage of empirical therapy was 51% and could not be enhanced compared to our previous study (PEG I). However, these RRs are similar to the results of first line therapy reported by other groups [12–15].

After second line therapy, patients with FUO had a RR of 94%. Therefore, one aim of the study, to shorten the time period until patients respond to an empirical treatment, was successful. In the previous study (PEG I) nearly 20% of FUO patients were still febrile after second line therapy. Here, antifungal therapy was delayed until the third phase of empirical treatment. Therefore, one can suggest, that improvement in RR for FUO patients achieved in PEG II study, was due to early antifungal therapy in patients unresponsive to initial antibacterial drugs. That points to a causative role of fungi for a significant subpopulation of FUO patients as early as 3 or 4 days after onset of fever [16,17]. This assumption is strengthened by the significant lower RR of antibacterial drugs compared to supplementation of the same drugs with amphotericin-B (Table 3).

In the reported PEG II study also the RR of patients, who developed pneumonia, could be improved (76%, table 5). This seems a consequence of earlier usage of amphotericin-B in these patients. In PEG I study antifungal therapy was delayed until the third phase of empirical therapy resulting in a RR of only 63%. Although patient numbers are relatively low, there was no statistically significant difference between amphotericin-B with or without addition of 5-FC. Therefore, in the particular situation of development of lung infiltrates, prompt antifungal therapy in addition to an antibiotic regimen seems to improve results, however supplementation with 5-FC seems not to be necessary. This might be important since 5-FC is associated with severe hematological and gastrointestinal toxicity.

Based on these results the PEG study group recently initiated a new study (PEG III) with the following objectives:

1. Can the results of the first line therapy be improved by using piperacillin/tazobactam in combination with aminoglycosides and will the RR be the same with monotherapy (carbapenem or cefepime) [18]?
The piperacillin/tazobactam combination was chosen for first line empirical therapy since in vitro studies have shown that tazobactam expands the activity of piperacillin to include distinct ß-lactamase producing bacterial strains (i. e. S. aureus, H. influenzae, Enterobacteriae) [19]. In addition, in the study published by Cometta et al. the combination of piperacillin/tazobactam and amikacin was found to be significantly more active (61% RR) than the reference combination ceftazidim and amikacin (54% RR) [20–22].

2. Since in PEG II study the important role of antifungal drugs for non responders as second line treatment has already been demonstrated, in the next study it should be investigated, whether the use of amphotericin-B with its high incidence of infusion related complications and nephrotoxicity is necessary, or fluconazole with its smaller antifungal spectrum and lower toxicity is equivalent.

## References

1. Estey EH, Keating MJ, McCredie KB, Bodey GP, Freireich EJ (1982) Causes of initial remission induction failure in acute myelogenous leukemia. Blood 60:309–15.
2. Bodey GP (1986) Infection in cancer patients. A continuing association. (Review). Am J Med 81(1A):11–26.
3. Bodey GP, Buckley M, Sathe YS, Freireich EJ (1966) Quantitative relationships between circulating leukocytes and infection in patients with acute leukemia. Ann Intern Med 64:328.
4. Bodey GP (1993) Empirical antibiotic therapy for fever in neutropenic patients. Clin Infect Dis 17 Suppl 2:S378–84.
5. Rubin M, Hathorn JW, Pizzo PA (1988) Controversies in the management of febrile neutropenic cancer patients. Cancer Invest 6(2):167–84.
6. Chanock S (1993) Evolving risk factors for infectious complications of cancer therapy. Hematol Oncol Clin North Am 7:771–93.
7. Walsh TJ, Hiemenz J, Pizzo PA (1994) Evolving risk factors for invasive fungal infections — all neutro-

penic patients are not the same. Clin Infect Dis 18:793–8.

8. Wilhelm M, Kantarjian HM, Obrien S, et al. (1996) Pneumonia during remission induction chemotherapy in patients with AML or MDS. Leukemia. Dec 10(12):1870–1873.

9. De Pauw BE, Dompeling EC (1996) Antibiotic strategy after the empiric phase in patients treated for a hematological malignancy. Ann Hematol 72(4): 273–9.

10. Maschmeyer G, Link H, Hiddemann W, et al. (1994) Pulmonary infiltrations in febrile patients with neutropenia. Cancer 73:2296–304.

11. Link H, Maschmeyer G, Meyer P, et al. (1994) Interventional antimicrobial therapy in febrile neutropenic patients. Study Group of the Paul Ehrlich Society for Chemotherapy. Ann Hematol 69(5): 231–43.

12. Winston DJ, Ho WG, Bruckner DA, Champlin RE (1991) Beta-lactam antibiotic therapy in febrile granulocytopenic patients. A randomized trial comparing cefoperazone plus piperacillin, ceftazidime plus piperacillin, and imipenem alone [see omments]. Ann Intern Med 115(11):849–59.

13. Rolston KV, Berkey P, Bodey GP, et al. (1992) A comparison of imipenem to ceftazidime with or without amikacin as empiric therapy in febrile neutropenic patients. Arch Intern Med 152(2): 283–91.

14. Anaissie EJ, Fainstein V, Bodey GP, Rolston K, Elting L, Kantarjian H (1988) Randomised trial of beta-lactam regimens in febrile neutropenic cancer patients. Am J Med 84:581–9.

15. Pizzo PA (1993) Management of fever in patients with cancer and treatment-induced neutropenia [see comments]. N Engl J Med 328(18):1323–32.

16. DeGregorio MW, Lee WM, Linker CA, Jacobs RA, Ries CA (1982) Fungal infections in patients with acute leukemia. Am J Med 73(4):543–8.

17. Gold JW (1984) Opportunistic fungal infections in patients with neoplastic disease. Am J Med 76(3):458–63.

18. Behre G, Link H, Maschmeyer G, et al. (1998) Meropenem monotherapy versus combination therapy with ceftazidime and amikacin for empirical treatment of febrile neutropenic patients. Ann Hematol 76(2):73–80.

19. Nishida K, Higashitani F, Hyodo A (1997) Superior effect of tazobactam/piperacillin compared to piperacillin on beta-lactamase-producing Pseudomonas aeruginosa. Chemotherapy 43(3):171–8.

20. Cometta A, Zinner S, de Bock R, et al. (1995) Piperacillin-tazobactam plus amikacin versus ceftazidime plus amikacin as empiric therapy for fever in granulocytopenic patients with cancer. The International Antimicrobial Therapy Cooperative Group of the European Organization for Research and Treatment of Cancer. Antimicrob Agents Chemother 39(2):445–52.

21. Hess U, Bohme C, Rey K, Senn HJ (1998) Monotherapy with piperacillin/tazobactam versus combination therapy with ceftazidime plus amikacin as an empiric therapy for fever in neutropenic cancer patients. Support Care Cancer 6(4):402–9.

22. Bohme A, Shah PM, Stille W, Hoelzer D (1998) Piperacillin/tazobactam versus cefepime as initial empirical antimicrobial therapy in febrile neutropenic patients: a prospective randomized pilot study. Eur J Med Res 3(7):324–30.

# Multivariate Analysis of Prognostic Factors in Patients with Refractory and Relapsed Acute Myeloid Leukemia Undergoing Sequential High-Dose Cytosine Arabinoside and Mitoxantrone (S-HAM) Salvage Therapy: Significance of Cytogenetic Abnormalities

W. Kern,[1] C. Schoch,[1] T. Haferlach,[1] J. Braess,[1] M. Unterhalt,[1] B. Wörmann,[2] T. Büchner,[3] and W. Hiddemann[1] for the German AML Cooperative Group

*Abstract.* To serve a basis for the refinement of the biologically determined stratification of patients with refractory and relapsed acute myeloid leukemia (AML), univariate and multivariate analyses of prognostic factors were performed in patients having received S-HAM salvage chemotherapy during two consecutive prospective trials of the German AML Cooperative Group. Two-hundred-fifty-four patients (median age 50 years, range 18–74) were analyzed, in 104 of whom karyotyping prior to first line therapy had been performed. In the multivariate analyses, duration of the first complete remission (CR) was the only factor associated with time to treatment failure (p=0.0223). Disease-free survival was influenced by a short duration of the first CR of less than six months (p=0.0001), WBC (p=0.0018), blast count (p=0.0037), neutrophil count (p=0.0119), and duration of the first CR (p=0.0457). The achievement of a CR following salvage treatment was related to the hemoglobin level only (p=0.0457), the early death rate was related to age only (p=0.0109), and survival was related to the bilirubin level only (p=0.0166). Unfavorable chromosome abnormalities were associated with a lower CR rate (univariate analysis, p=0.0342; CR 24% versus 53%) and were the only factor related to survival in the multivariate analysis of the 104 patients with karyotyping prior to first-line therapy. These analyses warrant the further evaluation of the impact of cytogenetic abnormalities on the outcome of patients with advanced AML in order to improve the characterization of distinct subgroups of patients with differing prognosis as a basis for the stratification in future trials.

## Introduction

The stratification of patients with acute myeloid leukemia (AML) is increasingly becoming incorporated into treatment strategies in order to account for the heterogeneity of biologic features between specific subgroups of this disease which are the basis for substantial differences in response to chemotherapy and long-term outcome [1–3]. Among the most important prognostic factors, chromosome abnormalities may indicate these differences in the biology of various AML subtypes most appropriately [4,5]. Along this line, treatment with all-trans retinoic acid specifically induces complete remissions in patients with promyelocytic leukemia [6–8] and cases with core binding factor-leukemias seem to specifically benefit from high-dose cytosine arabinoside (AraC) [2]. On the other hand, AML accompanied by complex chromosome abnormalities remains a therapeutic dilemma with nearly all of the currently used regimens and therefore may be most appropriately treated by experimental therapies [9]. In patients receiving second-line treatment for AML, however, considerably less effort has been made to refine the biologically determined stratification, which has mainly been based yet on the duration of the first complete remission [10–12]. Furthermore, previous analyses, alt-

[1] Klinikum Großhadern, Medizinische Klinik III, Ludwig-Maximilians-Universität, München;
[2] Städtisches Klinikum, Medizinische Klinik, Braunschweig;
[3] Medizinische Klink A, Westfälische-Wilhelms-Universität, Münster; Germany.

hough including a large number of patients, were hampered by the heterogeneity of the salvage regimens having been applied to the patients [11, 12]. Especially, AraC has been used at different dose levels which may have obscured the analysis of prognostic factors due to the interaction of treatment regimen and prognosis [13, 14]. The current analysis of the prognostic significance of pretreatment factors for response to chemotherapy and long-term outcome was performed in 254 patients from two consecutive prospective trials of the German AML Cooperative Group who uniformly had received the sequential high-dose AraC and mitoxantrone (S-HAM) regimen[15] as second-line therapy for AML [16].

## Patients and Methods

### Patients

Consecutive patients at ages 18 or older with relapsed and refractory AML who were admitted at the participating centers between september 1987 and january 1996 were eligible for the two studies. The diagnosis of AML was based on the revised French-American-British (FAB) Group criteria [17]. Refractoriness against standard chemotherapy was defined according to previously established criteria [10]: These included
a) primary resistance against two cycles of induction therapy;
b) first early relapse with a remission duration of less than six months;
c) second and subsequent relapse.

Patients with first relapses after six months remission duration were not considered refractory to standard therapy and were included as relapsed AML.

All patients were recruited from the first line trials of the German AML Cooperative Group and had thus received a standardized first line treatment. In patients less than 60 years of age first line therapy consisted in double induction therapy with either the repetitive application of the 9 day regimen of thioguanine, AraC, daunorubicin (TAD-9/TAD-9) or the sequential application of TAD-9 followed by HD-AraC and mitoxan-

trone (HAM). Older patients all received one course of TAD-9 and were treated by a second TAD-9 or HAM course only upon inadequate response to the first TAD-9 cycle. Patients of all ages who achieved a complete remission (CR) subsequently received TAD-9 for consolidation and monthly maintenance therapy for three years [18, 19].

Patients with a preceding allogeneic bone marrow transplantation were excluded from the study. Further exclusion criteria comprized coronary heart disease; heart failure; cardiomyopathy; severe arterial hypertension; abnormal liver function tests (aspartate aminotransferase [AST], alanine aminotransferase [ALT], or alkaline phosphatase [AP] more than three times the upper normal limits; total bilirubin $> 2.0$ mg/dl); impaired renal function (serum creatinine $> 2.0$ mg/dl); severe infections; or pregnancy.

### Antileukemic Therapy

Patients meeting the entry criteria were enrolled into the current study and were treated by S-HAM [15] comprizing AraC every 12 hours by a 3-hour infusion on days 1, 2, 8, and 9 and mitoxantrone 10 mg/m$^2$/day as a 30-min infusion on days 3, 4, 10, and 11, respectively. During the first study period from september 1987 to september 1992 patients younger than 60 were randomized to receive AraC at a dose of 3 g/m$^2$ or 1 g/m$^2$ per application while older patients were randomized to receive AraC at a dose of 1 g/m$^2$ or 0.5 g/m$^2$ per application. Based on the results of this comparison [20], during the second study period from september 1992 to january 1996 patients younger than 60 years with refractory disease, early relapse following a first CR of less than six months, or second and subsequent relapses received AraC at doses of 3.0 g/m$^2$ per application while all other patients were treated with 1.0 g/m$^2$ AraC per single dose. Only during this second study period, patients were randomly assigned to receive antifungal prophylaxis with fluconazole or not which had no effect on the outcome following S-HAM therapy [21]. These patients also received granulocyte-colony stimulating factor (G-CSF) 5 µg/m$^2$ subcutaneously starting on day 14, i.e. two days following the completion of chemotherapy as supportive therapy [22]. G-CSF was stopped in case of persistance of more than 5% leukemic blasts on a day 18 bone marrow examination or upon recovery of granulocytes to more than 1500/µl. To avoid imbalances in the patients' risk profile the respective randomization procedures were stratified for the following criteria:

a) primary resistance against two cycles of induction therapy,
b) first early relapse with a remission duration of less than six months,
c) first relapse with a remission duration of more than six months but less than 18 months,
d) first relapse with a remission duration of more than 18 months,
e) second and subsequent relapse.

Patients in CR after S-HAM therapy were scheduled to undergo an allogeneic transplant when available or to receive no further therapy.

## Study Parameters

Bone marrow examinations were carried out on day 18, i.e. one week after the end of chemotherapy, and upon full recovery of peripheral blood counts. Response to therapy was assessed according to CALGB criteria [23]. CR was defined as a normal cellular bone marrow with normal erythroid and myeloid elements and less than 5% myeloblasts, and with peripheral blood counts of more than 100,000/µl platelets and more than 1,500/µl granulocytes for at least four weeks. Patients with regenerated peripheral blood values but more than 5% and less than 25% myeloblasts were considered to be in partial remission (PR), as were patients fulfilling the bone marrow criteria of CR but without full recovery of peripheral blood platelet and/or white blood cell counts. Patients with persisting leukemic blasts in the bone marrow or blood or with leukemic regrowth within four weeks after initial response were considered as non-responders (NR). Patients dying within six week after the end of antileukemic therapy without evidence of leukemic regrowth were classified as early deaths (ED).

Survival and time to treatment failure (TTF) were measured by the time from the beginning of treatment to death, documentation of persisting leukemia, or relapse, respectively. Disease-free survival (DFS) was measured by the time from achievement of CR to relapse or death during CR. Actuarial values for time-dependent variables were calculated by the Kaplan Meier method [24].

Cytogenetic evaluations were performed both at diagnosis and at relapse. Karyotype abnormalities were classified according to definitions previously established for the German AML Cooperative Group first line trilas [25–28]. Favorable abnormalities included t(8;21), t(15;17), and inv(16)/t(16;16) while unfavorable karyotypes were inv(3)/t(3;3), -5/5q-, t(6;9), -7/7q-, 11q23 abnormalities, 17p abnormalities, and complex chromosomal changes ($\geq$3 numeric and/or structural changes). All other karyotypes, including normal cases, were considered intermediate.

## Statistics

Univariate and multivariate analyses were performed to evaluate the dependence of the variables CR, NR, ED, survival, TTF, and DFS on pretreatment factors including age, duration of first CR (duration set to zero months for patients with refractory disease), white blood cell count (WBC), blast count, neutrophil count, thrombocyte count, hemoglobin level, bilirubin level, lactate dehydrogenase (LDH) level, and date of therapy as continuous covariates and age below or higher than 60 years, disease status (refractory, first CR shorter than six months, first CR between six and 18 months, first CR more than 18 months, second or higher relapse), FAB subtype (M0 to M7), WHO performance status (0 to 3), extramedullary disease, sex, dose of AraC (3 g/m$^2$, 1 g/m$^2$, 0.5 g/m$^2$), prior application of high-dose AraC, scheduled application of supportive G-CSF, and treatment period (september 1987 to august 1989, september 1989 to september 1992, october 1992 to november 1993, december 1993 to january 1996) as dichotomous covariates. A separate set of univariate and multivariate analyses was performed for 104 patients with determinations of karyotypes before first-line therapy to evaluate the influence of chromosome abnormalities (favorable, intermediate/normal, unfavorable; dichotomous variables) on the dependent variables.

Univariate and multivariate analyses were performed for time-dependent variables by a proportional hazards model and for dichotomous variables by a logistic regression model using the PC-Statistik computer program (O. Hoffmann, Gießen, Germany).

## Study Conduct

Prior to therapy all patients gave their informed consent for participation in the current evaluation after having been advised about the purpose and investigational nature of the study as well as of potential risks. The study design adhered to the declaration of Helsinki and was approved by the ethics committees of the participating institutions prior to its initiation.

## Results

### Patient Characteristics

Two-hundred-fifty-four evaluable patients were entered into the two studies from 33 centers in Germany and Austria. The patients' ages ranged from 18 to 74 years (median 50 years), the sex distribution was even (127/127). All patients had received prior chemotherapy for their disease as indicated above. In 107 patients high-dose AraC had been applied as part of the first-line chemotherapy. Overall, 32 (13%) patients had primary refractory disease and 60 (24%) had early relapses after a first CR of less than six months duration. In 102 (40%) and 44 (17%) cases the relapses occured after a CR of more than six but less than 18 months and of more than 18 months duration, respectively; 16 (6%) patients suffered from second or subsequent relapses (Table 1). AML subtypes were predominantly M1, M2, M4, and M5. WHO performance status was 0 in 23 (9%) patients, 1 in 96 (38%), 2 in 125 (49%), and 3 in 9 (4%) cases. Pretreatment WBC values ranged from 400 to 21200/μl (median, 3500/μl) and extramedullary disease was present in 32 (13%)

**Table 1.** Univariate analyses of prognostic factors

| Dependent Variable | Covariate | p-Value |
|---|---|---|
| Survival | WBC | 0.0001 |
| | Blast count | 0.0002 |
| | Bilirubin | 0.0055 |
| | Duration of first CR <6 months | 0.0074 |
| | LDH | 0.0087 |
| | Duration of first CR | 0.0117 |
| | Age | 0.0221 |
| Time to treatment failure | Blast count | 0.0002 |
| | WBC | 0.0003 |
| | Duration of first CR <6 months | 0.0006 |
| | Duration of first CR | 0.0078 |
| | Duration of first CR >6<18 months | 0.0449 |
| Disease-free survival | WBC | <0.00005 |
| | Duration of first CR <6 months | <0.00005 |
| | Neutrophil count | 0.0004 |
| | Blast count | 0.0006 |
| | LDH | 0.0197 |
| | Duration of first CR | 0.0239 |
| Complete remission | Refractory disease | 0.0118 |
| | Duration of first CR | 0.0176 |
| | Hemoglobin | 0.0197 |
| | WBC | 0.0296 |
| | Blast count | 0.0315 |
| Non-response | Duration of first CR <6 months | 0.0048 |
| | Duration of first CR >6<18 months | 0.0058 |
| | Refractory disease | 0.0070 |
| | Duration of first CR | 0.0098 |
| Early death | Age | 0.0109 |

patients. Cytogenetic analyses were performed prior to first-line therapy in 104 patients. Karyotypes were classified favorable, normal/intermediate, and unfavorable in 17, 70, and 17 patients, respectively. All 254 patients received one course of S-HAM therapy only. Median follow-up interval for surviving patients is 10.7 months from start of salvage therapy.

### Antileukemic Activity

Overall, 126 (50%) and 10 (4%) of the 254 evaluable patients achieved a CR and a PR, respectively, while 55 (22%) cases were NR.

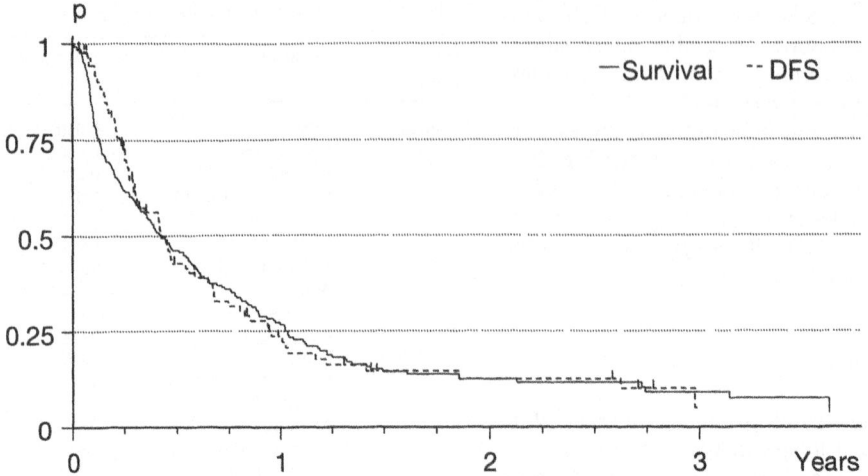

**Fig. 1.** Survival and time to treatment failure in 254 patients undergoing S-HAM salvage therapy

Sixty-three (25%) patients suffered from ED. Median actuarial values for disease-free survival, time to treatment failure, and survival are 5.1, 3.0, and 5.1 months, respectively (Fig. 1).

## Univariate Analyses

End points directly related to the response to treatment or to relapse of the disease, i.e. TTF, DFS, achievement of CR, and NR, were dependent on factors directly related to the status of the disease prior to salvage therapy, i.e. blast count, WBC, duration of first CR, neutrophil count, LDH, hemoglobin (Table 1). In contrast, the early death rate was dependent only on the patients' age. Accordingly, overall survival was influenced by age and bilirubin levels in addition to leukemia-related factors, i.e. WBC, blast count, duration of first CR, and LDH. Factors without an impact on any of the analyzed end points included FAB subtype, WHO performance status, sex, extramedullary manifestation of AML, thrombocyte count, date of salvage therapy, and administration of high-dose AraC during first-line therapy.

The evaluation of the 104 patients with karyptype analysis prior to first-line therapy revealed a dependence of survival and achievement of CR on the diagnosis of an unfavorable karyotype. In these 104 patients, factors influencing survival were WBC

(p=0.0191), blast count (p=0.0323), WHO performance status 3 (p=0.0412), and unfavorable karyotype (p=0.0583). The achievement of CR was dependent on the duration of first CR of more than six months and less than 18 month (p=0.0213), unfavorable karyotype (p=0.0342; CR 24% versus 53%), and WHO performance status 2 (p=0.0414) in these patients.

## Multivariate Analyses

The strongest association in the multivariate analyses was found for DFS with a duration of the first CR of less than six months (Table 2). Further covariates significantly related to DFS were WBC, blast count, neutrophil count, and

**Table 2.** Multivariate analyses of prognostic factors

| Dependent Variable | Covariate | p-Value |
| --- | --- | --- |
| Survival | Bilirubin | 0.0166 |
| Time to treatment failure | Duration of first CR | 0.0223 |
| Disease-free survival | Duration of first CR <6 months | 0.0001 |
| | WBC | 0.0018 |
| | Blast count | 0.0037 |
| | Neutrophil count | 0.0119 |
| | Duration of first CR | 0.0457 |
| Complete remission | Hemoglobin | 0.0457 |

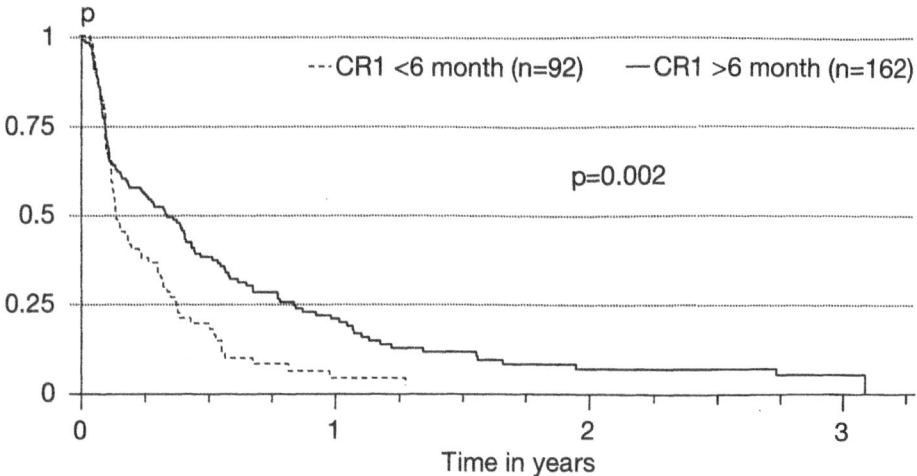

**Fig. 2.** Time to treatment failure according to duration of first CR

duration of first CR. Survival was dependent on bilirubin only and TTF was dependent on the duration of first CR only (Fig. 2). The only significant association for the achievement of CR following salvage therapy was found for hemoglobin while no significant association was found for NR in the multivariate analysis.

The multivariate analyses in the 104 patients with karyoptype analysis prior to first-line therapy revealed an unfavorable karyotype as the only factor significantly associated with survival (p=0.0360). No factor was found to be significantly related to the achievement of CR in the multivariate analysis in these patients.

## Discussion

The current analyses of prognostic factors in patients receiving S-HAM salvage therapy for refractory and relapsed AML revealed that in addition to parameters reflecting the stage and the status of the disease, i.e. WBC, blast count, neutrophil count, and duration of first CR, and to patient-related characteristics, i.e. age and bilirubin, the karyotype prior to first-line therapy significantly influences the overall outcome. Hence, the diagnosis of unfavorable chromosome abnormalities was the only factor significantly related to overall survival in the multivariate analysis. These data are in accordance to reports on the prognostic sig-

nificance of karyptype abnormalities for the response to first-line therapy [3, 9, 21, 2 8–31] and furthermore stress the results of a previous analysis in patients receiving second-line therapy which revealed the duration of the first CR and unfavorable chromosome abnormalities to be the most important prognostic factors in these patients [11, 12].

Until recently, the main criterion to estimate the prognosis of patients undergoing salvage therapy has been the duration of the first CR [10]. These data were generated from 150 patients having received standardized first-line [18] and second-line [10] therapies and thus provided the basis to analyze the patients' prognosis idependently from possibly confounding therapeutic effects. Hence, cases with refractory disease and cases with early relapses, i.e. following a first CR of less than six months duration, had a significantly poorer response to therapy (CR rate 28% versus 59%) and overall outcome as compared with patients in relapse after a first CR of more than six months duration.

Similar results were obtained in analyses performed in 243 patients at the M.D. Anderson Cancer Center in Houston, USA, which also indicated that the duration of the first CR is the most important prognostic factor for response to salvage therapy with age and level of LDH being additional significant factors in a multivariate analysis [12]. However, the best cut-off point in this analysis was 12 months duration of the first CR with 19% versus 60% of the patients achieving a second CR. As in the current data bilirubin was the most important factor for overall survival with other patient-related factors (age, alkaline phosphatase) and leukemia-related factors (duration of first CR, percentage of blasts and promyeleocytes) being significant in a multivariate analysis. However, 41 different salvage regimens were applied to the analyzed patients. As a consequence, it cannot be ruled out, that individual risk factors might have influenced the decision which therapy to apply and that the significance of other possible prognostic factors, i.e. cytogenetics, might have been underestimated.

Another analysis from the M.D. Anderson Cancer Center on 806 patients with refractory and relapsed AML confirmed the prognostic significance of the duration of the first CR and in addition stressed the importance of chromosome abnormalities for patients with a first CR of less than one year [11]. However, besides the use various treatment regimens the lack of a multivariate analysis hampered this evaluation and no final conclusion can be drawn about the significance of cytogenetics as compared with the duration of the first CR on the basis of these data.

Further evidence for the relevance of the six-months cut-off point of duration of first CR came from a French study in which 240 patients receiving uniform salvage treatment according to the EMA protocol were evaluated for prognostic factors [32, 33]. The rates of CR following EMA therapy were 44% versus 78% for the respective groups while only refractory disease and hemoglobin level were significant in a multivariate analysis. Refractory disease and a hemorrhagic syndrom were associated with a short DFS and refractory disease, initial fever, and bone marrow blasts at 80% were predictive of short survival in multivariate analyses, respectively. No analyses, however, were performed on the relevance of cytogenetic abnormalities.

Unfortunately, further multivariate analyses of prognostoc factors in this group of patients have not yet been reported on, mainly due to relatively small sample sizes [34–44] in studies evaluating salvage regimens.

Thus, on the basis of the current analyses, the assignment of salvage regimens to patients with refractory and relapsed AML should be stratified not only with regard to the duration of the first CR but also with regard to chromosome abnormalities. Further patients should be evaluated to add on the current data and to also clarify the role of chromosome abnormalities determined directly prior to salvage therapy which are different to the initial karyotype in about 60% of cases [45] and might be a tool to more exactly estimate these patients' prognosis. The results of these further analyses sholud be the basis for further trials that analyze in a randomized fashion different treatment strategies in the respective subgroups of patients. In addition, the negative results of the current analyses should be kept in mind, e.g. the lack of influence of the application of high-dose AraC during first-line treatment on the outcome following S-HAM salvage therapy. Furthermore, age was a prognostic factor for ED only, which might indicate that not age per se but a higher freuquency of unfavorable leukemia-specific characteristics is the basis for the worse prognosis of elderly patients [46]. Hence, the study strategies outlined above should be evaluated in a large number of patients including cases refractory to high-dose AraC containing regimens and elderly patients.

## References

1. Russell NH: Biology of acute leukaemia. Lancet 349:118–122, 1997
2. Bloomfield CD, Lawrence D, Byrd JC, et al: Frequency of prolonged remission duration after high-dose cytarabine intensification in acute myeloid leukemia varies by cytogenetic subtype. Cancer Res 58:4173–4179, 1998
3. Grimwade D, Walker H, Oliver F, et al: The importance of diagnostic cytogenetics on outcome in AML: analysis of 1,612 patients entered into the MRC AML 10 trial. The Medical Research Council Adult and Children's Leukaemia Working Parties. Blood 92:2322–2333, 1998
4. Mrozek K, Heinonen K, Lawrence D, et al: Adult patients with de novo acute myeloid leukemia and t(9; 11)(p22; q23) have a superior outcome to patients with other translocations involving band 11q23: a cancer and leukemia group B study. Blood 90:4532–4538, 1997
5. Dreyling MH, Schrader K, Fonatsch C, et al: MLL and CALM are fused to AF10 in morphologically distinct subsets of acute leukemia with translocation t(10;11): both rearrangements are associated with a poor prognosis. Blood 91:4662–4667, 1998

6. Fenaux P, Le Deley MC, Castaigne S, et al: Effect of all transretinoic acid in newly diagnosed acute promyelocytic leukemia. Results of a multicenter randomized trial. European APL 91 Group. Blood 82:3241–3249, 1993

7. Tallman MS, Andersen JW, Schiffer CA, et al: All-trans-retinoic acid in acute promyelocytic leukemia [see comments] [published erratum appears in N Engl J Med 1997 Nov 27; 337(22):1639]. N Engl J Med 337:1021–1028, 1997

8. Lo Coco F, Nervi C, Avvisati G, et al: Acute promyelocytic leukemia: a curable disease. Leukemia 12:1866–1880, 1998

9. Schoch C, Haferlach T, Haase D, et al: Complex chromosome aberrations in patients with de novo AML are associated with a very poor prognosis despite intensive treatment: a study of 90 patients. Blood 90:62a, 1997

10. Hiddemann W, Martin WR, Sauerland CM, et al: Definition of refractoriness against conventional chemotherapy in acute myeloid leukemia: a proposal based on the results of retreatment by thioguanine, cytosine arabinoside, and daunorubicin (TAD 9) in 150 patients with relapse after standardized first line therapy. Leukemia 4:184–188, 1990

11. Estey E: Treatment of refractory AML. Leukemia 10:932–936, 1996

12. Keating MJ, Kantarjian H, Smith TL, et al: Response to salvage therapy and survival after relapse in acute myelogenous leukemia. J Clin Oncol 7:1071–1080, 1989

13. Buchner T, Hiddemann W, Wormann B, et al: Double induction strategy for acute myeloid leukemia: The effect of high-dose cytarabine with mitoxantrone instead of standard-dose cytarabine with daunorubicin and 6-thioguanine: A randomized trial by the German AML Cooperative Group. Blood 93:4116–4124, 1999

14. Rowe JM, Liesveld JL: Treatment and prognostic factors in acute myeloid leukaemia. Baillieres Clin Haematol 9:87–105, 1996

15. Kern W, Schleyer E, Unterhalt M, et al: High anti-leukemic activity of sequential high dose cytosine arabinoside and mitoxantrone in patients with refractory acute leukemias. Results of a clinical phase II study. Cancer 79:59–68, 1997

16. Kern W, Schoch C, Haferlach T, et al: Significance of cytogenetic abnormalities in a multivariate analysis of prognostic factors in patients with refractory and relapsed acute myeloid leukemia. Blood 92:78a, 1998

17. Bennett JM, Catovsky D, Daniel MT, et al: Proposed revised criteria for the classification of acute myeloid leukemia. A report of the French-American-British Cooperative Group. Ann Intern Med 103:620–625, 1985

18. Buchner T, Urbanitz D, Hiddemann W, et al: Intensified induction and consolidation with or without maintenance chemotherapy for acute myeloid leukemia (AML): two multicenter studies of the German AML Cooperative Group. J Clin Oncol 3:1583–1589, 1985

19. Buchner T, Hiddemann W, Wormann B, et al: Longterm effects of prolonged maintenance and of very early intensification chemotherapy in AML: data from AMLCG. Leukemia 6 Suppl 2:68–71, 1992

20. Kern W, Aul C, Maschmeyer G, et al: Superiority of high-dose over intermediate-dose cytosine arabinoside in the treatment of patients with high-risk acute myeloid leukemia: results of a age-adjusted prospective randomized comparison. Leukemia 12:1049–1055, 1998

21. Kern W, Behre G, Rudolf T, et al: Failure of fluconazole prophylaxis to reduce mortality and the requirement of systemic amphotericin B therapy during treatment for refractory acute myeloid leukemia: results of a prospective randomized phase III study. Cancer 83:291–301, 1998

22. Patt YZ, Peters RE, Chuang VP, et al: Effective retreatment of patients with colorectal cancer and liver metastases. Am J Med 75:237–240, 1983

23. Yates J, Glidewell O, Wiernik P, et al: Cytosine arabinoside with daunorubicin or adriamycin for therapy of acute myelocytic leukemia: a CALGB study. Blood 60:454–462, 1982

24. Kaplan EL, Meier P: Nonparametric estimation from incomplete estimations. Am Stat Assoc J 53:457–481, 1958

25. Schoch C, Haase D, Fonatsch C, et al: The significance of trisomy 8 in de novo acute myeloid leukaemia: the accompanying chromosome aberrations determine the prognosis. German AML Cooperative Study Group. Br J Haematol 99: 605–611, 1997

26. Schoch C, Haase D, Haferlach T, et al: Fifty-one patients with acute myeloid leukemia and translocation t(8;21)(q22;q22): an additional deletion in 9q is an adverse prognostic factor. Leukemia 10:1288–1295, 1996

27. Schoch C, Haase D, Haferlach T, et al: Incidence and implication of additional chromosome aberrations in acute promyelocytic leukaemia with translocation t(15;17)(q22; q21): a report on 50 patients. Br J Haematol 94:493–500, 1996

28. Buchner T, Hiddemann W, Wormann B, et al: Threapeutic outcome in AML is mainly determined by cytogenetics, LDH in serum, early response and, in a poor risk subgroup, by intensified induction treatment. Blood 90:504a, 1997

29. Byrd JC, Lawrence D, Arthur DC, et al: Patients with isolated trisomy 8 in acute myeloid leukemia are not cured with cytarabine-based chemotherapy: results from Cancer and Leukemia Group B 8461. Clin Cancer Res 4:1235–1241, 1998

30. Bloomfield CD, Shuma C, Regal L, et al: Long-term survival of patients with acute myeloid leukemia: a third follow-up of the Fourth International Workshop on Chromosomes in Leukemia. Cancer 80: 2191–2198, 1997

31. Lowenberg B, Suciu S, Archimbaud E, et al: Use of recombinant GM-CSF during and after remission induction chemotherapy in patients aged 61 years and older with acute myeloid leukemia: final report of AML-11, a phase III randomized study of the Leukemia Cooperative Group of European Organisation for the Research and Treatment of Cancer and the Dutch Belgian Hemato-Oncology Cooperative Group. Blood 90:2952–2961, 1997

32. Archimbaud E, Thomas X, Leblond V, et al: Timed sequential chemotherapy for previously treated patients with acute myeloid leukemia: long-term follow-up of the etoposide, mitoxantrone, and cytarabine-86 trial [see comments]. J Clin Oncol 13:11–18, 1995

33. Archimbaud E, Leblond V, Fenaux P, et al: Timed sequential chemotherapy for advanced acute myeloid leukemia. Hematol Cell Ther 38:161–167, 1996

34. Montillo M, Mirto S, Petti MC, et al: Fludarabine, cytarabine, and G-CSF (FLAG) for the treatment of poor risk acute myeloid leukemia. Am J Hematol 58:105–109, 1998

35. Sierra J, Granena A, Bosch F, et al: Mitoxantrone and intermediate-dose cytosine arabinoside for poor-risk acute leukemias: response to treatment and factors influencing outcome. Hematol Oncol 10:301–309, 1992

36. Harousseau JL, Milpied N, Briere J, et al: Mitoxantrone and intermediate-dose cytarabine in relapsed or refractory acute myeloblastic leukemia. Nouv Rev Fr Hematol 32:227–230, 1990

37. Smits P, Schoots L, de Pauw BE, et al: Prognostic factors in adult patients with acute leukemia at first relapse. Cancer 59:1631–1634, 1987

38. Herzig RH, Lazarus HM, Wolff SN, et al: High-dose cytosine arabinoside therapy with and without anthracycline antibiotics for remission reinduction of acute nonlymphoblastic leukemia. J Clin Oncol 3:992–997, 1985

39. Hiddemann W, Kreutzmann H, Straif K, et al: High-dose cytosine arabinoside and mitoxantrone: a highly effective regimen in refractory acute myeloid leukemia. Blood 69:744–749, 1987

40. Walters RS, Kantarjian HM, Keating MJ, et al: Mitoxantrone and high-dose cytosine arabinoside in refractory acute myelogenous leukemia. Cancer 62:677–682, 1988

41. Martiat P, Ghilain JM, Ferrant A, et al: High-dose cytosine arabinoside and amsacrine or mitoxantrone in relapsed and refractory acute myeloid leukaemia: a prospective randomized study. Eur J Haematol 45:164–167, 1990

42. Carella AM, Carlier P, Pungolino E, et al: Idarubicin in combination with intermediate-dose cytarabine and VP-16 in the treatment of refractory or rapidly relapsed patients with acute myeloid leukemia. The GIMEMA Cooperative Group. Leukemia 7:196–199, 1993

43. Spadea A, Petti MC, Fazi P, et al: Mitoxantrone, etoposide and intermediate-dose Ara-C (MEC): an effective regimen for poor risk acute myeloid leukemia. Leukemia 7:549–552, 1993

44. Vogler WR, McCarley DL, Stagg M, et al: A phase III trial of high-dose cytosine arabinoside with or without etoposide in relapsed and refractory acute myelogenous leukemia. A Southeastern Cancer Study Group trial. Leukemia 8:1847–1853, 1994

45. Garson OM, Hagemeijer A, Sakurai M, et al: Cytogenetic studies of 103 patients with acute myelogenous leukemia in relapse. Cancer Genet Cytogenet 40:187–202, 1989

46. Kern W, Schoch C, Fonatsch C, et al: Treatment of acute myeloid leukemia in the elderly. Home Health Care Consultant 6:2–13, 1999

338

# Incidence of Central Venous Catheter (CVC)-Infections in Patients with Acute Leukemia

M. Karthaus, T. Doellmann, T. Klimasch, J. Krauter, G. Heil, and A. Ganser

Central venous catheters have become an essential tool for an appropriate management of patients with acute leukemia. CVC-related infections may cause significant morbidity as a source of nosocomial infections. Data regarding the incidence are rare in patients with acute leukemia and neutropenia (<500/µl).

*Patients and Methods.* We analyzed non-tunneled CVC in 58 patients with acute leukemia (22 m/36 f) within 119 chemotherapy cycles from 4/96 to 1/98. Proven CVC-related infection was the isolation of the same organism from peripheral blood and CVC-tip. CVC-infection was suspicious, respectively possible when exit-site inflammation and positive blood culture respective organisms typical for CVC-infection were observed.

*Results.* Mean neutropenia/cycle was 16,3 days (SD 8,0). 178 CVC with 2576 CVC days (mean 14,5d, SD 7,2d) were used in 119 cycles. Fever occurred in 87 cycles (73%). Bloodstream infection was proven in 31 out 87 episodes (26,1%) with 40 isolates (8 gram-negative 31 gram-positive, 1 *candida ssp*.). Colonization of the CVC-tip was observed in 24 CVC-lines with 28 isolates (27 gram-positive, 1 gram-negative), however, proven CVC-related infections were observed in 5 episode only, all with coag.-positive Staphylococci. In another 6 episodes CVC-related infection was assumed (local inflammation and gram-pos. blood culture). Six further episodes had typical isolates (4 coag-positive staphylococci, 1 *Candida ssp*) from the blood and were considered possible CVC related infections. In none of the remaining afebrile 32 cycles a CVC-infection was observed or suspected.

*Conclusion.* Gram-positive organisms contributed to the majority of CVC-related infections (16 out 17 CVC-infections), however, overall incidence of CVC-infection in acute leukemia patients is low 6,5/1000 CVC-days (1,9 proven/2,3 suspected/2,3possible/1000 CVC-days).

## Introduction

Central venous catheters are an important tool in the appropriate management of patients treated for acute leukemia. These devices provide reliable access for administration of chemotherapeutic drugs, blood products as well as parenteral feeding or antimicrobial agents during intensive treatment of acute leukemia. Bloodstream infections related to a CVC can result in serious medical complications [1–3]. Infectious complications are reported to be CVC-related in 4% to 14% in patients with febrile neutropenia and acute leukemia. Neutropenia has been shown an independent risk factor for infection related to tunneled central venous catheters [4].

The skin, the insertion site and the catheter hub are considered to be important sources of CVC colonization and subsequent CVC-related bacteremia [5]. The major pathogens that cause CVC-related infections are the gram-positive cocci, mainly coagulase-negative staphylococci [6].

Local inflammation at the insertion site is a common observation in patients with acute leukemia and fever. Localized infection may lead to CVC removal, however, prospective data regarding a relation between local inflammation at insertion site and the incidence of CVC-related bacteremia are rare in

---

Medizinische Hochschule Hannover, Department of Hematology and Oncology

acute leukemia patients. In a prospective trial, we studied CVC-related infections in patients treated for acute leukemia with nontunneled CVCs.

## Patients and Methods

The trial was conducted between April 1996 and January 1998. Patients were recruited from the Department of Hematology and Oncology at the Hannover Medical School. Hospitalized adults who had a nontunneled CVC and who were treated with intensive chemotherapy for acute leukemia were eligible. All patients had an expected severe neutropenia (<100/μl) with a duration of >10 days. Patients were excluded if they had microbiological evidence of infection or were receiving already intravenous antibiotics at the time of CVC insertion.

## Catheter insertion and care

Consecutive patients with a nontunneled, triple-lumen polyurethane CVC (Arrowguard blue, Arrow Inc., Reading, Pa.) were included in the trial. Catheters were inserted into the subclavian or jugular vein using maximal sterile-barrier precautions. To avoid the potential confounding effect of the controversial practice of catheter exchange over a guide wire, we determined to study only catheters inserted through a new vein puncture. At the time of catheter insertion and at each dressing time, the insertion site was disinfected with 10% povidine-iodine. CVC care included changing of the dressing at least every 48h by registered nurses or by physicians, who followed maximal barrier precautions. The insertion site was softly scrubbed with sterile gauze saturated with povidine-iodine. The dressing was changed and the insertion site was inspected five to seven days a week. The decision to remove the catheter was made solely by the patient's physician, who kept the catheter in place until it was no longer needed or until an adverse event, such as a CVC-related infection or CVC occlusion, necessitated its removal.

## Cultures

The outer surfaces of the catheter tips of the aseptically removed CVC were cultured by the roll-plate method as described previously (Maki-technique) [7]. The criteria for positively of the CVC tip culture were counts of ≥15 CFU by the roll plate method. In patients with a febrile episode (≥38,5°C or two times 38,0°C within 12 hours), blood cultures were taken from peripheral veins and from the CVC. Recovered microorganisms were identified by standard microbiologic methods. In addition, cultures from the exit site were recommended in case of inflammation.

## Definitions

We adopted the definitions of catheter colonization and infection proposed by the Centers for Disease Control and Prevention. CVC-related bloodstream infection was defined as the isolation of the same microorganism from the colonized catheter and the peripheral blood in a patient with clinical manifestation or sepsis and no other apparent source of bloodstream infection.

CVC-colonization was defined as the growth of 15 or more colony-forming units in culture of catheter segments prepared by roll-plate method.

CVC-infection was suspicious when exit-site inflammation and positive blood culture or micro-organisms typical for CVC-infection were observed. CVC-infection was possible when an infection with microbiologically proven microorganisms typical for CVC-infection without any other apparent clinical focus was observed.

## Results

We included 58 consecutive patients who were treated with 119 cycles of intensive chemotherapy for acute leukemia. A total of 178 CVCs were documented with a duration of 2576 days of catheterization. Catheters remained in place for a mean of 14.5 days (SD 7.2) with a minimum of 2 days and a maximum of 43 days. Mean duration of neutropenia per treatment cycle was 16.3 days (SD 8.0). The

**Table 1.** Patient characteristics

| Patients/chemotherapy cycles | 58/119 |
|---|---|
| Median age /range (years) | 47/19–76 |
| Sex (male/female) | 22/36 |
| Underlying disease and chemotherapy cycles | |
| AML (patients/cycles) | 44/97 |
| ALL (patients/cycles) | 13/19 |
| AUL (patients/cycles) | 1/3 |
| Mean duration of neutropenia/cycle (days) | 16,3 (SD 8,0) |
| Total number of central venous lines (CVC) | 178 |
| one CVC/cycle | 119 |
| two CVC/cycle | 47 |
| three CVC/cycle | 12 |
| Total number of CVC-days | 2576 |
| Mean duration of CVC placement (days) | 14,5 (SD 7,2) |
| Range (days) | 2–43 |

**Table 2.** Characteristics of treatment cycles

| Total number of chemotherapy cycles | n=119 (100%) |
|---|---|
| Number of cycles with fever | 87 (73%) |
| Origin of fever unknown (FUO) | 24 |
| Episodes with clinically defined infection (CDI) | 22 |
| Episodes with CDI and microbiological results | 17 |
| Episodes with MDI | 22 |
| n.a. | 2 |
| Number of cycles without fever | 32 (27%) |

baseline characteristics of the patients are shown in Table 1.

Within 119 cycles, a total of 87 cycles (73%) with fever were observed (Table 2). Inflammation at insertion site was documented in a total of 57 insertion sites out of 87 cycles of chemotherapy with febrile episodes (65,5%). Blood cultures were positive in 31 out of 87 febrile episodes (26.1%). A total of 40 isolates (31 gram-positive, 8 gram-negative, 1 Candida ssp.) were obtained. The CVC-tip was colonized in 24 CVC-lines with 28 isolates (27 gram-positive, 1 gram-negative). In 21 out of these 24 colonized CVC-lines, febrile neutropenia was observed. A proven CVC-

**Table 3.** Relation of microbiological results, culutre of the CVC-tip and exit site infection in patients with febrile neutropenia

| | Bloodculture | CVC culture | Exit site infection |
|---|---|---|---|
| Proven CVC related infections: n= 5 | 1. Staphylococcus epidermidis | Staphylococcus epidermidis | positive |
| | 2. Staphylococcus epidermidis | Staphylococcus epidermidis | positive |
| | 3. Staphylococcus epidermidis | Staphylococcus epidermidis | positive |
| | 4. Staphylococcus epidermidis | Staphylococcus epidermidis/ Staphylococcus coag.neg | n.a. |
| | 5. Staphylococcus epidermidis/ Corynebacter spp. | Staphylococcus epidermidis/ Staphylococcus coag.neg | positive |
| Assumed CVC related infections: n= 6 | 1. Stomatococcus mucilaginosus | negative | positive |
| | 2. Streptococcus aginosus/ Streptococcus viridans spp. | negative | positive |
| | 3. Staphylococcus epidermidis | negative | positive |
| | 4. Enterococcus faecium | negative | positive |
| | 5. Streptococcus viridans spp. | negative | positive |
| | 6. Streptococcus oralis | negative | positive |
| Possible CVC related infections: n= 6 | 1. Staphylococcus epidermidis | negative | negative |
| | 2. Staphylococcus epidermidis | negative | negative |
| | 3. Staphylococcus coag.neg./ Staphylococcus epidermidis | negative | negative |
| | 4. Candida tropicalis | negative | negative |
| | 5. Staphylococcus epidermidis/ Staphylococcus coag.neg./ Enterococcus faecalis | negative | negative |
| | 6. Staphylococcus epidermidis/ negative Streptococcus mitis/ Pseudomonas aeruginosa | negative | |

related infection as defined, however, was observed in 5 febrile episodes only. These CVC-infections related to coagulase-negative staphylococci in all cases. In another 6 episodes, a CVC-related infection was suspicious, characterized by a local inflammation and a positive blood culture (Table 3).

Six further febrile episodes were considered to be a possible CVC-related infection (Table 3). In these episodes, positive blood cultures with microorganisms typical for a CVC-infection were observed without any other apparent clinical focus. The overall incidence of CVC-infection in acute leukemia patients was found to be 6,5/1000 CVC-days (1,9 proven/2,3 suspected/2,3possible/1000 CVC-days).

Within 32 out of 119 cycles of chemotherapeutic treatment, no febrile episode occurred. A total of 42 CVC had been inserted in these cycles. A local inflammation at the insertion site of the CVC had been documented in 19 of these CVCs.

## Discussion

Despite important advances in preventive measures, CVC-related infections are considered to be a significant source of bacteremia in cancer patients [8]. Data regarding the incidence of CVC-related infections are rare in patients with acute leukemia. Our prospective study focuses on patients at high risk for infectious complications because of a long and severe neutropenia. Although local inflammation at insertion site was commonly found in more than half of the patients with febrile neutropenia, colonization of the CVC-tip was observed less often (24,1%) with a proven CVC-related infection documented in 5,7% of febrile episodes only. The incidence of CVC-related colonization and bacteremia in our study was comparable with the control arm of a trial recently reported by Carratala et al. who found an incidence of catheter colonization of 15.8% and a CVC-related bacteremia of 7.0% in cancer patients with a neutropenia of <500/µl [9]. In the trial of Carratala et al., no data are stated on local inflammation. Raad et al. [10] reported a 2.6% rate of inflammation at the insertion site for short subclavian CVCs. Local inflammation at insertion site was considerably higher in our study. This may be due to a more severe and longer lasting neutropenia or our common practice of the jugular vein for insertion. Our data, however, confirm the observation of Raad et al. [10] that most of the exit-site inflammations did not predispose patients to catheter bacteremia. Since prospective data on nontunneled CVCs in acute leukemia patients are lacking, we compared the incidence of CVC-related bacteremia to a trial on tunneled CVCs. Engelhard et al [11] reported on a 5-year prospective study with 242 bone marrow transplant patients with a tunneled Hickman/Broviac catheter. They showed a septicemia incidence of 7.0% with a colonization incidence of 7%. There was, however, a remarkable low incidence of exit site infection (3.7%) in that trial [11].

## Conclusion

Although exit-site infection in patients with acute leukemia undergoing intensive chemotherapy was common, a CVC-related bacteremia was low. Nontunneled CVCs offer a safe alternative to surgically implantable tunneled catheters in patients with acute leukemia.

## References

1. Carratala J, Gudiol F: Changing epidemiology of bacterial infections in neutropenic patients with cancer; in Karthaus M, Ganser A (eds): Supportive Care in Cancer Patients- Recent Developments. Basel, Karger, 1999, pp 1–9.
2. Gonzalez Barca E, Fernandez Sevilla A, Carratala J, et al: Prospective study of 288 episodes of bacteremia in neutropenic cancer patients in a single institution. Eur J Clin Microbiol Infect Dis 1996; 15:291–296.
3. Salwender HJ, Egerer G, Bach A, et al: Central venous catheter-related complications; in Karthaus M, Ganser A (eds): Supportive Care in Cancer Patients. Recent Developments. Basel, Karger, 2000, pp 133–143.
4. Howell PB, Walters PE, Donowitz GR, et al: Risk factors for infection of adult patients with cancer who have tunnelled central venous catheters. Cancer 1995;75:1367–1375.
5. Raad I: Intravascular-catheter-related infections. Lancet 1998;351:893–898.
6. Kappers Klunne MC, Degener JE, Stijnen T, et al: Complications from long-term indwelling central venous catheters in hematologic patients with special reference to infection. Cancer 1989; 64: 1747–1752.

7. Maki DG, Weise CE, Sarafin HW: A semiquantitative culture method for identifying intravenous-catheter-related infection. N Engl J Med 1977; 296: 1305–1309.
8. Garaventa A, Castagnola E, Dallorso S, et al: Sepsis in children with malignant neoplasia, equipped with a Broviac-type venous catheter. Pediatr Med Chir 1995;17:147–150.
9. Carratala J, Niubo R, Fernandez-Sevilla A, et al: Randomized, double-blind trial of an antibiotic-lock technique for prevention of gram-positive central venous catheter-related infection in neutropneic patients with cancer. Antimicrobial Agents and Chemotherapy 1999;43:2200–2204.
10. Raad I, Davis S, Becker M, et al: Low infection rate and long durability of nontunneled silastic catheters. A safe and cost-effective alternative for long-term venous access. Arch Intern Med 1993; 153: 1791–1796.
11. Engelhard D, Elishoov H, Strauss N, et al: Nosocomial coagulase-negative staphylococcal infections in bone marrow transplantation recipients with central vein catheter. A 5-year prospective study. Transplantation 1996;61:430–434.

# Do we Need a Triple Antibiotic Therapy?

G. Heussel, C.P. Heussel, A. Ullmann, D. Domkin, M. Klousche, G. Derigs and K. Kolbe

## Purpose

To compare the efficacy and toxicity of triple antibiotic therapy in patients undergoing autologous peripheral blood-stem-cell transplantation (PBSCT) with literature data.

## Patients

138 patients (66 female, 72 male) were treated with high dose chemotherapy followed by stem cell support for non Hodgkin lymphoma (30%), breast cancer (25%), multiple myeloma (16%), chronic myeloic leukemia (10%) and other diseases (19%). Quinolones were administrated prophylactically. After

developing fever, the patient received triple therapy of Piperacillin-Tazobactam, Netilmycin, and Vancomycin.

## Results

Bacteriemia was detected in 45% of patients. Pneumonia was diagnosed in 14% of the patients using high-resolution computed tomography. 138 microorganisms were identified.

Overall response defined by defervescence of the patients was seen in 75% after 48h to first line antibiotic therapy Piperacillin-Tazobactam, Netilmycin, and Vancomycin. 14% of the patients responded after adding Ampho-

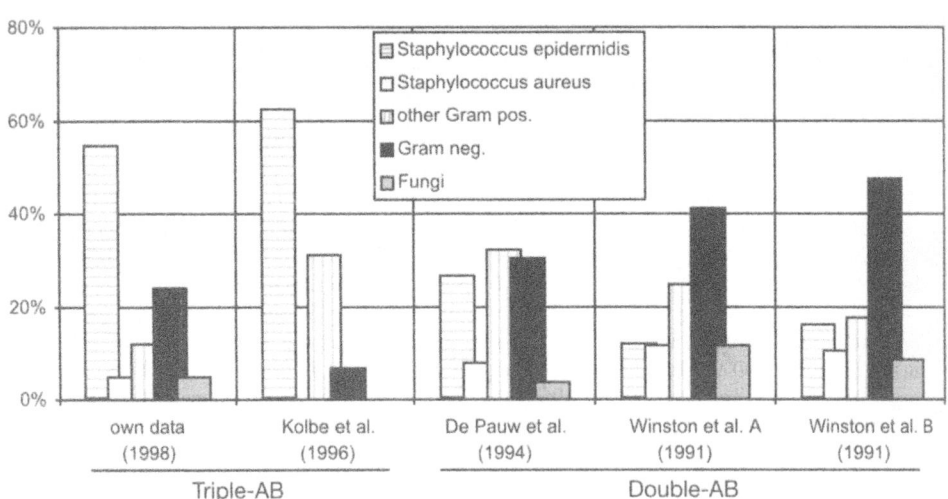

**Fig. 1.** Relative frequency of microorganisms detected in the different studies. The frequency of staphylococcus aureus is comparable in all studies.

Internal Medicine III, Johannes Gutenberg-University, Mainz, Germany

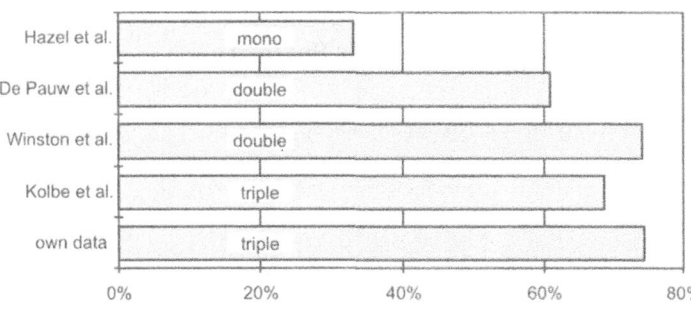

**Fig. 2.** The overall response to antibiotic therapy is comparable to data given in literature for double antibiotic therapy. A relevant advantage can be seen in comparison to a mono antibiotic therapy strategy.

**Table 1.** Frequency of identified microorganisms.

| Identified Microorganisms | total: 83 |
|---|---|
| **Gram positive** | 59 (71%) |
| Staphylococcus epidermidis | 45 |
| Oxacilline resistant | 29 / 45 |
| Oxacilline sensitive | 16 / 45 |
| Staphylococcus aureus (sensitive) | 4 |
| Streptococcus viridans | 4 |
| Corynebacteroids | 2 |
| Micrococci | 2 |
| Clostridium difficile | 1 |
| non-differentiated | 1 |
| **Gram negative** | 20 (25%) |
| Pseudomonas aeruginosa | 7 |
| Escherichia coli | 4 |
| Enterobacter cloacae | 4 |
| Acinetobacter lwolfii | 2 |
| Xantomonas maltophilia | 1 |
| Serratia marzescens | 1 |
| Fusobacterium nucleatum | 1 |
| **Fungi** | 4 (5%) |
| Candida species | 3 |
| Aspergillus species | 1 |

**Table 2.** Clinical outcome and patient' data.

| Febrile episodes after autologous PBSCT | | n=138 |
|---|---|---|
| | Tazobac | 102 (74%) |
| frequency of | Amphotericin B | 20 (14%) |
| response to | other AB | 6 (4%) |
| | reconstitution | 5 (4%) |
| | change of CVC | 2 (1%) |
| duration of fever [d] | | 4.5 (1–19) |
| duration of neutropenia (ANG < 1000/µl) [d] | | 9.9 (5–21) |
| duration of hospitalization [d] | | 26.9 (17–81) |
| duration of antibiotic therapy [d] | | 8.0 (1–23) |
| frequency of allergic reactions (erythema) | | 5 (4%) |

The large number of gram pos. bacteriemia with S. epidermidis associated with line contamination underlines the point of not applying Vancomycin in the first line therapy of neutropenic patients.

tericin B (after a total of 96h), another 4% responded after changing the antibiotics, after hematological reconstitution or after reinserting a new central venous catheter 4% respectively 1% defervesced.

## Conclusion

Compared with literature data, Piperacillin-Tazobactam, Netilmycin, and Vancomycin was as effective as Piperacillin / aminoglycoside or cephalosporin with overall response in patients with autologous peripheral blood-stem-cell transplantation of approximately 75%.

## References

1. De Pauw BE, Deresinski SC, Feld R, Lane-Allman EF, Donnelly JP. Ceftazidime compared with piperacillin and tobramycin for the empiric treatment of fever in neutropenic patients with cancer. A multicenter randomized trial. The Intercontinental Antimicrobial Study Group. Ann Intern Med. (1994) 120: 834–844
2. Hazel DL, Graham J, Dickinson JP, Newland AC, Kelsey SM. Piperacillin-tazobactam as empiric monotherapy in febrile neutropenic patients with hematological malignancies. J Chemother (1997) 9: 267–272
3. Kolbe K, Domkin D, Derigs HG, Bhakdi S, Huber C, Aulitzky WE. Infectious complications during neutropenia subsequent to peripheral blood stem cell transplantation. BMT (1997) 19: 143–147
4. Winston DJ, Ho, WG, Bruckner DA, Champlin RE. Beta-Lactam Antibiotic Therapy in Febrile Granulocytopenic Patients: A Randomized Trial Comparing ceroperazone plus Piperacillin, Ceftazidime plus Piperacilin, and Imipenem Alone. Ann Intern Med (1991) 115: 849–859

# Study of G-CSF Influences on CD10 and CD64 Distribution on Neutrophils in Leukemic Patients

S. Wehner, S. Weber, E. Niegemann and U. Ebener

*Abstract.* Following chemotherapy the regeneration of granulopoiesis as well as the expanding of peripheral blood stem cells nowadays is supported by the administration of granulocyte-colony stimulating factor (G-CSF). This cytokine is known to alter the immunological profile of granulocytes and to activate neutrophils. CD10 (NEP/CALLA), found on the membrane of about 90% of polymorphonuclear granulocytes (PMNs) is responsible for degrading oligopeptides (i.e. fMLP). CD64 (IgG receptor FcγRI) verifiable on nearly 50% of mature PMNs is mainly involved in the presentation of antigens and decisive participates the oxidative burst.

The present study was initiated to distinguish the effects of antigenic pattern referring to CD10 and CD64 performing FACS-analysis in patients suffering from hematological and oncological diseases (n = 19). For a control we analysed PMNs derived from healthy donors (n = 36) as well as umbilical cord blood (UCB; n = 33).

Compared to the control subjects, G-CSF treatment diminished CD10 antigen expression significantly, whereas CD64 is significantly increased. After finishing application of hematopoetic growth factor, percentages of CD10 and CD64 again reached values of donors. Most interestingly, UCB-PMNs of newborns likewise showed reduced CD10 values, too, similar to the effect of G-CSF therapy (29/33). In the contrary only 50% of investigated infants showed increased expression of CD64 (16/33).

The observation of likewise diminished CD10 expression on PMNs in cord blood may indicate an immature state of phagocytic system in newborns. We therefore presume that down regulation of CD10 in G-CSF treated patients could be justified due to a shortened maturation time of neutrophils under G-CSF therapy. Its functional consequences still remain to be investigated.

## Introduction

Granulocyte colony-stimulating factor (G-CSF) is a predominantly lineage-specific hematopoietic growth factor that acts upon cells of the neutrophil lineage [1]. This cytokine has been shown ton increase the production of neutrophils, to accelerate neutrophil recovery through amplification in the bone marrow maturation compartment and to demonstrate clinical benefits in patients receiving intensive cytotoxic chemotherapy [2, 3]. It stimulates neutrophil function by both amplifying the cell number of cell divisions and by accelerating the maturation of neutrophils to enter the blood. Current data indicate that neutrophils produced following stimulation with G-CSF have normal or near normal functional capacities [4, 5, 6, 7]. G-CSF is involved to effects such as priming on neutrophil superoxide production activated by N-formyl-Met-Leu-Phe (fMLP) [4, 8] as well as the enhancement of phagocytic and cytotoxic capacity and chemotaxis [9]. As recently demonstrated, apart from regeneration of granulopoiesis, application of G-CSF causes changes in the immunological marker profile of granulocytes, too [10, 11, 12, 13].

Dedicated to Prof. Dr. Dr. h.c. Bernhard Kornhuber

J. W. Goethe University, Clinic of Pediatrics-III, Department of Hematology and Oncology, Theodor-Stern-Kai 7, D-60590 Frankfurt/M., Germany

## Objective

Alterations in neutrophil pheontype, so the up-regulation of intracellular located CD10 following in-vitro stimulation using fMLP and other activating chemokines, have been described yet [14, 15, 16]. The common acute lymphoblastic leukemia antigen called CALLA (CD10) in the meantime is known to be a neutral endopeptidase (NEP), expressed on the surface of subsets of ALL blasts, on a minor population of bone marrow precursor cells and on about 95% of neutrophils. CD10 antigen cooperates with the aminopeptidase N (CD13) in degrading N-formyl-methionine-leucyl-phenylalanine (fMLP), an oligopeptide, which itself upregulates CD10 and CD13 (Fig. 1) [17]. The present study was initiated to distinguish the effects of G-CSF therapy on the expression of CD10/NEP on granulocytes. Moreover we were interested in the antigenic pattern of CD64 (IgG receptor Fc gamma RI), present on nearly 50% of quiescent polymorphonucleated cells (PMNs). Fcγ receptor I, a 72 kDa-Glycoprotein, acts as an high affinity receptor for IgG immunoglobulins' Fc-fragments. These molecules mediate functions such as antibody-dependent cellular cytotoxicity (ADCC), phagocytosis, degranulation and immune complex clearence. The main task of CD64 (FcγRI) is the presentation of antigens and the generation of oxidative burst [10, 13, 18, 19, 20].

## Material and Methods

### Patients

To the present study 19 pediatrics from our department and clinic of internal medicine Frankfurt/Main suffering from various malignancies were comprised. The patients group consisted of the following diseases: acute leukemias, lymphoma, neuroblastomas, aplastic anaemias, rhabdomyosarcomas, eppendymoma, hemophagocytosis syndrome, medulloblastima and M. Hodgkin's disease. The distribution of patients to various malignancies is summarized in Table 1. Because of neutro-

**Table 1.** Patients and Control Subjects Enrolled to the Present Study

| Patients undergoing G-CSF therapy, n = 19 | | |
|---|---|---|
| Children (n = 15) | Adults (n = 4) | |
| Aplastic Anaemia | 2 | | |
| Acute Leukemia | 4 | | |
| B-Lymphoma | 1 | | |
| Eppendymoma | 1 | AML | 2 |
| Hemophagocytosis | 2 | ALL | 1 |
| Syndrome | | M. Hodgkin's | 1 |
| Medulloblastoma | 1 | Disease | 1 |
| Neuroblastoma | 3 | | |
| Rhabdomyosarcoma | 1 | | |

| Controls n = 69 | |
|---|---|
| Adults | 26 |
| Children | 10 |
| Newborns | 33 |

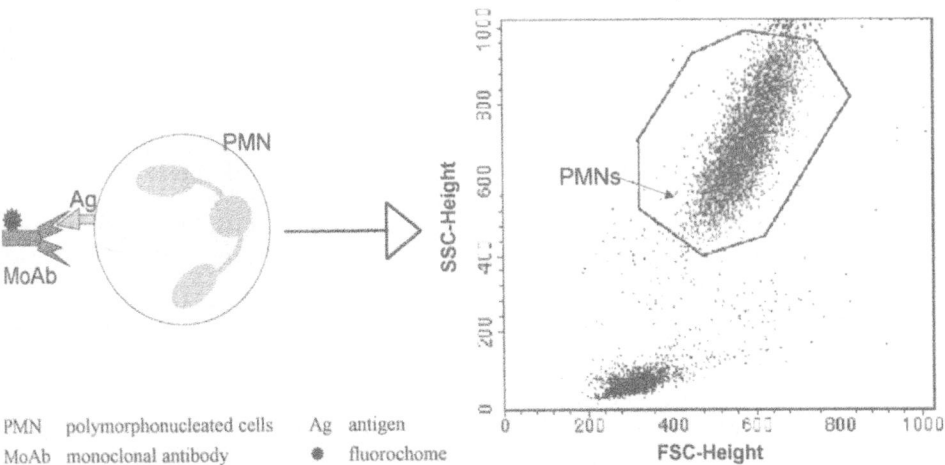

| PMN | polymorphonucleated cells | Ag | antigen |
|---|---|---|---|
| MoAb | monoclonal antibody | ● | fluorochome |

**Fig. 1.** Direct Immunofluorescence-Technique (FACS-analysis; whole lysed blood procedure)

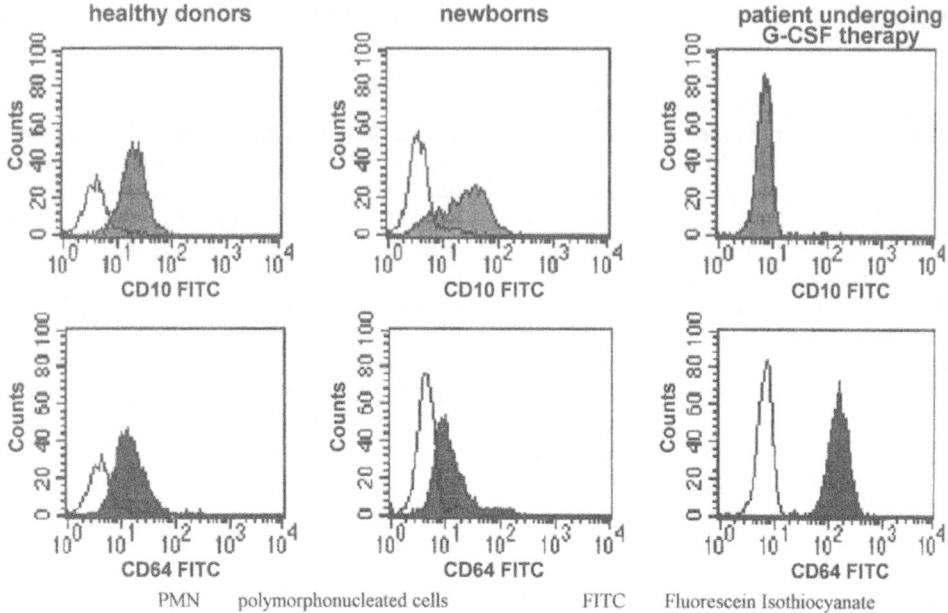

**Fig. 2.** Expression of CD10 and CD64 antigens on PMNs (FACS-analysis of various specimens)

penia due to chemotherapy all patients were undergoing rhG-CSF treatment (Amgen, Thousand Oaks, USA). As a control we chose PMNs form hematologically healthy children (n = 10) and adults (n = 26), as well as from cord blood (n = 33).

## Methods

Freshly derived heparinized peripheral blood was collected and immediately used for immunophenotyping by using saturating concentrations of FITC- or PE-conjugated monoclonal antibodies. Monoclonal antibodies (MoAbs) used in this study were obtained from Coulter/Immunotech, Hamburg/Germany and Becton Dickinson, Heidelberg/Germany. As a nonspecific fluorescence control, cells were incubated with isotype control (IgG1 Becton Dickinson, Heidelberg/Germany). Following an incubation time of 30 min in the dark at room temperature, 2 ml of lysing solution (Becton Dickinson, Heidelberg/Germany) were added. After a 10 min incubation period cells were washed out twice with phosphate buffered saline (PBS) at 300 g. The pellet was resuspended in 500 μl of

PBS and stored at 4°C in the dark until FACS.analysis.

Multidimensional flow cytometry was performed according to standard techniques on a FACScan cytometer (Becton Dickinson, Heidelberg) with serial filter configuration. Data from whole lysed peripheral blood from patients and healthy donors were collected using Cell Quest software. Electronic compensation was used between the FITC and PE fluorescence channels to correct spectral overlay of applied fluorochromes. Polymorphonucleated cells (PMNs) were identified in FSC vs. SSC Dot-plots (Fig. 1), gated, in order to subsequently analyse PMNs selectively for expression of CD10 and CD64 antigens in SSC vs. FL1-H respectively SSC vs. FL2-H Dot plots or FL1-H; FL2-H histograms (Fig. 2). A total of 10.000 events was acquired routinely and list mode files were evaluated using Cell Quest Software.

## Results

Representative FL1-H histograms (FACS-analysis) for the expression of CD10 and CD64 in healthy controls and umbilical cord blood as

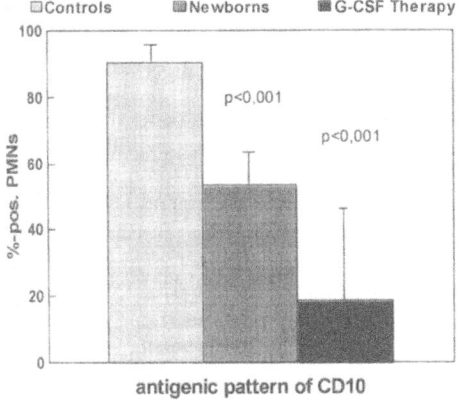

**Fig. 3.** Expression of CD10 on PMNs

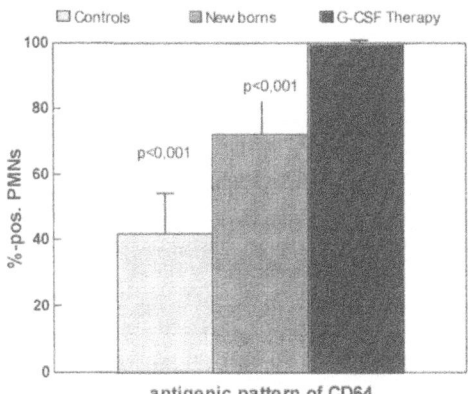

**Fig. 4.** Expression of CD64 on PMNs.

well as on neutrophils from patients under the influence of G-CSF are displayed in Figure 2. A summary of our results is given in Figure 3 and Figure 4. In peripheral blood derived from healthy donors, CD10 was found on nearly 95% of mature PMNs (Fig. 2/3). On the other hand CD64 regularly was detectable on approximately 50% of controls PMNs (Fig. 2/4). Compared to the control subjects, G-CSF treatment diminished CD10 antigen expression significantly (95% vs. 32%), whereas CD64-positivity is significantly increased (50% vs. 99%; Fig. 2/3/4. This strong expression of FcγRI (CD64) on neutrophils from patients during G-CSF treatment is in confirmation with reports previously described by Repp et al. [10]. Most interestingly, umbilical cord blood-PMNs of newborns likewise showed diminished CD10 values, too, mimicking the effect of G-CSF therapy. In the contrary only 50% of investigated infants showed increased CD64 expression (Fig. 2/3/4.

In order to proof the appearance of CD10-negative PMN-subpopulations during application of G-CSF, we started chronological studies. The results of those kinetic investigations are given in Figure 5. In advance to a treatment with hematopoietic growth factor G-CSF, PMNs, positive for CD10 antigen, dominate unequivocally. Subsequently on the 4th day of G-CSF application a marked reduction of CD10 and a continual increase in the number of CD10 negative neutrophils as well can be demonstrated (Fig. 5). After finishing G-CSF therapy, percentages of CD10 and

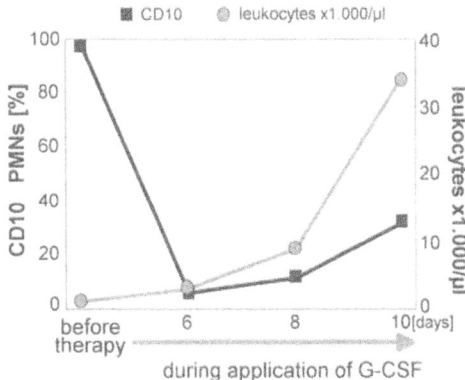

**Fig. 5.** CD10-Expression and Leukocyte Content during G-CSF Therapy

CD64 again reached values of donors (data not shown).

## Discussion

In the primary defense against invading micro-organisms neutrophil polymorphonucleated cells (PMNs) play a key role. Following stimulation, neutrophils leave the circulation and enter the inflamed site. For this purpose they express receptors on their plasma membranes for IgG antibodies and complement fragments present on opsonized bacteria. Certain cytokines have shown to be able to induce PMNs to express the high affinity FcγRI (CD64). In consens with others we found that neutrophils likewise under the influence of G-CSF are different from those of healthy donors [11, 12, 21, 22]. Our results verify that in addition to the expression of neutrophil endopeptidase (CD10) the FcγRI (CD64) is changed under hematopoietic growth factor [23, 24]. While CD64 is increased significantly, CALLA/NEP (CD10) is decreased markedly compared to healthy donors. Comparable results referring to the distribution of antigens CD10 and CD64 can be shown for UCB-PMNs, not treated with G-CSF. Those mimicking effects in PB-PMNs from patients administered with G-CSF and UCB-PMNs might be justified by similar effects. Both materials might be characterized by one corresponding correlation; it is a similarity in immaturity of PMNs released from the bone marrow into the circulation. G-CSF is shown to be primarily responsible for differentiation of myeloid precursors into neutrophils and the shortening of the maturation [9]. This assumption is emphasized by several authors, who indicate, too, other mechanisms, i.e. release of partially immature granulocytes from the bone marrow or indirect activation of the cells, might be responsible for those alterations found rather than direct influence of G-CSF [11, 12, 25, 26]. They confirm, that during differentiation from metamyelocytes towards mature granulocytes, for example a continuous downregulation of FcγRI expression can be observed, too. Experimental results derived from long-term cultures of CD34+ progenitors during application of G-CSF have shown that the induced mature neutrophils remain positive for FcγRI, whereas this receptor is regularly lost in the metamyelocyte stage [26, 27]. On the other hand, an activation of granulocytes can also induce profound alterations in surface antigen expression, namely an upregulation of FcγRI, even thought G-CSF is known to be a weak activator of neutrophils in vitro.

CD10, the antigen we were interested in the present study, too, was originally defined as the "common acute lymphoblastic antigen" (CALLA), a marker for "null" ALL [28]. Since this time CD10 turned out to be an important marker in the diagnosis and classification of acute leukemias and characterization of the immature types of the B-lineage ALLs (i.e. pre-B-ALL) [29]. CD10 as well as shown to be expressed in a variety of cells including a small subpopulation of bone marrow cells from healthy donors [30], renal cells [31] and cultured fibroblasts [32]. In addition nearly all granulocytes from healthy donors demonstrate CD10 [32]. Following identification of CALLA as a neutral endopeptidase 24.11 (NEP) the expression of CD10 on neutrophils was correlated with endopeptidase activity [33, 34]. NEP/CD10 divides several oligopeptides, i.e. chemotactical fMLP, and therefore functions as an immunomodulating protein. Additionally other peptides, f.e. natriuretical factor (ANF) are divided, as well [35].

Even though there are reports not only concerning antigen expressions but also functional activations of PMNs is following G-CSF application, i.e. an enhancement of superoxide anion release or an increased adherence to the endothelium of the blood vessels shortly after administration [4, 11, 20]. Authors report about an amplification of cytotoxicity of G-CSF-primed neutrophils, too, not to be blocked completely by antibodies directed against FcγRII binding site and may be an indication for an involvement of CD64. Other researchers have recently described influences concerning a decreased motility/migration of G-CSF-induced granulocytes in vitro as well as in vivo [10, 36]. The clinical consequences of such altered immunophenotype and function are not clear yet.

## Summary

In the present study neutrophils from 19 patients receiving G-CSF therapy were studied in-vitro for surface antigenic pattern and compared to PMNs derived from healthy donors and umbilical cord blood. We found that the expression of CD10 was strongly diminished during treatment with hematopoietic growth factor, whereas the expression of CD64 significantly was enhanced in these patients. The observation of likewise reduced CD10 expression on polymorphonucleated cells in cord blood, may indicate an immature state of phagocyte system in newborns. We therefore presume, that down-regulation of CD10 in G-CSF treated patients could be justified due to a shortened maturation time of granulocytes under G-CSF therapy. Its functional consequences still remain to be investigated.

*Acknowledgement.* This work was supported by "Hilfe für Krebskranke Kinder Frankfurt e.V.".

# References

1. Demetri GD, Griffin JD (1991) Granulocyte colony-stimulating factor and its receptor. Blood 78 (11): 2791–2808
2. Bensinger W, Price TH, Dale DC, Appelbaum FR, Clift R, Lilleby K, Williams B, Storb R, Thomas ED, Buckner CD (1993) The effects of daily recombinant human granulocyte colony-stimulating factor administration on normal granulocyte donors undergoing leukapheresis. Blood 81 (7): 1883–1888
3. Lieschke GJ, Burgess AW (1992) Granulocyte colony-stimulating factor and granulocyte-macrophage colony-stimulating factor (in two parts). New England Journal of Medicine 327 (1): 28–35 and 327 (2): 99–106
4. Lindemann A, Herrmann F, Oster W, Haffner G, Meyenburg W, Souza LM, Mertelsmann R (1989) Hematologic effects of recombinant human granulocyte colony-stimulating factor in patients with malignancy. Blood 74 (8): 2644–2651
5. Bronchud MH, Potter MR, Morgenstern G, Blasco MJ, Scarffe JH, Thatcher N, Crowther D, Souza LM, Alton NK, Testa NG (1988) In vitro and in vivo analysis of the effects of recombinant human granulocyte colony-stimulating factor in patients. British Journal of Cancer 58 (1): 64–69
6. Rösler J, Emmendörffer A, Elsner J, Zeidler C, Lohmann-Matthes M, Welte K (1991) In vitro functions of neutrophils included by treatment with rhG-CSF in severe congenital neutropenia. European J of Haematology 46 (2): 112–118
7. Welte K, Zeidler C, Reiter A, Mueller W, Odenwald E, Souza L, Riehm H (1990) Differential Effects of Granulocyte-Macrophage Colony-Stimulating Factor and Granulocyte Colony-Stimulating Factor in Children With Severe Congenital Neutropenia. Blood 75 (5): 1056–1063
8. Yuo A, Kitagawa S, Ohsaka A, Oht M, Miyazono K, Okabe T, Urabe A, Saito M, Takaku F (1989) Recombinant Human Granulocyte Colony-Stimulating Factor as an Activator of Human Granulocytes: Potentiation of Responses Triggered by Receptor-Mediated Agonists and Stimulation of C3bi Receptor Expression and Adherence. Blood 74 (6): 2144–2149
9. Welte K, Gabrilove J, Bronchud MH, Platzer E, Morstyn G (1996) Filgrastin (r-metHuGCSF): The first 10 years. Blood 88 (6): 1907–1929
10. Repp R, Valerius T, Sendler A, Gramatzki M, Iro H, Kalden JR, Platzer E (1991) Neutrophils express the high affinity receptor for IgG (Fc gamma RI, CD64) after in vivo application of recombinant human granulocyte colony-stimulating factor. Blood 78 (4): 885–889
11. Spiekermann K, Roesler J, Elsner J, Link H, Freund M, Welte K, Lohmann-Matthes M-L, Emmendoerffer A (1994) Kinetic of Human Neutrophil Surface Marker Expression and Chemotaxis During Granulocyte Colony-Stimulating Factor Treatment. In: Freund/Link/Schmidt/Welte (eds) Cytokines in Hematopoiesis, Oncology, and Immunology III. Springer, Berlin-Heidelberg, pp 103–113
12. Spiekermann K, Emmendoerffer A, Elsner J, Raeder E, Lohmann-Matthes M-L, Prahst A, Link H, Freund M, Welte K, Roesler J (1994) Altered surface marker expression and function of G-CSF-induced neutrophils from test subjects and patients under chemotherapy. British J of Haematology 87 (1): 31–38
13. Valerius T, Repp R, de Wit TP, Berthold S, Platzer E, Kalden JR, Gramatzki M, van de Winkel JG (1993) Involvement of the high-affinity receptor for IgG (FcγRI, CD64) in enhanced tumor cell cytotoxicity of neutrophils during granulocyte-colony stimulating factor therapy. Blood 82 (3): 931–939
14. Werfel T, Sonntag G, Weber MH, Gotze O (1991) Rapid increases in the membrane expression of neutral endopeptidase (CD10), aminopeptidase N (CD13), tyrosine phosphatase (CD45) and Fc gamma-RIII (CD16) upon stimulation of human peripheral leukocytes with human C5a. J Immunol 147 (11): 3909–3914
15. Connelly JC, Chambless R, Holiday D, Chittenden K, Johnson AR (1993) Up-regulation of neutral endopeptidase (CALLA) in human neutrophils by granulocyte-macrophage colony-stimulating factor. J Leukoc Biol 53 (6): 685–690
16. Shipp MA, Stefano GB, Switzer SN, Griffin JD, Reinherz EL (1991) CD10 (CALLA)/neutral endopeptidase 24.11 modulates inflammatory peptide-induced changes in neutrophil morphology, migration, and adhesion proteins and is itself regulated by neutrophil activation. Blood 78 (7): 1834–1841
17. Shipp MA, Look At (1993) Hemapoietic differentiation antigens that are membraneassociated enzymes: cutting is the key! Blood 82 (4): 1052–1070
18. Gergely J, Sarmay G (1990) The two binding-site models of human IgG binding Fcγ receptors. Federation of American Societies for Experimental Biology (FASEB). Journal 4 (15): 3275–3283
19. Ravetch JV, Kinet JP (1991) Fc receptors. Annual Review of Immunology 9: 457–492
20. Elsner J, Roesler J, Emmendorffer A, Zeidler C, Lohmann-Matthes ML, Welte K (1992) Altered function and surface marker expression of neutrophils induced by rhG-CSF treatment in severe congenital neutropenia. Eur J Haematol 48 (1): 10–19
21. Anderlini P, Przepiorka D, Champlin R, Korbling M (1996) Biologic and Clinical Effects of Granulocyte Colony-Stimulating Factor in Normal Individuals. Blood 88 (8): 2819–2825
22. Hansen PB, Kjaersgaard E, Johnson HE, Gram J, Pedersen M, Nikolajsen K, Hansen NE (1993) Different membrane expression of CD11b and CD14 on blood neutrophils following in vivo administration of myeloid growth factors. Br J Haematol 85 (1): 50–56
23. Zarco MA, Ribera JM, Villamor N, Balmes A, Urbano Ispizua A, Feliu E (1998) Phenotypic changes in neutrophil granulocytes after G-CSF administration in patients with acute lymphoblastic leukemia under chemotherapy. [letter] Haematologica 83 (6): 573–575

24. Hoglund M, Hakansson L, Venge P (1997) Effects of in vivo administration of G-CSF on neutrophil functions in healthy volunteers. European J of Hematology 58 (3): 195–202

25. Maeda M, van Schie RC, Yuksel B, Greenough A, Fanger MW, Guyre PM, Lydyard PM (1996) Differential expression of Fc receptors for IgG by monocytes and granulocytes from neonates and adults. Clinical & Experimental Immunology 103 (2): 343–347

26. Kerst JM, van de Winkel JG, Evans AH, de Haas M, Slaper-Cortenbach IC, de Wit TP, von dem Borne AE, van der Schoot CE, van Oers RH (1993) Granulocyte colony stimulating factor induces hFc gamma RI (CD64 antigen)-positive neutrophils via an effect on myeloid presursor cells. Blood 81 (6): 1457–1464

27. Olweus J, Lund-Johansen F, Terstappen LW (1995) CD64/Fc gamma RI is a granulomonocytic lineage marker on CD34+ hematopoietic progenitor cells. Blood 85 (9): 2402–2413

28. Ritz J, Pesando M, Notis-McConarty J, Larzarus J, Schlossman SF (1980) A monoclonal antibody to human acute lymphoblastic leukaemia antigen. Nature 283 (5747): 583–585

29. Bene MC, Castoldi G, Knapp W, Ludwig WD, Matutes E, Orfao A, van't Veer MB (1995) Proposals for the immunological classification of acute leukemias. European Group for the Immunological Characterization of Leukemias (EGIL). Leukemia 9 (10): 1783–1786

30. Greaves M, Delia D, Janossy G, Rapson N, Chessells J, Woods M, Prentice G (1980) Acute lymphoblastic leukemia associated antigen. IV. Expression on non-leukaemic "lymphoid" cells. Leukemia Research 4 (1): 15–32

31. Metzgar RS, Borowitz MJ, Jones NH, Dowell BL (1981) Distribution of common acute lymphoblastic leukemia antigen in nonhematopoietic tissues. J Exp Med 154 (4): 1249–1254

32. Braun MP, Martin PJ, Ledbetter JA, Hansen JA (1983) Granulocytes and Cultured Human Fibroblasts Express Common Acute Lymphoblastic Leukemia-Associated Antigens. Blood 61 (4): 718–725

33. Shipp MA, Vijayaraghavan J, Schmidt EV, Masteller EL, D'Adamio L, Hersh LB, Reinherz EL (1989) Common acute lymphoblastic leukemia antigen (CALLA) is active neutral endopeptidase 24.11 ("enkephalinase"): Direct evidence by cDNA transfection analysis Proceedings of the National Academy of Sciences of the United States of America 86 (1): 297–301

34. Iwamato I, Kimura A, Ochiai K, Tomioka H, Yoshida S (1991) Distribution of neutral endopeptidase activity in human blood leukocytes. J Leukoc Biol 49 (2): 116–125

35. Seymour AA, Abboa-Offei BE, Smith PL, Mathers PD, Asaad MM, Rogers WL (1995) Potentiation of natriuretic peptides by neutral endopeptidase inhibitors. Clinical & Experimental Pharmacology & Physiology 22 (1): 63–69

36. Price TH, Chatta GS, Dale DC (1992) The effect of recombinant granulocyte-colony stimulating factor (G-CSF) on neutrophil kinetics in normal human subjects. Blood 80: 350a (abstract)

# RHuGM-CSF (Molgramostim) in the Treatment of Children and Adolescents with Acute Myeloid Leukemia

S. Donska, J. Bazaluk and O. Ryzhak

## Introduction

Intensive chemotherapy protocols for treating patients with acute myeloid leukemias (AML) made it possible to achieve high remission rates (80–90%) and a 5-year EFS of about 50–60% in children and adolescents with these diseases (Leverger G. et al., 1994; Creutzig U. et al., 1999). However, the high intensity of induction and intensification courses led to long periods of severe bone marrow aplasia with an increased risk of morbidity and mortality due to infectious and bleeding complications.

From 1987 onward, hematopoetic growth factors – G-CSF and GM-CSF – have been used in clinical trials for reducing the duration of neutropenia and decreasing the number of infectious problems. Initial promising results notwithstanding, the safety of using these growth factors in patients with AML (Büchner T. et al, 1991)had to be confirmed by special prospective trials, since it had earlier been demonstrated that myeloid blast cells express receptors to G-CSF and GM-CSF (Kellner C.A. et al., 1988; Murohashi J. et al., 1989; De Gentile A. et al., 1992) and "in vitro" exposition to these factors could stimulate leukemic cell proliferation (Bradbury D. et al, 1992; Horicoshi A. et al., 1995). Some investigators utilized this fact by stimulating leucemic cells "in vivo" and eventually re-introducing them into the cell cycle prior to AraC chemotherapy. Several controlled studies in recent years have confirmed the beneficial effects and safe use of CSF in AML patients (Büchner T. et al., 1994; Rowe J. et al., 1995; Stone R. et al., 1995). These trials were, however, carried out in adult patients, and recent reports on the use of CSF in children and adolescents with AML are lacking. The introduction of a modern type protocol for the treatment of children and adolescents with de novo AML within the framework of the Cooperative AML Study in the Pediatric Group of Leukemias and Lymphomas in the Ukraine (PGLLU) – AML-PGLLU-95/97 – made it desirable to apply GM-CSF in order to reduce the rate of infectious problems in patients during intensive chemotherapy.

## Patients and Methods

MOLGRAMOSTIM, the recombinant human GM-CSF (Leucomax, "Novartis") was used in 12 children and adolescents with newly diagnosed AML from December 1995 to November 1998. AML variants were classified based on morphocytochemical and immunocytologic data according to FAB criteria. All patients were treated according to protocols AML-PGLLU-95 (Pilot) and -97 (modified AML-BFM-93) in the Pediatric Oncology-Hematology Department at the Kiev Regional Oncologic Dispensary.

GM-CSF therapy was considered indicated if:

1. neutropenia was<1000/µl later than day 21 from the start of induction (all patients had ≤5% bone marrow blasts on days 15 and 21 after induction),
2. febrile neutropenia arose during the consolidation phase and, as a result, protocol therapy had to be interrupted for more than 2 weeks
3. neutropenia was <1000/µl on days 6 to 8 after the start of intensification treatment.

Department of Pediatric Oncology-Hematology, Kiev Regional Oncologic Dispensary, Ukraine

**Table 1.** Patients with AML under GM-CSF therapy

| No. | Age | Sex | FAB variant | Risk group | Phase of protocol therapy | Daily Dose and duration of GM-CSF therapy |
|-----|-----|-----|-------------|------------|---------------------------|-------------------------------------------|
| 1. | 12 y | f | M6 | HRG 1 | Intensification I<br>Intensification II | 5 µg/kg; 4 days<br>5 µg/kg; 14 days |
| 2. | 5 y | f | M0 | HRG 2 | Induction II<br>Consolidation<br>Intensification I<br>Intensification II | 5 µg/kg; 9 days<br>5 µg/kg; 10 days<br>5 µg/kg; 8 days<br>5 µg/kg; 6 days |
| 3. | 10 y | f | M3 | SRG | Induction I<br>Intensification I | 5 µg/kg; 9 days<br>10 µg/kg; 9 days |
| 4. | 16 y | f | M3 | SRG | Intensification I<br>Maintenance | 5 µg/kg; 6 days<br>5 µg/kg; 6 days |
| 5. | 6 y | f | M4 | HRG 2 | Intensification I | 5 µg/kg; 9 days |
| 6. | 15 y | m | M4 | HRG 1 | Induction I<br>Intensification I | 5 µg/kg; 6 days<br>5 µg/kg; 5 days |
| 7. | 15 y | f | M5a | HRG 2 | Induction I<br>Induction II<br>Consolidation<br>Intensification I | 5 µg/kg; 6 days<br>5 µg/kg; 5 days<br>5 µg/kg; 2 days<br>5 µg/kg; 6 days |
| 8. | 17 y | m | M1 | HRG 1 | Consolidation<br>Intensification I<br>Intensification II | 5 µg/kg; 11 days<br>5 µg/kg; 14 days<br>5 µg/kg; 6 days |
| 9. | 5 y | f | M4 | HRG 1 | Induction I<br>Consolidation<br>Intensification I^<br>Intensification II | 5 µg/kg; 4 days<br>10 µg/kg; 14 days<br>5 µg/kg; 10 days<br>5 µg/kg; 10 days |
| 10. | 8 y | m | M1 | HRG 2 | Consolidation | 5 µg/kg; 7 days |
| 11. | 8 y | f | M1 | HRG 2 | Induction I<br>Consolidation | 5 µg/kg; 2 days<br>5 µg/kg; 5 days |
| 12. | 7 y | m | M7 | HRG 1 | Consolidation<br>Intensification I<br>Intensification II | 5 µg/kg; 5 days<br>5 µg/kg; 5 days<br>5 µg/kg; 11 days |

MOLGRAMOSTIM was used at a standard dose of 5µg/kg/day s.c. until recovery of the neutrophil count to above 1000/µl. 2 patients received GM-CSF at a dose of 10 µg/kg i.v. (as 6 h infusion) due to insufficient response to the initially given standard dose. Details on patients and episodes of GM-CSF use are given in Table 1.

## Results

A total of 12 patients received GM-CSF in 29 neutropenic episodes, for the most part (15 cases) following intensification courses; in 7 children, Leucomax was used during the consolidation phase of the protocol, 6 times it was given after the first and/or second induction, and 1 patient received GM-CSF during maintenance therapy due to agranulocytosis caused by viral hepatitis B. Leucomax was used for periods of 2 to 14 days (median: 6 days).

All of these patients achieved complete remission of AML. We did not register any sign of leukemic proliferation during or after any of 29 GM-CSF treatment episodes. After an observation period of 3 to 34 months (median: 17.5 months), there has been no AML relapse in this group. Only one patient died in remission due to fulminant anaerobic infection during maintenance therapy. The probability for event-free survival (pEFS) at 34 months in this group is 0.89 (SD = 0.1).

## Discussion

Our preliminary results show safety of rHuGM-CSF administration in children and adolescents with de novo AML under all phases of intensive chemotherapy, induction therapy included.

The comparably high level of pEFS in our group of children and adolescents with AML, even considering the large proportion of high risk patients, might be not only due to the decreased risk of severe infectious complications, but also to some contribution of rHuGM-CSF to the antileukemic effects of chemotherapy as demonstrated by some studies using different CSFs in adult patients (Bassan R. et al., 1994, Bettelheim P. Valent P. 1991 ).

Our preliminary results suggest high efficacy and safety of rHuGM-CSF application in children and adolescents with de novo AML and could be the basis of future controlled trials.

## References

1. Bassan R, Rambaldi A (1994) Unexpected remission of acute myeloid leukemia after GM-CSF. Brit J Haematol 87:835–838.
2. Bettelheim P, Valent P, et al (1991) granulocyte-macrophage colony-stimulating factor in combination with standard induction chemotherapy in de novo acute myeloid leukemia. Blood 77: 700–711.
3. Bradbury D, Rogers S (1992) Role of autocrine and paracrine production of granulocyte-macrophage colony-stimulating factor and interleukin-1b in the autonomous growth of acute myeloblastic leukemia cells-Studies using purified CD34-positive cells. Leukemia 6: 562–566.
4. Büchner T, Hiddeman W (1991) Recombinant human granulocyte-macrophage colony-stimulating factor after chemotherapy in patients with acute myeloid leukemia at higher age or after relapse Blood 78: 1190–1197.
5. Büchner T, Hiddemann W (1994) GM-CSF multiple course priming and long-term administration in newly diagnosed AML. Hematologic and therapeutic effects. Blood 84 (suppl 1): 27a
6. Creutzig U, Ritter J (1999) AML-BFM 93: Risk - adapted therapy and randomization in children with AML: Preliminary results. Ann Hematol 78 (Suppl II): 12
7. De Gentile A, Schlageter M.N. )1992) Djnnees actuelles sur les recepteurs du GM-CSF dans les leucemies aigues myeloides. Bulletin du Cancer 79: 123–131.
8. Horicoshi A, Sawada S (1995) Relationship between responsiveness to colony stimulation factors (CSFs) and surface phenotype of leukemic blasts. Leukemia Research 19: 195–201.
9. Kelleher C.A., Wong G.G. (1998) Binding of iodinated recombinant human GM-CSF to the blast of acute myeloblastic leukemia. Leukemia 2: 211–215.
10. Leverger G, Leblanc T, et aut (1994) Leucemies aigues myeloblastiques (LAM) de l'enfant amelioration du prognostic par l'intensification therapeutique. Resultats preliminaires du protocole LAME 89/91. Nouv. Rev. Fr. Hematol 36 (Supp II): 144.
11. Murobashi J, Thoda S (1989) Specific binding of radioiodinated human GM-CSF to the blast cell of acute myeloblastic leukemia. Leukemia Research 13: 599–604.
12. Rowe J, Andersen J.W. (1995) A randomized placebo-controlled Phase III study of granulocyte-macrophage colony-stimulating factor in adult patients ( > 55 to 70 years of age) with acute mayelogenouse leukemia: A study of the Eastern Cooperative Oncoloy Group (E1490). Blood 86: 457–462.
13. Ryzhak O, Donska S, et al. (1999): Preliminary results of a multicentre therapy study for the treatment of children and adolescents with AML in the Ukraine, in Acute Leukemias, Treatment Strategies and Risk Factors VIII, Ed: Büchner T, et al (2000) ....
14. Stone R.M., Berg D.T. (1995): Granulocyte-macrophage colony-stimulating factor after initial chemotherapy for elderly patients with primary acute myelogenouse leukemia. New Engl J Med 332: 1671–1677.

**ALL in Children**

# CCG Experience with the Augmented BFM Regimen

J. B. NACHMANN

## Introduction

In 1981, the Children's Cancer Group (CCG) first utilized a chemotherapy program modeled after the Berlin-Frankfurt-Munster 76-79 protocol in an effort to improve event free survival for children with acute lymphoblastic leukemia (ALL) and high risk features (WBC >50,000 and/or lymphomatous features) [1].

BFM studies utilized a seven day prednisone prophase in conjunction with measurement of peripheral blood blast count on day 7 to assess early response to therapy. Patients with >1000 blasts/mm³ in peripheral blood on day 7 were categorized as poor responders to prednisone (approximately 10% of patients).

Approximately 20–25% of ALL patients entered on CCG trials had <1000 peripheral blasts/mm3 at diagnosis and thus would derive no prognostic information from a prednisone prophase. Because of this finding, CCG investigators chose to give patients full induction therapy from day one and assess a day 7 marrow aspirate to measure early response. Patients with <25% blasts on a day 7 marrow aspirate were classified as rapid early responders (RER) while patients with >25% blasts were considered slow early responders (SER). The outcome for patients treated on the CCG-BFM pilot trial are shown in Table 1.

Patients with SER had a lower induction rate and a very poor EFS compared to patients with RER [2].

Utilizing four weeks of re-induction in protocol II resulted in prolonged myelosuppression and an unacceptable incidence of fungal infection. Therefore, in subsequent trials utilizing CCG modified BFM (C-BFM), a 3 week reinduction was used during protocol II. The post induction schema for C-BFM is shown in Table 2. In an effort to improve the outcome for high risk SER patients, CCG investigators developed the augmented BFM (A-BFM) chemotherapy program, also shown in Table 2.

### Early Use of C-BFM in CCG Trials

In 1989, CCG completed two randomized trials (106,123), which showed significant improvement in outcome for standard high risk patients (WBC >50,000: no lymphomatous features CCG 106) and for patients with lymphomatous features treated with C-BFM therapy [3]. The CCG 105 average risk showed that patients >10 years of age, WBC <50,000 and no lymphomatous features had a significant improvement in outcome utilizing C-BFM treatment compared to less aggressive treatment [4].

Therefore, a new definition for standard high risk was developed which included patients with age 1-9 and >50,000 WBC or age >10 and any WBC. Patients with lymphomatous features were excluded.

### The CCG 1882 Trial

The schema for the CCG 1882 standard high risk study is shown in Figure 1. Patients were

**Table 1.** Results of BFM Pilot by Early Response

|  | ≤25% Blasts Day 7 Marrow | >25% Blasts Day 7 Marrow |
| --- | --- | --- |
| # of Patients | 97 | 31 |
| Induction Rate | 96% | 90.3% |
| 4 Year EFS | 77% | 28% |

**Table 2.** The standard-therapy and augmented-therapy regimens.*

| Phase | Standard therapy Treatment | Dose | Phase | Augmented therapy Treatment | Dose |
|---|---|---|---|---|---|
| Consolidation (5 wk) | Prednisone | 7.5 mg/m²/day 0; 3.75 mg/m²/day days 1, 2 | Consolidation (9 wk) | Cyclophosphamide | 1000 mg/m²/day IV days 0, 28 |
| | Cyclophosphamide | 1000 mg/m²/day IV days 0, 14 | | Cytarabine | 75 mg/m²/day SQ or IV days 1–4, 8–11, 29–32, 36–39 |
| | Mercaptopurine | 60 mg/m²/day PO days 0–27 | | Mercaptopurine | 60 mg/m²/day PO days 0–13, 28–41 |
| | Vincristine | 1.5 mg/m²/day IV days 14, 21, 42, 49 | | Vincristine | 1.5 mg/m²/day IV days 14, 21, 42, 49 |
| | Cytarabine | 75 mg/m²/day IV days 1–4, 8–11, 15–18, 22–25 | | Asparaginase | 6000 U/m2/day IM days 14, 16, 18, 21, 23, 25, 42, 44, 46, 49, 51, 53 |
| | Methotrexate † | IT days 1, 8, 15, 22 | | Methotrexate † | IT days 1, 8, 15, 22 |
| | Radiotherapy ‡ | Cranial, 1800 cGy | | Radiotherapy‡ | Cranial, 1800 cGy |
| | | Cranial, 2400 cGy, and spinal, 600 cGy | | | Cranial, 2400 cGy, and spinal, 600 cGy |
| | | | | | Testicular, 2400 cGy |
| Interim maintenance (8 wk) | Mercaptopurine | 60 mg/m²/day PO days 0–41 | Interim maintenance I (8 wk) | Vincristine | 1.5 mg/m²/day IV days 0, 10, 20, 30, 40 |
| | Methotrexate | 15 mg/m²/day PO days 0, 7, 14, 21, 28, 35 | | Methotrexate | 100 mg/m²/day IV days 0, 10, 20, 30, 40 (escalate by 50 mg/m²/dose) |
| | | | | Asparaginase | 15,000 U/m²/day IM days 1, 11, 21, 31, 41 |
| Delayed intensification (7 wk) | | | Delayed intensification I (8 wk) | | |
| Reinduction (4 wk) | Desamethasone | 10 mg/m²/day PO days 0–20, then taper for 7 days | Reinduction (4 wk) | Desamethasone | 10 mg/m²/day PO days 0–20, then taper for 7 days |
| | Vincristine | 1.5 mg/m²/day IV days 0, 14, 21 | | Vincristine | 1.5 mg/m²/day IV days 0, 14, 21 |
| | Dosorubicin | 25 mg/m²/day IV days 0, 7, 14 | | Dosorubicin | 25 mg/m²/day IV days 0, 7, 14 |
| | Asparaginase | 6000 U/m²/day IM days 3, 4, 7, 10, 12, 14 | | Asparaginase | 6000 U/m²/day IM days 3, 4, 7, 10, 12, 14 |
| Reconsolidation (3 wk) | Vincristine | 1.5 mg/m²/day IV days 42, 49 | Reconsolidation (4 wk) | Vincristine | 1.5 mg/m²/day IV days 42, 49 |
| | Cyclophosphamide | 1000 mg/m²/ IV day 28 | | Cyclophosphamide | 1000 mg/m²/ IV day 28 |
| | Thioguanine | 60 mg/m²/day PO days 28–41 | | Thioguanine | 60 mg/m²/day PO days 28–41 |
| | Cytarabine | 75 mg/m²/day SQ or IV days 29–32, 36–39 | | Cytarabine | 75 mg/m²/day SQ or IV days 29–32, 36–39 |
| | Methotrexate† | IT days 29, 36 | | Methotrexate‡ | IT days 29, 36 |
| | | | | Asparaginase | 6000 U/m²/day IM days 42, 44, 46, 49, 51, 53 |
| | | | Interim maintenance II (8 wk) | Vincristine | 1.5 mg/m²/day IV days 0, 10, 20, 30, 40 |
| | | | | Methotrexate | 100 mg/m²/day IV days 0, 10, 20, 30, 40 (escalate by 50 mg/m²/dose) |
| | | | | Asparaginase | 15,k000 U/m²/day IM days 1, 11, 21, 31, 41 |
| | | | | Methotrexate† | IT days 0, 20, 40 |
| | | | Delayed intensification II (8 wk) | Same as for delayed intensification I | |
| Maintenance (12 wk) § | Vincristine | 1.5 mg/m²/day IV days 0, 28, 56 | Maintenance (12 wk)§ | Vincristine | 1.5 mg/m²/day IV days 0, 28, 56 |
| | Prednisone | 40 mg/m²/day PO days 0–4, 28–32, 56–60 | | Prednisone | 60 mg/m²/day PO days 0–4, 28–32, 56–60 |
| | Mercaptopurine | 75 mg/m²/day PO days 0–53 | | Mercaptopurine | 75 mg/m²/day PO days 7, 14, 21, 28, 35, 42, 49, 56, 63, 70, 77 |
| | Methotrexate | 20 mg/m²/day PO days 7, 14, 21, 28, 35, 42, 49, 56, 63, 70, 77 | | Methotrexate† | IT day 0 |
| | Methotrexate† | IT day 0 | | | |

* *IV* denotes intravenously, *PO* orally, *IT* intrathecally, *SQ* subcutaneously, and *IM* intremuscularly.
† The doses were age-adjusted as follows: age 1 to 1.9 years, 8 mg; age 2 to 2.9 years, 10 mg; age ≥3 years, 12 mg. Patients without central nervous system disease at diagnosis did not receive intrathecal methotrexate on days 15 an 22 of consolidation therapy.
‡ During the first two weeks of consolidation therapy, patients without central nervous system disease at diagnosis received 1800 cGy of cranial radiotherapy in 10 fractions; patients with central nervous system disease at diagnosis received 2400 cGy to the cranial midplane in 12 fractions and 600 cGy to the spinal cord in 3 fractions. In the augmented-therapy goutp, patients with resticulomegaly at diagnosis received 2400 cGy bilateral testicular radiation in 8 fractions.
§ The cycles of maintenance therapy were repeated until the total duration of therapy, beginning with the first interim maintenance period, reached two years for girls and three years for boys.

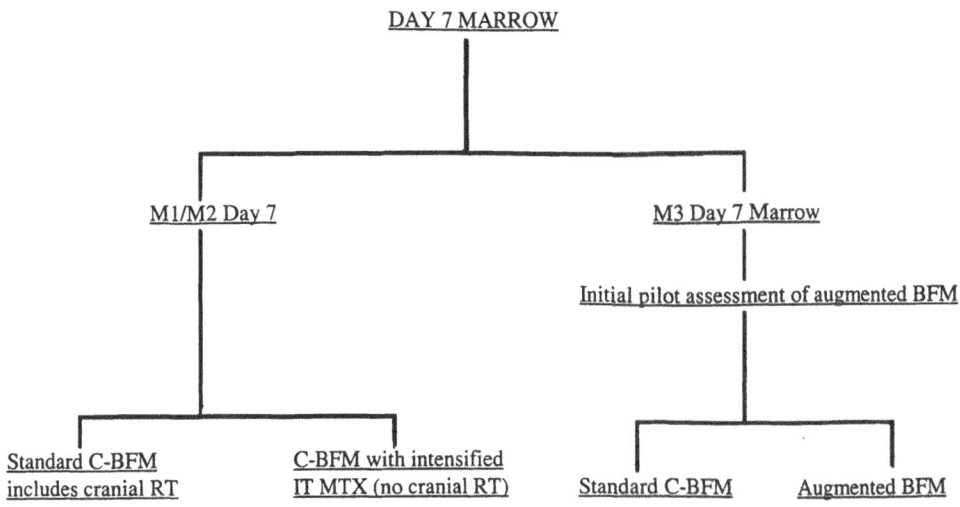

DAY 7 MARROW

M1/M2 Day 7

M3 Day 7 Marrow

Initial pilot assessment of augmented BFM

Standard C-BFM
includes cranial RT

C-BFM with intensified
IT MTX (no cranial RT)

Standard C-BFM

Augmented BFM

**Fig. 1.** CCG 1882 study design all patients receive 4 agent induction

stratified into two groups based on early marrow response. Rapid early responders were randomized to receive either C-BFM with IT MTX and cranial RT or C-BFM with intensified IT MTX alone for CNS prophylaxis. Slow early responders were initially assigned to a new treatment program designated augmented BFM (A-BFM).

In developing A-BFM, CCG investigators examined prior German BFM trials in which intensification of therapy was utilized in an effort to improve the EFS for prednisone poor responders. Utilization of chemotherapy blocks consisting of high dose cytosine arabinoside, high dose methotrexate, ifosfamide/VP-16, and mitoxantrone failed to improve EFS for prednisone poor responders. Since addition of new drug combinations had failed to improve outcome for prednisone poor responders, CCG investigators chose to intensify the use of standard drugs for ALL in an effort to improve outcome. Thus, A-BFM incorporated increased amounts of vincristine (VCR); L-asparaginase (L-ASP), and steroids during the first year. A-BFM also utilized intravenous MTX without rescue. Increased dose intensity was accomplished by adding a two week course of VCR (weekly x 2) and L-ASP (three times/week x 2 weeks) on day 14 of each consolidation and reconsolidation course. Chemotherapy during interim maintenance was changed from 6MP PO qd

and MTX PO q week to courses of VCR, IV MTX and L-ASP repeated at 10 day intervals x 5 with escalation of MTX dose with each course to toxicity. A second interim maintenance and second protocol II were also added. Number of doses for various chemotherapeutic drugs administered during the first year for C-BFM and A-BFM are shown in Table 3.

Induction results for patients entered on 1882 are shown in Table 3. The incidence of slow early response was 30%. Initially, SER patients were non-randomly assigned to receive A-BFM to determine whether the regimen would have acceptable toxicity. When 100 patients had completed the first year of therapy and no unanticipated side effects were noted, subsequent SER patients were randomized to receive either C-BFM (N = 156) or A-BFM (N = 155).

For SER pilot patients non-randomly treated with A-BFM, 5 year EFS was 70.9% [5]. Results for the randomized comparison of

**Table 3.** Standard VRS "augmented" therapy comparison of dose intensity in first year

|  | VCR | L-ASP | CTX | ARA-D courses | IV MTX |
|---|---|---|---|---|---|
| Standard | 15 | 15 | 3 | 6 | 0 |
| Augmented | 30 | 53 | 4 | 8 | 10 |

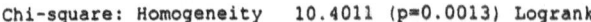

Chi-square: Homogeneity    10.4011 (p=0.0013) Logrank

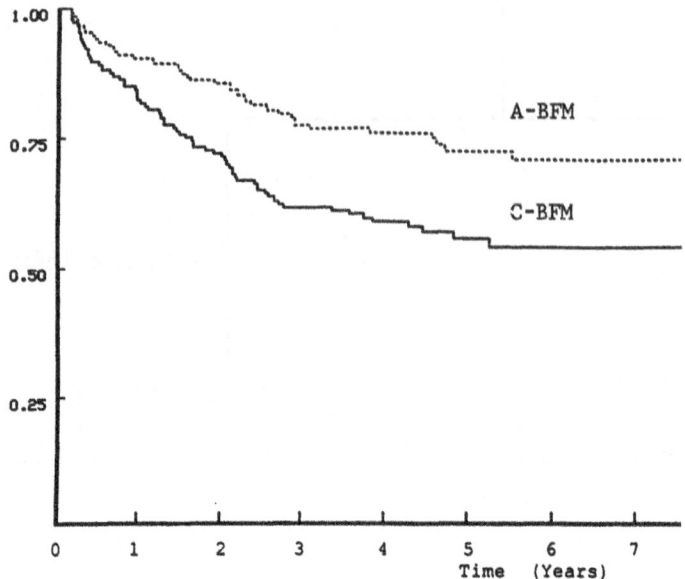

A-BFM

C-BFM

Time (Years)

**Fig. 2.** Randomized comparison of C-BFM and A-BFM for patients with slow early response

SER patients treated with A-BFM or C-BFM are shown in Figure 2. Five year EFS was 72.6% for patients treated with A-BFM vrs 55.6% for patients treated with C-BFM (P = .0013) [6].

SER patients <10 years of age showed the most benefit from A-BFM therapy. Five year EFS for patients <10 years of age was 80% for SER patients receiving A-BFM and 45% for patients receiving standard BFM. Although 5 year EFS was better for SER patients >10 years of age who received A-BFM compared to those who received C-BFM (68.4% vrs 60.3%), the difference was not statistically significant. A combined analysis of all SER patients who received A-BFM was undertaken to determine prognostic factors in this subgroup. WBC >200,000 was a significant adverse prognostic factor, particularly in patients >10 years of age. Patients with T-ALL and SER had a 5 year EFS of 86.3% vrs 63.6% for B lineage ALL.

There were 2 major toxicities associated with the use of A-BFM. Approximately 45% of patients developed an allergic reaction to E Coli L-ASP and had to be switched to either Erwinia L-ASP or PEG L-ASP. Approximately 20% of patients who switched L-ASP products had a second allergic reaction. There

was no difference in EFS for patients manifesting or not manifesting L-ASP allergy.

The second major toxicity noted was avascular necrosis of bone (AVN). AVN was seen almost exclusively in patients >10 years of age. It was more common in females than in males. There was a higher incidence of AVN in patients receiving two delayed intensification phases of therapy (A-BFM), probably related to the extra 21 day course of Dexamethasone.

## CCG 1961

The successor study to CCG 1882, CCG 1961, opened to patient accrual in 1987. Eligibility criteria were amended to include patients who met 1882 high risk criteria, but had lymphomatous features. The decision to include patients with lymphomatous features on CCG 1961 was based on the fact that patients with lymphomatous features had a good outcome when treated with standard BFM (CCG 123). EFS at 10 years was 66.6%. Slow early response was an important prognostic factor for patients with lymphomatous features treated with C-BFM. The excellent outcome for standard high risk T cell patients with SER treated

**Table 4.** 1882 – Final Induction Results By Day 7 Marrow Status (N = 1516)

|                  | M1/M2 Day 7   | M3 Day 7     |
|------------------|---------------|--------------|
| No               | 1047 (69.1%)  | 469 (30.9%)  |
| Remission Day 28 | 1035 (98.9%)  | 437 (93.2%)  |
| M3 Day 28        | 1             | 25           |
| Toxic Death      | 11            | 7            |
|                  | P <0.001      |              |

with A-BFM on 1882 suggested that outcome for patients with lymphomatous features and SER might be significantly improved with A-BFM.

As in CCG 1882, patients were divided into two treatment strata based on early response. For RER patients, the standard ARM was C-BFM with intensified IT MTX as CNS prophylaxis. The therapeutic questions for RER patients were based on incorporating components of A-BFM in an effort to improve EFS. A-BFM incorporated a second interim maintenance and delayed intensification (increased length) and intensification during consolidation reconsolidation courses and interim maintenance phases (increased strength). Three experimental arms were developed; full A-BFM, standard BFM plus a second interim maintenance and delayed intensification, and standard BFM with intensified consolidation, reconsolidation courses, and interim maintenance therapy.

For SER patients, the control ARM was A-BFM. Experimental interventions included the use of an immunotoxin B-43 PAP in induction and the use of an idarubicin/CTX based reinduction element.

An early comparison of outcome for CCG 1961 versus CCG 1882 (standard high risk) and CCG 1901 (lymphomatous features) shows an early improvement in EFS for CCG 1961. EFS at 18 months is 89.5% for patients treated on 1961 versus 83.9% for patients treated on 1882 or 1901.

## Conclusion

A-BFM had significant improved the outcome for standard high risk patients showing a slow early response to induction therapy. Preliminary analyses suggest that elements of A-BFM may benefit high risk rapid responder patients as well.

## References

1. Gaynon PS, Bleyer WA, Steinherz PG et al. (1988) Modified BFM therapy for children with previously untreated acute lymphoblastic leukemia and unfavorable prognostic features: report of Children's Cancer Study Group Study CCG-193P. Am J Pediatr Hematol Oncol 10: 42–50
2. Gaynon PS, Bleyer WA, Steinherz PG et al. (1990) Day 7 marrow response and outcome for children with acute lymphoblastic leukemia and unfavorable presenting features. Med Pediatr Oncol 18: 273–279
3. Gaynon PS, Steinherz PG, Bleyer WA et al. (1993) Improved therapy for children with acute lymphoblastic leukemia and unfavorable presenting features: A follow-up report of the Children's Cancer Group study CCG-106. J Clin Oncol 11: 2234–2242
4. Tubergen D, Gilchrist G, O'Brien RT et al. (1993) Improved outcome with delayed intensification for children with acute lymphoblastic leukemia and intermediate presenting features: a Children's Cancer Group phase III trial. J Clin Oncol 11: 527–537
5. Nachman J, Harland SN, Gaynon PS, Lukens JN, Wolff L, Trigg ME et al. Augmented Berlin-Frankfurt-Munster therapy abrogates the adverse prognostic significance of slow early response to induction chemotherapy for children and adolescents with acute lymphoblastic leukemia and unfavorable presenting features: A report from the Children's Cancer Group
6. Nachman J, Harland SN, Sensel MG, Trigg ME, Cherlow JM, Lukens JN, Wolff L, Uckun FM and Gaynon PS et al. Augmented post-induction therapy for children with high-risk acute lymphoblastic leukemia and a slow response to initial therapy

# Pharmacodynamics in Childhood Acute Lymphoblastic Leukemia

Ching-Hon Pui, M. V. Relling, J. T. Sandlund, D. Campana and W. E. Evans

*Abstract.* Pharmacokinetic variability clearly influences the outcome of treatment for acute lymphoblastic leukemia (ALL), but its utility as a clinical risk factor is limited when patients receive complex multiagent regimens of chemotherapy. However, judicious use of pharmacodynamic measures can increase the precision of risk assessment and guide the selection of therapy. For example, patients with slow reduction of their initial leukemic cell burden are excellent candidates for intensified chemotherapy. Also, recent studies indicate that the level of minimal residual leukemia, as measured by immunological or molecular methods at the time of remission induction, is highly predictive of treatment outcome. Patients achieving a "molecular" or "immunologic" remission, defined as leukemic involvement of less than 0.01% of mononucleated bone marrow cells, are predicted to have a better clinical outcome than those in whom remission is identified solely by blast cell morphologic criteria. A related approach is to measure specific biochemical endpoints that correlate closely with drug-induced cytotoxicity.

This is well illustrated by experience with methotrexate, whose accumulation as polyglutamates (active metabolites) in leukemic blast cells correlates positively with antileukemic responses.

Ongoing studies will determine the optimal dosage of methotrexate for the major phenotypic or genotypic subtypes of ALL. Although the erythrocyte concentration of 6-thioguanine nucleotides, the active metabolites of 6-mercaptopruine, correlates positively with long-term event-free survival, a recent study shows that the dose intensity of oral 6-mercaptopurine is an even more important determinant of clinical outcome, particularly among patients with a homozygous wild-type thiopurine methyltransferase phenotype, a cytosolic enzyme that inactivates 6-mercaptopurine and 6-thioguanine. Consistent administration of full protocol doses of daily oral 6-mercaptopurine is important in achieving optimal clinical responses; however, care must be taken to avoid excessive neutropenia, which can decrease dose intensity overall, leading to a poorer clinical outcome. For patients who tolerate thiopurine therapy poorly, molecular methods are available to diagnose a deficiency of thiopurine methyltransferase, allowing rational adjustment of drug dosages. Prospective clinical trials are needed to determine the optimal integration of pharmacodynamic measurements with more conventional predictors of the clinical relapse hazard in patients with ALL.

## Introduction

Childhood acute lymphoblastic leukemia (ALL) has long served as a paradigm for the development of treatment strategies for cancers of all types. Careful laboratory study of ALL has revealed many of the principles underlying current knowledge of tumor cell biology. Contemporary ALL treatment protocols are based on the principle of early intensive multiagent chemotherapy designed to

Supported in part by the following NIH grants: R37 CA 36401, P 30 CA 21765, RO1 CA 78224 and RO1 CA 60419, by a Center of Excellence grant from the State of Tennessee, and by the American Lebanese Syrian Associated Charities (ALSAC).

St. Jude Children's Research Hospital, and The University of Tennessee, Memphis, College of Medicine, TN, USA

ensure maximal leukemic cell kill and to avoid selection of drug-resistant mutants. Although pharmacokinetic variability (e.g. drug concentration) has been shown to influence the efficacy of ALL treatment [1, 2], the utility of conventional pharmacokinetic measures to predict response to individual chemotherapeutic agents can be confounded in the context of multi-agent chemotherapy. A complementary approach is to use pharmacodynamic endpoints to improve the risk assessment based on presenting clinical features and biological characteristics of leukemic cells. Moreover, pharmacodynamic studies may be useful to optimize therapy. In this brief review, we illustrate the utility of pharmacodynamic studies to monitor treatment response and to adjust chemotherapy to maximize efficacy while minimizing late sequelae in recent Total Therapy Studies for Childhood ALL.

## Materials and Methods

From 1988 to 1998, 620 consecutive children with newly diagnosed ALL were admitted to four successive clinical trials at St. Jude Children's Research Hospital: Total Therapy Study XII (1988–1991, n=188), Study XIIIA (1991–1994, n=165), Study XIIIB (1994–1998, n=247), and Study XIV (1998-present, n=20). Details of the treatment of the first three studies are given in earlier publications [2–4] and the last study will be provided upon request. Informed consent was obtained from the parent or guardian (as appropriate) and all research procedures were approved by our institutional review board.

Minimal residual leukemia was measured by flow cytometry [5] or polymerase chain reaction amplification of the clone-specific rearranged immunoglobulin heavy chain genes [6]. Intracellular concentrations of 6-thioguanine, other metabolites of 6-mercaptopurine and methotrexate polyglutamates were assayed by methods described previously [7–9]. Thiopurine methyltranferase (TPMT) activity in erythrocytes and TPMT genotype from somatic cell DNA were determined as previously described [10, 11]. The concentrations of purine bases from hydrolyzed nucleotides and the rate of de novo purine synthesis in leukemic blast cells were simultaneously determined by quantifying the unlabelled and radiolabeled purine bases (adenine, guanine, and hypoxanthine) after acid hydrolysis of a 2-h ex vivo incubation of $5 \times 10^6$ lymphoblasts with $^{14}C$ formate [12].

## Results and Discussion

### Cytoreduction response to remission induction therapy

Among pharmacodynamic endpoints that might be used to guide the selection of treatment, early treatment response, as indicated by the rate and degree of clearance of leukemic cells from blood or bone marrow during the early phase of remission induction therapy, is one of the most important and easily measured endpoints. Slow early response in general confers a poor prognosis and has variously been defined as the presence of any number of circulating blasts or more than 25% blasts in bone marrow after 7 days of multiagent remission induction, more than 1 blasts x $10^9$/L after 7 days of prednisone plus one dose of intrathecal methotrexate, or more than 5% blasts in bone marrow after 14 days of multiagent induction chemotherapy [13].

We recently correlated the persistence of lymphoblasts in bone marrow on day 15 and day 22–25 of remission induction with poor treatment outcome in patients treated on Total Therapy Studies XI and XII [14]. Altogether 397 patients had evaluable bone marrow exams on day 15 and 218 on day 22–25. Persistence of lymphoblasts was found in 14% of patients on day 15 and 7% on day 22–25. The complete remission rate was significantly lower in patients with persistent lymphoblasts on day 15 than in other patients (89% vs. 99%), p = 0.001. The remission rate for patients with persistent blasts on day 22–25 was even lower (59%). More importantly, the 5-year event-free survival (EFS) rates (±SE) for patients with and without lymphoblasts on day 15 were 40% ± 6% and 78% ± 2%, respectively (p<0.001), and on day 22–25 were 4% ± 13% and 76% ± 2%, respectively (p<0.001). A worse prognosis was observed even for patients with a low percentage of persistent lymphoblasts (i.e. 1–4%) on either day 15 (5-year EFS = 56% ± 18%) or day 22 (5-year EFS = 0%) compared to those who did not have persistent lymphoblasts at these time points (p<0.001 for both comparisons). The prognostic impact of persistent lymphoblasts on day 15 or day 22–25 marrow remained significant after adjusting for treatment, age, presenting leukocyte count, DNA index, leukemic cell immunophenotype and CNS status. Hence, persistence of morphologically identifiable lymphoblasts (even <5%) on day 15 was correlated with a poor prognosis and on day 22–25 signified a particularly dismal outcome. Because morphologic examination is subjective and can not reliably detect residual leukemia if lymphoblasts comprise only 1% or less of a cell population, more sensitive strategies may be even more informative in predicting outcome. In this regard, we and others, using immunologic methods or semiquantitative polymerase chain reaction analyses of clone-specific immunoglobulin or T-cell receptor gene rearrangement, have correlated higher levels of minimal residual disease (e.g. leukemic involvement of >0.01% of nucleated bone marrow cells) in the immediate post-induction period with an increased likelihood of relapse [5, 6, 15, 16]. However, neither of these assays can be applied to all patients, a prerequisite for the introduction of routine minimal residual disease detection in risk assessment in clinical protocols. Conceivably, the simultaneous application of both assays would allow the study of all patients [17]. To evaluate the comparability of the two assays, we have used both methods to study 56 bone marrow samples collected from patients in clinical remission. The immunologic method (sensitivity = 1:10^4) was applicable to approximately 80% of the cases and the molecular method (sensitivity = 1:10^5) to approximately 85% of cases. All patients can be studied by one or both methods. Percentages of leukemic cells as measured by either method correlated strongly. We now apply both methods in tandem in our current Total Therapy Study XIV. Patients with residual leukemia cells in the bone marrow at a level of 0.01% or more on remission date receive more intensive therapy than those with a lower level or no detectable leukemia.

## Intracellular Biochemical Response to Antileukemic Therapy

Another approach to assess the pharmacodynamics of antileukemic therapy is to measure specific biochemical endpoints that reflect the mechanism of cytotoxicity of individual drugs or combination chemotherapy. In this regard, such studies are instrumental in our studies to establish the optimal dosages of methotrexate and 6-mercaptopurine, antimetabolites that constitute an important component of chemotherapy in childhood ALL.

### Methotrexate

Until recently, relatively little was known about the intracellular disposition of methotrexate in leukemic lymphoblasts. Selection of drug dosage and schedule were based largely on imprecise clinical observations and suboptimal preclinical models. Total Therapy Studies XIIIA, XIIIB, and XIV were designed to address some of these issues in patients.

After entering cells via the reduced folate carrier and by passive diffusion at higher extracellular concentrations, methotrexate is metabolized by folylpolyglutamate synthetase (FPGS) to polyglutamated metabolites, with up to five additional glutamates sequentially added to the molecules in leukemic lymphoblasts [9]. Methotrexate binds directly to the target enzyme, dihydrofolate reductase, disrupting folate metabolism. Long chain methotrexate polyglutamates are retained longer in cells and inhibit additional target enzymes when compared to methotrexate (e.g. 5-aminoimidazole-4-carboxamide ribonucleotide transformylase – a key enzyme in de novo purine biosynthesis) [18]. Our in vivo studies have shown that B-lineage lymphoblasts accumulate higher intracellular concentrations of methotrexate polyglutamates compared to T-lineage lymphoblasts [9], partly due to higher activity of FPGS in the former [19]. Among B-lineage cases, hyperdiploid (>50 chromosomes) blasts accumulate higher methotrexate polyglutamates compared to non-hyperdiploid blasts [9], partly due to increased expression of the reduced folate carrier [20], located on human chromosome 21 (21q22.2-q22.3), suggesting a gene-dose effect (hyperdiploid B-lineage lymphoblasts almost always have at least one extra copy of chromosome 21) [21].

We also found that methotrexate polyglutamate concentrations in leukemic blasts were significantly higher in patients who have immediate onset of antileukemic effects, as evidenced by a decrease in circulating blast cell count within 24 hours of treatment, and also in those who had complete clearance of circulating blasts within 4 days of single-agent therapy with methotrexate [22]. Consistent with these findings, a significant correlation was found between the extent of inhibition of de novo purine synthesis in leukemic blasts and the degree of accumulation of methotrexate polyglutamates [22]. Our recent data also indicate that the degree of inhibition of de novo purine synthesis correlates with the extent of clearance of circulating blasts and that T-lineage lymphoblasts have a higher baseline level of de novo purine synthesis as compared to B-lineage lymphoblasts [23], consistent with clinical data indicating that T-cell ALL requires a higher dosage of methotrexate to achieve outcome comparable to B-lineage ALL [24].

It is not known whether very high-dose methotrexate (e.g. $\geq 5$ g/m$^2$) would yield methotrexate polyglutamate levels in T-lineage or non-hyperdiploid B-lineage blasts comparable to those in hyperdiploid B-lineage blasts. Administering very high doses of methotrexate to all patients is not an acceptable strategy to avoid suboptimal exposure, not only because of the increased cost of therapy but more importantly the increased risk of toxicities. Hence, it is important to establish the dosage of methotrexate that results in optimal accumulation in the target tissue (lymphoblasts) and to avoid unnecessarily high dosages. In Study XIV, we are rigorously defining the relation between steady-state plasma concentration and intracellular methotrexate polyglutamate accumulation in specific lineage and genetic subtypes of childhood ALL.

## 6-mercaptopurine

6-mercaptopurine is metabolized to nucleotide intermediates by hypoxanthine-guanine-phosphoribosyltransferase and then further metabolized to the principal active metabo-lites, 6-thioguanine nucleotides [25]. Nucleotide metabolites can be methylated by thiopurine S-methyltransferase (TPMT), yielding inactive S-methylated metabolites, thereby decreasing the amount of drug available for activation to 6-thiogranine [26]. Previous studies have correlated erythrocyte 6-thioguanine nucleotide and methotrexate polyglutamate concentrations positively with long-term event-free survival [27, 28]. However, since both methotrexate and 6-mercaptopurine were given orally, the association may reflect patient compliance in taking oral medications. In addition, in patients with TPMT deficiency, dosages of methotrexate may have been unnecessarily reduced along with those of 6-mercaptopurine.

In our Study XII, we prospectively measured erythrocyte 6-thioguanine and methotrexate polyglutamates, as well as plasma exposure to every dose of pulse therapy with either high-dose methotrexate or teniposide plus cytarabine. We have also documented the exact dosage of weekly parenteral methotrexate and daily oral 6-mercaptopurine for the entire 120 weeks of continuation treatment for all patients. Among pharmacologic variables analyzed, including average or maximal concentration of 6-thioguanine, thioinosine monophosphate, methylated metabolites of thioinosine monophosphate and methotrexate polyglutamates in erythrocytes; average plasma area under the concentration–times–time curve of methotrexate, teniposide or cytarabine; TPMT phenotype; and dose intensity (ratio of cumulative dosage administered to planned protocol dosage per week for all scheduled treatment until elective cessation of therapy or an adverse event) of 6-mercaptopurine or methotrexate, only higher dose intensity of 6-mercaptopurine (p=0.02) was a significant predictor of superior event-free survival [29]. Lower TPMT activity also appeared to correlate with better outcome (p=0.096). Dose intensity of 6-mercaptopurine was also correlated with outcome when the analysis was restricted to only those patients with homozygous wild-type TPMT phenotype (p=0.007). Lower dose intensity of 6-mercaptopurine was primarily due to missed weeks of therapy and not to reduction in daily dose, suggesting that increasing intensity of therapy such that neutropenia precludes administration of subsequent chemotherapy may be counterproductive.

In Study XII, we also observed a high incidence of malignant brain tumor in patients who had received cranial irradiation (5 of 52 children; 8-year cumulative incidence = 12.4% ± 5.5%, SE) [30]. This incidence was significantly higher than that (0%) of patients treated in the same study who did not receive irradiation (p=0.003) and those of patients in Total Therapy Studies X and XI that included cranial irradiation (p<0.0001). Compared to other Total Therapy Studies, Study XII incorporated more systemic antimetabolites during and prior to cranial irradiation. Of the five patients with brain tumor, four had erythrocyte levels of 6-thioguanine nucleotides above the 70th percentile for the entire cohort, and three were either heterozygous or homozygous deficient for TPMT activity. The 8-year cumulative incidence of brain tumors among children with 6-thioguanine nucleotides >800 vs. <800 pmol/8 x $10^8$ RBCs was 35.4% ± 19.4% vs. 8.0% ± 5.8% (p=0.035). The incidence was also higher among those with the *TEL-AML1* fusion in their leukemic lymphoblasts (28.6% ± 15%) compared to those with germline *TEL* (8.2% ± 5.8%) (p=0.036). These studies indicate that there are underlying genetic characteristics and treatment variables associated with enhanced risk of radiation-associated brain tumor. Toward this end, molecular genetic methods have been developed to diagnose TPMT-deficient patients by use of genomic DNA [11]. TPMT illustrates the clinical importance of genetic polymorphisms in drug metabolism as determinants of toxicity and efficacy of anticancer therapy [31].

# References

1. Evans WE, Crom WR, Abromowitch M, et al (1986) Clinical pharmacodynamics of high-dose methotrexate in acute lymphocytic leukemia. N Engl J Med 314:471–477
2. Evans WE, Relling MV, Rodman JH, et al (1998) Conventional compared with individualized chemotherapy for childhood acute lymphoblastic leukemia. N Engl J Med 338:499–505
3. Pui C-H, Mahmoud HH, Rivera GK, et al (1998) Early intensification of intrathecal chemotherapy virtually eliminates central nevous system relapse in children with acute lymphoblastic leukemia. Blood 92:411–415
4. Pui C-H, Rivera GK, Hancock ML, et al (1997) Risk-adapted treatment for acute lymphoblastic leukemia: findings from St. Jude Children's Research Hospital. In Bhchner et al (eds) Acute Leukemias VI. Prognostic Factors and Treatment Strategies. Springer-Verlag Berlin Heidelberg, pp. 629–637
5. Coustan-Smith E, Behm FG, Sanchez J, et al (1998) Immunological detection of minimal residual disease in children with acute lymphoblastic leukaemia. Lancet 351:550–554
6. Gruhn B, Hongeng S, Yi H, et al (1998) Minimal residual disease after intensive induction therapy in childhood acute lymphoblastic leukemia predicts outcome. Leukemia 12:675–681
7. Lennard L (1987) Assay of 6-thioinosinic acid and 6-thioguanine nucleotides, active metabolites of 6-mercaptopurine in human red blood cells. J Chromatogr 423:169–178
8. Lennard L, Singleton HJ (1992) High-performance liquid chromatographic assay of the methyl and nucleotide metabolites of 6-mercaptopurine: quantitation of red blood cell 6-thioguanine nucleotide, 6-thioinosinic acid and 6-methylmercaptopurine metabolites in a single sample. J Chromatogr 583:83–90
9. Synold TW, Relling MV, Boyett JM, et al (1994) Blast cell methotrexate-polyglutamate accumulation in vivo differs by lineage, ploidy, and methotrexate dose in acute lymphoblastic leukemia. J Clin Invest 94:1996–2001
10. McLeod HL, Lin JS, Scott EP, et al (1994) Thiopurine methyltransferase activity in American white subjects and black subjects. Clin Pharmacol Ther 55:15–20
11. Yates CR, Krynetski EY, Loennechen T, et al (1997) Molecular diagnosis of thiopurine S-methyltransferase deficiency: genetic basis for azathioprine and mercaptopurine intolerance [see comments]. Ann Intern Med 126:608–614
12. Masson E, Synold TW, Relling MV, et al (1996) Allopurinol inhibits *de novo* purine synthesis in lymphoblasts of children with acute lymphoblastic leukemia. Leukemia 10:56–60
13. Pui C-H (1998) Recent advances in the biology and treatment of childhood acute lymphoblastic leukemia. Curr Opin Hematol 5:292–301
14. Sandlund JT, Harrison P, Rivera G, et al (1997) Persistence of lymphoblasts in bone marrow on day 15 and day 22-25 of remission induction predicted a poorer treatment outcome in children with acute lymphoblastic leukemia. Blood 90 (suppl 1):560a
15. CavJ H, van der Werff Ten Bosch J, Suciu S, et al (1998) Clinical significance of minimal residual disease in childhood acute lymphoblastic leukemia. N Engl J Med 339:591–598
16. van Dongen JJM, Seriu T, Panzer-Grhmayer ER, et al (1998) Prognostic value of minimal residual disease in acute lymphoblastic leukaemia in childhood. Lancet 352:1731–1738
17. Neale GAM, Coustan-Smith E, Pan Q, et al (1998) Detection of minimal residual disease in childhood acute lymphoblastic leukemia with immunologic and molecular methods: a comparative study. Blood 92 (suppl 1):394a
18. Gorlick R, Goker E, Trippett T, et al (1996) Intrinsic and acquired resistance to methotrexate in acute leukemia. N Engl J Med 335:1041–1048

19. Barredo JC, Synold TW, Laver J, et al (1994) Differences in constitutive and post-methotrexate folyl-polyglutamate synthetase activity in B-lineage and T-lineage leukemia. Blood 84:564–569

20. Belkov VM, Krynetski EY, Schuetz JD, et al (1999) Reduced folate carrier expression and methotrexate accumulation are increased in hyperdiploid acute lymphoblastic leukemia and related to chromosome 21 copy number. Blood (in press)

21. Raimondi SC, Pui C-H, Hancock ML, et al (1996) Heterogeneity of hyperdiploid (51–67) childhood acute lymphoblastic leukemia. Leukemia 10:213–224

22. Masson E, Relling MV, Synold TW, et al (1996) Accumulation of methotrexate polyglutamates in lymphoblasts is a determinant of antileukemic effects in vivo. A rationale for high-dose methotrexate. J Clin Invest 97:73–80

23. Hon YY, Evans WE, Sandlund JT, et al (1998) *De novo* purine synthesis (DNPS) in childhood acute lymphoblastic leukemia (ALL). Proc Am Assoc Cancer Res 39:188

24. Pui C-H, Evans WE (1998) Acute lymphoblastic leukemia. N Engl J Med 339:605–615

25. Krynetski EY, Tai HL, Yates CR, et al (1996) Genetic polymorphism of thiopurine S-methyltransferase: clinical importance and molecular mechanisms. Pharmacogenetics 6:279–290

26. Krynetski EY, Krynetskaia NF, Yanishevski Y, et al (1995) Methylation of mercaptopurine, thioguanine and their nucleotide metabolites by heterologously expressed human thiopurine S-methyltransferase. Mol Pharmacol 47:1141–1147

27. Lennard L, Lilleyman JS, Van Loon J, et al (1990) Genetic variation in response to 6-mercaptopurine for childhood acute lymphoblastic leukaemia. Lancet 336:225–229

28. Schmiegelow K, Schrrder H, Gustafsson K, et al (1995) Risk of relapse in childhood acute lymphoblastic leukemia is related to RBC methotrexate and mercaptopurine metabolites during maintenance chemotherapy. J Clin Oncol 13:345–351

29. Relling MV, Hancock ML, Boyett JM, et al (1999) Prognostic importance of 6-mercaptopurine dose intensity in acute lymphoblastic leukemia. Blood (in press)

30. Relling MV, Rubnitz JE, Rivera GK, et al (1999) High incidence of secondary brain tumors related to irradiation and antimetabolite therapy. Lancet (in press)

31. Krynetski EY, Evans WE (1998) Cancer Genetics '98. Pharmacogenetics of cancer therapy: getting personal. Am J Hum Genet 63:11–16

# The Late Effects of Prophylactic CNS Treatment*

TH. LANGER, P. KRAPPMANN, S. KOCHENDÖRFER, M. KUSCH, E. GÖBEL, W. HUK, P. MARTUS and J. D. BECK for the Late Effects Working Group in the Gesellschaft für Pädiatrische Onkologie und Hämatologie

*Abstract.* Approximately 9,000 survivors of childhood ALL are living in Germany nowadays with an additional of almost 550 every year. The Late Effects Working Group of the GPOH performs investigations of major late sequelae in collaboration with the German Registry of Cancer in Childhood and the ALL-study groups.

Secondary tumors after successful ALL treatment were documented in a group of 7032 ALL survivors by the German Childrens Cancer Registry in Mainz since 1980. 103 patients out of these survivors developed secondary malignancies. 33 patients with a brain tumor were the largest group in the cohort of secondary malignancies. Most of the 33 patients were cranial irradiated for the CNS prophylaxis.

In a cross-sectional multicenter study 107 subjects, asymptomatic long-term survivors of childhood ALL were evaluated for structural alterations of the brain, intellectual, cognitive and psychosocial impairments. 7.3 years ago, the subjects were treated as standard/low or medium risk patients according to ALL-BFM 81/83 resp. COALL 82 protocols.

Corresponding to the method of CNS-prophylaxis a chemotherapy group (MTX-group) and a radiotherapy group (RT-group), receiving cranial irradiation of 18 Gy in combination with chemotherapy, were investigated. Demographical and clinical data at diagnosis were compared between both treatment groups. The performance was evaluated according to age, gender and treatment group by using analysis of variance.

We detected structural brain alterations, signs of leukoencephalopathy, intellectual and cognitive impairments especially in the irradiated group. Survivors with a detectable leukoencephalopathy showed significant impairments of attention, concentration and psychosocial adjustment. Prophylactic CNS irradiation with 18 Gy carries a higher risk for disturbances of the cognitive and psychosocial functioning in ALL survivors. Our results confirm the strategy of avoiding prophylactic CNS irradiation with a dose of 18 Gy in low/medium risk patients.

A prospective, standardized long-term follow-up program is currently underway to observe and to improve the health related quality of life of children treated for ALL.

## Introduction

More efficient therapy studies and the improved ability to treat complications have contributed to the better survival rates of children with acute lymphoblastic leukemia (ALL). The central nervous system (CNS) prophylaxis is an essential component of the treatment. In the past the central nervous system (CNS) was a frequent site of relapses in children with ALL. Therefore an effective preventive CNS therapy had to be developed [1]. Large clinical trials confirmed that the prophylactic cranial irradiation (CI) combined with periodic systemical and intrathecal chemotherapy, mostly methotrexate (MTX), reduced the CNS relapse rates very effectively [2, 3]. By increasing the dose of the systemic MTX in the treatment of low and medium risk patients, the CI can be avoided in these groups without increased CNS relapse rates [4]. However CNS prophylaxis occurs in the context of complex treatment protocols that include a variety of neurotoxic agents and the outcome has to be evaluated to detect major toxicities especially in the CNS.

*Supported by grants of the Deutsche Krebshilfe and Deutsche Leukämieforschungshilfe.

Secondary tumors, intellectual and cognitive deficits, morphological impairments of the CNS and growth disturbances become more relevant as late effects with the growing number of long-term survivors.

Our study group is part of the Late Effects Working Group founded by the Gesellschaft für Pädiatrische Onkologie und Hämatologie to study late effects in former pediatric cancer patients [5, 6].

## Methods

Secondary tumors after successful ALL treatment were documented in a group of 7032 ALL survivors by the German Childrens Cancer Registry in Mainz since 1980.

In 1992 the Late Effects Working Group initiated a cross-sectional, multicenter study in Germany and Austria to evaluate CNS late effects after ALL therapy in childhood (Fig. 1). ALL patients in first continuous remission, treated between 1981 and 1986 as standard- or medium risk patients according to comparable and highly standardized treatment protocols were examined. We compared in respect of the CNS prophylaxis the neuroradiological, neuropsychological, neurophysiological and auxological measurements between a radiotherapy (RT) and a MTX group.

### Patient Sample

Based on information which we have gathered by investigations from the German Childrens Cancer Registry we invited long-term survivors of ALL to participate in our study.

*Eligibility requirements:* All patients were treated according to the protocols of the BFM study group ALL-BFM-81/83, or to the corresponding COALL protocol COALL-82 between 1981 and 1986 in the eleven participating hospitals in Germany and Austria. Only patients with a standard/low or medium risk (risk factor** (RF) <1.7) without CNS involvement, in first continuous remission after the completed therapy were enrolled. They had to be older than 6 years at the time of investigation, had visited or were visiting a German school and were fluent in German.

*Exclusion criteria:* Patients with a secondary malignancy were excluded. The patients did not have a meningeal or encephalitic infection before the investigation nor had been suffering from the effect of a perinatal hypoxia. In addition a pre-existent neurological and/or psychiatric disease excluded patients from participation. Patients with somatical numeric or structural chromosomal aberration were excluded also.

The follow-up trial was carried out according to the Declaration of Helsinki (1975, revised in 1989). After the consent of the Medical Ethics Committee of the University Erlangen-Nuremberg (Germany), using the

---

** risk factor, tumor mass index, was calculated: 0.2 x log (peripher blasts/$\mu$l + 1) + 0.06 x liver size under the costal arch [cm] + 0.04 x spleen size under the costal arch [cm] [7].

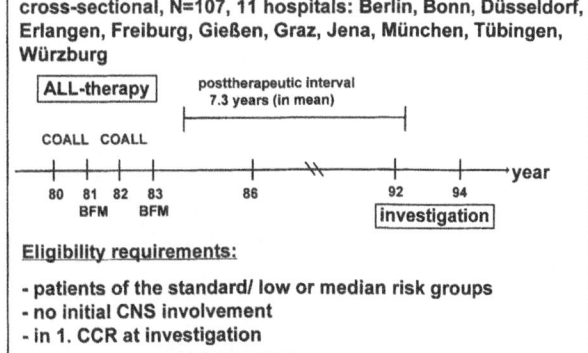

**Fig. 1.** Study design. Overview about the study design, the number of participating hospitals and the eligibility requirements.

**Table 1.** Sample Description. In Table 1 the sample description is presented. The demographic and clinical data at diagnosis, the morphology of leukemic cells (FAB; French-American-British-Group classification), methods of therapy and treatment branches of the performed treatment protocol (BFM; Berlin-Frankfurt-Münster therapy study group for acute lymphoblastic leukemia, COALL; German Cooperative study group for acute lymphoblastic leukemia) are shown for the MTX- and the RT-group. P-values present the results of a t-test for independent pairs or Chi-square-Test.

| | All subjects | Treatment Groups | | p |
| | | MTX-group | RT-group | |
|---|---|---|---|---|
| *Demographic Data* | | | | |
| Number of patients | 107 | 38 | 69 | |
| Age at diagnosis (yrs.) | 6.0 ± 4.0 | 6.6 ± 4.5 | 5.7 ± 3.7 | 0.27 |
| Age at investigation (yrs.) | 15.1 ± 4.3 | 15.4 ± 4.8 | 14.9 ± 4.1 | 0.59 |
| Post-therapeutic interval (yrs.) | 7.3 ± 1.8 | 7.0 ± 1.7 | 7.5 ± 1.8 | 0.14 |
| Gender (male/female) | 57 f/50 m | 19 f/19 m | 38 f/31 m | 0.69 |
| *Clinical Data at Diagnosis* | | | | |
| Hemoglobin (g/dl) | 7.8 ± 2.5 | 6.9 ± 2.0 | 8.4 ± 2.0 | < 0.01 |
| Risk Factor # | 1.0 ± 0.4 | 0.7 ± 0.2 | 1.1 ± 0.3 | < 0.001 |
| *Morphology* | | | | |
| FAB 1 (%) | 68 | 77 | 64 | |
| FAB 1-2 (%) | 14 | 8 | 16 | 0.68 |
| FAB 2 (%) | 18 | 15 | 19 | |
| *Treatment* | | | | |
| Mean total dose (Gy) | | – | 18 | |
| Mean dose/fraction (Gy) | | – | 1.8 – 0.4 | |
| Cumulative ITMTX (mg) | 80.0 ± 21.3 | 80.8 ± 17.0 | 79.5 ± 23.5 | 0.75 |
| Cumulative SMHHDMTX (mg/m$^2$) | 1 x 500,67 x 2000 | 38 x 2000 | 1 x 500, 29 x 2000 | |
| Duration (months) | 22.0 ± 2.9 | 22.1 ± 2.8 | 22.0 ± 2.8 | 0.84 |
| *Treatment protocols* | | | | |
| BFM-branches (year/branch) | | 81/SR-B (n = 15) | 81/SR-A (n = 23), | |
| | | 83/SR-L 1/2 (n = 22) | 83/SR-H 2 (n = 14) | |
| | | | 81/MR (n = 12), | |
| | | | 83/MR (n = 16) | |
| COALL-branches (year/branch) | | 82/LR (n = 1) | 82/MR (n = 4) | |

informations of the GCCR and using the criteria of our eligibility requirements, 163 subjects and their families agreed to participate in the follow-up investigation. From the total of 163 patients, 15 could not perform the follow-up trial because they did fulfil at least one of the study exclusion criteria. 27 cases were separated because their follow-up trials were not performed according to the recommendiations of the CNS late effects study group.

In the analysis we concentrated on a homogenous subject group, receiving either only chemotherapy (MTX-group) or the combination of chemotherapy, and cranial irradiation with the dose of 18 Gy (RT-group).

Therefore 107 patients (57 female, 50 male) were enrolled. These patients had stopped receiving antileukemic therapy for at least 4.5 years (mean: 7,3 yrs., maximum: 10.6 yrs.). The mean age at the time of diagnosis was 6.0 years (0.3 – 16.1 yrs.), the mean age at investi-

gation was 15.1 years (9.0 – 27.8 yrs.). Written informed consent for participation was obtained from the patients or their parents. Relevant data with respect to initial clinical features, illness and treatment parameters of the investigated subjects are summarized in Table 1.

**Treatment**

In the early 1980s, the patients had been consecutively enrolled into ALL-BFM 81, 83 or COALL 80, 82 protocols and were assigned to different prophylactic CNS regimens. At the time of investigation, the subjects were asymptomatic long-term survivors. For statistical analysis all treatment branches were divided into two treatment groups disregarding minor chemotherapeutic differences between the protocol branches and their influence on CNS prophylaxis (Fig. 2). The MTX-group

| MTX-group: (n=38) | MTX cumulative: i.th. (mean: 81 mg) + i.v. (2000 mg/m$^2$) without cranial irradiation |
|---|---|
| RT-group: (n=69) | MTX cumulative: i.th. (mean: 80 mg) +/- i.v. MTX (2000 mg/m$^2$) with cranial irradiation (18 Gy) |

**Fig. 2.** CNS-prophylactic treatment. Description of the both treatment groups and their CNS prophylactic therapy.

(n = 38) received only systemic MTX (SMTX) (cumulative dose 2000 mg/m$^2$ body surface area (BSA) in 4 infusions) and intrathecal MTX (ITMTX) (cumulative mean dose 81 mg (58 – 132 mg age dependent) in 6 to 8 injections) for CNS prophylaxis. The RT-group (n = 69) was treated with 18 Gy cranial irradiation combined with ITMTX (cumulative mean dose 80 mg (36 –156 mg dependent on age in 6–8 injections) with or without SMTX (cumulative dose 2000 mg/m$^2$ BSA in 4 infusions). The MTX-group included the treatment branches of the ALL-BFM-protocols BFM-81/SR-B, BFM-83/SR-L1/2 and COALL-protocol 82/LR, RT-group the branches BFM-81/SR-A, BFM-81/MR, BFM-83/SR-H2, BFM-83/MR and COALL-protocol 82/MR (Table 1). The CNS relapse incidence of the different treatment branches are: Patients of the BFM-study group receiving a chemotherapeutic CNS-prophylaxis exhibited a relapse rate with CNS-involvement of 11.9% and the corresponding patients of the COALL-study group of 12.1%. patients of the BFM-study group receiving CI for CNS-prophylaxis presented a relapse rate with CNS-involvement of 6.7% and the corresponding patients of the COALL-study group of 11.9% (Schrappe for the BFM-group, 1997 and Janka-Schaub for the COALL group, 1998 personalcommunications).

## Study Design

The study was carried out as a multicenter and cross-sectional examination. An extensive examination included the patients' case history and social background in order to estimate the socialpsychological and educational factors. The neurological examination was performed using the Touwen pattern. Neurophysiological investigations with electroencephalogram(EFG), visual evoked potentials (VEP) and event-related potentials (ERP) were carried out whenever available.

Magnetic resonance imaging (MRI) or computertomography (CCT) scans of the CNS were obtained for the neuroradiological examination. Pathologic criteria were: widening of the sulci or ventricles, findings believed to indicate brain atrophy. Low-density areas in CCT scans resp. hyperintensive areas in MRI seen in the white matter were judged as white matter necrosis (leukoencephalopathy). High-density in CCT scans resp. hypointensive areas in MRI and grey matter changes are possible signs for necrosis. Calcifications detectable in CCT are indicators for calcified focal brain necrosis.

For neuropsychological testing, the German version of the Hamburg-Wechsler Intelligence Scales for Children in Revision (HAWIK-R ,aged from 6–15 11/12 years) and the Hamburg-Wechsler Intelligence Scale for Adults in Revision (HAWIE-R, patients older than 15 11/12 years) were used. The scales are divided in two parts: Verbal IQ (VIQ) and Performance IQ (PIQ), forming the Full Scale IQ (FSIQ). Each part subsume specific subtests: for VIQ: "Information (I)", "Comprehension (c)", "Arithmetics (A)", "Similarities (S)", "Vocabulary (V)" and "Digit Span (DS)" and for PIQ: "Coding (Co)", "Picture Completion (PC)", "Picture Arrangement (PA)", "Block Design (BD)" and "Object Assembly (OA)". FSIQ, VIQ and PIQ score with a mean of 100 and a standard deviation (SD) of 15, all subtests of 10 resp. 3.

In addition to the Wechsler Scales, the Kaufman factor Freedom from Distractiblity (FD) was investigated which reflects attention, concentration, memory and the ability of processing and sequencing as defined by Kaufmann [8]. It is based on the subtests "A", "DS" and "Co". As described by Gutkin [9] a simple formula for the conversion of this factor score into a deviation quotient (mean of 100, SD of 15) was developed with the aid of procedures proposed by Tellegen and Briggs [10]: FD = 2.2* (A+DS+Co)+34,0 [9, 11].

For culture independent intelligence measuring, the German version of the Culture Fair Test (CFT) by Cattel, Weiß and Osterland was used, age dependent CFT-1 for 5–9 years old patients and CFT-20, if the patients were 8 1/2–18 years or older.

Recurring Figures Test (RFT) for memory functioning by Kimura were used, measuring nonverbal, visual memory in children aged four years or older.

Test d2 by Brickenham, testing attention, concentration and speed, usable for children older than 6 years was employed.

For CFT, RFT and Test d2 the 50. Percentile were calculated as the mean.

## Evaluation

The results of each of these sections were evaluated by experienced investigators (neurologist: K. Berger-Jones, Berlin, neurophysiologists: M. A. Ueberall, Erlangen und R. Korinthenberg, Freiburg, neuroradiologist: W. J. Huk, Erlangen, psycologist. W. Meier, Marburg) who had no knowledge of the patient's medical history.

## Statistical analysis

Categorial variables were compared between the treatment groups with the Chi-square-test. After inspection for normal distribution and for equality of the variances, test for independent samples ware used. Multivariate analysis of risk factors between both treatment groups was performed using logistic regression. Effect of age, gender and treatment group was evaluated by using three-factorial analysis of variance. The level of significance for the statistical tests was 5% (two-sided).

## Results

### Secondary Tumors

According to data of the German Childrens Cancer Registry in Mainz (Prof. Dr.Michaelis, Dr. Kaatsch), the cumulative risk for secondary tumors after antineoplastic therapy is estimated up to 2–3% for all malignancies. Second tumors after successful ALL treatment occurred in a group of 7032 ALL survivous in 103 cases, 33 brain tumors, 26 AML, 16 lymphomas were documented since 1980.

## CNS toxicity after ALL treatment

### Clinical data at diagnosis

With the exception of "platelets at diagnosis", in univariate analysis all disease related clinical data were significantly different between both treatment groups. However, in multivariate analysis only the tumor mass index, as defined in the methods ("risk factor"), remained significant:

## CNS Morphology

The subjects in the MTX-group showed in 39% one or more morphological alteration, the subjects in the RT-group in 58%.

In details: brain atrophy was found in 20–30% in both treatment groups, there was no statiticall significant difference. Neuroradiological signs of leukoencephalopathy were found in 15 subjects of the RT-group (24%), but only in one subject in the MTX-group (3%) (p<0.01). Subjects with signs of leukoencephalopathy exhibited significant P100 latency prolongations in the visual evoked potentials. Calcifications, only detectable in the CT (n = 46), were found in 3 subjects in the RT-group. These results are published elsewhere [12].

### Intellectual and cognitive performance

In the Hamburg-Wechsler Intelligence Teest, the RT-group showed a lower full scale IQ (FSIQ) than the MTX-group, in mean 9.0 IQ points lower (109.9 ± 14.9 vs. 100.9 ± 16.2, p = 0.005). In the Kaufman factor, Freedom from Distractibility (FD) die RT-group showed the lowest scores (105.5 ± 12.6 vs. 96.5 ± 14.0, p = 0.003) (Table 2).

Using a multiple regression analysis, the tumor mass index ("risk factor") was not significant for the reduction of the scores in the intellectual and cognitive test (especially

**Table 2.** Neuropsychological results in both treatment groups. The neuropsychological test results in the Wechsler Scales Full Scale-IQ, Verbal-IQ and Performance-IQ, the Kaufman factors Visual Comprehension, Perceptual Organisation and Freedom from Distractibility are shown in regard to the MTX- and RT-groups. P-values present the results of a t-test for independent pairs. P-values are adjusted to the recommendations by Bonferroni.

|  | MTX-group (n = 38) | p* | RT-group (n = 69) |
|---|---|---|---|
| Full scale IQ | 109.9 ± 14.9 | 0.005 | 100.9 ± 16.2 |
| Verbal IQ | 110.6 ± 16.6 | 0.04 | 103.0 ± 15.6 |
| Performance IQ | 106.6 ± 14.8 | 0.02 | 98.3 ± 16.2 |
| Kaufman Factors |  |  |  |
| VC | 107.2 ± 16.2 | 0.12 | 100.9 ± 16.2 |
| PO | 106.5 ± 15.1 | 0.06 | 98.7 ± 16.3 |
| FD | 105.5 ± 12.6 | 0.003 | 96.5 ± 14.0 |
| CFT (%) | 55.6 ± 26.0 | 0.4 | 51.2 ± 26.6 |
| D2 (%) | 56.8 ± 29.1 | 0.15 | 47.9 ± 31.4 |
| RFT (%) | 31.8 ± 30.7 | 0.08 | 22.0 ± 25.1 |

FSIQ and PD). Only the treatment modality of the RT-group including CI and MTX-applications exhibited a statistically significance.

### Effect of Different Single Cranial Irradiation Dosages

Regarding the RT-group there was a range in single irradiation dose between 1.0 and 3.6 Gy. Subjects receiving a single dose larger than 2 Gy exhibited a FSIQ of 96.0 ± 17.2, n = 27, compared with subjects receiving a single dose lower than 2 Gy (103.4 ± 15.0, n = 27). This difference was not statistically significant (p = 0.10).

### Comparisons of neuropsychological test results with morphological CNS abnormalities

Patients with reduced FD scores (-ISD = < 85 points) (n = 13) presented "leukoencephalopathy" more often (in 38.5%)) than patients with FD scores > 85 points (12.6%, 11/87) (p = 0.02) There was no difference between both groups concerning "brain atrophy": 46.2% (6/13) vs 33/82.

### Psychosocial and Behavior Problems

We used the Child Behavior Checklist (CBCL) for the investigation of somatic complaints, attention problems, anxiety, depression, aggressive behavior, deliquent behavior, social problems and withdrawal. Especially a young age at diagnosis (< 5 yrs.) was significant associated with attention and social problems and withdrawal. Subjects with neuroradiological signs of leukoencephalopathy exhibited significantly more often attention problems compared with a norm populatoion (5.8 vs. 2.6, p < 0,01).

### Neurophysiological Data

In the conventional EEG the results did not differ between the MTX- and the RT-group. But using a quantitative EEG analysis subjects of the RT-group showed significant more impairments than subjects of the MTX-group. Furthermore 13 subjects of the RT-group, investigated with event related potentials only in Erlangen, exhibited significant prolongations in the P300 latencies, compared to healthy controls and to the subjects of the MTX-group. These results are discussed and published elsewhere [13, 14, 15, 16, 17].

### Auxological Data

We detected that 40% of the subjects in both treatment groups are overweighted (body weight above the 97 percentile). Microcephaly was observed in 4 subjects only in the RT-group (head circumference lower than the 3 percentile). There was no abnormal body height in both groups, but we did not measure the sitting height.

### Discussion

#### Secondary Tumors

In the investigation of the GCCR, analysing 7032 ALL survivors since 1980, 103 secondary tumors including 33 brain tumors were documented. Neglia and collegues described in a cohort study of 9720 children, treated for ALL between 1972 and 1988, 43 secondary tumors, including 24 neoplasms of the CNS [18]. This represented a 22-fold excess of neoplasms of the CNS. This is comparable to the data of the German ALL-BFM group (chairman: Dr. Schrappe, Hannover). They report on a 19-fold increase for neoplasms of the CNS [19].

## CNS toxicity After ALL Treatment

In our cross-sectional study of 107 ALL long-term survivors we have had the opportunity to analyse a homogenous group of ALL patients cranial irradiated with 18 Gy (RT-group) and to compare their results with a group of patients with chemotherapy (MTX-group) only. The preventive irradiation of the CNS with 18 Gy in combination with systemical and intrathecal MTX promotes neuroradiological and neurophysiological alterations, neuropsychological and neurological deficits more pronounced than MTX alone.

In our cohort survivors, there was statistically significant difference before therapy in hematological and clinical data between both groups. Differences between both groups in neuropsychological performance might have been related to these differences in the study population. Therefore, we examined univariately the relations between clinical data and subsequent test results resp. neuropsychological performance, and in a multivariate model, we examined, whether adjusted for initial values, the significance concerning the test results disappeared. However, our analyses showed that there was no relation between clinical data and subsequent test results and that also multivariately the significance found for the test results persisted.

We detected that 40% of the subjects in both treatment groups are overweighted. This is comparable to other published data [20, 21]. But for further investigation we have to recommend to measure the body-mass-index and to compare the index of the patients with the index of their parents.

The results of several studies investigating the CNS of former ALL patients differ widely. For example, no brain damage, especially no white matter changes, was described in the study of Kramer et al. [22], even if patients were irradiated with 18 Gy or 24 Gy, contra-dictory to the investigation by Peylan-Ramu et al. [23]), who reported more than 50% abnormal CCT findings such as white matter changes, widening of the ventricles and sulci or calcifications in patients receiving ITMTX or intrathecal cystosine arabinosid an cranial irradiation with 24 Gy, comparable with our observations, using CI with 18 Gy.

However there are three distinct pathological entities that are believed to be the consequences of prophylactic CNS therapy on CNS morphology.

## Leukoencephalopathy

Leukoencephalopathy is correlated to myelin degeneration [24]. Using the protocols of the late 60s, children who had received cranial irradiation with more than 20 Gy and both intrathecal and systemic MTX treatment are at a greater risk to develop leukoencephalopathy [25]. The clinical symptoms of leukoencephalopathy can be seizures, ataxia, lethargy, slurred speach, spasticity, dysphasia, lowered IQ scores, memory impairments and confusion. It is reported that these symptoms occurred later than four months after irradiation. Possible correlating CCT findings are periventricular hypodensity, dilatation of the ventricles and subarachnoid spaces [26]. Most children recover completely. However the changes can be progressive also and some children survive with signs of permanent neurological deficits. These serious complications are found rarely in the context of modern treatment protocols. We can confirm this observation with our own findings.

The subclinical form of leukoencephalopathy is more common, as the results of Peylan-Ramu et al. [23] have shown, finding CCT abnormalities in 8 (57%) of 14 non-symptomatic patients who received 24 Gy irradiation and intrathecal MTX. Our own results confirm these investigations. Therefore we conclude that the lower irradiation doses (18 Gy) combined with MTX used in our patient sample is able to cause anatomical brain alterations, especially signs of subacute leukoencephalopathy.

## Mineralizing Microangiopathy

This alteration affects the grey matter of the CNS, mainly the region of the basal ganglia, the cerebral cortical sulci and, less frequently, the cerebellar grey matter [27]. Histologically, a deposition of calcium is found in the small blood vessels, with a particular occlusion of the lumens by precipitated mineralized debris. This is accompanied by a dystrophic calcification in the surrounding neural tissue. The prophylactic irradiation of the brain is assumed to be the main cause in developing these changes. Namely, patients who were younger than 10 years at the time of irradiation, a dose higher than 15 Gy, a post-irradiation interval of more than 10 months and CNS leukemic relapses with more intensive therapy are further variables of risk for mineralizing microangiopathy [28]. Other investigations believe that additional doses of MTX and cytosine arabinosid may influence the progression of these lesions [29]. Possible clinical manifestations of these alterations are headaches, seizures, EEG abnormalities, dyscoordination, gait abnormalities, memory deficits, learning disorders, declines in IQ scores and various behavioral difficulties [30]. These findings appear with a latency of about 10 months up to several years after the irradiation. The calcifications can be detected more clearly using CCT scans than MRI scans, mainly in the region of the basal ganglia or in the grey matter of the cortex. The more chronic form of mineralizing microangiopathy seem to occur only if a combination of both CT and ITMTX is used.

In our group of patients receiving CCT scans 3/46 had detectable calcifications. Noteworthy, all calcifications were detected in the RT-group (3/28 (11%)) whereas no calcification was seen in the MTX-group. One reason for this low incidence of calcifications could be the relatively low dose of irradiation used (18 Gy). However, it is significant that 2 from 3 patients belonged to the group with the intrathecal MTX dosages applied before CI and with the highest cumulative dose in intrathecal MTX. Therefore, a higher intrathecal MTX dose in combination with cranial irradiation may cause a higher risk for calcifications. Similar results are formerly reported in a review by Ochs et al. [31], who listed the frequency of anatomical abnormalities of the brain in relation to type of CNS prophylaxis and found that a chemoprophylaxis alone causes no brain calcifications in contrast to the irradiated patients (18 Gy) which present up to 7% calcifications. Another explanation for these findings could be the additional therapy using systemical MTX in this subgroup of the RT-group. These results confirm the review of Bleyer at al. [32] who described this alteration as usually seen after combined chemotherapy and CI.

## Subacute Necrotizing Leukomyelopathy

Patients receiving cranial or cranial-spinal irradiation followed by intrathecal MTX applications, displayed alteration of the spinal cord in the investigations conducted by Price [33]. These children presented a focal meyelin necrosis in the posterior and/or lateral columns of the spinal cord, extensive cervical and lumbar, milder in the thoracic section. He hypothesized that a folate deficiency resulting from the intrathecal MTX treatment with cumulative doses > 200 mg and a treatment duration longer than 2 years may be the cause. This injury of spinal cord radiation is related to neurological findings to the cord level of the radiation field [34].

Serious neurological impairments as clinical signs for leukomyelopathy were not found in our subject group.

## Neuropsychological Functioning after Therapy

Prospective as well as retrospective studies, investigating at different time periods after finishing CI, describe a progressive disturbance in neuropsychological abilities: just after irradiation there are often no impairments, but lengthening the time, irradiated patients show reductions in neuropsychological functions [35, 36]. Especially Jankovice et al. reported retrospectively on irradiated patients, showing a decline of 3.7 FSIQ points per year after diagnosis [37]. Ochs et al. in their prospective investigation lasting over six years presented progressive reductions in VIQ and FSIQ especially in the cranial irradiated group but also in patients treated with systemic and intrathecal chemotherapy (MTX) [38].

In our study cranial irradiated long-term survivors are impaired in cognitive development in mean 4.5–10.6 years after cessation of treatment. This finding confirms results describing a late manifestation of neuropsychological sequelae up to seven year after CI [39]. But in our study there is no significant decline of neuropsychological impairments over time. Within the period of 7 years after treatment reduced IQ-scores as well as disturbances in attention and memory were stable [40].

### Effect of Age at Diagnosis on Neuropsychological Performance

Children younger than 5 to 8 years at the time of diagnosis [41, 42] or even under an age of two or three years [43, 44] who received CI with 18 or 24 Gy show the lowest scores in intelligence performance. In our subject group, patients younger than 5 years show lower scores in intellectual ability than older patients, especially if they were cranial irradiated.

### Comparison of CNS-Morphology and Neuropsychology

Rubin and Casseret reported about the increased sensitivity of the white matter to develop structural changes after irradiation of the CNS by analysing autopsy findings and CCT scans [45]. Fletcher and Copeland [46] discussed correlations between morphological and intellectual and/or cognitive impairments: they stated that white matter alterations are typically manifested in a deterioration of nonverbal tasks, including attention, nonverbal memory and arithmetical computations. Further Rouke [47] concluded an interference between white matter abnormalities and right hemisphere dysfunction and Brouwers et al. [48] reported relations to frontal lobe dysfunction. In our investigation patients with a reduced Kaufman factor "Freedom from Distractibility (FD)" score below 85 points showed morphologically more often leukoencephalopathy – mainly in the frontal lobe. Therefore white matter alterations seem to be decisive for impairments in short-term memory, speed of processing, visuomotor coordination and sequencing ability [49], all components of mental speed measured with FD.

In outcome studies it is important to compare the benefits and the late effects of the treatment. Our MTX-group had a relapse rate with CNS involvement of 12% and intellectual impairments (IQ <85) in 5%. Our RT-group had a calculated relapse rate with CNS involvement of 7% and intellectual impairments (IQ <85) in 17%. Therefore the difference in relapse rates with CNS involvement is 5%. Now, if one reduces the RT-group for the 5% of the worst patients and if one compares again, the difference between the MTX- and the RT-group is still statistically significant present. Furthermore, if one compares only standard-risk patients in the RT-group with standard-risk patients in the MTX-group, the difference between the MTX- and the RT-groups is still significantly present.

## Prospective Study "CNS toxicity during and after ALL therapy in childhood"

A prospective, multicenter study, is in Germany and Austria underway, investigating CNS toxicity during and after ALL therapy in a study population of ALL patients, receiving CNS prophylactic therapy only by chemotherapy according to the ALL-BFM 95 and CoALL 97 trials. We expect a group of 150 patients in 23 hospital in Austria and Germany to be enrolled. The aims are the evaluation of the neuropsychological performance and the health related quality of life in this long-term follow-up for 8 years. The investigations will be performed within 2 weeks after diagnosis, after reinduction therapy, after maintenance therapy and 2 and 5 years after completing chemotherapy.

First results concern 48 patients, which were investigated at diagnosis, and 8 patients were evaluated after reinduction therapy. At diagnosis we detected normal intellectual and cognitive performance. In the Child Behavior Checklist parents describe more often somatic complaints, anxiety, depression and an aggressive behavior. After reinduction, until now no significant impairments in intellectual and cognitive performance were detected. However the group is too small for any conclusion and the follow-up is too short.

## Conclusion

Our findings and other reports propose, that impairments after CI with 18 Gy are a primary damage of the neuroglia, which influences secondary other specific functions, i.e. psychomotoric speed, attention-concentration, ability in learning, in planning and in coordinating psychomotoric and sequencing ability. CI applied with the techniques of the 80s appears to influence the long-term survivors' cognitive capacity of processing described as mental speed. Mental speed is represented in specific achievements as objectified in the Kaufman factor Freedom from Distractibility (FD) [8]. Long-term survivors of ALL in childhood often report about short attention span, distractibility, immaturity and learning disabilities [33] and exhibit significantly reduced scores in FD, if they were cranial irradiated with 24 Gy [50]. Noteworthy a CI with 18 Gy results in significant impairments in FD, as a result of deficits in attention, concentration, memory and the ability of cognitive processing, also. Therefore, some former ALL patients need assistance for a smooth re-entry into school and an identification of cognitive dysfunctions in school for a proper help in their academic achievements [51, 52]. However as stated by Cousens et al. [49], children are able to learn and to compensate, but they may be slower to require new material.

## References

1. Pochedly C (1979) Prophylactic CNS therapy in childhood acute leukemia. Review of methods used. Am J Pediatr Hematol Oncol 1: 119 –126
2. Dritschilo A, Cassady JR, Camitta B et al. (1976) The role of irradiation in central nervous system treatment and prophylaxis for acute lymphoblastic leukemia. Cancer 37: 272–2735
3. Simone J, Aur R, Hustu H et al. (1975) Combined modality therapy of acute lymphoblastic leukemia. J Natl Cancer Inst 32: 1333 –1341
4. Freeman AI, Weinberg V, Brecher ML et al. (1983) Comparison of intermediate-dose methotrexate with cranial irradiation for the post-induction treatment of acute lymphoblastic leukemia in children. N Engl J Med 308: 477–484
5. Beck JD, Winkler K, Niethammer D et al. (1995) Die Nachsorge der von einer Krebserkrankung geheilten Kinder und jungen Erwachsenen. Erste Empfehlungen der Arbeitsgemeinschaft Spätfolgen. Klin Padiatr 207: 186 –192
6. Langer T, Hertzberg H, Dörr HG et al. (1998) Prinzipien zur Erfassung von Spätfolgen. In: Creutzig U, Henze G (Hrsg.) Diagnostische und therapeutische Standards in der pädiatrischen Onkologie. Gesellschaft für Pädiatrische Onkologie und Hämatologie. W. Zuckschwerdt-Verlag, München, Bern, Wien, New York, pp 15 –23
7. Schrappe M, Beck JD, Brandeis WE et al. (1987) Die Behandlung der akuten lymphoblastischen Leukämie im Kindes- und Jugendalter: Ergebnisse der multizentrischen Therapiestudie ALL-BFM 81. Klein Padiatr 199: 133 –150
8. Kaufman AS (1975) Factor analysis of the WISC-R at eleven age levels between 6 1/2 and 16 1/2 years. J Consult Clin Psychol 43: 135 –147
9. Gutkin TB (1978) Some useful statistics for the interpretation of the WISC-R. J Consult Clin Psychol 46: 1561–1563
10. Tellegen A, Briggs PF (1967) Old wine in new skins: Grouping Wechsler subtests into new scales. J Consult Psychol 31: 499 –506
11. Sattler J (1974) Assessment of children's intelligence. Saunders, Philadelphia
12. Hertzberg H, Huk WJ, Überall MA et al. (1997) CNS late effects after ALL-therapy in childhood I: Neuroradiological findings in long-term survivors of childhood ALL. An evaluation of the interferences between morphology an neuropsychological performance. Med Pediatr Oncol 28: 387–400
13. Überall MA, Wenzel D, Hertzberg H et al. (1997) CNS late-effects after ALL therapy in childhood Part II: Conventional EEG recordings in asymptomatic long-term survivors of childhood ALL. An evoluation of the interferences between neurophysiology, neurology, psychology and CNS morphology. Med Pediatr Oncol 29: 121 –131
14. Überall MA, Haupt K, Hertzberg H et al. (1996) P300 abnormalities in long-time survivors of acute lymphoblastic leukemia in childhood – Side effects of CNS prophylaxis? Neuropediatrics 27: 130 –135
15. Überall MA, Haupt K, Hertzberg H et al.: Visual-Evoked potentials in long-term survivors of acute lymphoblastic leukemia in childhood. Neuropediatrics 27: 194 –196
16. Überall MA, Haupt K, Hertzberg et al. (1996) Quantitative EEG in long-term survivors of acute lymphoblastic leukemia. Pediatr Neurol 15: 293 –298
17. Überall MA, Skirl G, Straßburg HM et al. (1998) Neurophysiological findings in long-term survivors of acute lymphoblastic leukaemia in childhood treated with the BFM-protocol 81 SR-A/B. Eur J Pediatr 156: 727 –733
18. Negla JP, Meadows AT, Robinson LL et al. (1991) Second neoplasms after acute lymphoblastic leukemia in childhood. N Engl Med 325: 1330–1336
19. Löning L, Kaatsch P, Riehm H, Schrappe M for the ALL-BFM Group (1999) Secondary neoplasms after therapy of childhood ALL: Significantly risk without cranial irradiation. Ann Hematol 78: S40

20. Groot-Loonen JL, Otten BJ, van't Hof MA, Lippens RJJ, Stoelinga GBA (1996) Influence of treatment on body weight in acute lymphoblastic leukemia. Med Pediatr Oncol 27: 92–97

21. Sainsbury CPQ, Newcombe RG, Huges IA (1985) Weight gain and height velocity during prolonged first remission from acute lymphoblastic leukaemia. Arch Dis Child 60: 832–836

22. Kramer JH, Norman D, Brant-Zawadzki M, Ablin A, Moore IM (1988) Absence of white matter changes on magnetic resonance imaging in children treated with CNS prophylaxis therapy for leukemia. Cancer 61: 928 –930

23. Peylan-Ramu N, Poplack DG, Pizzo PA, Adornato BT, Di Chiro G (1978) Abnormal CT-scans of the brain in asymptomatic children with acute lymphocytic leukemia after prophylactic treatment of the central nervous system with radiation and intrathecal chemotherapy. N Engl J Med 298: 815 –818

24. Price RA, Jamieson PA (1975) The central nervous system in childhood leukemia: II. Subacute leukoencephalopathy. Cancer 35: 306 –318

25. Price RA (1983) Therapy related central nervous system diseases in children with acute lymphocytic leukemia. In Mastrangelo R, Poplack DG, Riccardi R (eds) "Central nervous system leukemia – prevention and treatment." Boston, Martinus Nijhoff Publishers, pp 71 –83

26. Valk PE, Dillon WP (1991) Diagnostic imaging of central nervous system radiation injury. In Gutin PH, Leibel SA, Sheline GE (eds) "Radiation injury to the nervous system." New York, Raven Press, pp. 211 –237

27. Price RA (1979) Histopathology of CNS leukemia and complications of therapy. Am J Pediatr Hematol Oncol 1: 21–30

28. Price RA, Birdwell DA (1978) The central nervous system in childhood leukemia. III. Mineralizing microangiopathy and dystrophic calcification. Cancer 42: 717 –728

29. McIntosh S, Fischer DB, Rothman S, Rosenfield N, Lobel JS, O'Brien RT (1977) Intracranial calcifications in childhood leukemia. J Pediatr 91: 909 –913

30. Stehbens JA, Kaleita TA, Noll RB, MacLean WE, O'Brien RT, Waskerwitz MJ, Hammond GD (1991) CNS prophylaxis of childhood leukemia: What are the long-term neurological, neuropsychological and behavioral effects? Neuropsychological Review 2: 147 –177

31. Ochs JJ (1989) Neurotoxicity due to central nervous system therapy for childhood leukemia. Am J Pediatr Hematol Oncol 11: 93 –105

32. Bleyer WA, Griffin TW (1980) White matter necrosis, mineralizing microangiography, and intellectual abilities in survivors of childhood leukemia: Associations with central nervous system irradiation and methotrexate therapy. In Gilbert HA, Kagan AR (eds) "Radiation damage to nervous system." New York, Raven Press, pp 155 –174

33. Price RA (1979) Histopathogenesis of meningeal leukaemia and complications of therapy. In Whitehouse JMA, Kay HEM (eds) "CNS complications of malignant disease." Baltimore, University Park Press

34. Pallis CA, Louis S, Morgan RL (1961) Radiation myelopathy. Brain 84: 460 –479

35. Meadows AT, Massari DJ, Fergusson J et al. (1981) Declines in IQ scores and cognitive dysfunctions in children with acute lymphocytic leukaemia treated with children with cranial irradiation. Lancet 7: 1015 –1018

36. Stehbens JA, Kisker CT (1884) Intelligence and achievement testing in childhood cancer. Three years post diagnosis. J Dev Behav Pediatr 5: 184–188

37. Jankovic M, Brouwers P, Valsecchi MG et al. Association of 1800 cGy cranial irradiation with intellectual function in children with acute lymphoblastic leukemia. Lancet 344

38. Ochs J, Mulhern RK, Rairclough D et al. (1991) Comparison of neuropsychologic functioning and clinical indicators of neurotoxicity in long-term survivors of childhood leukemia given cranial radiation or parenteral methotrexate: a prospective study. J Clin Oncol 9: 145 –151

39. Twaddle V, Britton P, Craft A et al. (1983) Intellectual function after treatment for leukemia or solid tumors. Arch Dis Child 58: 949 –952

40. Brouwers P, Poplack D (1990) Memory and learning sequelae in long-term survivors of acute lymphoblastic leukemia. Association with attention deficits. Am J Pediatr Hematol Oncol 12: 174 –181

41. Goff JR, Anderson HR, Cooper PF (1980) Distractability and memory deficits in long-term survivors of acute lymphoblastic leukemia. J Dev Behav Pediatr 1: 158 –163

42. Copeland DR, Fletcher JM, Pfefferbaum-Levine B et al. (1985) Neuropsychological sequelae of childhood cancer in long-terms survivors. Pediatrics 75: 745 –753

43. Jannoun L (1983) Are cognitive and educational development affected by age at which prophylactic therapy is given in acute lymphoblastic leukemia? Arch Dis Child 58: 953–958

44. Mulhern RK, Kovnar E, Lnagston J et al. (1992) Long-term survivors of leukemia treated in infancy: factors associated with neuropsychologic status. J Clin Oncol 10: 1095–1102

45. Rubin P, Casseret GW (1968) Central nervous system (Vol. 2). Saunders, Philadelphia

46. Fletcher JM, Copeland DR (1988) Neurobehavioral effects of central nervous system prophylactic treatment of cancer in children. J Clin Exp Neuropsychol 10: 495 –538

47. Rourke BP (1982) Central processing deficiencies in children: Toward a developmental neuropsychological mode. J Clin Neuropsychol 4: 1 –18

48. Brouwers P, Riccardi R, Fedio P et al. (1985) Long-term neuropsychologic sequelae of childhood leukemia: Correlation with CT brain scan abnormalities. J Pediatr 106: 723–728

49. Cousens P, Ungerer JA, Crawford JA et al. (1991) Cognitive effects of childhood leukemia therapy: a case for four specific deficits. J Pediatr Psychol 16: 475 –488

50. Rowland JH, Glidewell OJ, Sibley RF et al. (1984) Effects of different forms of central nervous system prophylaxis on neuropsychologic function in childhood leukemia. J Clin Oncol 2: 1327 –1335

51. Deasy-Spinetta P, Spinetta JJ (1980) The child with cancer in school: Teacher's appraisal. Am J Pediatr Hematol Oncol 2: 89 –94

52. Deasy-Spinetta P (1993) School issues and the child with cancer. Cancer 71: 3261 –3264

# The Use of PEG-Asparaginase in Leukemic Children with Prior Hypersensitivity to Native L-Asparaginase

B. Sikorska-Fic[1], K. Makowska[2] and R. Rokicka-Milewska[1]

*Abstract.* The aim of the study was to examine the results of PEG-L-Asparaginase administration in children with acute lymphoblastic leukemia and the symptoms of intolerance to L-Aspa E. Coli or Erwinase .

L-Asparaginase is widely used in the treatment of patients with acute lymphoblastic leukaemia. Use of L-Aspa E. Coli as well as Erwinase is not possible in all cases because of the side effects, mainly allergic reactions and dysfunction of pancreas. Recently, the new form of the enzyme, PEG-L-Asparaginase, was introduced. Binding L-Asparaginase E. Coli to poliethylene glycol has decreased its toxicity, extended its plasma half-live not significantly affecting the efficacy. PEG-Asparaginase (Oncaspar) was administred to three children with newly diagnosed ALL and three children with first relapse of ALL, treated according to New York Protocol and BFM 90 Protocol for ALL relapses respectively. Oncaspar was given at the dose of 2500 IU/m$^2$ in the first five patients and after that, according the new consideration, 1000 IU/m$^2$ . Six children received 16 doses of Oncaspar, the number of doses for individual patient varied from one to six. The short-lived nettlerash was observed in one patient during two subsequent infusions of the drug, which disappeared after hydrocotisone and anti-histamine drugs administration. Treatment with PEG-Asparaginase was discontinued in one child, who developed dyspnea, nausea, vomiting and face rash during the third dose of the drug.

*Conclusion:* Oncaspar is the valuable drug, which enabled continuation of treatment according to protocol in five out of six children with bad tolerance to routinly used L-Asparaginase preparations.

## Introduction

L-Asparaginase (L-Aspa) is an essential and durable constituent of polychemotherapy of acute lymphoblastic leukaemia (ALL) in children and adults [5,6,11]. Lack of direct bone marrow toxicity of L-Aspa allows for administration of the drug in periods of expectant myelosuppression caused by the disease or by concomitant chemotherapy [4]. L-Aspa acts by lowering extracellular concentration of L-Asparagine. L-Asparagine is an amino acid whose presence in the blood is necessary for some neoplastic cells, particularly lymphoblasts for DNA synthesis [3]. Two natural forms of the enzyme are produced by the Escherichia coli (E. coli) and Erwinia chrysanthemi (Erwinia) bacteria. Their plasma half-life (t $\frac{1}{2}$) is 1.2 and 0.6 days respectively [4]. Thus it is necessary to administer the drug every 2–3 days. There are a few preparations of L-Aspa derived from E.coli (Kidrolase, Rhone-Poulenc; L-Asparaginase, Medac; Elspar, MSD) and a preparation of L-Aspa derived from Erwinia (Erwinase, Porton). Each preparation administered in equal doses varies in enzymatic activity, plasma t $\frac{1}{2}$ and resulting L-Asparagine depletion level. The most effective form of L-Aspa derived from E.coli seems to be L-Asparaginase (Medac) [2]. Erwinase, administered in a dose equal to one dose of L-Aspa E.coli is considered less toxic but also less effective [9]. Administration of L-Aspa is not possible in all cases, because of adverse effects, mainly

---

[1] Dept. of Pediatric Hematology/Oncology, University Medical School, Warsaw , Poland
[2] Dept. of Hematology/Oncology, Childrens Hospital, Olsztyn, Poland

allergic reactions, dysfunction of pancreas and coagulopathy. When antibodies against L-Aspa are produced with or without symptoms of allergy, the effectiveness of consecutive doses of the drug decreases because of shortened t $\frac{1}{2}$ and lower asparagine depletion ability [1, 2]. In cases of allergic reactions to natural L-Aspa it is possible to administer Erwinase. However in some patients allergic to L-Aspa who were given Erwinase, the lack of asparagine depletion was found, so some authors question such a procedure. Allergy to both natural forms of L-Aspa makes it impossible to treat patients according to protocol. Recently, a new preparation PEG-Asparaginase has become available. In this preparation L-Aspa derived from E. coli is bound to polyethylene glycol. This has prolonged plasma t $\frac{1}{2}$ to 5,7 days, has made it possible to administer the drug every 2 weeks and has decreased its toxicity [4]. The drug was registered in the USA in 1994 and in Germany in 1997 as a preparation for patients allergic to native forms of L-Aspa [7]. Clinical investigations performed mostly in patients with relapse of ALL, confirmed a lower frequency of allergic reactions in comparison with reactions to the native form and indicates its effectiveness [10].

## Aim

The aim of the study is to present the results of PEG-Asparaginase administration in 6 children suffering from ALL. All children developed intolerance symptoms after administration of L-Aspa E.coli or Erwinase.

## Material and methods

PEG-Asparaginase (Oncaspar, Medac) was administered intravenously in 1 hour infusions of 2500 IU/m$^2$ in first five patients. Then the drug was administered in doses of 1000 IU/m$^2$ in accordance with the recommendations of the BFM group. The interval between consecutive doses has been determined in the treatment protocol and in one treatment cycle the interval was 2 weeks. The drug was administered to 6 patients (2 girls and 4 boys) aged 4–10 years, suffering from ALL. In 3

children high risk common-ALL was diagnosed and the patients were treated in accordance with the New York protocol [10]. In the other 3 children a relapse of ALL (common ALL in 2, pre B-ALL in 1) was diagnosed and they were treated according to the BFM 90 protocol for relapses. The number of doses in individual patients varied from 1 to 6. In patients receiving PEG-Asparaginase morphologic and biochemical parameters of the blood and coagulation parameters were estimated twice a week to evaluate the tolerance of treatment.

## Results

Six children were given 15 full doses of Oncaspar. In 2 children clinical adverse effects were observed. In one of these two children short-time urticaria appeared during second administration of the drug. This withdrew after hydrocortisone and antihistamine were administered. During the third administration of Oncaspar the second child developed violent symptoms: face rash, dyspnea, nausea and vomiting. Therefore, administration of the drug was discontinued. Laboratory abnormalities were noticed in 5 patients. There was an increase of aminotranspherases (twice the normal values), mild hypoalbuminaemia and hypofibrynogenaemia. In one child leucopenia lasting 10 days was noticed.

## Discussion

Allergic reactions as an reaction to xenogenic protein are the most frequent adverse effects during treatment with Asparaginase and occur in about 20–35% patients [7]. In some of them these allergic reactions result in a discontinuation of the treatment. Other adverse effects connected with decreased protein synthesis, such as pancreatitis, hyperglycaemia, impaired liver function, coagulopathy with symptoms of bleeding and/or thrombosis are less frequent. They are sometimes the reasons for withdrawal of L-Asparaginase. In two out of six of our patients treated with PEG-Asparaginase we observed allergic reactions and therefore administrartion of the drug was withdrawn in one child. Laboratory abnormalities were subclinical and shortlasting. Thus, the drug was well tolerated and allowed for the treatment protocols to be put into the practice. In patients treated with preparations of L-Aspa it is possible to monitor levels of drug activity and serum asparagine levels. Such tests enable better control of therapy and the readjustment of consecutive doses to different levels of asparagine depletion [1, 4]. In accordance with BFM group studies, doses of 1000 IU/m$^2$ appeared to be effective. This dose ensures asparagine depletion in most patients for 3 weeks after administration of the drug [8]. On the basis of BFM group comparative pharmacokinetic studies of different forms of L-Aspa, PEG-Aspa is administered as second-line drug, in cases of L-Aspa E.coli intolerance without administering Erwinase. [2].

## Conclusions

1. Administration of PEG-Aspa enabled a continuation of the treatment according to protocol in five out of six children with intolerance of routinely administered preparations of L-Aspa.
2. The drug was well tolerated, with the exception of one case when the treatment was discontinued after two doses of PEG-Aspa.
3. Laboratory abnormalities were transient and were not the reason for discontinuing the treatment.

4. PEG-Aspa is a valuable drug, which can replace L-Aspa E.coli and Erwinase in the cases of intolerance.

## References

1. Asselin B., at al.: "Comparative Pharmacokinetic Studies of Three Asparaginase Preparations". Journal of Clinical Oncology, 1993, 11, 1780–1786
2. Boos J., at al.: Monitoring of asparaginase activity and asparaginase levels in children on different asparaginase preparations. Eur J Cancer 1996, 32A, 1544–1550.
3. Broome J.D.: L-Asparaginase: Discovery and development as a tumor-inhibitory agent. Cancer Treat Rep 1981, 65 (Suppl.4), 111–114
4. Ettinger L.J., at al.:Acute Lymphoblastic Leukaemia – A Guide to Asparaginase and Pegaspargase Therpay. BioDrugs 1997 Jan 7 (1), 30–39
5. Henze G., at al.: BFM group treatment results in relapsed childhood acute lmphoblastic leukemia. Hematol Bluttransfus 1990, 33, 619–626
6. Holland J.F., Ohnuma T.: Asparaginase and amino acids in cancer therapeutics. Cancer Treat Rep 1981, 65 (Suppl. 4), 123–130
7. Holle L.M.: Pegaspargase:an alternative?. The Annals of Pharmacotherapy, 1997, 31, 616–624
8. Muller H.J., Boos J.: Use of L-Asparaginase in childhood ALL. Crit Rev Oncol Hematol, 1998, 28, 97–113
9. Otten J., at al.: The importance of L-Asparaginase(A'ASE) in the treatment of acute lymphoblastic leukemia (ALL) in children: Results of the EORTC 58881 randomized phase III trial showing efficiency of Escherichia coli (E.coli) as compared to Erwinia (ERW) A' ASE. Blood 1996, 88 (Suppl I):669
10. Patel S.S., Benfield P.: Pegaspargase (Polyethylene Glycol-L-Asparginase). Clin Immunother 1996 Jun: 5 (6), 492–496
11. Steinherz P.G., at al.: Improved disease free survival of children with acute lymphoblastic leukemia at high risk for early relaps with the New York regimen- a new intensive therapy protocol: a raport from the Children' s Cancer Study Group. J Clin Oncol 1986, 4, 744–752

# The Importance of MRI in Detection of Primary CNS Involvement in Leukaemic Children

E. Wagiel, K. Wagiel* and R. Rokicka-Milewska

*Abstract.* Magnetic resonance (MRI) of the central nervous system (CNS) was carried out in 36 children aged from 1.5 to 17 years with newly diagnosed leukaemia before treatment administration. In 25 patients MRI of the head and in 11 MRI of both the head and spine were performed. The results were compared with cerebro-spinal fluid (CSF) cytology and neurological examination. Leukaemic CNS infiltration was detected in 7 children (19,5%). CSF blasts were not found in any of the 36 examined children. Neurological examination revealed minimal symptoms in 2 patients. The results of the study implicate the importance of early routine MRI screening of CNS in leukaemic children. The range of examination should include MRI of the head and spine. In our study MRI was more sensitive than CSF examination in detecting CNS leukaemic involvement

## Introduction

CNS prophylaxis (primarily intrathecal methotrexat and radiotherapy) dramatically reduced CSN relapses (from 75% in patients with ALL to 5–10%) [1, 2, 3] .However for children with CNS leukaemia at diagnosis, the risk CNS relapse ( and subsequent hematologic relapse) is even higher, and can be observed in up to 25–30 % patients [3]. Therefore the detection of primary CNS involvement may have a profound implication for the prognosis and accurate stratification of CNS prophylactic therapy. Cytologic confirmation is necessary for diagnosis, but false-negative cytologies are common; initial CSF examina-tion reveals malignant cells in only 50–60% of patients with carcimatous meningosis [4]. Imaging, especially magnetic resonance ima-ging (MRI), can play an important role.

The aim of our study was to determine the usefulness of MRI in the detection of leukae-mic infiltrates within the brain and spinal canal in children with newly diagnosed leu-kaemia.

## Material and methods

Magnetic resonance were performed in 36 children, 24 boys and 12 girls, aged 1.5–17 years (median 6.9 years), with newly dia-gnosed leukaemia, hospitalized in the Department of Paediatrics, Haematology and Oncology in Warsaw in 1996,1997 and 1998. ALL was diagnosed in 30 children (83.4%), AML in 4 children (11.1%). and CML in 2 (5.5%). In 25 patients MRI of the head and in 11 patients MRI of both the head and spine were performed. The scans were performed using the following MRI units: Toshiba MRT (0.5 T) and Magnetom Siemens (1.5 T). The examinations were conducted in SE sequence in T1, T2 and PD-weighted images, before and after contrast enhancement (Gd DTPA). Brain examinations were performed in axial and coronary planes, while vertebral column examinations were carried out in saggital and axial planes .

CNS infiltration was detected as abnormal diffuse or nodullar dural thickening on pre-contrast images and as abnormal enhance-ment of the dura, subarachnoid , cisternal or pial on postcontrast T1 -images

Dept.of Paediatric Haematology and Oncology, Medical School, Warsaw, Poland
*Dept. of Diagnostic Imaging, Central Railway Hospital

In all examined children a lumbar puncture and a complete neurological examination (including EEG) were performed as a standard procedure in leukaemic children. Spinal fluid was analyzed for glucose, protein content and WBC count. The CNS disease was diagnosed on the basis of the WBC count above 5/mm³ and a presence of leukaemic cells in the spinal fluid.

## Results

Leukaemic CNS infiltrates were detected in MRI in 7 children (19.5%). In 4 cases the infiltrates were localized only intracranially. Involvement of the meninges of the brain in 3 cases were detectable: in 1 case before the contrast as a marked thickening of the meninges (up to 3 mm), in 2 cases after administration of Gd GTPA, as segmental or diffuse meninges contrast enhancement (Fig. 1); In 1 case leukaemic infiltrates were observed within the nervous tissue as hyperintensive regions in the deep structures of both hemispheres with a weak mass-effect which underwent intense irregular enhancement after contrast injection. Within the spi-

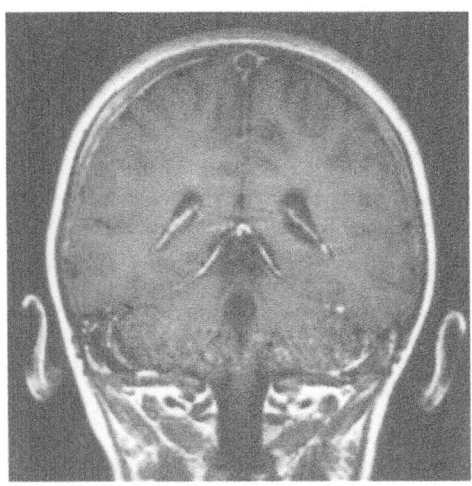

**Fig. 1.** 12-years old boy with ALL. In MRI (T1 weighted images) diffuse meninges contrast enhancement after Gd-DTPA

nal canal leukaemic infiltrates were detected in 2 children. They had the form of a diffuse infiltration of the meninges (Fig. 2a, 2b ). One child had a massive leukaemic CNS involvement localised intracranially and intraspinally (Fig. 3).

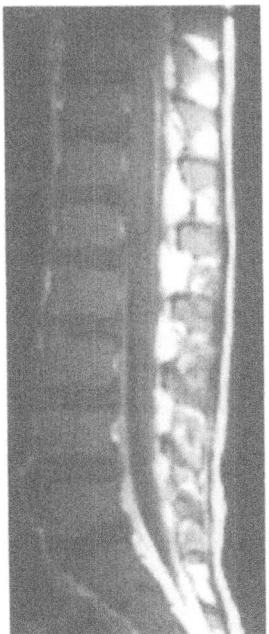

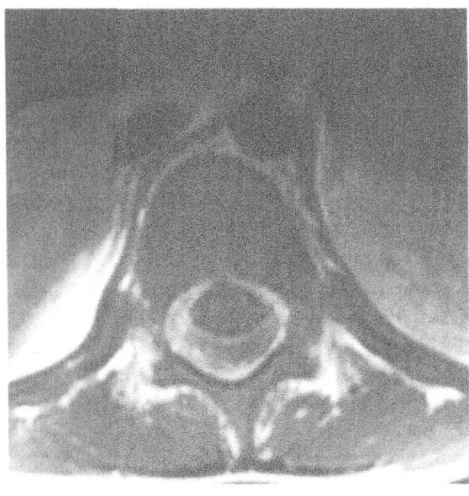

**Fig. 2.** 7-years old boy with ALL. **a)** MRI (T1 weighted images), saggital plane. Meningeal leukaemic infiltration at the Th10/L2 level. **b)** Axial plane. The extradural infiltration in the posterior part of spinal canal

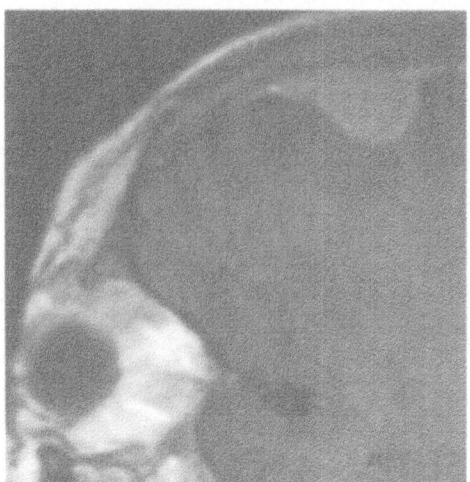

**Fig. 3.** 14-years old boy with AML. MRI (T1-weighted images with contrast enhancement) shows thickening of the meninges (up to 3 mm) with formation of meningeal tumour (a diameter of 2,5 cm) pressing on the adjacent nervous tissue;leukemic infiltration of the orbit and the soft tissues of the front

Neither blast cells in the CSF and not the WBC count above 5/mm³ were found in any of the 36 examined children. Neurological examination revealed minimal symptoms in 2 patients.

The detectability of CNS infiltrates depends on the range of MRI. In the group of 25 patients who underwent MRI of the head the detectability of leukaemic infiltrates was arround 16%

Two of the 7 children with initial MRI abnormalities (28.5%) died during the course of the disease. The remaining 5 are alive and are on maintenance therapy. In 29 patients, without leukaemic CNS involvement in initial MRI, 1 child (3.4%) died, 3 children (10.3%) developed CNS relapse. In two of them the first MRI showed a prolonged T1 relaxation time of the bone marrow of vertebral bodies. Treatment has been completed in 4 patients and and the reste are still being treated.

## Discussion

It is estimated that CNS leukaemia at diagnosis occurs in fewer than 5% of leukaemic children [1]. In our study leukaemic infiltrates of the CNS were detected in MRI in 19,5% newly diagnosed children. None of these children, including a child with massive infiltrates involving the brain meninges and spinal canal in the thoracic and sacro-lumbar regions had blasts in the CSF or WBC count above 5/mm³.

Some authors have also reported that CSF examination may give false negative results and as in the present cases, a negative finding of lymphoblasts in the cerebrospinal fluid does not exclude CNS leukaemic involvement. Diagnosis should rely on CT or MRI scans of the brain and spinal cord [5–8].

We regard MRI as a valuable method of detection of leukaemic infiltrates in the brain and the spinal canal. The results of our study implicate the importance of early routine MRI screening of CNS in leukaemic children at the moment of diagnosis, also in the asymptomatic patients, without blasts in CSF. The range of examination should include MRI of the head and spine.

Supported by grant KBN nr 4 PO5E

## References

1. Bleyer AW. Central nervous system leukaemia. In HendersonHS, Lister TA, eds,
2. Riehm H. et all: Acute lymphoblastic leukaemia. In: Voute PA, Barrett A.Bloom HJG, Lemerle J, Neidhardt MK (eds) Cancer in Children. Berlin; Springer, 101–118, 1986
3. Pinkel D, Woo S: Prevention and treatment of meningeal leukaemia in children. Blood 84, 355–366, 1994
4. Caimcross JG,Macdonald DR: Lumbar puncture In: Wittes RE ed.Manual of oncologic therapeutics. Philadelphia, Lippincott, 305–307, 1991Leukaemia, 5ᵗʰ ed. Philadelphia, Saunders, 207–224, 1990
5. H.Nielsen: Fatal intramedular tumor of the cervical cord during remission of acute lymphoblastic leukaemia. J of Neuro-Oncol 7, 315–317,1989
6. Marra R. et all: Solid leukaemic intracerebral deposits in patients with acute leukaemia. Haematologica 71, 303–306, 1986
7. Wendling LR. et all: Computed tomography of intracerebral masses. AJR 132, 217–220, 1979
8. Wu CY. et all: Detection of dural involvement by magnetic resonance imaging in adult patients with acute leukaemias- preliminary experiece. Ann Haematol 70, 243–249, 1995

**ALL in Adults**

# Treatment of Adult Acute Lymphoblastic Leukemia Long Term Results of a Prospective Study: LALA 87

D. Fière, J.P. Vernant, M. Michallet, L. Degos, V. Leblond, N. Olteanu, C. Boucheix, C. Charrin, B. Varet, F. Rigal Huguet, A. Delannoy, N. Gratecos, E. Lepage and C. Sebban

Treatment of adult acute lymphoblastic leukemia (ALL) remains unsatisfactory [1–4]. Different strategies such as allogenic, autologous transplantation or more intensive chemotherapy may improve the outcome. Their exact place is still controversial according to the stage (first or second remission) or to the aggressiveness of the disease (high or standard risk).

The purpose of the prospective multicentric study reported here comparing three different treatment regimens in first post induction was to better define indications and exact value of these strategies. Protocol and results with a shorter follow up have been already published [5–8].

## Material and Methods

The prospective study LALA 87 included patients aged 15 to 60 years with the diagnosis of de novo ALL, excepted L3 FAB subtype. From November 1986 to July 1991, 634 patients for 43 hematological centers, localized in France and Belgium, were included. 572 were evaluable from final analysis. There were 274 initial analyzable karyotypes and 562 immunophenotyping characterisations.

For induction treatment, patient were randomized between Daunorubicine and Zorubicine associated with Prednisone, Vincristine and cyclophosphamide. A second salvage chemotherapy course could be added if complete remission (CR) was not achieved at day 28 with Amsacrine and Aracytine.

After achievement of remission, patients were included in different study arms.

– patients over 50 received the chemotherapy arm with a first phase of 3 consolidation courses: once per month with one day randomized anthracycline followed by Aracytine for 5 days and L Asparaginase for 5 days.

Between consolidation and maintenance period a cranial irradiation was performed in prevention of meningeal leukemia. The maintenance phase consisted of 8 alternative courses of L10 modified maintenance regimen administred during 18 months.

## Allogeneic Bone Marrow Transplantation (BMT) Trial

Patients in CR aged 15–40 years, with at least one sibling were included in the trial and according to the result of HLA typing were in BMT arm if they had an identical sibling. Other patients without identical sibling were in the control arm.

Allogeneic BMT had to be performed before day 90 after a short consolidation course using Cyclophosphamide, Vincristine and Prednisone (CVP). The conditioning regimen was the Seattle one with 2 days of Cyclophosphamide and total body irradiation (TBI).

## Autologous – Chemotherapy Trial

Patient aged 40–50 years, included in the control group of allo BMT trial, patients without any sibling or patients without HLA typing, in remission, received the first and second consolidation courses. At this point they were randomized between autologous or chemotherapy arms.

The chemotherapy arm has been described for older patient. In autologous BMT

Hôpital Edouard Herriot - Lyon France

389

arm, 20 to 30 days after consolidation 2, bone marrow harvest was performed. Graft were purged according to the initial phenotype with B, T lineage antibodies, or Mafosfamide in other cases.

Patient received the same conditioning regimen as in allo BMT arm and no any further treatment.

## Analysis

Final analysis has been done after a median follow up of 10 years and on an intention to treat basis. Allogeneic arm was compared with the control group constituted as a genetic randomization, and for autologous arm classicaly randomized with chemotherapy arm.

Patients were stratified in two groups of standard or high risk criteria of relapse according to the Hoelzer's criteria [9]. Kaplan Meier product-limit estimates were used to assess the probability of overall survival and disease free survival and differences between groups were tested using log rank test [10–11].

## Results

### Result of Induction of Remission

There were no statistical difference between the two Anthracycline Daunorubicine and Zorubicine arms. In Daunorubicine arm 78% achieve CR and 74% in Zorubicine arm. Overall 76% were in CR, 15% failed to obtain remission after 2 courses and 9% died during induction period. 436 patients were in CR. The overall survival of 572 included patient at 10 years is 27% and the survival of patients achieving CR is 30%.

### Allogenic BMT Trial

257 patients in CR with at least one sibling had HLA typing. 116 had an identical donor and were in the BMT arm, 141 had no donor and formed the control group. Due to early relapses (14) and other causes (8) 94 were actually transplanted according to the proto-

col in CR1. In the control group, due to early relapses (13) and other causes (11), 117 patients were actually randomized between auto BMT (57) and chemotherapy arms (58) during the second consolidation. Distribution of patients in high risk (HR) and standard risk (SR) was as followed: in allo BMT arm 41 HR and 75 SR, in control arm 55 HR and 86 SR. No difference appears between the two arms.

For all patients the percentage of survival at 10 years is 46 in allo BMT arm against 31 in control arm. The difference is just significant with p : 0.04. In standard risk the results are 49% in allo BMT arm versus 43% in control group without any difference (p = 0.6) but in high risk group, the difference is highly significant (p = 0.009) with 44% of survival in allo BMT versus 11% in control group.

### Autologous Versus Chemo Trial

262 patients after achievement of CR were potentially incluable in this trial. During the time between CR achievement and the second consolidation, there were 21 early relapses and 50 exclusions. 191 patients were randomized, 96 in chemo arm and 95 in auto arm with 63 patients actually transplanted.

The survival at ten years is 34% for auto BMT and 29 for chemotherapy arm. There are no statistical difference in the whole group as well in the standard or high risk group. Survival is 49% versus 40% in standard risk and 11% versus 16% in high risk group.

## Discussion

The analysis of the results of a prospective study on the treatment of adult ALL allows to draw some data about possible better therapeutic strategy.

Allogeneic BMT with an identical sibling give a better long term outcome than other therapies. The benefit is evident and hightly significant for high risk ALL with 44% versus 11% of surviving patients at ten years. There is no benefit with only a trend favouring allogeneic BMT for patients with standard risk criteria. This result differs from studies comparing allogeneic BMT in first remission with chemotherapy. ALL included in the database of the IBMTR, and paired with patients treated in first remission by chemotherapy prospective protocols [12]. In these two studies outcome was not statistically different. A difference appeared only in the type of failure: more relapses in the chemotherapy arm, more death related to transplantation in the allogeneic arm.

The second trial comparing autologous BMT in first remission and chemotherapy does not show difference in the long term outcome. A difference may only appears in the quality of life with a shorter period of treatment and may be in the total cost. Most of the published papers on autologous BMT performed in CR1 give with a shorter follow up, results better than those of the present study, with often a survival of more than 50%. This may be due to a selection of patients: the pronostic is better if the time elapsing between CR achievement and transplantation is shorter.

The results of this protocol allow us to propose a new prospective study running now according to the following prospective indications:

- allogeneic bone marrow transplantation
  - should be recommended in high risk adult ALL in first complete remission
  - should be evaluable in standard risk adult ALL in second complete remission (no benefitfor allo BMT in SR ALL in CR1)
- autologous bone marrow (or peripheral stem cells) transplantation
  - has at least similar outcome than classical chemotherapy in adult ALL in first com-

plete remission (with a trend in favour of auto arm)
  - needs to be further evaluated
  - should be prospectively tested mainly in high risk adult ALL
- chemotherapy
  - more optimal chemotherapy regimens must be prospectively tested in adult ALL in first remission for standard risk ALL.

## References

1. Hoelzer D (1994) Treatment of acute lymphoblastic leukemia. Seminars in Hematol 31:1–15
2. Preti A and Kantarjian HM (1994) Management of adult acute lymphocytic leukemia : present issues and key challenges. J Clin Oncol 12:1312–1322
3. Cortes E, Kantarjian HM (1995) Acute lymphoblastic leukemia. A comprehensive review with emphasis on biology and therapy. Cancer 76: 2393–2417
4. Laport GF and Larson RA (1997) Treatment of adult acute lymphoblastic leukemia. Semin Oncol 24:70–82
5. Fière D, Lepage E, Sebban C, Boucheix C, Gisselbrecht C, Vernant JP, Varet B, Broustet A, Hervé P, Rigal-Huguet F, Michaux JL, Witz F, Michallet M, Reiffers J, Reporting for the French Group of Therapy of Adult ALL (1993) Adult acute lymphoblastic leukemia. A multicentric randomized trial (LALA 87 protocol). Autologous bone marrow transplantation as consolidation therapy in adult patients. J Clin Oncol 11:1990–2001
6. Sebban C, Lepage E, Vernant JP, Gluckman E, Attal M, Reiffers J, Sutton C, Racadot E, Michallet M, Maraninchi D, Dreyfus F, Fière D. Allogenic bone marrow transplantation in adult acute lymphoblastic leukemia in first complete remission. J Clin Oncol 12/2580–2587
7. Boucheix C, David B, Sebban C, Racadot E, Bene MC, Bernard A, Campos L, Jouault H, Sigaux F, Lepage E, Hervé P, Fière D (1994) Immunophenotype of adult acute lymphoblastic leukemia, clinical parameters and outcome and analysis of a prospective trial including 562 tested patients (LALA87). Blood 84:1603–1612
8. Sebban C, Browman GP, Lepage E, Fière D (1995) Prognostic value of early response to chemotherapy assessed by the day 15 bone marrow aspiration in adult acute lymphoblastic leukemia: a prospective analysis of 437 cases and its applications of designing induction chemotherapy trials. Leukemia Res 19:861–868
9. Hoelzer D, Thiel E, Loffler H, Buchner T, Ganser A, Heil G, Koch P, Freund M, Diedrich H, Ruhl H, Maschmeyer G, Lipp T,Nowrousian MR, Burkert M, Gerecke D, Pralle H, Muller U, Lunscken Ch, Fulle H, Ho AD, Kuchler R, Busch FW, Schneider W, Gorg Ch, Emmerich B, Braumann D, Vaupel HA, Von Paleske A, Bartels H, Neiss A and Messerer D (1988) Prognostic factors in a multicenter

**Table 1.** Long term results of adult ALL treated in first remission in percentage. a) allogeneic BMT versus control group; b) autologous BMT versus chemotherapy

| A | ALLO | control | p |
|---|---|---|---|
| All patients | 46 | 31 | 0.04 |
| Standard risk | 49 | 43 | 0.6 |
| High risk | 44 | 11 | 0.009 |

| B | Auto | Chemo | p |
|---|---|---|---|
| All patients | 34 | 29 | 0.65 |
| Standard risk | 49 | 40 | 0.7 |
| High risk | 11 | 16 | 0.7 |

study for treatment of acute lymphoblastic leukemia in adults. Blood 71:123–131

10. Horowitz MM, Messerer D, Hoelzer D, Gale R, Neiss A, Atkinson K, Barret J, Buchner T, Freund M, Heil G, Hiddermann W, Kolb HJ, Loffler H, Marmont A, Maschmeyer G, Rimm AA, Rozman C, Sobocinski KA, Speck B, Thiel E, Wersdorf DJ, Zwaan FE, Bortin MM (1991) Chemotherapy compared with bone marrow transplantation for adults with acute lymphoblastic leukemia in first remission. Ann Intern Med 115:13–18

11. Peto R, Pike ML, Armitage P, et al (1977) Design and analysis of randomized clinical trials requiring prolonged observation of each patient. Br J Cancer 35:1–39

12. Kaplan EL, Meier P (1958) Non parametric estimation from incomplete observations. J Am Stat Assoc 53:457–481

# Results of Recent Clinical Trials in Acute Lymphoblastic Leukemia by the Cancer and Leukemia Group B

R. A. Larson, R. K. Dodge, T. P. Szatrowski and S. R. Frankel

*Abstract.* Since 1988, the CALGB has enrolled 598 adults with untreated acute lymphoblastic leukemia (ALL) onto 4 clinical trials using intensive multi-agent therapy. The median age was 35 years (range, 16–81 years); 15% were >60 years old. Seventy-one percent were B/BMy and 19% were T/TMy by immunophenotyping. Of 334 studied, 28% were Philadelphia chromosome positive or BCR/ABL positive; 8% had t(4;11). Overall, complete remission (CR) was achieved in 85%. The median disease-free survival (DFS) was 2.1 years (95% confidence interval (CI), 1.7–2.4 years), and the median survival was 2.2 years (95% CI, 1.9–3.0 years). At 3 years, 41% (95% CI, 37–46%) remained in continuous CR, and 45% (95% CI, 41–50%) were alive. In CALGB study 9111, filgrastim (G-CSF) was shown to reduce the median time to recover 1000 neutrophils/ml during treatment from 22 days to 16 days (p<.001), but without improvement in DFS or overall survival. Importantly, the CR rate for patients >60 years old improved from 55% to 81%. In CALGB study 9311, B-lineage ALL patients received two postremission courses of anti-B4-blocked ricin, an anti-CD19 immunotoxin, over 7 days each. Toxicity was minimal, but neither clinical outcome nor molecular monitoring for unique antigen receptor genes suggested efficacy. T-cell ALL patients received high-dose cytarabine consolidation. CALGB study 9511 explored the pharmacokinetics of PEG-asparaginase. One dose (2000 U/m$^2$) resulted in asparagine depletion for 14 days in the majority of patients. An additional 24 patients with Burkitt-type ALL-L3 were enrolled on CALGB study 9251, a 17-week intensive regimen that included cranial irradiation. The median age for these patients was 45 years (range, 20–71 years); 21% were >60 years old. The CR rate was 75%. The median DFS was >1.7 years, and the median survival was 2.1 years. At 3 years, 53% (95% CI, 29–76%) remained in continuous CR, and 44% (95% CI, 25–65%) were alive. The current study for adult ALL (CALGB 19802) evaluates higher doses of daunorubicin during induction and higher doses of cytarabine and methotrexate during consolidation in lieu of cranial irradiation. Patients with relapsed or refractory T-cell ALL are enrolled on a phase 2 trial (CALGB 19801) evaluating GW506U78, the prodrug for 9-D-arabinofuranosylguanine (ara-G). Our risk-adapted strategy recommends allogeneic stem cell transplantation in first remission for patients with t(9;22) or t(4;11).

The Cancer and Leukemia Group B (CALGB) has performed a series of studies evaluating different aspects of induction and post-remission treatment in adults with acute lymphoblastic leukemia (ALL). In recent years, these clinical trials have been supplemented by systematic morphologic, immunophenotyping, cytogenetic and molecular genetic studies, leading to the identification of different risk groups of patients who may warrant individualized treatments. Importantly, these protocols have enrolled all adult patients older than 15 years with ALL without an upper age restriction and did not exclude Philadelphia (Ph) chromosome positive patients.

The University of Chicago, Chicago, IL; the Cancer and Leukemia Group B (CALGB) Statistical Center, Durham NC; Weill Medical College of Cornell University – New York Presbyterian Hospital, New York, NY; Georgetown University Medical Center, Washington, D.C.; and the CALGB, Chicago, IL.

## CALGB Study 8811

Intensive multi-agent chemotherapy programs produce complete remissions (CR) in the majority of adults with ALL [1]. CALGB study 8811 built upon observations by the CALGB and others that a more intensive remission induction program might produce more durable responses [2]. A single dose of cyclophosphamide (1200 mg/m$^2$) was added to a modification of the 4 drug regimens (daunorubicin, vincristine, prednisone, L-asparaginase) used in earlier CALGB studies (7612 and 8011) [3, 4]. The treatment schema is shown in Table 1. In addition, a more intensive program of L-asparaginase administration was used during induction and the first 2 months of post-remission consolidation because of reports suggesting the importance of intensive asparaginase therapy in children with high-risk ALL. Other aspects of post-remission therapy were patterned after that used by the adult German multicenter ALL (GMALL) study group and included a total of 2 years of scheduled chemotherapy [5].

In this trial, 85% of the 197 evaluable patients (median age, 32 years; range, 16–80 years) achieved a CR, including 94% of patients less than 30 years old, 85% of patients aged 30–59 and 39% of patients ≥60 years old. The median duration of CR was 2.4 years (95% confidence interval (CI), 2.0–5.3 years) and was also age-related. Improved results were noted in patients with T-cell ALL (estimated 3 year survival, 69%) compared to B-lineage ALL (estimated 3 year survival, 38%). At the most recent follow-up, 43% of patients had survived >5 years (95% CI, 36–50%), and 42% (95% CI, 35–50%) were in continuous CR (CCR).

In contrast to earlier CALGB studies, there was no adverse impact on outcome associated with the coexpression of myeloid antigens [6]. Although the CR rate was very high, remission induction treatment was complicated by prolonged granulocytopenia requiring an average of 26 days of hospitalization. In particular, the mortality in patients >60 years of age was unacceptably high, and a dose reduction in the cyclophosphamide and the daunorubicin was implemented for these patients. Similarly, the first course of con-solidation therapy was also quite myelosuppressive, requiring an average of 14 days of hospitalization during this 2-month treatment.

## CALGB Study 9111

The major cause of treatment-related morbidity and mortality for patients with ALL is infection due in part to bone marrow suppression by cytotoxic therapy. Therefore, the CALGB designed a study (9111) to test the effectiveness of filgrastim (granulocyte colony stimulating factor, G-CSF) in reducing the complications of treatment by potentially shortening the time to neutrophil recovery following courses of remission induction chemotherapy and post-remission consolidation treatment [7].

The primary objectives of this randomized, double-blind, placebo-controlled clinical trial were to compare the time to bone marrow recovery, the incidence of infections, the days of hospitalization, and the side-effects of treatment following intensive chemotherapy for ALL in patients receiving either G-CSF or placebo. In addition, we determined the impact of G-CSF on the rate and duration of CR and the incidence of death during treatment. We also compared the dose-intensity of chemotherapy that was delivered to patients assigned to receive G-CSF or placebo during the first 3 months of treatment. Finally, we continued to investigate the prognostic significance of disease and patient entry characteristics for disease-free survival (DFS) using this treatment program.

We randomly assigned 198 adults with untreated ALL (median age, 35 years; range, 16–79 years) to receive either placebo or G-CSF (5 µg/kg/day) subcutaneously, beginning 4 days after starting the intensive remission induction chemotherapy and continuing until the neutrophil count was ≥1000/µl for 2 days. The study assignment was unblinded as individual patients achieved a CR. Patients initially assigned to G-CSF then continued to receive G-CSF through 2 monthly courses of consolidation therapy. Patients assigned to placebo received no further study drug.

The median time to recover neutrophils ≥1000/µl during the remission induction course was 16 days (interquartile range (IQR), 15–18 days) for the patients assigned to receive G-CSF and 22 days (IQR, 19–29 days) for the patients assigned to placebo (p<0.001). Patients in the G-CSF group had significantly shorter durations of neutropenia (<1000/µl) and of thrombocytopenia (<50,000/µl) and fewer days in hospital (median, 22 days vs 28 days, p=0.02) compared to patients receiving placebo. The patients assigned to receive G-CSF had a higher CR rate (87% vs 77%) and fewer deaths during remission induction (5% vs 11%) than did those receiving placebo (p=0.04 by the chi-square test for trend). During Courses IIA and IIB of consolidation treatment, patients in the G-CSF group had significantly more rapid recovery of neutrophils ≥1000/µl than did the control group by approximately 6–9 days. However, the patients in the G-CSF group did not complete the planned first 3 months of chemotherapy any more rapidly than did the patients in the placebo group. Overall toxicity was not lessened by the use of G-CSF.

After a median follow-up of 4.7 years, there was no significant difference in the DFS for the patients assigned to G-CSF (median, 2.3 years) compared to those assigned to placebo (median, 1.7 years; p=0.53). Nor was there a significant difference in overall survival between the two groups (medians, 2.4 years with G-CSF and 1.8 years with placebo; p=0.25). Adults who received intensive chemotherapy for ALL benefited from G-CSF treatment, but its use did not markedly affect the ultimate outcome.

Older age (>60 years) was associated with a lower CR rate, slower neutrophil and platelet recovery, and longer hospitalization during induction, all of which were improved by G-CSF therapy. There was no adverse effect of G-CSF on the outcome of patients with myeloid antigen positive or Ph+ ALL. It was concluded that the addition of G-CSF to the CALGB induction treatment reduced the duration of hematologic toxicity and improved some measures of clinical outcomes, particularly in older patients. An economic analysis of the use of G-CSF in this clinical trial will soon be completed [8]. G-CSF was therefore added as part of the induction regimen in subsequent trials.

## CALGB Study 9311

Half of all adults with B-lineage ALL have Ph+ disease, and most of these are not able to undergo allogeneic bone marrow transplantation (BMT). In addition, there is considerable room for improving the outcome for the remaining patients with B-lineage ALL. Clinical experience using the immunotoxin, anti-B4 blocked ricin (anti-B4-bR), had demonstrated reduction in tumor size in patients with B-cell lymphoproliferative disorders [9]. There was also evidence that this immunotoxin might be useful in bone marrow purging for patients with follicular lymphomas undergoing autologous bone marrow transplant. Anti-B4-bR (ImmunoGen, Inc., Cambridge, MA) is comprised of an anti-CD19 monoclonal antibody conjugated to blocked ricin, which has cytotoxic activity in lymphoid malignancies and is capable of killing malignant cells resistant to chemotherapy.

The Leukemia Committee of the CALGB therefore explored the use of anti-B4 blocked ricin in B-lineage ALL during a minimal disease state. In CALGB study 9311, two 7-day courses of the immunotoxin were given after completion of the first two months of intensive therapy given as in the 9111 protocol and prior to the central nervous system (CNS) prophylaxis phase [10, 11].

A total of 82 patients with previously untreated ALL were enrolled on CALGB 9311, of whom 4 were deemed to have AML (FAB M0) and were thus ineligible. For the remaining 78, the median age was 35 years (range, 17–81 years); 56% were male, and 85% had B-lineage ALL. Qualitative polymerase chain reaction (PCR) assays for the *BCR/ABL* fusion gene and semi-quantitative PCR assays for T-cell receptor (*TCR*) and/or Ig heavy chain (*IGH*) gene rearrangements were performed at diagnosis and prospectively on bone marrow and peripheral blood at CALGB central reference laboratories to serve as markers of minimal residual disease [11]. At baseline, 22 (39%) of 57 evaluable patients were *BCR/ABL* positive, while 57 (79%) of 72 evaluable patients were TCR and/or IGH-positive. The CR rate was 85% overall and 87% in the B-lineage patients. At last follow-up, 41% (95% CI, 30–53%) of all eligible patients were estimated to be in remission at 3 years, and 45% (95% CI, 34–56%) were alive.

Forty-six B-lineage patients whose ALL cells expressed CD19 at baseline and who remained in CR after one consolidation course were treated with anti-B4-bR at 30 μg/kg/day during two continuous IV infusions (days 1–7 and 15–21). The most common toxicities were asymptomatic elevation of hepatic transaminases (33 patients) and lymphopenia (21 patients). Flu-like symptoms occurred in 17 patients, and two patients had serositis. Two patients developed anti-mouse or anti-ricin antibodies after the first week of anti-B4-bR. In all, 37 patients were able to receive all 14 days of anti-B4-bR.

PCR studies were repeated prior to each treatment course and then every 6 months, as well as at relapse. Eighteen of 22 BCR/ABL positive patients had post-treatment PCR studies, and 12 achieved BCR/ABL negative status, of whom 4 relapsed, one died, and 7 remain in CR, the duration of which ranges from 22 to 38 months [12]. Twelve of 55 TCR/IGH-positive patients were studied post-treatment, and 8 achieved PCR negative status, of whom 3 relapsed and 4 remain in CR (duration, 14+ to 28+ months); one died after an allogeneic BMT. Four remained PCR positive and all 4 remain in CR.

Eight patients who were BCR/ABL positive and 7 who were TCR/IGH positive at baseline had PCR studies immediately before and after courses of anti-B4-bR. Of the 8 BCR/ABL patients, 3 were positive prior to anti-B4-bR and remained positive after anti-B4-bR treatment; 5 were BCR/ABL negative prior to anti-B4-bR, of whom 4 remained negative and one converted from negative to positive. Of the 7 TCR/IGH patients, 4 remained positive, one converted from positive to negative, and 2 converted from negative to positive after anti-B4-bR. Thus, in a small number of patients, treatment with anti-B4-bR seemed to have little impact on these measurements of minimal residual disease in ALL. However, this protocol serves as a model for evaluating the effects of monoclonal antibody therapy or other novel therapies prior to conducting more definitive randomized trials.

Six patients enrolled on study 9311 had T-cell ALL and lacked the CD19 antigen. In place of the anti-B4-bR course, these patients received one course of high-dose cytarabine (2 gm/m$^2$ every 12 hours for 6 days) for post-remission consolidation. The toxicity of this course was acceptable. Four (67%) of these patients have remained in CCR for longer than 3 years.

## CALGB Study 9511

Two components of these more recent CALGB ALL trials differed from previous group trials: the more extensive use of asparaginase and the use of cyclophosphamide [13]. The addition of these agents appears to have led to improved CR rates and better DFS. CALGB 9511 was a phase II study of pegylated (PEG)-asparaginase as a replacement for E. coli asparaginase in previously untreated adult patients with ALL. The protocol otherwise used the same chemotherapy treatment schedule as delivered in CALGB studies 8811, 9111, and 9311.

Asparaginase hydrolyses asparagine to aspartate and ammonia. ALL cells lack asparagine synthetase and are thus dependent on exogenous asparagine for survival. Rapid depletion of asparagine results in selective killing of ALL cells since normal cells are able to synthesize asparagine. Because asparaginase is not markedly myelosuppressive, it is easily added to combination chemotherapy regimens.

Three preparations of asparaginase are available. One preparation is derived from Escherichia coli (E. Coli) and is commercially available for use in the United States. A second preparation is derived from Erwinia carotovora and is commercially available in Europe; it can be ordered in the U.S. only for patients with allergy to E. coli asparaginase. PEG-asparaginase is derived from E. coli L-asparaginase by covalently conjugating units of polyethylene glycol (PEG) to the protein. Currently, PEG-asparaginase is indicated for use in adult patients with hypersensitivity to native E. coli asparaginase at a dose of 2000 U/m$^2$ every 14 days.

Differences between PEG-asparaginase and the other two forms of the drug include decreased immunogenicity and a longer half-life [13]. The half-life of E. coli asparaginase is 1.2 days, Erwinia asparaginase 0.7 days, and

PEG-asparaginase 5.7 days [14]. The asparaginase levels that are produced from a single administration reportedly result in asparagine depletion for 7–10 days, 3–5 days, and 14–28 days, respectively.

No large trial of PEG-asparaginase had previously been initiated in adults with ALL. The use of PEG-asparaginase instead of E. coli asparaginase may decrease the incidence of neutralizing anti-asparaginase antibodies and improve the efficacy of this drug. The optimal dosing schedule of PEG-asparaginase in adults, however, remains to be determined. Studies in children have shown that a dose of 2000 U/m$^2$ delivered every 2 weeks produced asparagine depletion for 14 days in more than 70% of patients despite inclusion of some patients with neutralizing antibodies [15]. We therefore chose initially to test a dose of 2000 U/m$^2$ (maximum, 3750 U) administered SC or IM once during each of the first three courses of therapy in newly diagnosed patients [16]. PEG-asparaginase was given on Day 5 during Course I and Day 15 during Courses IIA and IIB (Table 1).

To assess the proper dosing of PEG-asparaginase in adult patients receiving multi-agent chemotherapy, pharmacokinetic stu-

**Table 1.** CALGB chemotherapy regimen for acute lymphoblastic leukemia in adults (2,7)

| Course I: Induction (4 weeks) | | | |
|---|---|---|---|
| Cyclophosphamide* | IV | 1200 mg/m$^2$ | Day 1 |
| Daunorubicin* | IV | 45 mg/m$^2$ | Days 1, 2, 3 |
| Vincristine | IV | 2 mg | Days 1, 8, 15, 22 |
| Prednisone* | PO/IV | 60 mg/m$^2$/d | Days 1–21 |
| L-Asparaginase (E. Coli) | SC/IM | 6000 IU/m$^2$ | Days 5, 8, 11, 15, 18, 22 |
| *For patients ≥60 years old: | | | |
| Cyclophosphamide | | 800 mg/m$^2$ | Day 1 |
| Daunorubicin | | 30 mg/m$^2$ | Days 1, 2, 3 |
| Prednisone | | 60 mg/m$^2$/d | Days 1–7 |

In CALGB studies 9311 and 9511, patients received G-CSF 5µg/kg subcutaneously once daily, starting on day 4 and continuing until the absolute neutrophil count was ≥ 1000/µl on two consecutive determinations > 24 hours apart (see text).

| Course IIA: Early Intensification (4 weeks; repeat once for Course IIB) | | | |
|---|---|---|---|
| Intrathecal methotrexate | | 15 mg | Day 1 |
| Cyclophosphamide | IV | 1000 mg/m$^2$ | Day 1 |
| 6-Mercaptopurine | PO | 60 mg/m$^2$/d | Days 1–14 |
| Cytarabine | SC | 75 mg/m$^2$/d | Days 1–4, 8–11 |
| Vincristine | IV | 2 mg | Days 15, 22 |
| L-Asparaginase (E. Coli) | SC/IM | 6000 IU/m$^2$ | Days 15, 18, 22, 25 |

| Course III: CNS prophylaxis and interim maintenance (12 weeks) | | | |
|---|---|---|---|
| Cranial irradiation | | 2400 cGy | Days 1–12 |
| Intrathecal methotrexate | | 15 mg | Days 1, 8, 15, 22, 29 |
| 6-Mercaptopurine | PO | 60 mg/m$^2$/d | Days 1–70 |
| Methotrexate | PO | 20 mg/m$^2$ | Days 36, 43, 50, 57, 64 |

| Course IV: Late intensification (8 weeks) | | | |
|---|---|---|---|
| Doxorubicin | IV | 30 mg/m$^2$ | Days 1, 8, 15 |
| Vincristine | IV | 2 mg | Days 1, 8, 15 |
| Dexamethasone | PO | 10 mg/m$^2$/d | Days 1–14 |
| Cyclophosphamide | IV | 1000 mg/m$^2$ | Day 29 |
| 6-Thioguanine | PO | 60 mg/m$^2$/d | Days 29–42 |
| Cytarabine | SC | 75 mg/m$^2$/d | Days 29–32, 36–39 |

| Course V: Prolonged maintenance (until 24 months from diagnosis) | | | |
|---|---|---|---|
| Vincristine | IV | 2 mg | Day 1 of every 4 weeks |
| Prednisone | PO | 60 mg/m$^2$/d | Days 1–5 of every 4 weeks |
| 6-Mercaptopurine | PO | 60 mg/m$^2$/d | Days 1–28 |
| Methotrexate | PO | 20 mg/m$^2$ | Days 1, 8, 15, 22 |

dies of asparaginase levels were also done. Asparaginase levels provided a surrogate measure of asparagine depletion since levels >0.03 U/ml produce complete asparagine depletion. The frequency of anti-asparaginase neutralizing antibodies was also measured using an enzyme linked immunoassay (ELISA) method.

Pharmacokinetic sampling of the first 21 patients studied in this trial showed that asparaginase levels were > 0.03 U/ml in all 21 patients at 7 days and in 16 of 20 patients (80%) at 14 days but in only 5 of 20 (25%) at 24 days after the initial dose of PEG-asparaginase (16). When the second dose was given on day 15 of the second chemotherapy course, 16 of 18 evaluable patients (83%) had complete asparagine depletion 7 days later, and 12 of the 18 (67%) had depletion at 14 days. A third dose was given on day 15 of the third chemotherapy course, and 14 of 16 patients (85%) had depletion at 7 days and 13 of 16 (79%) at 14 days following this final dose. Therefore, through all 3 doses, 67–80% of patients maintained sufficient asparaginase levels to deplete asparagine for 2 weeks. Antibodies to PEG-asparaginase developed in 3 patients but none before the end of the third course. No grade 3 or 4 allergic reactions or pancreatitis were observed. Hyperglycemia was reported in 38% of patients. Four patients (15%) had grade 3 phlebitis or thrombosis, and one patient had a deep vein thrombosis of the leg with embolization to the lung.

Preliminary retrospective analyses in pediatric ALL populations have suggested that the longer periods of asparagine depletion that result from the use of E. coli asparaginase are associated with better outcomes than the shorter periods of depletion that result from the use of Erwinia asparaginase. Therefore, a second cohort of patients was treated on the 9511 trial, and a second dose of PEG-asparaginase was added on day 22 of the induction course to extend the duration of asparagine depletion [17]. Pharmacokinetic analyses of this cohort of patients showed asparagine depletion in 18 of 20 patients (90%) at 14 days and 10 of 14 (71%) at 31 days. Further analyses are pending.

## CALGB Study 9251

Patients with mature B-cell ALL (Burkitt-type, ALL-L3, surface immunoglobulin positive, t(8q24)) fare poorly with conventional ALL chemotherapy approaches. Early CALGB data for patients with the t(8;14) showed that none of those patients were long-term disease-free survivors. Of the 8 patients with the L3 subtype enrolled on CALGB 8811, 2 failed to achieve CR and 5 relapsed after a median remission duration of only 3 months; all 5 developed CNS involvement.

CALGB study 9251 (High intensity, brief duration chemotherapy for diffuse small non-cleaved cell lymphoma and the L–3 subtype of ALL: A pilot study of a multidrug regimen) was derived from a series of reports, both in children and adults, which highlight a different approach to the treatment of these diseases [18–20]. Repeated short courses of cyclophosphamide and high-dose methotrexate led to CR rates of 85–95% and impressive long-term DFS in a large number of patients with Burkitt-type leukemia or lymphoma. All regimens contained aggressive CNS prophylaxis and some included an initial cytoreduction using modest doses of cyclophosphamide and corticosteroids. In CALGB 9251, therapy was given over a 17-week period of time, including the use of CNS irradiation [21]. We used a regimen similar to that used successfully by the German ALL study group for patients with L3 ALL [20]. The major differences between the 9251 regimen and Hoelzer's are the use of etoposide (VP–16) instead of teniposide (VM–26) and the use of cytarabine as a continuous infusion for 48 hours rather than as subcutaneous injections.

One hundred fourteen patients with either the L3 variant of ALL or small noncleaved cell lymphoma have been treated to date. Approximately 75% of patients with L3 ALL have achieved a CR. After a median follow-up of >2 years, the estimated CCR rate at 3 years is 53% (95% CI, 29–76%), and the survival is 44% (95% CI, 25–65%) [21].

Toxicity was significant with all patients having myelosuppression and most patients having grade 3 or 4 mucositis. Severe neurologic toxicity was observed in 10 of the first 70 patients, including transverse myelitis in 5 patients, cortical dysfunction in 3, and peripheral neuropathy in 2. In some of these patients the deficit has been persistent. As a consequence, the CNS prophylaxis therapy was changed. The intrathecal chemotherapy (methotrexate, cytarabine, and hydrocortisone) was reduced from 12 to 6 doses and the cranial irradiation was rescheduled to the end of treatment rather than between courses 2 and 3 to avoid concurrent administration with systemic chemotherapy.

## ALL in Relapse: CALGB Study 19801

There have been almost no new drugs introduced into the treatment of ALL in recent years. Compound 506U78 (Glaxo Welcome) is a pro-drug of 9-D-arabinofuranosylguanine (ara-G), a deoxyguanosine analog. Previous studies have demonstrated that immature T-lymphocytes are extremely sensitive to the cytotoxic effects of deoxyguanosine. The toxicity of deoxyguanosine to T-cells is related to the accumulation of deoxyguanosine triphosphate (dGTP) with subsequent inhibition of ribonucleotide reductase, inhibition of DNA synthesis, and resultant cell death. Recent information indicates that the rate of ara-GTP catabolism is similar in T-cells and B-cells, but that initial ara-G concentrations are higher in T-cells than B-cells for a given dose. Thus, T-cells have a greater intracellular exposure to ara-GTP than do B-cells.

In a phase I study, 506U78 was given as a one-hour intravenous infusion daily for 5 consecutive days [22, 23]. More than 90 adult and pediatric patients with refractory T-cell hematologic malignancies were enrolled. Neurotoxicity was dose-limiting. Signs and symptoms of neurotoxicity (e.g., drowsiness, muscle twitching, tremors, or ataxia) generally appeared on day 4 or 5 of therapy and resolved several days after drug discontinuation. Pharmacokinetic data suggested that drug clearance was related to age, with pediatric patients having a more rapid drug clearance than adult patients. A subsequent phase I study demonstrated that higher doses could be given safely using an alternate day schedule.

CALGB study 19801 is a phase II trial of GW506U78 in patients with relapsed or refractory T-cell ALL or T-lymphoblastic lymphoma that has recently been opened to accrual. Patients receive 506U78 at 2.2 g/m$^2$ over 2 hours on days 1, 3, and 5. If the activity of this agent were encouraging, we would plan to utilize 506U78 in a lineage-specific fashion for newly diagnosed T-cell patients analogous to our approach with high-dose cytarabine in CALGB 9311.

## Immunophenotyping and Cytogenetic Studies in ALL

Immunophenotyping has been a required feature of CALGB protocols since 1983 (CALGB study 8364) [24]. Approximately 19% of adults have T-lineage ALL, but this has varied from 8–28% between sequential studies. The outcome for this group of patients seems to be improving with more intensive programs, possibly because of the addition of cyclophosphamide to previous CALGB regimens. As was first reported by the CALGB, approximately 25% of adult patients with either B- or T-lineage ALL have the coexpression of at least one myeloid antigen detectable on their blast cells. This finding initially appeared to have an adverse impact on achievement of CR and on overall survival [6]. This adverse effect on CR or survival is no longer present with more intensive treatments [2, 24]. A small number of patients with morphologically apparent ALL have been found to have only myeloid antigens on the leukemia cell surface. Such "myeloid only" patients have what is now considered FAB subtype M0 (minimally differentiated AML), emphasizing the critical importance of immunophenotyping at the time of diagnosis in patients with ALL.

Immunophenotyping has been performed by multiparameter flow cytometry in a central CALGB laboratory, using a panel of monoclonal antibodies and indirect immunofluorescence [2, 7, 24]. The criterion for surface marker positivity was expression by at least 20% of the leukemia blast cell population. B-lineage was defined as CD19 or CD20 positivity. T-lineage was defined by CD2 or CD7 expression together with CD1, CD3, CD4, CD5, or CD8 reactivity. Myeloid (My) antigen expression included CD13 or CD33. Expression of the common ALL antigen

(CALLA) was assessed by CD10 reactivity. Cases co-expressing lymphoid and myeloid antigens (BMy or TMy) were generally classified according to their lymphoid lineage (B- or T-cell, respectively). The small number of cases expressing combinations of both B-lineage and T- lineage antigens were classified as BT, BTMy, or miscellaneous. Cases expressing surface membrane immunoglobulin (SmIg) were considered FAB-L3 (Burkitt-type ALL) and were not included among the other B-lineage cases in most analyses. Patients with myeloperoxidase negative blasts that expressed only myeloid antigens (and not B- or T-lymphoid antigens) were considered acute myeloid leukemia (AML), subtype M0, and thus not eligible for CALGB ALL trials.

Cytogenetic studies are performed on marrow specimens at CALGB local institutions and centrally reviewed by a committee of CALGB cytogeneticists (CALGB study 8461) [25]. Approximately 29% of the adults studied have had the t(9;22) detected cytogenetically. Using a combination of molecular probes for the BCR/ABL fusion protein, CALGB investigators identified the t(9;22) in 33% of CALGB patients with ALL [25, 26]. Importantly, molecular techniques detected the translocation in patients in whom cytogenetic studies were not diagnostic or were inadequate. Conversely, the molecular techniques were positive in essentially all patients in whom a Ph chromosome was found cytogenetically. Approximately one-third of the translocations were in the BCR/ABL region typical of CML (p210), whereas two-thirds produced the p190 variant. RT-PCR methods are now used as a necessary part of the evaluation of CALGB patients with ALL (CALGB study 9862).

Ph positive patients almost invariably had B-lineage ALL. Although three-quarters of these patients achieved a CR on CALGB treatment protocols and some have been rendered *BCR/ABL* negative as determined by PCR, the CR duration has been brief (approximately 11 months) and there will be few, if any, long-term disease free survivors using conventional chemotherapeutic approaches [1, 2, 7, 12, 26]. It still appears that there are no curative therapies for such patients other than allogeneic stem cell transplantation. For the present, these patients will continue to be treated on our frontline ALL studies with a recommendation for allogeneic transplantation while in first CR if a donor were available. It continues to be critical, however, to rigorously categorize patients by immunophenotype and cytogenetic and molecular genetic techniques and outcome results in ALL should be reported according to these groupings.

*Acknowledgements.* We thank the many physicians, nurses and data managers at each of the CALGB institutions and their affiliated hospitals for their assistance with the conduct of these clinical trials. We also thank Audrey McKinnon, CALGB data coordinator, for her expertise in central data management and quality assurance. This research was supported in part by grants from the National Cancer Institute to the Cancer and Leukemia Group B (CA31946 and CA37027), to the CALGB Statistical Center (CA33601), and to CALGB member institutions.

# References

1. Laport GF, Larson RA. Treatment of adult acute lymphoblastic leukemia. Sem Oncol 24: 70–82, 1997.
2. Larson RA, Dodge RK, Burns CP, Lee EJ, Stone RM, Schulman P, Duggan D, Davey FR, Sobol RE, Frankel SR, Hooberman AL, Westbrook CA, Arthur DC, George SL, Bloomfield CD, Schiffer CA. A five-drug remission induction regimen with intensive consolidation for adults with acute lymphoblastic leukemia: Cancer and Leukemia Group B study 8811. Blood 85: 2025–2037, 1995.
3. Gottlieb AJ, Weinberg V, Ellison RR, Henderson ES, Terebelo H, Rafla S, Cuttner J, Silver RT, Carey RW, Levy RN, Hutchinson JL, Raich P, Cooper MR, Wiernik P, Anderson JR, Holland JF: Efficacy of daunorubicin in the therapy of adult acute lymphocytic leukemia: a prospective randomized trial by Cancer and Leukemia Group B. Blood 64: 267–274, 1984.
4. Ellison RR, Mick R, Cuttner J, Schiffer CA, Silver RT, Henderson ES, Woliver T, Royston I, Davey FR, Glicksman AS, Bloomfield CD, Holland JF. The effects of postinduction intensification treatment with cytarabine and daunorubicin in acute lymphocytic leukemia: a prospective randomized clinical trial by Cancer and Leukemia Group B. J Clin Oncol 9: 2002–2015, 1991.
5. Hoelzer D, Thiel E, Löffler H, Büchner T, Ganser A, Heil G. Koch P, Freund M, Diedrich H, Rühl H, Maschmeyer G, Lipp T, Nowrousian MR, Burkert M, Gerecke D, Pralle H, Müller U, Lunscken CH, Fulle H, Ho AD, Kuchler R, Busch FW, Schneider W, Görg CH, Emmerich B, Braumann D, Vaupel HA, von Paleske A, Bartels H, Neiss A, Messerer D. Prognostic factors in a multicenter study for treat-

ment of acute lymphoblastic leukemia in adults. Blood 71: 123–131, 1988.

6. Sobol RE, Mick R, Royston I, Davey FR, Ellison RR, Newman R, Cuttner J, Griffin JD, Collins H, Nelson DA, Bloomfield CD: Clinical importance of myeloid antigen expression in adult acute lymphoblastic leukemia. N Engl J Med 316: 1111–1117, 1987.

7. Larson RA, Dodge RK, Linker CA, Stone RM, Powell BL, Lee EJ, Schulman P, Davey FR, Frankel SR, Bloomfield CD, George SL, and Schiffer CA. A randomized controlled trial of filgrastim during remission induction and consolidation chemotherapy for adults with acute lymphoblastic leukemia: CALGB study 9111. Blood 92: 1556–1564; 1998.

8. Smith TJ, Herndon JE, Larson RA, Schiffer CA, McDonald K, Penberthy L, Weeks JA. Measuring costs and clinical outcomes from prospective clinical trial and retrospective financial databases: experience gained from Cancer and Leukemia Group B study 9411. Proc Am Soc Clin Oncol 16: 420a, 1997.

9. Grossbard ML, Freedman AS, Ritz J, Coral F, Goldmacher VS, Eliseo L, Spector N, Dear K, Lambert JM, Blättler WA, Taylor JA, Nadler LM. Serotherapy of B-cell neoplasms with anti-B4-blocked ricin: a phase I trial of daily bolus infusion. Blood 79:576–585, 1992.

10. Szatrowski TP, Larson RA, George S, Dodge R, Hurd D, Kolitz J, Velez-Garcia E, Sklar J, Reynolds C, Westbrook CA, Frankel SR, Stewart C, Bloomfield CD, Schiffer CA. Anti-B4-blocked ricin as consolidation therapy for patients with B-lineage acute lymphoblastic leukemia (ALL): A phase II trial (CALGB 9311). Blood 86 (Suppl 1): 783a, 1995.

11. Szatrowski TP, Larson RA, Dodge R, Sklar J, Reynolds C, Westbrook CA, Hurd D, Kolitz J, Velez-Garcia E, Frankel SR, Stewart C, Bloomfield CD, Schiffer CA. The effect of anti-B4-blocked ricin (anti-B4-BR) on minimal residual disease (MRD) in adults with B-lineage acute lymphoblastic leukemia (ALL) (CALGB 9311, 8762, 8763). Blood 88 (Suppl 1): 669a, 1996.

12. Westbrook CA, Dodge R, Szatrowski TP, Horrigan SK, Kim SJ, Wu D, Jantzen N, Schiffer CA, Bloomfield CD. PCR monitoring of minimal residual disease identifies good outcome in BCR/ABL positive acute lymphoblastic leukemia (ALL): CALGB 8762. Blood 88 (Suppl 1): 477a, 1996.

13. Larson RA, Fretzin MH, Dodge RK, Schiffer CA. Hypersensitivity reactions to L-asparaginase do not impact on the remission duration of adults with acute lymphoblastic leukemia. Leukemia 12: 660–665, 1998.

14. Asselin BL, Whitin JC, Coppola DJ, Rupp IP, Sallan SE, Cohen HJ. Comparative pharmacokinetic studies of three asparaginase preparations. J Clin Onc 11: 1780–1786, 1993.

15. Kurtzberg J, Asselin B, Pollack B, Bernstein M, Buchanan G. The Pediatric Oncology Group: PEG-L-Asparaginase (PEGasp) vs native E coli asparaginase (asp) for reinduction of relapsed acute lymphoblastic leukemia (ALL): POG #8866 Phase II trial. Proc Am Soc Clin Oncol 12: 325, 1993.

16. Frankel SR, Kurtzberg J, DeOleivera D, Dodge R, Peterson B, Powell BL, Larson RA, Schiffer CA.

17. Frankel SR, Kurtzberg J, DeOliveria D. Dodge R, Peterson B, Powell BL, Kolitz J, Larson RA, and Schiffer CA. Toxicity and pharmacokinetics of PEG-asparaginase (PEG-asn) in newly diagnosed adult acute lymphoblastic leukemia (ALL): CALGB 9511. Blood 90 (Suppl 1): 334a, 1997.

18. Patte C, Philip T, Rodary C, Zucker J-M, Behrendt H, Gentet J-C, Lamagnère, Otten J, Dufillot D, Pein F, Caillou B, Lemerle J. High survival rate in advanced-stage B-cell lymphomas and leukemias without CNS involvement with a short intensive polychemotherapy: results from the French Pediatric Oncology Society of a randomized trial of 216 children. J Clin Onc 9: 123–132, 1991.

19. Schwenn MR, Blattner SR, Lynch E, Weinstein HJ. HiC-COM: A 2-month intensive chemotherapy regimen for children with stage III and IV Burkitt's lymphoma and B-cell acute lymphoblastic leukemia. J Clin Onc 9: 133–138, 1991.

20. Hoelzer D, Ludwig WD, Thiel E, Gabmann W, Loffler H, Fonatsch C, et al. Improved outcome in adult B-cell acute lymphoblastic leukemia. Blood 88: 495–508, 1996.

21. Lee EJ, Petroni GR, Freter CE, Johnson JL, Schiffer CA, Peterson BA. Brief duration high intensity chemotherapy for patients with small non-cleaved lymphoma (IWF J) and FAB L3 acute lymphocytic leukemia in adults: preliminary results of CALGB 9251. Proc Am Soc Clin Oncol 16: 24a, 1997.

22. Kurtzberg J, Keating M, Moore JO, Gandhi V, Blaney S, Gold S, Ernst T, Henslee-Downey J, Chang A, Kisor D, Plunkett W, Mitchell B. 2-Amino-9-B-D-arabinosyl-6-mthoxy-9H-guanine (GW 506U; Compound 506U) is highly active in patients with T-cell malignancies: results of a phase I trial in pediatric and adult patients with refractory hematological malignancies. Blood 88 (Suppl 1): 669a, 1996.

23. Gandhi V, Plunkett W, Rodriquez CO Jr, Nowak BJ, Du M, Ayres M, Kisor DF, Mitchell BS, Kurtzberg J, Keating MJ. Compound GW506U78 in refractory hematological malignancies: relationship between cellular pharmacokinetics and clinical response. J Clin Oncol 16: 3607–3615, 1998.

24. Czuczman MS, Dodge RK, Stewart CC, Frankel SR, Davey FR, Powell BL, Szatrowski TP, Schiffer CA, Larson RA, Bloomfield CD. Value of immunophenotyping in intensively treated adult acute lymphoblastic leukemia; Cancer and Leukemia Group B study 8364. Blood 1999, in press.

25. Wetzler M, Dodge RK, Mrozek K, Carroll AJ, Tantravahi RR, Block AMW, Pettenati, MJ, Le Beau MM, Frankel SR, Stewart CC, Szatrowski TP, Schiffer CA, Larson RA, Bloomfield CD. Prospective karyotype analysis in adult acute lymphoblastic leukemia – The Cancer and Leukemia Group B experience. Blood 1999, in press.

26. Westbrook CA, Hooberman AL, Spino C, Dodge RK, Larson RA, Davey F, Wurster-Hill DH, Sobol RE, Schiffer CA, Bloomfield CD. Clinical significance of the BCR-ABL fusion gene in adult acute lymphoblastic leukemia: A Cancer and Leukemia Group B study (8762). Blood 80: 2983–2990, 1992.

# Early Application of Anthracyclines in Adult Acute Lymphoblastic Leukemia (ALL)

R. Bassan, A.Z.S. Rohatiner, T. Lerede, M. Carter, E. Di Bona, E. Pogliani, G. Rossi, P. Fabris, S. Morandi, G. Lambertenghi-Deliliers, P. Casula, M. Vespignani, T.A. Lister and T. Barbui

## Introduction

### Unsolved questions

The anthracyclines (ANT) constitute a class of powerful antileukemic agents that exert their antiproliferative effects mainly through inhibition of nuclear topoisomerase II and the related induction of cellular apoptosis [1, 2]. The addition of ANT to prednisone (P), vincristine (V), and L-asparaginase (As) has significantly improved the outcome of patients with acute lymphoblastic leukemia (ALL) [3]. However, several questions remain. With regard to remission induction: which is the best drug (daunorubicin/DNR vs adriamycin/ADR vs idarubicin/IDR), schedule (weekly vs 3 consecutive days or other intensive schedule), and dose? With regard to the early postremission therapy: what is the best ANT containing regimen? Which subgroups of ALL are more sensitive to such therapy? How does resistance to ANT develop? And is it reversible? The results of ANT containing therapy were reviewed in a series of 328 adults with ALL who received either IDR or ADR as induction phase ANT in addition to V/P/As [4]. Once complete remission had been achieved, these patients received postremission therapy with multidrug regimens which contained ANT at high or low dose intensity (DI). High ANT DI was defined as delivery of a total ADR dose of 360–405 mg/m$^2$ during remission induction and the early consolidation cycles (72–100 mg/m$^2$/cycle) or, a total IDR dose of 116–132 mg/m$^2$ (24 mg/m$^2$/cycle). Low ANT DI was defined as a total ADR dose of 120 mg/m$^2$ (30 mg/m$^2$/cycle) or a total IDR dose of 58–80 mg/m$^2$ (10–12 mg/m$^2$/cycle). The results from these first studies are summarized as follows.

### Remission induction phase

The greatest experience is with IDR containing therapy. Compared with DNR and ADR, the favorable features specific to IDR are: more favorable pharmacokinetics/pharmacodynamics with faster and greater drug uptake by blast cells, release by the liver of a long-lived cytotoxic metabolite, and lesser sensitivity to the multidrug resistance type-1 (MDR1) mechanism [5]. The long-term outcome of 7 randomized trials conducted in acute myelogenous leukemia (AML) has confirmed the superioriority of IDR over DNR, while no conclusion is possible as yet as far as ADR is concerned [6]. Another large three-arm trial comparing IDR vs DNR vs mitoxantrone in AML patients aged >55 years has not revealed any significant difference [7]. Other controlled studies are ongoing. In our phase II studies IDR was highly effective in FAB L3/B-ALL and advanced Burkitt's lymphoma [8, 9] and in early B-lineage Philadelphia (Ph) chromosome/BCR-ABL-negative ALL [10], as evidentiated by lower resistance rates in these subtypes, in comparison with ADR-treated patients. However, a direct comparison with ADR at equimyelotoxic dosages has not been performed and refractory ALL remains a problem. The early IDR program was IVAP-1, a schedule consisting of IDR 12 mg/m$^2$ for 3 days plus V/P/As. This regimen was highly toxic and yielded a low remission rate (7/16, 44%) [11]. An amended regimen (IVAP-2) with IDR 10 mg/m$^2$ for 2 days and a delay of

Hematology Dpts. at Bergamo, Vicenza, Monza, Bolzano, Brescia, Cremona, Milan, Cagliari, and Venice Hospitals, Italy, and ICRF Medical Oncology Unit at St. Bartholomew's Hospital, London, U.K.

one week for As improved the remission rate (72/80, 90%; p=0.0001) [12, 13]. In elderly ALL, with only one IDR dose added to V/P/As (IVAP-3), the response rate was intermediate (13/22, 59%) [14]. Early recombinant granulocyte colony-stimulating factor (G-CSF) added early to IVAP-2 reduced significantly the length of absolute neutropenia, the rate of infectious complications, and the need for intravenous antibiotics and antifungals [15]. More recently, although the number of patients with disease refractory to IVAP-2 has remained low, fractionated cyclophosphamide (f-CY) was added in order to try and rescue the few resistant cases. The results obtained with IVAP-2 with or without f-CY and with a new intensive ADR-containing schedule developed at St. Bartholomew's Hospital [16] will be presented.

## Mechanisms of resistance

IDR was shown to be less vulnerable than other ANT to MDR1 [5]. Hence, IDR may be used when MDR1 is functionally (not just phenotypically) over expressed by blast cells, but there little information as regards both MDR1 activity and the expression of other resistance mechanisms (MRP, LRP, GST, altered topoisomerase-II MDR, altered CD95 expression, dysregulated apoptosis genes) able to interfere with ANT activity in adult ALL. At variance with in vitro studies which used IDR concentrations that cannot be obtained in vivo, we have shown that IDR 50–100 ng/ml, corresponding to peak plasma levels obtainable in vivo following an iv. injection of IDR 10–12 mg/m$^2$, exerts little pro-apoptotic and cytotoxic effects against MDR1+ ALL cells. Furthermore, the addition of the MDR1 inhibitor cyclosporin A 1500 ng/ml enhanced greatly the cytotoxic potential without the need for prolonged exposure to CsA, contrary to DNR (17,18). Because of these results, a clinical study was instituted in patients with refractory acute leukemia using an IDR dose (>12 mg/m$^2$) that results in a peak plasma level of about 100 ng/ml plus a short cyclosporin A infusion. The early results of this study are reported elsewhere in this volume.

## Postremission consolidation, dose intensity, and ALL subset specificity

With regard to postremission therapy, preliminary data suggested that some groups of patients who received high ANT DI protocols tended to have longer remissions than those who received low ANT DI regimens [4, 19, 20]. We postulated that assessing the long-term outcome of discrete ALL subsets treated with regimens at either high or low ANT DI could be a valid indicator of chemosensitivity as well as a new treatment-related prognostic variable. We found that early-B CD10+ Ph– ALL and Ph/BCR-ABL+ ALL were significantly more ANT sensitive than other ALL subtypes. We therefore have modified the definition of standard-risk ALL (disease-free survival rate ≥50% at 5 years), to include patients with pre-B CD10+ Ph/BCR-ABL– ALL with a low blast count (<10–25x10$^9$/l) who have received high ANT DI protocols. It is worth noting that the clinical results are in general agreement with recent in vitro studies showing a decreased chemosensitivity to ANT in pro-B ALL and T-ALL [21]. Following a 1992 report on 269 cases [22], this is the second analysis carried out on all patients treated by the 'L-B-V' (London-Bergamo-Vicenza) group and affiliated institutions.

## Patients and Methods

### Patient selection criteria, treatment regimens, ANT type and dose intensity

All patients with ALL treated with any of eight consecutive 'L-B-V' programs at the participating centres were included in the analysis. Depending on specific entry criteria, a few patients were younger or older than 15 and 60 years, respectively, or had advanced-stage lymphoblastic lymphoma of either B-cell or T-cell lineage. The study period ranged from 1972 to 1998. The general design of the eight regimens is shown in Table 1, with emphasis on ANT type and DI. All regimens included central nervous system prophylaxis. ANT DI was defined by the cumulative dose delivered during induction and early consolidation cycles, i.e. within the first 3–4 months of treatment. The total ADR dose was 120

**Table 1.** Overview of treatment regimens according to ANT type and DI

| Type of protocol[1] (No. of patients) | Induction drugs | | Early consolidation[2] | | Additional therapy |
|---|---|---|---|---|---|
| | ANT (mg/m$^2$) | other drugs | ANT mg/m$^2$/ cycle | other drugs | |
| **ADR, Low DI:** | | | | | |
| OPAL | ADR (60) | V, P, As | 30, x2 | V | MAINT |
| OPAL-HDAC | ADR (60) | V, P, As | 30, x2 | V, HDAC | MAINT |
| **ADR, High DI:** | | | | | |
| HEAV'D | ADR (55) | V, P, As | 75–100, x4 | V, CY | MAINT |
| R-HEAV'D | ADR (60) | V, P, As | 75, x4 | V, CY | V, CY, T, AC, MAINT |
| Short-term | ADR (90) | V, P, As, +/-GM | 90, x3 (total 5) | IDAC, E, V, P | MAINT (no T-ALL) |
| **IDR, Low DI:** | | | | | |
| IVAP-3 | IDR (10) | V, P, As, G | 12, x4 | V, CY, As | V, CY, T, AC, MAINT |
| 07–93 | IDR (20) | V, P, As, G | 10, x6 | V, CY, E, IDAC | ABCT, MAINT |
| 08–96 HR-B | IDR (20) | V, P, As, +/-CY, G | nil | V, Dx, HD-CY/AC/MTX, ABCT | |
| **IDR, High DI:** | | | | | |
| IVAP-1 | IDR (36) | V, P, As | 24, x4 | V, CY, As | ABMT, V, CY, T, AC, MAINT |
| IVAP-2 | IDR (20) | V, P, As, G | 24, x4 | V, CY, As | as IVAP-1 |
| 08–96 SR-B | IDR (20) | V, P, As, +/–CY, G | 24, x4 | V, CY | HD-MTX, V, CY, T, AC, MAINT |
| 08–96 T | IDR (20) | V, P, As, +/–CY, G | 24, x4 | V, CY, HDAC | HD-MTX, V, CY, T, AC, MAINT |

[1] With regard to ANT type (induction +consolidation) and DI (early consolidation); 08–96 SR/HR-B: standard/high-risk B-lineage ALL, T: T-ALL
[2] Cycles at approximately three-week intervals, total no. of early consolidation cycles is indicated for each protocol
Abbreviations excluding ANT/V/P/As: GM, GM-CSF; G, G-CSF; CY, cyclophosphamide; HDAC, high-dose ara-C; IDAC, intermediate-dose ara-C; E, etoposide; Dx, dexamethasone; T, teniposide; HD-MTX, high-dose methotrexate; MAINT, low-dose maintenance; ABMT/ABCT, myeloablative regimen with marrow/blood cell autograft

mg/m$^2$ in the low DI protocols OPAL and OPAL-HiDAC [23, 24]. The total IDR dose ranged from 58–80 mg/m$^2$ in the low DI programs IVAP-3 for elderly ALL and 07–93 [8, 9, 14], characterized by a single dose of IDR per cycle (every 21 days, 4 and 6 times respectively). No ANT was used during the brief highly intensive postremission schedule of program 08–96 for high-risk B-lineage (HR-B) ALL. All other programs included more ADR (75–100 mg/m$^2$ per course) or IDR (24 mg/m$^2$ per course) during early consolidation, hence they were defined as high DI protocols [11–13, 25–27]. In the short-term therapy regimen, ADR 90 mg/m$^2$ was given on consolidation cycles 1, 3 and 4, but not in cycles 2 and 5 (only intermediate/high-dose ara-C and etoposide). Nonetheless, the total ADR administered after course 1 was 270 mg/m$^2$, with a high DI in the ADR cycles (90 mg/m$^2$) and a mean DI of 54 mg/m$^2$/cycle if all five cycles are considered [16].

## Methods

### Definitions and statistics

The criteria used to define a condition of complete remission (CR) and recurrent ALL have previously been described [11–15, 22–27]. Early deaths were those occurring within day 40 from the start of chemotherapy, in relation to complications of treatment and/or disease. Resistant ALL (RES ALL) is defined as progression occurring during or after the induction course(s), or a failure to respond after day 40. Disease-free survival (DFS) was the interval from CR to relapse at any site, death in CR from any cause, or date of last follow-up. CR rates and DFS for different clinico-prognostic groups were determined and compared using the chi-square method with Yate's correction, the Kaplan-Meier method and the log-rank method. Significant variables from univariate analysis (U/V) were entered into multivariate analyses (M/V) using the Cox's proportional hazards procedure. Data analysis was by 'intention-to-treat'. Results were analyzed as of January, 1999.

## Study design

This retrospective study aimed to correlate clinical outcome with the use of ANT during remission chemotherapy (ADR vs IDR) and postremission therapy (ADR vs IDR, high vs low ANT DI). The analysis was carried out for the whole patient series and for specific ALL subsets. Prognostic determinants were first identified by U/V and M/V analyses. The factors assessed for prognostic significance were age, gender, disease characteristics such as absolute blast count, FAB morpholgy (L1, L2, L3), immunophenotype (T-cell, mature B-cell, early-B cALLA/CD10+, early-B cALLA/CD10–), cytogenetics/molecular study results, presence of lymphadenopathy and hepato-splenomegaly, and treatment-dependent factors such as time to CR, myeloablative therapy in first remission (with hematopoietic stem cell allograft/autograft), ANT type and early consolidation DI (Table 2), and the use of other drugs during consolidation: high/intermediate/conventional-dose cytarabine, vincristine (no. of injections), cyclophosphamide, podophyllotoxins (VP-16 and VM-26), and high-dose methotrexate. The factors found to be significant in U/V analysis were then entered into M/V analyses. Eventually, the cumulative incidence of risk factors positive in M/V analysis served to identify groups of patients with different DFS probabilities, in whom the effects of ANT DI could be tested separately. A further analysis evaluated ANT-related effects in the main ALL subtypes identifiable by morphologic, immunophenotypic, and cytogenetic features: FAB L3/B-ALL, T-ALL, Ph/BCR-ABL+ ALL, early-B Ph/BCR-ABL– CD10+ and CD10– ALL. The prognostic impact of ANT type and DI was then tested in these subgroups, with additional stratification for other factors found to be positive on M/V analysis.

## Results

### Patients and treatments

Data were available on 689 patients treated between 1972 and 1998. Six hundred and

**Table 2.** Clinical characteristics of 676 patients

| Variables | Units, Range/Cut-off | Results |
|---|---|---|
| Age | years, median (range) | 32 (12–78) |
| | no., <15 yr / >65 yr | 14 / 36 |
| Gender | no., M / F | 401 / 275 |
| Blast count | x10⁹/l, median (range) | 6.4 (0–999+) |
| FAB morphology | no., L1 / L2 / L3 / N/A | 148 / 481 / 34 / 13[1] |
| Immuno-phenotype[2] | no., B / EB CD10+ / EB CD10– / T / N/A | 31 / 291 / 138 / 122 / 92 |
| Cytogenetics[3] | no., Ph / t(4;11) / Abnormal / Normal / N/A | 88 / 12 / 86 / 194 / 296 |
| Hepato-splenomegaly | no., yes / no | 394 / 282 |

N/A, not available
[1] includes 10 cases with lymphoblastic lymphoma
[2] EB, early-B
[3] including gene rearrangement studies for Ph chromosome, t(4;11) and t(1;19)

seventy-six were evaluable, 11 received only V and P only, 2 did not receive any chemotherapy. Clinical characteristics of evaluable patients are shown in Table 2. With regard to chemotherapy (Table 2), 105 patients initially received OPAL, 132 HEAV'D, 79 OPAL-HDAC, 39 reinforced (R) HEAV'D, 119 IVAP regimens, 24 the short-term regimen, 91 07–93, and 87 08–96 risk-adapted regimens.

### Induction of complete remission

### Results with recently developed regimens

The IVAP-2, IVAP plus fractionated cyclophosphamide (f-CY), and ADR-containing short-term regimens are depicted in Table 3 together with treatment outcome. In study 08–96, f-CY was added to IVAP at a cumulative dose of 1200 or 600 mg/m². Eventually f-CY was omitted so that, despite minor structural differences between IVAP-2 and f-CY-IVAP, 27 patients not given f-CY in study 08–96 were included in the IVAP-2 group. Although f-CY could be added safely to IVAP, it did not reduce the incidence of RES ALL, suggesting a cross-resistance between f-CY and the IDR-containing regimen. The results obtained with the intensive ADR schedule were remarkably good, although the number of patient number was small. Time to was CR was longer than for IDR-treated cases; none of the patients was older than 49 years.

**Table 3.** Recently developed induction regimens for adult ALL (early intrathecal therapy not reported).

| | IVAP without f-CY | f-CY-IVAP | Short-term |
|---|---|---|---|
| **Drugs:** | | | |
| IDR, mg/m$^2$/d (days) | 10 (2,3) | 10 (1,2) | – |
| ADR, mg/m$^2$/d (days) | – | – | 30 (1–3) |
| f-CY, mg/m$^2$/bd (days) | – | 75–150 (–3 to 0)– | |
| V, tot mg (days) | 2 (1, 8) | 2 (1, 8, 15) | 2 (1, 8, 15) |
| As, U/m$^2$/d (days) | 10000 (8–14) | 6000 (8,10,12,14,16,18) | 10000 (1–14) |
| P, mg/m$^2$/d (days) | 40 (1–21) | 20 (–3 to 0), 60 (1–21) | 40 (until CR) |
| Growth factor | +/-G-CSF | G-CSF | +/–GM-CSF |
| **Patients:** | | | |
| No. | 197 | 61 | 24 |
| Age (yr), median (range) | 32 (14–66) | 37 (17–74) | 32 (15–49) |
| FAB L1 / L2 / L3 / N/A (no.) | 47 / 132 / 13 / 5[1] | 19 / 39 / 0 / 3[1] | 8 / 15 / 0 / 1[1] |
| Blast count (x10$^9$/l), median (range) | 5.6 (0–700) | 4.7 (0–234) | 11.5 (0.7–288) |
| **Treatment outcome:** | | | |
| CR, no. (%) | 164 (83) | 54 (88) | 21 (88) |
| Time to CR (days), median (range) | 27 (15–96) | 27 (22–58) | 49 (18–80)[2] |
| Early death, no. | 19 | 2 | 2 |
| RES ALL, no. (%) | 14 (7) | 5 (8) | 1 (4) |

N/A, not available
[1]including cases with lymphoblastic lymphoma
[2]p<0.0001 vs IVAP-treated groups

## Cumulative IDR vs ADR results

The results presented in section 3.2.1 refer to patients treated since 1991, for whom uniform diagnostic criteria and supportive care measures were used. However, some ALL subgroups were scarcely represented and the ADR-treated group comprised only 24 younger patients. Therefore the analysis was extended to all 'L-B-V' protocols, including all studies from 1972 to 1998. For ADR-based regimens (except STT) ADR was usually given on days 1 and 15 at the dosage reported in Table 1. The analysis included IDR-containing regimens IVAP-1 (associated with high toxicity and a low CR rate) and IVAP-3 for elderly ALL (associated with a suboptimal CR rate). In all IDR-containing studies the As dose was lower than in equivalent ADR-containing studies (diminished by 50% or more). Nevertheless, the results summarized in Table 4 confirm the high activity of IDR-containing protocols, in terms of increased CR rate, shorter time to CR and a lower incidence of RES ALL. The shorter time to CR with IDR was highly significant when considering the number of cases in whom a response was achieved later than day 40 from the start of treatment: 24/239 (10%) vs 117/277 (42%) with ADR (p=0.0001). In both ADR-treated and IDR-treated patient groups the incidence of early death and RES ALL was associated with higher patient age (median 45 and 44 years, respectively, vs 27 years in ADR-treated group (p<0.001), and 47 and 40 years, respectively, vs 33 years in IDR-treated group (p<0.001 and p=0.017)). No other pretreatment feature affected the probability of CR. The incidence of RES ALL in discrete ALL subtypes was then analyzed (Table 5). With IDR, RES ALL was significantly less frequent in FAB L3/B-ALL, early-B Ph/BCR-ABL– ALL and CD10– ALL, but not in T-ALL and Ph/BCR-ABL+ ALL. The lowest RES ALL rate was observed CD10+ Ph/BCR-ABL– ALL treated with IDR-containing regimens (3.8%), but this was not statistically significant in comparison with

**Table 4.** Induction results of ADR vs IDR based regimens (cumulative data).

| | ADR-containing | IDR-containing | p value |
|---|---|---|---|
| No. of patients | 379 | 297 | – |
| CR, no. (%) | 277 (73) | 239 (80) | 0.031 |
| Time to CR (days), median (range) | 35 (11–100+) | 27 (15–96) | <0.0001 |
| Early death, no. | 46 | 33 | NS |
| RES ALL, no. (%) | 56 (15) | 25 (8.4) | 0.0125 |

NS, non significant p value

**Table 5.** Comparative incidence of RES ALL by ANT regimen (ADR vs IDR) in ALL subsets.

| ALL subset | ADR-containing | IDR-containing | p value |
|---|---|---|---|
| B (SIg+) | 6/16 (37.5%) | 0/15 (0%) | 0.028 |
| T-cell | 12/62 (19.3%) | 6/60 (10%) | NS |
| Early-B | 34/211 (16.1%) | 17/218 (7.8%) | NS |
| Early-B subsets: | | | |
| CD10– | 15/71 (21) | 3/67 (4.4) | 0.0081 |
| CD10+ | 11/140 (7.8) | 14/151 (9.2) | NS |
| Ph/BCR-ABL– | 19/116 (16) | 6/139 (4.3) | 0.002 |
| Ph/BCR-ABL+ | 4/27 (14.8) | 9/61 (14.7) | NS |
| CD10+ Ph/BCR-ABL– | 4/46 (8.7) | 3/78 (3.8) | NS |
| CD10– Ph/BCR-ABL– | 15/70 (21.4) | 3/61 (4.9) | 0.013 |

NS, nonsignificant p value

ADR regimens (RES ALL 8.7%) because of the rather small number of patients. Altogether, the lack of advantage for IDR-based regimens in the entire early-B CD10+ subgroup can be explained by the high incidence of Ph/BCR-ABL positivity. The rates of RES ALL in early-B Ph/BCR-ALL— ALL, whether CD10 positive or not, were constantly below 5% and therefore distinctly lower than with ADR-based regimens. There were too few t(4;11) ALL patients to perform a subset analysis.

## DFS results

### Prognostic factors and role of ANT DI
The median DFS for all 516 patients in first CR was 1.4 years, with an actuarial proba-bility of 0.28 at 5 years and 0.25 at 10 years. The factors correlating with DFS duration that were found to retain a statistical signifi-cance in U/V and then M/V analyses were an age >35 years (p=0.036), a blast count >25x10⁹/l (p<0.0001), and Ph/BCR-ABL posi-tivity (p=0.001). According to cumulative incidence of these three risk factors in indivi-dual patients, the following prognostic sub-groups were identified (Figure 1): standard-risk (no adverse factor: median DFS 2.29 years, 37.7% at 5 years), intermediate-risk (any one factor; median DFS 1.1 years, 27.7% at 5 years), and poor-risk (two or three fac-tors; median DFS 0.67 years, 7.2% at 5 years). Among treatment-related variables, only high-dose therapy supported by hematopoietic cell allograft/autograft (p=0.010; neither graft procedure was significant when considered alone) and a high ANT DI (p=0.004) were found to correlate favorably with DFS on both U/V and M/V analyses. Neither ANT type nor the use of other drugs considered isolatedly (+/–high-dose or conventional-dose cytara-bine, +/–podophyllotoxins, +/–cyclophospha-mide, +/–high-dose methotrexate, +/–vincri-stine ≥6 times) exerted any significant effect on DFS duration. The prognostic effect of a high ANT DI (median DFS 1.74 vs 1.13 years, 34% vs 21.8% at 5 years) is shown in Figure 2. In the three different risk groups, the use of a high ANT DI protocol was found to increase the DFS rate further only in standard-risk cases (median DFS 4.52 vs 1.89 years, 47% vs 24.8% at 5 years; Figure 3), while it had minor and statistically nonsignificant effects in intermediate-risk (30% vs 25% at 5 years) and high-risk (11% at 5 years vs 4% at 4 years) groups (data not shown).

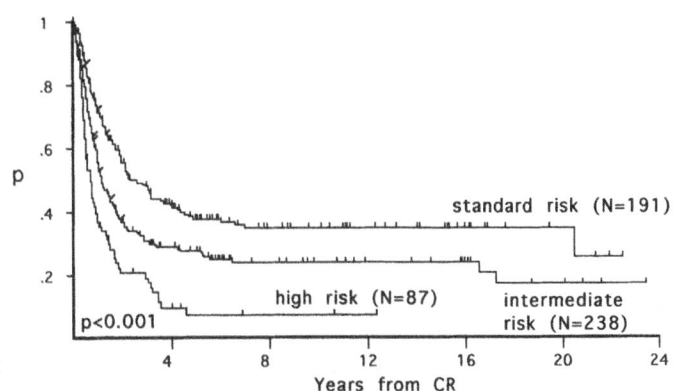

**Fig. 1.** Duration of DFS according to risk class.

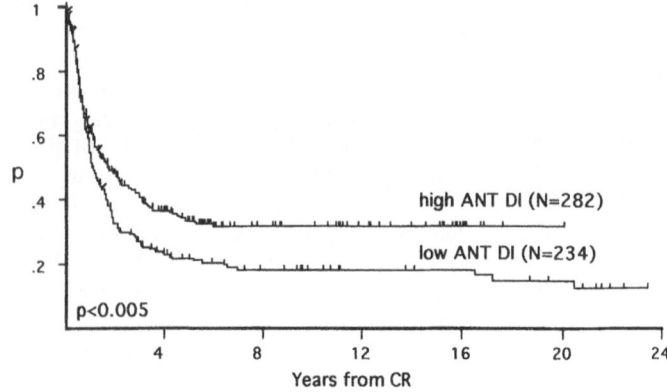

**Fig. 2.** Duration of DFS according to high/low anthracycline dose intensity (ANT DI).

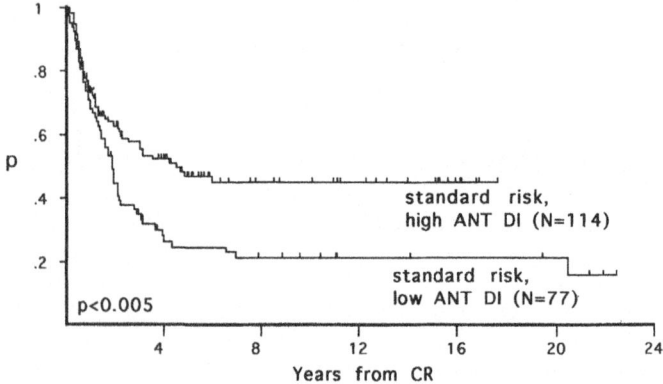

**Fig. 3.** Duration of DFS in standard-risk cases according to high/low anthracycline dose intensity (ANT DI).

## DFS according to ANT DI and ALL subtypes

The analysis of ANT DI-related effects in discrete ALL entities was restricted to cases with a known immunophenotype and concerned, in early B-lineage cases with successful cytogenetic or gene rearrrangement stu-

**Table 6.** Comparative DFS results in ALL subtypes by high/low anthracycline dose intensity (ANT DI).

| ALL subset | ANT DI | No. of patients | Median DFS (years) | 5-year DFS rate | p value |
|---|---|---|---|---|---|
| B-ALL | Low | 11 | 1.34 | 36.4% | NS |
| | High | 6 | 0.4 | 16.7% | |
| T-ALL | Low | 46 | 1 | 27.1% | NS |
| | High | 53 | 1.1 | 32.8% | |
| Early-B[1] | Low | 155 | 1.26 | 20.7% | <0.005 |
| | High | 188 | 2.1 | 33.4% | |
| Early-B subsets: | | | | | |
| Ph/BCR-ABL+ | Low | 36 | 0.75 | 0% | <0.01 |
| | High | 34 | 1.45 | 16.7% | |
| Ph/BCR-ABL– | Low | 61 | 1.64 | 17.8% | <0.025 |
| | High | 98 | 2.7 | 39% | |
| Ph/BCR-ABL– subsets: | | | | | |
| CD10+ | Low | 38 | 1.26 | 19.4% | <0.025 |
| | High | 69 | 2.68 | 42.8% | |
| CD10– | Low | 23 | 0.89 | 0% | NS |
| | High | 29 | 2.1 | 30.7% | |

[1]includes all cases CD10+ and CD10– regardless information about Ph/BCR-ABL status
NS, nonsignificant p value

408

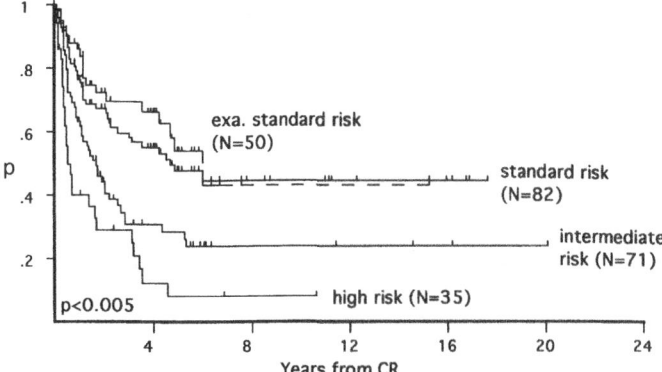

**Fig. 4.** DFS by risk class in high ANT DI-treated early-B ALL, including cases with no high-risk factors (exa. standard).

Figure labels: exa. standard risk (N=50); standard risk (N=82); intermediate risk (N=71); high risk (N=35); p<0.005; Years from CR; p

dies, a further subdivision according to CD10 antigen expression and Ph/BCR-ABL status. The results are reported in Table 6, and show a significantly degree of chemosensitivity to ANT in early-B ALL (DFS significantly improved with high ANT DI) as opposed to B-ALL and T-ALL (DFS no or minimally improved by high ANT DI). The prognostic advantage correlated with a high ANT DI was observed in both Ph/BCR-ABL+ and Ph/BCR-ABL– CD10+ ALL. The difference was not significant in CD10– ALL because of the small number of patients in the subgroups.

### High ANT DI and other prognostic variables in early-B ALL

One-hundred eighty-eight early-B ALL patients received high ANT DI. Because of the favorable prognostic effect of high ANT DI in this patient subset, an additional sub-analysis was performed to include other independent risk factors such as presenting blast count, patient age and Ph/BCR-ABL status (Table 7). The results confirmed the previous analysis for the whole patient series, since patients

with standard risk early-B ALL had the best median and long-term DFS rates (Figure 4). Because in the standard risk group there were several cases in whom the with Ph/BCR-ABL status was unknown (lack of cytogenetics/molecular study), we next examined the 50 patients known to have no high risk factor, including Ph/BCR-ABL negativity. For this group, the median DFS and 5-year rate were in excess of 5 years and 50%, respectively, as shown in the Table and Figure. The best results were achieved in the group of 38 cases with standard risk Ph/BCR-ABL– CD10+ ALL, with a 5-year DFS projection at about 60%.

## Discussion

This analysis focused on the role of anthracyclines in the treatment of ALL. The treatment programs considered in this study have been developed from 1972 to 1998, and have included either ADR or IDR during induction and early consolidation courses, with both

**Table 7.** DFS by risk factors in high ANT DI-treated early-B ALL.

| Category[1] | No. of patients | Median DFS (years) | 5-year DFS rate | p value |
|---|---|---|---|---|
| **Risk:** | | | | |
| Standard | 82 | 4.68 | 47.5% | <0.005 |
| Intermediate | 71 | 1.73 | 26.4% | |
| High | 35 | 0.59 | 8.3% | |
| **Standard risk:** | | | | |
| Ph/BCR-ABL– | 50 | 5.97 | 54% | NS |
| Ph/BCR-ABL– CD10+ | 38 | 5.97 | 59% | |
| Ph/BCR-ABL– CD10– | 12 | 4.68 | 45.8% | |

[1]risk class by age, blast count, Ph/BCR-ABL status; Ph/BCR-ABL– when exactly known

409

drugs given at either high or low DI. The concept of DI for ANT in adult ALL was first introduced in 1994 by the Verona University Hospital team (28). In that report, the patients able to receive DNR >21 mg/m$^2$/week during the first three months of treatment fared considerably better than the rest. Depending on the different drugs and lay-out of the protocols, we adopted a slightly different definition of DI. However, excluding the induction course, patients treated according to the HEAV'D/R-HEAV'D, STT, IVAP-2, and 08–96 standard-risk and T-ALL regimens (Table 1), were to receive ADR 15–39 mg/m$^2$/week or IDR 10.6 mg/m$^2$/week during the first 9–12 weeks of postremission therapy. These figures, considering an approximate drug ratio (vs DNR) of 1.5 for ADR and >3 for IDR, fit well with the high ANT DI range proposed by Todeschini et al [28]. Hence we were able to perform, with the limitations of a retrospective study, a comparative analysis of the results obtained with two different drugs (ADR vs IDR) during induction chemotherapy, and two different DI (high vs low) during early consolidation therapy. We evaluated these issues in a large patient series with long follow-up, and for the first time were therefore able to to look at ANT-related effects in different risk groups and ALL subtypes.

## Remission induction:
## IDR vs ADR, ALL subsets

With regard to the remission induction phase, the overall results were in favor of intensified ANT treatment. In general, our results (IDR vs ADR) were similar to those reported in AML phase III trials, where the use of IDR was associated with a better CR rate, shorter time to CR, and a lower incidence of refractory AML in comparison with DNR [6]. The cumulative CR rate achieved with the IVAP-2 schedule employing a total IDR dose of 20 mg/m$^2$ was 84% (218/258), and the RES ALL rate was 7% (18/258). These figures were significantly better than those achieved with the use of ADR-based regimens. In the single study adopting an intensive ADR treatment (STT, Table 3), the CR rate was comparably high but patient age and

number were lower and smaller, respectively, and time to CR was longer. We underline that, in the single AML study comparing IDR vs ADR, no major difference was found between the two study arms, but again the number of patients was rather small for a randomized trial [6]. The interpretation of these results is however complicated by two facts. First, the equivalent therapeutic doses of IDR, ADR, and DNR are not exactly known. Furthermore, since we were forced to reduce the total IDR dose from 36 to 20 mg/m$^2$ because of toxicity, it would seem that, in terms of clinical activity, this IDR dose is clinically equivalent to and hence comparable with an ADR dose of up to 30 mg/m$^2$/d for three consecutive days, as employed in the STT regimen. Second, because CR rates are usually higher in ALL than in AML (due to the high activity of the V/P/As combination), it may be more difficult to detect any significant therapeutic difference abscribable to ANT type. The IDR-based IVAP-2 regimen was associated with a high CR rate in a large, unselected patient population including some aged >60 years or with unfavorable disease such as FAB L3/B-ALL, and the response was obtained quickly. Most importantly, with IDR-containing regimens, the incidence of RES ALL was significantly reduced in B-ALL and CD10– early-B ALL but not in T-ALL and CD10+ early-B ALL. This was in part related to the high incidence of Ph/BCR-ABL+ cases in the latter subset (Table 5), since RES ALL rate was lowest (3.8%) in CD10+ Ph/BCR-ABL– patients treated with IDR. These results are difficult to explain, given the lack of preclinical information on IDR activity in discrete ALL subsets. Greater cytotoxicity in MDR-1+ cases may be anticipated, but it is not known to what extent this is clinically significant in adult ALL. In chemosensitive ALL cases, IDR may simply optimize the response rate by virtue of its improved lypophilicity that warrants a greater and faster uptake by blast cells. The combination of these two effects could explain the improved outcome observed in B-ALL and Ph/BCR-ABL– early-B ALL. T-ALL and Ph/BCR-ABL+ ALL would appear relatively IDR-resistant. It is worth noting how the addition of cyclophosphamide for a cohort of patients receiving the IDR protocol did not modify the incidence of

RES ALL. This suggests that IDR-resistant (and by definition also V/P/As-resistant) cases are likely to express truly pleiotropic multidrug resistance, that may be due to more than one mechanism, as reported in advanced-stage ALL [29]. One alternative (or complementary) explanation may be an insufficient IDR dosage, but this is unlikely in view of high CR rate obtained with this regimen. However, because IDR resistance may be dose-dependent, as ascertained by *in vitro* studies on MDR1+ ALL cells [17], increased-dose IDR may find a place in the treatment of patients with documented MDR1+ and probably MRP+ ALL [30], with or without the additional use of an inhibitor of MDR1 function [17–18, 31].

## Postremission consolidation: role of ANT DI, risk class and ALL subset

In multivariate analysis, DFS of CR patients was found to be strongly influenced by some treatment-unrelated risk factors (age, blast count, Ph/BCR-ABL status) and, among treatment-related variables, by ANT DI more than by high-dose regimens supported by hematopoietic stem cell transplantation. DFS was not influenced by ANT type, and not by allograft or autograft separately and by other drug classes singularly considered. Based on the analysis of classic risk factors, we developed a three-stage prognostic system. The prognostic effects of a high or low ANT DI could then be tested separately in each risk category, in specific ALL syndromes and, in the most ANT-sensitive ALL subtype (early-B ALL), in relation to other risk factors. In contrast to the remission induction phase, DFS was the same for ADR- and IDR-treated patients. This is not a discrepant finding because, once a response is achieved (IDR better), patients initially responsive to both ADR and IDR may continue to respond well to the same ANT delivered during early consolidation, but those given less ANT, whether IDR or ADR, will do worse if ANT DI matters. Indeed, in AML studies comparing IDR vs DNR, the difference in favor of IDR mostly concerned CR rates and time to CR, as in our case, while DFS was marginally affected (p=0.07) [6]. In keeping with these results, it was ANT DI rather than ANT type which significantly affected the probability of long-term DFS. Evaluating different risk groups, we found that standard risk patients (age <35 years, blast count <25x10$^9$/l, Ph/BCR-ABL–) with early-B ALL (regardless CD10 antigen expression) were those who benefitted most from a high ANT DI. The high ANT DI-related effect was particularly in the subgroup of patients with known Ph/BCR-ABL negativity, the DFS rate approaching 60% at 5 years. The outcome of Ph/BCR-ABL+ cases was interesting too, given that an intensive ANT-containing therapy was associated with a significantly improved outcome in a fraction of patients [10]. In this very poor-risk category, neither age <35 years nor a blast count <25x10$^9$/l conferred any prognostic advantage, but we have previously found that patients aged <50 years fared better [10]. The results obtained in T-ALL, in contrast, are consistent with what was observed in the induction phase, and did not confirm any positive prognostic effect of an increased ANT DI. Subset analyses were not attempted in T-ALL, since neither age nor blast count affected outcome significantly (data not shown).

## Conclusions

A major concern of this study was the difficulty in extrapolating data inherent to single drugs (i.e. ANT type and DI) from increasingly complex multidrug programs such as those developed for adult ALL by the 'L-B-V' group and affiliated centres over the past 26 years. The task is even harder if we consider the subsequent changes in diagnostic methodology, ALL classification systems, and general patient care and management. However, if the objective is a more rational use of these drugs, there is no easy way out. Practically speaking, we have shown that IDR is highly active as an induction drug for adult ALL, its use being associated with a low incidence of RES ALL and short time to response. The issue of postremission therapy is perhaps more important. We have substantially confirmed early observations on the role of ANT DI [4, 5, 10, 19, 20, 28] and further developed the issue of the patterns of chemosensitivity according to patient and disease characteristics. In accordance with our clinical results, *in vitro* chemosensitivity to ANT has been reported to be low in T-ALL and pro-B ALL and higher in pre-B ALL [21]. We now look forward to differentiating pro-B from pre-B ALL, in order to assess this hypothesis and offer these patients alternative forms of treatment. It also emerges that a high ANT DI during early postremission therapy could be considered a good prognostic co-factor for DFS. Our current definition of standard-risk ALL considers thiat. This is a new proposal but, not surprisingly, treatment itself has always been prognostically relevant because it is the only means to alter the fatal course of this illness. The ever increasing complexity (and toxicity) of modern treatments raises the question of which components of treatment matter most and in which cases. In our studies, an high ANT DI played a significant role in the achievement of improved results in the standard risk category and particularly in the patients with early-B ALL.

# References

1. Richardson DS, Johnson SA (1997) Anthracyclines in haematology: preclinical studies, toxicity and delivery systems. Blood Rev 11:201–223.
2. Johnson SA, Richardson DS (1997) Anthracyclines in haematology: pharmacokinetics and clinical studies. Blood Rev 12:52–71.
3. Gottlieb AJ, Weinberg V, Ellison RR, et al (1984) Efficacy of daunorubicin in the therapy of adult acute lymphocytic leukemia: a prospective randomized trial by Cancer and Leukaemia Group B. Blood 64:267–274.
4. Bassan R, Lerede T, Rambaldi A, et al (1996) The role of anthracyclines in adult acute lymphoblastic leukaemia. Leukemia 10 (Suppl 2): S58-S61.
5. Bassan R, Chiodini B, Lerede T, et al (1997). The role of idarubicin in adult acute lymphoblastic leukemia: from drug resistance studies to clinical application. Leuk Lymphoma 26 (Suppl 1):89–97.
6. The AML Collaborative Group (1998) A systemic collaborative overview of randomized trials comparing idarubicin with daunorubicin (or other anthracyclines) as induction therapy for acute myeloid leukaemia. Br J Haematol 103:100–109.
7. Rowe JM, Neuberg D, Friedenberg W, et al (1998) A phase II study of daunorubicin vs idarubicin vs mitoxantrone for older adult patients (>55 yrs) with acute myelogenous leukemia (AML): a study of the Eastern Cooperative Oncology group (E3993). Blood 92 (Suppl 1):313a (Abstract).
8. Lerede T, Bassan R, Rossi A, et al (1996) Therapeutic impact of adult-type acute lymphoblastic leukemia regimens in B-cell/L3 acute leukemia and advanced-stage Burkitt's lymphoma. Haematologica 81:442–9.
9. Lerede T, Bassan R, Viero P, et al (1998) Prolonged remission in adult B-ALL (L3) and advanced Burkitt's lymphoma using acute leukemia regimens: study of 34 patients. In Hiddeman W, Büchner T, Wörmann B, Ritter J, Creutzig U, Keating M, Plunkett W (eds): Acute Leukemias VII, Berlin, Springer-Verlag, pp 783–789.
10. Bassan R, Rohatiner AZS, Rambaldi, et al (1998) Clinical sensitivity to anthracyclines in Ph/BCR+ acute lymphoblastic leukemia. Leukemia 12:282 (Abstract).
11. Bassan R, Battista R, Corneo G, et al (1993) Idarubicin in the initial treatment of adults with acute lymphoblastic leukemia: the effect of drug schedule on outcome. Leuk Lymphoma, 11: 105–110.
12. Bassan R, Battista R, Viero P, et al (1993) Intensive therapy for adult acute lymphoblastic leukemia: preliminary results of the Idarubicin/Vincristine/L-asparaginase/Prednisolone regimen. Semin Oncol, 20 (Suppl 8):39–46.
13. Bassan R, Lerede T, Di Bona E, et al (1999) Induction-consolidation with an idarubicin-containing regimen, unpurged marrow autograft, and postgraft chemotherapy in adult acute lymphoblastic leukaemia. Br J Haematol (in press).
14. Bassan R, Di Bona E, Lerede T, et al (1995) Age-adapted moderate-dose induction and flexible outpatient postremission therapy for elderly patients with acute lymphoblastic leukemia. Leuk Lymphoma, 22:295–301.
15. Bassan R, Lerede T, Di Bona, et al (1997) Granulocyte colony-stimulating factor (G-CSF, Filgrastim) after or during an intensive remission induction therapy for adult acute lymphoblastic leukaemia: effects, role of patient pretreatment characteristics, and costs. Leuk Lymphoma 26: 153–161.
16. Papamicheal D, Andrews T, Owen D, et al (1993) Intensive chemotherapy for adult acute lymphoblastic leukaemia (ALL) given with or without granulocyte/macrophage colony stimulating factor (GM-CSF). Br J Haematol, 93 (suppl 2): 60 (Abstract).
17. Chiodini B, Bassan R, Barbui T (1999) Cellular uptake and antiproliferative effects of therapeutic concentrations of idarubicin or daunorubicin and their alcohol metabolites, with or without cyclosporin A, in MDR1+ humanleukemic cells. Leuk Lymphoma (in press).
18. Chiodini B, Bassan R, Borleri G, et al (1998) Idarubicin activity against multidrug-resistant (mdr1+) cells is increased by cyclosporin A. In Hiddeman W, Büchner T, Wörmann B, Ritter J, Creutzig U, Keating M, Plunkett W (eds): Acute Leukemias VII, Berlin, Springer-Verlag, pp 475–482.
19. Bassan R, Lerede T, Rambaldi A, et al (1995) The use of anthracyclines in adult acute lymphoblastic leukemia. Haematologica 80: 280–291.
20. Bassan R, Rambaldi A, Lerede T, et al (1997) Correlation beteween early anthracycline dose intensity and clinical outcome identifies specific chemoresistance patterns in adult acute lymphoblastic leukemia. in Pieters R, Kaspers GJL, Veerman AJP

(eds): Drug resistance in leukemia and lymphoma II. Harwood Academic Publishers, Amsterdam, pp 395–402.

21. Den Boer ML, Pieters R, Veerman AJP (1998). Mechanisms of cellular anthracycline resistance in childhood acute leukemia. Leukemia 12: 1657–1670.

22. Bassan R, Battista R, Rohatiner AZS, et al (1992) Treatment of adult acute lymphoblastic leukaemia (ALL) over a 16 year period. Leukemia 6 (Suppl 2):186–190.

23. Lister TA, Whithouse JMA, Beard MEJ, et al (1978) Combination chemotherapy for acute lymphoblastic leukaemia in adults. Br Med J 1:199–203.

24. Rohatiner AZS, Bassan R, Battista R, et al (1990) High dose cytosine arabinoside in the initial treatment of adults with acute lymphoblastic leukaemia. Br J Cancer 62:454–458.

25. Barnett MJ, Greaves MF, Amess JAL, et al (1986) Treatment of acute lymphoblastic leukaemia in adults. Br J Haematol 64:455–468.

26. Bassan R, Battista R, D'Emilio A, et al (1991) Long-term results of the HEAVD protocol for adult acute lymphoblastic leukaemia. Eur J Cancer Clin Oncol 27:441–447.

27. Bassan R, Battista R, Montaldi A, et al (1993) Reinforced HEAV'D therapy for adult acute lymphoblastic leukemia: improved results and revised prognostic criteria. Hematol Oncol 11:169–177.

28. Todeschini G, Meneghini V, Pizzolo G, et al (1994) Relationship between daunorubicin dosage delivered during induction therapy and outcome in adult acute lymphoblastic leukemia. Leukemia 8: 376–381.

29. Beck J, Handgretinger R, Dopfer R, et al (1995) Expression mdr1, mrp, topoisomerase IIa/b, and cyclin A in primary or relapsed states of acute lymphoblastic leukaemias. Br J Haematol 89: 356–363.

30. Ross D, Tong Y, Cornblatt (1993) Idarubicin (IDA) is less vulnerable to transport mediated multidrug resistance (MDR) than its metaboliteidarubicinol (IDAol) or daunorubicin (DNR). Blood (suppl 1) 82:257a (Abstract).

31. Chiodini B, Bassan R, Barbui T. (1998) Apoptosis by anthracyclines at therapeutic concentrations in MDR1+ human leukemic cells. Leukemia 12:269 (Abstract).

# Allogeneic Bone Marrow Transplantation for BCR-ABL Positive Acute Lymphoblastic Leukemia

D. S. Snyder[1], A. P. Nademanee[1], M. R. O'Donnell[1], P. M. Parker[1], A. S. Stein[1], K. Margolin[1], G. Somlo[1], A. Molina[1], R. Spielberger[1], A. Kashyap[1], H. Fung[1], N. Vora[2], M. L. Slovak[3], J. Niland[4], J. Palmer[4], R. S. Negrin[5], M. D. Amylon[6], K. G. Blume[5] and S. J. Forman[1]

*Abstract.* The prognosis for patients with bcr-abl positive acute lymphoblastic leukemia (ALL) treated with chemotherapy is extremely poor. Allogeneic bone marrow transplantation (BMT) may offer a curative option for patients who have appropriate donors available. Between 1984 and 1998, 76 consecutive patients with bcr-abl positive ALL were treated with allogeneic BMT from HLA-matched donors: 26 patients in 1st complete remission (CR) with matched sibling donors (group A), 35 patients >1st CR with matched sibling donors (group B), and 15 patients (1st CR or more advanced) with matched related (MRD) or unrelated donors (MUD) (group C). The age range for all patients was from 3 to 56 years. Surviving patients have been followed for a median of four years. For patients in group A, the two-year probabilities of disease-free survival (DFS) and relapse are 68.6 % and 10.8 %, respectively. For patients transplanted after 1992, these probabilities are 81 % and 11% respectively. The relatively low relapse rate in this group of patients compared to published reports may reflect the enhanced anti-leukemic activity of etoposide in combination with FTBI compared to other conditioning regimens. The enhancement in overall survival for patients transplanted after 1992 may reflect improvements in supportive care, in particular, the prophylaxis of serious fungal and viral infections. For patients in Group B, the two-year probabilities for DFS and relapse are 36.7% and 38.2% respectively; and for Group C, the two-year probabilities for DFS and relapse are 6.7% and 59.4% respectively. Significant prognostic factors for DFS and risk of relapse include: disease status, allogeneic vs. MUD/MRD BMT, the occurrence of Grade II-IV acute GVHD, and the detection of p190 bcr-abl post-BMT.

## Introduction

The Philadelphia chromosome (Ph) is found in 20–30% of adults and 3–5% of children with acute lymphoblastic leukemia (ALL) [1–3]. Patients with Ph+ ALL have an extremely poor prognosis for long-term survival [4]. Allogeneic bone marrow transplantation (BMT) has been utilized as a post-induc-tion therapy to try to improve disease-free survival (DFS) for these patients [5]. The IBMTR has reported a 38% disease-free survival rate for patients transplanted with Ph+ ALL in first CR, 41% for patients transplanted after relapse, and 25% for patients with induction failure [6].

The bcr-abl oncogene, which is the molecular counterpart of the Ph chromosome, is detected in two variant forms, either p190 or p210 by sensitive polymerase chain reaction (PCR) techniques. In adults with Ph+ ALL, the p190 form is detected in about 50% of cases, whereas in pediatric cases, the p190 is the dominant variant and is detected in about 90% of cases [2,7]. Generally, there are no significant differences in the biology or response to chemotherapy between p190+ vs. p210+ ALL [8]. However, a recent report on allogeneic BMT for Ph+ ALL suggested that the

[1] Division of Hematology/Bone Marrow Transplantation,
[2] Division of Radiation Oncology,
[3] Division of Pathology,
[4] Division of Information Sciences, City of Hope National Medical Center, Duarte, CA;
[5] Departments of Medicine and
[6] Pediatrics, Division of Bone Marrow Transplantation, Stanford University Medical Center, Stanford, CA

expression of p190 bcr-abl after BMT was associated with a significantly increased risk of relapse compared to the expression of the p210 variant [9].

We now report the results for a group of 76 patients who have been followed for a median of 4 years (surviving patients). Risk factors such as type of transplant, stage of disease, bcr-abl PCR results, and year of transplant are reviewed.

## Patients and Methods

### Patient characteristics

The patient characteristics are presented in Table 1. All patients were Ph+ either by classic cytogenetics or by PCR. The patients were treated with a variety of induction chemotherapy regimens, often at outside institutions before they were referred for BMT. For the majority of patients, a combination of vincristine, prednisone, daunorubicin, and L-asparaginase was used to induce a remission. Twenty-six patients in 1st CR were transplanted utilizing matched sibling donors (Group A), 35 patients >1st CR were transplanted utilizing matched sibling donors (Group B), and 15 patients at various stages of disease (4 in 1st

**Table 1.** Patient Demographics

| Total no. of patients | 76 | |
|---|---|---|
| Diagnosis | ALL – 73 | BPL-3 |
| Age range (median) | 3.5–56.6 yrs (29.6) | |
| Gender | Female – 18 (23.7%) Male- 58 (76.3%) | |
| Type of transplant | Allo sib – 60 Syngeneic – 1 MUD – 11 MRD – 4 | |
| Group A | 1st CR Allo – 26 | |
| Group B | >1st CR Allo- 35 | |
| Group C | MUD/MRD – 15 | |
| Year of Transplant | 1984–1992 1993–1998 | 28 pts (36.8%) 48 pts (63.2%) |
| Stem Cell Source | Bone marrow – 74 Primed PBSC- 1 Cord blood- 1 | |

BPL- biphenotypic leukemia; Allo sib- allogeneic transplant from matched sibling donor; MUD- matched unrelated donor; MRD- partly mismatched related donor; Primed PBSC- G-CSF primed peripheral blood stem cells

CR, 11 >1st CR) were transplanted utilizing either partially-matched relatives (MRD-4) or matched unrelated donors (MUD-11) (Group C). The date of analysis was December 31, 1998.

### Polymerase Chain Reaction

The bcr-abl mRNA was detected by PCR pre-BMT and after BMT for many of the patients. The method for PCR was a single-step amplification of 30–33 rounds as previously described [10].

### Bone Marrow Transplantation

For patients in Group A, the conditioning regimen consisted of fractionated total body irradiation (FTBI) 1320 cGy delivered in 11 fractions over 4 days, followed by etoposide (VP16) at 60mg/kg [11,12] in 22/26 patients; FTBI followed by cyclophosphamide (CY) at 120mg/kg given over 2 days in two patients; busulfan/CY in one patient; and a combination of FTBI/VP16/CY in one patient [13]. For Group B patients, 14/35 were conditioned with FTBI/VP16; 11/35 with FTBI/VP16/CY; 6/35 with BU/FTBI/VP16; 2 with BU/CY; and 2 with other combinations. For patients in Group C, 14/15 patients were conditioned with FTBI/CY, and one patient received FTBI/VP16/CY. (See Table 2)

All patients except two received hematopoietic cells in the form of unmanipulated bone marrow from HLA-matched sibling donors. One patient received G-CSF primed peripheral blood stem cells from her HLA-matched sister, and one patient received cord

**Table 2.** Conditioning Regimens

| | Group A (n = 26) | Group B (n = 35) | Group C (n = 15) |
|---|---|---|---|
| F/VP | 22 | 14 | |
| F/CY | 2 | | 14 |
| F/VP/CY | 1 | 11 | 1 |
| BU/CY | 1 | 2 | |
| BU/F/VP | | 6 | |
| Other | | 2 | |

F – fractionated total body irradiation; VP- etoposide (VP-16); CY- cyclophosphamide; BU- busulfan; Other- F/melphalan (1); BU/VP/CY (1)

blood cells from a matched sibling. Graft vs. host disease (GVHD) prophylaxis consisted of: cyclosporine A (CSA) plus methotrexate (MTX) (8 patients); CSA/methylprednisolone (PSE) (38 patients), CSA/MTX/PSE (27 patients), or MTX/PSE (3 patients) as per institutional trials conducted during this time period [14–16].

Supportive care was provided as previously described [12]. The preemptive utilization of ganciclovir based on shell vial positivity from bronchoalveolar lavage or peripheral blood samples was introduced as standard care starting in 1991 [17]. Routine fungal prophylaxis with low dose IV amphotericin B at 0.15 mg/kg/d was instituted in 1992 [18]. Patients were treated in hepa-filtered isolation rooms until engraftment of neutrophils. All patients were treated on protocols approved by the Institutional Review Boards at City of Hope National Medical Center or at Stanford University Medical Center.

## Statistical Analysis

The log-rank test was used to determine significant differences in survival curves for the various parameters tested. Kaplan-Meier plots [19] were used to calculate probabilities of DFS, overall survival (OS), and relapse rates.

## Results

### Overall and Disease-free Survival

The median follow-up time for all patients is 8.9 mos. (range of 0.6–158.8 mos.), and for living patients, the median follow-up time is 48 mos. (range of 3.2–158.8 mos). The probability of 2-yr. DFS (95% confidence intervals) for all patients is 40.9% (30.3–52.5%), and the probability of relapse is 30.0% (20.1–44.8 %). The probabilities for 2-yr DFS and relapse for groups A, B, and C are presented in Table 3. These differences are statistically significant as shown by the p values in the table. For Group A patients, there is a significant difference in DFS for patients transplanted between 1984–1992 compared to those transplanted between 1993–1998 with a 3 yr.

**Table 3.** Outcomes

| | 2-yr DFS (95% CI)[a] | 2-yr Risk of Relapse (95% CI)[b] |
|---|---|---|
| Group A | 68.6% (48.5–83.5%) | 10.8% (3.6–34.6%) |
| Group B | 36.7% (22.4–53.7%) | 38.2% (20.9–59.2%) |
| Group C | 6.7% (0.9–35.2%) | 59.4% (21.6–88.5%) |

DFS – disease-free survival; CI- confidence intervals; a- log rank, p=0.0016, comparing the three groups; b- log rank, p=0.0333, comparing the three groups

probability of DFS of 81% (48–95%) for the group transplanted after 1993 compared to 45% (20–73%) for the earlier cohort. (p=0.04 by the log-rank test). When Group A and B patients are combined, there is a similar trend (60% vs. 40% 2-yr DFS), though it is not significant.

At the time of this analysis, 27 of the patients are alive in remission (35.5%), one is alive in relapse (1.3%), 16 died of relapse (21.1%), and 32 died from other causes (42.1%). The main causes of death other than relapse were: GVHD +/- infection (6 patients); pneumonitis (6 patients); and other (VOD, hemorrhage, organ failure, other – 16 patients).

### Graft vs. Host Disease

The incidence of acute GVHD Grade 0-I was 64.5% (46.1% had Grade 0), and Grade II-IV was 35.5%. Of the 50 patients who survived to day 100, 19 (38%) developed chronic GVHD (12/19 extensive; 7/19 limited). There was a significant advantage in 2-yr DFS for patients with Grade 0-I vs Grade II-IV aGVHD ( 55.9% vs 18.5%, p=0.0001). However, there was no significant difference in DFS for patients who did or did not develop cGVHD.

### Polymerase Chain Reaction results

The impact of PCR findings was analyzed. For patients who had a positive PCR result post-BMT, there was a significant increase in the risk of relapse for those patients who expressed either p190 alone (relapse risk of 33% of 12 patients) or p190 plus p210 (100% of 3 patients), compared to patients who expressed p210 alone (14% of 7 patients) (p=0.0252).

## Discussion

In this report, we present the results for DFS and relapse rates for a three groups of patients with Ph+ ALL treated with allogeneic BMT at two institutions. These results compare favorably to previous reports from the IBMTR [6]. Other centers have reported results that include patients at various stages of disease with lower DFS rates and higher relapse rates than our results [20–22]. In those reports, most of the patients were conditioned with regimens of TBI/CY or busulfan/CY. A group from Germany [20] described their results for 10 patients transplanted for Ph+ ALL from either sibling, matched related, or matched unrelated donors. All patients were conditioned with a regimen of TBI/CYT/VP16. Only two of the 10 patients relapsed. In a more recent report from this group, [23] the 3-yr DFS rate for 15 patients transplanted from allogeneic donors while in 1st CR was 46%, and for all 24 patients ( 5 autologous, 13 allo-related, and 6 allo-unrelated) it was 38%. We speculate that the use of high-dose etoposide in the conditioning regimen may be important in explaining the lower relapse rates observed both in our study and in the German studies compared to the other reports.

The impact of bcr-abl patterns of expression post-BMT was evaluated. Though the numbers of patients with samples post-BMT was small, the results support the observations of Radich et al. [9] who found a significantly increased risk of relapse for patients who expressed the p190 bcr-abl mRNA post-BMT.

For Groups A and B, there was a difference in survival rates for patients transplanted after 1992 compared to those transplanted before 1992. The mortality rate from causes other than relapse was lower for the more recent cohort of patients. This improvement in treatment related mortality may reflect the impact of a variety of innovations in supportive care that have been introduced since the early 1990's. Most notably perhaps is the pre-emptive use of ganciclovir in patients with early evidence of activated CMV to prevent the development of CMV pneumonitis [17]. In addition, the routine use of low-dose prophylactic intravenous amphotericin B [18] may account for a reduction in mortality due to systemic fungal infections.

The detection of minimal residual disease after BMT by PCR may predict a higher risk of relapse if the p190 bcr-abl gene is found.

The results of this study indicate that allogeneic BMT from matched sibling donors is a very effective treatment for patients with Ph+ ALL in first CR (Group A). As expected, the relapse rates for patients >1st CR transplanted from sibling donors (Group B) are higher than for Group A, but the results are still encouraging. On the other hand, the results for patients transplanted from MRD or MUD donors (Group C) are very discouraging. These patients had a significantly higher risk of relapse and death compared to the other two groups of patients. The inclusion of high-dose etoposide (VP-16) along with FTBI (Groups A and B) may have reduced the risk of relapse and increased survival compared to Group C. We would recommend that any patient with Ph+ ALL should have HLA typing performed and potential sibling donors identified early in their course, and that allogeneic BMT should be offered soon after a 1st CR is achieved. MRD or MUD BMTs as currently performed do not seem to offer a significant chance of DFS for patients with Ph+ ALL that lack a matched sibling donor.

*Acknowledgements.* We gratefully acknowledge the dedicated work of our nurse coordinators, Rodrigo Nunez, Pilar Fonbuena, and Kathryn Tierney who provided critical support for our patients and physicians.

## References

1. Grp Français de Cytogénétique Hématol (1996) Cytogenetic abnormalities in adult acute lymphoblastic leukemia: correlations with hematologic findings and outcome. A collaborative study of the Groupe Francais de Cytogenetique Hematologique. Blood 87:3135–3142
2. Maurer J, Janssen JWG, Thiel E, Van Denderen J, Ludwig W-D, Aydemir U, Heinze B, Fonatsch C, Harbott J, Reiter A, Riehm H, Hoelzer D, Bartram CR (1991) Detection of chimeric bcr-abl genes in acute lymphoblastic leukaemia by the polymerase chain reaction. Lancet 337:1055–1058
3. Tuszynski A, Dhut S, Young BD, Lister TA, Rohatiner AZ, Amess JAL, Chaplin T, Dorey E, Gibbons B (1993) Detection and significance of bcr-abl mRNA transcripts and fusion proteins in Philadelphia-positive adult acute lymphoblastic leukemia. Leukemia 7:1504–1508

4. Beyermann B, Adams HP, Henze G (1997) Philadelphia chromosome in relapsed childhood acute lymphoblastic leukemia; A matched-pair analysis. J.Clin.Oncol. 15:2231–2237

5. Blume KG, Forman SJ, Snyder DS, Nadamanee AP, O'Donnell MR, Fahey JL, Krance RA, Sniecinski IJ, Stock AD, Findley DO, Lipsett JA, Schmidt GM, Nathwani MB, Hill LR, Metter GE (1987) Allogeneic bone marrow transplantation for acute lymphoblastic leukemia during first complete remission. Transplantation 43:389–392

6. Barrett AJ, Horowitz MM, Ash RC, Atkinson K, Gale RP, Goldman JM, Henslee-Downey PJ, Herzig RH, Speck B, Zwaan FE, Bortin MM (1992) Bone marrow transplantation for Philadelphia chromosome- positive acute lymphoblastic leukemia. Blood 79:3067–3070

7. Suryanarayan K, Hunger SP, Kohler S, Carroll AJ, Crist W, Link MP, Cleary ML (1991) Consistent involvement of BCR gene by 9;22 breakpoints in pediatric acute leukemias. Blood 77:324–330

8. Kantarjian HM, Talpaz M, Dhingra K, Estey E, Keating MJ, Ku S, Trujillo J, Huh Y, Stass S, Kurzrock R (1991) Significance of the P210 versus P190 molecular abnormalities in adults with Philadelphia chromosome-positive acute leukemia. Blood 78: 2411–2418

9. Radich J, Gehly G, Lee A, Avery R, Bryant E, Edmands S, Gooley T, Kessler P, Kirk J, Ladne P, Thomas ED, Appelbaum FR (1997) Detection of *bcr-abl* transcripts in Philadelphia chromosome-positive acute lymphoblastic leukemia after marrow transplantation. Blood 89:2602–2609

10. Snyder DS, Rossi JJ, Wang J-L, Sniecinski IJ, Slovak ML, Wallace RB, Forman SJ (1991) Persistence of bcr-abl gene expression following bone marrow transplantation for chronic myelogenous leukemia in chronic phase. Transplantation 51:1033–1040

11. Blume KG, Forman SJ, O'Donnell MR, Doroshow JH, Krance RA, Nadamanee AP, Snyder DS, Schmidt GM, Fahey JL, Metter GE, Hill LR, Findley DO, Sniecinski IJ (1987) Total body irradiation and high-dose etoposide: A new preparatory regimen for bone marrow transplantation in patients with advanced hematologic malignancies. Blood 69:1015–1020

12. Snyder DS, Chao NJ, Amylon MD, Taguchi J, Long GD, Negrin RS, Nadamanee AP, O'Donnell MR, Schmidt GM, Stein AS, Parker PM, Smith EP, Stepan DE, Molina A, Lipsett JA, Hoppe RT, Niland JC, Dagis AC, Wong RM, Forman SJ, Blume KG (1993) Fractionated total body irradiation and high-dose etoposide as a preparatory regimen for bone marrow transplantation for 99 patients with acute leukemia in first complete remission. Blood 82: 2920–2928

13. Long GD, Amylon MD, Stockerl-Goldstein KE, Negrin RS, Chao NJ, Hu WW, Nadamanee AP, Snyder DS, Hoppe RT, Vora N, Wong R, Niland J, Reichardt VL, Forman SJ, Blume KG (1997) Fractionated total-body irradiation, etoposide, and cyclophosphamide followed by allogeneic bone marrow transplantation for patients with high-risk or advanced-stage hematological malignancies. Biology of Blood and Marrow Transplantation 3:324–330

14. Chao NJ, Schmidt GM, Niland JC, Amylon MD, Dagis AC, Long GD, Nadamanee AP, Negrin RS, O'Donnell MR, Parker PM, Smith EP, Snyder DS, Stein AS, Wong RM, Blume KG, Forman SJ (1993) Cyclosporine, methotrexate, and prednisone compared with cyclosporine and prednisone for prophylaxis of acute graft- versus-host disease. N.Engl.J.Med. 329:1225–1230

15. Forman SJ, Blume KG, Krance RA, Miner PJ, Metter GE, Hill LR, O'Donnell MR, Nadamanee AP, Snyder DS (1987) A prospective randomized study of acute graft-v-host disease in 107 patients with leukemia: methotrexate/prednisone v cyclosporine A/prednisone. Transplant.Proc. 19:2605–2607

16. Schmidt GM, Snyder DS, Nadamanee AP, O'Donnell MR, Parker P, Stein A, Chao NJ, Amylon MD, Blume KG, Forman SJ (1989) A prospective randomized study: Cyclosporine A/Prednisone/Methotrexate (CSA/PSE/MTX) versus CSA/PSE for prevention acute graft versus host disease (GVHD). Blut 59(3):299

17. Schmidt GM, Horak DA, Niland JC, Duncan SR, Forman SJ, Zaia JA, City of Hope-Stanford-Syntex CMV Study Group (1991) A randomized, controlled trial of prophylactic ganciclovir for cytomegalovirus pulmonary infection in recipients of allogeneic bone marrow transplants. N.Engl.J.Med. 324:1005–1011

18. O'Donnell MR, Schmidt GM, Tegtmeier BR, Faucett C, Fahey JL, Ito J, Nademanee A, Niland J, Parker P, Smith EP, Snyder DS, Stein AS, Blume KG, Forman SJ (1994) Prediction of systemic fungal infection in allogeneic marrow recipients: impact of amphotericin prophylaxis in high risk patients. J.Clin.Oncol. 12:827–834

19. Kaplan G, Meier P (1958) Non-parametric estimations from incomplete observations. J.Am.Stat.Ass 53:457-481

20. Stockschlader M, Hegewisch-Becker S, Kruger W, tom Dieck A, Mross K, Hoffknecht M, Berger C, Kohlschutter B, Martin H, Peters S, Kabisch H, Kuse R, Weh H, Zander A (1995) Bone marrow transplantation for Philadelphia-chromosome-positive acute lymphoblastic leukemia. Bone Marrow Transplant 16:663–667

21. Dunlop LC, Powles R, Singhal S, Treleaven JG, Swansbury GJ, Meller S, Pinkerton CR, Horton C, Mehta J (1996) Bone marrow transplantation for Philadelphia chromosome-positive acuty lymphoblastic leukemia. Bone Marrow Transplantation 17:365–369

22. Annino L, Ferrari A, Cedrone M, Giona F, Lo Coco F, Meloni G, Arcese W, Mandelli F (1994) Adult Philadelphia-chromosome-positive acute lymphoblastic leukemia: Experience of treatments during a ten-year period. Leukemia 4:664

23. Kröger N, Krüger W, Wacker-Backhaus G, Hegewisch-Becker S, Stockschläder M, Fuchs N, Rüssmann B, Renges H, Dürken M, Bielack S, De Wit M, Schuch G, Bartels H, Braumann D, Kuse R, Kabisch H, Erttmann R, Zander AR (1998) Intensified conditioning regimen in bone marrow transplantation for Philadelphia chromosome-positive acute lymphoblastic leukemia. Bone Marrow Transplantation 22:1029–1033

# Preliminary Results of a Risk-Oriented Program for B-Lineage Adult Acute Lymphoblastic Leukemia (ALL): The Collaborative Italian Study 08/96

R. Bassan, A. Rambaldi, E. Pogliani, G. Rossi, P. Fabris, S. Morandi, P. Casula, G. Lambertenghi-Deliliers, M. Vespignani, T. Lerede, A. Personeni, P. Bellavita and T. Barbui

## Introduction

In an effort to improve the prognosis of patients with B-precursor ALL, we recently introduced a new risk-oriented postremission treatment policy (collaborative ALL study 08–96). Standard-risk (SR) cases were defined by CD10 positivity, blast cell count $<10 \times 10^9/l$, and lack of t(9;22)/t(4;11) or the corresponding gene rearrangements. These patients, according to our previous studies, had a relatively good long-term outcome (24 patients, minimum follow-up 3 years, disease-free survival at 5+ years 52%) with the use of moderately intensive consolidation therapies including anthracyclines and excluding very high-dose treatments supported by hematopoietic cell graft [1]. Therefore, in the new 08–96 prospective phase II trial, SR patients initially responsive to a combination of idarubicin+vincristine+asparaginase+prednisone+/–cyclophosphamide (IVAP+/–C) were to receive a multidrug program with early dose-intensive idarubicin, meningeal prophylaxis, high-dose methotrexate, rotational vincristine-cyclophosphamide and cytarabine-teniposide pulses, plus 2-year low-dose maintenance with 6-mercaptopurine and methotrexate. High-risk (HR) cases, i.e. those not satisfying the above mentioned criteria, fared much less well, with an overall long-term DFS rate of 24% (257 patients), that could vary depending on the cumulative incidence of high-risk features such as hyperleukocytosis, older age, and adverse immunobiologic ALL characteristics. Hence, HR cases with HLA and DR histocompatible donors were eligible to allogeneic bone marrow transplant (allo-BMT) in first remission, while those without donor were allocated to receive a brief all-high-dose sequence with cyclophosphamide, cytarabine, methotrexate, and then melphalan plus total body irradiation (TBI) followed by a highly purified autologous blood cell transplant (HP-ABCT). This latter treatment plan was adapted from a successful schedule developed at Istituto Nazionale Tumori (Milan) for the treatment of aggressive non-Hodgkin's lymphomas [2]. The difference consisted in the introduction of high-dose cytarabine, the limited folinic-acid rescue after high-dose methotrexate, the withdrawal of etoposide, the additional use of vincristine, dexamethasone and triple intrathecal therapy, and the refinement of the myeloablative regimen with high-dose melphalan and TBI. The *ex vivo* purging of autologous CD34+ cells was performed by a new and highly effective two-step immunomagnetic method specific for B-lineage disease, able to eliminate contaminating ALL cells with a sensitivity level between $10^{-4}$ and $10^{-6}$ cells on nested polymerase chain reaction [3]. Therefore, the HR regimen would allow to evaluate, in a patient subgroup with a globally poor prognosis, the therapeutic potential of an innovative, brief high-dose chemoradiotherapy sequence including HP-ABCT and excluding maintenance. Notably, HR patients not fit enough to receive the planned all-high-dose sequence were shifted to the SR program. We report and discuss the results obtained with this new risk-oriented postremission strategy in the firts 59 patients with early B-lineage ALL.

Hematology/Radiotherapy/Blood Service Units: Bergamo, Monza, Brescia, Bolzano, Cremona, Milan, and Cagliari Hospitals, Italy.

## Patients and methods

### Patients and diagnosis

ALL study 08–96 started in November, 1995. As of October, 1998, 88 adult ALL patients were registered and were evaluable for response. The presenting features of these cases are illustrated in Table 1.

Early B-lineage ALL was defined by morphology (FAB L1 or L2 myeloperoxidase negative blast cells) and immunophenotype (negative expression of surface immunoglobulin light chain, CD19+, CD10+ or negative, CD20+ or negative, HLA-DR+, intracytoplasmic CD22 and CD79a as necessary, nuclear TdT+). A cytogenetic evaluation or gene rearrangement studies for the detection of t(9;22)/Philadelphia chromosome (Ph/BCR-ABL+), t(4;11), and t(1;19) were available in most cases.

### Treatment regimens

The IVAP induction regimen (all drugs by intravenous route unless differently stated) consisted of idarubicin 10 mg/m²/d on days 1 and 2; vincristine 2 mg total dose on days 1, 8, and 15; L-asparaginase 6000 U/m² on alternate days x6 starting on day 8; prednisone 60

**Table 1.** Demographic and diagnostic features of 88 patients with ALL.

| Presentation features | Results |
|---|---|
| Patient age (yr), median (range) | 37 (15–74) |
| Gender (M/F), no. | 52/36 |
| Blast count (x10⁹/l), median (range) | 3.2 (0–240) |
| FAB class (L1, L2, L3, other), no. | 31, 51, 2, 4[1] |
| Phenotype (B, T, early-B CD10+, CD10–) | 2, 14, 49, 19 |
| t(9;22)/BCR-ABL+, no. | 13 |
| Other chromosome changes, no. | 17 |
| Risk class (SR/HR)[2], no. | 25/63 |

[1] 4 pts. with advanced-stage lymphoblastic lymphoma (also not included in phenotype results)
[2] SR, standard risk: early-B CD10+, <10x10⁹/l blast cells, Ph/BCR-ABL and t(4;11) negative; HR, high risk

mg/m²/d on days 1–21; recombinant G-CSF 5 mcg/kg/d subcutaneously from day 3 to a stable neutrophil count recovery following the neutropenic nadir; and intrathecal chemoprophylaxis on days 1 and 15 with methotrexate 12.5 mg+cytarabine 50 mg+prednisone 40 mg). Fractionated cyclophosphamide was initially added to this schedule but lately removed because, with regard to incidence of primary refractory ALL, results were not improved over historical IVAP-treated patients. Two different cyclophosphamide schedules were employed: 150 or 75 mg/m²/bd for 4 consecutive days before IVAP. Postremission consolidation regimens for SR and HR pa-

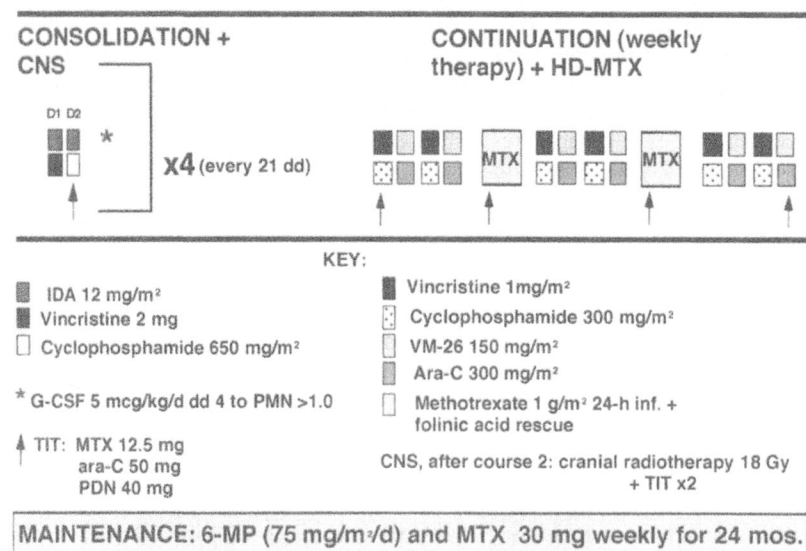

**Fig. 1.** Standard risk consolidation regimen.

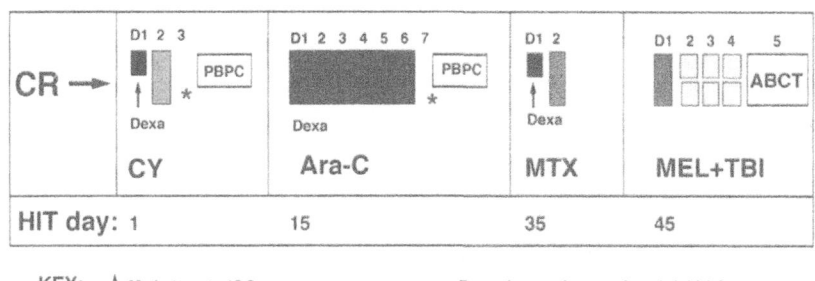

**Fig. 2.** High risk consolidation regimen.

KEY:  ↑: Methotrexate 12.5 mg + ara-C 50 mg + PDN 40 mg IT

\* G-CSF 5 mcg/kg/d

PBPC: autologous peripheral CD34+ cell collection and super-purification

ABCT: highly purified blood cell autograft

Dexa, dexamethasone 4 mg bd dd 1-6

■ Vincristine 2 mg

□ Cyclophosphamide 7 g/m²

■ Ara-C 2 g/m² bd 2-h infusion

■ Methotrexate 1.5 g/m² 24-h infusion + limited folinic acid rescue

■ Melphalan 140 mg/m²  □ TBI 2 Gy bd

tients are illustrated in detail in Figures 1 and 2, respectively. At one centre where TBI was not available, combinations of high-dose busulfan+cyclophosphamide or high-dose mitoxantrone+melphalan were used as preparative myeloablative regimens before autograft. For autograft purposes, G-CSF-primed peripheral CD34+ blood cells were collected after high-dose cyclophosphamide as well as after high-dose cytarabine. If possible, only the latter were used to support the autograft phase *in vivo*. The SR protocol was employed as pre-graft therapy in HR patients waiting to have an allo-BMT, and was also prescribed to HR cases who, for variuos reasons, did not continue with the intensive autograft program.

### Definitions and statistics

A CR was defined by the disappearance of ALL cell infiltration in the bone marrow (blast cell content <5%) with simultaneous recovery of normal trilineage hemopoiesis, near-normal blood counts with no need for transfusional support, and absence of clinical signs related to leukemia and/or extramedullary involvement. Refractory ALL was defined by the persistence in the bone marrow of greater than 5% ALL cells after the first induction course. A relapse was defined by the detection of greater than 5% ALL cells in the bone marrow of CR patients or by an extramedullary involvement. Death was the interval from diagnosis to death by any cause

or last follow-up, and disease-free survival (DFS) was the interval from CR to relapse in any site, death by any cause, or last follow-up. Comparisons between different prognostic groups were by means of the chi-squared test with Yate's correction and the log-rank test. DFS estimates were calculated by the standard life-table method.

## Results

### Achievement of CR

Seventy-six of 88 patients achieved a CR after a single IVAP+/-C course (86%). Median time to CR was 27 days with C and 22 days without C (p=0.0003). Median duration of neutropenia <0.500 was 15 days with C and 12 days without C (nonsignificant p value). Six patients had refractory ALL (7%) and 6 other succumbed to pancytopenic complications. Out of 76 CR patients, 22 had SR early B-lineage ALL (CD10+, blast count <10x10⁹/l, Ph/BCR and t(4;11) negative) and 38 had HR early B-lineage ALL, 10 of whom with Ph/BCR-ABL+ disease.

### Allocation to postremission protocol

Consolidation for 22 SR patients was SR protocol 21 and SR protocol followed by allo-BMT 1 (violation). Out of 38 HR patients, 16 had a matched sibling for allo-BMT and 22 did not. However, only 9 of the patients with a

421

donor actually had an allo-BMT. Exclusions were due to: too early, toxicity, early relapse, and physician's choice because of young age with mild hyperleukocytosis. Therefore, consolidation for 38 HR patients was nil 1 (toxicity and age >60 years with early loss to follow-up, patient presumably dead), allo-BMT 9, intensive HR program completed 15, shift to SR protocol 10, and waiting to complete autograft or allograft phase 3.

## DFS results

With a median follow-up of about 1.5 years, the outcome of the different risk and actual treatment groups is summarized in Table 2. The rather short follow-up does not allow to detect, at this time, any relevant prognostic difference between HR patients undergoing autograft or allograft and those shifted to SR treatment. SR patients, on the contrary, incurred in a lower relapse rate (5/22, 23%), and one late relapse was an isolated meningeal recurrence in a patient who had not received cranial irradiation as part of the prophylactic regimen, that has been successfully managed until now.

With regard to the new high-dose sequential treatment with HP-ABCT, we performed a preliminary analysis of intercycle times, toxicity, collection and purification of CD34+ circulating cells, and outcome according to disease subtype and to whether the *ex vivo* purging procedure had been performed or not. The results are reported in Table 3. Hence, the median time needed to complete postremission therapy from date of CR is the sum of the single intercycle times given, i.e. 83 days (range 62–109). This lapse of time is

**Table 2.** Treatment outcome by risk class and postremission protocol.

| Risk class (no.) | Protocol (no.) | Events (no.) | CCR (no.) | 1.5-yr DFS rate |
|---|---|---|---|---|
| SR (22) | SR (22)[1] | 6[2] | 16 | 67% |
| HR (38) | overall | 17[3] | 20 | 43% |
| HR evaluable by treatment: | | | | |
| | allo-BMT (9) | 5[4] | 4 | 56% |
| intensive+autograft (15) | | 7 | 8 | 43% |
| | shift to SR (10) | 4 | 6 | 49% |

[1] plus subsequent allo-BMT in 1 pt.
[2] relapse 5 (bone marrow 3, late meningeal 1, meningeal+marrow 1), CR death 1
[3] plus 1 pt. lost early to follow-up (not evalauble)
[4] relapse 3, CR death by toxicity 2

greater than that planned initially (Figure 2). It is interesting to note how enough CD34+ peripheral blood cells were collected following the Ara-C phase in 7 patients. This autologous product was used for ABCT in these cases. The day of CD34+ cells collection ranged from +9 to +15 after CY and from +17 to +23 after Ara-C. It is also interesting to note that, despite the rather short absolute neutropenic period after CY, Ara-C and ABCT, there were documented infections which tended to recur in the same patient (4 patients with subsequent infectious episodes and 2 patients with isolated infectious complication). Other complications were rare and mainly represented by gut and mucosal toxicity during the autograft phase (only WHO grade >II is indicated in Table 3). No patient died of the transplant procedure and all were discharged home without major complications and transfusion-free.

With regard to clinical outcome of HR autografted patients, we report in Table 4 the principal patient characteristics as well as

**Table 3.** Details of high-dose consolidation plus HP-ABCT program in 15 HR B-lineage ALL.

| Study parameters | High-dose phase (see Figure 2) | | | |
|---|---|---|---|---|
| | CY | Ara-C | MTX | Myeloablative regimen |
| Intercycle (days), median (range) | 10 (3–50) | 22 (14–41) | 17 (17–35)[1] | 18 (11–35) |
| CD34+ cells (x10^6/kg), median (range) | 7.1 (2.2–22)[2] | 9 (7.4–42)[3] | – | 5.9 (3.7–20)[4] |
| Neutropenia <0.500 (days), median (range) | 6 (3–12) | 9 (6–18) | 0 | 8 (6–13) |
| Toxicities[5], no. | IF 7, M 1 | IF 8 | IF 1, GI 2 | IF 3, GI 6, H 1 |

[1] 3 pts. excluded from MTX phase
[2] CD34+ cell collection not performed in 2 pts.
[3] CD34+ cell collection not performed in 8 pts.
[4] reinfused CD34+ cells; HP-ABCT in 11 pts.
[5] IF, infection; M, metabolic; GI, gastrointestinal; H, hemorragic

422

**Table 4.** Patients and outcome in high-dose HP-ABCT protocol for high-risk B-lineage ALL

| UPN | Age (yr) | Blast count (x10⁹/L) | Ph/BCR-ABL | ABCT | Outcome (DFS yr) |
|-----|----------|---------------------|------------|------|------------------|
| BG15 | 47 | 18.6 | – | HP | CR (1.4+) |
| BG31 | 17 | 0.9 | – | HP | CR (0.2+) |
| BZ4 | 40 | 0 | – | not HP | Relapse (1.6) |
| MZ6 | 49 | 0 | – | HP | CR (1.5+) |
| MZ12 | 52 | 22.8 | – | HP | Relapse (0.5) |
| MZ15 | 33 | 8.7 | – | HP | CR (0.4+) |
| MZ16 | 47 | 20 | – | HP | CR (0.4+) |
| BS1 | 35 | 19.3 | – | HP | Relapse (0.8) |
| CA6 | 44 | 16 | unknown | not HP* | CR (0.8+) |
| BG22 | 50 | 25.1 | + | HP | CR (0.7+) |
| CA3 | 19 | 19.5 | + | not HP* | Relapse (1) |
| CA7 | 42 | 4.4 | + | not HP* | Relapse (0.4) |
| MZ13 | 26 | 29 | + | HP | Relapse (0.7) |
| BS7 | 55 | 10.6 | + | HP | Relapse (0.8) |
| CR3 | 39 | 0.16 | + | HP | CR (1.4+) |

*without TBI

their respective outcome. It is evident how, despite the small number of cases, post-graft relapse tended to occur more frequently in patients with Ph/BCR-ABL+ ALL (4/6 vs 3/9) and in those in whom the autologous graft had not undergone the "HP" *ex vivo* purging procedure (4/11 in HP-ABCT group vs 3/4 in ABCT group). Hence, by combining Ph/BCR-ABL status and "HP" purging method, the relapse rate of different patient groups decreased from 100% (2/2, Ph/BCR-ABL+ and ABCT) to 50% (2/4 Ph/BCR-ABL+ and HP-ABCT; and 1/2 Ph/BCR-ABL– and ABCT) to 28% (2/7 Ph/BCR-ABL– and HP-ABCT).

## Discussion

The principle of regulating length and intensity of postremission therapy according to disease- and host-related risk factors has long been applied, often with successful results, in childhood ALL studies but seldom in adult ALL. With regard to adult patients, most recent and larger series have identified some independent prognostic factors such as patient age, presentation blast count, and chromosome abnormalities, although with variable cut-offs and ranges in relation to clinical outcome and type or intensity of treatment itself. In our case, the patients with the best DFS (52% at 5 years and beyond) were those with CD10+ pre-B ALL with a blast cell count <10–25x10⁹/l and without t(9;22)/BCR-ABL-

rearrangements or t(4;11), who were treated with anthracycline-containing consolidation regimens plus low-dose standard maintenance. In accordance with that, we do not prescribe very high-dose treatments including allograft or autograft to SR patients in first remission. The prospects for long-term control of the disease have been strikingly different for the HR group. It is for these reasons that ALL study 08–96 was begun. In this trial, SR patients were to receive a modified version of previous SR protocols, while HR patients, once in CR, were allocated to undergo allo-BMT when a donor was available or to enter a short intensive all-high-dose program ending with a myeloablative phase supported by HP-ABCT. Because the results being achieved in the SR category do not appear to differ from the previous ones, we do not discuss further this matter at this point. The allo-BMT results so far obtained in HR patients, on the contrary, are rather disappointing in terms of relapse rate and toxic death rate, but the patient number is small. The general experience with allo-BMT in adult ALL indicates a relatively high incidence of recurrent disease with a long-term DFS rate of about 50%. These are usually patients aged less than 50–55 years including SR cases. Allo-BMT studies limited to HR cases only were performed retrospectively [4] or are ongoing [5], and the results may be worse. The prototypic HR disease is Ph/BCR-ABL+ ALL. In this subset, allo-BMT results are poorer, but an improvement seems possible using more aggressive conditioning regimens [6, 7]. Thus, while it is reasonable to try and improve the allo-BMT procedure for HR patients with matched family donors and to find an unrelated donor for those without, the same effort should be directed towards an improved treatment of the patients without compatible siblings who are at great risk of very early relapse. For HR patients lacking a marrow donor, the news in study 08–96 is represented by the brief intensive high-dose plus HP-ABCT arm. Even if the number of the patients treated is small and the follow-up is short, we think this early report is worthwhile for a number of reasons. First, the use of high-dose regimens supported by a transplant but without prolonged consolidation and/or maintenance phases was pioneered by the cooperative SAKK/Swiss group [8]. However, early intensification beyond a certain level was accompanied by increased toxicity [9], so that in the most recent SAKK study the patients were elected to proceed to allograft or autograft immediately after CR [10]. The final results of this therapeutic strategy are not yet known. A recent study from Rome is investigating a similar approach; the results are too preliminary to allow any conclusion [11]. In the first 15 patients of our study we have demonstrated that the chosen high-dose sequence was safe to administer. Only high-dose methotrexate was omitted in few cases, because of reactivation of hepatitis C-type virus or impossibility to defer a close date for TBI. Likewise, some of the abnormally long intervals between any two subsequent high-dose cycles were due to problems inherent to the hospitalization of patients rather than toxicity. Because we have previously shown that undue treatment delay can alter the probability of DFS in adult ALL [12], the attenuation of treatment intensity in programs such as 08–96 is potentially very dangerous, but we have no data as yet to confirm this claim. We are now trying to adhere as strictly as possible to the original treatment plan. Apart from feasibility and the heterogeneous pattern of protocol realization, there are two additional problems in this study, concerning autologous CD34+ cells preparation and the intensity of the conditioning regimen for autograft, respectively. Although conceptually correct, the clinical role of *ex vivo* purging for autologous marrow transplantation in adult ALL is still undefined. Some evidence in favor of purging has emerged from studies in recurrent disease [13]. The purging procedure herein denominated "HP" is very effective and problably among the best methods to date available [3]. However, since we are treating HR patients, the risk of relapse caused by *in vivo* disease rather than inoculum of unpurged ALL cells is very high, and must be evaluated by a parallel study on minimal residual disease. Such study is ongoing in cases with Ph/BCR-ABL+ ALL. Altogether, given the limited amount of data, we can assume that the achievement of a negative BCR-ABL status post-graft (cases BG22 and CR3, Table 4) be the combined result of the high-dose sequence plus the reinfusion of a molecularly clean product at autograft. The problem of treatment type and intensity may be crucial as well. The three high-dose cycles before HP-ABCT were intended to exert and *in vivo* purging effect before the final step with HP-ABCT. All three high-dose drugs (CY, Ara-C, MTX) are effective in ALL and are expected to be mutually noncross-resistant. Myelotoxicity was mitigated by the concurrent use of G-CSF and the two more toxic courses (Ara-C and HP-ABCT) were spaced with the two less toxic ones (CY and MTX). Whether this protocol is any better than other brief high-dose regimens reviewed [8–11] is not known, but it preserves the patient from accumulating intolerable degrees of systemic toxicity and at the same time it allows the exposure to many active anti-ALL drugs (Figure 2), some of which at the maximum tolerated dose. We do not know if, given the study circumstances, the autograft schedule is optimal or not. TBI regimens may be superior to nonTBI ones in adult ALL with HR features [14, 15]. There remain the problems of TBI dose and associated drugs. Ph/BCR-ABL+ ALL and other HR subsets might benefit from a total TBI dose >12 Gy [16, 17], but we are presently unwilling to increase over this dosage, not to compromise the feasibily of the whole program and then the interpretation of results. On the contrary, once it proved feasible, the melphalan dose was increased from 110 to 140 mg/m$^2$. We now look forward to expanding this experience especially in Ph/BCR-ABL+ ALL, to give treatment cycles without unnecessary delays, and to adopt the "HP" procedure in as many cases as possible. Patient accrual in risk-oriented protocol 08–96 will continue during 1999.

# References

1. Bassan R, Lerede T, Rambaldi A, et al (1996) The role of anthracyclines in adult acute lymphoblastic leukaemia. Leukemia 10 (Suppl 2): S58-S6.
2. Gianni AM, Bregni M, Siena S, et al (1997) High-dose chemotherapy and autologous bone marrow transplantation compared with MACOP-B in aggressive B-cell lymphoma. N Engl J Med 336: 1290–1297.
3. Rambaldi A, Borleri G, Dotti G, et al (1998) Innovative two-step negative selection of granulocyte colony-stimulating factor-mobilized circulating progenitor cells: adequacy for autologous and allogeneic transplantation. Blood 91: 2189–2196.
4. Zikos P, Van Lint MT, Lamparelli T, et al (1998) Allogeneic hemopoietic stem cell transplantation for patients with high risk acute lymphoblastic leukemia: favorable impact of chronic graft-versus-host disease on survival and relapse. Haematologica 83:896–903.
5. Ribera JM, Ortega JJ, Oriol A, et al (1998) Treatment of high-risk acute lymphoblastic leukemia. Preliminary results of the protocol PETHEMA ALL-93. In: Hiddeman W, Büchner T, Wörmann B, Ritter J, Creutzig U, Keating M, Plunkett W (eds): Acute Leukemias VII, Berlin, Springer-Verlag, pp 755–765.
6. Kröger N, Krüger W, Wacker-Becker G, et al (1998) Intensified conditioning regimen in bone marrow transplantation for Philadelphia chromosome-positive acute lymphoblastic leukemia. Bone Marrow Transplant 22:1029–1033.
7. Snyder DS, Nademanee AP, O'Donnell MR, et al (1998) Allogeneic bone marrow transplantation for Philadelphia chromosome-positive acute lymphoblastic leukemia in first complete remission: long-term follow-up. Blood 92 (suppl 1): 657a (abstract).
8. Wernli M, Tichelli A, von Fliedner V, et al (1994) Intensive induction/consolidation therapy without maintenace in adult acute lymphoblastic leukaemia: a pilot assessment. Br J Haematol 87:39–43.
9. Wernli M, Fey MF, Tobler A, et al (1994) The limit of dose-intensification in the treatment of adult acute lymphoblastic leukemia despite growth factor therapy. Blood 81 (suppl 1):144a (abstract).
10. Wernli, M., Bargetzi, M., Hoffman, T., et al. (1996) DV-ICE followed immediately by BMT: a new therapeutic strategy in adult acute lymphoblastic leukemia (ALL). Blood 89 (Supp JJ):375a (abstract).
11. Buccinasco F, Del Poeta G, Venditti A, et al (1998) Dose-intensive, Ara-C/mitoxantrone-based chemotherapy followed by hematopoietic stem cell transplantation for adult acute lymphoblastic leukemia. Blood 92 (suppl 1):84a (abstract).
12. Bassan R, Lerede T, Di Bona E, et al (1998) An index of treatment intensity highly correlated with outcome in adult acute lymphoblastic leukemia (ALL). Blood 92 (suppl 1):401a (abstract).
13. Bassan R, Lerede T, Barbui T (1996) Strategies for the treatment of recurrent acute lymphoblastic leukemia in adults. Haematologica 81:20–36.
14. Ringden O, Labopin M, Tura S, et al (1996) A comparison of busulfan versus total body irradiation combined with cyclophosphamide as conditioning for autograft and allograft bone marrow transplantation in patients with acute leukaemia. Br J Haematol 93:637–645.
15. Camara R, Granados E, Gil JJ, et al (1998) Bone marrow transplantation in acute lymphoblastic leukemia (ALL): comparison of busulfan versus total body irradiation (TBI) as conditioning. Bone Marrow Transplat 21 (Suppl 1):359a (abstract).
16. Clift RA, Buckner CD, Appelbaum FR, et al (1991) Allogeneic marrow transplantation in patients with chronic myeloid leukemia in the chronic phase: a randomized trial of two irradiation regimens. Blood 77: 1660–1665.
17. Deconinck E, Cahn JY, Milpied N, et al (1997) Allogeneic bone marrow transplantation for high risk acute lymphoblastic leukemia in first remission: long-term results for 42 patients conditioned with an intensified regimen (TBI, high-dose ara-C and melphalan). Bone Marrow Transplant 20: 731–735.

# Prognostic Factors in Philadelphia+/BCR-ABL+ Acute Lymphoblastic Leukemia

R. Bassan, A. Zs Rohatiner, E. Di Bona, T. Lerede, M. Carter, A. Rambaldi, E. Pogliani, G. Rossi, P. Fabris, S. Morandi, G. Lambertenghi-Deliliers, T. A. Lister and T. Barbui

## Introduction

Adult patients with acute lymphoblastic leukemia (ALL) expressing the t(9;22)/Philadelphia chromosome (Ph+) or the corresponding BCR-ABL rearrangements (BCR+, P190 and P210) constitute the prognostically worst ALL subtype [1, 2]. Although complete remission (CR) rates are 56%–96%, the median duration of CR and survival is one year or less and <20% of patients survive disease-free for >2 years. Disease-free survival can be improved by allogeneic bone marrow transplantation, while the role of high-dose treatments supported by autograft is presently less well defined [3–7]. However Ph/BCR+ ALL behaves heterogeneously, and some patients may benefit from chemotherapy alone. Longer remissions have been reported in cases with hyperdiploid karyotype and in other selected subgroups [8–10]. We noted that, using Anthracycline-based consolidation, outcome was improved in a fraction of cases [11]. In another study, some patients who converted to BCR negative status after intensive treatment without allogeneic transplantation were in remission for >3 years [12]. Prolonged remissions were also described in subsets of childhood Ph/BCR+ ALL treated with aggressive modern-type chemotherapy regimens [13, 14]. In the light of these reports, we review the long-term outcome of an unselected patient population of 76 adults with Ph/BCR+ ALL, treated over a 25-year period with regimens developed by the L-B-V Group (St. Bartholomew's Hospital, London, UK; Ospedali Riuniti, Bergamo, Italy; Ospedale Civile, Vicenza, Italy).

## Materials and methods

### Diagnosis

ALL was defined by French-American-British (FAB) criteria. ALL immunophenotype was determined by automated cytofluorimetry or immunofluorescence microscopy, to assess the expression by blast cells of nuclear TdT, "common" ALL antigen, surface immunoglobulin, HLA-DR, CD19, and T-cell and myeloid cell antigens. The cytogenetic analysis was performed by means of standard Giemsa banding. BCR-ABL rearrangements (BCR+) were identified by reverse-transcriptase PCR (RT-PCR). Ph/BCR positivity was defined by cytogenetic analysis, RT-PCR, or both assays.

### Treatment programs

Patients received one of seven consecutive regimens adopted between 1972 and 1996. OPAL consisted of a four-drug induction schedule with moderate-dose consolidation and long-term maintenance [15]. HEAV'd and reinforced HEAV'd were characterized by the 'early' administration of dose-intensive Anthracycline (doxorubicin 360–405 mg/m$^2$) [16, 17]. OPAL/high-dose Cytarabine (OPAL/HiDAC) included Cytarabine 2 g/m$^2$/b.d. for 6 days as early consolidation, without prophylactic cranial irradiation (18). IVAP comprised intensive, Idarubicin-based induction and early consolidation therapy (total Idarubicin = 116 mg/m$^2$) followed by high-dose treatment (BCNU-Etoposide-Melphalan in patients <50 years old) with autologous

Depts. of Hematology at Bergamo, Vicenza, Monza, Brescia, Bolzano, Cremona, an Milan Hospitals (Italy); and ICRF Medical Oncology Unit, St. Bartholomew's Hospital, London (England).

bone marrow transplantation (ABMT). Subsequently, patients received weekly continuation therapy and standard low-dose maintenance [19]. A less intensive IVAP schedule was adopted for patients aged >60 years. STT (short-term therapy) consisted of a total of 6 cycles of treatment comprising Vincristine-Doxorubicin-Prednisone alternating with high-dose Cytarabine-Etoposide, supported by granulocyte/macrophage colony-stimulating factor (GM-CSF) and without maintenance [20]; the total Doxorubicin dose equalled 360 mg/m$^2$. 07/93 consisted of IVAP-type induction followed by 6 Idarubicin-Vincristine-Cyclophosphamide and intermediate-dose Cytarabine-Etoposide pulses, followed by high-dose treatment (Cyclophosphamide-Etoposide-Melphalan) supported by peripheral blood progenitor cells (PBPC). This was followed by low-dose maintenance (unpublished data). Allogeneic bone marrow transplantation (allo-BMT) was offered in first remission to younger patients with a histocompatible sibling donor.

## Definitions and statistics

The definitions of complete remission (CR) and refractory ALL were previously given [15–20]. A recurrence was defined by the detection of >25% leukemic blast cells in the bone marrow, CSF, or elsewhere (biopsy proven). Survival was taken from the date of diagnosis to death by any cause and relapse-free survival (RFS) from date of CR to first relapse at any site or death in CR from any cause. For statistical analysis, unmodifiable prognostic factors were patient age and gender and disease characteristics such as FAB morphology, immunophenotype, P190 or P210 transcript, blast count, hepatosplenomegaly, extramedullary involvement, and serum LDH level. Modifiable prognostic factors were type of induction and consolidation protocol, anthracycline type and dose intensity (high: HEAV'd, R-HEAV'd, IVAP, STT; and low: OPAL, OPAL-HiDAC, IVAP for elderly ALL, 07–93) [11], autograft and allograft. Data were were compared using the chi-squared test with Yate's correction. RFS and overall survival curves were plotted by the standard Kaplan and Meier method and compared by

the log-rank method. Multivariate analyses were carried out by means of Cox's linear regresssion model.

## Results

### Identification and clinical features of Ph/BCR+ ALL

A total of 562 adult patients with ALL were evaluable. No patient with T-ALL or mature-type B-ALL was found to be Ph/BCR+ among those studied. Blast cells from 234 with pre-B ALL were successfully screened for Ph and/or BCR-ABL rearrangements. Seventy-six cases were Ph/BCR+ (32%). All exhibited FAB-L1/L2 morphology with myeloperoxidase negative blasts. Nearly half of the Ph/BCR+ cases were identified by the cytogenetic study (49%) and 18 (24%) by RT-PCR only. The majority of RT-PCR+ cases expressed P190 (27/38, 69%). Higher patient age (median 43 years) and blast count, and CD10 positivity were strongly associated with Ph/BCR positivity. Considering the entire group of 234 pre-B ALL cases evaluated, the combination of age >40 years plus concurrent CD10+ phenotype plus blast count >50x10$^9$/l conferred a 77% chance (10/13) of Ph/BCR positivity, compared with 51% (38/73) in patients with any two features, 21% in those with any one (26/122), and only 4% in those with none (1/24) (p=0.0001). No other significant difference was found between Ph/BCR positive and negative cases and, within the former group, between P190+ and P210+ cases.

### CR, RFS and overall survival

The overall response rate of the Ph/BCR+ group was 79% (60/76), similar to that observed in Ph/BCR– cases.Six patients died early of pancytopenic complications and 10 proved to have refractory ALL. Although the incidence of refractory disease was significantly lower in Ph/BCR– patients receiving Idarubicin-containing regimens (not shown), this was not the case for the Ph/BCR+ group (Table 1).Sixty CR patients were evaluable for RFS after an actual observation time to relapse, death, or last follow-up of 1 month to 10+years (median 10 months). Median and

**Table 1.** Refractory Ph/BCR+ ALL by induction regimen and blast count, no. and (%).

| Blast count x10⁹/l | Induction: All treatments | Adriamycin-based | Idarubicin-based |
|---|---|---|---|
| 0–49 | 4/54 (7)[1] | 1/19 (5) | 3/35 (8) |
| 50–100 | 3/14 (21) | 1/5 (20) | 2/9 (22) |
| >100 | 3/8 (37) | 2/4 (50) | 1/4 (25) |
| Cumulative | 10/76 (13) | 4/28 (14) | 6/48 (12) |

[1]p=0.051 vs hyperleukocytic groups

5–year RFS rates were 10.5 months and 10%, respectively, compared with 1.8 years and 30% in Ph/BCR– cases (p<0.005). Most relapses occurred in the bone marrow (43/48, 89%), 3 in the CNS, and two in the testes. The median survival from the time of recurrence was 4.2 months.The median survival for all 7 patients was 1.15 years; 14% were alive at 5 years, compared with 1.6 years and 30% in Ph/BCR– cases (p <0.005).Six patients (8%) remained alive in first remission between 5.2 and 9.6 years. Three of these patients had undergone an allo-BMT and 3 had received an intensive Anthracycline combination plus ABMT in one case.

## Prognostic factors in Ph/BCR+ ALL

### Response to therapy

The incidence of primary refractory ALL correlated to some extent with a high blast cell count at presentation (p=0.051, Table 1). With regard to RFS, only younger age (<50 years) predicted for a better outcome in both univariate (p<0.005) and multivariate (p=0.02) analyses. The median RFS was 1.1 years and the 5-year RFS was 17% vs 0.7 years and 0% in patients older than 50 years (Figure 1a). On analysing treatment-related variables, patients who received intensive Anthracycline therapy during early consolidation had longer RFS intervals than those receiving less intensive Anthracycline consolidation (OPAL, OPAL-HiDAC, 07/93 and IVAP >60 years): median and 5-year RFS rates 1.4 vs 0.7 years and 21% vs 0%, respectively (Figure 1b). This difference was significant in the log-rank test (p<0.025) as well as in the regression analysis (p=0.039), even censoring allo-BMT patients (p<0.05). The combined effect of age <50 years and intensive Anthracycline consolidation (i.e. the best prognostic subgroups) was then assessed (Figure 1c): 23 patients with both favorable variables had a median RFS of

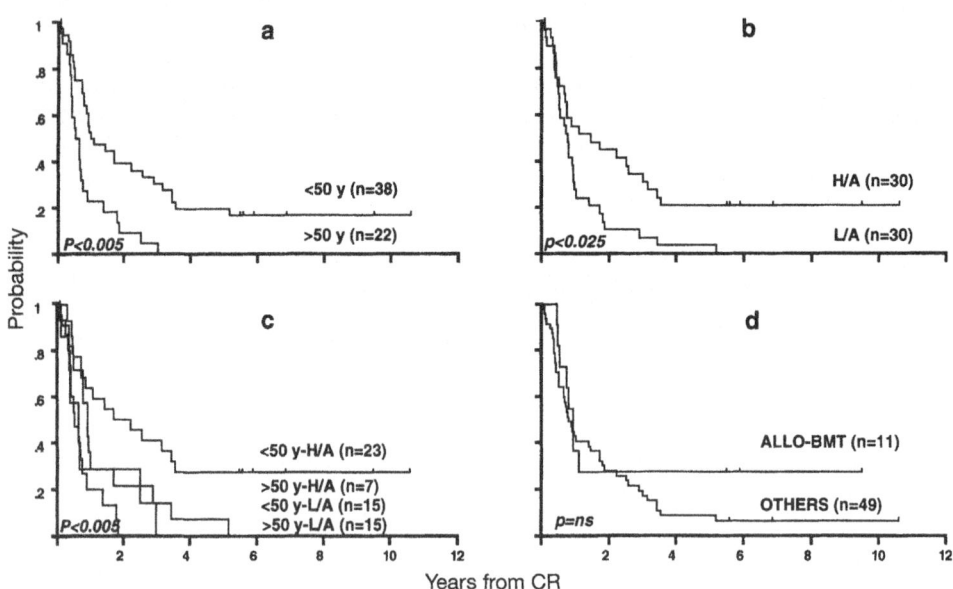

**Fig. 1.** Relapse-free survival in Ph/BCR+ ALL by (**a**) age +/–50 years, (**b**) early anthracycline dose-intensiti (H/A, high v L/A, low), (**c**) age and Anthracycline dose-intensity in combination, and (**d**) allogeneic hematopoietic cell transplantation.

**Table 2.** Cumulative incidence of favorable prognostic factors (FPF) and RFS.

| No. FPF | No. of patients | FPF | | | RFS[1] | |
|---|---|---|---|---|---|---|
| | | Age <50 | H/A | allo-BMT | median | 5-year rate |
| 3 | 5 | 5 | 5 | 5 | NR | 60% |
| 2 | 23 | 23 | 18 | 5 | 1 | 14% (32% at 2 yr)* |
| 1 | 18 | 10 | 7 | 1 | 0.8 | 0% (23% at 2 yr)* |
| 0 | 14 | 0 | 0 | 0 | 0.7 | 0% at 1.9 yr |

[2]Median in years
NR, not reached
*Unified in RFS model (Figure 2a)

**Table 3.** Cumulative incidence of favourable prognostic factors (FPF) and overall survival (OS).

| No. of FPF | No. of patients | FPF | | | | OS[1] | |
|---|---|---|---|---|---|---|---|
| | | Blasts <50 | Age <50 | H/A | allo-BMT | median | 5-year rate |
| 4 | 5 | 5 | 5 | 5 | 5 | NR | 60% |
| 3 | 15 | 14 | 14 | 14 | 1 | 1.8 | 7%* |
| 2 | 27 | 18 | 21 | 11 | 4 | 1.3 | 19%* |
| 1 | 26 | 16 | 7 | 2 | 1 | 0.9 | 0% (11% at 2 yr)** |
| 0 | 3 | 0 | 0 | 0 | 0 | 0.7 | 0% at 1.1 yr** |

H/A denotes high anthracycline dose intensity
[1]Median in years
NR, not reached
*/**Unified in overall survival model (Figure 2b)

2.2 years, with a 5-year RFS rate of 27%, compared with significantly inferior results in patients with either one or no favorable factor (p<0.005). Again, even excluding allo-BMT cases, the prognostic difference remained significant (p<0.025). With regard to allo-BMT patients, the relapse rate was lower (p=0.019) in 11 allografted patients than in chemotherapy treated and/or ABMT/PBPC (6 cases) treated patients, but transplant-related mortality led to a 5-year RFS rate of only 27% (Figure 1d).

### Prognostic model in Ph/BCR+ ALL

Because CR rate, RFS and, by extrapolation, overall survival rates could vary according to the presence (or absence) of four distinct favorable prognostic factors (FPF: presenting blast count $<50 \times 10^9$/l, age <50 years, consolidation with intensive Anthracycline-containing regimen, allo-BMT), we tested the cumulative prognostic effect exerted by these 4 FPF in individual patients.

Blast count, affecting only the probability of CR and hence survival, was excluded from RFS evaluation. The results, shown in Tables 2

and 3, document increasing probabilities of RFS and overall survival according to the cumulative incidence of FPFs. In the final RFS model three distinct prognostic categories were recognized (Figure 2a). In the overall survival analysis, including all four FPFs, there were also three homogeneous prognostic subgroups (Figure 2b).

### Discussion

The long-term results from this retrospective survey in adult Ph/BCR+ ALL are in accordance with the concept of a clinically heterogeneous syndrome. Although the initial CR rate was 79%, patients with a blast count $>50 \times 10^9$/l were likely to have refractory disease. In the context of a globally poor therapeutic outlook, an elevated blast cell count at onset might correlate with an early expansion of drug-resistant subclones. Prior reports are in agreement with a drug resistance/blast cell count direct relationship in Ph/BCR+ ALL [13, 14], a link that appears to be even tighter in cases expressing a minor

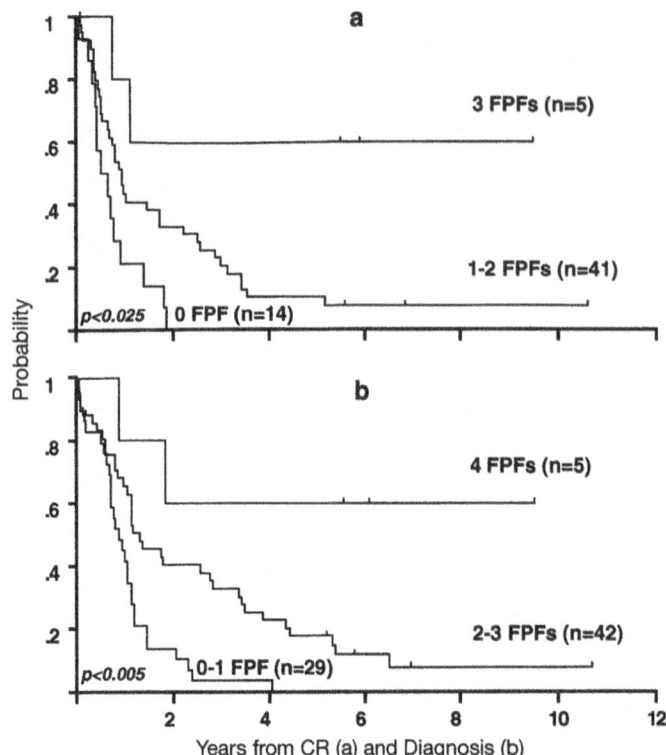

**Fig. 2.** Relapse free-survival (a) and overall survival (b) according to cumulative incidence of favorable prognostic factors (FPFs): blast count <50x10$^9$/l (only overall survival analysis), age <50 years, high Anthracycline dose-intensity, allogeneic hematopoietic cell transplantation.

myeloid cell component [9] or additional abnormalities of chromosomes 7 and 9 [8]. The analysis of RFS and overall survival results documented a positive impact from an allo-BMT in first CR, however only 11 out of 60 patients were transplanted and few survived disease-free. Allo-BMT result in adult Ph/BCR+ ALL are rather poor with standard transplantation regimens and might be improved by the application of newer conditioning schemes [21]. Autografting with ABMT or PBPC is an alternative way to deliver high-dose treatments outside the setting of allo-BMT and the related immune toxic reactions. This approach is therefore being investigated with improved treatment and autograft preparation regimens, but data are still scanty as concerns an improvement of long-term RFS results [7, 22]. Apart from allo-BMT, we saw a positive effect on RFS and overall survival from an early intensive consolidation with Anthracycline-containing regimens. The reasons for this pattern of drug sensitivity are unknown, but it may correlate

with a pre-B immunophenotype [23]. Although the Anthracycline-related effect was transitory, in a few cases it was associated with a very prolonged control of the disease and, moreover, it acted in concert with younger patient age. This may reflect either intrinsic characteristics of blast cells or changes in drug metabolism that can occur with ageing, since the best results so far obtained with chemotherapy alone in Ph/BCR+ ALL have been reported in children [13, 14]. Our best results were achieved in patients aged <50 years who were treated with intensive Anthracycline-containing protocols. Because the younger patients are those considered eligible for transplant procedures, an Anthracycline-related prolongation of RFS might allow more patients to reach this phase or to complete a search for a marrow unrelated donor. For instance, only 1 of 17 CR patients treated with the low-dose Anthracycline protocol 07/93 was autografted, compared with 5 of 19 in the high-dose Anthracycline IVAP study, in spite of the exclusion of patients older than 50 years in the latter trial. In summary, adult Ph/BCR+ ALL is heterogeneous with regard to clinical response to Anthracyclines. The subset of patients aged <50 years may respond very well to intensive Anthracycline-containing consolidation and may experience median RFS rates very close to those reported in Ph/BCR− ALL. Further research on the mechanisms of resistance and sensitivity to Anthracyclines is indicated.

# References

1. Faderl S, Kantarjian HM, Talpaz M, et al (1998) Clinical significance of cytogenetic abnormalities in adult acute lymphoblastic leukemia. Blood 91: 3995–4019.
2. Hoelzer D (1998) Therapy of acute lymphoblastic leukemia. In: Freireich EJ, Kantarjian HM (eds), Medical management of hematological malignant diseases, New York, Marcel Dekker, pp 19–58.
3. Barrett AJ, Horowitz MM, Ash RC, et al (1992) Bone marrow transplantation for Philadelphia chromosome-positive acute lymphoblastic leukemia. Blood 79: 3067–3070.
4. Sierra J, Radich J, Hansen JA, et al (997) Marrow transplants from unrelated donors for treatment of Philadelphia chromosome-positive acute lymphoblastic leukemia. Blood 90: 1410–1414.
5. Grigg AP (1993) Approaches to the treatment of Philadelphia-positive acute lymphoblastic leukemia. Bone Marrow Transplant 12: 431–435.
6. Martin H, Hoelzer D, Atta J, et al (1993) Autologous bone marrow transplantation in Ph-positive/BCR-ABL positive acute lymphoblastic leukemia. Blood 82 (Suppl 1): 167a (abstract).
7. Stryckmans P, Suciu S, Annino L, et al (1997) Molecular evaluation of consolidation theraphy and early allograft or autograft for BCR-ABL[pos] adult acute lymphoblastic leukaemia (ALL) patients: A pilot study of EIGLE (European intergroup of GIMEMA, French LALA and EORTC). Blood 90 (Suppl 1): 183a (abstract).
8. Rieder H, Ludwig WD, Gassmann W, et al (1996) Prognostic significance of additional chromosome abnormalities in adult patients with Philadelphia chromosome positive acute lymphoblastic leukaemia. Br J Haematol, 95: 678–691.
9. Cuneo A, Demuynck H, Ferrant A, et al (1994) Minor myeloid component in Ph chromosome positive acute lymphoblastic leukaemia: correlation with cytogenetic pattern and implication for poor response to therapy. Br J Haematol 87: 515–522.
10. Secker-Walker LM, Craig JM (1993) Prognostic implications of breakpoint and lineage heterogeneity in Philadelphia-positive acute lymphoblastic leukaemia: a review. Leukemia 7: 147–151.
11. Bassan R, Lerede T, Rambaldi A, et al (1996) The role of anthracyclines in adult acute lymphoblastic leukaemia. Leukemia 10 (Suppl 2): S58-S61.
12. Annino L, Ferrari A, Meloni G, et al (1997) RT-PCR monitoring and treatment outcome in BCR/ABL-positive acute lymphoblastic leukemia (ALL): persistence of PCR positivity in some long term survivors. Blood, 90 (Suppl 1): 183a (abstract)
13. Ribeiro RC, Broniscer A, Rivera GK, et al (1997) Philadelphia chromosome-positive acute lymphoblastic leukaemia in children: durable responses to chemotherapy associated with low initial white blood cell counts. Leukemia 11: 1493–1496.
14. Aricò M, Schrappe M, Harbott J, et al (1997) Prednisone good response (PGR) identifies a subset of t(9;22) childhood acute lymphoblastic leukemia (ALL) at lower risk for early leukemia relapse. Blood 90: 560a (abstract).
15. Lister TA, Whithouse JMA, Beard MEJ, et al (1978) Combination chemotherapy for acute lymphoblastic leukaemia in adults. Br Med J 1, 199–203.
16. Barnett MJ, Greaves MF, Amess JAL, et al (1986) Treatment of acute lymphoblastic leukaemia in adults. Br J Haematol, 64: 455–468.
17. Bassan R, Battista R, Montaldi A, et al (1993) Reinforced HEAV'D therapy for adult acute lymphoblastic leukaemia: improved results and revised prognostic criteria. Hematol Oncol 11: 169–177.
18. Rohatiner AZS, Bassan R, Battista R, et al (1990) High dose cytosine arabinoside in the initial treatment of adults with acute lymphoblastic leukaemia. Br J Cancer 62: 454–458.
19. Bassan R, Battista R, Viero P, et al (1993) Intensive therapy for adult acute lymphoblastic leukemia: preliminary results of the Idarubicin/Vincristine/L-asparaginase/Prednisolone regimen. Semin Oncol 20 (Suppl 8): 39–46.
20. Papamicheal D, Andrews T, Owen D, et al (1993) Intensive chemotherapy for adult acute lymphoblastic leukaemia (ALL) given with or without granulocyte/macrophage colony stimulating factor (GM-CSF). Br J Haematol 93 (Suppl 2): 60 (abstract).
21. Snyder DS, Nademanee AP, O'Donnell MR, et al (1998) Allogeneic bone marrow transplantation for Philadelphia chromosome-positive acute lymphoblastic leukemia in first complete remission: long-term follow-up. Blood 92 (Suppl 1), 657a (abstract).
22. Laporte JP, Labopin M, Gorin NC (1998) Comparison of the outcome of Philadelphia+ versus Phi- acute lymphoblastic leukemia (ALL) following stem cell transplantation: an EBMT survey. Bone Marrow Transplant 21 (Suppl 1): S12 (abstract).
23. Den Boer ML, Pieters R, Veerman AJP (1998) Mechanisms of cellular anthracycline resistance in childhood acute leukemia. Leukemia 12: 1657–1670.

# High-Dose Cytarabine Combined to Mitoxantrone in the Treatment of Refractory and Relapsed Acute Lymphoblastic Leukemia

X.Thomas, N.Bouheddou and D.Fière

*Abstract.* We summarize here our experience in a cohort of 20 patients (median age: 31 years, range: 17–64) with either refractory acute lymphoblastic leukemia (ALL) (11 patients) or relapsing ALL (9 patients) treated with a combination of high-dose cytarabine (HD-AraC) and mitoxantrone after a first line therapy according to LALA protocols. HD-AraC was administered at 1 g/m²/12 hours from day 1 to day 4, and mitoxantrone was given at 10 mg/m²/day from day 3 to day 5. Ten patients had B-lineage ALL, 9 had T-lineage ALL. One patient had undifferentiated ALL. Philadelphia chromosome was identified in 4 cases. Complete remission (CR) was achieved in 11 cases (55%, 95% confidence interval, [CI] 31%–77%) (6 relapsed patients and 5 refractory patients). Seven patients (35%) did not respond to treatment and 2 (10%) died during induction. All of these patients experienced profound myelosuppression. Median time to recovery of neutrophils > 0.5 x 10⁹/l and of platelets > 50 x 10⁹/l was 29 days (range 20–42). Although severe infectious complications (WHO grade ≥ 3) were common (13 patients), few patients developed severe cardiac toxicity (2 patients), severe hepatic toxicity (1 patient), severe gastrointestinal toxicity (1 patient), or severe neurological complications (2 patients). Among patients achieving CR, 4 patients received chemotherapy alone as post-remission therapy, 2 patients received autologous and 3 patients allogeneic transplants. Two patients did not receive any consolidation because of severe toxicity of reinduction therapy. The median disease-free survival (DFS) and median overall survival were 7.4 months and 6.7 months respectively. DFS was significantly longer in resistant ALL comparatively to relapsing ALL (9 months versus 1.7 months; p = 0.05) and in patients aged less than 35 years (7.4 months versus 1.3 months; p = 0.03). Regarding immunophenotypic patterns, no differences were noted in terms of outcome. We conclude that our schedule combining HD-AraC and mitoxantrone allows CR achievement in more than half of patients with an acceptable toxicity in adult ALL. However, long-term results argue in favor of individualization of therapy according to risk factors.

## Introduction

Despite substantial progress in the treatment of acute lymphoblastic leukemia (ALL), only 20% to 35% of adults treated with chemotherapy alone are long-term leukemia-free survivors (Laport et al. 1997). Patients who relapse or are resistant to remission induction generally have a poor prognosis (Welborn 1994, Weiss 1997). The question of what to do with patients whose initial treatment failed or in whom relapse occurred during or shortly after therapy remains unanswered. Many chemotherapy reinduction protocols have been tested in the setting of relapsed ALL. High-dose regimens appear to result in a greater incidence of second complete remissions (CRs) compared with reinduction with standard vincristine, prednisone, anthracycline-based regimens. Escalation to high-dose cytarabine (HD-AraC) is an approach to overcome cellular resistance against this substance and proved active as a single drug treatment (Rudnick et al. 1979, Kantarjian et al. 1986, Marsh et al. 1987). A similar single drug salvage effect was shown for mitoxantrone (Paciucci et al. 1984). HD-AraC combined with an anthracycline or an anthracenedione has the greatest likelihood of achieving a first CR in ALL patients with refractory disease or a second CR in relapsed patients. This combination was designed in order to combine both single drug effects and has demonstrated an improvement of the "quality of remission" (Hiddemann et al. 1990, Arlin et al. 1991).

Data reported here summarize our experience in patients with relapsed or refractory ALL treated with HD-AraC and mitoxantrone. This study has been initiated in order to assess the efficacy and side effects of this combination.

## Patients and Methods

### Patients

Between November 1987 and March 1998, 20 adult patients (13 males and 7 females) with relapsed (9 first relapses of which 6 occurred "on therapy") or refractory (11 patients) ALL were treated in our institution with an intensive chemotherapy combining mitoxantrone and HD-AraC. At diagnosis, relapsed patients were treated according to the design of two successive LALA protocols (Fiere et al. 1993, Thomas et al. 1995). The median of first CR was 18.3 months (range 3.6–26.5 months). Refractory patients were initially treated with a combination of anthracycline, vincristine, cyclophosphamide, and prednisone according to the induction schedule of LALA94 protocol (Dombret et al. 1998). Only patients with a performance status of 2 or less and no major organ failure, according to the World Health Organization (WHO) grading system, could entered the study. ALL were morphologically classified according to the French-American-British (FAB) criteria (Bennett et al. 1976). Immunophenotyping of leukemic cells, defined according to Boucheix et al. (Boucheix et al. 1994), was attempted in all patients to classify ALL. Cytogenetic study was performed in 19 patients on BM or seldom on peripheral blood cells before initiation of therapy, using short unstimulated cultures and RHG banding.

### Treatment regimen

The reinduction phase included HD-AraC, 1 g/m$^2$/12 hours from day 1 to day 4, and mitox-antrone, 10 mg/m$^2$/day from day 3 to day 5. For prophylaxis of HD-AraC-induced photophobia and conjunctivis, all patients received glucocorticoid eye drops every 12 hours. All patients received gastrointestinal decontamination and prophylactic red blood cell and platelet transfusions. Broad spectrum empirical antibiotherapy was initiated as soon as the patient became febrile. Intra-thecal administration of AraC, methotrexate, and soludecadron was performed in patients with central nervous system (CNS) leukemic involvement. Response to reinduction treatment was evaluated after one course. After achieving CR, 4 patients received consolidation courses, 3 patients with a familial sibling donor were allografted, and 2 patients received autologous stem cell transplantation. Two patients did not receive any more treatment after induction because of severe toxicity.

### Response criteria

To assess response to therapy, bone marrow aspirations were made around day 28 of reinduction therapy. Patients were considered in CR if there was less than 5% leukemic blast cells in bone marrow (BM) aspirate at time of evaluation, no symptoms or physical findings suggestive of leukemia, and normal blood cell counts (Ellison et al. 1968).

### Statistical methods

95% confidence intervals on proportions of CR patients and toxic deaths were calculated using the exact binomial formula. Overall survival and DFS were estimated by the Kaplan-Meier method. Patients undergoing BM transplantation while in CR were conventionally censored at the time of grafting.

## Results

### Patient population

Main clinical and laboratory characteristics of patients are shown in Table 1. Nineteen patients presented with blast cell bone marrow involvement and 4 with CNS involvement. Median age was 31 years (range 17–64 years). There was 13 males and 7 females. Fourteen patients could be classified according to FAB criteria. Seven presented with ALL 1, 6 with ALL 2, and 1 with ALL 3. Immunophenotypic analysis was realized in all patients. Ten patients were diagnosed as B-cell lineage ALL, and 9 as T-cell lineage ALL. One patient had undifferentiated leukemia. Karyotypes were analyzable in 18 cases. Among them, 4 patients presented with Philadelphia chromosome positive ALL.

## Efficacy of therapy

Eleven patients (55%, 95% CI 31–77%) achieved CR: 6 of the 9 relapsed patients and 5 of the 11 refractory patients (Table 1). All 4 patients with CNS involvement achieved CR. Seven patients (35%) did not respond to treatment and 2 (10%, 95% CI 1–31%) died during aplasia, of whom one died from severe infection and one from hepatic complications. The median time for CR achievement was 30 days (range 24–42 days). Nine of the 11 patients who achieved CR received consolidation therapy: 3 underwent allogeneic BM transplantation, 2 autologous stem cell transplantation, and 4 consolidation and maintenance chemotherapy. Two patients did not receive any consolidation therapy because of a WHO grade 3 performance status after reinduction treatment. Median DFS for the entire cohort was 7.4 months. One patient died while in CR. Seven patients relapsed. Median time of relapse was 6.3 months (range 2.6–12.1 months). After retreatment, two of them achieved a new CR. Median overall survival for the entire cohort was 6.7 months.

## Toxicity

Chemotherapy-related toxicity was mainly hematologic. All patients experienced profound myelosuppression. Median duration of aplasia was 29 days (range 20–42 days). The most important extrahematologic toxicity was severe infections. Sepsis was documented in 10 cases (50%), and pneumonia in 4 cases (20%) of which one patient died from aspergillosis. Severe gastrointestinal toxicity (grade

**Table 1.** Main characteristics and outcome of patients

|  | Refractory ALL (n=11) | Relapsed ALL (n=9) |
|---|---|---|
| Age (years) | 28 (18–50)* | 39 (25–64) |
| Sex (M/F) | 9 / 2 | 4 / 5 |
| FAB classification |  |  |
| L1 | 5 | 2 |
| L2 | 3 | 3 |
| L3 | 0 | 1 |
| unclassable | 2 | 2 |
| Immunophenotype |  |  |
| B-cell lineage | 5 | 5 |
| T-cell lineage | 5 | 4 |
| unclassable | 1 | 0 |
| BM involvement | 11 | 8 |
| CNS involvement | 0 | 4 |
| Aplasia (days) | 28 (20–35) | 31 (27–42) |
| Toxicity of chemotherapy: |  |  |
| infection (WHO grade ≥ 3) | 8 | 5 |
| CNS (WHO grade ≥ 3) | 1 | 1 |
| cardiac (WHO grade ≥ 3) | 2 | 0 |
| liver (WHO grade ≥ 3) | 0 | 1 |
| gastro (WHO grade ≥ 3) | 0 | 1 |
| CR achievement | 5 | 6 |
| Median DFS (months) | 9 | 1.7 |
| Median overall survival (months) | 20.5 | 5.6 |
| Post-induction treatment: |  |  |
| chemotherapy alone | 2 | 2 |
| allogeneic BMT | 3 | 0 |
| autologous BMT | 0 | 2 |
| no therapy | 0 | 2 |
| Relapse | 2 | 5 |

* median (range)

3 or more) as severe hepatic toxicity both occurred in only 1 patient. Two patients (10%) developed neurotoxicity (grade 3 or more) and 2 patients (10%) developed cardiac toxicity (grade 3 or more). No patient had severe renal complications.

## Prognostic factors for outcome

Patients aged less than 35 years had a better prognosis. Their median DFS was 7.4 months versus 1.3 months in patients aged more than 35 years (p = 0.03) and their median overall survival was 6.7 versus 1.7 (p = 0.03). There was no statistical difference between B-cell and T-cell lineage ALL. Median DFS was significantly longer in the group of refractory patients comparatively to that of relapsed patients (9 months versus 1.7 months, p = 0.05).

## Discussion

The prognosis of refractory and relapsing adult ALL is generally considered to be poor. All therapeutic experiences are based on small and heterogeneous patient populations (Welborn 1994). However, salvage therapy in adult ALL remains unsatisfactory. A second CR occurred generally in 25 to 50% of patients with a probability of long-term DFS very poor, even when patients are subsequently consolidated with allogeneic or autologous stem cell transplantation. The increased dosage of chemotherapy has been proposed with the objective of overcoming drug resistance. HD-AraC has been extensively used in relapsed acute leukemia, either alone (Herzig et al. 1983, Kantarjian et al. 1986, Marsh et al. 1987) or in combination with an anthracycline (Giona et al. 1990), L-asparaginase (Capizzi et al. 1984), amsacrine (Arlin et al. 1988), fludarabine (Suki et al. 1993, Montillo et al. 1997), or mitoxantrone (Hiddemann et al. 1987). HD-AraC gives also a good penetration into the cerebral fluid and could then prevent further relapses (Morra et al. 1993). Our current data showed antileukemic efficacy of mitoxantrone combined to HD-AraC in both B-cell and T-cell lineage ALL with an overall CR rate of 55%. The predominant side effect was profound myelosuppression, which caused one fatal infection. However, hematologic toxicity remained easily manageable, and extra-hematologic toxicity was acceptable. Regarding CR rate, our results are similar to those of earlier reports using the same drug combination (Table 2) (Kantarjian et al. 1990, Lejeune et al.

1990, Hiddemann et al. 1990, Rosmyslowicz et al. 1990). Surprisingly, refractory patients had a better outcome than relapsed patients. This suggests the persistence of drug sensitivity, and also a possible inadequate induction treatment for those high risk ALL patients. A previous study has shown a high sensitivity of Philadelphia chromosome-positive ALL to that drug combination (Weiss et al. 1996) suggesting the use of such a combination as first line chemotherapy in those patients. There was apparently no difference between our results and those from groups using higher doses of cytarabine (Hiddemann et al. 1987, Hiddemann et al. 1990). This tend to encourage the use of cytarabine at 1 gr/m$^2$ comparatively to cytarabine at 2 or 3 gr/m$^2$ because of less severe toxicity related to chemotherapy, although these doses were never compared in a randomized trial. Similar results have also been reported with mitoxantrone and cytarabine combination using continuous infusion of a standard dose of AraC (Liso et al. 1992, Keskin et al. 1994). However, this could be explain by biases related to patient selection and by patient and tumor characteristics in those small series. The addition of etoposide to HD-AraC and mitoxantrone combination did not improve the CR rate. It has even been reported increased deaths attribuable to toxicity associated with the chemotherapy (Mazza et al. 1996). In our study, age, known as a prognostic factor at diagnosis, appears also of prognostic value when considering refractory and relapsed patients.

We confirm here that the mitoxantrone and HD-AraC combination is extremely active in refractory and relapsed ALL setting with a high CR rate and an acceptable toxicity. These data support its application as salvage treatment during first line ALL therapy. However, the major problem remains the

**Table 2.** Results of studies combining HD-AraC and mitoxantrone in refractory or relapsed ALL

| References | Patients | CR(%) | DFS(months) | HD-AraC + mitoxantrone |
|---|---|---|---|---|
| Lejeune et al. 1990 | 20 | 80 | 6 | 2 g/m$^2$ x 8 + 12 mg/m$^2$ x 2 |
| Rozmyslowicz et al. 1990 | 18 | 33 | 3 | 1 g/m$^2$ x 8 + 12 mg/m$^2$ x 2 |
| Hiddemann et al. 1990 | 24 | 50 | 3.5 | 3 g/m$^2$ x 8 + 10 mg/m$^2$ x 4 or 5 |
| Kantarjian et al. 1991 | 25 | 36 | 3 | 3 g/m$^2$ x 6 + 5 mg/m$^2$ x 5 |
| Our study | 20 | 55 | 7.4 | 1 g/m$^2$ x 8 + 10 mg/m$^2$ x 3 |

limited duration of DFS in relapsing ALL. There is no study with markedly different results in this respect.

# References

Arlin ZA, Feldman E, Kempin S, Ahmed T, Mittelman A, Savona S, Ascensao J, Baskind P, Sullivan P, Fuhr HG, Mertelsmann R (1988) Amsacrine with high-dose cytarabine is highly effective therapy for refractory and relapsed acute lymphoblastic leukemia in adults. Blood 72:433–455

Arlin ZA, Feldman EJ, Finger LR, Ahmed T, Mittelman A, Cook P, Puccio C, Baskind P, Arnold P, Razis ED, et al. (1991) Short course high dose mitoxantrone with high dose cytarabine is effective therapy for adult lymphoblastic leukemia. Leukemia 5:712–714

Bennett JM, Catovsky D, Daniel MT, Flandrin G, Galton DAG, Gralnick HR, Sultan C (1976) Proposals for the classification of acute leukaemias. Br J Haematol 33:451–458

Boucheix C, David B, Sebban C, Racadot E, Bené MC, Bernard A, Campos L, Jouault H, Sigaux F, Lepage E, Hervé P, Fiere D, for the French Group on Therapy for Adult Acute Lymphoblastic Leukemia (1994) Immunophenotype of adult acute lymphoblastic leukemia, clinical parameters, and outcome: An analysis of a prospective trial including 562 tested patients (LALA87). Blood 84:1603–1612

Capizzi RL, Poole M, Cooper MN, Richards F II, Stuart JJ, Jackson DV, White DR, Spurr CL, Hopkins JO, Muss HB, Rudnick SA, Wells R, Gabriel D, Ross D (1984) Treatment of poor risk acute leukemia with sequential high-dose Ara-C and asparaginase. Blood 63:694–700

Dombret H, Thomas X, Blaise D, Huguet F, Boiron JM, Buzyn A, Stamatoulas A, Delannoy A, Bradstock K, Boucheix C, Charrin C, Gabert J, Lebbé G, Lhéritier V, Fiere D, for the LALA Group (1998) Intensive therapy in 100 patients with Ph1 and/or BCR-ABL positive acute lymphoblastic leukemia (ALL): First interim analysis of the French-Belgian-Australian LALA-94 trial. Br J Haematol 102:270

Ellison RR, Holland JF, Weil M, Jacquillat C, Boiron M, Bernard J, Sawitsky A, Rosner F, Gussoff B, Silver RT, Karanas A, Cuttner J, Spurr CL, Hayes DM, Bloom J, Leone LA, Haurani F, Kyle R, Hutchinson JL, Forcier RJ, Moon JH (1968) Arabinosyl cytosine: A useful agent in the treatment of acute leukemia in adults. Blood 32:507–523

Fiere D, Lepage E, Sebban C, Boucheix C, Gisselbrecht C, Vernant JP, Varet B, Broustet A, Cahn JY, Rigal-Huguet F, Witz F, Michaux JL, Michallet M, Reiffers J, for the French Group on Therapy for Adult Acute Lymphoblastic Leukemia (1993) Adult acute lymphoblastic leukemia: a multicentric randomized trial testing bone marrow transplantation as postremission therapy. J Clin Oncol 11:1990–2001

Giona F, Testi AM, Amadori S, Meloni G, Carotenuto M, Resegotti L, Corella R, Leoni P, Carella AM, Grotto P, Miniero R, Mandelli F (1990) Idarubicin and high-dose cytarabine in the treatment of refractory and relapsed acute lymphoblastic leukemia. Ann Oncol 1:51–55

Herzig RH, Wolff SN, Lazarus HM, Phillips GL, Karanes C, Herzig GP (1983) High-dose cytosine arabinoside therapy for refractory leukemia. Blood 62:361–369

Hiddemann W, Kreutzmann H, Straif K, Ludwig WD, Mertelsmann R, Planker M, Donhuijsen-Ant R, Lengfelder E, Arlin Z, Buchner T (1987) High-dose cyosine arabinoside in combination with mitoxantrone for the treatment of refractory acute myeloid and lymphoblastic leukemia. Sem Oncol 14:73–77

Hiddemann W, Buchner T, Heil G, Schumacher K, Diedrich H, Maschmeyer G, Ho AD, Planker M, Gerith-Stolzenburg S, Donhuijsen-Ant R, Lengfelder E, Hoelzer D (1990) Treatment of refractory acute lymphoblastic leukemia in adults with high dose cytosine arabinoside and mitoxantrone (HAM). Leukemia 4:637–640

Kantarjian HM, Estey EH, Plunkett W, Keating MJ, Walters RS, Iacoboni S, McCredie KB, Freireich EJ (1986) Phase I-II clinical and pharmacologic studies of high-dose cytosine arabinoside in refractory leukemia. Am J Med 81:387–394

Kantarjian HM, Walters RL, Keating MJ, Estey EH, O'Brien S, Schachner J, McCredie KB, Freireich EJ (1990) Mitoxantrone and high-dose cytarabine for the treatment of refractory acute lymphocytic leukemia. Cancer 65:5–8

Kantarjian HM, Estey EH, O'Brien S, Anaissie E, Beran M, Rios MB, Keating MJ, Gutterman J (1992) Intensive chemotherapy with mitoxantrone and high-dose cytosine arabinoside followed by granulocyte-macrophage colony-stimulating factor in the treatment of patients with acute lymphocytic leukemia. Blood 79:876–881

Keskin A, Tombuloglu M, Atamer MA, Buyukkececi F (1994) Mitoxantrone and standard dose cytosine arabinoside therapy in refractory or relapsed acute leukemia. Acta Haematol 92:14–17

Laport GF, Larson RA (1997) Treatment of acute lymphoblastic leukemia in adults. Semin Oncol 24:70–82

Lejeune C, Tubiana N, Gastaut JA, Maraninchi D, Richard B, Launay MC, Sainty D, Sebahoun G, Carcassone Y (1990) High-dose cytosine arabinoside and mitoxantrone in previously-treated acute leukemia patients. Eur J Haematol 44:240–243

Liso V, Specchia G, Capalbo S, Pavone V, Iacobazzi A, Iaculli ML, Dione R, Pansini N (1992) Mitoxantrone and continuous infusion of cytosine arabinoside in refractory and relapsed acute lymphoblastic leukemia. Acta Haematol 87:54–57

Marsh W, Wozniak A, McCarley D (1987) Therapy of relapsed acute lymphocytic leukemia: A 5-year experience with high-dose ara-C. Proc Am Soc Clin Oncol 6:147

Mazza JJ, Leong T, Rowe JM, Wiernick PH, Cassileth PA (1996) Treatment of adult patients with acute lymphoblastic leukemia in relapse. Leuk Lymph 20:317–319

Montillo M, Tedeschi A, Centurioni R, Leoni P (1997) Treatment of relapsed adult acute lymphoblastic leukemia with fludarabine and cytosine arabinoside followed by granulocyte colony-stimulating factor (FLAG-GCSF). Leuk Lymph 25:579–583

Morra E, Lazzarino M, Brusamolino E, Pagnucco G, Castagnola C, Bernasconi P, Orlandi E, Corso A, Santagostino A, Bernasconi C (1993) The role of systemic high-dose cytarabine in the treatment of central nervous system leukemia. Clinical results in 46 patients. Cancer 72:439–445

Paciucci PA, Cuttner J, Holland JF (1984) Mitoxanrone as a single agent and in combination chemotherapy in patients with refractory acute leukemia. Semin Oncol 11(suppl.1):36–40

Rozmyslowicz T, Palynyczko G, Mazur J, Konecki R, Appel D, Marianska B, Maj S, Holowiecki J, Konopka L, Pawelski S (1990) Mitoxantrone in treatment of refractory acute leukemias. Blood 76(suppl.1):315a

Rudnick SA, Cadman EC, Capizzi RL, Skeel Rt, Bertino JR, McIntosh S (1979) High dose cytosine arabinoside (HDARAC) in refractory acute leukaemia. Cancer 44:1189–1193

Suki S, Kantarjian H, Gandhi V, Estey E, O'Brien S, Beran M, Rios MB, Plunkett W, Keating M (1993) Fludarabine and cytosine arabinoside in the treatment of refractory or relapsed acute lymphocytic leukemia. Cancer 72:2155–2160

Thomas X, Danaïla C, Bach QK, Dufour P, Christian B, Corront B, Bosly A, Bastion Y, Gratecos N, Leblay R, Sebban C, Archimbaud E, Fiere D (1995) Sequential induction chemotherapy with vincristine, daunorubicin, cyclophosphamide, and prednisone in adult acute lymphoblastic leukemia. Ann Hematol 70:65–69

Weiss M, Maslak P, Feldman E, Berman E, Bertino J, Gee T, Megherian L, Seiter K, Scheinberg D, Golde D (1996) Cytarabine with high-dose mitoxantrone induces rapid complete remissions in adult acute lymphoblastic leukemia without the use of vincristine or prednisone. J Clin Oncol 14:2480–2485

Weiss MA (1997) Treatment of adult patients with relapsed or refractory acute lymphoblastic leukemia (ALL). Leukemia 11(suppl.4):S28-S30

Welborn JL (1994) Impact of reinduction regimens for relapsed and refractory acute lymphoblastic leukemia in adults. Am J Hematol 45:341–344

# Split-Course High-Dose ARA-C Plus Idarubicin and Multidrug Blockade by short Cyclosporin-A Infusion for Refractory Acute Myeloid Leukemia

R. Bassan, T. Lerede, B. Chiodini, A. Rossi, M. Buelli and T. Barbui

## Introduction

Refractory acute myeloid leukemia (R-AML), defined as primary resistance to induction chemotherapy, early relapse (within 6–12 months from remission), and second or subsequent relapse, is typically a multidrug-resistant illness, for which effective treatment is presently lacking. We have treated R-AML patients with a combination of intermediate-dose ara-C, carboplatin and either mitoxantrone or idarubicin in a cross-over design, obtaining an encouraging response rate (46%) in a small group of 13 R-AML patients who were given an amended, low-toxicity regimen [1]. Five more patients were treated with a similar carboplatin-containing schedule delivered in a sequential manner, but only one remission was achieved, to an overall response rate of 33% (6/18). This result prompted a further change in retreatment strategy. In R-AML, clinical multidrug resistance is often associated with functional overexpression of the MDR1 drug efflux machinery and/or other mechanisms such as LRP (lung-related protein) and MRP (multidrug resistance-associated protein) [2–11]. Theoretically, in view of the high incidence of MDR1 activation in R-AML and its adverse clinical significance, functional MDR1 inhibition with cyclosporin A (CsA), verapamil, tamoxifen, PSC 833, quinine [12–19] or the use of drugs scarcely (Idarubicin=IDR) or not (high-dose ara-C=HiDAC, carboplatin) MDR1-sensitive could underlie therapeutic improvement. In preclinical in vitro studies on a MDR1+ human leukemic cell line [20, 21], we found that both cellular uptake and pro-apoptotic effects of IDR used at the-

rapeutic concentration (50–100 ng/ml, corresponding to the ranges of peak plasma level obtainable after rapid intravenous administration of IDR 10–12 mg/m$^2$) were significantly increased by co-incubation with CsA 1500 ng/ml. Interestingly, CsA enhanced IDR-related cytotoxicity only in the early phase of IDR-blast cell interaction while, contrary to daunorubicin, 12-hour IDR retention by blast cells was not modified by CsA. The study conclusion was that both cellular uptake of and related biologic effects from IDR can be up-regulated by CsA in MDR1+ cells but, partly because IDR is highly lypophilic and partly because it is less vulnerable to MDR1, this effect does not require a prolonged CsA exposure. On this basis we initiated a new clinical study, using CsA and aiming to determine the upper IDR concentration tolerated by patients with R-AML. This new sequential regimen included HiDAC 3 g/m$^2$ every 12 hours for two consecutive days followed by IDR 12.5 mg/m$^2$ as starting dose level (both drugs were given for two times on days 1–3 and 8–10) together with CsA 6 mg/kg over 1 hour and then 7.5 mg/kg over 11 hours according to the List schedule [22]. IDR was delivered 4 hours after starting CsA. The three-day sequence was repeated on days 8–10. Recombinanat human granulocyte colony-stimulating factor (G-CSF) was administered from day 11 until response evaluation. We report the therapeutic results obtained in the first 10 patients, who received IDR from 12.5 to 17.5 mg/m$^2$/dose.

Hematology Department, Ospedali riuniti, Bergamo, Italy

## Materials and methods

### Patient eligibility and prior treatments

All adult patients with a diagnosis of R-AML and life expectancy >3 months were eligible to the study. Very stringent criteria were used to define R-AML within the highly experimental context of this study. Patients with R-AML were those initially refractory to current induction/salvage protocols and those who relapsed after a complete remission lasting <6 months or who were at second or subsequent relapse. Primary refractory patients were those failing to respond to a single induction course. For these patients, the remission rate upon repetition of the same induction schedule is 34–38% [23, 24] and therefore needs to be improved. Prior treatments were as follows. Induction therapy for patients aged 15–60 years comprised IDR 10 mg/m²/d on days 1–3, etoposide 100 mg/m²/d on days 1–5, ara-C 200 mg/m²/d on days 1–7, G -CSF from day 8, and with or without all-trans retinoic acid (ATRA) 45 mg/m²/d on days 1–14 and 25 mg/m²/d on days 15–28

(ICE+G+/-ATRA). Induction therapy for patients aged >60 years consisted of mitoxantrone 10 mg/m²/d on days 1–5, etoposide 100 mg/m²/d on days 1–5, ara-C 200 mg/m²/d on days 1–5, and G -CSF from day 6. Postremission consolidation consisted, in younger patients, of one more ICE course followed by HiDAC and then a myeloablative regimen with reinfusion of peripheral blood stem cells in selected instances. In patients aged >60 years, postremission consolidation was attempted with induction-like course(s) or HiDAC. AML diagnosis and characterization was according to institutional guidelines (morphology, cyctochemistry, immunophenotype, cytogenetics). Multidrug resistance was defined clinically as R-AML; the expression of specific multidrug resistance mechanisms by blast cells was not looked for.

### Retreatment regimen

The preclinical basis for this study is summarized in Figure 1. The *in vitro* experiments showed a time-independent (at 12 hours) but

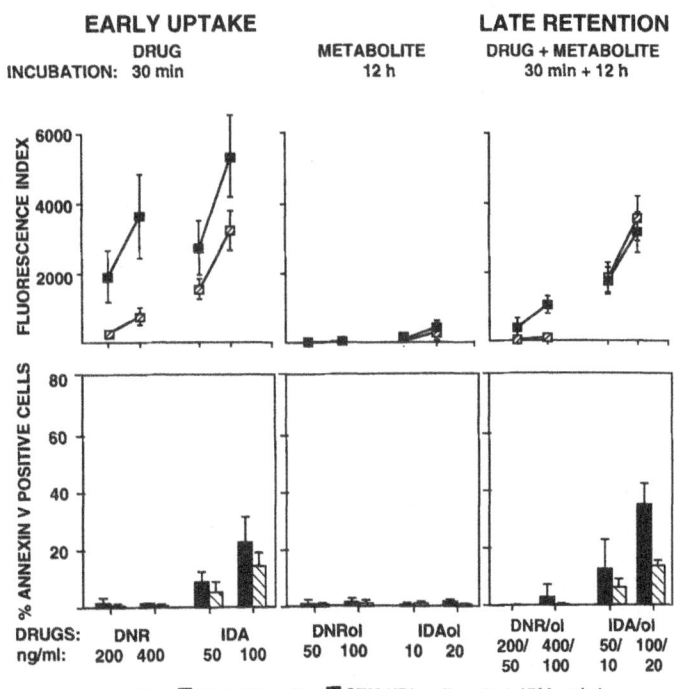

**Fig. 1.** Preclinical evaluation of IDR with or without CsA in MDR1+ CEM-VBL human leukemic cell line: early cellular uptake (after 30' incubation) and late retention (12 h) of IDR and daunorubicin (DNR), their metabolites, and drug plus metabolite combinations at equivalent therapeutic concentrations (Fluorescence index); and related induction of apoptosis (FITC-annexin V binding assay, subtracted of values from control experiments with untreated cells).

439

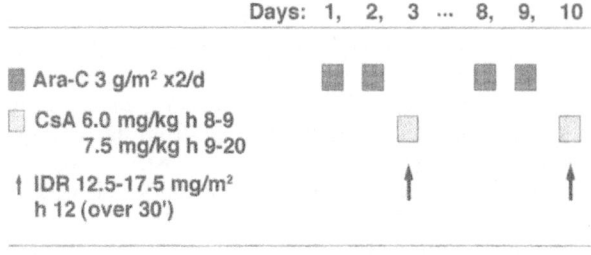

Days: 1, 2, 3 ... 8, 9, 10

Ara-C 3 g/m² x2/d

CsA 6.0 mg/kg h 8-9
7.5 mg/kg h 9-20

IDR 12.5-17.5 mg/m²
h 12 (over 30')

Bone marrow on days 11 and 28
G-CSF 5 µg/kg/d from day 11 to response

**Fig. 2.** Sequential regimen for R-AML.

early CsA-dependent (after 30' incubation) cellular uptake of IDR, with related induction of apoptosis, in MDR1+ blast cells (human leukemic CEM-VBL T-lymphoblastic cell line) challenged with therapeutic concentrations of the drug. Compared with daunorubicin, both effects were significantly increased (p<0.05). The treatment protocol developed in accordance to that is reported in Figure 2. The study design is very similar to the sequential retreatment regimen developed by the German AML Cooperative Group (25), differing for the use of escalating dosages of IDR plus CsA instead of mitoxantrone. All drugs were given intravenously through a central venous line. This was a phase I trial, in which IDR dose was increased starting from 25 mg/m² (cumulative dose to be divided in two administrations), with 5 mg/m² increments. Three patients were to be entered on each dose level. The maximum tolerated dose (MTD) was defined as the IDR dose preceding that associated with the development of life-threatening complications according to the common toxicity criteria scale (CTC grade 3 and 4). When, however, the occurrence of these complications was not clearly abscribable to the retreatment regimen itself, other patients were accrued at the same or higher IDR dose level. This adjustment was necessary because some patients were already critically ill (disease, infections, hemorrhages, toxicity related to prior treatment), so that the salvage protocol could not totally account for the observed toxic complications. The CsA schedule was that proposed by List et al. [22], by which means it is possible to obtain a plasma concentration >1500 ng/ml that warrants the functional downregulation of MDR1 in patients with MDR1+ R-AML. To avoid

acute side-effects by CsA, patients were medicated with dexamethasone 8 mg, clorphenamine 4 mg, and lorazepam 1–2.5 mg (orally) 1 hour before starting the CsA load. IDR was administered over 30' on days 3 and 10 as shown in Figure 2. During the period of marrow hypoplasia and drug-induced mucositis, patients were routinely supported by total parenteral nutrition. Fluconazole and ciprofloxacin were given prophylactically. Early neutropenic fever or documented infections were treated empirically with ceftazidime (or cilastatin-imipenen), amikacin and teicoplanin. Changes in empiric antimicrobial therapy were made according to the results of diagnostic assays, or in the case of unremitting fever for 48–72 hours (amphotericin-B 0.75 mg/kg or lipid encapsulated amphotericin B 3 mg/kg).

**Evaluation of response and postremission therapy**

Bone marrow morphology was checked on days 11 and 28. A complete hematologic remission (CHR) was defined as the clearance of marrow blast cells (<5%) with reappearance of normal trilineage hematopoiesis in a regenerating normocellular or slightly hypocellular bone marrow. With regard to postremission therapy, an allogeneic hematopoietic stem cell transplantation was the preferred option. In patients without a suitable donor, a second chemotherapy course of the same type and intensity was attempted. Regimen-related toxicity (RRT) was determined according to common toxicity criteria. In view of the very high-risk setting of R-AML, only severe (CTC grade 3 and 4), potentially life-threatening toxicity was considered informative for this study and hence reported.

## Results

### Patients with R-AML

Ten patients were treated between May '98 and January '99. All cases but one satisfied the criteria for R-AML, and no patient had acute promyelocytic leukemia. A patient at first relapse after 9 months was included because at high-risk by age (63 years), prior consolidation therapy (including HiDAC), and disease karyotype (monosomy 7). Median patient age was 43.5 years. All patients had been treated according to institutional protocols. The main patient characteristics, status of disease, previous treatments and, when applicable, length of prior response at time of salvage therapy are shown in Table 2. Of note, most cases were severely neutropenic (median and range: 0.5 and 0–10x10⁹/l) and thrombocytopenic (median and range: 28 and 6–86x10⁹/l), with 0–20 (median 2.2) x10⁹/l blast cells. Very high-risk prognostic features were additionally present in some patients and are referred because of their potential contribution to the incidence of RRT. Case no. 1 had a resistant relapse. Case no. 2 had suffered from an extensive fungal pneumonia during early treatment, for which front-line therapy had been curtailed. Case no. 4 was that detailed above. Case no. 3 had

R-AML after second-line therapy and was febrile and infected with an very poor performance status. Case no. 5 had suffered from life-threatening drug-induced liver injury during treatment for first relapse and had diabetes and serious multiple dental and parodontal problems. Case no. 6 was in a very poor physical condition because of an associated central nervous system relapse, and had also received reduced-dose consolidation due to inadequate performance status. Case no. 8 was in very early relapse after allogeneic hematopoietic stem cell transplantation for primary refractory AML (to ICE regimen).

### Treatment outcome

The results are summarized in Table 2. The first four patients were entered onto the lower IDR level (12.5 mg/m²/dose). A positive hematologic response was achieved in three patients (no. 1, 2 and 4), while case no. 3 died early of uncontrolled infections. This patient had remained severely neutropenic for >2 months and was already infected at start of treatment. Patient no. 2 had only a brief response, after which the disease progressed rapidly and she was lost to follow-up. Patient no. 4, who obtained a CHR, developed a progressive liver impairment and died of liver failure and pneumonia without evidence of leukemic relapse. Because the toxicities observed in cases no. 4 and especially no. 3 were not exclusively put in relation with the re-

**Table 1.** Pretreatment characteristics of patients with R-AML

| Patient no. | Age | Sex | AML diagnosis | Status of disease | Prior treatment* | Prior remission |
|---|---|---|---|---|---|---|
| 1 | 41 | F | M5, del11(p14) | 2nd relapse | ICE+HDT, CHAM | 1 mo. |
| 2 | 46 | F | M2 | 1st relapse | ICE | 3.3 mos. |
| 3 | 38 | M | M1 | Refractory | ICE, CHAM | – |
| 4 | 63 | F | M2, –5 | 1st relapse | MEC+HDT | 9 mos.** |
| 5 | 56 | M | M2, inv(16) | 2nd relapse | ICE+HDT, CHAM | 15 mos. |
| 6 | 58 | M | M1 | 1st relapse | ICE | 3.5 mos. |
| 7 | 52 | M | M6+MDS | Refractory | ICE | – |
| 8 | 31 | M | M2 | Refractory | ICE, allo-BMT | – |
| 9 | 17 | F | M6+MDS | Refractory | ICE | – |
| 10 | 28 | M | M4 | Refractory | ICE | – |

*ICE, idarubicin-cytarabine-etoposide; HDT, high-dose treatments +/-hematopoietic stem cell support; CHAM, carboplatin-intermediate/high-dose cytarabine-mitoxantrone; MEC, mitoxantrone-etoposide-cytarabine; allo-BMT: pt. no. 8 refractory to ICE
and relapsed after allogeneic bone marrow transplantation
MDS, associated myelodysplasia
**included because aged >60 and with monosomy 5

**Table 2.** Retreatment results

| Patient no. | IDR dose (mg/m$^2$) | Bone marrow d 11 | Bone marrow d 28 | Further therapy | Outcome |
|---|---|---|---|---|---|
| 1 | 12.5 | Blasts cleared | CHR | 1 cycle + allogeneic BMT | CHR 8+ mos. |
| 2 | 12.5 | – | Blasts <10% | – | Progression, lost to FUP |
| 3 | 12.5 | – | – | – | Death by infection d +14 |
| 4 | 12.5 | – | CHR | – | Death d +40 |
| 5 | 15 | Blasts cleared | – | – | Death by infection d +24 |
| 6 | 15 | Blasts cleared | – | – | Death by hemorrhage d +16 |
| 7 | 15 | Blasts cleared | CHR | 1 cycle | CHR 3+ mos. |
| 8 | 15 | Few blasts | CHR | too early | too early |
| 9 | 15 | Blasts cleared | CHR* | too early | too early |
| 10 | 17.5 | Blasts cleared | CHR | None (lung infection) | CHR 3+ mos. |

*Autologous CD34+ blood cells collected at remission (454 x10$^6$) to support consolidation cycle

treatment regimen and, in any case, no acute RRT from IDR-CsA had been observed, the next patients were entered onto the subsequent IDR dose level (15 mg/m$^2$/dose). Two patients with very poor-risk pretreatment characteristics died early of cerebral bleeding (case no. 6 with concurrent central nervous system relapse) and fulminating soft tissue infection of head and neck (case no. 5 with uncontrolled hyperglycemia and severe parodontopathy), while a CHR was obtained in patients no. 7–9. Finally, the single case so far entered onto the third dose level (IDR 17.5 mg/m$^2$/dose) achieved a CHR too. Altogether, on examination day 28 six of 10 patients obtained a CHR (60%) and one (case no. 2) a significant reduction (>50%) of bone marrow blast cell content. If the three patients who died early are not considered, the response rate was high among fully evaluable cases: 6/7 (86%) or 5/7 (71%) excluding the case who died of complications in CHR. Considering the 7 cases who had their bone marrow examined early on day 11, 6 of them (86%) showed a complete clearing of blast cells on a background of marrow hypocellularity, and this was associated with a complete hematologic and clinical response in those who did not succumb to complications. With regard to postremission therapy, only cases no. 1 and 7 received a single, identical consolidation cycle. Eventually, while in early relapse, case no. 1 underwent an allograft from an HLA-mismatched sibling donor. In case no. 9, G-CSF-primed autologous CD34+ blood cells were collected at remission in order to support the myelotoxicity of the

planned consolidation course. The patient is then expected to undergo an unrelated donor bone marrow transplantation.

### Analysis of RRT

The results are summarized in Table 3, including the data inherent to CsA plasma levels determined at time of IDR administration (noon) and at end of CsA infusion (20.00 p.m.). CsA was >1500 ng/ml in all 10 patients when IDR was infused, and it was still above that threshold in 9/10 at end of infusion. IDR peak plasma levels will be determined, to assess whether a concentration equal to or greater than 100 ng/ml was achieved in accordance with study objectives. No serious side effect developed acutely during IDR plus CsA infusion. Neurologic symptoms resembling alcoholic intoxication, due to ethanol present in CsA preparation, were seen in the first two patients treated. In subsequent cases, the premedication schema was highly effective. The degree of myelosuppression has been remarkable but not intolerable, with a median period of severe absolute granulocytopenia of 24 days. The most common extrahematologic symptom was a transient hyperbilirubinemia, observed in nearly all cases, but so far independent of IDR dose. Gastrointestinal symptoms and oral mucositis were severe but reversible. Life-threatening infections were observed in the patients presenting with the worst prognostic profile (cases no. 3, 5, and 6). Apart from that, the regimen was rather well tolerated by the younger patients in be-

**Table 3.** Analysis of RRT and CsA concentrations.

| Patient no. | IDR (mg/m²) | CSA (ng/ml) h-12 | h-20 | Hematologic toxicity[1] ANC <0.5 | PTL <20 | PRC (x) | PC (x) | Nonhematologic toxicity (grade 3 and 4) |
|---|---|---|---|---|---|---|---|---|
| 1 | 12.5 | 2548 | 1614 | 30 | 45 | 3 | 12 | Hepatic (bilirubin), infection (VZV) |
| 2 | 12.5 | 3180 | 1780 | 25 | 41 | 2 | 4 | Infection (Gram -ve sepsis) |
| 3 | 12.5 | 1766 | 1097 | 14 | 14 | 4 | 7 | Hepatic, gastrointestinal, infection (death by infection) |
| 4 | 12.5 | 2589 | 1636 | 35 | 47+ | 8 | 25 | Hepatic, infection (pneumonia) gastrointestinal, cardiac (arrythmia) |
| 5 | 15 | 2715 | 2397 | 25 | 22 | 5 | 8 | Metabolic (hyperglicemia), hepatic, gastrointestinal, skin rash, infection (death by infection) |
| 6 | 15 | 2465 | 1857 | 11 | 11 | 1 | 6 | Hepatic, gastrointestinal, neurologic, infection (pneumonia + Gram +ve sepsis) (death by hemorrhage/infection) |
| 7 | 15 | 2878 | 1832 | 24 | 24 | 14 | 6 | Hepatic, infection (pneumonia) |
| 8 | 15 | 3370 | 1882 | 23[2] | 30 | 6 | 12 | Gastrointestinal, infection (fungal pneumonia) |
| 9 | 15 | 2508 | 2005 | 9 | 21 | 4 | 7 | – |
| 10 | 17.5 | 2105 | 2149 | 25 | 30 | 4 | 11 | Gastrointestinal, infection (fungal pneumonia) |

[1]ANC <0.5, absolute neutrophil count $<0.5 \times 10^9/L$ (days); PTL <20, platelet count $<20 \times 10^9/l$ (days); PRC, transfusion with packed red cells (times); PC, transfusion with platelet concentrates (times)
[2]Reinfused with allogeneic hematopoietic stem cells

tter physical shape. In view of the clinical results in the first 10 patients treated, the MTD for IDR has not been determined and appears to be ≥15 mg/m²/dose.

## Discussion

Adult patients with R-AML as defined in this report have a very poor outlook, owing to expression of high-risk biologic characteristics such as chromosome abnormalities and multidrug resistance mechanisms MDR1, MRP, and LRP [2–11]. Attempts to improve the prognosis of these very poor-risk cases have met with only partial success. One of the most active regimens to date available is s-HAM (sequential high-dose Ara-C at 3 g/m²/dose, plus mitoxantrone) [25]. With s-HAM, 46% of R-AML patients aged 60 years and less entered a complete remission, as opposed to generally inferior results adopting less intensive regimens (reviewed in the same paper). Because MDR1 is often overexpressed in refractory/relapse states of adult AML ]2–11], we introduced a modified s-HAM regimen in order to take advantage of the minor vulnerability of IDR to MDR1 [26]. Because it was already known from previous in vitro studies that such favorable feature is

less evident at clinically relevant drug concentrations [20, 21], we took into consideration the adjunct of CsA as MDR1 downregulator as well as an increase of IDR dose, given that cellular IDR uptake does vary in a fashion that is proportional to the drug's peak plasma level [27]. The use of the less MDR1-sensitive compound at the highest tolerated dose, instead of highly MDR1-sensitive drugs at conventional dosage, has been advocated as a strategy to counteract MDR1 overexpression by neoplastic cells [28]. The feasibility of this approach was to be determined in a phase I clinical trial. Since we had documented, in in vitro studies, only short-term effects by CsA on IDR cellular uptake and related biologic effects (Figure 1 and refs. 20 and 21), we designed the current, brief CsA schedule in support of IDR activity (Figure 2). This was probably one of the reasons by which overall RRT remained within an acceptable range even with an IDR dose of 17.5 mg/m². On the contrary, prolonged CsA infusions are toxic to the patients, as previously shown with IDR [29] and other MDR1-sensitive drugs, essentially because the MDR1 mechanism is normally expressed in several tissues and organs. Therefore, even if blocking of MDR1 can be attained in AML cells, a prolonged inhibition of this function in non-neoplastic MDR1+

cells (in first place liver and kidney and bone marrow stem cells) can lead to significant RRT with reduction of drug dosages (sometimes reported with daunorubicin, mitoxantrone and etoposide) [13, 15, 17]. In the current study we have not observed any of these untoward side effects. Rather, we have obtained a very encouraging response rate in a small cohort of patients with R-AML and, as yet, have not been able to define the MTD for IDR used from 12.5 to 17.5 mg/m$^2$/dose. Unlike some other study adopting prolonged CsA infusions, we have been able to increase the anthracycline dose and to attain an appreciale response rate without exacerbating toxicity. However, phase I trials of this type appears difficult to perform in R-AML, because some patients can be at very high risk of treatment failure for reasons partially unrelated to RRT. We have underlined this fact and shown how this treatment was applicable with success only to patients featuring an adequate performance status, without severe co-morbid diseases, unininfected before treatment, and aged <60 years. Only understanding this difference we were able to introduce the second and third IDR dose level. In the more favorable cases (no. 1, 2 and 7–10) a positive hematologic response was induced in all those treated with IDR 15–17.5 mg/m$^2$/dose, and in one of two treated with IDR 12.5 mg/m$^2$/dose. Thus, even if MDR1 expression was not determined in this limited clinical sample, sequential HiDAC plus IDR 15–17.5 mg/m$^2$/dose plus short-course CsA was a feasible protocol that exerted a considerable clinical activity. With regard to study proposal, we do not know yet whether the latter IDR dose represents the study endpoint (MTD). Apart from the expected toxicities seen in the four very poor-risk patients, all cases suffered from transient mucosal and gastrointestinal drug-related damage including hyperbilirubinemia, that may be an indicator of CsA activity, as suggested [22]. Myelotoxicity was severe, with a median absolute neutropenia <0.5 x10$^9$/l lasting 24 days that was associated with documented bacterial or fungal infections in 8 out of 10 patients. This degree of myelosuppression was however inferior to that reported in the German s-HAM study, in which the median neutropenic period was as long as 41 days,

and the difference may lie in the use of G-CSF in our study. This may be an useful information, because of the extremely high risk for the development of serious infectious complications present in these patients. We had no clinical evidence that G-CSF given from day 11 stimulated the growth of AML blast cells. In order to reduce further the myelotoxic effects of this therapy we are now considering the additional use of the marrow-protectant amifostine. Also, the planned postremission cycle will be supported, in responsive patients lacking a histocompatible donor, by G-CSF-primed autologous CD34+ hemopoietic blood cells collected after the induction course.

## References

1. Bassan R, Lerede T, Buelli M et al (1998) A new combination of carboplatin, high-dose cytarabine and cross-over mitoxantrone or idarubicin for refractory and relapsed acute acute myeloid leukemia. Haematologica 83:422–427.
2. Filipits M, Pohl G, Stranzl T et al (1998) Expression of the lung resistance protein predicts poor outcome in de novo acute myeloid leukemia. Blood 91:1508–1513.
3. Del Poeta G, Stasi R, Aronica G et al (1996) Clinical relevance of P-glycoprotein expression in de novo acute myeloid leukemia. Blood 87:1997–2004.
4. List AF, Spier CS, Grogan TM et al (1996) Overexpression of the major vault transporter protein lung-resistance protein predicts treatment outcome in acute myeloid leukemia. Blood 87: 2464–2469.
5. te Boekhorst P, Löwenberg B, van Kapel J et al (1995) Multidrug resistance cells with high proliferative capacity determine response to therapy in acute myeloid leukemia. Leukemia 9:1025–1031.
6. Nüssler V, Pelka-Fleischer R, Zwierzina H et al (1996) P-glycoprotein expression in patients with acute leukemia – clinical relevance. Leukemia 10 (Suppl 3):S23-S31.
7. Leith CP, Chen IM, Kopecky KJ et al (1995) Correlation of multidrug resistance (MDR1) protein expression with functional dye/drug efflux in acute myeloid leukemia by multiparameter flow cytometry: identification of discordant Mdr$^-$/efflux$^+$ and MDR1$^+$/efflux$^-$ cases. Blood 86: 2329–2342.
8. Ross DD, Doyle LA, Schiffer CA et al (1996) Expression of multidrug resistance-associated protein (MRP) mRNA in blast cells from acute myeloid leukemia (AML) patients. Leukemia 10: 48–55.
9. Guerci A, Merlin JL, Missoum N et al (1995) Predictive value for treatment outcome in acute myeloid leukemia of cellular daunorubicin accumulation and P-glycoprotein expression simultaneously determined by flow cytometry. Blood 85: 2147–2153.

10. Campos L, Guyotat D, Archimbaud E et al (1992) Clinical significance of multidrug resistance P-glycoprotein expression on acute nonlymphoblastic leukemia cells at diagnosis. Blood 79:473–476.

11. Schneider E, Cowan KN, Bader H et al (1995) Increased expression of the multidrug resistance-associated protein gene in relapsed acute leukemia. Blood 85:186–193.

12. Wattel E, Solary E, Hecquet B et al (1998) Quinine improves the results of intensive chemotherapy in myelodysplastic syndromes expressing P glycoprotein: results of randomized study. Br J Haematol 102:1015–1024.

13. Kornblau SM, Estey E, Madden T et al (1997) Phase I study of mitoxantrone plus etoposide with multidrug blockade by SDZ PSC-833 in relapsed or refractory acute myelogenous leukemia. J Clin Oncol 15:1796–1802.

14. Solary E, Caillot D, Chauffert B et al (1992) Feasibility of using quinine, a potential multidrug resistance-reversing agent, in combination with mitoxantrone and cytarabine for the treatment of acute leukemia. J Clin Oncol 10:1730–1736.

15. Solary E, Witz B, Caillot D et al (1996) Combination of quinine as a potential reversing agent with mitoxantrone and cytarabine for the treatment of acute leukemias: a randomized multicenter study. Blood 88:1198–1205.

16. Berman E, McBride M, Lin S et al (1995) Phase I trial of high-dose tamoxifen as a modulator of drug resistance in combination with daunorubicin in patients with relapsed or refractory acute leukemia. Leukemia 9:1631–1637.

17. Bartlett NL, Lum BL, Fisher GA et al (1994) Phase I trial of doxorubicin with cyclosporine as a modulator of multidrug resistance. J Clin Oncol 12:835–842.

18. Ross DD, Wooten PJ, TongY et al (1994) Synergistic reversal of multidrug-resistance phenotype in acute myeloid leukemia cells by cyclosporine A and cremophor EL. Blood 83:1337–1347.

19. Ross DD, Wooten PJ, Sridhara R et al (1993) Enhancement of daunorubicin accumulation, retention, and cytotoxity by verapamil or cyclosporin A in blast cells from patients with previously untreated acute myeloid leukemia. Blood 82:1288–1299.

20. Chiodini B, Bassan R, Borleri G et al (1998) Idarubicin activity against multidrug- resistant (mdr-1+) cells is increased by cyclosporin A. In: Hiddemann W, Büchner T, Wörmann B, Ritter J, Creutzig U, Keating M, Plunkett W (eds) Acute Leukemias VII. Springer-Verlag Berlin Heidelberg: pp 475–482.

21. Chiodini B, Bassan R, Barbui T (1999) Cellular uptake and antiproliferative effects of therapeutic concentrations of idarubicin or daunorubicin and their alcohol metabolites, with or without cyclosporin A, in MDR1+ human leukemic cells. Leuk Lymph ( in press).

22. List AF, Spier C, Greer J et al (1993) Phase I/II trial of cyclosporine as a chemotherapy-resistance modifier in acute leukemia. J Clin Oncol 11: 1652–1660.

23. Liso V, Iacopino P, Avvisati G et al (1996) Outcome of patients with acute myeloid leukemia who failed to respond to a single course of first-line induction therapy: a GIMEMA study of 218 unselected consecutive patients. Leukemia 10: 1443–1452.

24. Anderlini P, Ghaddar HM, Smith TL et al (1996) Factors predicting complete remission and subsequent disease-free survival after a second course of induction therapy in patients with acute myelogenous leukemia resistant to the first. Leukemia 10:964–969.

25. Kern W, Aul C, Maschmeyer G et al (1998) Superiority of high-dose over intermediate-dose cytosine arabinoside in the treatment of patients with high-risk acute myeloid leukemia: results of an age-adjusted prospective randomized comparison. Leukemia 12:1049–1055.

26. Bassan R, Chiodini B, Lerede T et al (1997) The role of idarubicin in adult acute lymphoblastic leukaemia: from drug resistance studies to clinical application. Leuk Lymph 26 (Suppl 1):89–97.

27. Speth PA, Minderman H, Haanen C (1989) Idarubicin v daunorubicin: preclinical and clinical pharmacokinetic studies. Semin Oncol 16 (Suppl 2): 2–9.

28. Lehnert M (1996) Clinical multidrug resistance in cancer: a multifactorial problem. J Clin Oncol 32A:912–920.

29. Damiani D, Michieli M, Ermacora A et al (1998) Adjuvant treatment with cyclosporin A increases the toxicity of chemotherapy for remission induction in acute non-lymphoblastic leukemia. Leukemia 12:1236–1240.

# AML in Adults

# Recent Genetic Studies of Adult Patients with Acute Myeloid Leukemia Performed by the Cancer and Leukemia Group B

J. C. Byrd[1], A. J. Carroll[2], M. A. Caligiuri[3], R. A. Larson[4] and C. D. Bloomfield[3]

*Abstract.* The Cancer and Leukemia Group B (CALGB) has performed prospective cytogenetic and molecular genetic studies concurrent with their acute myeloid leukemia (AML) treatment trials for the past 15 years. Results from these studies presented herein describe recently published data that form the basis for stratifying post-remission therapy based upon cytogenetics. Specifically we discuss the impact of cytogenetics on results of post remission dose intensification with cytarabine, the adverse prognostic significance of trisomy as a sole abnormality (i.e. isolated trisomy 13, 8 and 11) in patients with AML and the adverse clinical consequences of a partial tandem duplication of the MLL gene in patients with normal cytogenetics. In addition, factors affecting outcome of patients with specific translocations are discussed including the impact of secondary cytogenetic abnormalities in patients with t(15;17) and t(9;11), and the impact of the presence of extramedullary leukemia, CD56 blast expression and multiple cycles of post induction high dose cytarabine therapy in patients with t(8;21). Based upon the studies described herein, karyotype specific directed therapy is proposed, concurrent with additional molecular studies, to better define factors involved in leukemogenesis.

## Introduction

Advances in understanding the pathogenesis and improvement in the treatment of acute myeloid leukemia (AML) have occurred during the last two decades. This has occurred in part through identification of new therapies for patients with AML, such as administration of high-dose cytarabine therapy, allogeneic stem cell transplantation, and all-trans-retinoic acid therapy. Concomitant with the introduction of these therapies has been the perceived need to better stratify patients with AML based both upon clinical features (e.g. age) and genetic features. Over the past 15 years the Cancer and Leukemia Group B (CALGB) has had an active correlative laboratory research program that has investigated cytogenetics and dysregulation of genes involved in the pathogenesis of AML. Herein, we describe some recent discoveries related to studies performed by CALGB in AML.

## Patients and Methods

### Patients

Patients included in the studies performed were 16 years or older with primary AML as

This work was supported by National Cancer Institute Grants 26806, 31946, 77658, 16058 and the Coleman Leukemia Research Fund.
The opinions or assertions contained herein are the private views of the authors and are not to be construed as official or as reflecting the views of the U.S. Army or Department of Defense.
[1] Hematology Oncology Service, Walter Reed Army Medical Center Washington D.C.
[2] Laboratory of Medical Genetics, University of Alabama at Birmingham, Birmingham AL.
[3] Division of Hematology and Oncology, Department of Internal Medicine and the Comprehensive Cancer Center, The Ohio State University, Columbus, OH.
[4] Section of Hematology/Oncology, Department of Medicine and Cancer Research Center, University of Chicago Medical Center, Chicago IL.

defined by the French-American-British (FAB) classification system [1] and were participants in treatment trials conducted by the CALGB between June 1984 and November 1995. Of the 1,561 patients included in this group, 1,353 (87%) received similar daunorubicin and cytarabine for induction therapy. [2-6] Patients with a prior history of myelodysplasia, other antecedent hematological malignancies, prior non-steroidal cytotoxic chemotherapy or radiation therapy, pre-existing liver disease as previously defined, [2-6] or uncontrolled infection were excluded. Central review of the pathologic diagnosis was performed.

## Cytogenetics

Chromosomal analysis of bone marrows were performed in institutional CALGB cytogenetics laboratories and karyotypes were centrally reviewed biannually by an expert panel of CALGB cancer cytogeneticists. Specimens were obtained at diagnosis from all patients. Specimens were processed using direct methods and unstimulated short term (24, 48, and 72 hour) cultures. G-banding was usually done although Q banding was acceptable for inclusion in this series. A minimum of 20 bone marrow metaphase cells was analyzed in each patient designated as having a normal karyotype. The criteria used to describe a cytogenetic clone and description of karyotype followed the recommendations of the International System for Human Cytogenetic Nomenclature [7].

## Evaluation

During treatment, patients underwent a bone marrow aspiration following completion of each consolidation or intensification and at completion of maintenance therapy (if relevant). Thereafter, patients were followed with bone marrow testing every three months for one year, every six months for two years, and then every year for two additional years. Patients were followed yearly after five years of remission with bone marrow examinations being performed only if the blood counts suggested relapse of AML.

## Criteria for Response and Definition of Relapse

A complete remission (CR) was defined as the presence of a morphologically normal bone marrow and at least 1,500/ĨL granulocytes and 100,000/ĨL platelets in the blood. Relapse was defined as greater than five percent leukemic cells in bone marrow aspirates or new extramedullary leukemia in patients with a previously documented CR utilizing the previously published NCI guidelines [8]

## Major Results

### Remission Duration After High-Dose Cytarabine Varies by Cytogenetics

The CALGB was the first cooperative group to define the importance of pre-treatment cytogenetics in predicting the frequency of long-term remission after treatment with high-dose cytarabine intensification. [9,10] A total of 285 newly diagnosed patients with primary AML who had adequate karyotypes were randomly assigned to post-remission treatment with standard, intermediate or high-dose cytarabine intensification. [2] Patients were categorized to one of three cytogenetic groups: core binding factor type (CBF) [i.e. t(8;21)(q22;q22), inv(16)(p13q22), t(16;16) (p13q22) and del(16)]; normal; and other abnormality karyotype. The patient population included 57 CBF AML, 140 normal karyotype AML, and 88 with other cytogenetic abnormalities. Treatment outcome of CBF AML was superior with an estimated 50% still in continuous CR after five years as compared to 32% and 15% for the normal and other abnormality AML patients, respectively (p<0.001).

Univariate analysis showed the following non-karyotype factors to predict prolonged CR duration: younger age (p<0.008), lower leukocyte count (p=0.01), presence of Auer rods (p=0.004), and lower percentage of bone marrow blasts (p=0.001) at the time of diagnosis and higher post-remission cytarabine dose (p< 0.001). The impact of cytarabine dose on long-term remission was most marked in the CBF AML group (after 5 years, 78% still in CR with $3g/m^2$, 57% with $400 mg/m^2$, and 16% with $100 mg/m^2$, p<0.001) followed by normal karyotype AML (after 5 years, 40% still in CR with 3g/m², 37% with 400 mg/m², and 20% with 100 mg/m² p=0.01). In contrast, cytarabine at all doses produced a 21% or less chance of long-term continuous CR for patients with other cytogenetic abnormalities.

A multivariate analysis of CR duration assessed the independent impact of each of these variables upon cure. Significant factors entering this model in descending order of importance were cytogenetic group (CBF > Normal > Other Abnormality) [p= 0.00001], cytarabine dose (3g/m² > 400 mg/m² > 100 mg/m²) [p=0.00001], logarithm of leukocyte count at time of diagnosis (p=0.0005) and FAB subtype of AML (p=0.005). This study [10] demonstrated that the curative impact of cytarabine intensification varies significantly among cytogenetic groups and results in substantial prolongation of CR among patients with CBF and normal karyotypes but not in those with other karyotypic abnormalities. These findings provided support for the use of pre-treatment cytogenetics in risk stratification of post-remission AML therapy that is currently being performed by the CALGB [11].

## Sole Numerical Karyotype Abnormalities Predict for Inferior Outcome in AML

Addition of a sole chromosome (i.e. trisomy) is not uncommon in AML. CALGB studies were among the first to demonstrate that AML patients with trisomy 13, 8, and 11 do quite poorly with standard therapeutic approaches.

**Trisomy 13:** Isolated Trisomy 13 is a rare, recurring chromosomal abnormality whose clinical features were described initially by CALGB investigators [12]. At the time of this initial publication, this abnormality was found in approximately 1.3% of patients with acute leukemia enrolled in the prospective cytogenetic study CALGB 8461. Of the 8 patients initially described in this report, 5 had AML, 1 mixed (myeloid and lymphoid) leukemia, 1 acute lymphoblastic leukemia, and 1 undifferentiated leukemia. Six of these patients were male and two were female with no distinguishing clinical features with the exception of a high predisposition to leukocytosis (5 of 8 with leukocyte count > 50 x 10⁹/L) at presentation. Induction therapy was successful in three of the patients; only one of the 5 patients with isolated trisomy 13 and AML attained a CR. All patients with trisomy 13 attaining a CR relapsed. The overall survival of patients with acute leukemia and isolated trisomy 13 or the subset group with both this abnormality and AML was statistically inferior to those patients without this abnormality. Based upon these data, consideration of alternative approaches in AML patients with isolated trisomy 13 should be considered.

**Trisomy 8:** Trisomy 8 is the most common isolated trisomy noted in patients with AML. Despite this, there are limited data reporting the prognostic significance of this cytogenetic abnormality in adult patients with *de novo* AML. A total of 42 patients with isolated trisomy 8 (3.03%) were identified from five treatment studies performed by the CALGB [13] and treatment outcome reviewed relevant to other previously published reports related to this specific cytogenetic abnormality. Patients identified had a median age of 64 (range, 16–79) years with 81% being younger than 70 years old. There was an equivalent number of men and women and a low frequency of organomegaly. Classification of this group by FAB criteria revealed 2% M0, 26% M1, 19% M2, 21% M4, 14% M5, and 5% M6 with 7% of patients being unclassifiable. No patient with isolated trisomy 8 had FAB M3 or M7 morphology.

Treatment outcome for these patients with trisomy 8 was poor, with a CR rate of 59%. The median duration of remission was 13.5 months, with a 3 year Kaplan Meier estimate of continuous remission of only 16%. Of the four patients remaining in continuous CR, 3 had an autologous stem cell transplant in first CR. Treatment after relapse was ineffective, with all patients dying as a consequence of AML. The median survival for this whole group of patients was 13.1 months, with a 3-year Kaplan Meier estimate of survival of 17%.

Examination of the impact of age within this cytogenetic group demonstrated that older age adversely affected outcome. Specifically, the CR rate was 40% for those patients greater than the age of 60 as compared to 88% for those younger than 60 (p=0.004). Similarly, the overall median survival was only 4.8 months for those patients over the age of 60 as compared to 17.5 months for those younger than 60 years of age (p=0.01). There were no long-term survivors in the 25 trisomy 8 patients aged 60 and older as compared to 4 of the 17 patients younger than the age of 60. These findings demonstrate that few patients with isolated trisomy 8 and AML can expect long term disease-free survival with standard treatment approaches, thus providing support for exploring novel therapeutic approaches in both young and elderly AML patients with this abnormality.

**Trisomy 11:** Trisomy 11 is the third most frequent isolated trisomy noted in AML and is the only one for which a specific molecular defect has been identified. Work by CALGB investigators and other colleagues demonstrated that a partial tandem duplication of the MLL gene was present in 90% of patients with isolated trisomy 11. [14] Indeed, this represented the first identification of a specific gene rearrangement associated with a recurrent trisomy in human cancer. The clinical data related to 13 patients with isolated trisomy 11 have been reported by the CALGB. [15] Patients with trisomy 11 had a median age of 64 and a high predisposition to having FAB M1 or M2 AML. Outcome in this group was uniformly poor with all relapsing except for a single patient who underwent an allogeneic stem cell transplant in first CR. These findings provide support for exploring novel therapeutic approaches in both young and elderly AML patients with sole trisomy 11.

## Tandem Duplication of the MLL Gene Predicts For Poor Outcome in Patients with Normal Cytogenetics

Approximately 45% of patients with AML have normal cytogenetics which place them in an intermediate risk group when treated with high-dose cytarabine intensification as defined previously.[10] Identification of a molecular aberration in this group of patients that predicted for poor outcome would facilitate improved risk stratification and potentially allow molecularly targeted therapy. Caligiuri

and colleagues[14,16] were the first to demonstrate that a subset of patients without cytogenetic evidence of an 11q23 chromosomal translocation (with normal cytogenetics or sole trisomy 11) had a partial tandem duplication of the MLL gene. Examination of a larger cohort of 98 AML patients with normal cytogenetics revealed that 11 (11%) had evidence of this tandem duplication.[17] Seven of these patients were examined for trisomy 11 utilizing fluorescence *in situ* hybridization or comparative genomic hybridization which failed to demonstrate either evidence of +11 or DNA copy number changes suggestive of this abnormality.

Among the 98 AML patients with normal cytogenetics, the clinical features of the patients with the MLL rearrangement (MLL1+) were not different than those of patients without this abnormality. The MLL1+ patients had a median age of 41 years with nine patients being female. FAB criteria included two M1, six M2, and two M4. The CR rate for this group was 70% which did not differ from those patients without this abnormality. In contrast, remission duration was shorter (median 7.1 versus 23.2 months; p=0.01) with all but one of the MLL1+ patients relapsing. The overall survival for MLL+ patients was also shorter (13.8 versus 20.1 months; p=0.06). Investigation by CALGB investigators and others to elucidate the mechanism by which this partial tandem duplication contributes to the leukemogenesis and poor outcome of patients is ongoing. As this tandem duplication maintains an in frame reading sequence, it is possible that the resultant mRNA could be translated into a full length functional protein. Demonstration of such a finding could form the basis for developing anti-sense therapies for this target gene.

## Outcome for Specific Translocations in Acute Myeloid Leukemia

### AML Patients with t(9;11)(p22;q23) have a Superior Outcome Compared to Other

**Patients with Translocations involving Band 11q23:** The outcome of adult AML patients with translocations involving the 11q23 band has not been well described. Investigators in

CALGB sought to determine if outcome of adults with translocations involving the 11q23 band varied based on the partner chromosome (i.e. chromosome 9 or another chromosome) [18]. A total of 24 patients with t(9;11)(p22;q23) and 23 patients with other 11q23 translocations were identified from patients enrolled on the prospective cytogenetic study CALGB 8461. The clinical features between these two groups of patients were similar, except patients with t(9;11)(p22;q23) had both a higher frequency of M5 morphology (83% versus 43%; p=0.006) and higher frequency of secondary abnormalities involving chromosome 8 (46% versus 9%; p=0.008). Of note, the leukocyte count was elevated above 50 x 10⁹/L in 33% and 43% of patients with t(9;11)(p22;q23) and other 11q23 translocations, respectively.

Examination of treatment outcome between the two groups revealed patients with t(9;11)(p22;q23) have an improved outcome as compared to those with other 11q23 translocations. The CR rate was similar (79% versus 57%; p=0.13) but remission duration (median 10.7 months versus 8.9 months; p=0.02) and overall survival (median 13.2 months versus 7.7 months; p=0.009) were superior for those patients with t(9;11) (p22;q23). Examination of treatment outcome relative to intensity of post-remission therapy in the patients with t(9;11)(p22;q23) was informative. All seven of those patients not receiving high-dose cytarabine or stem cell transplantation as part of their post-remission therapy have relapsed. In contrast, of the 11 patients receiving stem cell transplant (n=2) or intensification therapies including high-dose cytarabine therapy or high-dose cytarabine combined with other therapies (n=9), seven remain in continuous first remission. –

All 13 of the patients with other 11q23 translocations have relapsed, including seven who received intensification including high-dose cytarbine therapy or high dose cytarabine combined with other therapies. In summary, these findings demonstrate that adult patients with AML and the t(9;11)(p22;q23) have an improved outcome when compared to patients with other 11q23 translocations and may be cured with intensive high-dose cytarabine and etoposide-based therapies.

**Impact of Secondary Cytogenetic Abnormalities in Patients with t(15;17)(q22;q11-12) and t(9;11)(p22;q23):** A variety of common translocations in *de novo* AML, including t(15;17)(q22;q11-12), t(9;11)(p22;q23), and t(8;21)(q22;q22), have secondary chromosomal changes that include addition of a whole chromosome or another secondary abnormality. Examination of the prognostic significance of secondary chromosomal changes in specific subsets of AML patients has been limited to date. In two separate papers reported by the CALGB, the prognostic significance of secondary abnormalities for both patients with t(9;11)(p22;q23) and t(15;17) (q22;q11-12) was examined [18,19]. In patients with the t(9;11)(p22;q23) [18] where trisomy 8 was the most frequent secondary abnormality, no clinical feature was associated with this or any other secondary abnormality. Furthermore, no difference in treatment outcome was appreciated among patients who possessed secondary abnormalities as compared to those with the isolated translocation.

For the 161 patients enrolled on CALGB 8461 with the t(15;17)(q22;q11-12), the frequency of secondary cytogenetic abnormalities was 32% with abnormalities involving chromosome 8 being the most frequent [19]. Presenting clinical features among the patients with and without secondary cytogenetic abnormalities were similar. Examination of PML/RAR· isoform type in 56 patients demonstrated a high predisposition for developing secondary cytogenetic abnormalities among the S isoform type (12 of 20; 60% of patients) as compared to those with the L isoform (4 of 32; 12.5%) (p<0.001). Patients with t(15;17)(q22;q11-12) and secondary abnormalities had a similar CR rate and overall survival when compared to those with sole t(15;17)(q22;q11-12). Surprisingly, the event free survival was superior (17 months versus 12.2 months; p=0.03) for patients with t(15;17)(q22;q11-12) and secondary abnormalities as compared to those with t(15;17)(q22;q11-12) alone. Examination of the impact of secondary cytogenetic abnormalities in other cytogenetic groups is planned. Data published by the CALGB thus far suggest that secondary abnormalities do not impact on the long-term outcome of AML patients with t(15;17)(q22;q11-12) or t(9;11) (p22;q23) translocations.

**Outcome in t(8;21)(q22;q22) Patients Varies by Presence of Extramedullary Leukemia and Blast Expression of CD56:** Patients with AML and the t(8;21)(q22;q22) translocation are young and have a high frequency of attaining a CR with standard induction therapy. Long-term outcome of these patients has improved markedly with the introduction of post-remission high-dose cytarabine, with the 5-year disease-free survival being 78% [10,20]. However, a proportion of these patients fail to attain a first remission or relapse and die as consequence of their leukemia. Recent reports by the CALGB have identified both extramedullary disease at presentation [21] and blast expression of CD56 [22] as predictors of poor outcome in this favorable cytogenetic group.

In the first report, [21] 84 consecutive patients with t(8;21)(q22;q22) enrolled on the prospective cytogenetic study CALGB 8461 were examined. Of these patients, 8 (9.5%) possessed extramedullary leukemia at diagnosis including granulocytic sarcomas (paraspinal, n=5; breast, n=1; and subcutaneous, n=1) or symptomatic meningeal leukemia (n=1). The pre-treatment clinical variables between patients with and without extramedullary leukemia were similar. The CR rate (50% versus 92%; p=0.006) was significantly lower for those patients with extramedullary leukemia at diagnosis, and overall survival was similarly shorter (median 5.4 months versus 59.5 months; p=0.002). This poor outcome in patients with t(8;21) with extramedullary leukemia may have related to inadequate local therapy directed at spinal or meningeal leukemia which resulted in recurrent extramedullary leukemia at time of relapse (n=2) or permanent neurologic deficits (n=4) thus predisposing to other infectious related complications. Examination of the impact of high-dose cytarabine on this group of patients was not possible as only one patient with extramedullary leukemia was assigned to this post-remission therapy and remains in continuous CR at 74.7 months. In summary, these data suggest that patients with t(8;21)(q22;q22) may have a higher predisposition to developing extramedullary leukemia, especially paraspinal disease. Given the poor outcome observed, aggressive local and systemic therapy should be considered for this subset of patients. The effectiveness of high-dose cytarabine therapy in t(8;21) patients with extramedullary leukemia is uncertain, and warrants further study.

In the second study, [22] CALGB investigators examined if expression of CD56 (neural cell adhesion molecule) was associated with poor outcome in patients with t(8;21) (q22;q22). This study was initiated based upon the fact that CD56 had been previously associated with both extramedullary disease and multidrug resistance in acute leukemia and was frequently expressed in patients with t(8;21)(q22;q22). A total of 29 consecutive patients who were enrolled on both the prospective CALGB cytogenetic study CALGB 8461 and the CALGB immunophenotyping study CALGB 8361 had CD56 blast expression assessment performed. Of these 29 patients, 16 (55%) demonstrated blast expression of CD56. Pre-treatment clinical features were similar for CD56 positive and CD56 negative patients. Two of the 16 patients with CD56 blast expression had extramedullary leukemia as compared to no patients whose blasts failed to express this antigen. The CR rate was similar for patients whose blasts did and did not express CD56 (88% versus 92%; p=1.0). However, disease-free (median 8.7 months versus not reached; p=0.01) and overall survival (median 16.5 months versus not reached; p=0.008) was shorter for patients with blast expression of CD56. Although these results are based on a small number of patients and will require confirmation by other groups, they suggest that patients with t(8;21) (q22;q22) who have blast expression of CD56 may have a poor outcome.

**Treatment Outcome in t(8;21)(q22;q22) Patients Varies by Number of Cycles of High-Dose Cytarabine Treatment:** A recently reported study by the CALGB[23] examined the effect of single compared to repetitive (at least 3) cycles of high-dose cytarabine post-induction therapy for AML patients with the t(8;21)(q22;q22) karyotype. Patients included in this study were those with AML and t(8;21) who attained a CR on four successive CALGB studies. These studies either administered ≥ 3 cycles of high-dose cytarabine or one cycle of high-dose cytarabine followed by sequential cyclophosphamide/etoposide and mitoxantrone/diaziquone/filgrastim. Clinical characteristics and outcome of these two groups of t(8;21) patients were compared. Of 50 patients with centrally reviewed AML and t(8;21), 29 were assigned to receive one and 21 to ≥ 3 cycles of high-dose cytarabine as postinduction therapy. The clinical features of these two groups of patients were similar. Initial remission duration for t(8;21) patients assigned to one cycle of high-dose cytarabine was significantly inferior (p=0.016), with 62% of patients relapsing with a median disease-free survival of 10.4 months, as compared to those patients receiving ≥ 3 cycles where only 19% have relapsed and disease-free survival is estimated to be greater than 28 months. Furthermore, overall survival was also significantly compromised (p=0.028) in patients assigned to one cycle of high-dose cytarabine, with 59% having died as a consequence of AML as compared to 24% in those receiving ≥ 3 cycles of high-dose cytarabine. These data demonstrate that disease-free survival and overall survival of patients with t(8;21)(q22;q22) may be compromised by treatment approaches that do not include sequential high-dose cytarabine therapy, emphasizing the importance of cytogenetically stratified treatment in AML.

## Conclusions and Future Directions

Prospective cytogenetics studies over the past 15 years in AML patients have yielded many new findings that are now being translated into approaches that stratify treatment. In addition, refinement of molecular techniques are now allowing transition from stratifying post-remission therapy based upon morphologic or classical cytogenetic findings to one involving confirmation of the specific molecular defect. An example of this is risk stratified therapy based upon identification of the fusion transcript in patients with t(8;21)(q22;q22) and inv(16)(p13q22) and t(16;16)(p13;q22) concurrent with cytogenetics that is currently being performed by the CALGB as part of a prospective clinical treatment trial in untreated adults with de novo AML. [11] Similarly, utilization of new techniques such as those described by Marcucci

and colleagues may allow determination of what constitutes a sufficient amount of minimal residual disease following therapy to predict relapse. [24] These advances in the biology combined with new therapies directed specifically at molecular defects in the leukemia cells will hopefully improve the outcome of adult patients with AML.

## References

1. Bennett JM, Catovsky D, Daniel MT, Flandrin G, Galton DAG, Gralnick HR, Sultan C. Proposed revised criteria for the classification of acute myeloid leukemia: A report of the French-American-British Cooperative Group. Ann Intern Med 103: 626–629, 1985.
2. Mayer RJ, Davis RB, Schiffer CA, Berg DT, Powell BL, Schulman P, Omura GA, Moore JO, McIntyre OR, Frei E. Intensive postremission chemotherapy in adults with acute myeloid leukemia. N Engl J Med 331: 896–903, 1994.
3. Moore JO, Dodge RK, Amrein PC, Kolitz J, Lee EJ, Powell B, Godfrey S, Robert F, Schiffer CA: Granulocyte-colony stimulating factor accelerates granulocyte recovery after intensive postremission chemotherapy for acute myeloid leukemia with aziridinyl benzoquinone and mitoxantrone: Cancer and Leukemia Group B Study 9022. Blood 89: 780–788, 1997.
4. Moore JO, Powell B, Velez-Garcia E, Kolitz J, George S, Dodge R, Rizzieri DA, Schiffer C: A comparison of sequential non-cross resistant therapy or Ara-C consolidation following complete remission in adult patients < 60 years with acute myeloid leukemia: CALGB 9222. Proc Am Soc Clin Oncol 16:14a, 1997 (abstr)
5. Mayer RJ, Schiffer CA, Petterson BA, Silver RT, Cornwell GG, McIntyre OR, Rai KR, Budman DR, Ellison RR, Maguire M, Davis RB, Frei E III: Intensive postremission therapy in adults with acute nonlymphocytic leukemia using various dose schedules of Ara-C: A progress report from the CALGB. Semin Oncol 14 (Suppl. 1): 25–31, 1987.
6. Stone RM, Berg DT, George SL, Dodge RK, Paciucci PA, Schulman P, Lee EJ, Moore JO, Powell BL, Schiffer CA. Granulocyte-macrophage colony-stimulating factor after initial chemotherapy for elderly patients with primary acute myelogenous leukemia. N Eng J Med 331: 1671–1677, 1995.
7. ISCN (1995): An international system for human cytogenetic nomenclature, Mitelman F (ed); S. Karger, Basel 1995.
8. Cheson BD, Cassileth PA, Head DR, Schiffer CA, Bennett JM, Bloomfield CD, Brunning R, Gale RP, Grever MR, Keating MJ, Sawitsky A, Stass S, Weinstein H, Woods W. Report of the National Cancer Institute– sponsored workshop on definitions of diagnosis and response in acute myelogenous leukemia. J Clin Oncol 8: 813–819, 1990.
9. Bloomfield CD, Lawerence D, Arthur DC, Berg DT, Schiffer CA, Mayer RJ: Curative impact of intensification with high-dose cyarabine in acute

myeloid leukemia varies by cytogenetic group. Blood 84:111a, 1994 (abstr).

10. Bloomfield CD, Lawrence DL, Byrd JC, Carroll A, Pettenati MJ, Tantravahi R, Patil SR, Davey FR, Berg DT, Schiffer CA, Arthur DC, Mayer, RJ: Frequency of prolonged remission duration following high-dose cytarabine intensification in acute myeloid leukemia varies by cytogenetic subtype. Cancer Res 58: 4173–4179, 1998.

11. Mrózek K, Prior TW, Edwards C, Snyder PJ, Carroll AJ, Koduru PRK, Pettenati MJ, Archer KJ, Caligiuri MA, Kolitz J, Larson RA, Bloomfield CD. A comparison of cytogenetic and molecular genetic detection of t(8;21)(q22;q22) and inv(16)(p13q22) in adults with de novo acute myeloid leukemia (AML): A Cancer and Leukemia Group B (CALGB) study. Blood 92: 77a, 1998 (abstr).

12. Döhner H, Arthur DC, Ball ED, Sobol RE, Davey FR, Lawrence D, Gordon L, Patil SR, Surana RB, Testa JR, Verma RS, Schiffer CA, Wurster-Hill DH, Bloomfield CD. Trisomy 13: A new recurring chromosome abnormality in acute leukemia. Blood 76: 1614–1621, 1990.

13. Byrd JC, Lawrence D, Arthur DC, Pettenati MJ, Tantravahi R, Qumsiyeh M, Stamberg J, Davey FR, Schiffer CA, Bloomfield CD. Patients with trisomy 8 in acute myeloid leukemia are not cured with cytarabine-based chemotherapy: Results from Cancer and Leukemia Group B 8461. Clin Cancer Res 4: 1235–1241, 1998.

14. Caligiuri MA, Strout MP, Schichman SA, Mrózek K, Arthur DC, Herzig GP, Baer MR, Schiffer CA, Heinonen K, Knuutila S, Nousiainen T, Ruutu T, Block AW, Pedersen-Bjergaard J, Croce CM, Bloomfield CD. Partial tandem duplication of ALL1 as a recurrent molecular defect in acute myeloid leukemia with trisomy 11. Cancer Res 56: 1418–1425, 1996.

15. Heinonen K, Mrózek K, Lawrence D, Arthur DC, Pettenati MJ, Stamberg J, Qumsiyeh MB, Verma RS, MacCallum J, Schiffer CA, Bloomfield CD: Clinical characteristics of patients with de novo acute myeloid leukaemia and isolated trisomy 11: a Cancer and Leukemia Group B study. Br J Haematol 101: 513–520, 1998.

16. Caligiuri MA, Schichman SA, Strout MP, Mrózek K, Baer MR, Frankel SR, Barcos M, Herzig GP, Croce CM, Bloomfield CD. Molecular rearrangement of the ALL-1 gene in acute myeloid leukemia without cytogenetic evidence of 11q23 chromosomal translocations. Cancer Res 54: 370–373, 1994.

17. Caligiuri MA, Strout MP, Lawrence D, Arthur DC, Baer MR, Feng Y, Knuutila S, Mrózek K, Oberkircher AR, Marcucci G, de la Chapelle A, Elonen E, Block AM, Rao PN, Herzig GP, Powell BL, Ruutu T,

Schiffer CA, Bloomfield CD: Rearrangement of ALL1 (MLL) in acute myeloid leukemia with normal cytogenetics. Cancer Res 58: 55–59, 1998.

18. Mrózek K, Heinonen K, Lawrence D, Carroll AJ, Koduru PRK, Rao KW, Strout MP, Hutchison RE, Moore JO, Mayer RJ, Schiffer CA, Bloomfield CD. Adult patients with de novo acute myeloid leukemia and t(9;11)(p22;q23) have a superior outcome to patients with other translocations involving band 11q23: A Cancer and Leukemia Group B Study. Blood 90: 4532–4538, 1997.

19. Slack JL, Arthur DC, Lawrence D, Mrózek K, Mayer RJ, Davey FR, Tantravahi R, Pettenati MJ, Bigner S, Carroll AJ, Rao KW, Schiffer CA, Bloomfield CD. Secondary cytogenetic changes in acute promyelocytic leukemia–Prognostic importance in patients treated with chemotherapy alone and association with the intron 3 breakpoint of the PML gene: A Cancer and Leukemia Group B Study. J Clin Oncol 15: 1786–1795, 1997.

20. Bloomfield CD, Shuma C, Regal L, Philip PP, Hossfeld DK, Hagemeijer AM, Garson OM, Peterson BA, Sakurai M, Alimena G, Berger R, Rowley JD, Ruutu T, Mitelman F, Dewald GW, Swansbury J: Long-term survival of patients with acute myeloid leukemia. Cancer 80: 2191–2198, 1997.

21. Byrd JC, Weiss RB, Arthur DC, Lawrence D, Baer MR, Davey F, Trikha ES, Carroll AJ, Tantravahi R, Qumsiyeh M, Patil SR, Moore JO, Mayer RJ, Schiffer CA, Bloomfield CD: Extramedullary leukemia adversely affects hematologic complete remission rate and overall survival in patients with t(8;21)(q22;q22): Results from the Cancer and Leukemia Group B 8461. J Clin Oncol 15:466–475, 1997.

22. Baer MR, Stewart CC, Lawrence D, Arthur DC, Byrd JC, Davey FR, Schiffer CA, Bloomfield CD. Expression of the neural cell adhesion molecule CD56 is associated with short remission duration and survival in acute myeloid leukemia with t(8;21)(q22;q22). Blood 90:1643–1650, 1997.

23. Byrd JC, Dodge R, Carroll A, Baer MR, Edwards C, Stamberg J, Qumsiyeh M, Moore JO, Mayer RJ, Schiffer CA, Bloomfield CA. Patients with t(8;21)(q22;q22) and acute myeloid leukemia have a superior disease-free and overall survival when repetitive cycles of high-dose cytarabine are administered. J Clin Oncol 17:3767–3775, 1999.

24. Marcucci G, Livak KJ, Bi W, Strout MP, Bloomfield CD, Caligiuri MA. Detection of minimal residual disease in patients with AML1/ETO-associated acute myeloid leukemia using a novel quantitative reverse transcription polymerase chain reaction assay. Leukemia 12: 1482–1489, 1998

456

# The Impact of Treatment on the Outcome of Cytogenetic Subgroups in Acute Myeloid Leukemia – Results of the German AML Cooperative Group

W. Hiddemann and T. Büchner for the AMLCG

## Introduction

In recent years, the prognosis of patients with acute myeloid leukemia (AML) has gradually increased. This development results particularly from the intensification of therapy both during induction and postremission. A major component of intensification was the introduction of high-dose cytosine-arabinoside (HD Ara-C) which proved superior to conventional dose treatment in several prospective randomized trials [1–4].

In addition to intensification of therapy, the definition of cytogenetic subgroups had a major impact on defining subgroups of patients with different prognoses. Based on cytogenetics, three different subgroups of patients can be discriminated anticipating a favorable, intermediate, or poor prognosis [5–7]. A pending and still unanswered question is in how far cytogenetics and the underlying biology are independent determinants of overall outcome or whether treatment may influence the prognostic significance of karyotype abnormalities. This question was addressed as part of the AMLCG study 92 which applied double induction therapy randomly assigning patients to either the sequence of TAD-TAD or TAD-HAM [8].

## Patients, Material and Methods

### Treatment protocol

The AMLCG study 92 comprised the prospective randomized comparison of double induction therapy randomly assigning patients below 60 years of age either to TAD9-TAD9 or TAD9 followed by HAM as second induction course (Figure 1).

TAD 9 consisted of cytosine-arabinoside (AraC) 100 mg/m² per day by a four hour continuous infusion followed by short-term infusions of 100 mg/m² Ara-C q12 hours from days 3–8, daunorubicine 60 mg/m² per day from day 3 – 5 and 6 thioguanine 200 mg/m² per day orally from day 3 to 9. HAM comprised HD Ara-C 3 g/m² q 12 hours from days 1 – 3 and mitoxantrone 10 mg/m² per day by 30 minute infusion on days 3 – 5.

Patients achieving a complete remission obtained one additional TAD9 course for consolidation followed by monthly maintenance for three years comprising a sequence of Ara-C / daunorubicine, Ara-C / thioguanine, Ara-C / cyclophosphamide, Ara-C / thioguanine etc.

## Cytogenetics

Cytogenetic analysis was performed by G-banding following conventional preparation techniques. For the association with clinical

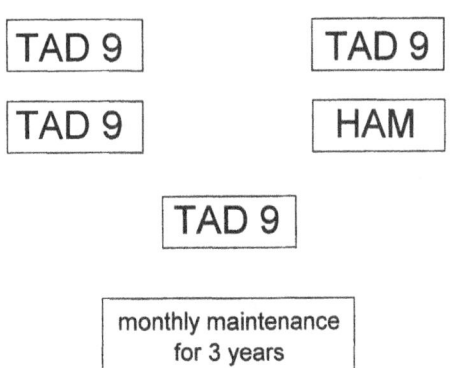

**Fig. 1.** German AML Cooperative Group Double Induction Therapy in Patients ≤60 Years

outcome and therapeutic response patients were grouped into categories of favorable karyotypes comprising t(8;21), t(15;17) and inv [16]. Patients with an unfavorable karyotype were defined as having complex karyotype abnormalities or numeric aberrations including −5,5q-, -7,7q-, +8, t(9;11) and t(6;9). Patients with a normal karyotype and other karyotypic abnormalities were considered to represent the subgroup of intermediate prognosis.

## Statistical analysis

Comparisons between two independent variables were carried out by the chi-square test and the students' t-test.

The study was approved by the local ethical committees at the participating institutions and adhered to the updated declaration of Helsinki

## Results

A total of 704 patients entered the study from 29 participating institutions in Germany. The

**Table 1.** German AML Cooperative Group: Double Induction Therapy in Patients ≤ 60 Years.

|    | Total | | TAD/TAD | | TAD/HAM | |
|----|-------|--|---------|--|---------|--|
| n  | 704 | (100%) | 347 | (100%) | 357 | (100%) |
| CR | 483 | (69%) | 228 | (66%) | 255 | (71%) |
| NR | 146 | (20%) | 77 | (22%) | 69 | (19%) |
| ED | 75 | (11%) | 42 | (12%) | 33 | (10%) |

overall response rate was 69 % complete remissions (CR), 20 % of patients were non-responders (NR) and 11 % of cases died during the treatment period and were considered as early deaths (ED). Analysis of the two double-induction arms indicated a slightly higher response rate for the TAD-HAM sequence which was not statistically significant however (Table 1, Figure 2). The global analysis of all patients according to the defined cytogenetic subgroups revealed a significant increase particularly in non-responders in patients with unfavorable karyotypes as compared to favorable cytogenetics and a corresponding decrease in the rate of complete remissions (Table 2). A more detailed evaluation according to the type of treatment however revealed striking differences bet-

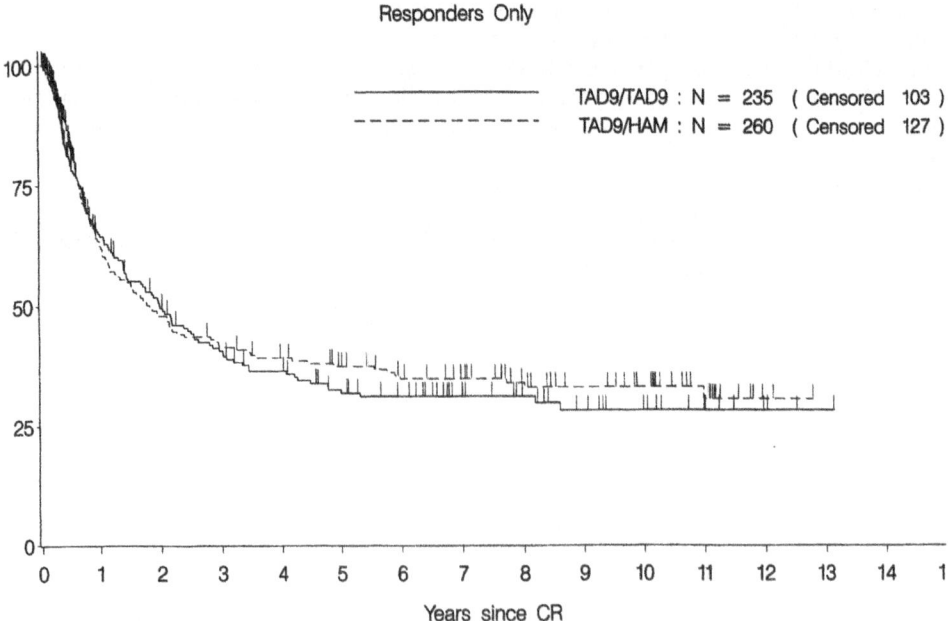

Responders Only

TAD9/TAD9 : N = 235 ( Censored 103 )
TAD9/HAM : N = 260 ( Censored 127 )

Years since CR

**Fig. 2**

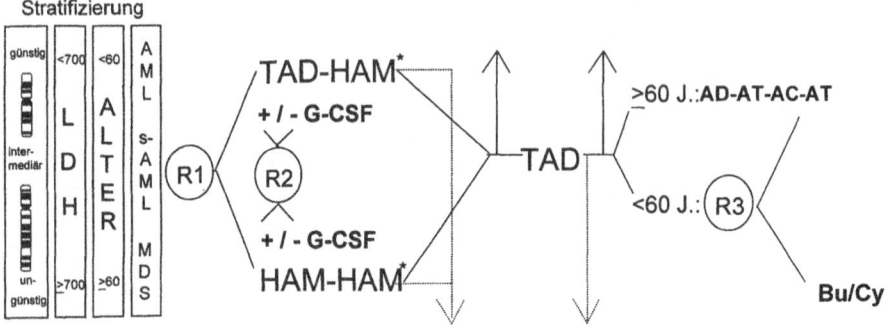

**Fig. 4**

demonstrating a beneficial effect of high-dose Ara-C when applied during post-remission treatment (10). This beneficial effect was in contrast to the data from AMLCG particularly prominent in patients with good prognostic karyotypes. From the currently available data it can be concluded that biology and therapy are both of influence on treatment outcome and prognosis and must be considered as non-independent variables on clinical results. Further analyses are certainly needed to identify the most appropriate treatment for distinct cytogenetic subgroups which are best gained from well designed prospective randomized evaluations. Hence, in the current AMLCG study cytogenetics are used for treatment stratification to assess the impact of priming with G-CSF, intensification of induction therapy by comparing the new standard of TAD-HAM with HAM-HAM and finally by analyzing the therapeutic value of myeloablative chemotherapy followed by blood stem cell transplantation (Figure 4).

# References

1. Hoyle CF, de Bastos M, Wheatley K, et al. (1989) AML assiciated with previous cytotoxic therapy. MDS or myelo-proliferative disorders: results from the MRC's 9th AML trial. British Journal of Haematology 72:45 – 53.
2. Bishop JF, Matthews JP, Young GA et al. (1996) A randomized study of high-dose cytarabine in induction in acute myeloid leukemia. Blood 87: 1710 – 7

3. Weick JK, Kopecky KJ, Appelbaum FR et al. (1996) A randomized investigation of high-dose versus standard dose cytosine arabinoside with daunorubicin in patients with previously untreated acute myeloid leukemia: A Southwest Oncology Study Group. Blood 88:2841 – 51.
4. Mayer RJ, Davis RB, Schiffer CA et al. (1994) Intensive postremission chemotherapy in adults with acute myeloid leukemia. New England Journal of Medicine 6:896 – 942.
5. Rigal F, Stoppa A-M, Marit G, Molina L, Michallet M., Maraninchi D, Attal M, and Reiffers J. (1995) Prognostic significance of karyotype in de novo adult acute myelogenous leukemia. Leukemia (Baltimore) 9: 1491 – 1498
6. Mrózek K, Heinonen K, de la Chapelle A et al. (1997) Clinical significance of cytogenetics in acute myeloid leukemia. Semin. Oncol. 24: 17 – 31
7. Stasi R, Del Poeta G, Masi M et al. (1993) Incidence of chromosome abnormalities and clinical significance of karyotype in de novo acute myeloid leukemia. Cancer Genet. Cytogenet. 167: 28 – 34
8. Büchner T, Hiddemann W, Löffler H et al (1994) Double induction strategy in AML comparing high with standard dose AraC. Hematotoxicity and antileukemic efficiacy. Blood, 84 Suppl 1: 232a
9. Büchner T, Hiddemann W, Wörmann B et al. (1999) Double induction strategy for acute myeloid leukemia: The effect of high-dose cytarabine with mitoxantrone instead of standard-dose cytarabine with daunorubicin and 6-thioguanine. A randomized trial by the German AML Cooperative Group. Blood 93: 4116–24
10. Bloomfield C, Lawrence D, Byrd J et al. (1998) Frequency of prolonged remission duration after high-dose cytarabine intensification in acute myeloid leukemia varies by cytogenetic subtype. Cancer Research 58; 4173–4179

# High Dose Cytosine Arabinoside Combined with an Anthracycline as Remission Induction in Acute Myeloid Leukemia

S. Fekete and S. Lueff

Beside the better supportive care the substantial improvement reached in the treatment of AML is due to the intensified chemotherapy. This approach can be used as conditioning in transplant setting, early in the postremission period (4), as a double induction (2) or upfront as proposed among others by James Bishop [1].

In the present paper we summarize our results and discuss the experience gained with high-dose cytosine arabinoside combined with an anthracyclin given in standard dose as an induction therapy.

## Patients

Twenty two newly diagnosed AML patients all under 55 were included (Table 1. ). No patient with myelodysplastic related or secondary AML were excluded, only a few with serious organ failure or significant comorbidity. The diagnosis of AML was based on morphological and immunological data and in every case an efford was made to get evaluable cytogenetical information (Karyotyping of minimum 20 mitoses with G-banding were performed).

Less than 5% of blasts in the bone marrow and no blasts in the blood, irrespective of the normalisation of blood cell counts satisfied the criteria of CR in our study.

The survival data which was analysed by Kaplan-Meier method.

The side effects were evaluated according the WHO classification.

**Table 1.** Patients' characteristics

| Patient No | Male/ Female | Age years | FAB | Cytogenetics | Previous MDS |
|---|---|---|---|---|---|
| 1 | M | 30 | M7 | 46,XY | no |
| 2 | M | 41 | M2 | 46,XY | no |
| 3 | F | 47 | M2 | 46,XY | yes |
| 4 | M | 44 | M4 | 48,XY, -4,del(11q),+8+21+M | yes |
| 5 | F | 35 | M1 | 46,XY | no |
| 6 | M | 39 | M2 | 46,XY | yes |
| 7 | M | 52 | M2 | 46,X,t(8;21) | no |
| 8 | F | 42 | M2 | 46,XX,t(8;21) | no |
| 9 | F | 36 | M2 | 46,XX | no |
| 10 | M | 45 | M4 | 46,XY | no |
| 11 | F | 53 | M4 | 46,XY | no |
| 12 | M | 20 | M5 | 46,XY | no |
| 13 | F | 25 | M4 | 46,XXt(6;11), complex abnormality | no |
| 14 | M | 50 | M2 | 46,XY,-3,del(5),+8,del(12) | yes |
| 15 | M | 39 | M4 | unsuccessfull | no |
| 16 | M | 51 | M5 | 46,XY | no |
| 17 | M | 18 | M4Eo | 46,XY,inv16 | no |
| 18 | M | 47 | M4 | 46,XY | no |
| 19 | M | 40 | M0 | 46,XY | no |
| 20 | M | 28 | M5 | 46,XY | no |
| 21 | M | 47 | M1 | 46,XY,inv(9), del 18 | yes |
| 22 | F | 25 | M2 | 46,XX | yes |

## Treatment

Ara-C 2–3 g twice a day on the first, 3rd, 5th and 7th day combined with 45mg/m² daunorubicine or 12mg/m² idarubicin on the day 1–3 in short infusion was the induction therapy. In CR high dose ara-C monotherapy similar to the CALGB protocoll (4) was applied two-, three- or maximum four times and no further treatment were given. In cases of less than CR after the first cycle the induction treatment was repeated once and followed HD-ara-C monotherapy or a different type of salvage therapy accoring its efficacy.

## Results

17/22 patients reached CR after one cycle of HD-ara-C + anthracyline therapy. The median of relapse free survival is not reached yet because all patients except four are living in their first remission (a median follow up of 20 months) (Fig. 1). The patients who went to remission only after the second cycle relapsed more likely and belonged into an unfavorable prognostic group ( secondary cases and unfavourable kariotype ).

During the induction phase only 1 of 22 patients died. The early death of this patient was not connected with the leukaemic process itself nor to the type of treatment.

The analyses of side effects showed neither more frequent nor more serious than those experienced in connection with standard dose chemotherapy. Hematological recovery made the continuation of the treatment possible after maximum of 34 days. Fortunately no CNS side effect was seen in this patient population. Most patients in remission continue their original work.

## Discussion

This paper summarizes our treatment experiencies using HD-ara-C combined with an anthracycline upfront in induction of a relatively younger AML patient population. These patients would be ideal candidates for allogeneic BMT, being young and healthy enough, without significant comorbidity and organ dysfunction, but they had no potential or -as later revealed- suitable sibling donors.

Because of the limited number of patients, the different doses of cytosine arabinoside and type of anthracycline used as well as the lack of randomisation our data are not suitable to draw any firm conclusion, still our impression was -as it was recently demonstrated (3) – that high dose chemotherapy can produce at least as good therapautic resuslts as BMT does. In this context we would like to stress the relatively short period of treatment,

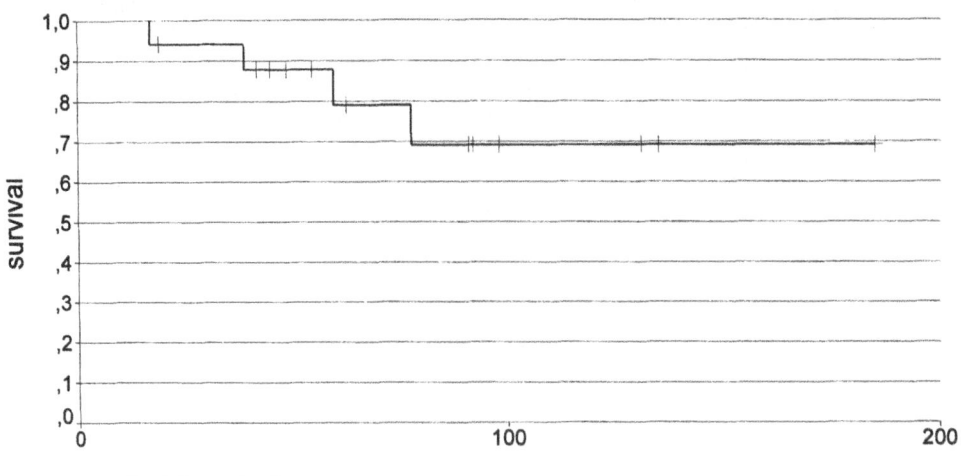

**Fig. 1.** Disease-free survival of 17 complete responders

the acceptable number and severity of side effects, the excellent quality of life and durable relapse free survival (median not reached) among patients who reached CR after the first induction cycle.

## References

1. Bishop JF et al (1996) A randomized study of high-dose cytarabine in induction in acute myeloid leukemia. Blood 87:1710–1717.
2. Büchner T et al. (1994) Double induction in AML comparing high with standard dose ara-C. Hematotoxicity and antileukemic efficacy. Blood 84 (Suppl 1) 232a
3. Cassileth PA et al (1998) Chemotherapy compared with autologous or allogeneic bone marrow transplantation in the management of acute leukemia in first remission N Engl J Med 339:1649–1656.
4. Mayer RJ et al (1994) Intensive postremission chemotherapy in adults with acute myeloid leukemia N Engl J Med 331: 896–903.

# Comparison of the Efficacy of TAD–TAD and "7+3"Regimens in Adult AML, the Role of Dose Intensity and Mdr-1 Gene Expression

A.Zaritskey[1,2], N.Anikina[2], N.Medvedeva[2], O.Marinets[1], Yu.Ogorodnikova[1], T.Bykova[1], O.Frolova[1], L.Peskina[4], A.Klimovitch[2], T.Zabelina[1], L.Zoubarovskaya[1], E.Kuchinskaya[3] and B.Afanasiev[1]

*Abstract.* The combination of ARA-C and anthracyclines is a stantard for AML treatment. Although addition of another drugs, dose intensification are unequivocal. Prognostic significance of mdr-1 gene expression and its protein product still remains doubtful according to prognosis of adult AML patients.

The aims of the study were comparison of survival data of patients treated with TAD–TAD or "7+3" regimens with impact of the role of dose reduction and mdr–1 gene expression. The predominance of patients were of intermediate cytogenetic prognostic group. It appeared that EFS, CCR, DFS were superior in patients treated by TAD–TAD in comparison to "7+3". AutoBMT did not improve the results of survival. Reduction of dose intensity resulted in inferior results. Mdr-1 gene expression in de novo patients had no impact on their survival. Although its expression in remission may be a marker of following relapse.

Conclusion. TAD–TAD regimen is superior to "7+3" in OS, EFS, and CCR. AutoBMT in first remission does not improve these data. Mdr-1 gene expression in de novo patients has no prognostic significance, although may a marker of forthcoming relapse.

## Introduction

There are a lot of novel variants of treatment of adult AML. All of them remain to be based on standard combinations of Ara-C and different anthracyclines [1, 2, 3]. Most of new programs are based on the use of newly developed anthracyclines [3, 4, 5]. Meanwhile combination of Ara-C and daunorubicine appeared to be a golden standard. Addition of etoposide [6, 7] or thioguanine [1] to this combination may significantly improve the results. Increase of dose intensity [2,3,8] due to shortened intervals between cycles of chemotherapy appeared to become a new approach to the treatment of AML (TAD-TAD, TAD-HAM). According to the recent data TAD-HAM has advantage only in poor cytogenetic group – complex abnormalities of chromosomes 5 and 7 [9]. Moreover, it was shown the –5, –7 chromosome aberrations had adverse effect only in case of preceding hematological abnormalities (10). Autologous hematopoietic cell transplantation in first remission, as a tool of early intensification, is being actively discussed (11). Another approach to obtain better results in treatment is the use of modifiers of mdr-1 gene activity (12) which is expressed in some de novo AML patients (13–15). Although the prognostic significance of mdr-1 gene expression in primary AML is controversial (12, 16). The aim of the study was the comparison of the results of TAD-TAD and "7+3" treatment, the role of reduced dose intensity and prognostic significance of mdr-1 gene expression.

## Patients and methods

53 primary AML patients were included in the study (age 17–68). Standard treatment

Centre of Haematology and BMT Department, StPsb. State Medical University[1],
Centre for Advanced Medical Technologies[2],
Health Committee of StPetersburg[3] Administration, St. Petersburg, Inst. of Pediatric Haematology, Moscow[4],
Russia

comprised "7+3" (19 patients), TAD-TAD with maintenance (22 patients). Nonstandard treatment (reduced dose intensity due to decrease of doses, number of cycles, and prolongation of periods between cycles) – 12 patients. Patients undergone autotransplantation were censored at the time of transplantation. Autologous transplantation was performed in 7 patients in first early remission.

Cytogenetic studies were done in 27 patients by routine and G-banding methods. The results were stratified according to cytogenetic prognostic score [9,11].

Mdr-1 gene expression was studied by in situ hybridization [17]. CD34-positive blast cells were counted by immunofluorescense with appropriate antibodies.

Statistics.Survival analysis was estimated by Kaplan and Meier [18], using log-rank test. Fisher exact test and chi-square were also used [19].

## Results and discussions

### Patient characteristics

Patients in the studied groups did not differ in their age ("7+3" – 15–68, mean 41.4, TAD-TAD – 17–55, mean 36.8, nonstandard group –16–68, mean 45.8, p > 0.05). There were no difference in the number of CD34-positive blast cells in these groups(p>0.05). The predominant FAB subtype was M4-5 – 60%. In the group of nonstandard therapy cytogenetics was performed only in two patients, both were of intermediate prognosis. In "7+3" group 7/8 of cytogenetically studied patients

belonged to intermediate prognosis, one had fafourable cytogenetics. 13/14 of TAD-TAD treated patients were of intermediate prognostic group, 1 had unfavourable cytogenetics: –5, –7, 5q+, +21, +22, +14, 6q+, 3q–. The latter patient was resistant to standard and intensified programs of treatment.

3 patients with favourable cytogenetics (8,21 translocation) and 1 with unfavourable(Ph+) were involved in another clinical trials. The latter patient was successfully treated by "7+3",followed by maintenance according to Buechner [2] – survival 7..5+ years.

### Comparison of the results of TAD-TAD and "7+3" regimens

CR rate on both regimens was comparable(90% and 72%, Chi square p= 0.08). Thereafter we have compared the postremission period in these groups. CCR appeared to be superior in patients treated by TAD-TAD(Fig. 1, p < 0.05). The difference was significant only in M1-2 subtypes (Fig. 2), whereas no difference was revealed in M4-5 subtypes(p=0.44). The peculiarity of M4-5 patients treated with TAD-TAD was CNS relapse(2/4 patients). So, CNS prophilactic treatment in this subgroup should be useful. The overall survival was also superior in patients treated by TAD-TAD (Fig. 3). To exclude the influence of early deaths, deaths in complete remission, rate of relapses EFS was compared in these groups. It appeared to be superior in patients treated by TAD-TAD (Fig. 4).

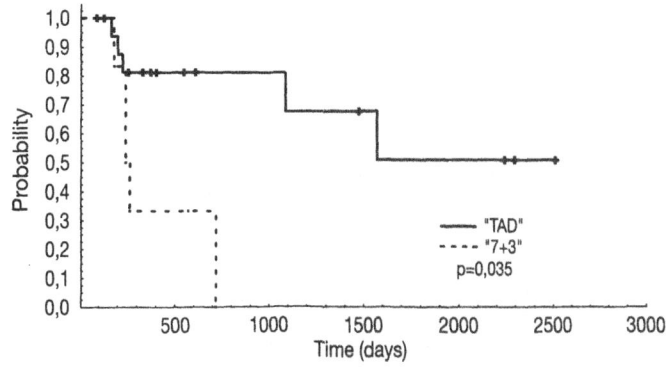

**Fig. 1.** CCR in patients treated by TAD-TAD (——) and "7+3" (-----). p<0,05

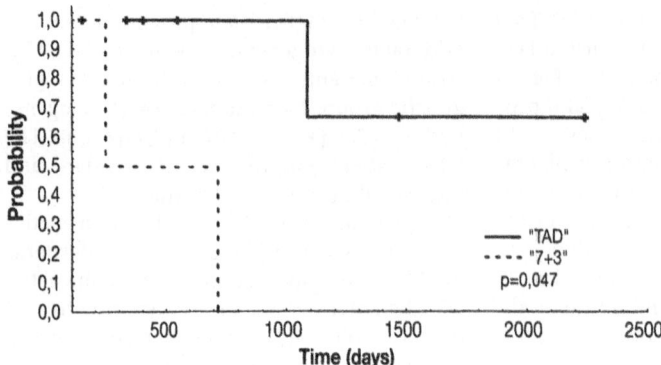

**Fig. 2.** CCR in M1-2 subtypes treated by TAD-TAD (——) and "7+3" (------). p<0,05

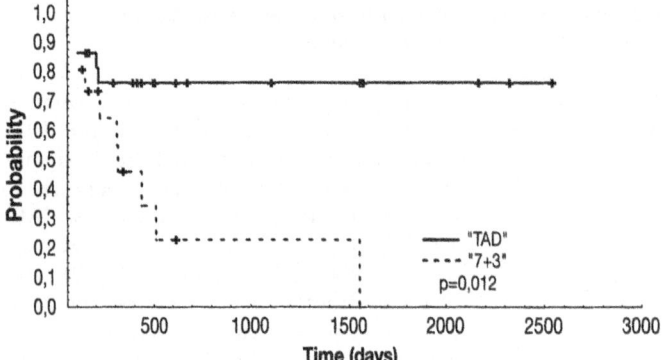

**Fig. 3.** Overall survival in patients treated by TAD-TAD (——) and "7+3" (-----). p=0,012

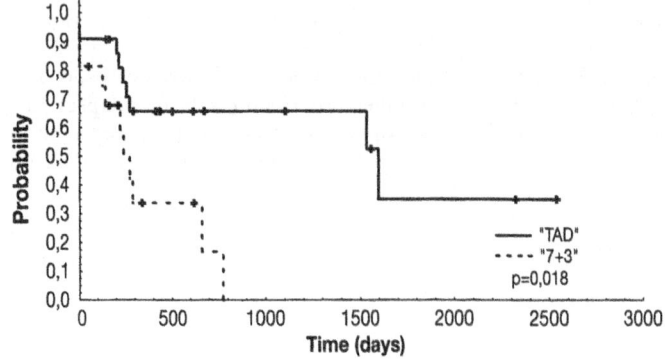

**Fig. 4.** EFS in patients treated by TAD-TAD (——) and "7+3" (-----). p=0,018

## Comparison of standard and nonstandard modes of treatment

CR rate in the nonstandard group was 50% that is significantly inferior to TAD-TAD (p=0.007) and did not differ significantly from "7+3"(p=0.28) and the whole group of standard treated patients(p=0.06). All main criteria of survival were superior on standard treatment. They include CCR(Fig.5), overall survival (Fig. 6), EFS (Fig. 7). Better CCR and EFS in standard group means that the quality of remission is poorer in nonstandard group.

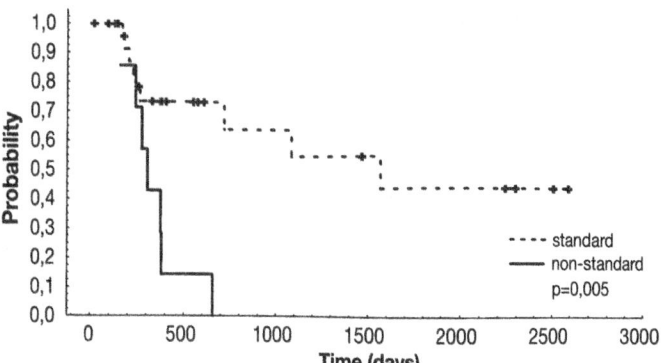

**Fig. 5.** CCR in patients treated standardly TAD-TAD or "7+3"(----) and with decreased dose intensity (——). p=0,005

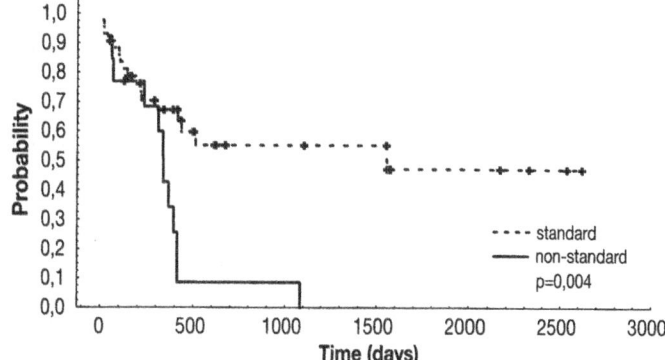

**Fig. 6.** Overall survival in patients treated standardly TAD-TAD or "7+3"(----) and with decreased dose intensity (——). p=0,004

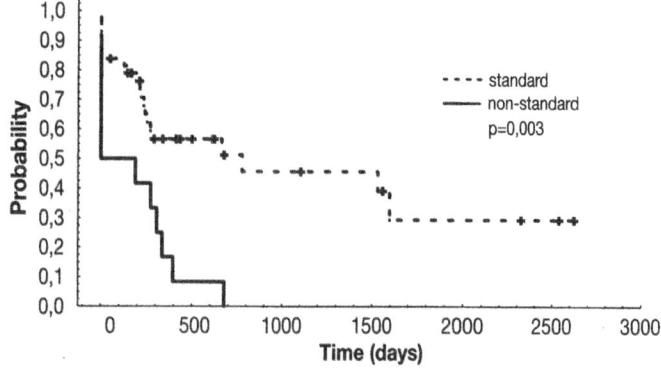

**Fig. 7.** EFS. in patients treated standardly TAD-TAD or "7+3"(----) and with decreased dose intensity (——). p=0,003

## Comparison of TAD-TAD regimen and autoBMT in first early remission

Patients undergone autoBMT were previously treated with "7+3", "7+3+VP", TAD-TAD. Some of them were consolidated by HD-Ara-C before transplantation. CCR and EFS in this group appeared to be comparable to patients treated by TAD-TAD(p>0.05). The data are coincident with the recently published data of Cossileth et al [20], which are extensively reviewed by A.Burnett [11]. Cost efficiency may be discussed.

### Mdr-1 gene expression in AML patients

Mdr-1gene expression was studied in AML *de novo* patients and in CR. Expression of mdr-1 gene was detected in bone marrow samples of 5/17 *de novo* patients (29%). Four patients with mdr-1 positive phenotype achieved CR while one patient did not achieve CR not due to resistance. Expression of mdr-1 gene in *de novo* AML patients had now effect on the probability of CR (p>0.05) and one can propose the multiple mechanisms of resistance of leukemic cells in majority cases of AML [16]. Knowing that primary therapy of AML may select resistant clones which could be responsible for further relapse we compared the mdr-1 expression level and the duration of CR. In our study correlation between primary mdr-1 positive phenotype and duration of remission was not revealed (p>0.05).

Twelve patients were investigated in early remission just after consolidation therapy and the mdr-1 gene expression have been detected in nine patients (75%). We examined the possibility of mdr-1 positive cells to impact remission duration. There was now significant correlation between mdr-1 gene expression and remission duration (p>0.05), and probably it may be related to mdr-1 gene expression in normal haemapoietic cells undergone intensive chemotherapy. For example, survival of one patient with 30% mdr-1 positive cells just after chemotherapy is 7.5+ years.

Mdr-1 positive phenotype in remission (more than 3 months after consolidation therapy) was detected in 5/11 patients (45%). The quantity of mdr-1 positive cells in these patients was not high (not more than 3%) but the level of expression was strong. The 5-year survival of mdr-1 positive patients was significantly lower compared mdr-1 negative. 5/6 mdr-1 negative patients were long-lived while 4/5 mdr-1 positive had relapses earlier than 5 years after the begining of treatment (p<0.05).

So, according to obtained data it is possible to conclude the following: TAD-TAD regimen is superior to "7+3", predominantly in M1-2 subtypes of AML. M4-5 patients treated by TAD-TAD need CNS prophilaxis. Reduction of dose intensity results in poorer outcome. Neither primary or early postremission mdr-1 gene expression has impact on prognosis, although high expression of this gene in late remission may be a sign of relapse.

### References

1. Yates J. et al (1983). Cytosine arabinoside and daunorubicin therapy in acute nonlymphocytic leukemia. Cancer Chemoter Rep 57: 485
2. Buechner T. et al (1992). Combined effect of very early intensification and prolonged postremission chemootherapy in patients with AML. Leukemia 5. Suppl 4: 68–70
3. Buechner T. et al (1998). Intensified therapy of AML – the role of the HAM Combination In: Hiddemann W, Buechner T. (eds) Acute leukemias. Spriger, pp. 821–823
4. Keating M. et al (1998). FLAG-Ida, on effective regimen for high risk AML. In: Hiddemann W, Buechner T. (eds) Acute leukemias. Springer pp. 828–833
5. Estey E. et al (1998). Recenf studies in AML, RAEB-t, and RAEB at M.D.Anderson Hospital. In: Hiddemann W, Buechner T. (eds) Acute leukemias. Springer pp. 824–827
6. Bichop J, (1991). Etoposide in the management of leukemia: review. Seminars in oncology 18. Suppl. 2: 62–67
7 Savchenco B. et al (1994). The results of multicenter cooperative study in AML treatment in adults. Ther. Arch. (Rus) 7: 11–17
8. Buechner T. et al (1994). Double induction in AML comparing high with standard dose Ara-C. Hematotoxicity and antyleukemicefficaci. Blood 84 Suppl. 1:232 a
9. Buechner T. et al (1997). Therapeutic autcome in AML is mainly determined by cytogenetics, LDH in serum early response and, in a poor risk subgroup, by intensified induction treatment. Blood 90. Suppl. 1: 504a
10. Ravandi F, et al (1997). Identification of a relatively favorable group within AML/MDS pts with cromosome 5 and/or 7 abnormalities. Blood 90. Suppl. 1:64a
11. Burnett A, (1998). Transplantation in first remission of acute myeloid leukemia N Engl j Med 339: 1698–1700
12. List A. Pharmacological modulators and alternate mechanisms of multidrug resistance. In: Hiddemann W, Buechner T. (eds) Acute leukemias. Springer pp.422–430
13. Campos L. et al (1992). Clinical significance of multidrag resistance P-glycoprotein expression on acute non-lymphoblastic leukemia cells at diagnosis. Blood 79: 473–476
14. Hunault M. et al (1997). Multidrug resistance gene expression in acute myeloid leukemia: major prognosis significance for in vivo drug resistance to induction treatment. Ann Hematol. 74:65–71
15. Wood P. et al (1994). P-glycoprotein expression on acute myeloid leukemia blast cells at diagnosis predicts response to chemotherapy and survival. Br j Haematol. 87: 509–514

16. Kasimir-Bauer S. et al (1998). In acute myeloid leukemia only the coexpression of at least two proteins including P-glucoprotein, the multidrug resistance-related protein MRP, bcl-2, mutant p53 and heat-shock protein 27 is predictive for the response to induction chemotherapy. In: Hiddemann W, Buechner T. (eds) Acute leukemias. Springer pp 444–453

17. Kanz L. et al (1988). Detection of messenger RNA within single hemopoietic cells by in situ hibridization on small slide areas. Exp. Hematol. 16: 394–399

18. Kaplan E., Meier P. (1958). Nonparametric estimation from incomplete observations. J Am Stat Assoc 53: 457–481

19. Cox D., Sheel E. (1989). The analysis of binary data 2 nd ed. New-York; Chapman, Holl

20. Cassileth P. et al (1998). Chemotherapy compared with autologous or allogenetic bone marrow transplantation in the management of acute myeloid leukemia in first remission. N Engl JE Med 339: 1649–1656

# Stratification of Postremission Therapy in Patients with Acute Myeloid Leukemia ≤ 60 Years According to the Karyotype: Results of the German Multicenter Treatment Trials AML HD93 and AML HD98-A

R.F. Schlenk[1], S. Fröhling[1], F. Del Valle[2], F. Hartmann[3], A. Glasmacher[7], J.Th. Fischer[5],
W. Grimminger[9], C. Weber[4], W. Weber[8], U. Gunzer[6], K. Götze[10], C. Waterhouse[11], A. Benner[12],
K. Döhner[1], R. Haas[1], A.D. Ho[1] and H. Döhner[1]

## Summary

The objective of our treatment trial AML HD93 was to evaluate the impact of different postremission therapies in genetically defined subgroups of acute myeloid leukemia (AML). All patients except those with AML FAB M3 received a double induction therapy with ICE followed by a first consolidation therapy was given according to the HAM protocol. A bone marrow harvest or a peripheral blood progenitor cell collection was performed during hematological reconstitution after the first consolidation. For second consolidation therapy the patients were stratified in three risk groups: *Low-risk* [t(8;21), abn(16q22), t(15;17)]: HAM; *intermediate-risk* [normal karyotyp]: allogeneic transplantation (AlloSCT), if an HLA-identical sibling was available, or S-HAM; *high-risk* [all other abnormalities]: AlloSCT, if an HLA-identical sibling was available, or autologous transplantation (AutoSCT). Between September 1993 and January 1998, 246 patients, aged 16 to 60 years, entered the AML HD93 trial. Complete remission rates after double induction significantly differed between the three risk groups; low-risk: 92%, intermediate-risk: 82%, high-risk: 59%. The overall survival for patients with refractory disease was very poor with 12% at 2 years and all patients, who survived, had received AlloSCT. The disease free survival (DFS) for low, intermediate and high-risk was 67%, 49% and 34% at 2 years, respectively. There was a marked difference in the low-risk group between patients either exhibiting t(8;21) or t(15;17) and those exhibiting abn(16q22) with an DFS of 78% and 44%, respectively. In the high-risk group, patients exhibiting abn(11q23) did better than those exhibiting abn(3q), -5/5q-, -7/7q-, abn(12p), abn(17p), and complex karyotypes with a DFS of 38% and 28%, respectively. Based on the results of the AML HD93 trial and on published data from large multicenter study groups, in February 1998 we initiated our new trial AML HD98-A. Two major objectives of this ongoing trial are
- to evaluate in a randomized manner the impact of AutoSCT compared to HAM in patients exhibiting a normal karyotype and
- to study the feasibility and efficacy of AlloSCT either from HLA-identical siblings or matched unrelated donors in high-risk patients.

## Introduction

Advances in the understanding of the pathogenesis in acute myeloid leukemia (AML) has

[1] Medizinische Klinik and Poliklinik V, Universität Heidelberg
[2] Städtisches Klinikum, Oldenburg
[3] Medizinische Klinik I, Universität Homburg
[4] Medizinische Klinik, Universität Giessen
[5] Städtisches Klinikum, Karlsruhe
[6] Medizinische Klinik I, Universität Würzburg
[7] Medizinische Klinik, Universität Bonn
[8] Krankenhaus der Barmherzigen Brüder, Trier
[9] Bürgerhospital, Stuttgart
[10] Medizinische Klinik, Technische Universität München
[11] Städtisches Krankenhaus, München-Schwabing
[12] Abteilung "Biostatistik", Deutsches Krebsforschungszentrum, Heidelberg

led to the improvement of treatment. In particular, the prognostic value of the karyotype has opened the possibility to identify patients with a high-risk of relapse early in the treatment course. About 65 to 80% of patients, 60 years of age or younger, achieve a complete remission (CR) following induction therapy consisting of cytarabine in combination with an anthracycline (Stone et al 1993). However, the majority of these patients relapse despite conventional consolidation or maintenance therapy. In several randomized multicenter treatment trials it has been shown that dose intensification of cytarabine significantly improves the disease-free survival (DFS) (Mayer et al 1994, Weik et al 1996). Bloomfield and coworkers (1998) showed that the curative impact of dose intensification of cytarabine in postremission therapy varied significantly among the different cytogenetic groups. The remission duration for patients exhibiting t(8;21), abn(16q22) or normal karyotypes was significantly improved by using high-dose instead of standard-dose cytarabine. In contrast, for patients exhibiting other cytogenetic abnormalities the remission duration was short irrespective of the dose of cytarabine given.

Based on these results we performed a multicenter treatment trial in which postremission therapy was stratified according to the karyotype. The stratification in three different risk groups was based on the cytogenetic criteria proposed by the Cancer and Leukemia Study Group B (CALGB) (Bloomfield et al 1998). Patients exhibiting t(8;21) or abn(16q22) were assigned to high-dose cytarabine in combination with mitoxantrone (HAM) (low-risk); patients exhibiting a normal karyotype were assigned either to allogeneic stem cell transplantation (AlloSCT), if an HLA-matched sibling was available, or an intensified high-dose cytarabine based regimen (S-HAM) (intermediate-risk); patients exhibiting other abnormalities were assigned either to AlloSCT, if an HLA-matched sibling was available, or to autologous stem cell transplantation (AutoSCT) (high-risk). The study was designed to evaluate whether autologous or allogeneic transplantation in high-risk patients results in an improved DFS and whether AlloSCT is superior to intensified chemotherapy in patient exhibiting a normal

karyotype. Based on the results of the AML HD93 study, in February 1998 we initiated our new treatment trial AML HD98-A. In the following we present the results of the AML HD93 study and first data of the AML HD98-A study.

## Methods

### AML HD93

*Patients*: The study opened in September 1993 and closed in Jauary 1998. Eligible patients were 16 to 60 years old and had either de novo AML of French-American-British (FAB) types M0 to M7, or secondary AML following treatment of a primary malignant disease. In all patients cytogenetic analysis, including conventional G-banding and interphase cytogenetics using fluorescence in-situ hybridization, was performed in a central reference laboratory (Fischer et al 1996). The study was approved by the local Ethics Review Committee. A written informed consent was obtained from all patients at entry of the study.

*Treatment plan of the AML HD93 study*: All patients, except those with AML FAB M3, received a first induction cycle with ICE (idarubicin 12 mg/m$^2$ i.v., day 1,3,5; cytarabine 100 mg/m$^2$ continuously i.v., day 1–7; etoposide 100 mg/m$^2$ i.v., day 1–3). Patients with AML FAB M3 were treated according to the AIDA protocol (Avvisati et al 1996) (all-trans retinoic acid 45 mg/m$^2$ p.o., day 1–28; idarubicin 12 mg/m$^2$ continuously i.v., day 2,4,6,8). Bone marrow was evaluated between day 21 and 28 by aspiration. Patients with refractory disease after ICE received a second induction cycle according to the HAM protocol (cytarabine 3 g/m$^2$/12hr i.v., day 1–3; mitoxantrone 12 mg/m$^2$ i.v., day 2–3). Patients achieving complete (CR) or partial (PR) remission following ICE received a second induction cycle according to the ICE protocol. For first consolidation therapy all patients in CR received HAM. After hematological reconstitution a peripheral blood progenitor cell collection or a bone marrow harvest was performed (Schlenk et al 1997). Bone marrow was treated with mafosfamid in a dose adapted manner prior to cryopreservation (Martin et al 1993). For second consolidation therapy patients 54 years of age or younger were stratified according to the karyotype at diagnosis: patients exhibiting abn(16q22), t(8;21) or t(15;17) received a second consolidation with HAM (low-risk), patients exhibiting a normal karyotype received either an AlloSCT, if an HLA-matched sibling was available, or a second consolidation with S-HAM (Hiddemann et al, 1988) (intermediate-risk), and patients with any other cytogenetic abnormality were assigned to autologous or allogeneic transplantation (high-risk). The preparative regimen for both autologous and allogeneic transplantation consisted of either hyperfractioned total body irradiation (12,2 to 14,4 Gy) or busulfan (1mg/kg/6h p.o.) followed by cyclophosphamid (120–200mg/kg i.v.). Bone marrow or peripheral blood progenitor cell grafts were reinfused after 1 or 2 days of rest. Patients 55 years of age or older were not stratified but received a second consolidation with HAM.

## AML HD98-A

*Patients*: The inclusion criteria are identical to those of the AML HD93 protocol with one exception: patients with refractory anemia with excess of blasts in transformation (RAEB-t) and secondary AML after myelodysplastic syndrome are included in the AML HD98-A protocol. The study was approved by the local Ethics Review Committee. A written informed consent was obtained from all patients at entry of the study.

*Treatment plan of the AML HD98-A study*: The study design is shown in Figure 1. Double induction and first consolidation therapy are identical to the AML HD93 protocol with one exception: patients with refractory disease following ICE receive A-HAM (cytarabine 3 g/m$^2$/12hr i.v., day 1–3; mitoxantrone 12 mg/m$^2$ i.v., day 2–3, all-trans retinoic acid 45mg/m$^2$, day 3–5, and 15mg/m$^2$, day 6–28). Major changes to the AML HD93 protocol regard the definition of the risk groups and the treatment assigned as second consolidation following stratification. In contrast to the AML HD93 protocol all patients up to the age of 60 years are stratified.

*Low-risk* [t(8;21), t(15;17)]: These patients are assigned to a second cycle of HAM.

*Intermediate-risk*: Patients with an HLA-identical sibling are assigned to AlloSCT. If no HLA-identical sibling is available the treatment plan is as follows:

[normal karyotype]: patients are randomly assigned to either a second cycle of HAM or AutoSCT, with peripheral blood progenitor cells or bone marrow collected after the first consolidation with HAM.

[abn(16q22), abn(11q23), other abnormalities]: These patients are assigned to AutoSCT.

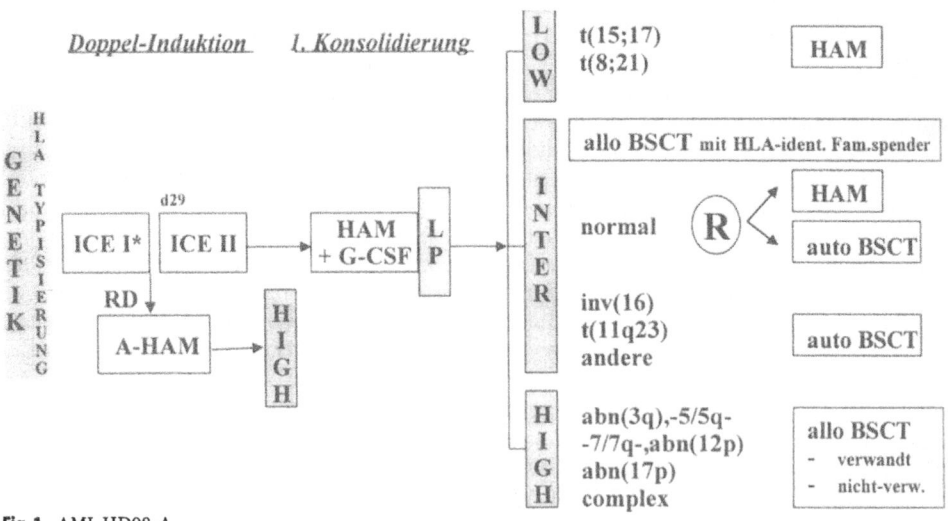

**Fig. 1.** AML HD98-A

*High-risk* [abn(3q), -5/5q-, -7/7q-, abn(12p), abn(17p), complex karyotype ( ̰ 3 abnormalities)]: All patients are assigned to AlloSCT. The algorithm includes both transplantation from an HLA-identical sibling and from an unrelated donor. Patients who are ineligible for a myeloablative regimen may receive a less intense conditioning.

## Statistical Analysis

DFS was defined as the time from date of CR until date of relapse or of death from any cause. Overall survival was defined as the time from date of diagnosis until date of death. Statistical computations were performed using the statistical software packages SAS, Version 6.11 (SAS Institute Inc., 1995). The data were analyzed on an intention-to-treat basis. Survival curves were estimated using the Kaplan-Meier product-limit method. DFS and overall survival data were stated at 2 years.

## Results

### AML HD93

278 patients were enrolled in the study. 246 patients were eligible; the reasons for ineligibility were as follows: 20 patients had diagnoses other than AML, 9 patients were excluded because of protocol violation, and 3 patients had concomitant disease (lung cancer, Wegener´s disease with renal insufficiency, cardiac insufficiency). The cytogenetic analysis was successful in 240 of 246 patients (97%). Six patients without adequate karyotype were excluded from further consideration. The patients characteristics at diagnosis are shown in Table 1. The median follow-up time was 35 months ranging from 13 to 72 months.

*Remission rates:* Of the 240 eligible patients, 187 patients achieved a CR (78%), 30 patients had refractory disease (12%), and 23 patients died (10%) during the first induction therapy (early death: ED). Remission rates significantly differed among the three cytogenetic risk groups. The CR rates in the low, intermediate and high-risk groups were 92%, 82% and 59%, respectively. In the low-risk

**Table 1.** Patient Characteristics (AML HD93 study)

| | |
|---|---|
| No. of patients | 246 |
| Male/female | 125/121 |
| Age (yrs) (median, range) | 46 (16–60) |
| No. of secondary leukemias (after cured cancer) | 16 |
| Hematological parameters at diagnosis (median, range) | |
| Hemoglobin (g/dl) | 8.9 (4.3 – 16.5) |
| WBC (x 10⁹/l) | 13.2 (0.38–369.0) |
| Platelets (x 10⁹/l) | 54 (5–488) |
| LDH (U/l) | 396 (89–6430) |
| Blasts in BM (%) | 90 (3–100) |

group, there was no induction failure due to resistant disease. In the intermediate and high-risk groups, the rates of refractory disease were 8% and 30%, respectively. Of the 45 patients with refractory disease, 39 received a second induction chemotherapy with HAM (n=33) or ICE (n=6): 14 patients achieved a CR (31%). Five patients received AlloSCT with refractory disease after ICE and HAM; all of them achieved a CR. The survival of the ICE refractory patients was poor with 12% and only patients after AlloSCT survived.

*Survival data analysis.* The DFS and overall survival of the whole study population was 52% and 50% respectively. In the three risk groups the DFS was as follows: low-risk 67%, intermediate-risk 49%, high-risk 34%. In the low-risk group, patients exhibiting abn(16q22) showed a markedly inferior DFS of 44% compared to those exhibiting t(8;21) or t(15;17) with a DFS of 78%. In the intermediate-risk group, the intention to treat analysis for second consolidation of chemotherapy compared to AlloSCT revealed a DFS of 48% and 60% respectively. In the high-risk group, patients with abn(3q), -5/5q-, -7/7q-, abn(12p), abn(17p) or complex karyotypes had a DFS of 28%, and patients with abn(11q23) or other abnormalities a DFS of 38%.

### AML HD98-A

Since February 1998, 111 patients were registered. Thirteen were ineligible, 7 because of protocol violation and 6 because of diagnosis other than AML. The median age is 48 years ranging from 18 to 60. So far, data on remission rates are available from 82 patients: 54 (66%) patients achieved a CR, 18 (22%) patients had refractory disease, and there were 10 ED (12%).

*Intermediate-risk:* So far, 18 patients exhibiting a normal karyotype achieved a CR after double induction with ICE. For second consolidation, 3 patients received AlloSCT, 13 were randomized to either HAM (n=6) or AutoSCT (n=7). Two patients refused randomization and received HAM. Of the 7 patients exhibiting abn(16q22), 2 received AlloSCT, 1 AutoSCT, 1 died in CR during the second induction therapy, and 3 patients are scheduled for AutoSCT. Two patients exhibiting abn(11q23) received AutoSCT.

*High-risk:* So far, 22 patients either with refractory disease after ICE or exhibiting abn(3q), -5/5q-, -7/7q-, abn(12p), abn(17p) or complex karyotype are in the high-risk group. Twelve patients received AlloSCT, 7 from an HLA-identical sibling and 5 from a matched unrelated donor (MUD). Three patients are scheduled for MUD transplantation. Four patients were older than 55 years and were considered ineligible for AlloSCT. Three patients with refractory disease died shortly after induction therapy.

## Discussion

The central element of the AML HD93 study was the stratification of the second consolidation therapy according to the cytogenetically defined risk of relapse. We used the classification for risk groups proposed by Bloomfield and coworkers (1998): low-risk [t(8;21), inv(16)], intermediate-risk [normal karyotype], high-risk [all other abnormalities].

Consistent with the results from other studies (for review see Mròzek et al 1997), we found a significant difference in the remission rates between the three risk groups, ranging from no induction failure in the low-risk group to 30% resistant disease in the high-risk group. One third of the patients, who had resistant disease after the first cycle of ICE, achieved CR after consecutive therapy with HAM (dosage of cytarabine 6 x 3g/m²). However, there was no difference in overall

survival between responders and non-responders to this high-dose cytarabine containing salvage induction regimen [data not shown]. The overall survival of the ICE refractory patients was very poor, but there were some (approximately 10 to 20%) long term survivors and all of them had received AlloSCT. Therefore in these patients the value of such additional dose-intensified second induction therapy seems questionable. Rather early high-dose chemotherapy followed by transplantation from a sibling or a MUD should be envisaged for this subgroup of patients (Biggs et al 1992, Forman et al 1991).

The outcome of the patients with low-risk abnormalities was excellent, with a DFS of 63% at 2 years for the group of patients with either t(8;21) or abn(16q22). This result is consistent with the data published recently by the CALGB showing a DFS of 78% at 2 years in the group of patients who had received repetitive cycles of high-dose cytarabine (Bloomfield et al 1998). In our study, the DFS for patients exhibiting abn(16q22) was markedly inferior compared to that of the patients with t(8;21) indicating differences in cytarabine sensitivity of these two leukemia subtypes. The patients in our study received only 2 cycles of high-dose cytarabine in postremission therapy compared to 4 cycles in the CALGB study. This difference in cumulative cytarabine dosage may account for the difference in DFS seen for patients with abn(16q22). In analogy to our study, Grimwade and coworkers (1998) reported a higher risk of relapse for patients exhibiting abn (16q22) compared to those exhibiting t(8;21).

The results of the CALGB study also demonstrated a significant benefit of cytarabine dose intensification in the group of patients exhibiting a normal karyotype. The data for DFS of our patients following chemotherapy according to the S-HAM protocol are comparable to those of the CALGB and the MRC-10 trial (Bloomfield et al 1998, Grimwade et al 1998). Consistent with the data from the MRC-10 trial we observed an improved DFS for patients, who received AlloSCT, but the difference did not reach statistical significance.

For high-risk patients the data from the CALGB trial showed that dose intensification of cytarabine did not result in an improved

DFS (Bloomfield et al 1998). One objective of our trial was to evaluate whether myeloablative conditioning followed by Auto/Allo-SCT can improve the outcome of these patients.

For patients exhibiting t(11q23) Mròzek and coworkers (1997) showed in a retrospective meta-analysis of several CALGB trials a significant better DFS and overall survival for patients exhibiting t(9;11) compared to patients exhibiting other t(11q23), in particular if they had received high-dose cytarabine for consolidation. In our trial we prospectively stratified all patients with t(11q23) to either allogeneic or autologous transplantation and 81% of the patients in CR received the assigned treatment. Our results with a DFS plot reaching a plateau at 38% are encouraging. However it remains open whether high-dose cytarabine or Auto/Allo-SCT should be recommended in these patients.

Among the patients exhibiting abn(3q), -5/5q-, -7/7q-, abn(12p), abn(17p) or complex karyotypes only a minority achieved a CR following ICE. Only 4 patients received AutoSCT and all these patients rapidly relapsed. The outcome of this group was dismal, comparable to that of the patients with ICE refractory disease. All patients exhibiting one of these high-risk chromosomal alterations who survived had received AlloSCT. Our data are at variance to those of the MRC-10 trial suggesting a possible role for AutoSCT (Grimwade et al 1998). The overall survival of these high-risk patients following AutoSCT was 46%.

Based on the results of the AML HD93 trial and on published data from large multicenter study groups (Bloomfield et al 1998, Grimwade et al 1998), in February 1998 we initiated our new trial AML HD98-A. Major changes regard the definition of the risk groups and the type of consolidation therapy assigned following stratification.

The low-risk group is defined by t(8;21) or t(15;17). The second consolidation therapy consists of HAM and is unchanged. The objective in this treatment arm is to confirm the good results of the AML HD93 trial.

The intermediate-risk group is defined by normal karyotype, t(11q23), abn(16q22) or various abnormalities. All patients with an HLA-identical sibling are assigned to AlloSCT. Although there was a high anti-leu-kemic efficacy of the S-HAM regimen in our AML HD93 trial, this therapy was associated with unacceptable hematological toxicity (data not shown). Therefore we decided to use HAM instead of S-HAM for the randomized comparison with AutoSCT for patients exhibiting a normal karyotype. This approach will provide prospective data on the impact of AutoSCT in a genetically defined subgroup of AML patients compared to a high-dose cytarabine based regimen, which is currently considered as a standard consolidation therapy. To achieve an in-vivo purging, stem cells will only be collected following 3 cycles of intensive chemotherapy, i.e. 2 cycles of ICE and 1 cycle of HAM. We previously showed that a sufficient amount of stem cells can be collected after such an intensive therapy in the majority of patients (Schlenk et al 1997).

In the subgroup of patients exhibiting abn(16q22) or t(11q23), those lacking an HLA-identical sibling are assigned to AutoSCT. A desirable randomization between HAM and AutoSCT in this group cannot be performed because of insufficient patient numbers in each subgroup. Therefore, intergroup studies are necessary in these subgroups to evaluate the impact of various treatment strategies in a randomized fashion.

The high-risk group is defined by abn(3q), -5/5q-, -7/7q-, abn(12p), abn(17p) or complex karyotypes as well as by refractory disease after ICE. Despite significant improvements in some genetically defined subgroups, the outcome of patients with these aberrations remains very poor. Since in the AML HD93 trial AutoSCT failed to demonstrate an improvement in this subgroup, all patients are now assigned to AlloSCT. With the advent of new treatment modalities, such as allogeneic transplantation after less intense conditioning, and given the encouraging data from transplantation studies using matched unrelated donors, we anticipate that the majority of our patients will actually receive the assigned treatment. This will allow us to study the impact of AlloSCT given early in the treatment course to these high-risk patients.

## References

Avvisati G, Coco FL, Diverio D, Falda M, Ferrara F, Lazzarino M, Russo D, Petti MC, Mandelli F (1996)

AIDA (all-trans retinoic acid + idarubicin) in newly diagnosed acute promyelocytic leukemia: a gruppo italiano malattie ematologiche maligne dell'adulto (GIMEMA) pilot study. Blood 88:1390–1398

Biggs JC, Horowitz MM, Gale RP, Ash RC, Atkinson K, Helbig W, Jacobsen N, Phillips GL, Rimm AA, Ringden O, et al (1992) Bone marrow transplants may cure patients with acute leukemia never achieving remission with chemotherapy. Blood 80:1090–1093

Bloomfield CD, Lawrence D, Byrd JC, Carroll A, Pettenati MJ, Tantravahi R, Patil SR, Davey FR, Berg DT, Schiffer CA, Arthur DC, Mayer RJ. (1998) Frequency of Prolonged Remission Duration after High-Dose Cytarabine Intensification in Acute Myeloid Leukemia Varies by Cytogenetic Subtype. Cancer Res 58:4173–4179

Burnett AK, Goldstone AH, Stevens RM, Hann IM, Rees JK, Gray RG, Wheatley K (1998) Randomized comparison of addition of autologous bone-marrow transplantation to intensive chemotherapy for acute myeloid leukaemia in first remission: results of MRC AML 10 trial. UK Medical Research Council Adult and Children's Leukaemia Working Parties. Lancet 351:700–708

Fischer K, Scholl C, Salat J, Fröhling S, Schlenk R, Bentz M, Stilgenbauer S, Lichter P, Döhner H (1996) Design and validation of DNA probe sets for a comprehensive interphase cytogenetic analysis of acute myeloid leukemia. Blood 88: 3962–3971

Forman SJ, Schmidt GM, Nademanee AP, Amylon MD, Chao NJ, Fahey JL, Konrad PN, Margolin KA, Niland JC, O'Donnell MR, et al (1991) Allogeneic bone marrow transplantation as therapy for primary induction failure for patients with acute leukemia. J Clin Oncol 9:1570–4

Grimwade D, Walker H, Oliver F, Wheatley K, Harrison C, Harrison G, Rees J, Hann I, Stevens R, Burnett A, Goldstone A (1998) The importance of diagnostic cytogenetics on outcome in AML: analysis of 1,612 patients entered into the MRC AML 10 trial. Blood 92:2322–33

Hiddemann W, Büchner Th, Essink M, Koch O, Stenzinger W, van de Loo J (1988) High-dose cytosine arabinoside and mitoxantrone: preliminary results of a pilot study with sequential application (S-HAM) indicating a high antileukemic activity in refractory acute leukemias. Oncologie 11:10–12

Martin H, Bruecher J, Claudé R, Hoelzer D (1993) Cumulative chemotherapy increases mafosfamide toxicity for normal progenitor cells in AML patients: rationale for cryopreserving adapted-dose purged marrow early in first complete remission. Bone Marrow Transplantation 12:495–499

Mayer RJ, Davis RB, Schiffer CA, Berg DT, Powell BL, Schulman P, Omura GA, Moore JO, McIntyre OR, Frei E (1994) Intensive post remission chemotherapy in adults with acute myeloid leukemia. New Engl J Med 331:896–903

Mròzek K, Heinonen K, Lawrence D, Carroll AJ, Koduru PR, Rao KW, Strout MP, Hutchison RE, Moore JO, Mayer RJ, Schiffer CA, Bloomfield CD (1997) Adult patients with de novo acute myeloid leukemia and t(9;11)(p22;q23) have a superior outcome to patients with other translocations involving band 11q23: a Cancer and Leukemia Group B study. Blood 90:4532–4538

Mròzek K, Heinonen K, de la Chapelle A, Bloomfield CD (1997) Clinical significance of cytogenetics in acute myeloid leukemia. Semin Oncol 24:17–31

Schlenk RF, Döhner H, Pförsich M, Benner A, Fischer K, Hartmann F, Fischer JT, Weber W, Gunzer U, Pralle H, Haas R (1997) Successful collection of peripheral blood progenitor cells in patients with acute myeloid leukaemia following early consolidation therapy with granulocyte colony-stimulating factor-supported high-dose cytarabine and mitoxantrone. Br J Haematol. 99:386–93

Stone RM, Mayer RJ (1993) Treatment of the newly diagnosed adult with de novo acute myeloid leukemia. Hematol Oncol Clin North Am 7:47–64

Weick JK, Kopecky KJ, Applebaum FR, Head DR, Kingsbury LL, Balcerzak SP, Bickers JN, Hynes HE, Welborn JL, Simon SR, Grever M (1996) A randomized investigation of high-dose versus standard-dose cytosine arabinoside with daunorubicin in patients with previously untreated acute myeloid leukemia: A Southwest Oncology Group Study. Blood 88:2841–2851

# Phase I Trial of Docetaxel (Taxotere) for Patients with Relapsed or Refractory Acute Myeloid Leukemia (AML)

T. P. Szatrowski[1], M. L. Hensley[2] and S. Ely[1]

## Background and Rationale

While complete remissions (CR) are obtained in 60–80% of patients with *de novo* acute myeloid leukemia (AML), in poor-prognosis AML the CR rate is much lower. There is about a 30% chance of achieving CR in secondary AML, refractory *de novo* AML, and AML in second relapse[1]. Thus the treatment of the poor-prognosis secondary AML patients, and early relapse or second relapse *de novo* AML, remains a major challenge in leukemia therapy. Investigation of new agents with potential anti-leukemic activity is therefore warranted in these groups.

Docetaxel is a member of the taxane family of chemotherapeutic agents. The stabilizing effect of docetaxel (Taxotere) on tubulin results in inhibition of mitotic and interphase cellular functions.

Three characteristics of docetaxel make it potentially well-suited for use in poor-prognosis AML. First, docetaxel has profound activity against normal myeloid cells. Second, docetaxel has been shown to be relatively platelet-sparing. Prolonged thrombocytopenia and bleeding events may therefore be avoidable. Third, docetaxel has activity in tumors that are anthracycline-resistant. Each of these points may be illustrated by the example of a single clinical trial: when docetaxel was given at a dose of 100 mg/m[2] to patients with anthracycline-resistant breast cancer, 94.5% of patients developed grade 4 neutropenia[2] but none developed grade 4 thrombocytopenia. Its activity in anthracycline-resistant tumors implies that it may have potential activity against cells that express the multi-drug resistance (MDR) gene product, a common mechanism for drug resistance in leukemia cells [3–6].

The use of G-CSF in this setting may be particularly appropriate in that infectious complications are a frequent cause of early mortality in the treatment of patients with poor-prognosis AML. Prolonged neutropenia is poorly tolerated, particularly in older patients[78]. Moreover, the duration of the neutropenia can be shortened in the older population with the use of myeloid growth factors [9].

The maximum tolerated dose (MTD) of docetaxel in phase I studies in pediatric patients with solid tumors has been 125 mg/m[2] without granulocyte colony stimulating factor (G-CSF), and 185 mg/m[2] with G-CSF support [10], which is 85% higher than the MTD determined for adult patients. Dose-limiting toxicity (DLT) in both pediatric and adult patients is neutropenia. The use of G-CSF allowed a higher MTD. However, a generalized, desquamating skin rash was the DLT at 235 mg/m[2]. The starting dose level for this study was chosen to be 100 mg/m[2], the MTD defined in previous Phase I studies in adults with solid tumors [11], with subsequent dose levels escalating by 30mg/m[2].

We have instituted this phase I clinical trial in order to: [1] determine the MTD of docetaxel given with G-CSF in relapsed and refractory AML; (2) describe the dose-limiting non-hematologic effects of docetaxel when given at myelosuppressive doses; and (3) describe the anti-leukemic activity of docetaxel. The determination of marrow expression of the MDR gene product, p53,

---

[1] Weill Medical College of Cornell University, New York Presbyterian Hospital, New York, NY, U.S.A.
[2] Memorial Sloan Kettering Cancer Center, New York, NY, U.S.A.

and bcl-2 and how they correlate with clinical response will be reported separately.

## Methods

The following eligibilty criteria were used. Patients were required to have an unequivocal diagnosis of:

1. AML in relapse less than 6 months after initial remission for *de novo* or secondary AML;
2. resistant *de novo* or secondary AML (failed to achieve complete remission with two cycles of anthracycline and/or cytarabine-containing therapy);
3. AML in second or subsequent relapse;
4. AML with a preceding myelodysplastic syndrome or other antecedent abnormal bone marrow; or
5. AML as a complication of prior chemo-therapy or radiation therapy.

In addition, patients were required to have a bilirubin level less than or equal to institutio-nal upper limit of normal, a creatinine less than twice the institutional upper limit of normal. All patients signed, written, informed consent, and the study was approved by our institutional review board (IRB). Patients were required to be age 18 years or older, to have no active, uncontrolled infection, and to be non-pregnant.

In order to determine the MTD of doceta-xel in this patient population and describe the grade 3 and 4 hematologic and non-hemato-logic toxicities, we entered at least 3 new patients at each dose level. We defined dose limiting toxicity (DLT) as the occurrence in any one patient of any one of the following: death before day 15, or grade 3 non-hemato-logic or non-infectious toxicity, or bone mar-row hypoplasia persisting until day 42. If one patient at a given dose level developed DLT, then 3 additional patients would be added to that dose level. If a second patient developed any of these endpoints at that same dose level, then the previous dose level would be defined as the MTD for this patient population.

Patients were treated as follows (Figure 1). On days −1, 0, and +1, dexamethasone, 8 mg, was given orally or intravenously twice a day. On day 0, docetaxel was given intravenously over one hour. On day +2, G-CSF, 5 µg per kg was given subcutaneously, daily until the absolute neutrophil count was at least 500 per µl for three days.

On day +21, bone marrow aspiration and biopsy were performed. Patients whose bone marrow cellularity was greater than 15% and who had more than 5% blasts in the bone marrow could receive a second course of docetaxel at 75% of the initial dose. Any patients achieving complete remission (CR, fewer than 5% blasts in the bone marrow, with an absolute neutrophil count greater than 1000 per µl and a platelet count greater than 100,000 per µl) after either one or two cycles of docetaxel were to be observed for relapse. Patients who achieved a partial remission (PR, between 5 and 24% blasts in the marrow, with recovery of peripheral blood counts as for CR) were observed for disease progression. Patients who had more than 5% bone marrow blasts or who did not have recovery of peripheral blood counts after two courses of docetaxel were conside-red treatment failures and did not receive fur-ther study drug.

Patients whose white blood cell count was above 50,000 per µl during day −1, 0, or +1 were given hydroxyurea, one gram orally every six hours, until the white count was less than 40,000 per µl or until day +2, whichever came first. Patients who achieved a CR after either one or two courses of docetaxel were eligible to receive further treatment, inclu-ding stem cell transplantation, at the discre-tion of their treating physicians. The treat-ment schema is shown in Figure 1.

Observed toxicity was graded using Natio-nal Cancer Institute Common Toxicity Crite-ria [12].

## Results

To date, five patients have been treated according to the above protocol, three at the initial dose level of 100 mg/m$^2$, two at the second dose level, 130 mg/m$^2$. Patients ranged in age from 31 to 75. All had been previously treated.with refractory or relapsed were either secondary to myleoproliferative or myelodysplastic syndromes or heavily pre-treated.

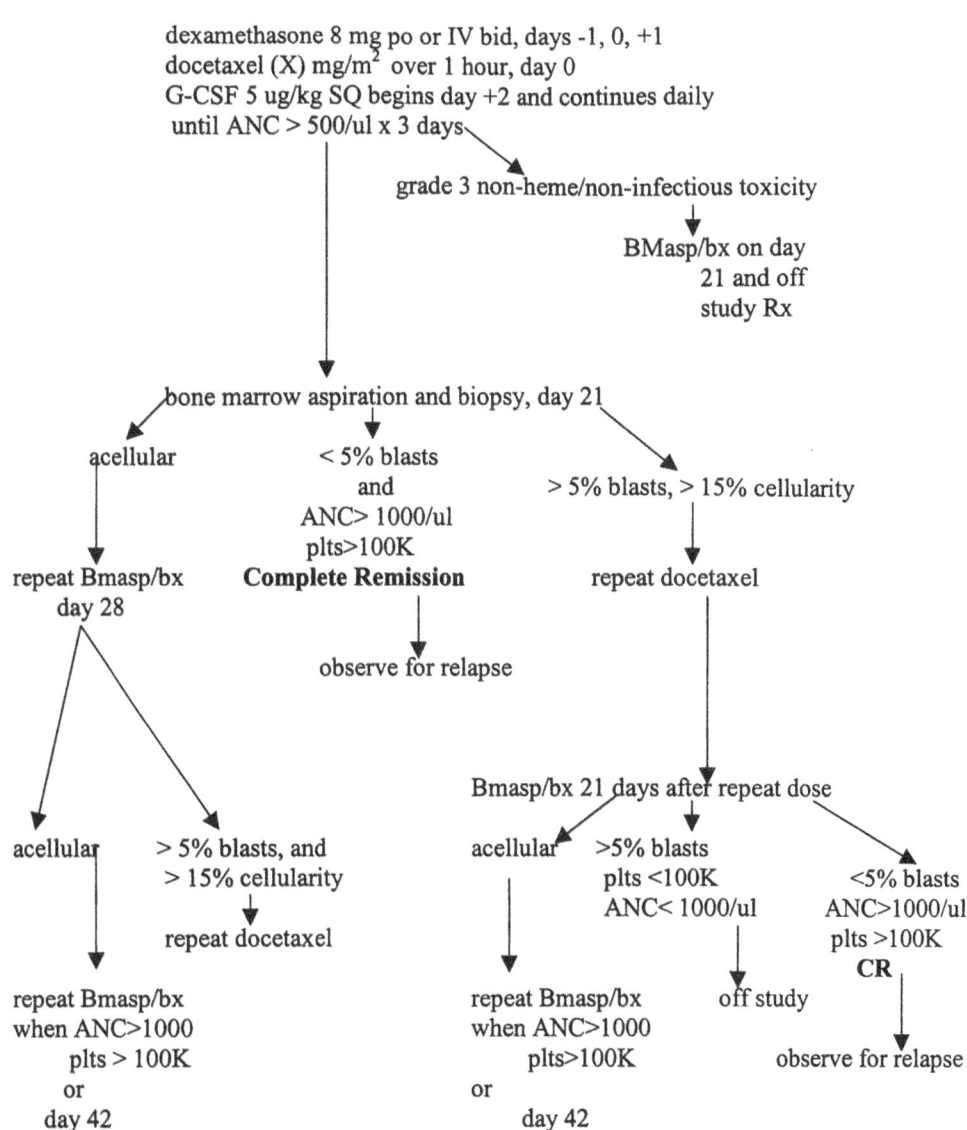

**Fig. 1.** The treatment schema for treatment of patients with relapsed of refractory AML with docetaxel.

Specific results in these patients are shown in Table 1. Two patients were able to receive 2 courses of docetaxel. All patients were thrombocytopenic prior to receiving docetaxel. Hematologic toxicity was manageable, and there were no major hemorrhagic events. Observed non-hematologic toxicity consisted primarily of mucositis, rash, and edema.

No dose-limiting toxicity was observed in the first cohort of patients (dose level = 100 mg/m²). No clear toxicity patterns were apparent. Docetaxel decreased peripheral blast counts in 4 patients.

## Discussion

The optimal therapeutic approach to patients with poor-prognosis secondary AML or with relapsed or refractory *de novo* AML remains a

479

**Table 1.** Results

| Dose Level | # | ID | Prior Treatment | Pre-Docetaxel Blood & Marrow | Treatment & Toxicity | Post-Docetaxel Blood & Marrow | Survival |
|---|---|---|---|---|---|---|---|
| $100mg/m^2$ | 1 | age:49, M AML relapse@9mo, refract | Ara-C/DNR; HiDAC; Mitox/VP-16; antiCD33 | wbc 138 96%bl plt 47 BM:88%bl | 1 course gr1 mucositis | wbc 10.9 68%bl plt 13 | d. day 21 |
| $100mg/m^2$ | 2 | age:74, M refract AML -5, 7q-, +8 | Ara-C/Ida | wbc 1.1 plt 21 BM:13%bl | 1 course gr2 rash | wbc 0.5 BM:87%bl | d. day 97 |
| $100mg/m^2$ | 3 | age:31, F M0 AML relapsed 11 mo. s/p allo-BMT | Ara-C/Ida/ Vcr/pred/ L-asp/Mtx; alloBMT | wbc 2.6 plt 41 BM:88%bl | 2 courses gr5 infect | wbc 0.8 0%bl plt 49 BM:80%bl | d. day 38 |
| $130mg/m^2$ | 4 | age:59, M MPDx5yr; AML refractory | Ara-C/DNR | wbc 5.8 76%bl plt 26 | 2 courses; gr2 edema; gr2 cellulitis | wbc 3.7 53%bl plt 32 | d. day 39 |
| $130mg/m^2$ | 5 | age:75, F AML, 6-yr remission; MDS6AML refractory | Ara-C/DNR; Ara-C/mitox/ VP-16 | wbc 9.8 plt 72 BM: | too early | | alive day 6 |

formidable challenge. In this situation, drug resistance on the part of leukemic cells commonly plays an important role; these cells often express the MDR gene product, p-glycoprotein [3–6]. Moreover, in a patient population that may be quite heavily pre-treated or elderly, the inability to tolerate myelosuppression may make the delivery of therapeutically active doses of cytotoxic treatment problematic. New agents with properties circumventing these obstacles might have promise in this clinical setting.

The taxane docetaxel is semi-synthetic drug derived from a precursor extracted from the needles of the European yew tree *Taxus baccata*. Docetaxel is an antimitotic agent, which acts as a spindle poison. *In vitro*, docetaxel promotes microtubule assembly and inhibits disassembly, thus stabilizing microtubules. This mode of action is essentially the opposite of that of the vinca alkaloids [13–15]. Importantly, docetaxel has demonstrated acitivity in tumors that are anthracycline-resistant[2]. In addition, in patients with solid tumors, it has been shown to be relati-

vely platelet-sparing, while producing significant neutropenia, suggesting considerable activity against normal myeloid cells[2].

In the first cohorts of the present Phase I/II trial of the use of docetaxel for patients with acute myeloid leukemia, docetaxel appears to be well tolerated. No dose-limiting toxicity has been observed to present. In addition, dexamethasone pre-treatment and G-CSF support have been well-tolerated in patients with relapsed and refractory AML.

Decreases in peripheral blast counts have been observed even in the limted numbers of patients treated to date. On the other hand, prolonged cytopenias in the patients treated at 100 mg/m² and 130 mg/m² have not been seen.

It appears that docetaxel doses of at least 100 mg/m² can be safely administered to patients with refractory or relapsed AML, and dose escalation continues. Docetaxel may be potentially well suited for use in patients with poor-prognosis AML, and further phase I/II testing is warranted.

# References

1. Hiddeman W and Büchner T (1991) Treatment strategies in acute myeloid leukemia (AML). Blut 60: 163–171.
2. Docetaxel (Taxotere) package insert, Rhône-Poulenc Rorer.
3. Ma DDF, Davey RA, Harman DH, Isbister JP, Scurr RD, Mackertich SM, Dowden G, Bell DR (1987) Detection of a multidrug resistant phenotype in acute non-lymphocytic leukaemia. Lancet 1: 135–137.
4. Marie J-P (1995) P-glycoprotein in adult hematologic malignancies. Hematol Oncol Clin North Am 9: 239–249.
5. Zhou DC, Marie J-P, Suberville AM, et al. (1992) Relevance of mdr1 gene expression in acute myeloid leukemia and comparison of different diagnostic methods. Leukemia 6: 879–885.
6. Sonneveld P, van Rens GL, de Boevere MJ, et al. (1995) Molecular and functional multidrug resistance phenotypes in poor-risk AML with 7q/7q-karyotype. Proc Am Soc Hematol 86: 517a.
7. Mayer RJ, Davis RB, Schiffer CA, et al. (1994) Intensive postremission chemotherapy in adults with acute myeloid leukemia. N Engl J Med 331: 896–903.
8. Stone RM, Mayer RJ (1993) The approach to the elderly patient with acute myeloid leukemia. Hematol Oncol Clin North Am 7: 65–79.
9. Stone RM, Berg DT, George SL, et al. (1995) Granulocyte-macrophage colony-stimulating factor after initial chemotherapy for elderly patients with primary acute myelogenous leukemia. N Engl J Med 332: 1671–1677.
10. Seibel NL, Blaney SM, O'Brien M, et al. (1997) Pediatric phase I trial of docetaxel (D) with G-CSF: collaborative pediatric branch, NCI and Children's Cancer Group trial. Proc Am Soc Clin Oncol 16: 769a.
11. Tange UB, Lung B, Hansen HH, Dombernowsky P, Le Bail N (1994) Phase I study of Taxotere (docetaxel) in patients with solid tumors. Proc Am Soc Clin Oncol 13: 1388a.
12. Miller AB, Hoogstraten B, Staquet M, et al. (1981) Reporting results of cancer treatment. Cancer 47: 207–214.
13. Ringel I, Horwitz S (1991) Studies with RP56976 (Taxotere): a semisynthetic analogue of Taxol. J Natl Cancer Inst 83: 288–291.
14. bissery MC, Guenard D, Gueritte-Voegelein F, et al. (1991) Experimental antitumor activity of Taxotere (RP56976, NSC 628503), a Taxol analogue. Cancer Res 51: 4845–4852.
15. Verwiej J, Clavel M, Chevalier B (1994) Paclitaxel (Taxol) and docetaxel (Taxotere): not simply two of a kind. Ann Oncol 5: 495–505.

# Including Quality of Life as an Important End Point in Evaluating Intensive and Prolonged Treatment for Acute Myeloid Leukemia (AML)

A. Schumacher, D. Wewers, T. Büchner and W.E. Berdel

## Aims

Intensification of treatment for AML resulted in a substantial improvement in longterm prognosis (Büchner 1997). As intensive therapy might be associated with high morbidity and most patients with AML eventually relapse, quality of life (QL) of patients has become an important parameter to be assessed. This study was designed to evaluate QL in patients with AML treated according to the protocol of the German AML-Cooperative Group.

## Measurements of Quality of Life

An individual's health related QL is not observable in a direct way, but can only be concluded from different components. Therefore, an instrument to measure QL should be multidimensional and should comprise the relevant categories of variables: physical complaints, psychological distress, social interaction and functional status.

Based on conceptual, methodological and practical criteria, we used the QL-questionnaire developed by the European Organization for Research and Treatment of Cancer: EORTC QLQ- C 30 (Aaronson et al. 1993). The EORTC QLQ-C 30 is a well-validated 30-item self-report questionnaire composed of multi-item scales and single items that reflect the multidimensionality of the QL construct. (Table 1). In addition to the core questionnaire QLQ-C 30 and according to EORTC guidelines, a novel leukemia specific module was developed by our study group. The module was constructed to assess diagnosis-

**Table 1.** EORTC-QLQ C 30 Subscales

| Functional Scales | Symptom Scales |
| --- | --- |
| Physical Functioning | Fatigue |
| Role Functioning | Nausea and Vomiting |
| Emotional Functioning | Pain |
| Cognitive Functioning | Dyspnea |
| Social Functioning | Sleep Disturbance |
| Global Health Status/ | Appetite Loss |
| Qualitiy of Life | Constipation |
| | Diarrhea |
| | Financial Impact |

**Table 2.** Leukemia-Specific-Module Subscales

| | |
| --- | --- |
| General Symptoms | Pain Medication |
| Diagnosis-Specific Symptoms | Treatment Strain |
| Pain | Hope/Confidence |

specific and treatment-related symptoms. (Table 2)

## Design of the study

QL has been analysed throughout induction therapy, consolidation and maintenance therapy over 3 years, evaluating defined specific parameters at 12 sequential time points. The questionnaires were administered in the first 4 courses of chemotherapy (double induction, consolidation, first and second cycle of maintenance therapy) during inpatient treatment, before and after drug-induced myelo-aplasia. Every six months during outpatient treatment patients assessed a set of mailed questionnaires up to the end of their treatment. Patients' individual perception of

Dept. Internal Med. Hematology/Oncology, University of Münster, FRG

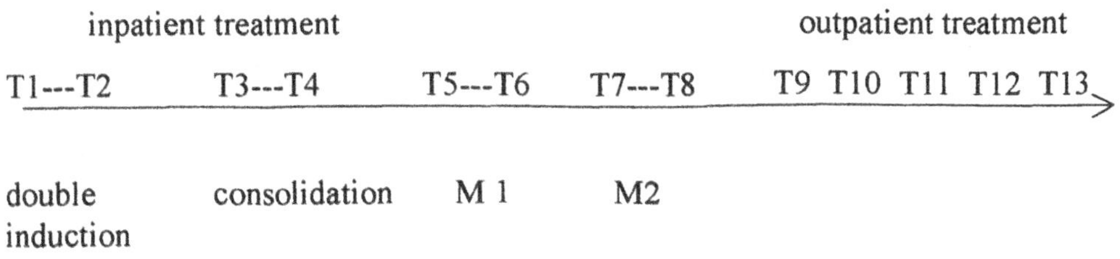

| inpatient treatment | | | | outpatient treatment |
|---|---|---|---|---|

T1---T2　　　　T3---T4　　　　T5---T6　　　T7---T8　　T9 T10 T11 T12 T13⟶

double　　　　consolidation　　M 1　　　M2
induction

**Fig. 1.** Design of the study

their disease and therapy was evaluated by a semi-structured interview during the first cycle of maintenance therapy (Fig. 1).

The design of the study was approved by the Ethical Committee of the School of Medicine, University of Münster.

## Patients

The study was conducted at the Department of Internal Medicine (Hematology/Oncology) at the University of Münster, FRG. All patients, aged 16 to 70, admitted with newly diagnosed acute myeloid leukemia were approached to participate in the study.

Out of 101 patients being enrolled in the protocol, 37 patients were able to complete inpatient treatment.

Exclusions from the study:

27 patients: relapse during inpatient treatment phase
26 patients: death during inpatient treatment phase
15 patients: excluded from AMLCG-protocol due to therapy associated complications
6 patients: bone marrow transplantation after achieving CR
5 patients: participation ceased
5 patients: lost to follow up

As the aim of the study was to assess the impact of this specific kind of prolonged and intensive therapy on patients' subjective well-being over time, it was necessary to consider a subset of patients with full data sets and a sufficiently long follow-up period (Hopwood et al. 1994).

## Statistical Analyses

Changes in patients' assessments of the various EORTC-subscales were evaluated by doing multivariate analyses of variance for repeated measurements (SPSS Win 6.0.1) which is the appropriate procedure recommended by the EORTC.

## Results

### Inpatient treatment phase

For those patients having completed the courses of inpatient treatment (n=37), self-assessed *Physical Functioning* (p<.001), *Role Functioning* (p<.001), *Emotional Functioning* (p<.001) and *Social Functioning* (p<.001) improved significantly from beginning of chemotherapy to the end of inpatient treatment (Fig. 2). This means: at the end of inpatient treatment, patients' physical fitness had improved and patients didn't worry that much anymore. Patients' ability to fullfill minor tasks in and around the house had improved and the impairment of their social activities was decreasing. Individual assessment of *Global Health Status and Subjective QL* improved significantly over the same time. (Fig. 3)

At the end of inpatient treatment, patients felt significantly less distressed by *General Symptoms* – e.g. weight loss or fever – (p<.001) and by *Specific Symptoms* – e.g. bleeding or infections by central venous catheter – (p<.001). (Fig. 4)

Accordingly, patients suffered significantly less from *Fatigue* (p<.001), *Appetite loss* (p=.012), *Dyspnea* (p=.001) and *Pain* (p=.024). (Fig. 5)

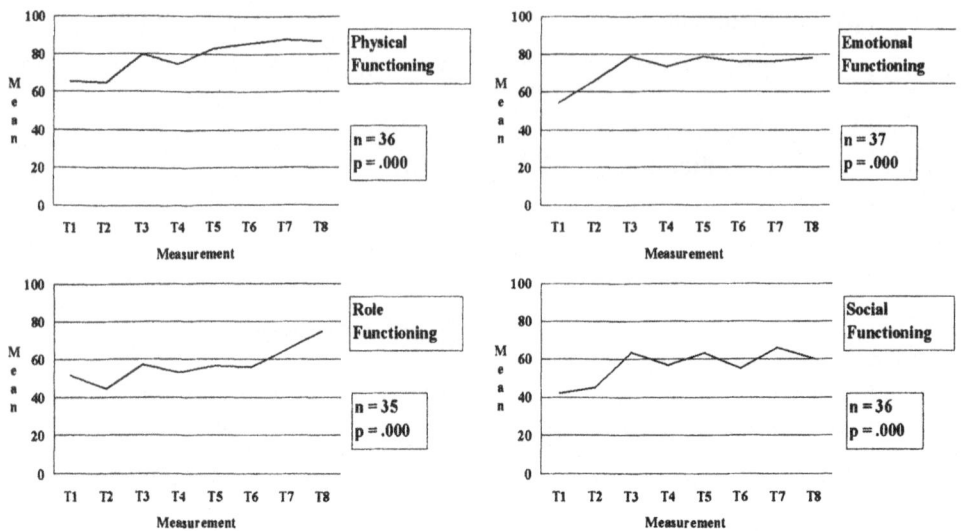

**Fig. 2.** EORTC-QLQ C 30 Subscales; A higher score indicating better functioning

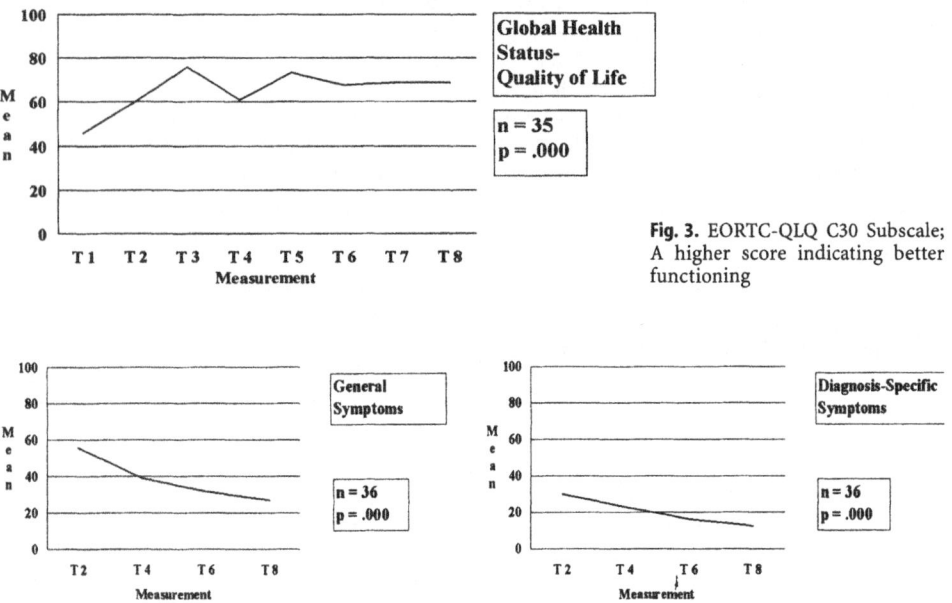

**Fig. 3.** EORTC-QLQ C30 Subscale; A higher score indicating better functioning

**Fig. 4.** Leukemia-Specific-Module Subscales; A higher score indicating a higher degree of symptoms

### Outpatient treatment phase

During outpatient treatment phase, patients' assessment of Subjective QL and the various functional scales revealed no significant changes compared to the end of inpatient therapy. Compared to the beginning of treatment, patients evaluated their *Physical Functioning*, *Emotional Functioning* and *Global Health Status and Subjective QL* as significantly better (Fig. 6, Fig. 7).

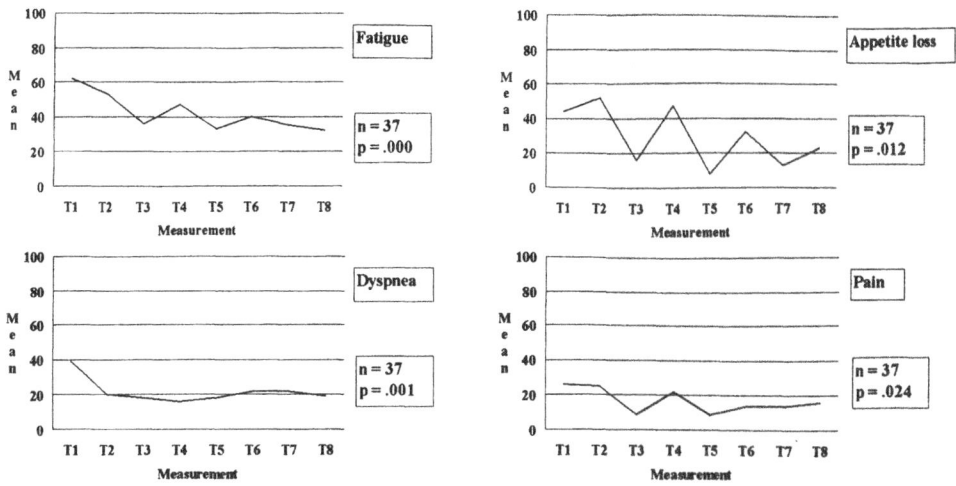

**Fig. 5.** EORTC-QLQ C30 Subscales; A higher score indicating a higher degree of symptoms

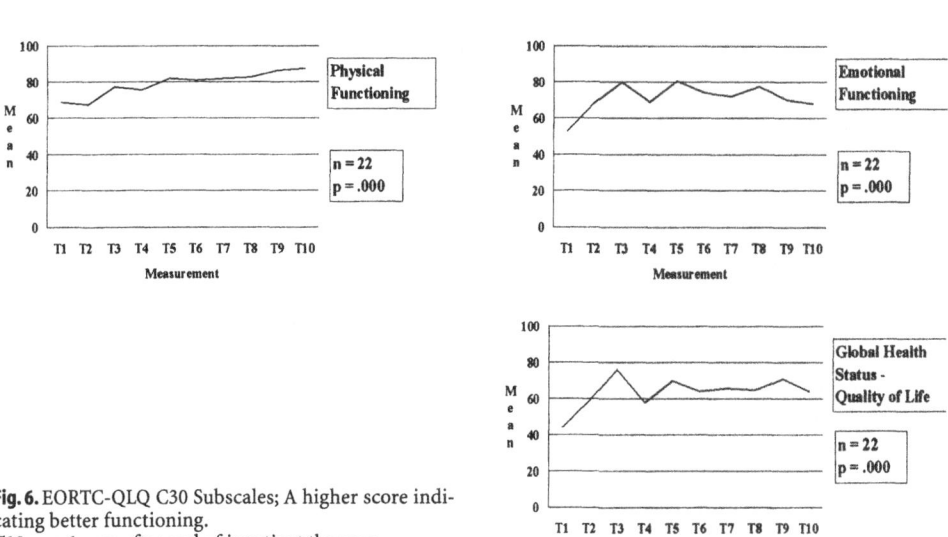

**Fig. 6.** EORTC-QLQ C30 Subscales; A higher score indicating better functioning.
T10 app. 1 year after end of inpatient therapy.

## Discussion

The German AML-Cooperative Group (Büchner et al. 1992, Büchner 1997) has shown that a multiple-step chemotherapy combining double induction, intensified consolidation and long-term maintenance can improve both treatment response and longterm prognosis. The aim of the study was to evaluate QL in patients undergoing treatment as an important parameter. In order to assess the impact of prolonged and intensive AML-therapy on patients' subjective QL, only patients with CR and disease-free survival throughout inpatient treatment were included in the analysis. Due to the severity of the disease and the treatment associated symptoms, uncertainty about their individual prognosis is common to all patients undergoing treatment. So it is not to be expected that patients who fail to complete treatment successfully, might experience a different

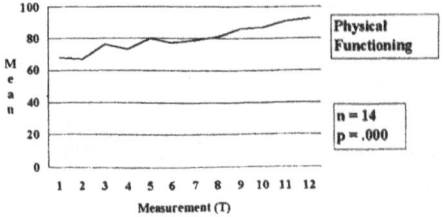

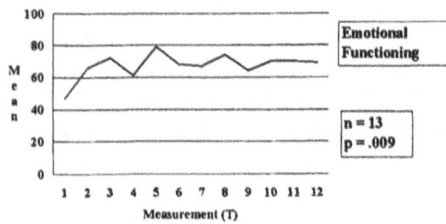

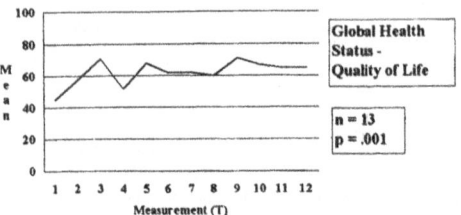

**Fig. 7.** EORTC-QLQ C30 Subscales; A higher score indicating better functioning.
T12 app. 2 years after end of inpatient therapy.

kind of QL from the very beginning of therapy. As shown by a one-way analysis, patients who subsequently went off protocol due to relapse or death or therapy associated complications did not differ significantly in their self-assessed QL while still under treatment when compared to patients who completed therapy.

## Conclusion

The results of our study clearly show that at the end of inpatient treatment, patients assessed their physical, psychological and functional status as better than at the beginning of therapy. As well patients suffered significantly less from various symptoms, mostly side-effects of chemotherapy. During outpatient treatment, patients' assessment revealed no further significant changes in the QL domains. This might seem to be unexpected since one would assume that treatment toxicity and poor prognosis would be associated with poor QL. The qualitative data highlight the fact that patients set different priorities in defining their individual QL compared to what doctors and nurses would consider, e.g. patients may trade more toxicity for a brief extension of life (Richards et al. 1992, Slevin et al. 1990). In the interviews a substantial number of patients (70% out of 37) reported a *secondary benefit* they experienced from the disease, despite the uncertainty of a longterm

remission and the duration of therapy: those patients claim they get a different perspective on life, being ill makes them readjust their priorities, life has become more valuable to them and therefore they are able to enjoy it in a very intensive way.

*Due to advances in treatment for AML an increasing minority of patients will be cured. The inclusion of QL as an outcome parameter shows that intensive and prolonged therapy is not associated with poor QL and patients'subjective benefits outweigh the adverse effects of antileukemic therapy.*

## References

Büchner T, Hiddemann W, Wörmann B, Löffler H, Maschmeyer G, Hossfeld D, Ludwig WD, Nowrousian M, Aul C, Schaefer UW, Sauerland C, Heinecke A (1992) Longterm effects of prolonged maintenance and of very early intensification chemotherapy in AML: data from AMLCG. Leukemia 5 (suppl 4): 68–70

Büchner, T (1997) Treatment of adult acute leukemia. Current Opinion in Oncology: 18–25

Aaronson NK, Ahmedzai S, Bergman B, Bullinger M, Cull A, Duerz NJ, Filiberti A, Flechtner H, Fleishman SB, de Haes J, Kaasa S, Klee M, Osoba D, Razavi D, Rofe PB, Schraub S, Sneeuw K, Sullivan M, Takeda F (1993) The European Organization for Research and Treatment of Cancer, QLQ-C 30: A quality-of-life instrument for use in international clinical trials in oncology. J Nat Cancer Inst 85: 365–376

Hopwood P, Stephens RJ, Machin D (1994) Approaches to the analysis of quality of life data: experiences gained from a Medical Research Council Lung Cancer Working Party palliative chemotherapy trial. Quality of Life Research 3: 339–352

Richards MA, Hopwood P, Ramirez AJ, Twelves CJ, Ferguson J, Gregory WM, Swindell R, Scrivener W, Miller J, Howell A, Rubens RD (1992) Doxorubicin in advanced breast cancer: influence of schedule on response, survival and quality of life. Eur J Cancer 28A: 1023–1028

Slevin ML, Stubbs L, Plant H, Wilson P, Gregory WM, Armes PJ, Downer SM (1990) Attitudes to chemotherapy: comparing views of patients with cancer with those of doctors, nurses and general public. BMJ 300: 1458–1460

# The 10.000/µl Morning Trigger for Prophylactic Platelet Transfusion is Safe: Prospective Experience in 411 AML Patients

H. Wandt, M. Frank, Th. Denzel, W. Aulitzky, H. Bodenstein, N. Brack, H. Duerk, R. Engberding, A. Fauser, Th. Geer, B. Germann, M. Gramatzki, J. Kaesberger, J. Kisro, O. Knigge, G. Köchling, R. Kuse, H. Link, A. Neubauer, S. Öhl, P. Pflüger, J. Saal, U. Schäkel, K. Schalk, H. Schmidt, S. Soucek, T. Wagner, K. Wilms, R. Winter and G. Ehninger for the Cooperative AML 96 Study, Süddeutsche Hämoblastosegruppe (SHG)

## Introduction

There is an increasing demand for platelet transfusions and it remains an ongoing challenge for most blood centers to maintain an adequate platelet inventory. Platelet transfusions doubled in the US and in Canada from 1980 to 1987[1-3]. Between 1989 and 1992 the number of platelet concentrates decreased in the US by 8.9 % while the number of apheresis platelets administered increased by 75 % [4] There is no doubt that platelet transfusions are beneficial and they have permitted the use of more aggressive chemotherapy and bone marrow transplantation. However, there is still controversy regarding when platelets should be administered to maximize their benefit while minimizing the risk of bleeding [5-12].

In the 1960s studies demonstrated a relationship between hemorrhage and platelet count in patients with acute leukemia [13]. Since that time, most hematologists have used a 20 x $10^9$/l platelet trigger for giving prophylactic platelet transfusions with a considerable inter-institutional heterogeneity in transfusion policies. A study performed in 1992 by the Transfusion Practice Committee of the American Association of Blood Banks reported the current practice for prophylactic platelet transfusion. More than 70 % of hospitals transfused platelets primarily for prophylaxis. Eighty percent of these hospitals set the threshold for prophylactic transfusion at 20 x $10^9$/l or even higher [3]. During the last ten years, there has been increasing debate based on both old and more recent data that have

brought into question the traditional platelet transfusion policy [7-11, 14]. Those data indicate that there is no real threshold for bleeding complications. Other factors affect bleeding risk like platelet function, rapid platelet consumption during febrile episodes, plasma coagulation factor deficiencies and local factors such as vascular lesions or organ infiltrations.

We and two other groups have recently shown in prospective studies that the 10.000/µl trigger is safe and cost effective[15, 16, 17]. In the ongoing AML SHG study the 10.000/µl trigger was therefore used for all patients of any age. The objective was to see whether the results gained in the previous studies with maximal 125 patients could be confirmed in a larger AML population.

## Methods

Daily morning blood counts were performed as long as patients were receiving platelet transfusions or until the platelet count was self-supporting of > 25 x $10^9$/l for 2-3 days. Blood counts were performed on EDTA-anticoagulated blood using a flow cytometer. The patients were examined daily for evidence of hemorrhage. Fundoscopy was done only in case of impairment of vision.

Hemoglobin levels were maintained at > 80 g/l by packed red cell transfusions.

During each course of chemotherapy bleeding complications according to WHO-criteria (0 = none; 1 = petechial, 2 = mild blood loss, 3 = gross blood loss, 4 = debilita-

Medical Clinic 5, Institut for Medical Oncology and Hematology, Nürnberg, Germany

ting blood loss) were recorded as well as the number of red cells and platelet transfusions given. The bleeding complication scores were recorded in parallel to the treatment of each patient by the treating physician and controlled by a board certified hematologist, responsible for the study at each center. Major bleeding complications (WHO grade 3 and 4) were verified by chart review performed by the study coordinator. Platelet transfusions were given at the discretion of each center as pooled random donor platelet concentrates (normally 4-6) or as apheresis single donor products. The use was determined by the standard of each center and the actual availability of the different platelet products. It was recommended but not a study requirement that platelets be leuco-reduced by filtration at the bedside. Random ABO-compatible (non HLA-typed) platelet transfusions were given until a major bleeding episode and alloimmunisation necessitated HLA-matched platelet transfusions.

All patients were followed from the beginning of each chemotherapy cycle until discharge with a stable platelet count > 25 x $10^9$/l, treatment failure or death.

### Platelet transfusion protocol

Prophylactic platelet transfusions were given routinely for morning platelet counts below 10 x $10^9$/l. Platelet transfusions were given for morning platelet counts of < 15 x $10^9$/l, if patients had a fever of > 38,5°C and a rapid decrease in platelet count (> 10 x $10^9$/l), plasma coagulation factor deficiencies due to sepsis or leukemia, or when hyperleucocytosis (> 50 x $10^9$/l) was present at the start of chemotherapy. The platelet counts were maintained at > 20 x $10^9$/l in both groups, when biopsies (bone marrow biopsies excluded) were performed and in case of major bleeding. Major bleeding was defined as melaena, haematemesis, macrohematuria, hemoptysis, vaginal bleeding, epistaxis for more than one hour with gross blood loss, retinal haemorrhages with impairment of vision or soft tissue bleeding requiring blood transfusion.

### Results

We report on our prospectively gained experience in 411 AML patients. We recorded 32 clinically, relevant hemorrhages (WHO grade 3 [14 patients] and WHO grade 4 [18 patients]) in these patients during induction and consolidation chemotherapy (incidence of bleeding 7.8 %). Patients' age with major bleeding complication ranged from 24 to 83 years without any increased risk for elderly patients. 29 hemorrhages (91 %) occurred during the first weeks of induction therapy. Platelet count at bleeding event ranged from < 5 to 146 x $10^9$/l. Bleeding happened in 80 % with platelets counts > 10 x $10^9$/l. Major causes of bleeding were plasmatic coagulation disorders and leukemia (10x), local factors at bleeding site (24x), pneumonia and sepsis (6x), refractoriness (3x). The outcome of 18 patients was fatal. Death was related to plasmatic coagulation problems in parallel with uncontrolled leukemia and sepsis (9/18 patients) or pneumonia/ARDS and multiorgan failure (6/18 patients) or because patients were refractory to platelet transfusion (3/18 patients). Bleeding could be stopped by therapeutic platelet transfusions only if the underlying cause of hemorrhage could be treated effectively at the same time.

### Conclusion

This study in 411 AML patients confirms the safety of the 10.000/μl trigger for routine prophylactic platelet transfusion in a multicenter trial. No fatal outcome was related to the stringent trigger we used. This report underlines once more that major bleeding complications in leukemia patients are not primarily due to the degree of thrombocytopenia. They are mainly the consequence of other factors as plasmatic coagulation problems, pneumonia or local factors. Relevant hemorrhages happened mostly (91 %) during induction therapy. This observation is in parallel with our published study showing that most hemorrhages occurred during induction chemotherapy even with the traditional 20.000/μl trigger [17].

# References

1. Surgenor DM et al. (1990) Collection and Transfusion of Blood in the United States, 1982-1988. N Engl J Med 322(23):16
2. Davey M (1988) Trends in platelet utilization in Canada, 1981-1987. Curr Stud Hematol Blood Transfus 54:89
3. Pisciotto PT et al. (1995) Prophylactic versus therapeutic platelet transfusion practices in hematology and/or oncology patients. Transfusion 35:498
4. Wallace EL et al. (1995) Collection and transfusion of blood and blood components in the United States, 1992. Transfus 35:802
5. Schiffer CA (1992) Prophylactic platelet transfusion. Transfus 32:295
6. Baer MR, Bloomfield CD (1992) Controversies in transfusion medicine. Prophylactic platelet transfusion therapy. Pro Transfus 32:381
7. Solomon J et al. (1978) Platelet prophylaxis in acute non-lymphoblastic leukemia. Lancet 1:267
8. Murphy S et al. (1982) Indications for platelet transfusion in children with acute leukemia. Am J Hematol 12:347
9. (1987) Platelet transfusion therapy. Consensus conference. Jama 257:1777
10. Beutler E (1993) Platelet transfusions: the 20 000 µl trigger. Blood 81:1411
11. Slichter SJ et al. (1986) Transfusion Medicine – Newer Approaches to Platelet Transfusion Therapy. In McArthur JR (ed): Hematology, Orlando, American Society of Hematology, 1996, p 119
12. Patten E (1992) Controversies in transfusion medicine. Prophylactic platelet transfusion revisited after 25 years. Con Transfus 32:381
13. Gaydos LA et al. (1962) The quantitive relation between platelet count and haemorrhage in patients with acute leukemia. N Engl J Med 266:905
14. Gmür J et al. (1991) Safety of stringent prophylactic platelet transfusion policy for patients with acute leukemia. Lancet 338:1223
15. Heckmann KD et al. (1997) Randomized study of prophylactic platelet transfusion treshhold during induction therapy for adult leukemia 10.000/µl versus 20.000/µl. JCO 15:1143
16. Rubella P et al. (1997) The treshhold for prophylactic platelet transfusion in adults with acute myeloid leukemia. N Engl J Med 337:1870
17. Wandt H et al. (1998) Safety and cost effectiveness of a 10 x $10^9$/l trigger for prophylactic platelet transfusion compared to the traditional 20 x $10^9$/l trigger: a prospective comparative trial in 105 patients with acute myeloid leukemia. Blood 91, 10:6301

# AML in Children

# Prognostic Factors and Patterns of Failure in Childhood Acute Myeloid Leukemia: Experience on Pediatric Oncology Group Study # 8821

Y. Ravindranath[1], M. Chang[2], S. Raimondi[3], A.J. Carroll[4], C.P. Steuber[5], B. Camitta[6] and H. Weinstein[7], for the Pediatric Oncology Group

## Introduction

Risk Group-based therapy in Childhood Acute Lymphoblastic Leukemia is now standard and has allowed for tailored intensification of therapy based on risk for relapse [1]. Risk group definitions in childhood AML, on the other hand, have proven to be more complex because of the morphologic and cytogenetic diversity, frequent occurrence of extramedullary disease, the presence of a myelodysplastic prodrome and the differences in etiology (de novo versus secondary). Nevertheless, emerging data suggests that there may be distinct cytogenetic and morphologic subgroups with high probability of good outcome. It is now clear that AML children with Down syndrome (DS) have a superior outcome with regimens that include high-dose cytarabine early in consolidation [2]. The use of All-transretinoic acid along with chemotherapy has significantly improved the results in patients with Acute Promyelocytic Leukemia (APL) [3]. Thus, it is now necessary to develop therapeutic strategies for improving the therapy for the remaining large group of children with AML.

With this in mind, we conducted a retrospective univariate and multivariate analysis of a large cohort of children with AML treated on the Pediatric Oncology Group (POG) AML Study # 8821.

## Methods

The POG 8821 study evaluated the role of purged autologous bone marrow transplantation (ABMT) early in remission in comparison to an intensive multiagent consolidation therapy [4]. The results were analyzed by the intent to treat principle and showed the outcome to be similar in the two groups. The study required a central FAB morphology review. In this study, based on prior POG studies (8101), patients with $M_1$ and $M_2$ were grouped in to one category, and $M_4Eo$ was not separately tracked. Cytogenetics were performed in one of the central reference laboratories at the University of Alabama (A.J. Carroll) or at the St. Jude Research Hospital (S. Raimondi).

## Statistical Analysis

Patients with either $M_1$ marrow (< 5% blasts) or $M_2A$ marrow (< 15% blasts) at the end of two induction courses were considered to have achieved remission. Event-free survival (EFS) was calculated from the date of registration until the (earlier of ) date of not achieving remission, first relapse or the date of death. Disease-free survival (DFS) was calculated from the date of randomization, the date of first relapse, or the date of death. Overall survival was calculated from the date of registration or the date of death.

[1] Barbara Ann Karmanos Cancer Institute and Wayne State University, Detroit MI
[2] POG Statistical office, University of Florida Gainesville, FL
[3] St Jude Children's Research Hospital, Memphis, TN
[4] University of Alabama, Birmingham, AL;
[5] Baylor College of Medicine, Houston, TX
[6] Midwest Children's Hospital, Milwaukee, WI and
[7] Massachusetts General Hospital and Harvard University, Boston, Ma

The following covariates were analyzed for univariate and multivariate methods for their correlation of EFS: age at entry; WBC at diagnosis; gender; FAB; cytogenetics (inv(16); t(8;21) and other abnormalities); blast cells in CSF and non-CNS extra-medullary disease. The remission rates were compared by the CHI-Square test and the various survival rates were compared by the log rank test [5]. Survival estimates were made by the method of Kaplan and Meier [6].

## Results

Between June, 1988 and March, 1993, 666 patients younger than 21 years, with previously untreated AML were registered on the POG 8821 AML study. Informed consent was obtained from each patient and/or guardian at their local institution. Of the 666 patients enrolled on the protocol, 649 were evaluable for treatment response. Ten patients were ineligible for study and 7 were not evaluable for response. Fifty-six patients (including 1 DS patient) had t(15;17) and were deleted from this analysis. Thirty-four children with Down syndrome were analyzed separately. Thus, this analysis comprises 560 patients. In 478 (76%) patients, the bone marrow samples were adequate for complete cytogenetic analysis [7]. A patient was classified as having a normal karyotype only after 20 normal meta-phases were analyzed. Of the 478 children with complete cytogenetics, 109 (22.8%) had an apparently normal karyotype (see Figure 1). Of the remaining 369 cases with an abnormal karyotype (77.2% of the study population), 280 (75.9%) had consistent or recurrent abnormalities, and 89 (24.1%) had miscellaneous chromosomal changes. We then categorized patients into five cytogenetic groups: inv(16), t(8;21), 11q23 abnormality and rare chromosomal abnormalities, and those with normal karyotype (see Tables 1 and 2).

Table 1 summarizes the initial response and survival data by prognostic categories. For comparison, the results on Down syndrome patients are included. Female gender, inv(16) and t(8;21) were positive predictors for initial response, whereas age under 2yrs and 11q23 or other rare abnormalities and $M_5$ predicted for poor response. Of these, only the presence of inv(16) / t(8;21) was predictive at a p-value of < 0.01. With regard to EFS, inv(16)/t(8;21) were positive predictors at a p-value of 0.0003 and normal cytogenetics was a positive predictor at a p-value of 0.03. The negative predictors at p-value < 0.01 were age under 2 years, 11q23 or other rare abnormalities, and $M_5$ subtype. The presence of non-CNS EMD was a negative predictor at a p-value of 0.043.

The causes of failure are listed by each prognostic category in Table 2. A striking observation was the rather substantially different

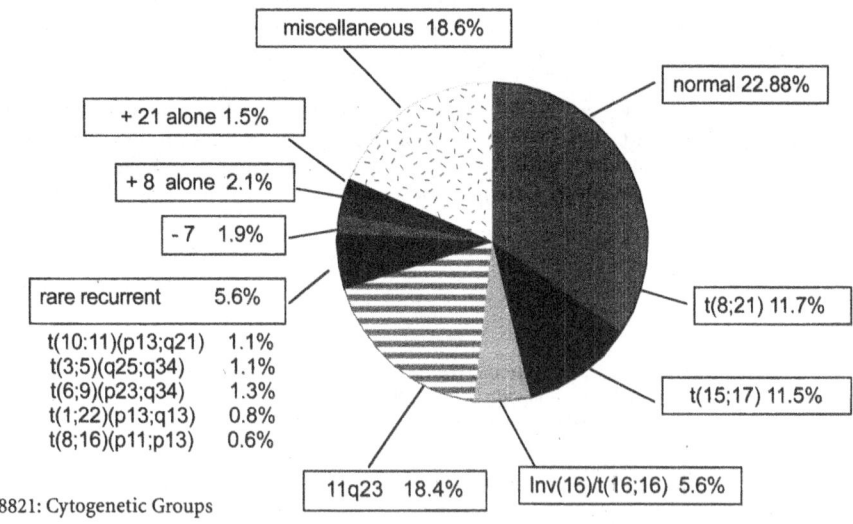

**Fig. 1.** POG 8821: Cytogenetic Groups

**Table 1.** POG 8821 AML Study: Initial Response and Survival by Prognostic Categories

| Category | N | Remission Rate | CHI-Square P-value | EFS% | Log Rank P-Value | DFS% | OS% |
|---|---|---|---|---|---|---|---|
| Whole Group | 560 | 480 (85.7%) | | 32.7 (2.2) | | 38.1 (2.4) | 41.6 (2.2) |
| Down Syndrome | 34 | 31(91.2%) | | 66.4 (9.1) | | 66.9 (9.3) | 67.6 (8.6) |
| Female | 260 | 231 (89%) | + 0.049 | 35.7 (3.2) | 0.092 | 40.2 (3.5) | 43.6 (3.2) |
| Male | 300 | 249 (83%) | | 30.1 (2.9) | | 36.1 (3.4) | 39.6 (3.1) |
| Age <2yrs | 119 | 94 (79 %) | −0.018 | 22.9 (4.2) | −0.0004 | 29.0 (5.1) | 32.8 (4.5) |
| Age >2yrs | 441 | 386 (87.5%) | | 35.3 (2.5) | | 40.3 (2.8) | 43.9 (2.5) |
| Non-CNS EMD | 19 | 15 (78.9%) | 0.15 | 20.0 (8.9) | −0.043 | 25.3 (10.9) | 26.7 (9.3) |
| WBC  < 50K | 393 | 344 (87.5%) | | 32.2 (5.0%) | | 37.2 (5.7%) | 39.9 (5.1%) |
|       > 50K | 167 | 136 (81.4%) | −0.059 | 30.4 (3.9) | 0.12 | 37.4 (4.6%) | 40.1 (4.0%) |
| Inv(16) | 29 | 29 (100%) | | 59.7 (10.5) | | 59.7 (10.5) | 75.9 (8.6) |
| t(8;21) | 57 | 55 (96.5%) | + 0.002 | 44.3 (7.6) | + 0.0003 | 44.1 (7.6) | 50.7 (7.6) |
| 11q23 | 91 | 76 (83.5%) | | 23.3 (4.7) | −<0.0001 | 23.3 (4.8) | 32.7 (5.2) |
| Rare | 27 | 21 (77.8%) | −0.035 | 19.7 (8.8) | | 19.7 (8.8) | 29.6 (10.1) |
| Normal | 109 | 93 (85.5%) | 0.69 | 43.1 (5.0) | 0.03 | 43.1(5.1) | 53.8 (5.0) |
| M1/M2 | 213 | 187 (87.8%) | 0.32 | 34.4 (3.8) | 0.11 | 34.4 (3.8) | 42.3 (3.7) |
| M4 | 94 | 85 (90.4%) | 0.17 | 36.1 (5.3) | 0.26 | 36.1 (5.4) | 47.8 (5.5) |
| M5 | 88 | 69 (78.4%) | −0.023 | 21.2 (4.7) | −0.0002 | 21.2 (4.7) | 28.9 (5.3) |
| M7 | 32 | 26 (81.2%) | 0.42 | 28.1 (8.4) | 0.14 | 28.1 (8.4) | 34.4 (8.4) |
| Other | 52 | 45 (86.5%) | 0.91 | 43.0 (7.5) | 0.24 | 43.0 (7.5) | 47.9 (7.2) |

EFS= Event free survival from study entry; DFS= event free survival from remission; OS= Overall survival

**Table 2.** POG 8821 AML Study: Patterns of Failure

| Category | N | Early Death | No Response | Deaths in CR | Relapses | Deaths in Rel. | Total deaths | Alive[#] |
|---|---|---|---|---|---|---|---|---|
| Whole Group | 560 | 21 | 57 | 33 | 252 | 219 | 333 | 213 |
| Down Syndrome | 34 | 2 | 1 | 3 | 3 (10%) | 3 | 11 | 22 |
| Female | 260 | 10 | 18 | 17 | 116 (44.6%) | 101 | 149 | 109 |
| Male | 300 | 11 | 39 | 16 | 136 (54.6%) | 118 | 184 | 108 |
| Age <2yrs | 119 | 8 | 16 | 4 | 61 (64.9%) | 55 | 81 | 37 |
| Age >2yrs | 441 | 13 | 41 | 29 | 191 (49.5%) | 164 | 292 | 176 |
| Non-CNS EMD | 19 | 0 | 4 | 1 | 14 | 14 | 18 | 6 |
| WBC | | | | | | | | |
| < 50K | 393 | 13 | 33 | 28 | 177 | 156 | 231 | 153 |
| > 50K | 167 | 8 | 24 | 5 | 75 | 63 | 102 | 60 |
| Inv(16) | 29 | 0 | 0 | 1 | 9 ( 31%) | 5 | 7 | 20 |
| t(8;21) | 57 | 1 | 1 | 2 | 25 (40%) | 23 | 28 | 27 |
| 11q23 | 91 | 5 | 10 | 3 | 46 (60.5%) | 39 | 63 | 27 |
| Rare | 27 | 4 | 2 | 0 | 14 (66.6%) | 12 | 19 | 8 |
| Normal | 109 | 1 | 13 | 3 | 43 (39.5%) | 36 | 52 | 53 |
| M1/M2 | 213 | 6 | 18 | 17 | 93 | 82 | 126 | 80 |
| M4 | 94 | 2 | 6 | 2 | 46 | 36 | 49 | 44 |
| M5 | 88 | 7 | 13 | 8 | 38 | 33 | 63 | 24 |
| M7 | 32 | 1 | 6 | 1 | 16 | 15 | 22 | 9 |
| Other | 52 | 0 | 5 | 1 | 22 | 20 | 27 | 23 |

[#] 14 pts. were lost to follow up

overall survival rate between t(8;21) and inv(16) subgroups with the survival being considerably better in the inv(16) group. It is also noteworthy that, unlike in some adult studies, the EFS and overall survival rates of those with normal cytogenetics in childhood AML approaches that of t(8;21). In order to understand these differences better, we looked at the causes of failure by prognostic categories (summarized in Table 2). These data show that children with inv(16) had a lower relapse rate compared to other cytogenetic subgroups and also an apparently higher salvage rate post-relapse. The group with normal cytogenetics behaved essentially similar to those with t(8;21) in this study.

The poorer outcome in children under 2 years of age in this analysis (which excluded DS children) is largely accounted for by a somewhat higher frequency of the $M_5$ subtype, those with 11q23 and other rare cytogenetic abnormalities. The overall outcome of DS children treated on POG 8821 AML study was lower than what we reported with our previous AML study, POG # 8498.[2] This is in part due to a higher frequency of early deaths, and deaths in CR in this study (14.7%). Further, all three children with DS who relapsed died of disease.

## Summary and Discussion

POG 8821 AML study represents one of the largest cohorts of cases of childhood AML with complete cytogenetic data. The results show that excluding children with DS and APL, inv(16) is the best predictor for positive outcome. In this group the EFS is 59.7% and the overall survival is 75.9%. The subgroup with t(8; 21) and normal cytogenetics have an intermediate level of outcome with an EFS of 44.1% and 43.15 and overall survival of 50.7% and 53.8% respectively. Those with 11q23 or other rare abnormalities have the poorest outcome. Female gender is associated with a trend towards superior outcome. DS children continue to do well with high-dose Ara-C containing regimens, but in this group, reduction of mortality from toxicity should be the primary goal of therapeutic strategies.

Considerable controversy exists on the two sides of Atlantic with regard to the role of allogeneic BMT in first remission for AML patients (DS and APL excluded). In this study it was not possible to evaluate the interaction of different post remission treatment strategies because of the relatively small patient population in each of the randomized groups and multiplicity of prognostic variables.

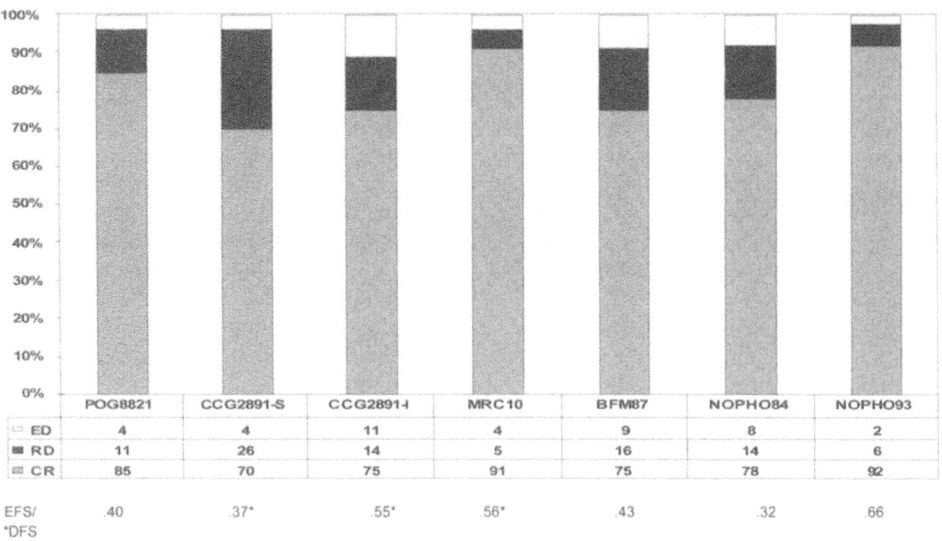

| | POG8821 | CCG2891-S | CCG2891-I | MRC10 | BFM87 | NOPHO84 | NOPHO93 |
|---|---|---|---|---|---|---|---|
| ED | 4 | 4 | 11 | 4 | 9 | 8 | 2 |
| RD | 11 | 26 | 14 | 5 | 16 | 14 | 6 |
| CR | 85 | 70 | 75 | 91 | 75 | 78 | 92 |
| EFS/ *DFS | .40 | .37* | .55* | .56* | .43 | .32 | .66 |

ED= Early deaths; RD= Resistant disease; CR= Remission

**Fig. 2.** Childhood AML: Response, Induction Toxicity and Survival

Nevertheless, the high overall survival in inv(16) subgroup suggests that, allo-BMT could be delayed in this group until after relapse. With regard to the t(8;21) subgroup, the outcome in this study is lower than reported in some adult and pediatric studies.[8-11] A contributing factor was the unexpected biphasic and delayed platelet recovery following the first consolidation course which utilized the drug combination of etoposide and 5-Azacytidine and the resulting significant delay in initiating the next phase of therapy [4].

An important prognostic variable in leukemia therapy is the efficacy of and response to the first induction course. The results of several recent pediatric studies are summarized in the Figure 2.[11-14] While exact comparisons are not possible there are significant differences in the first induction course

The following POG institutions participated in the POG 8821 AML study.

| Institution | Grant Number | Institution | Grant Number |
|---|---|---|---|
| Alberta Children's Hospital | | Rush-Presbyterian | CA-07431 |
| All Children's Hospital | | SPOG Basel | |
| Baylor | CA-03161 | SPOG Bern | |
| Boston Floating Hospital | | SPOG Geneva | |
| Cancer Center of Hawaii | | SPOG Lausanne | |
| Carolinas Medical Center | CA-69177 | SPOG Zurich | |
| Children's Hospital Greenville System | CA-69177 | SUNY Syracuse | |
| Children's Hospital Michigan | CA-29691 | Sacred Heart Hospital | |
| Children's Hospital New Orleans/LSU CCOP | | San Antonio MPC & BDC | |
| | | San Jorge Children's Hospital | |
| Children's Memorial Hospital (Chicago) | CA-07431 | St. Christopher's Hospital | |
| UC/San Diego | CA-28439 | St. Francis Regional | |
| Christ Hospital | CA-07431 | St. Johns Hospital | CA-29691 |
| City of Hope | | St. Mary's Hospital | |
| Cook-Ft. Worth Children's Medical Center | CA-33625 | St. Vincent Hospital | |
| | | Stanford University | CA-33603 |
| Dana-Farber Cancer Institute | CA-41573 | Tampa Children's Hospital | |
| Dartmouth Hitchcock | CA-29293 | Tripler Army Medical Center | |
| Duke University | CA-15525 | University of Alabama | CA-25408 |
| East Carolina University | CA-69177 | University of Arizona | CA-33603 |
| Emory University | CA-20549 | University of Arkansas | |
| Fairfax Hospital | CA-28476 | University of Florida | |
| Hackensack Medical Center | | University of Kansas | |
| Hurley Medical Center | CA-29691 | University of Massachusetts | CA-69428 |
| Joe DiMaggio Children's | | University of Miami | |
| Johns Hopkins University | CA-28476 | University of Mississippi Medical Center | CA-15989 |
| Kaiser Permanente/San Diego | CA-28439 | | |
| Kaiser/Santa Clara | CA-33603 | University of Missouri | CA-05587 |
| Keesler AFB Hospital | CA-15898 | University of Rochester | |
| Medical University of South Carolina | CA-69177 | University of South Alabama | |
| Maine Children's | CA-41573 | University of South Florida | |
| Operations Office | CA-30969 | University of Vermont | CA-29293 |
| Statistical Office | CA-29139 | University of Virginia | |
| Massachusetts General Hospital | CA-29293 | UC/Davis | |
| McGill University | CA-33587 | UC/San Diego | CA-28439 |
| Medical College Virginia | | Southwestern Medical School | CA-33625 |
| Miami Children's Hospital | | UT/Galveston | CA-03161 |
| Midwest Children's Cancer Center | CA-32053 | UT/San Antonio | |
| Mount Sinai Medical School (N.Y.) | CA-69428 | Wake Forest University School of Medicine | |
| Naval Medical Center, SD | | | |
| Nemours Children's Clinic | | West Virginia University, Charleston | CA-15525 |
| Nemours/Orlando | | West Virginia University, Morgantown | CA-15525 |
| Oklahoma University | CA-11233 | Walt Disney Memorial Cancer Institute | |
| Presbyterian Hospital | CA-69177 | Walter Reed Army Medical | |
| Puerto Rico POG | | Warren Clinics | CA-11233 |
| Rhode Island Hospital | CA-29293 | Washington University | CA-05587 |
| Roswell Park Cancer Institute | CA-28383 | Yale University | CA-69428 |

in each of the studies. The MRC and BFM regimens utilize 10 days of cytarabine (Ara-C) in the first induction course and the MRC /BFM and CCG include etoposide as well. In preliminary studies of in-vitro drug sensitivity studies (data not shown here) we have observed that sensitivity to Ara-C is highly predictive of initial response and that there is a positive correlation of Ara-C sensitivity with that for daunorubicin and etoposide. Thus the choice of drugs and the dosage schedule in the first induction course may be critical for the eventual outcome.

*Acknowledgements.* The authors wish to thank Ms Julie Nucci for her help in preparing this manuscript.

# References

1. Smith M , Arthur D, Camitta B et al: Uniform approach to classification and treatment assignment for children with acute lymphoblastic leukemia. J Clin Oncol. 14:18-24, 1996
2. Ravindranath Y, Abella E, Krischer JP, et al: Acute myeloid leukemia (AML) in Down's Syndrome is highly responsive to chemotherapy: experience on Pediatric Oncology Group AML Study 8498. Blood 80:2210-2214,1992.
3. Degos L, Dombret H, Chomianne C, Daniel M-T, Miclea J-M, Chastang C, Castaigne S, Fenaux P. All-trans-retinoic acid as a differentiating agent in the treatment of acute promyelocytic leukemia. Blood 85:2643-2653, 1995
4. Ravindranath Y, Yeager AM, Chang MN, Steuber CP, Krischer J, Graham-Pole J, Carroll A, Inoue , Camitta B, Weinstein HJ. Autologous bone marrow transplantation versus intensive consolidation chemotherapy for Acute Myeloid Leukemia in childhood. N Eng J Med 334:1428-1434, 1996
5. Cox DR. Regression models and life-tables. J.R. Stat. Sec {B} 1992; 34: 187-220
6. Kaplan EL, Meier P. Non parametric Estimation From Incomplete Observations. Journal of the American Statistical Association. 1958; 53, 475-481.
7. Raimondi SC, Chang M, Ravindranath Y et al. Chromosomal abnormalities in 478 children with Acute Myeloid Leukemia: Clinical characteristics and Treatment Outcome in a Cooperative Pediatric Oncology Group study-POG 8821. Blood (in press)
8. Bloomfield C, Lawrence D, Byrd JC, et al. Frequency of prolonged remission duration after high dose cytarabine intensification in acute myeloid leukemia varies by cytogenetic subtype. Cancer Res 58:4173-9, 1998
9. Wheatley K, Burnett A, Goldstone A, Hann I, Stevens R, Rees J, Gray R. A simple robust and highly predictive prognostic index for the determination of risk directed therapy in Acute Myeloid Leukemia (AML) derived from the United KingdomMedical Research Council (MRC) AML10 trial. Blood 86: 598a (abs#2381, suppl 1) 1995.
10. Creutzig U, Ritter J, Schellong G. Identification of two risk groups in childhood acute myelogenous leukemia after therapy intensification in the study AML-BFM-83 as compared with study AML-BFM-78. Blood 75:1932, 1990
11. Creutzig U, Harbott J, Sperling C, Ritter J, Zimmerman M, Loffler H, Riehm J, Schellong G, Ludwig W-D. Clinical significance of surface antigen expression in children with acute myeloid leukemia: Results of study AML-BFM-87. Blood 86:3097-3108, 1995
12. Woods WG, Kobrinsky N, Buckley JD, Lee JW, Sanders J, Neudorf S, Gold S, Barnard DR, De Swarte J, Dusenberry K, Kalousek D, Arthur DC, Lang B. Timed-sequential induction therapy improves post-remission outcome in Acute Myeloid Leukemia: A report from Children's Cancer Group. Blood 87: 4979-4989, 1996
13. Hann I, Stevens RF, Goldstone AH, Rees JKH, Wheatley K, Gray RG, Burnett AK . Randomized comparison of DAT versus ADE as induction chemotherapy in children with acute myeloid leukemia. Results of the Medical Research Council's AML trial (MRC AML-10). Blood 89:2311-2318, 1997
14. Lie S, Jonmundsson G, Mellander L, Siimes MA, Yssing M, Gustafson G. A population based study of 272 children with acute myeloid leukemia treated on two consecutive protocols with different intensity: best outcome in girls, infants and children with Down's syndrome. Brit J Haematol 94: 82-89, 1996

# Early Response to Therapy is the Strongest Prognostic Factor in Childhood AML

S. O. Lie[1], N. Clausen[2], G. Jonmundsson[3], L. Mellander[4], M. A. Siimes[5] and G. Gustafsson[6]
on behalf of the Nordic Society of Pediatric Hematology and Oncology (NOPHO)

*Abstract.* From July 1984 the five Nordic countries (Denmark, Finland, Iceland, Norway and Sweden) have registered all children with AML and treated them on three consecutive protocols of different intensity (NOPHO-84, NOPHO-88 and NOPHO-93). We probably have information on every child with this diagnosis in our region. We have found an annual incidence of AML of 0.7 new cases per 100,000 children less than 16 years of age. We observe a distinct age peak incidence in the two first years of life. Children with Down's syndrom account for 13–15% of all cases.

The NOPHO-93 protocol continued the elements of NOPHO-88 but allowed time for recovery after the first induction block. This made it possible to distinguish between children entering complete remission (CR) after the first block and those children who had not, and who then received an alternative and more intensive induction approach.

Analysis in October 98 have given the following results of NOPHO-93: Among the 148 children entered up to Jan. 1, 1998, 21 (14%) had Down's syndrome (DS). 136/148 (92%) went into complete remission. In children with DS, the 5 year pEFS was 0.86 versus 0.53 in non-DS children (p = 0.02). DS-children are thus excluded in the following analysis for prognostic factors: Children who went into remission on one block only (n = 84; 66%) had a significant (p <0.01) better outcome (pEFS = 0.61) than children who required additional and more aggressive therapy to go into remission (n = 43, pEFS = 0.32). WBC >50 correlated with a worse prognosis (p = 0.05) while age and gender had no significant impact in this protocol.

*Conclusion.* The results of NOPHO-93 are significantly better than what we have achieved previously. Down's syndrome is associated with a »good-risk« AML. In non-DS children, the strongest prognostic factor is early response to therapy.

## Introduction

Acute myeloid leukemia (AML) is a much more complex and resistent disease than acute lymphocytic leukemia (ALL) [1–3]. However, progress in recent years has been quite impressive and long term survival now close to 50% has been reported in some recent published studies [4–9]. This has certainly not been achieved because of the introduction of new drugs, but because of a more aggressive use of »old« drugs and better supportive care. Modern protocols therefore are among the most aggressive and life threatening therapies in pediatric oncology.

In the Nordic countries (Denmark, Finland, Iceland, Norway and Sweden) we have since 1984 registered all children with AML and treated them on 3 consecutive protocols of different intensity (NOPHO-84, NOPHO-88, NOPHO-93). The results of the two first studies have been published [9]. The focus of this paper is the results of our latest protocol

[1] Dept. of Pediatrics, National Hospital of Norway, Oslo
[2] Depr. of Pediatrics, University Hospital, Arhus, Denmark
[3] Dept. of Pediatrics, Landspitalinn, Reykjavik, Iceland
[4] Dept. of Pediatrics, Östra sjukhuset, Gothenborg, Sweden
[5] Dept. of Pediatrics, University of Helsinki, Helsinki, Finland
[6] Dept. of Pediatrics, Karolinska Hospital, Stockholm, Sweden

(NOPHO-93). In principle, the therapeutic blocks in this study are the same as in NOPHO-88. However, in NOPHO-88 the first two blocks were given with a short interval in order to achieve an »up-front-loading«. The toxicity of this approach was close to unacceptable. In NOPHO-93 the children have been given time to recovery after the first block and thereby allowed us to identify the children who had gone into remission and these who had not. Subsequent therapy was different for the two groups. This approach has reduced therapy related morbidity and mortality and has resulted in a significant improved outcome.

## Patients and Methods

NOPHO-84 recruited 105 patients and NOPHO-88 118 patients. Patient characteristics and treatment results have been published earlier [9].

Between January 1993 and January 1998, 148 children less than 16 years of age with AML were registered in NOPHO-93. Out of these 21 (14.2%) had Down's syndrome. This is a proportion similar to what has been reported in NOPHO-84 and NOPHO-88. Patient characteristics are presented in Table 1.

The diagnosis of AML was based on the presence of more than 25% abnormal blasts or promyelocytes as defined by regular staining, histochemistry, immunophenotyping or chromosome analysis when possible. With 5 countries involved, it was impossible to have a central review, but the diagnostic criteria were the same in all countries. Therapy was centralized to the University Hospitals and included 21 centers.

## Therapy

NOPHO-84 induction therapy consisted of three series including bolus ara-C (100 mg/m$^2$ i.v. q12 h days 1, 2, 3, 4), 6-thioguanine (100 mg/m$^2$ p.o. q12h days 1, 2, 3, 4) and adriamycin 75 mg/m$^2$ given i.v. as infusion on day 5. Consolidation therapy consisted of high-dose ara-C (2 g/m$^2$ q12h days 1, 2, 3) repeated four times with a 3- to 4-week interval (total length of therapy, 7–9 months).

Table 1. Characteristics of Patients Enrolled on NOPHO-84, NOPHO-88 and NOPHO 93

| | | NOPHO-88 n | NOPHO-84 NOPHO-93 n | n |
|---|---|---|---|---|
| Gender | F | 61 | 60 | 79 |
| | M | 44 | 58 | 69 |
| Age | < 1 year | 12 | 15 | 13 |
| | 1–< years | 16 | 27 | 27 |
| | 2–< 10 years | 45 | 42 | 66 |
| | > = 10 years | 32 | 34 | 42 |
| FAB | M-1 | 19 | 23 | 22 |
| | M-2 | 30 | 30 | 33 |
| | M-3 | 8 | 6 | 4 |
| | M-4 | 19 | 17 | 28 |
| | M-5 | 11 | 19 | 19 |
| | M-6 | 6 | 4 | 4 |
| | M-7 | 3 | 6 | 22 |
| | Unknown/ missing | 9 | 11 | 16 |
| WBC | < 20 | 57 | 72 | 79 |
| | 20– <50 | 18 | 22 | 35 |
| | > = 50 | 29 | 24 | 34 |
| | Unknown | 1 | 0 | 0 |
| Platelet count | < 20 | 27 | 23 | 40 |
| | 20–< 50 | 26 | 35 | 46 |
| | 50–< 150 | 33 | 38 | 40 |
| | > = 150 | 17 | 18 | 19 |
| | Unknown | 3 | 0 | 3 |
| Hgb, g/l | < 75 | 33 | 34 | 60 |
| | 75– < 100 | 49 | 59 | 59 |
| | > = 100 | 21 | 22 | 27 |
| | Unknown | 2 | 0 | 2 |
| CNS disease | | 5 | 4 | 9 |
| Down | | 9 | 14 | 21 |
| Total | | 105 | 118 | 148 |

The therapy in NOPHO-88 was intensified through the addition of etoposide and mitoxantrone both during induction and consolidation. If the condition of the child allowed, the second course (block B) in induction should be given not more than 2 weeks after course 1.

The details of NOPHO-93 are shown in Figure 1. The blocks are identical to those in NOPHO-88 where all patients received blocks A→B→C in sequence. However, in NOPHO-93 time to recovery was allowed after course A. Children who were in remission after block A then received another identical block. For those children that failed remission, course B was given as soon as persistence of leukemic cells was demonstrated. For those still not in remission after course B, course C was given as the third induction course.

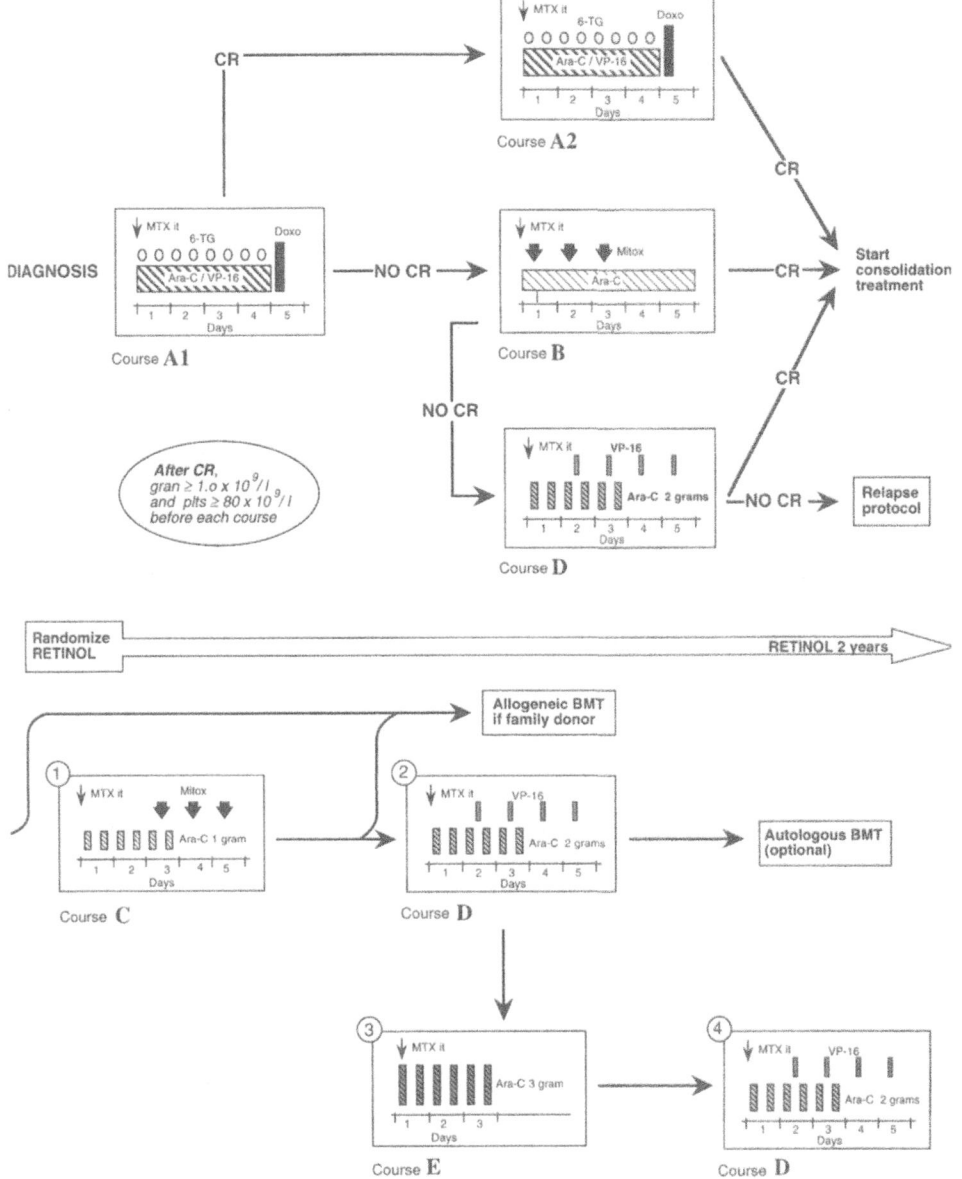

**Fig. 1.** Outline of protocol NOPHO-93
Footnote to the figure:

| | | Doxorubicin (Doxo): | 75 mg/m²/d |
|---|---|---|---|
| Cytarabine (Ara-C): | 200 mg/m²/d continous infusion | Methotrexate i.t.: | < 1 year 6 mg, 1–2 years 8 mg |
| Etoposide (VP-16): | 100 mg/m²/d continous infusion | | 2–3 years 10 mg, >3 years 12 mg |
| 6-thioguanine (6-TG): | 100 mg/m² twice daily | | 75 mg/m² |
| Mitoxantrone (Mitox): | 10 mg/m²/d i.v. | | |

Consolidation therapy in NOPHO-88 and NOPHO-93 was identical and consisted of four additional blocks.

Transplantation with allogeneic bone marrow was offered to all patients where an HLA identical family donor was available. During the course of study, some centers started to do autologous bone marrow transplantation, but never before the second consolidation course. A conditioning regime consisting of busulfan and cyclophosphamide was used in the majority of the patients with the remaining receiving TBI and cyclophosphamide according to the protocol of the bone marrow transplant center involved. Patients with Down's syndrome were offered the same chemotherapy as other children, but never transplantation.

## Statistical and Methods

Statistical analyses were performed with SPSS statistical software [10]. Survival curves were performed using the Kaplan-Meier method [11] and remission durations for subgroups were compared with the log-rank test [12]. Cox multivariate proportional hazard regression analyses were performed for evaluating prognostic factors [13].

## Results

### Remission Induction

The results of the 3 studies are presented in Table 2. The CR induction rate overall in NOPHO-93 is now 92%. Of the 21 children with Down's syndrome 20 went into remission after course A. Of the remaining 127 non-Down's patients, 84 (66%) went into remission after course A, while 2 children died (1 in aplasia and 1 early death before

therapy). The remaining non-responding 43 children received course B, after which 5 children died (2 in aplasia, 3 resistant deaths), while 24 went into remission. Of the 14 remaining children who received block D, 4 died of persistent resistant disease, while 10 went into remission.

## Outcome after CR

Figure 2 compares the event free survival curves of our studies. The results of NOPHO-93 is clearly superior to what we have achieved in our previous NOPHO trials. A pEFS of 0.57 compares very favourably with our previous studies and all recently published reports [2–8].

Children with Down's syndrome (DS) did very well. Their survival curves are compared with those of non-DS patients as shown in Figure 3. Of the 21 children with DS, 20 went into remission and only 2 have relapsed during the first year, resulting in an EFS of 0.86. For subsequent analysis of prognostic factors the Down's syndrome patients have therefore been excluded in order to compare with other studies where the proportion of children with Down's is much smaller.

The survival curve of the non-DS patients resulted in an EFS at 5 years of 0.53, 5 children died in remission and we have experienced 20 relapses, mostly in the bone marrow. Relapses after the second year is very rare. We saw only 1 relapse at three years after diagnosis. Five children died in CR, 4 after BMT and 1 after chemotherapy.

## Prognostic Factors

Figure 4a shows the event free survival curves of children according to the sensitivity of their disease during induction. Eighty-four of the 127 non-DS-patients went into remission on block A. pEFS in this group is 0.61 and significantly better than for those who needed more than one induction course. There was no difference between children who went into remission on two courses (pEFS = 0.29), and those who needed three courses (pEFS = 0.36). This is in accordance with recently published English experience [7]. This diffe-

**Table 2.** Results of Induction Therapy

| | NOPHO-84 | Protocols NOPHO-88 | NOPHO-93 |
|---|---|---|---|
| n | 105 | 118 | 148 |
| Death in aplasia | 8 | 14 | 4 |
| RD | 15 | 4 | 8 |
| CCR (n) | 82 | 100 | 136 |
| CCR (%) | 78 | 84 | 92 |
| | NOPHO-84 | NOPHO-88 | NOPHO-93 |
| Death in aplasia | 7,6 | 11,8 | 2,7 |
| RD | 14,2 | 3,3 | 5,4 |
| CCR | 78 | 84 | 92 |

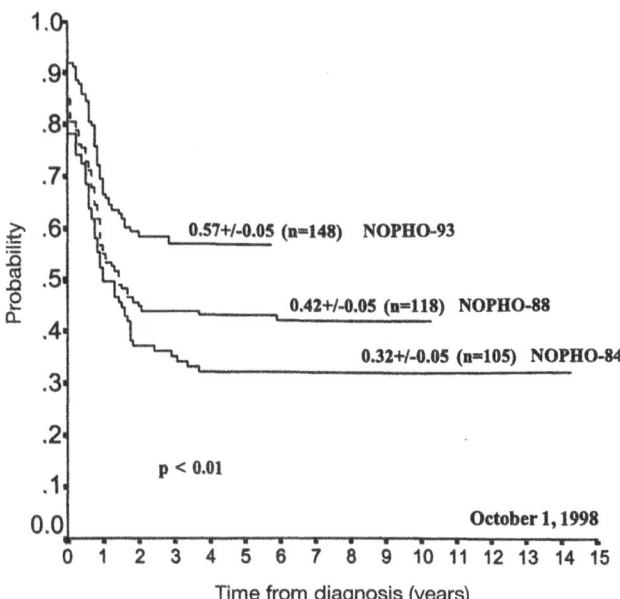

**Fig. 2.** Probability of event free survival in the three Nordic AML-studies

Probability

0.57+/-0.05 (n=148)   NOPHO-93

0.42+/-0.05 (n=118)   NOPHO-88

0.32+/-0.05 (n=105)   NOPHO-84

$p < 0.01$

October 1, 1998

Time from diagnosis (years)

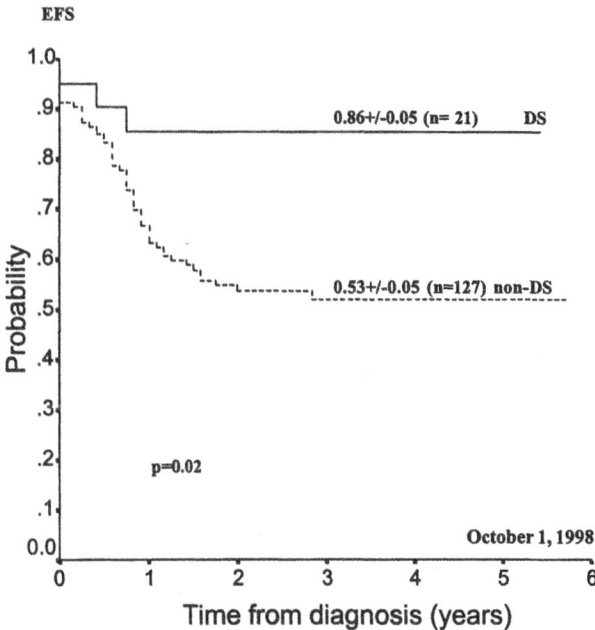

**Fig. 3.** Probability of event free survival in Downs syndrome children versus normal children.

EFS

0.86+/-0.05 (n= 21)   DS

0.53+/-0.05 (n=127) non-DS

Probability

$p=0.02$

October 1, 1998

Time from diagnosis (years)

rence is partly related to different induction rates, but is still present when analysing only children who achieved remission (Fig. 4b).

Figure 5 shows that WBC >50 at diagnosis carried an adverse prognostic factor. This is in contrast to what we have been able to demonstrate in our earlier studies, but in agreement with the observation of others. The main reason is difference in induction rates.

Figure 6a and b presents the results of various postinduction therapies. It should be

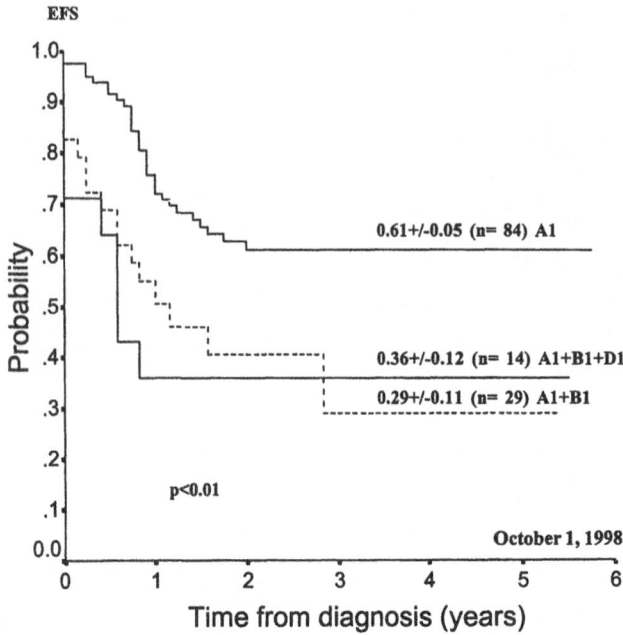

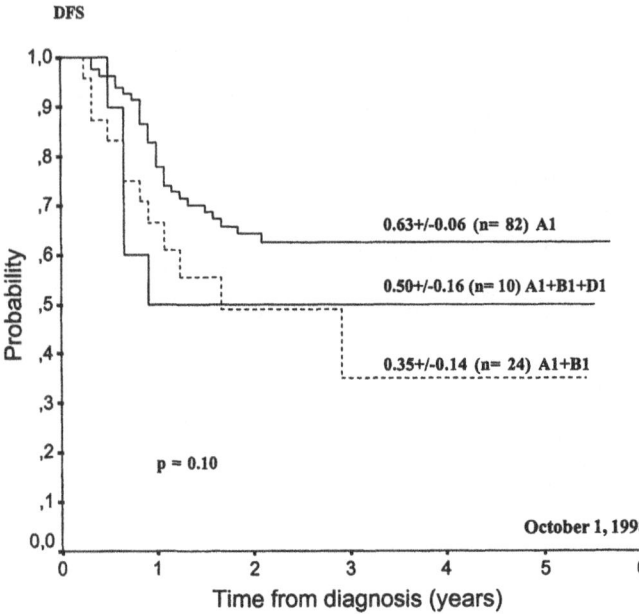

**Fig. 4.** Probability of event free survival (Fig. 4a) and disease free survival (Fig. 4b) according to the number of courses required to bring the child into remission.

underlined that these are not randomized studies. Figure 6a shows the results of all children achieving remission regardles of number of induction courses, while Figure 6b shows the outcome in those children who achieved remission after course A1 only. In both figures it is apparent that allogeneic transplant offers the best chance of survival, while there is no significant difference between chemotherapy only and autologous bone marrow transplant.

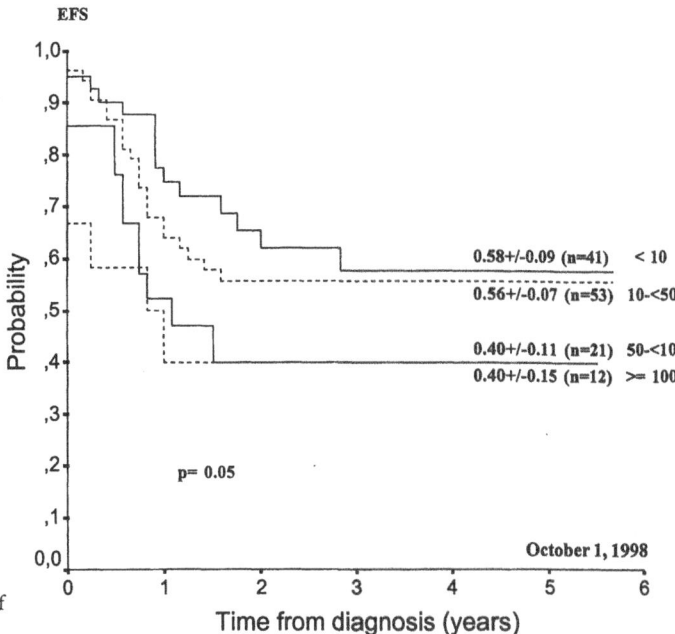

EFS

0.58+/-0.09 (n=41)  < 10
0.56+/-0.07 (n=53)  10-<50
0.40+/-0.11 (n=21)  50-<100
0.40+/-0.15 (n=12)  >= 100

p= 0.05

October 1, 1998

Time from diagnosis (years)

**Fig. 5.** Probability of event free survival according to number of white blood cells at diagnosis.

## Discussion

One of the most striking characteristics of the population of children with AML in the Nordic countries is the high proportion of children with Down's syndrome. A proportion of up to 15% has not been reported in any other series. In the recent large study from the UK Medical Research Council, only 16 out of 341 patients had this chromosomal abnormality [8]. In other cooperative groups the incidence has definitely increased. In the US Children Cancer Study Group the incidence has increased from 2.5% to 9% during the last 20 years [14–15]. This leukemia is most often of the megakaryoblastic type with markers from several lineages [16–18]. Given the good prognosis for children with Down's syndrome and AML (pEFS = 0.86) it has therefore been necessary to exclude these children from analysis of prognostic factors.

The event free survival of the 127 non-DS-children is 0.53 at 5 years, which compares favourably with other recently published surveys. The best reported results up to now is the Medical Research Council AML 10, which has the same CR-rate as that of our study and a pEFS of 0.49 at 5 years [8].

It is of interest to compare NOPHO-88 and NOPHO-93 since the basic components are the same. The main difference is that we can identify the chemosensitive leukemias by allowing time to recovery after the first block. Children who have a disease with a drug sensitivity to this combination are then given another identical block, while those children not in CR receive block B containing mitoxatrone as a new drug.

Close to 70% of the patients go into remission on one block only. This is a figure which is very similar to the recently published UK AML-10. Our analysis shows that these patients have a good prognosis with a pEFS of 0.61. This is no big surprise, but this upfront sensitivity has not influenced choice of further therapy in any other group study. In ALL, the BFM group has of course used prednisone responsiveness for many years as a prognostic factor that strongly influences choice of therapy [19]. Whether or not a change of protocol in a non-responding disease will influence the long term outcome, is not answered by our study. Again, comparing with the English experience, a repetition of the same course also induces additional children to go into remission and larger studies are needed

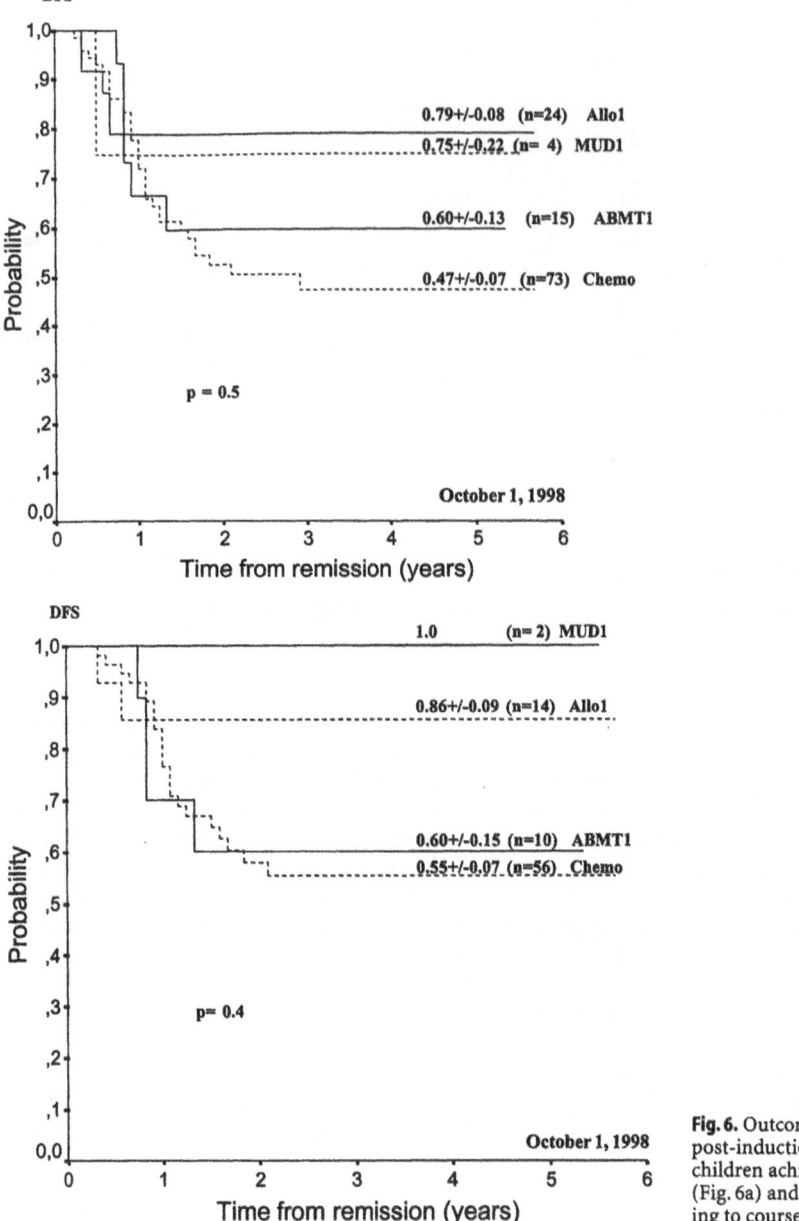

**Fig. 6.** Outcome according to post-induction therapy in all children achieving remission (Fig. 6a) and in those responding to course A (Fig. 6b).

to answer such a question. Probably the major benefit of the NOPHO-93 is in the reduction in toxicity. We have observed a reduced incidense of death in aplasia and even more importantly, death in CR has been reduced from 8% to 3% in the two studies. Four of the 5 deaths in CR in NOPHO-93 was after allo-

geneic bone marrow transplant, while 1 died after chemotherapy.

One report which has gained wide publicity recently is the report on intensively timed induction therapy from the US CCG group [6]. In this study a very intensive timed-sequential induction therapy was compared with a standard time induction in which a more conventional difference of some 28 days between block. The author claim that there is a significant improvement in the intensive arm not only on induction rate (although not significantly), but more importantly on the long term outcome. What makes this study hard to evaluate is that the overall results are clearly inferior to the European studies with an induction rate of about 70% and a pEFS of 0.42 in the intensive arm versus 0.27 on the standard timing arm at 3 years.

In 1994, Novakovic announced that AML is the »childhood tumor with the most dismal prognosis« [20]. In 1999 this certainly is not any longer the case.

# References

1. Lie SO (1995) Treatment of acute myelogenous leukemia in children. Bailléres Clin Paed 3: 757–778
2. Stevens R (1996) Acute myeloid leukaemia. Brit Med Bulletin 52 (4): 764–777
3. Vormoor J, Boos J, Stahnke K, Jürgens H, Ritter J, Creutzig U (1996) Therapy of childhood acute myelogenous leukemias. Ann Hematol 73: 11–24
4. Creutzig U, Ritter J, Schellong G (1990) Identification of two risk groups in childhood acute myelogenous leukaemia after therapy intensification in study AML-BFM-83 as compared with study AML-BFM-78. Blood 75: 1932–1940
5. Creutzig U, Ritter J, Zimmermann M, Schelling G (1993) Does cranial irradiation reduce the risk for bone marrow relapse in acute myelogenous leukaemia? Unexpected results of the childhood acute myelogenous leukaemia study BFM-87. J Clin Oncol 11: 279–286
6. Woods WG, Kobrinsky N, Buckley JD, Lee JW, Sanders J, Neudorf S, Gold S, Barnard DR, DeSwarte J, Dusenbery K, Kalousek D, Arthur DC, Lange BJ (1996) Timed-sequential induction therapy improves postremission outcome in acute myeloid leukemia: a report from the Children_s Cancer Group. Blood 87 (2): 4979–4989
7. Ravindranath Y, Yeager AM, Chang MN, Steuber CP, Krischer J, Graham-Pole J, Carroll A, Inoue S, Camitta B, Weinstein HW for the Pediatric Oncology Group (1996) Autologous bone marrow transplantation versus intensive consolidation chemotherapy for acute myeloid leukemia in childhood. New Engl J Med 334 (22): 1428–1438
8. Stevens RF, Hann IM, Wheatley K, Gray RG on behalf of the MRC Childhood Leukaemia Working Party (1998) Marked improvements in outcome with chemotherapy alone in paediatric acute myeloid leukaemia: results of the United Kingdom Medical Research Council_s 10th AML trial. Brit J Haematol 101: 130–140
9. Lie SO, Jonmundsson G, Mellander L, Siimes MA, Yssing M. Gustafssen behalf of the Nordic Society of Paediatric Haematology and Oncology (NOPHO) (1996) A population-based study of 272 children with acute myeloid leukaemia treated in two consecutive protocols with different intensity: best outcome in girls, infants, and children with Down_s syndrom. Brit J Haematol 94:82–88
10. Norusis MJ (1998) SPSS statistical software 8.0 for Windows. Chicago Il, SPSS inc.
11. Kaplan EL, Meier P (1958) Non-parametric estimation from incomplete observations. J Am Stat Ass 63: 457–481
12. Mantel N (1966) Evaluation of survival data and tow new rank order statistics arising in its consideration. Cancer Chemotherapy 50: 163–170
13. Cox D (1972) Regression models and life-tables. J Royal Stat Soc B4: 187–202
14. Robinson LL, Nesbit ME, Sather HN et al. (1984) Down syndrome and acute Leukaemia in children: A 10-year retrospective survey from Childrens Cancer Study Group. J Pediatr 105: 235–242
15. Lange BJ, Kobrinsky N, Barnard DR, Arthur DC, Buckley JD, Howells WB, Gold S, Sanders J, Neudorf S, Smith FO, Woods WG (1998) Distinctive demography, biology, and outcome of acute myeloid leukemia and myelodysplastic syndrome in children with Down syndrome. Children_s Cancer Group Studies 2861 and 2891. Blood 91 (2): 608–615
16. Slordahl SH, Smeland EB, Holte H, Gronn M, Lie SO, Seip M (1993) Leukemic blasts with markers of four cell lineages in Down_s syndrome (»megakaryoblastic leukaemia«). Med Ped Oncol 21: 254–258
17. Creutzig U, Ritter J, Vormoor J, Ludwig WD, Niemeyer C, Reinisch I, Stollmann-Gibbels B, Zimmermann M, Harbott J (1996) Myelodysplasia and acute myelogenous leukemia in Down_s syndrome. A report of 40 children of the AML-BFM Study Group. Leukemia 10 (11): 1677–1686
18. Ravindranath Y, Abella E, Krischer JP, Wiley J, Inoue S, Harris M, Chauvenet A, Alvarado CS, Dubowy R, Rithcey K et al. (1992) Acute myeloid leukemia (AML) in Down_s syndrome is highly responsive to chemotherapy: Experience on Pediatric Oncology Group AML Study 8498. Blood 80: 2210–2214
19. Riehm H, Reiter A, Schrappe M, Berthold F, Dopfer G, Gerein V, Ludwig R, Ritter J, Stollmann B, Henze G (1987) Die Corticosteroidabhängige Dezimierung der Leukämiezahl im Blut als Prognosefaktor bei der akuten lymphoblastischen Leukämie im Kindesalter (Therapiestudie ALL-BFM 83). Klin Pädiat 199: 151
20. Novakovic B (1994) US childhood cancer survival, 1973–1987. Medical & Pediatric Oncology 23: 480–486

# Long-Term Outcome and Prognostic Factors in Children's Cancer Group Study 2891 for Children and Adolescents with Previously Untreated Acute Myeloid Leukemia and Myelodysplastic Syndrome

B. J. Lange, F. O. Smith, N. Kobrinsky, J. Buckley, W. Howells, J.-W. Lee, J. E. Sanders, S. Neudorf, S. Gold, D. Barnard, J. DeSwarte, K. Dusenbery, D. C. Arthur and W. G. Woods for the Children's Cancer Group, Arcadia, CA

## Introduction

The primary objective of Children's Cancer Group (CCG) study 2891 is to improve the event-free survival (EFS), disease-free survival (DFS) and survival of children with acute myeloid leukemia (AML) or myelodysplastic syndrome (MDS). The secondary objective to identify prognostically discrete subsets of patients. To achieve these objectives CCG-2891 uses randomized comparisons of 2 induction strategies and 3 post-remission strategies and prospectively examines several patient subsets.

CCG-2891 compares remission induction rate and the long-term EFS, DFS and survival following an intensively scheduled 5-drug induction regimen outcomes following a conventionally timed induction. The rationale for intensively-timed induction derives from preclinical trials and clinical trials conducted by Burke Karp, et al. [1] Their laboratory studies showed that cytotoxic chemotherapy given for several days followed first by a 6-day rest and then by a second cycle of cytotoxic therapy achieved optimal reduction of AML blasts. An early pilot trial of this timed sequential therapy showed excellent results with a 42% EFS in adults with AML [2, 3], and CCG had shown the benefits of timed sequential high dose Ara-C in consolidation [4].

Secondly CCG-2891 compares post-remission outcomes among patients biologically assigned to a matched, related sibling or parental bone marrow transplantation (BMT) or randomly assigned to either 4-hydroperoxcyclophosphamide (4-HC)-purged autologous BMT (ABMT) or high-dose Ara-C based chemotherapy. Previous studies of CCG and others had shown an advantage to matched, related BMT [5-7] and the advantages of high-dose Ara-C-based therapy compared to conventional maintenance therapy [4, 8]. Because a number of studies had shown efficacy of ABMT in second remission,(9, 10) the CCG and other pediatric groups chose to test the efficacy and toxicity of ABMT in first remission in comparison with matched related BMT and high dose Ara-C based chemotherapy [11-17]. A pilot study, CCG-2861, demonstrated the feasibility of intensive timing of induction therapy followed by BMT or ABMT. CCG-2861 achieved a long-term EFS of 43% [11].

Third CCG-2891 assesses disease-related and host-related prognostic factors and to investigate prospectively subsets of patients already identified as having different outcomes than most pediatric AML patients, specifically those with MDS or a history of MDS, [18-21] with Down syndrome [22-25] or those with treatment related AML (t-AML) [26, 27] The ultimate goal of these subset analyses is to identify groups of patients who may benefit from more or less aggressive or entirely different therapy.

This manuscript presents the long-term outcome and subset analyses of CCG-2891 with a median follow-up of over 6 years.

## Patients and Methods

### Patients

CCG-2891 opened in October 1989 and closed in April 1995 to all patients but those with Down syndrome. Patients from birth through

---

The Childrens's Cancer Group Operations, 440 E. Huntington Drive, Suite 300, Arcadia, CA 91006

20 years of age with previously untreated AML or MDS were eligible for registration after Institutional Review Board approval and signed consent document. This report concerns 1089 eligible patients of 1098 patients registered through 10/12/95.

AML and MDS were classified according to French-American-and British (FAB) criteria. Morphology and histochemistry were centrally reviewed in 94 percent of patients as previously described [25, 28]. Karyotypes performed on stimulated and unstimulated cultures were centrally reviewed in 53 percent of patients with 83 percent acceptance.

## Treatment Plan

Figure 1 shows the schema of CCG-2891. The study compares a schedule of chemotherapy administration beginning with a 4-day cycle of 5 drugs (dexamethasone, cytosine arabinoside, 6-thioguanine, etoposide, rubidomycin, »DCTER«) given on days 0 to 3 and repeated on days 10 to 13 (intensive timing) or on days 0-3 and days 14-17 or later depending on day 14 bone marrow status (standard timing) (Figure 2) [11, 17] Upon marrow recovery patients receive a second course of intensively timed or standard DCTER. Patients in remission with a matched related donor are allocated to allogeneic BMT; the others are ran-

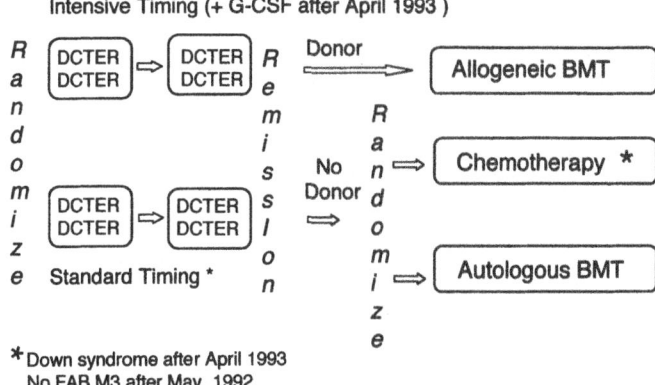

**Fig. 1.** Treatment schema for CCG-2891. DCTER is dexamethasone 6 mg/m²/day, PO for 4 days, cytarabine 100 mg/m²/day CI for 96 hours, 6-thioguanine, 50 mg/m²/day PO, BID for 4 days, etoposide 100 mg/m²/day CI for 4 days (96 hours), and rubidomycin 20 mg/m²/day CI IV for 96 hours. Chemotherapy consolidation consisted of Capizzi 2 high dose ara-C consists of ara-C 3000 mg/m² hours 0-3,12-14,24-27, and 36-39on days 1 and 2 and 7 and 8 and L-asparaginase, 6000

IU/m² IM on days 2 and 8 at hour 42. Continuation therapy consisted of daily 6-thioguaine and q 28 days 4 day pulses of Ara-C, 5-azacytidine, cyclophosphamide for 56 days followed by a final course of modified cycle DCTER. CNS prophylaxis was with intrathecal cytarabine.

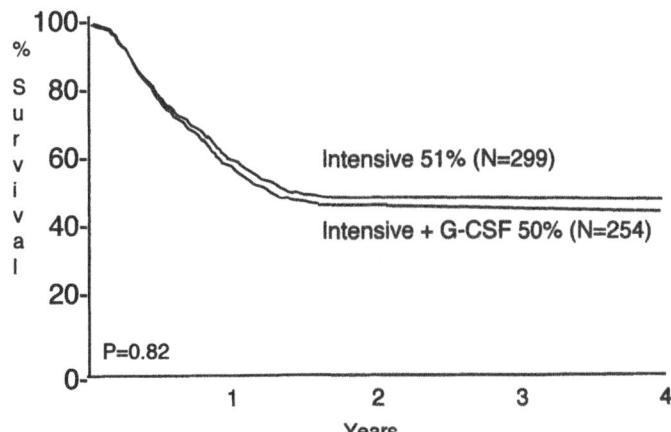

**Fig. 2.** Actuarial survival at 6 years in patients receiving intensively-timed induction therapy with or without G-CSF.

domly assigned to 4-HC purged ABMT or chemotherapy with Capizzi high dose Ara-C [29] 35, followed by 3 months of lower dose chemotherapy with daily 6-thioguanine and monthly pulses of 4 drugs as in previous CCG studies [5, 8, 17]. Central nervous system (CNS) prophylaxis is with intrathecal Ara-C. Chloromas are irradiated at the investigators' option with 20 cGy in 10 fractions with a 1 cm margin [17, 30].

Five amendments were introduced in the protocol:

1. as of August, 1990 patients with DS were excluded from the BMT regimens;
2. in July 1992 patients with DS were excluded from intensively timed induction;
3. in April 1993 patients randomized to intensive timing were assigned to receive granulocyte-colony-stimulating factor (G-CSF) at 5 mcg/kg/day from day 6 until the absolute neutrophil count (ANC) was >1500/mm$^2$ for 2 days.

Standard induction therapy was discontinued in February 1994 based on interim analyses showing unequivocal benefits of intensive therapy. After 1992, patients with acute promyelocytic leukemia were treated according to the Intergroup protocol [31].

## Statistical Methods

Sample size estimates were determined for a power of 0.88 to detect at 2 years a 10 percent difference in DFS between the 2 induction regimens [32]. The log-rank statistic was used to calculate significance of differences in survival, DFS and EFS [32]. Infants ≤2 years of age with M5 FAB morphology were stratified for induction and post-remission randomizations according to the induction regimen. As it is generally recognized that patients with Down syndrome, MDS, or t-AML have significantly different outcomes than patients with other forms of AML, these patients were stratified and their outcome parameters were analyzed separately from the large group of patients without trisomy 21, antecedent MDS or previous therapy for another malignancy. For patients with DS results of the pilot study CCG-2861 were combined with those of CCG-2891 as therapy was identical except for the lack of a chemotherapy randomization in CCG-2861.

Survival estimates were calculated by the method of Kaplan and Meier [33] with confidence intervals calculated by Greenwood's formula [34]. When sample size was small, Yates' contingency tables were used [35]. Significance of observed differences in properties were based on intent-to-treat. Data were also analyzed according to treatment-received [17].

Variables selected for univariate and multivariate analyses of prognostic factors are as follows: age (0-2, 3-10, 11 years), sex, race, neurofibromatosis type 1, chloromas, leukemia, cutis, gingival hypertrophy, liver size, spleen size, adenopathy by region (6 regions), extramedullary disease, meningeal leukemia, cranial nerve involvement, WBC (<20, 20-100, >100 x 10$^3$ cells/mm$^3$), percent of peripheral blasts, disseminated intravascular coagulation, serum fibrinogen and factor VIII levels, histochemistry, FAB morphology, karyotype, monoclonal antibody reactivity, percent marrow blasts at diagnosis and on day 7 (0-5, 6-30, >30%) and platelets on day 7.

## Results

There were 1098 patients registered on CCG-2891 up to April 1995; 1089 were eligible. Table 1 lists the characteristics of patients. Results and prognostic factors for patients with AML are presented below. Results of patients with MDS and DS and t-AML and isolated chloromas are presented as distinct populations.

**Table 1.** CCG-2891 Patient Characteristics

N=1098 registered patients; 1089 eligible

Diagnoses
|     |     |
|-----|-----|
| 890 | AML |
| 90  | MDS |
| 104 | Down syndrome (AML or MDS) |
| 24  | Treatment-related AML |
| 10  | Isolated chloroma |

Age: 1 day to 21 years (median 7.1 years)

Sex: m:f=1.04:1

**Table 2.** Toxicity of DCTER Induction ± G-CSF

| Regimen | N | Die | Fail | CR |
|---|---|---|---|---|
| Standard | 318 | 4% | 23% | 73% |
| P value | | <0.05 | <0.05 | NS |
| Intensive | 257 | 13% | 10% | 77% |
| P value | | 0.13 | 0.79 | 0.14 |
| Intensive + G-CSF | 299 | 8% | 10% | 82% |

## AML Patients

### Induction Outcomes
There are 890 eligible patients with AML randomized to induction therapy. Three hundred eighteen received standard timing, 299 received intensive timing, and 257 received intensive timing plus G-CSF (Table 2). Compliance with induction randomization was 98%. Patients receiving intensive timing are significantly less likely to fail induction (23% vs

10%, p=<.005)and more likely to succumb to toxicity (13% vs 4%) than those receiving standard timing. Introduction on day 6 of G-CSF before the second DCTER cycle as a potential recruiting and synchronizing agent does not reduce the failure rate. (Table 2) Continuation of G-CSF on days 14 until the ANC was >1500 for 2 days reduces the death rate from 13% to 8%, and allows a significant increase in dose intensity by shortening the duration of induction. However, neither of these presumed benefits translates into improved DFS or survival (Figure 2). Despite the higher mortality and greater toxicity in the intensive timing regimens, intensive timing achieved a significant improvement in EFS (44 ± 5% vs 28 ± 5%) and survival (49 ± 5% vs 36 ± 6%) at 6 years (Figure 3).

### Post-Remission Outcome
Compliance with post-remission randomization is 75%. Results are almost identical when

**Table 3.** Post Remission Survival and DFS at 6 Years According to Randomized Induction and Post-Remission Therapy

| All Patients | N | Survival | p values | DFS | p values |
|---|---|---|---|---|---|
| Allogeneic BMT | 179 | 64% | 0.003 | 59% | 0.06 |
| Chemotherapy | 180 | 54% | 0.001 | 47% | 0.0004- |
| Autologous BMT | 177 | 48% | 0.20 | 43% | 0.40 |
| | | | | | |
| Intensive ± G-CSF | | | | | |
| | | | | | |
| Allogeneic BMT | 111 | 75% | 0.005 | 70% | 0.008 |
| Chemotherapy | 109 | 57% | 0.002 | 53% | 0.001- |
| Autologous | 115 | 54% | 0.68 | 49% | 0.61 |

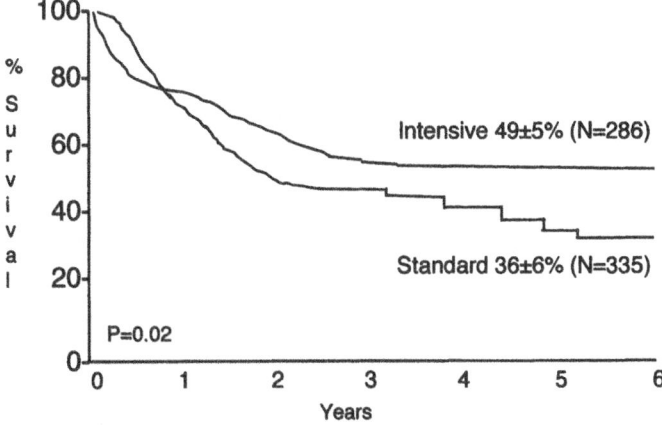

**Fig. 3.** Actuarial survival at 6 years in patients receiving standard-timing induction or intensive timing induction therapy with or without G-CSF

Intensive 49±5% (N=286)

Standard 36±6% (N=335)

P=0.02

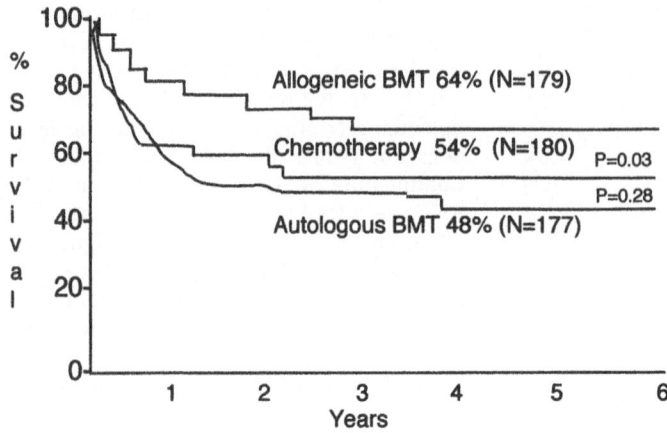

**Fig. 4.** Acturial post-remission survival at 6 years in all patients according to post-remission regimen assigned or randomized

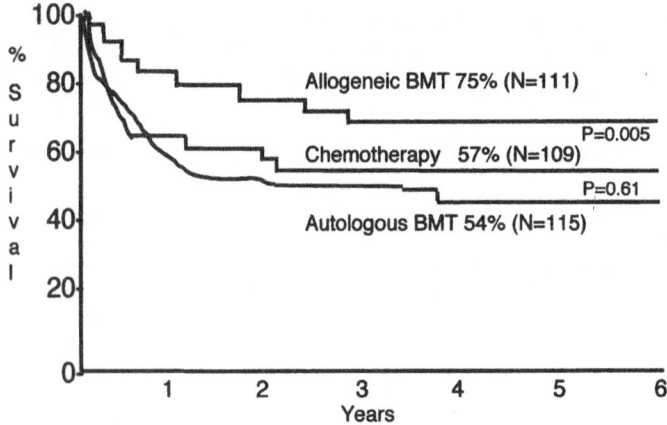

**Fig. 5.** Acturial post-remission survival at 6 years in patients according to post-remission regimen in patients who received intensive timing induction with or without G-CSF

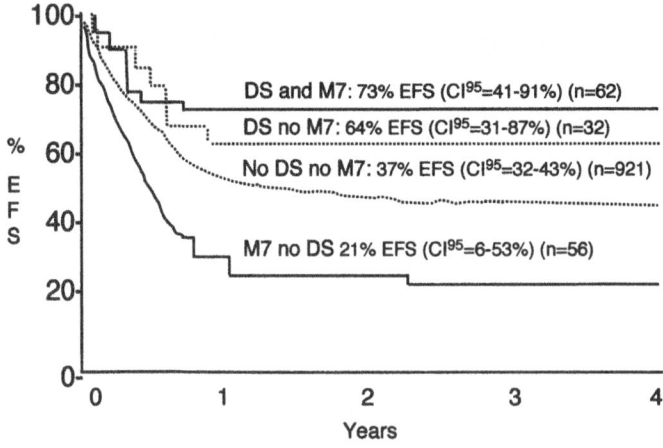

**Fig. 6.** Acturial event-free survival at 4 years in patients with Down syndrome with and without FAB M7 AML or MDS and in non Down syndrome patients with or without FAB M7 AML or MDS.

intent-to-treat outcome data were compared to the as-treated outcomes. Table 3 and Figure 4 illustrate survival for all patients according to the randomized regimens as determined by intent-to-treat analysis. Allogeneic BMT confers significantly higher survival (64%) than either chemotherapy (54%), or ABMT (48%). The most common event in all three regimens is leukemic relapse.

Table 3 and Figure 5 show post-remission survival according to the intensive timing induction regimen. Patients who received intensive timing have a significantly better DFS and survival than those receiving standard timing regardless of the post-remission regimen received. Furthermore, the respective order of superiority of the post-remission remains the same: i.e., allogeneic BMT is significantly superior to either chemotherapy or ABMT and chemotherapy is modestly better than ABMT.

## Prognostic Factors in de novo AML

Table 4 shows the multivariate analysis of EFS for 890 patients with AML according to variables which have been shown to have prognostic significance in the studies of CCG and others as listed in the methods. There are no important differences in the distribution of patients with these characteristics in randomization to either the induction or post-remission therapy. Table 4 shows that non-white race, white blood cell count >20,000/mm$^3$, FAB M7, and leukemia cutis are unfavorable but FAB M5 is favorable. Failure to show a reduction in blast percentage to

**Table 4.** Prognostic Factors: Multivariate Model for EFS from On Study

| Variable | N | Odds Ratio | p value |
|---|---|---|---|
| WBC >20-100k* | 337 | 1.4 | 0.005 |
| WBC >100k* | 226 | 1.9 | <0.0001 |
| Leukemia Cutis | 40 | 1.8 | 0.004 |
| Non White race* | 470 | 1.3 | 0.02 |
| FAB M5 | 90 | 0.6 | 0.03 |
| FAB M7 | 42 | 2.1 | 0.003 |
| Day 7 marrow | | | |
| >5% blasts | 397 | 1.4 | 0.004 |
| Increased blasts | 51 | 2.0 | 0.0002 |

*Indicates significance for DFS also

**Table 5.** Prognostic Factors for Cytogenetic Subset Multivariate Model for EFS (n=323)

| Variable | N | Odds Ratio | p value |
|---|---|---|---|
| WBC >100 k | 266 | 1.9 | 0.001 |
| FAB M7 | 19 | 2.7 | 0.001 |
| Day 7 marrow Blasts increase | 32 | 2.2 | 0.0006 |
| Monosomy 7, 7q- | 10 | 2.6 | 0.01 |

<5% on day 7 or to show an increased percentage of blasts on day 7 are also unfavorable. Age, specifically age <2 years, is not a prognostic factor for EFS. The only variables that are significantly associated with DFS were WBC >20,000/mm$^3$ and black race. There is a trend for extramedullary leukemia, liver enlargement and gingival hypertrophy to predict shorter DFS.

Cytogenetic studies were deemed acceptable in 323 of the 890 patients (37%). The only cytogenetic feature that is independently predictive of outcome is monosomy 7 or 7q- in univariate analysis. For none of these prognostic factors is it possible to show significant benefits of one post-remission regimen over another although the order of allogeneic BMT, chemotherapy, and ABMT is usually maintained.

## Subsets of Myeloid Leukemia

### Down Syndrome (DS)

In the combined CCG-2861 and 2891 studies there are 109 patients with Down syndrome. These patients are younger than those without DS with median age of 2 years compared to 7.1 years and are more likely than others to have FAB M7 (62% vs 6% p=<0.001).(25) EFS in patients with DS is 68% (C1$^{95}$ 47%-84%) and is 35% (C1$^{95}$ 30%-41%) in the others [25]. In contrast to patients without DS, FAB M7 in DS is not unfavorable in DS patients EFS of 73% (C1$^{95}$ 41%-91%) in DS FAB M7 and EFS 21% (C1$^{95}$ 6%-53%) in those without DS and FAB M7 [25]. Finally, in contrast to the non-DS population, patients with DS do not benefit from intensive timing of induction or allogeneic BMT.(25)

## Myelodysplastic Syndrome (MDS)

There are 89 patients with a history of antecedent MDS or MDS at time of study entry. Formal review of these patients reveals that 16 have what has been called low-blast count AML or early AML. Their outcome is similar to that of de novo AML patients. (Woods submitted). In contrast those with MDS as a group experienced an interior outcome. (Woods submitted) Of the FAB subsets of AML, those with JMML (n=13) had an EFS of 31 ± 26% and RAEB (n-33) fared least well with EFS 18 ± 31% while those with RAEB - t(n= 25) had a 35 ± 20% EFS. Small numbers preclude statistical significance.

## Isolated Chloromas

Ten patients presented with granulocytic sarcoma without marrow disease. Of these 7 are alive event-free suggesting that they may constitute a lower risk group. When the data from CCG-213, CCG-2861 and CCG-2891 are pooled, the 18 patients with isolated chloromas experience a significantly better EFS than 1633 patients without chloromas and with marrow disease [30]. Furthermore, among 96 patients with chloromas with or without marrow disease, local and systemic relapse rates are the same regardless of whether they received local irradiation or not. In contrast 103 patients with leukemia cutis experienced the worst EFS [30].

## Treatment-Related AML

Twenty patients had t-AML. The patients with t-AML were also an unfavorable group. Their remission induction rate was 50%. Induction therapy was compromised by limits on the amount of anthracycline they could receive and toxic death and induction failure. The actuarial EFS at 2 years approaches 0%.

## Discussion

CCG-2891 shows that in a large cohort of young patients with AML intensive timing of induction increases 6 year survival to 49 ± 5 percent, 36 ± 6 percent in standard timing, and intensive timing improves 6 year EFS to 44 ± 5 percent from 27 ± 5 percent, a clinically important difference of 17 percent. This improvement in outcome occurs despite a significantly higher induction mortality in patients receiving intensive timing: 13 percent vs 4 percent. To improve induction outcome, G-CSF was introduced on day 6 and continued through the second cycle of therapy in days 11-13 and discontinued when the ANC was 1500/mm$^3$. Although addition of G-CSF reduced induction mortality from 13 percent to 8 percent, it had absolutely no impact on survival or EFS. Furthermore, the use of G-CSF before and during the second cycle of therapy apparently did not recruit more blasts into the cell cycle as the failure rate remained 10 percent. These results are similar to many in the literature where early improvement in induction fail to translate into higher cure rates [36, 37].

The randomized comparisons of intensive and standard timing are consistent with the data in vitro showing that timed sequential therapy renders more AML cells susceptible to killing with Ara-C [1]. The results of CCG-2891 are similar to those of the timed sequential therapy pilot at Johns Hopkins [2, 3]. At the same time no one has been able to prove that recruitment and synchronization is actually occurring in vivo.

It is possible that intensive timing is superior to standard timing by virtue of sheer dose-intensity rather than timed-sequential kinetics. In CCG-2891 patients receiving intensive timing received twice as much therapy on day 14 as those receiving standard timing. In CCG-2891 patients randomized to standard timing who had >25 percent blasts on day 14 (slow early responders) went on to receive cycle 2 of therapy on days 14 through 17. Contrary to an expected inferior outcome, these slow early responding patients experienced an EFS that was marginally superior to the majority of patients receiving the second cycle of DCTER two or three weeks later [17]. The dose-intensity hypothesis also is supported by a number of recent trials such as the BFM '83 [13, 16, 38, 39], all of which use a dose-intensity of Ara-C and anthracycline that is substantially higher than that of standard«7 and 3«, and all of which have long-term EFS above 40 percent. Furthermore, it remains to be shown that etoposide, 6-thioguanine, dexamethasone or other agents add anything to Ara-C and an anthracycline. Maximal intensification of these two agents alone may achieve the best long-term outcome.

In CCG-2891 as in previous CCG studies, allogeneic BMT effects a significantly higher DFS and survival than either ABMT or chemotherapy [5, 8], and in this study chemotherapy is either the same as or marginally superior to ABMT. POG-8821 and LAME '89-'91 show similar results [12, 13]. The superiority of allogeneic BMT persists when the induction regimens are considered. In CCG-2891 DFS is 70 percent at 5 years in the intensive timing/allogeneic BMT regimen compared to 50 percent in the standard timing/BMT regimen. The poorest DFS is in the standard timing ABMT, 39 percent compared to 49 percent in intensive timing/BMT regimen. DFS is intermediate with intensive timing/chemotherapy, 53 percent. The implication of these findings is that the remission induction therapy influences post-remission outcome, no matter what the post-remission therapy is. In effect, not all remission are equal: those achieved with a more toxic, more intensive therapy are more durable. Similarly not all matched related allogeneic BMTs are equal: those preceded by an intensive induction therapy are more likely to succeed that those preceded by the least amount of therapy needed to achieve a remission. Hence both an intensive induction and post remission strategy are likely to produce the best long-term survival and EFS, provided that mortality and overwhelming morbidity do not eliminate a substantial number of patients early in treatment. Steven et al report that with 3 cycles of high-dose Ara-C based therapy, EFS at 7 years is 48%. (16) Subsequent addition of allogeneic BMT or autologous BMT in first remission reduce relapse but do not increase survival [16].

The purpose of analyzing prognostic factors is to identify subsets who may benefit from more or less therapy. A few prognostic factors are beginning to emerge in AML: Down syndrome [12, 23-25], and low white blood cell count [38, 40, 41], are generally accepted as favorable while high white blood cell count, induction failure and del (7) are unfavorable [42, 43], and t(9:11) and t(8:21) remain controversial [44]. Among the non-DS AML patients, multivariate analysis of the large cohort of pediatric patients in CCG-2891 found variables independently predictive EFS: WBC >20,000;/mm$^3$ leukemia cutis, non-white race, FAB M5 and M7, >5 percent blasts on day 7 and increase in blasts on day 7. Of these only FAB M5 was favorable, a noteworthy inversion of some earlier studies [40, 45] have recently noted »that patients with leukemia cutis have a remarkable propensity to relapse in extramedullary sites following marrow transplantation.« [45] While (inv) 16 and t(8:21) show a trend to be favorable in univariate analyses, in CCG-2891 they do not maintain their significance in multivariate analyses. Cytogenetics are available for only 37 percent of patients, but among this subset, WBC >100,000, FAB M7, increased blasts on day 7 and del [7] predict poor outcome and no variable predict a superior outcome. These discrepancies in defining prognostic variables between the findings of CCG-2891 and other cooperative studies emphasize the fact that treatment itself is a major prognostic variable.

Multivariate analysis of DFS showed only WBC >20,000;/mm$^3$ and black race to be predictive. Those factors that are predictive of EFS but not DFS identify a group of patients who may benefit from a more effective induction but who are less likely to benefit from a more effective post-remission therapy. (46) (Smith '98) Hence these analyses failed to uncover a group of patients in whom alternative donor BMT or stem cell transplant is likely to make a major impact, although those with high WBC and black patients may need both better induction and post-remission therapy.

Among the subsets of patients who prospectively stratified, those with isolated chloromas and those with Down syndrome have a significantly better outcome than the standard AML patients. Early in CCG-2891, randomization of patients with Down syndrome ceased: they non-randomly received standard timing and chemotherapy. This combination achieved 88 percent EFS at 4 years [25]. It is possible that those with isolated chloromas, particularly those with t(8;21) may require less substantial therapy than the larger group of AML patients with marrow disease [30]. However, even with so large a pediatric AML study, the small numbers of patients with isolated chloromas precludes reliable significance estimates. Pooling of data from three CCG studies is necessary to ascertain that patients with isolated chloromas constitute a favorable subset. Among the MDS patients is a subset who by history, morphology and blast percentage fit into the category of low blast count AML [47]. Their response and that of patients with RAEB-t to AML therapy is similar to that of patients with generic AML. They are probably well-served by AML therapy. Optimal treatment for the other MDS patients particularly those with myeloproliferative/myelodysplastic disorders and for those with t-AML awaits discovery.

# References

1. Karp, J. E., Donehower, R. C., Enterline, J. P., Dole, G. B., Fox, M. G., and Burke, P. J. In vivo cell growth and pharmacologic determinants of clinical response in acute myelogenous leukemia, Blood. 73(1): 24-30, 1989.
2. Vaughan, W. P., Karp, J. E., and Burke, P. J. Two-cycle timed-sequential chemotherapy for adult acute nonlymphocytic leukemia, Blood. 64(5): 975-80, 1984.
3. Burke, P. J., Karp, J. E., Geller, R. B., and Vaughan, W. P. Cures of leukemia with aggressive postremission treatment: an update of timed sequential therapy (Ac-D-Ac), Leukemia. 3(10): 692-4, 1989.
4. Woods, W. G., Ruymann, F. B., Lampkin, B. C., Buckley, J. D., Bernstein, I. D., Srivastava, A. K., Smithson, W. A., Benjamin, D. R., Feig, S. A., Kim, T. H., and al., e. The role of timing of high-dose cytosine arabinoside intensification and of maintenance therapy in the treatment of children with acute nonlymphocytic leukemia, Cancer. 66(6): 1106-13, 1990.
5. Nesbit, M. E., Jr., Buckley, J. D., Feig, S. A., Anderson, J. R., Lampkin, B., Bernstein, I. D., Kim, T. H., Piomelli, S., Kersey, J. H., Coccia, P. F., and al., e. Chemotherapy for induction of remission of childhood acute myeloid leukemia followed by marrow transplantation of multiagent chemotherapy: a report from the Children's Cancer Group, Journal of Clinical Oncology. 12(1): 127-35, 1994.
6. Amadori, S., Testi, A. M., Arico, M., Comelli, A., Giuliano, M., Madon, E., Masera, G., Rondelli, R., Zanesco, L., and Mandelli, F. Prospective comparative study of bone marrow transplantation and postremission chemotherapy for childhood acute myelogenous leukemia. The Associazione Italiano Ematologia ed Oncologia Pediatrica Cooperative Group, Journal of Clinical Oncology. 11(6): 1046-54, 1993.
7. Dahl, G. V., Kalwinsky, D. K., Mirro, J., Jr,, Look, A.T., Pui, C. H., Murphy, S. B., Mason, C., Ruggiero, M., Schell, M., Johnson, F. L., and al., e. Allogeneic bone marrow transplantation in a program of intensive sequential chemotherapy for children and young adults with acute nonlymphocytic leu-

8. Wells, R. J., Woods, W. G., Buckley, J. D., Odom, L. F., Benjamin, D., Bernstein, I., Betcher, D., Feig, S., Kim, T., Ruymann, F., and al., e. Treatment of newly diagnosed children and adolescents with acute myeloid leukemia: a Children's Cancer Group study, Journal of Clinical Oncology. 12(11): 2367-77, 1994.
9. Yeager, A. M., Kaizer, H., Santos, G. W., Saral, R., Colvin, O. M., Stuart, R. K., Braine, H. G., Burke, P. J., Ambinder, R. F., Burns, W. H., and al., e. Autologous bone marrow transplantation in patients with acute nonlymphocytic leukemia, using ex vivo marrow treatment with 4-hydroperoxycyclophosphamide, New England Journal of Medicine. 315(3): 141-7, 1986.
10. Dinndorf, P. and Bunin, N. Bone Marrow transplantation for children with acute myelogenous leukemia, Journal of Pediatric Hematology/Oncology. 17(3): 211-24, 1995.
11. Woods, W. G., Kobrinsky, N., Buckley, J., Neudorf, S., Sanders, J., Miller, L., Barnard, D., Benjamin, D., DeSwarte, J., Kalousek, D., and al., e. Intensively timed induction therapy followed by autologous or allogeneic bone marrow transplantation for children with acute meyloid leukemia or myelodysplastic syndrome: a Children's Cancer Group pilot study, Journal of Clinical Oncology. 11(8): 1448-57, 1993.
12. Ravindranath, Y., Yeager, A. M., Chang, M. N., Steuber, C. P., Krischer, J., Graham-Pole, J., Carroll, A., Inoue, S., Camitta, B., and Weinstein, H. J. Autologous bone marrow transplantation versus intensive consolidation chemotherapy for acute myeloid leukemia in childhood. Pediatric Oncology Group, New England Journal of Medicine. 334(22): 1428-34, 1996.
13. Michel, G., Baruchel, A., Tabone, M. D., Nelken, B., Leblanc, T., Thuret, I., Bordigoni, P., Bergeron, C., Esperou-Bourdeau, H., Perel, Y., Vannier, J. P., DeLumley, L., Dommergues, J. P., Lamagnere, J. P., Couillaud, G., Auvrignon, A., Schaison, G., and Leverger, G. Induction chemotherapy followed by allogeneic bone marrow transplantation or aggressive consolidation chemotherapy in childhood acute myeloblastic leukemia. A prospective study from the French Society of Pediatric Hematology and Immunology (SHIP), Hematology & Cell Therapy. 38(2): 169-76, 1996.
14. Vignetti, M., Rondelli, R., Locatelli, F., Lanino, E., Miniero, R., Rossetti, F., and Meloni, G. Autologous bone marrow transplantation in children with acute myeloblastic leukemia: report from the Italian National Pediatric Registry (AIEOP-BMT), Bone Marrow Transplantation. 18 Suppl 2: 59-62, 1996.
15. Ritter, J., Creutzig, U., and Schellong, G. Treatment results of three consecutive German childhood AML trials: BFM-78, -83, and -87. AML-BFM-Group, Leukemia. 6 Suppl 2: 59-62, 1992.
16. Stevens, R. F., Hann, I. M., Wheatley, K., and Gray, R. G. Marked improvements in outcome with chemotherapy alone in pediatric acute myeloid leukemia: results of the United Kingdom Medical Research Council's 10th AML trial. MRC Childhood Leukaemia Working Party, British Journal of Haematology. 101(1):, 1998.

17. Woods, W. G., Kobrinsky, N., Buckley, J. D., Lee, J. W., Sanders, J., Neudorf, S., Gold, S., Barnard, D. R., DeSwarte, J., Dusenbery, K., Kalousek, D., Arthur, D. C., and Lange, B. J. Timed-sequential induction therapy improved postremission outcome in acute myeloid leukemia: a report from the Children's Cancer Group, Blood. 82(12): 4979-89, 1996.

18. Castro-Malaspina, H., Schaison, G., Passe, S., Pasquier, A., Berger, R., Bayle-Weisgerber, C., Miller, D., Seligmann, M., and Bernard, J. Subacute and chronic myelomonocytic leukemia in children (juvenile CML), Cancer. 54: 675, 1984.

19. Wagelius, R. Bone marrow dysfunctions preceding acute leukemia in children: a clinical study, Leuk Res. 16: 71, 1992.

20. Passmore, S., Hann, C., Stiller, P., Ramani, G., Swansbury, B., Gibbons, B., Reeves, B., and Chessells, J. Pediatric myelodysplasia: a study of 68 children and a new prognostic scoring system, Blood. 85: 1742, 1995.

21. Luna-Fineman, S., Shannon, K. M., Atwater, S. K., Davis, J., Masterson, M., Ortega, J., Sanders, J., Steinherz, P., Weinberg, V., and Lange, B. J. Myelodysplastic and Myeloproliferative Disorders of Childhood: A Study of 167 Patients, BLood. 93(2): 459-466, 1999.

22. Ravindranath, Y., Abella, E., Krischer, J. P., Wiley, J., Inoue, S., Harris, M., Chauvenet, A., Alvarado, C. S., Dubowy, R., Ritchey, A. K., and al., e. Acute myeloid leukemia (AML) in Down's syndrome is highly responsive to chemotherapy: experience on Pediatric Oncology Group AML Study 8498, Blood. 80(9): 2210-4, 1992.

23. Creutzig, U., Ritter, J., Vormoor, J., Ludwig, W. D., Niemeyer, C., Reinisch, I., Stollmann-Gibbels, B., Zimmermann, M., and Harbott., J. Myelodysplasia and acute myelogenous leukemia in Down's syndrome. A report of 40 children on the AML-BFM Study Group, Leukemia. 10(11): 1677-86, 1996.

24. Lie, S. O., Jonmundsson, G., Mellander, L., Simes, M. A., Yssing, M., and Gustafsson, G. A population-based study of 272 children with acute myeloid leukaemia treated on two consecutive protocols with different intensity: best outcome in girls, infants, and children with Down's syndrome. Nordic Society of Paediatric Haematology and Oncology (NOPHO), British Journal of Haematology. 94(1): 82-8, 1996.

25. Lange, B. J., Kobrinsky, N., Barnard, D. R., Arthur, D. C., Buckley, J. D., Howells, W. B., Gold, S., Sanders, J., Neudorf, S., Smith, F. O., and Woods, W. G. Distinctive demography, biology and outcome of acute myeloid leukemia and myelodysplastic syndrome in children with Down syndrome: Children's Cancer Group Studies 2861 and 2891, Blood. 91(2): 608-15, 1998.

26. LeBeau, M., Applebaum, F. R., and Willman, C. L. Secondary leukemia, Hematology 33-47, 1996.

27. Rubin, C. M., Arthur, D. C., Woods, W. G., Lange, B. J., Howell, P. C., Rowley, J. D., Nachman, J., Bostrom, B., Baum, E. S., Suarez, C. R., and al., e. Therapy-related myelodysplastic syndrome and acute myeloid leukemia in children: correlation between chromosomal abnormalities and prior therapy, Blood. 78(11): 2982-8, 1991.

28. Barnard, D. R., Kalousek, D. K., Wiersma, S. R., Lange, B. J., Benjamin, D. R., Arthur, D. C., Buckley,

J. D., Kobrinsky, N., Neudorf, S., Sanders, J., Miller, L. P., Shina, D. C., Hammond, G. D., and Woods, W. B. Morphologic, Immunologic and cytogenetic classification of actue myeloid leukemia and myelodysplastic syndrome in childhood: a report from the Children's Cancer Group, Leukemia. 10(1): 5-12, 1996.

29. Capizzi, R. L., Davis, R., Powell, B., Cuttner, J., Ellison, R. R., Cooper, M. R., Dillman, R., Major, W. B., Dupre, E., and McIntyre, O. R. Synergy between high-dose cytarabine and asparginase in the treatment of adults with refractory and relapsed acute myelogenous leukemia-a Cancer and Leukemia Group B study, Journal of Clinical Oncology. 6(3): 499-508, 1988.

30. Dusenbery, K. E., Arthur, D. C., Howells, W., Lange, B. J., Lampkin, B., Buckley, J., Masterson, M., Lee, J. W., Nesbit, M. E., Wells, R. J., and Woods, W. G. Granulocytic sarcomas (chloromas) in pediatric patients with newly diagnosed acute myeloid leukemia (meeting abstract), Pro Annu Meet Am Soc Clin Oncol. 15: A1096, 1996.

31. Tallman, M. S., Andersen, J. W., Schiffer, C. A., Appelbaum, F. R., Feusner, J. H., Ogden, A., Shepherd, L., Willman, C., Bloomfield, C. D., Rowe, J. M., and Wiernik, P. H. All-trans-retinoic acid in acute promyelocytic leukemia, New England Journal of Medicine. 337(15): 1021-8, 1997.

32. Peto, R. and Peto, J. Asymptotically efficient rank in variant test procedures, J R STat Soc. (A) 135: 185, 1972.

33. Kaplan, E. L. and Meier, P. Nonparametric estimation from incomplete observations, J AM Stat Assoc. 53: 457, 1958.

34. Greenwood, M. The natural duration of cancer. Reports on Public Health and Medical Subjects, 33, London UK, Her Majesty's Stationery Office 1, 1926.

35. Yates, F. Contingency tables involving small numbers and the chi-square test, J of the Royal Statistical Soc. Supp 1: 217, 1934.

36. Schiffer, C. A. Hematopoietic growth factors as adjuncts to the treatment of acute myeloid leukemia, Blood. 88(10): 3675-85, 1996.

37. Estey, E. Hematopoietic growth factors in the treatment of actue leukemia, Current Opinion in Oncology. 10(1): 23-30, 1998.

38. Creutzig, U., Ritter, J., and Schellong, G. Identification of two risk groups in childhood acute myelogenous leukemia after therapy intensification in study AML-BFM-83 as compared with study AML-BFM-78. AML-BFM Study Group, Blood. 75(10): 1932-40, 1990.

39. Hann, I. M., Stevens, R. F., Goldstone, A. H., Rees, J. K., Wheatley, K., Gray, R. G., and Burnett, A. K. Randomized comparison of DAT versus ADE as induction chemotherapy in children and younger adults with acute myeloid leukemia. Results of the Medical Research Council's 10th AML trial (MRC AML10). Adult and Childhood Leukaemia Working Parties of the Medical Research Council, Blood. 89(7): 2311-8, 1997.

40. Grier, H. E., Gelber, R. D., Camitta, B. M., Delorey, M. N., Link, M. P., Price, K. N., Leavitt, P. R., and Weinstein, H. J. Prognostic factors in childhood acute myelogenous leukemia, Journal of Clinical Oncology. 5(7): 1026-32, 1987.

41. Hurwitz, C. A., Schell, M. J., Pui, C. H., Crist, W. M., Behm, F., and Mirro, J., Jr. Adverse prognostic features in 251 children treated for acute myeloid leukemia, Medical & Pediatric Oncology. *21(1):* 1-7, 1993.

42. Kalwinsky, D. K., Raimondi, S. C., Schell, M. J., Mirro, J., Jr.,, Santana, V. M., Behm, F., Dahl, G. V., and Williams, D. Prognostic importance of cytogenetic subgroups in de novo pediatric acute nonlymphocytic leukemia, Journal of Clinical Oncology. *8(1):* 75-83, 1990.

43. Woods, W. G., Nesbit, M. E., Buckley, J., Lampkin, B. C., McCreadie, S., Kim, T. H., Piomelli, S., Kersey, J. H., Feig, S., Bernstein, I., and al., e. Correlation of chromosome abnormalities with patient characteristics, histologic subtype, and induction success in children with acute nonlymphocytic leukemia, Journal of Clinical Oncology. *3(1):* 3-11, 1985.

44. Creutzig, U., Harbott, J., Sperling, C., Ritter J., Zimmermann, M., Löffler, H., Riehm, H., Schellong, G., and Ludwig, W. D. Clinical significance of surface antigen expression in children with acute myeloid leukemia: results of a study AML-BFM-87, Blood. *86(8):* 3097-3108, 1995.

45. Michel, G., Boulad, F., Small, T. N., Black, P., Heller, G., Castro-Malaspina, H., Childs, B. H., Gillio, A. P., Papadopoulos, E. B., Young, J. W., Kernan, N. A., and O'Reilly, R. J. Risk of extramedullary relapse following allogeneic bone marrow transplantation for acute myelogenous leukemia with leukemia cutis, Bone Marrow Transplantation. *20(2):* 107-12, 1997.

46. Neudorf, S., J.E., S., Howells, W., Gold, S., Lange, B. J., Kobrinsky, N., DeSwarte, J., Arthur, D. C., Barnard, D., Dunsenbery, K. E., Buckley, J., and Woods, W. G. The Beneficial Role of Autologous Bone Marrow Transplantations (ABMT) in the Treatment of Childhood Acute Myeloid Leukemia (AML): A Report From the Children's Cancer Group, ASH, 1998.

47. Chan, G. C., Wang, W. C., Raimondi, S. C., Behm, F. G., Krance, R. A., Chen, G., Freiberg, A., Ingram, L., Butler, D., and Head, D. R. Myelodysplastic syndrome in children: differentiation from acute myeloid leukemia with a low blast count, Leukemia. *11(2):* 206-11, 1997.

# Risk-Adapted Therapy and Randomization in Children with AML: Preliminary Results of Study AML-BFM 93

U. CREUTZIG[1], J. RITTER[1], M. ZIMMERMANN[1], J. HERMANN[2] and H. GADNER[3]
for the AML-BFM Study Group

## Introduction

Therapy results in AML in children and adults have improved considerably in the late 70s and 80s. Further progress was achieved by a more intensive therapy and bone marrow transplantation. This intensification has become feasible by improved management of infectious complications, a better comprehension of pharmakokinetics and the mechanisms of antileukemic agents such as cytosine arabinoside (Ara-C) and anthracyclines. Next to Ara-C, anthracyclines are the most effective drugs in AML treatment. For many years daunorubicin (DNR) was the preferred drug in AML, however since several trials in adults compared DNR with idarubicin (IDR) in induction regimens and achieved high remission rates in patients treated with IDR, this drug is used increasingly [1-3]. Especially in children the risk of anthracycline-induced cardiotoxicity limits the cumulative dose [4]. Therefore, one of our first aims was to compare DNR with IDR during induction therapy to study the efficacy and toxicity of these drugs.

Intensified regimens with HD-Ara-C have shown promising results in refractory disease [5] and were then introduced in first line therapy during induction [6] and postremission therapy [7,8]. Double induction with thioguanine, Ara-C, DNR (TAD) followed by TAD or TAD followed by HD Ara-C/mitoxantrone (HAM) have been used in the German adult AML Cooperative Group [9]. We introduced HAM as intensification therapy after induction either as 2nd or 3rd therapy block, and compared the efficacy and toxicity rate for early or late HAM.

## Patients and Methods

Patients: The entry criteria included: diagnosis of de novo AML, FAB classification M0 to M7, age between 0 to 17 years, and written informed consent of the patient or parent. According to these criteria 416 patients enrolled in study AML 93 between January 1993 to March 31, 1998. The study was closed for patient entry in June 98, follow up of the last patients (August 1998) however, was too short for this analysis.

### Treatment

The treatment protocol of study AML-BFM 93 (Fig. 1) evolved from study BFM 87 [10]. All patients were randomized initially to receive either ADE (= cytosine arabinoside [Ara-C] and VP-16 [etoposide] combined with daunorubicin [DNR]) or AIE (= Ara-C and VP-16 with idarubicin [IDR]). Therapy started with an 8-day induction ADE (Ara-C 100 mg/m²/day continuous infusion for 2 days followed by 30 min. infusion every 12 h/ days 3-8, DNR 30 mg/m² 30 min. infusion every 12 h/ days 3,4,5 and VP-16 150 mg/m² 120 min. infusion, days 6,7,8) or AIE (IDR 12 mg/m² 30 min. infusion every 24 h, days 3,4,5 instead of DNR).

Day 15 bone marrow was one of the most important prognostic factors, indicating early response to induction treatment. Patients were stratified by initial morphological criteria and blast cell reduction on day 15 in standard (SR) or high risk (HR) patients[11][1].

---

[1] Standard risk group: FAB M1/M2 with Auer rods, FAB M3 and FAB M4eo with ≤5% blasts in the bone marrow on day 15; high risk group: all others. Patients with FAB M3 were always treated as standard risk, regardless of their blast count on day 15.

University Children's Hospital, Dept. of Hematology/Oncology Münster[1], Jena[2], Germany[1,2], St. Anna Children's Hospital, Vienna[3], Austria[3]

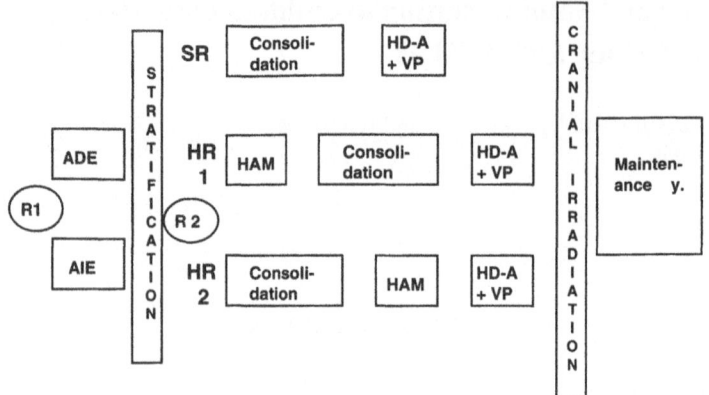

**Fig. 1.** Treatment schedule of Study AML-BFM 93

Further treatment consisted of consolidation therapy with 7 different drugs and intensification with high dose Ara-C together with VP-16 in SR patients, whereas HR patients were randomized to receive either HAM, followed by consolidation (HR1) or consolidation followed by HAM (HR2). This was followed in all patients with one block of HD-Ara-C plus VP-16 and cranial irradiation with 18 Gy (standard dose in children $\geq$3 years) and maintenance therapy with daily thioguanine 40 mg/m$^2$ orally and Ara-C 40 mg/m$^2$ s.c. for a total duration of 18 months. Allogeneic bone marrow transplantation (BMT) was recommended only for children in first CR in the HR group, if a sibling donor was available.

## Definition

Complete remission (CR) was defined according to the CALGB criteria [12]. Early death (ED) patients were those dying before or within the first 6 weeks of treatment. Life-table estimations were performed for survival, event-free survival (EFS) and disease-free survival (DFS).

## Results

Of 416 patients 341 (82%) have been randomized. Initial patient data of both groups were comparable (Table 1).

A comparison of overall results of study AML-BFM 93 with study AML-BFM 87 is presented in Table 2. In study AML-BFM 93, 345 (83%) of 416 patients achieved remission, estimated probability for 3-year EFS and DFS was 54%, SE 3% and 65%, SE 3%, respectively.

**Table 1.** Initial Patient Data - 1. Randomization ADE *vs* AIE

|  | ADE | AIE |
|---|---|---|
| Gender m:f | 1.40 | 1.11 |
| Age, median, range (years) | 8.9 (0.2–16.9) | 8.4 (0–10.8) |
| Leukocytes, median, range (/µl) | 18050 (800 - 336 000) | 17300 (400–520 000) |
| Favorable karyotypes (n)* | 25 (30%) | 21 (21%) |
| Standard risk (n) | 60 (36%) | 65 (37%) |
| High risk (n) | 106 (64%) | 110 (63%) |
| Total (n) | 166 | 175 |

*Favorable karyotypes = t(8;21), t(15;17) and inv16, the percentage of patients with cytogenetic data is indicated

**Table 2.** Overall Results of Studies AML-BFM 87 and 93

| Study | -87 | % | -93§ | % |
|---|---|---|---|---|
| Patients | 307 | | 416 | |
| ED# | 28 | 9 | 28 | 7 |
| NR | 49 | 16 | 43 | 10 |
| CR | 230 | 75 | 345 | 83 |
| Events in CCR | 8 | | 18 | |
| allog. BMT in 1st CR | 17 | | 36 | |
| 3yrs. pEFS (SE) | | 41 (3) | | 54 (3) |
| 3yrs. pEFI (SE) | | 55 (3) | | 65 (3) |
| 3yrs. pSurvival (SE) | | 49 (3) | | 60 (3) |

§ last patient entry 3/98, # ED before therapy included
Abbr.: allog. = allogeneic; BMT = bone marrow transplantation;
CR = complete remission; CCR = continuous complete remission;
ED = early death; NR = nonresponder

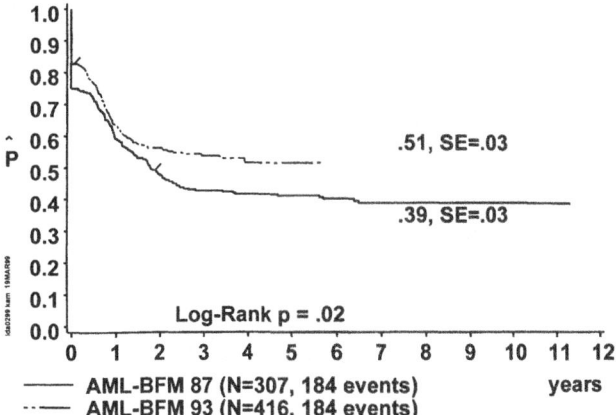

**Fig. 2.** Estimated probability for event-free survival in study AML-BFM 93 compared to study AML-BFM 87. Slash indicates last patient of the group

Figure 2 shows a comparison of pEFS with study AML-BFM 87.

### Results of first randomization ADE vs. AIE:

Results show no difference in outcome with a similar pEFS for ADE and AIE patients. The slightly higher early deaths rate in the AIE group might be explained by two early deaths

**Table 3.** Results by 1. Randomization ADE vs AIE

|  | ADE | AIE |
|---|---|---|
| Total | 166 | 175 |
| ED | 4 | 9* |
| PR/NR | 19 | 16 |
| CR | 143 (86%) | 150 (86%) |
| in CCR | 90 (54%) | 101(58%) |

Abbr.: CR = complete remission, CCR = continuous complete remission, ED = early death; NR = nonresponder; PR = partial responder

occurring in patients with hyperleukocytosis of >200.000/µl and one early death after HAM. The response rate was the same in each group (Figure 3, and Table 3).

The non-hematological toxicity regarding the infection rate was slightly higher in the AIE arm with a similar rate of other complications in both arms (percentage of patients without any infections in the ADE group 22%, and in the AIE group 10%, p-trend = 0.02).

Hematological toxicity measured by aplasia from induction until neutrophil recovery to 500/µl revealed a two day longer recovery time for patients in the AIE group (ADE, median 25 days, range 12-104 days; AIE, median 27 days, range 10–80 days, pU test =0.03). There was no significant difference in the platelet recovery time between the two arms (ADE median 23 days, range 7-71 days, AIE 25 days, range 7-83 days, pU test = 0.29).

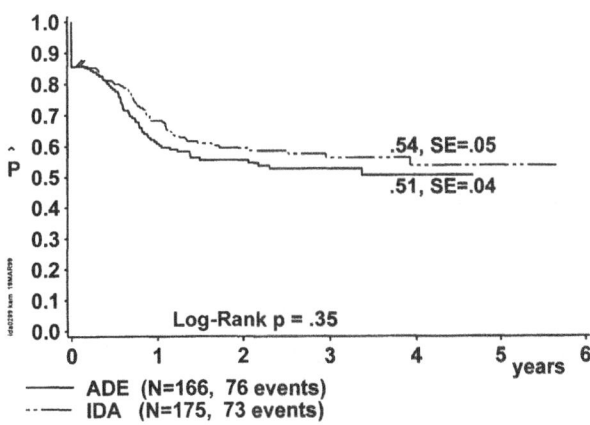

**Fig. 3.** Estimated probability for event-free survival for patients randomized for ADE and AIE in study AML-BFM 93. Slash indicates last patient of the group

**Table 4.** Results by Blast Cell Reduction on Day 15 - 1. Randomization ADE *vs* AIE

| 1. Rand. | Blasts Day 15 | N | % | CR % |
|----------|---------------|-----|------|------|
| ADE | ≤ 5% | 91 | 66 | 93 |
| | > 5% | 48 | 35* | 81 |
| AIE | ≤ 5% | 115 | 81 | 88 |
| | > 5% | 27 | 19* | 85 |

*p chi square 0.003

However, a significant better blast cell reduction on day 15 could be seen in patients treated with IDR. Eighty-one percent of patients of the AIE group presented with ≤5% blasts on day 15 compared to only 66% of the ADE group (Table 4), p chi² =0.003.

### Results by second randomization HR 1 vs HR2

One-hundred-ninety-four patients were randomized in either HR1 (n=95) or HR2 (n=99). Overall results were similar in both treatment groups regarding response and relapse rate. Figure 4 shows the pEFS of both groups. Non-hematological toxicity was also similar in both arms. Whereas patients of the HR 1 group treated initially with either ADE or AIE responded similarly, patients of the HR 2 group showed slightly inferior results

**Table 5.** Results by 2. Randomization HR1 *vs* HR2

| 2. Rand | Induction | n | CR (%) | EFS (%) |
|---------|-----------|-----|--------|---------|
| HR1 | ADE | 44 | 86 | 54 (8) |
| | AIE | 51 | 88 | 50 (7) |
| HR2 | ADE | 52 | 83 | 39 (7)* |
| | AIE | 47 | 89 | 56 (8) |

*p 0.11

when treated with ADE (Table 5). This indicates that early treatment with HAM can improve outcome, especially in patients treated with ADE during induction

Overall, significantly better results could be achieved in high risk patients of study AML-BFM 93 compared to study AML-BFM 87 (Figure 5). An improvement which has to be contributed mainly to the introduction of HAM, a treatment block which had not been given in study 87.

### Discussion

Several studies have demonstrated, that more intensive therapy can improve results [6,13,14]. The first randomization comparing ADE vs. AIE resulted in a better blast cell reduction on day 15, which, however, did not translate into a better outcome, partly due to the efficacy of HAM given either as 2nd or 3rd treatment course. Randomization of HR1 vs. HR2 did not show differences in outcome, however, the historical control between studies AML-BFM 87 (without HAM) and study 93 (with HAM in HR patients) showed better results in the latter study (Figure 5), indicating that HAM is effective and the time-point in the treatment may be less important. More distinctive analyses revealed HAM introduced late seems to be less effective, mainly for patients treated with ADE initially. Whereas similar remission rates were achieved in patients treated with AIE initially followed by late or early HAM and patients treated with early HAM after ADE.

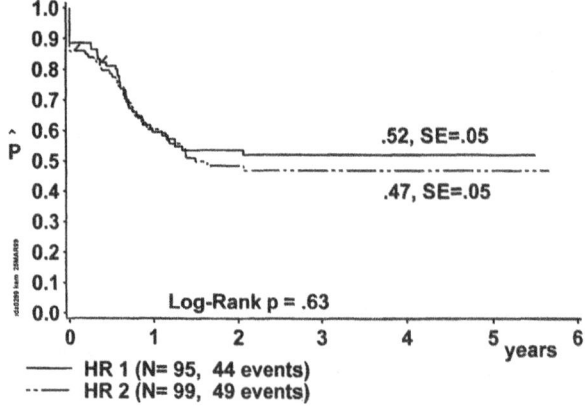

**Fig. 4.** Estimated probability for event-free survival for patients randomized for HR 1 and HR 2 in study AML-BFM 93. Slash indicates last patient of the group

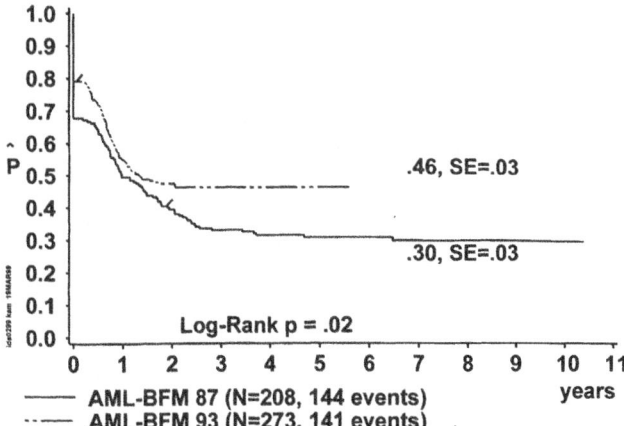

**Fig. 5.** Estimated probability for event-free survival for high risk patients of study AML-BFM 93 compared to study AML-BFM 87. Slash indicates last patient of the group

## Conclusion

Both randomizations have shown no significant differences in outcome, however, slightly better results in certain patient groups, especially after induction therapy with AIE and early HAM. Therefore, in the ongoing study AML-BFM 98 we introduced this treatment option for the majority of the patients.

*Acknowledgements: Principal investigators of Study AML-BFM 93 in Germany:* R. Mertens, Kinderklinik RWTH, Aachen; A. Gnekow, I. Kinderklinik des Klinikums, Augsburg; G.F. Wündisch, Universitäts-Kinderklinik, Bayreuth; G. Henze, CCVK-Kinderklinik Berlin; E. Hilgenfeld, Charité-Kinderklinik; W. Dörfel, II. Kinderklinik Berlin-Buch; N. Jorch Kinderklinik Gilead Bielefeld, U. Bode, Universitäts-Kinderklinik, Bonn; H.-J. Spaar/Th. Lieber Prof.-Hess-Kinderklinik, Bremen; W. Eberl, Städtische Kinderklinik, Braunschweig; I. Krause, Städtische Kinderklinik Chemnitz; E. Holfeld, Kinderklinik d. Carl-Thiem-Klinikums Cottbus; W. Andler/Th. Wiesel, Vestische Kinderklinik, Datteln; I. Lauterbach, Kinderklinik d. TU Dresden; V. Scharfe, Städtische Kinderklinik Dresden-Neustadt; U. Göbel/D. Körholz. Universitäts-Kinderklinik, Düsseldorf; G. Weinmann, Kinderklinik Erfurt; J.D. Beck, Universitäts-Kinderklinik, Erlangen; W. Havers Universitäts-Kinderklinik, Essen; B. Kornhuber, Universitäts-Kinderklinik, Frankfurt; Ch. Niemeyer, Universitäts-Kinderklinik, Freiburg; F. Lampert/R. Blütters-Sawatzki, Universitäts-Kinderklinik, Gießen; M. Lakomek/ A. Pekrun, Universitäts-Kinderklinik, Göttingen; H. Weigel, Universitäts-Kinderklinik Greifswald V. Gerein Kinderklinik Gummersbach, T. Reiß, Universitäts-Kinderklinik Halle/S; H. Kabisch, Universitäts-Kinderklinik, Hamburg; K. Welte/ P. Weinel, Kinderklinik der Medizinischen Hochschule, Hannover; B. Selle, Universitäts-Kinderklinik, Heidelberg; N Graf, Universitäts-Kinderklinik, Homburg/Saar; J. Hermann, Universitäts-Kinderklinik Jena; G. Nessler, Städtische Kinderklinik, Karlsruhe; Th. Wehinger, Städt. Kinderklinik, Kassel; M. Rister, Kinderklinik Kemperhof, Koblenz; F. Berthold, Universitäts-Kinderklinik, Köln; W. Sternschulte, Städtisches Kinderkrankenhaus, Köln; R. Schneppenheim, Universitäts-Kinderklinik, Kiel; K. Rieske, Universitäts-Kinderklinik Leipzig; P. Bucsky, Universitäts-Kinderklinik, Lübeck; H.Ch. Dominick Kinderklinik St. Annastift, Ludwigshafen; U. Kluba, Universitäts-Kinderklinik Magdeburg; W. Scheurlen, Städt. Kinderklinik, Mannheim; P. Gutjahr, Universitäts-Kinderklinik, Mainz; H. Christiansen, Universitäts-Kinderklinik, Marburg; R.J. Haas, v. Haunersches Kinderspital, München; St. Müller-Weihrich/L. Stengel-Rutkowski, Kinderklinik d. Technischen Universität, München-Schwabing; Ch. Bender-Götze/M. Führer, Universitäts-Kinderpoliklinik, München; H. Jürgens, Universitäts-Kinderklinik, Münster; A. Jobke, Cnopfsche Kinderklinik, Nürnberg; U. Schwarzer, Städtische Kinderklinik, Nürnberg; G. Eggers/M. Hagen, Universitäts-Kinderklinik Rostock; R. Schumacher, Kinderklinik Schwerin; R.

Dickerhoff, Johanniter Kinderklinik, St. Augustin; J. Treuner, Olgahospital, Stuttgart; D. Niethammer/H. Scheel-Walter, Universitäts-Kinderklinik, Tübingen; W. Behnisch, Universitäts-Kinderklinik, Ulm; J. Kühl, Universitäts-Kinderklinik, Würzburg

*Principal investigators of Austria:*
Ch. Urban, Universitäts-Kinderklinik d. Landeskrankenhauses Graz; F.M. Fink, Universitäts-Kinderklinik d. A.ö. Landeskrankenhauses Innsbruck; K. Schmitt/G. Ebetsberger Landes-Kinderkrankenhaus Linz; I. Slavc AKH-Universitäts-Kinderklinik Wien; G. Mann, St. Anna-Kinderspital Wien

*Principal investigators of Switzerland:*
R. Angst, Kinderklinik d. Kantonsspital Aarau; P. Imbach, P.A. Avoledo Universitäts-Kinderspital Basel; A. Feldges Ostschweizerisches Kinderspital St. Gallen; M. Nenadov-Beck/C. Desseng CHUV-Kinderklinik Lausanne; U. Caflisch Kinderspital Luzern; L. Nobile Buetti Kinderklinik Hospital La Carita Locarno; H.J. Plüss Universitäts-Kinderklinik Zürich

*The coordinators of studies AML-BFM 93 were:* J. Ritter, U. Creutzig, J. Hermann, H. Gadner, Universitäts-Kinderklinik, Münster, Jena und St. Anna Kinderspital Wien.

We thank P. Stappert, E. Kurzknabe and J. Meltzer for excellent technical assistance and Christa Lausch for her valuable assistance in the management of the AML studies.
Supported by the Deutsche Krebshilfe

# References

1. Berman E, Heller G, Santorsa J, et al. (1991) Results of a randomized trial comparing idarubicin and cytosine arabinoside with daunorubicin and cytosine arabinoside in adult patients with newly diagnosed acute myelogenous leukemia. Blood 77:1666-1674
2. Vogler WR, Velez-Garcia E, Weiner RS, Flaum MA, Bartolucci AA, Omura GA, Gerber MC, Banks PLC (1992) A Phase III trial comparing idarubicin and daunorubicin in combination with cytarabine in acute myelogenous leukemia: A Southeastern Cancer Study Group. Journal Cancer Research 10:1103-1111
3. Wiernik PH, Banks PLC, Case DCJr, Arlin ZA, Perlman PO, Todd MB, Ritch PS, Enck RE, Weitberg AB (1992) Cytarabine plus idarubicin or daunorubicin as induction and consolidation therapy for previously untreated adult patients with acute myeloid leukemia. Blood 79:313-319
4. Kesavan S, Lincoff AM, Young JB (1996) Anthracycline-induced cardiotoxicity. Ann Intern Med 125:47-58
5. Hiddemann W, Kreutzmann H, Straif K, Ludwig WD, Mertelsmann R, Donhuijsen Ant R, Lengfelder E, Arlin Z, Büchner T (1987) High-dose cytosine arabinoside and mitoxantrone: a highly effective regimen in refractory acute myeloid leukemia. Blood 69:744-749
6. Bishop JF, Matthews JP, Young GA, Szer J, Gillett A, Joshua D, Bradstock K, Enno A, Wolf MM, Fox R, et al (1996) A randomized study of high-dose cytarabine in induction in acute myeloid leukemia. Blood 87:1710-1717
7. Wolff S, Herzig R, Fay J, Phillips GL, Lazarus HM, Flexner JM, Stein RS, Greer JP, Cooper G, Herzig GP (1989) High dose cytosine arabinoside and daunomycin as consolidation therapy for acute non-myeloid leukemia in first remission: long term results. J Clin Oncol 7:1260-1267
8. Mayer RJ, Davis RB, Schifffer CA, Berg DT, Powell BL, Schulman P, Omura GA, Moore JO, McIntyre OR, Frei E (1994) Intensive postremission chemotherapy in adults with acute myeloid leukemia. N Engl J Med 331:896-903
9. Hiddemann W, Heinecke A, Büchner T (1997) Intensified therapy of acute myeloid leukemia: Results of the German AML Cooperative Group. Hematol Blood Transfus 38:769-773
10. Creutzig U, Ritter J, Zimmermann M, Schellong G, for the AML-BFM Study Group (1993) Does cranial irradiation reduce the risk for bone marrow relapse in acute myelogenous leukemia (AML): unexpected results of the childhood AML Study BFM-87. J Clin Oncol 11:279-286
11. Creutzig U, Zimmermann M, Ritter J, Henze G, Graf N, Löffler H, Schellong G (1999) Definition of a standard-risk group in children with AML. Br J Haematol 104:630-639
12. Cheson BD, Cassileth PA, Head DR, Schiffer CA, Bennett JM, Bloomfield CD, Brunning R, Gale RP, Grever MR, Keating MJ, Sawitsky A, Stass S, Weinstein H, Woods WG (1990) Report of the National Cancer Institute-sponsored workshop on definitions and response in acute myeloid leukemia. J Clin Oncol 8:813-819
13. Büchner T, Hiddemann W, Löffler G, Gassmann W, Maschmeyer G, Heit W, Hossfeld D, Weh H, Ludwig WD, Thiel E, Nowrousian M, Aul HC, Lengfelder E, Lathan B, Mainzer K, Urbanitz D, Emmerich B, Middelhoff G, Donhuijsen-Ant HR, Hellriegel H-P, Heinecke A (1991) Improved cure rate by very early intensification combined with prolonged maintenance chemotherapy in patients with acute myeloid leukemia: data from the AML Cooperative Group. Semin Hematol 28:76-79
14. Woods WG, Kobrinsky N, Buckley JD, Lee JW, Sanders J, Neudorf S, Gold S, Barnard DR, DeSwarte J, Dusenbery K, Kalousek D, Arthur DC, Lange BJ (1996) Timed-sequential induction therapy improves postremission outcome in acute myeloid leukemia: A report from the Children's Cancer Group. Blood 87:4979-4989

# Acute Myeloid Leukemia (AML) in Children: Results of the French Trials

G. Schaison, A. Auvrignon, G. Michel, T. Leblanc, A. Baruchel, J. Landman-Parker, I. Thuret, P. Bordigoni, H. Esperou, Y. Perel, J.P. Vannier, E. Le Gall, B. Nelken, J.L. Stephan, F. Mechinaud, G. Couillault and G. Leverger

## Introduction

During the past ten years major progress has been made in the treatment of childhood AML with the introduction of intensified induction therapy, followed by an aggressive post induction chemotherapy or an allogenic bone marrow transplantation.

We report here the outcome of 259 children with AML who were enrolled on the prospective French protocol LAME 89/91. This protocol was designed to assess the comparative value of BMT when an HLA compatible related donor was available versus an aggressive post remission intensification including high dose Cytarabine and Asparaginase, with respect to remission duration, relapse rate, death in remission and over all survival. A second objective was to compare patients with or without maintenance treatment. The therapeutic relevance of cytogenetic assessment was also evaluated.

As previous protocols have raised doubts about the value of initial prognostic factors, all patients received the same treatment omitting risk directed therapy. Other trials have suggested that induction with Mitoxantrone may be more effective than Daunorubicin (2, 3, 7), so all patients received the same induction containing Ara-C and Mitoxantrone. Mitoxantrone has also be reported to be less cardiotoxic than Daunorubicin. It is clear that more intensive treatment has provided better control of leukemia with substantially lower relapse rates. Sequential therapy with high dose Ara-C and Asparaginase has been extensively used in pediatric AML and is proven to be useful with an acceptable toxicity (4, 10, 12). It is assumed that allogenic BMT would benefit all children and therefore if a sibling was available, patients received an allograft.

## Patients and Methods (Fig. 1 and 2)

259 children, 126 boys, 133 girls entered the protocol between december 1988 and june 1996. Mean age was 7.2 y (0.1–18.3). Mean WBC were 67.300/mm³ (0.7–600.000).

Previously untreated AML with FAB subtype ranging from M1 to M6 and age less 20 years were eligible. Down syndrome children form a special group whose disease appears to respond very well to treatment: therefore they were excluded. Patients with M0 or M7 or biphenotypic leukemia, myelodysplasia and secondary AML were also excluded. Repartition in FAB Subtypes is given in Table 1.

Table 1. Répartition of 259 patients in FAB subtypes.

| M1 | 33 = 13 % |
|---|---|
| M2 | 73 = 28 % |
| M3 | 17 = 7 % |
| M4 | 40 = 15 % |
| M4 eosino | 16 = 6 % |
| M5 | 73 = 28 % |
| M6 | 7 = 3 % |

### Induction therapy

Induction therapy was a combination of Cytarabine (200 mg/m²/day by continuous intavenous infusion from day 1 to day 7) and Mitoxantrone (12 mg/m²/day 1 to day 5). These drugs were reduced to two thirds for children younger than one year of age. Bone marrow aspiration was performed on day 20 and patients who had more than 20 % blasts received additional chemotherapy consisting of Cytarabine 200 mg/m²/day by continuous IV infusion for 3 days and Mitoxantrone 12 mg/m²/day for 2 days. Complete remission was defined as less 5 % blasts in a normocel-

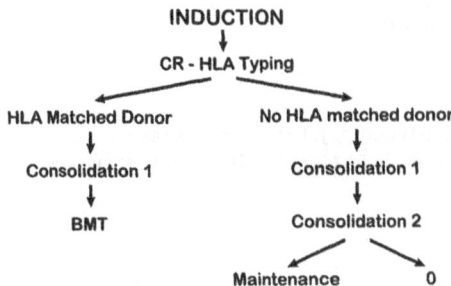

**Fig. 1.** Design of Protocol LAME 89-91

lular bone marrow and no evidence of extra-medullary leukemia.

## Post induction therapy

Consolidation chemotherapy. Two consolidations were given to patients without an HLA matched donor. Consolidation 1 was a combination of VP16 (100 mg/m²/day IV from 1 to day 4), Cytarabine (100 mg/m²/day as continuous IV infusion from day 1 to day 4), and Daunorubicin (40 mg/m²/day from day 1 to day 4). Consolidation 2 which was given after complete hematological recovery of consolidation 1 consisted of two cycles of Cytarabine infusion (1 g/m² every 12 hours x 4) administered at 7 days interval (first cycle on day 1 and day 2, second cycle on day 8 and 9) followed by one dose of Asparaginase at 6000 U/m². Between the two Cytarabine cycles children older than one year of age were treated with Amsacrine at 150 mg/m²/day IV on day 4, 5 and 6 whereas younger children did not receive this medication.

## Maintenance Chemotherapy

After consolidation chemotherapy patients were treated with an 18 month maintenance program consisting of continuous oral 6 Mercaptopurine 50 mg/m²/day and monthly pulses of subcutaneous Cytarabine 25 mg/m² twice a day for 4 days. In march 1991, a decision was made by the participating centers to randomize children to receive the maintenance treatment or not to receive any further treatment after consolidation 2. An interim

analysis revealed no difference in relapse rate or DFS between these two groups. Consequantly all patients treated on the chemotherapy arm were analysed as a single group for the purpose of comparison with BMT whether or not they received the maintenance program.

## CNS therapy

CNS prophylaxis was administered to patients with the M4 or the M5 FAB subtype and to patients with an initial WBC higher than 50 x 10⁹/l. These patients received intrathecal therapy (IT) with five doses of Cytarabine, Methotrexate and steroids. Two IT were performed during induction therapy (on day 1 and at time of hematological recovery and three during consolidation 1 (on day 1, 5 and 20).

Patients with initial CNS involvement received three additional IT doses (two during induction and one during consolidation 1) and 24 Gy cranial radiation for children over 2 years after hematologic recovery from consolidation 2.

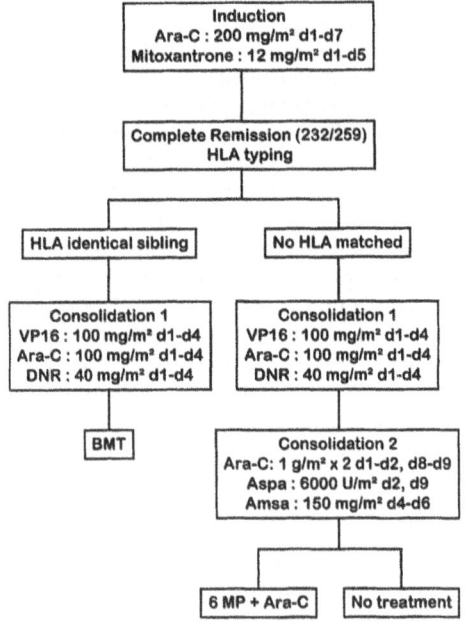

**Fig. 2.** Chemotherapy of Protocol LAME 89-91

## Bone Marrow Transplantation

All patients in complete remission after induction chemotherapy were assessed to the presence of an HLA compatible sibling donor. Among 232 patients who achieved a complete remission 60 (25.8 %) had an HLA identical sibling donor and were eligible to receive an allogenic BMT early in first CR. The preparative regimen for transplantation was a TBI containing regimen (with Cyclophosphamide or high dose Ara-C and Melphelan) in 16 cases and a Busulfan (BU) Cyclophosphamide (CY) regimen in 44 cases.

Cyclophosphamide was given IV at a dose of 60 mg/K/day for 2 days (n = 8) as described by Copeland (Bu Cy 120) [5] or at 50 mg/K/day for four days (n = 36) as described by Santos (Bu Cy 200) (11). Patients were transplanted just after induction in 4 cases, after consolidation 1 in 45 cases and after consolidation 2 in 11 cases. All recipients of HLA identical BMT received GVHD prophylaxis consisting of Cyclosporin A and short Methotrexate. Mean interval between CR and BMT was 82 ± 8 days.

## Statistical considerations

Probabilities of relapses, disease free survival, event free survival and therapy related mortality were estimated with the Kaplan Meyer method. Log Rank test was used to compare between the two regimen based on intention to treat. Multivariate analysis were performed using Cox proportional hazards regression model.

## Results

Among 259 patients included in the protocol, 232 (89 %) achieved complete remission. 235 of them received the standard 7 day induction whereas 24 required the additional induction chemotherapy course. 27 failures (11 %) were observed. The reasons for not entering remission were resistant disease (6 %) and death during induction therapy (5 %). Interval between the day 1 of treatment and complete remission was 36 ± 1.4 days. Mean duration of neutropenia, thrombocytopenia and hospitalization were respectively 33 ± 1.3, 29 ± 1.7 and 40 ± 1.5 d. Complete remission rate was only 66 % for children receiving the additional induction course.

## Long term follow up

Mean follow up is 5.3 years. Survival in first complete remission (EFS) is 47 ± 6 % for all 259 patients (Fig. 3). The 7 year DFS probability for all patients was 52 % ± 6 (Fig. 4). The 7 year DFS was only 27 % ± 20 for the subgroup of patients receiving additional induction course.

DFS is 60 % ± 12 for the BMT group (60 patients) as compared to 50 % ± 7 in the che-

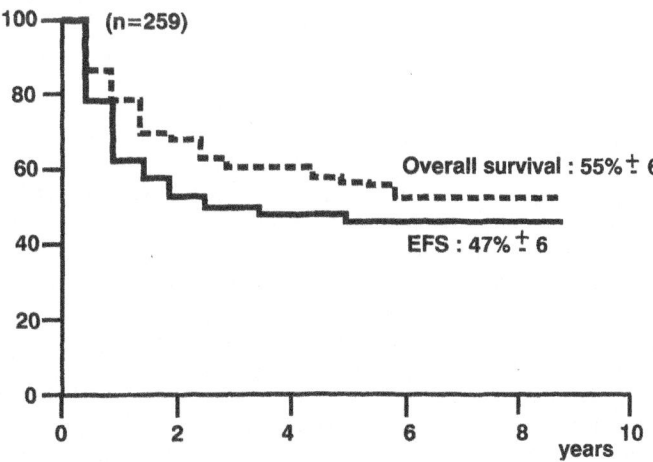

**Fig. 3.** EFS and overall survival

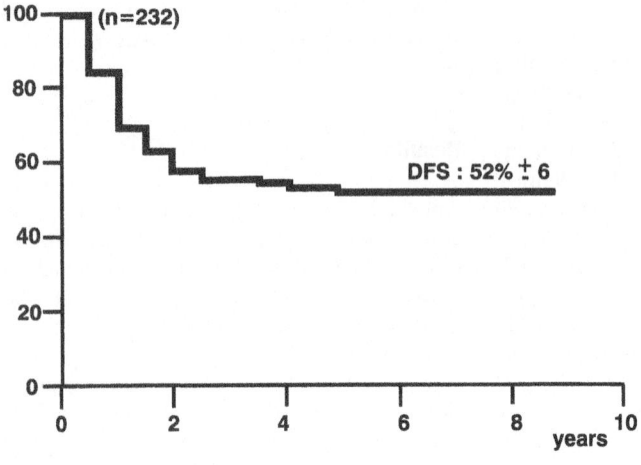

**Fig. 4.** DFS of Protocol LAME 89-91 (232 patients in complete remission).

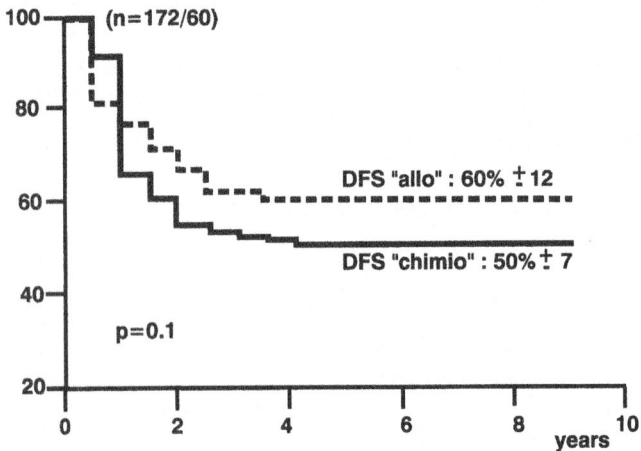

**Fig. 5.** DFS of chemotherapy group and DFS of patients receiving allogenic bone marrow transplantation.

motherapy group (172 patients) p = 0.1 (Fig. 5). The actuarial relapse rate was 34 % ± 12 for the BMT group and 46 % ± 6 for patients treated in the chemotherapy regimen. Time to relapse was 8.7 months for the chemotherapy arm and 17 months after BMT. The probability of death in complete remission was similar in both group 6.8 and 7 %. The second consolidation was more toxic with 40 % of severe infections as compared to 25 % after the first consolidation. Most relapses occured in the bone marrow except for 3 % of patients who had an extra-medullary relapse. Among 27 children with initial CNS involvement only 8 had received cranial irradiation. Half of relapsing patients treated in the chemotherapy regimen achieved a second remission.

DFS for patients randomized with or without a maintenance chemotherapy was respectively 70 ± 15 % and 49 ± 12 %, p = 0.16 and survival were 89 % ± 14 % and 55 % ± 17 %, p = 0.004. After intensive consolidation maintenance treatment does not increase DFS.

### Prognostic factors

Age, initial WBC, t(9;11), cytogenetics, tumor burden, CNS involvement were studied in a multivariate analysis. The impact of these differents factors on DFS and relapse is shown on Table 2. Meningeal involvement and bulky diseases did not affect relapse risk or DFS. Only two factors were statistically significant in the multivariate analysis, age less 1 year and WBC.

**Table 2.** Prognostic factors in the chemotherapy group using a COX model.

| | DFS | Relapses |
|---|---|---|
| Age less 1 y | p = 0.02 | p = 0.09 |
| WBC < or > 50.000 | NS (p = 0.11) | p = 0.02 |
| FAB M5 versus others | NS | NS |
| CNS involvement | NS | NS |
| Bulky disease | NS | NS |

**Karyotype analysis** was available at diagnosis in 220/250 children. 27 % of karyotypes are normal and 73 % are abnormal. 37 % have one for the four FAB related translocation/rearrangement t(8;21), t(15;17), inv(16) and t(9;11) and DFS were respectively 48, 57, 68 and 77 %. 17 % of patients have chromosomal rearrangement involving the 11q23 band and 58 patients have other various abnormalities. DFS of patients with t(9;11) and of patients with other rearrangement involving the 11q23 band are respectively 77 and 24 % (p = 0.007). There is no significant difference neither for mean age, nor for mean WBC within these two group. Among the patients with a chromosomal rearrangement involving the 11q23 band the prognosis is significantly better for those with t(9;11) than for patients with other 11q23 rearrangement.

**The prognostic value** of the conditioning regimen and of the pre transplant chemotherapy was as followed. The survival is 68 % ± 21 (n = 16) for patients receiving a TBI regimen 61 ± 15 % after the Bu Cy 200 (n = 36) and 37 + 28 % (n = 8) after the Bu Cy 120. There is no statistical difference but the later group is very small. The patients who had received 2 consolidations before transplant have 92 ± 17 % probability of survival in CR (n = 12) as compared to 50 ± 14 % for those receiving no or only one consolidation before transplant (n = 48), p = 0.019. Similarly the relapse rate for these patients is 8 % versus 43 % (p = 0.04).

## Discussion

The goals of protocol 89/91 include :
1. To improve the cure rate of patients with newly diagnosed AML.
2. To use a classical 7 + 3 backbone induction regimen omitting risk directed therapy.
3. To compare the value of allogenic bone marrow transplantation versus conventional consolidation.
4. To evaluate the efficacy of a maintenance regimen.

There have been only marginal increase in the CR rates for children with AML since the introduction of the so-called 7 + 3 regimen. Mitoxantrone and continuous infusion of Aracytine are an appropriate induction regimen giving 89 % remission rate and the results presented here demonstrate that Mitoxantrone is at least as effective as Daunomycin (2, 9, 13, 16).

10 % of patients have an initial CNS disease at diagnosis. CNS relapses, isolated or associated were less 3 % indicating that cranial irradiation don't seem necessary for patients receiving otherwise high dose Aracytine. The impact of maintenance treatment was also tested by CCG investigators (15). We confirmed that after two intensive consolidations including high dose Aracytine, VP16, Amsa, the maintenance treatment does not increase DFS and even appears to be a negative predictive factor for survival.

Many published studies have reported that the antileukemic effects of BMT was partially counter balanced by a 25 % risk of transplanted related mortality. The transplant related mortality was 7 % similar to that of chemotherapy. The use of myeloablative therapy followed by allogenic BMT rescue is one of the most important ways to improve long term survival in children with AML. Our results in the 60 patients receiving BMT are somewhat disappointing with only 60 % long term survivors demonstrating only a slight advantage for BMT.

DFS is similar for patients receiving a conditioning regimen with Busulfan and Cytoxan or including TBI. It is clear here that a very early BMT just after CR is followed by an important number of relapses. We observed very encouraging results in the small number of patients transplanted after 2 consolidations with a probability of survival and relapse rate respectively 90 % and 8 %. More intensive treatment before BMT has provided a better control of leukemia with substantially lower relapse rates after BMT. The impact of increasing the interval from CR to transplant must be confirmed in a larger number of patients [15].

It is unclear whether or not allo BMT is of benefit for patients associating good prognostic factors (ie age over 1 year, WBC less 50.000 and favourable karyotype).

Autologous transplantation was not tested in this study but results of POG or CCG (10, 14) did not show any clear advantage over conventional chemotherapy. However ABMT was used in second complete remission with a 3 year DFS of 40 %.

The multivariate analysis have identified only two clinical and laboratory parameters that appeared to be predictive of outcome. The multivariate analysis has shown that age less 1 year was associated with a lower 5 year DFS after exclusion of children with Down syndrome. Children less 1 year old have a higher risk of relapses and a lower DFS than older children.

A WBC count higher than $50 \times 10^9$ was associated a higher risk of relapses but the impact on DFS did not reach the level of statistical significance. None of the following variables affected the long term survival: Bulky disease, initial CNS involvement, FAB subtype.

There is correlation between karyotype and outcome (6). 72 % of children have cytogenetic abnormalities. Favourable karyotypes are inv(16) t(9;11) and t(15;17). But now patients with M3 subtype must be excluded from conventional therapy and treated with ATRA and intensive therapy. DFS for patients with t(8;21) is not significantly different from other patients and do not support the so called good prognosis related with this translocation.

# References

1. AMADORI S. et al. 1993. Prospective comparative study of bone marrow transplantation and post remission chemotherapy for childhood acute myelogenous leukemia. J. Clin. Oncol., 11 : 1046-1054.
2. ARLIN Z. et al. 1990. Randomized multicenter trial of Cytosine Arabinoside with Mitoxantrone or Daunorubicin in previously untreated adult patients with acute non lymphoblastic leukemia (ANLL). Leukemia, 4 : 177-183.
3. ARLIN Z. et al. 1994. Randomized multicenter trial of Cytosine Arabinoside with Mitoxantrone or Daunorubicin in previously untreated adult patients with acute myeloid leukemia. N. Engl. J. Med., 331 : 896.
4. CAPIZZI R.H., POOLE M., COPPER M.R. 1984. Treatment of poor risk acute leukemia with sequential high dose Ara-C and Asparaginase. Blood, 63 : 694-700.
5. COPELAND E.A. et al. 1991. Treatment for acute myelocytic leukemia with allogenic bone marrow transplantation following preparation with Bu Cy 120. Blood, 78 : 838-843.
6. LEBLANC T., BERGER R. 1997. Molecular cytogenetics of childhood acute myelogenous leukemias. Eur. J. Haematol., 59 : 1-13.
7. LÖWENBERG B. et al. 1991. Mitoxantrone versus Daunorubicin in induction of acute myelogenous leukemia in elderly patients and low dose Ara-C versus control as maintenance : An EORTC phase 3 trial (AML 9). Haematologica, 76 (suppl. 4) : 91.
8. NESBIT M.E. et al. 1994. Chemotherapy for induction remission of childhood acute myeloid leukemia followed by marrow transplantation or multiagent chemotherapy. A report from the Children's Cancer Group. J. Clin. Oncol., 12 : 127-135.
9. PREISLER H.D. et al. 1987. Comparison of three remission induction regimen and two post induction strategies for the treatment of acute non lymphocytic leukemia. A cancer and leukemia group B study. Blood, 69 : 1441.
10. RAVINDRANATH Y. et al. 1991. High dose Cytarabine for intensification of early therapy of childhood acute myeloid leukemia. A Pediatric Oncology Group Study. J. Clin. Oncol., 9 : 572-586.
11. SANTOS G.W. et al. 1983. Marrow transplantation : acute non lymphocytic leukemia after treatment with Busulfan and Cyclophosphamide. N. Engl. J. Med., 309 : 1347-1353.
12. WELLS R.J., WOODS D.G., LAMPKIN B.C. 1993. Impact of high dose Cytarabine and Asparaginase intensification on childhood acute myeloid leukemia : a report from the Children's Cancer Group. J. Clin. Oncol., 11 : 538-545.
13. WIERNIK P.H. et al. 1979. A comparative trial of Daunorubicin, Cytosine Arabinoside and Thioguanine and a combination of the three agents for the treatment of acute myelocytic leukemia. Med. Pediatr. Oncol., 6 : 261.
14. WOODS W.G. et al. 1990. The role of timing of high dose Cytosine Arabinoside intensification and of maintenance therapy in the treatment of children with acute non lymphoblastic leukemia. Cancer, 66 : 1106-1113.
15. WOODS W.G. et al. 1996. Timed sequential induction therapy improves post remission outcome in acute myeloid leukemia. A report from the Children's Cancer Group. Blood, 87 : 4979-4989.
16. YATES J. 1992. Cytosine Arabinoside with Daunorubicin or Adriamycin therapy for acute myelocytic leukemia. Blood, 60 : 454.

# AML in Children: The Medical Research Council Data

R. F. Stevens, I. M. Hann, K. Wheatley, and R. G. Gray.
On behalf of the MRC Childhood Leukemia Working Party

The United Kingdom Medical research Council's 10th Acute Myeloid Leukaemia trial for children (AML10) was opened in May 1988 and by March 1995, 364 children aged less than 15 years had been entered from 41 centres in the UK, Republic of Ireland, and New Zealand. In addition to patients with *de novo* AML, those with AML secondary to previous myelodysplasia (mds-AML) or to previous therapy for other diseases (s-AML) and those with aggressive myelodysplastic syndrome (RAEB-t) were also eligible. Five patients were excluded due to misdiagnosis: three with ALL, one with lymphoma and one with histiocytosis.

At the start of the trial, two centres made a policy decision not to take part in the induction randomisation but did register all children who were considered suitable for induction therapy for later randomisation to A-BMT or not. These 55 children are therefore included in the main outcome analysis together with the 286 randomised children giving a total of 341 evaluable for overall outcome. A further 18 patients from 7 centres were not randomised for induction therapy on an *ad hoc* basis and are not included in the overall outcome results as this could artificially inflate remission rates and survival, but they are included in transplant analyses where relevant.

## Treatment

The treatment outline for AML 10 is shown in Fig. 1. Treatment was the same for all children including those with secondary AML and Down syndrome. Patients were randomised to receive either two courses of DAT (daunorubicin, Ara-C and 6-thioguanine) or two courses of ADE (daunorubicin, Ara-C and etoposide). If remission was achieved with these two courses, two further consolidation courses (one MACE; amsacrine, Ara-C and etoposide, and one MidAC; mitoxantrone and Ara-C) were scheduled. Children not in CR after 2 courses were recommended to continue on protocol if a further attempt to induce CR was considered appropriate. In addition, triple intrathecal therapy with methotrexate, Ara-C and hydrocortisone was given as part of each course. For children with CNS disease at presentation, two courses of triple intrathecal chemotherapy were given each week until 2 weeks after CNS clearance. Matched sibling allogeneic transplantation (allo-BMT) was recommended for children with a HLA-matched sibling donor, whereas the remainder were randomised between A-BMT and stopping treatment. Condition for BMT was cyclophosphomide (60mg/kg/day for 2 days) plus total body irradiation. For children aged < 2 years the conditioning was busulphan (4mg/kg/day on days -8 to -5) and cyclophosphamide (50mg/kg/day on days -4 to -1).

## Statistical Methods

Remission rates were compared using chi-squared tests. For survival data, Kaplan-Meier life tables were constructed and the curves were compared by means of the log-rank test. Median follow up is 5.6 years. All p values are two-tailed.

The following definitions are used: overall survival is the time of entry to death; event free survival (EFS) is the time of entry until the first event; disease free survival is the time from CR to any event; relapse free survival (RFS) is the time from CR to relapse. Ranges in parentheses are 95% confidence limits.

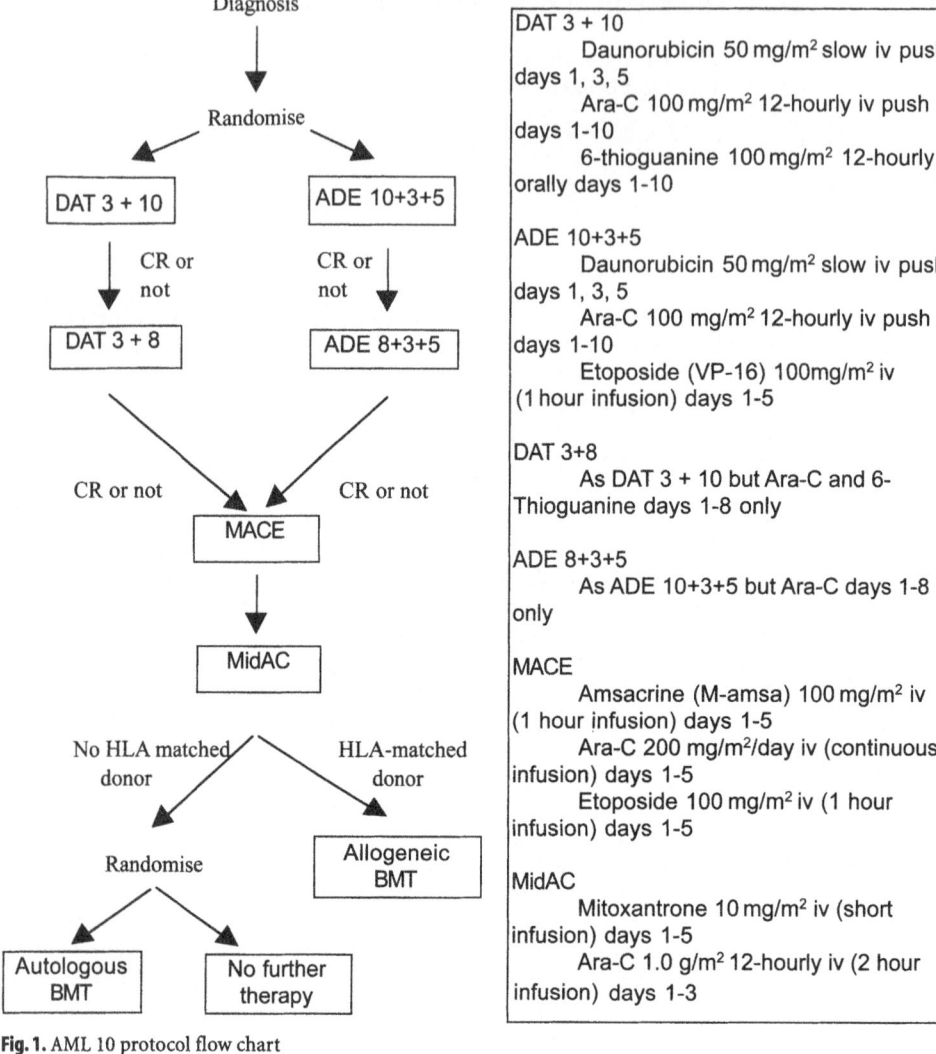

**Fig. 1.** AML 10 protocol flow chart

The text within the figure:

Diagnosis

Randomise

DAT 3 + 10

ADE 10+3+5

CR or not

CR or not

DAT 3 + 8

ADE 8+3+5

CR or not

CR or not

MACE

MidAC

No HLA matched donor

HLA-matched donor

Randomise

Allogeneic BMT

Autologous BMT

No further therapy

DAT 3 + 10
    Daunorubicin 50 mg/m² slow iv push days 1, 3, 5
    Ara-C 100 mg/m² 12-hourly iv push days 1-10
    6-thioguanine 100 mg/m² 12-hourly orally days 1-10

ADE 10+3+5
    Daunorubicin 50 mg/m² slow iv push days 1, 3, 5
    Ara-C 100 mg/m² 12-hourly iv push days 1-10
    Etoposide (VP-16) 100mg/m² iv (1 hour infusion) days 1-5

DAT 3+8
    As DAT 3 + 10 but Ara-C and 6-Thioguanine days 1-8 only

ADE 8+3+5
    As ADE 10+3+5 but Ara-C days 1-8 only

MACE
    Amsacrine (M-amsa) 100 mg/m² iv (1 hour infusion) days 1-5
    Ara-C 200 mg/m²/day iv (continuous infusion) days 1-5
    Etoposide 100 mg/m² iv (1 hour infusion) days 1-5

MidAC
    Mitoxantrone 10 mg/m² iv (short infusion) days 1-5
    Ara-C 1.0 g/m² 12-hourly iv (2 hour infusion) days 1-3

## Results

The presenting features of the 341 evaluable patients are shown in Table 1. FAB type was reviewed centrally in 82% of patients, otherwise the referring centre classification was used. 16 children had Down syndrome.

Most (79%) of children received 4 courses of chemotherapy as per protocol. The main reason for failure to complete protocol was treatment failure and in a few cases chemotherapy was stopped because of toxicity (n = 8) or early BMT (n = 8).

### Remission Induction

The overall CR rate was 92% (315/341). The remission rate was 63% after one course and 83% after two courses. Of the 26 remission failures, seven died of haemorrhage within 5 days of entry, seven deaths were due to infection and one due to haemorrhage while hypoplastic after chemotherapy. Eleven deaths were due to resistant disease.

Induction deaths fell as the study progressed with 6% (10/174) of children dying in the first half (1988 to 1991) compared with 3%

**Table 1.** Complete remission rates by presentation features

| Parameter | No.of children | % of children | CR rate (%) | p value for difference in CR rate |
|---|---|---|---|---|
| All children | 341 | 100 | 92 | |
| Age(years) | | | | |
| <1 | 25 | 7 | 92 | 0.9 |
| 1-4 | 113 | 33 | 94 | |
| 5-9 | 87 | 26 | 90 | |
| 10-14 | 116 | 34 | 93 | |
| Type of AML | | | | |
| *de novo* | 321 | 94 | 93 | 0.06 |
| mds-AML | 18 | 5 | 89 | |
| s-AML | 2 | 1 | 50 | |
| FAB Type | | | | |
| M0 | 5 | 1 | 100 | 0.01 |
| M1 | 57 | 17 | 96 | |
| M2 | 116 | 34 | 94 | |
| M3 | 27 | 8 | 100 | |
| M4 | 49 | 14 | 84 | |
| M5 | 43 | 13 | 95 | |
| M6 | 5 | 1 | 60 | |
| M7 | 21 | 6 | 95 | |
| RAEB-t | 13 | 4 | 85 | |
| (unclassifiable/ unknown) | 5 | 1 | 60 | |
| CNS involvement | | | | |
| No | 317 | 93 | 93 | 0.4 |
| Yes | 24 | 7 | 88 | |
| White cell count(x10 /l) | | | | |
| 0-9 | 138 | 40 | 95 | 0.001 |
| 10-99 | 149 | 44 | 93 | |
| 100-199 | 30 | 9 | 93 | |
| 200+ | 22 | 6 | 73 | |
| Cytogenetic group | | | | |
| Favourable | 85 | 25 | 94 | 0.5 |
| Intermediate | 207 | 61 | 92 | |
| Adverse | 31 | 9 | 87 | |

(5/167) entered in the second half (1992 to 1995). This difference is not significant (p = 0.2).

## Outcome after CR

Twenty children, 6% of remitters, died in remission during consolidation therapy. There was a suggestion that deaths in CR during consolidation became less frequent as the study progressed: 9% (14/158) of remitters entered in the first half of the trial died

compared with 4% (6/157) of those entered in the second half (p = 0.1). Considering both induction and consolidation therapy, there was a significant (p = 0.03) reduction in toxic deaths in the second half of the study (11/167, 7%) compared with the first (24/174, 14%).

There were 124 BMTs performed in first remission, including 61 allo-BMTs and 60 A-BMTs. There were 4 non-protocol matched unrelated donor (MUD) BMTs and one HLA-mismatched parental BMT. Of the A-BMTs, 44 were randomised, 8 were elected by the clinician and 8 at the parents request. There were

11 BMT procedure related deaths in CR: 8 after allo-BMT, one after A-BMT and 2 after MUD BMT. Transplant mortality was thus 13% after allo-BMT and 2% after A-BMT (p = 0.02). Survival after BMT at 7 years was 69% (57–81%) for allo-BMT and 73% (62–84%) for A-BMT, whereas survival from day 155 after CR (median time from CR to BMT) for chemotherapy only patients was 66% (58–74%). These differences are not significant, but are not based on randomised comparisons.

The relapse rate was low with a 26% chance of relapse in the first year from CR decreasing to 11%, 3% and 2% in years 2–4 respectively, with no relapses beyond year 4. This equates to a 7 year RFS of 58% (52–64%) (Fig. 2). Of the 118 relapses, the majority (n = 99) were isolated to the bone marrow, with others in the CNS (one), skin (three), testes (one), multiple sites (11) and unknown site (three). Four of the combined relapses included the CNS, so only 4% of relapses have involved the CNS.

DFS is 52% (47–57%) at 7 years from CR. DFS was best for those achieving CR after one course at 57% (51–63%) but worse for those taking two courses to CR at 37% (26–48%) than it was for those taking more than two courses at 48% (31–65%). This suggests that children who achieve CR late do not invariably do badly.

The high CR rate and low relapse rate combine to give an overall survival from entry of 56% (51 - 61%) at 7 years. There have been only four deaths beyond 4 years out of 360 child-years at risk.

The EFS at 7 years from entry is 48% ( 43 - 53%) (Fig. 2).

## Autologous BMT

One hundred children were randomised between A-BMT versus stop. Of those achieving CR but not randomised, 127 were not available for randomisation (30 achieved CR after more than 2 courses, 19 died in CR or relapsed before randomisation, and a further 78 had a matched donor available). 100 children eligible for randomisation were not randomised because physician (n = 5) or parent (n = 8) elected A-BMT or the clinician (n = 45) or

parent (n = 42) elected to stop therapy. Thus 50% of eligible children were randomised. Of the 50 children allocated A-BMT, 44 received it. The results of this randomisation, based on intention-to-treat analyses of all 100 patients, are summarised in Table 2 and Fig.3. The reduction in relapse risk in the A-BMT arm did not translate into a significant survival benefit, due to the worse outcome after relapse.

## Allogeneic BMT

To assess the effectiveness of allo-BMT, the tissue typing status of all 332 children who achieved CR was obtained. Children were classified into 3 groups: no siblings (n = 81), no HLA matched sibling available (n = 149) and HLA matched sibling available (n = 85). HLA status was unknown in 16 children, including 4 who died or relapsed before typing could be undertaken and 2 with Down syndrome who were not considered for allo-BMT.

The outcome of children with a donor available was compared to that of children with no donor. Of the 85 children with a donor, 61 actually received an allo-BMT. Of the 230 children in the no donor or no sibling groups, 60 received an A-BMT in first CR, 165 received chemotherapy only, 4 received a MUD BMT, and one a mismatched parental BMT.

There was no significant difference in survival (p = 0.1) between those with and without donors (Fig. 4). Fewer relapses (p = 0.02) in the matched donor group were counterbalanced by procedure related deaths (p = 0.001) ( Table 3).

## Prognostic Factors

Based on the entire AML 10 population, a simple prognostic index for outcome from CR has been developed (Wheatley et al, 1995). Good risk patients are those with favourable cytogenetic abnormalities – t(8;21), t(15;17), and inv(16) – or FAB type M3. Poor risk patients are those not in CR or PR after course 1 or with adverse cytogenetic abnormalities – monosomy of chromosomes 5 or 7, del (5q), abnormalities of 3q, or complex

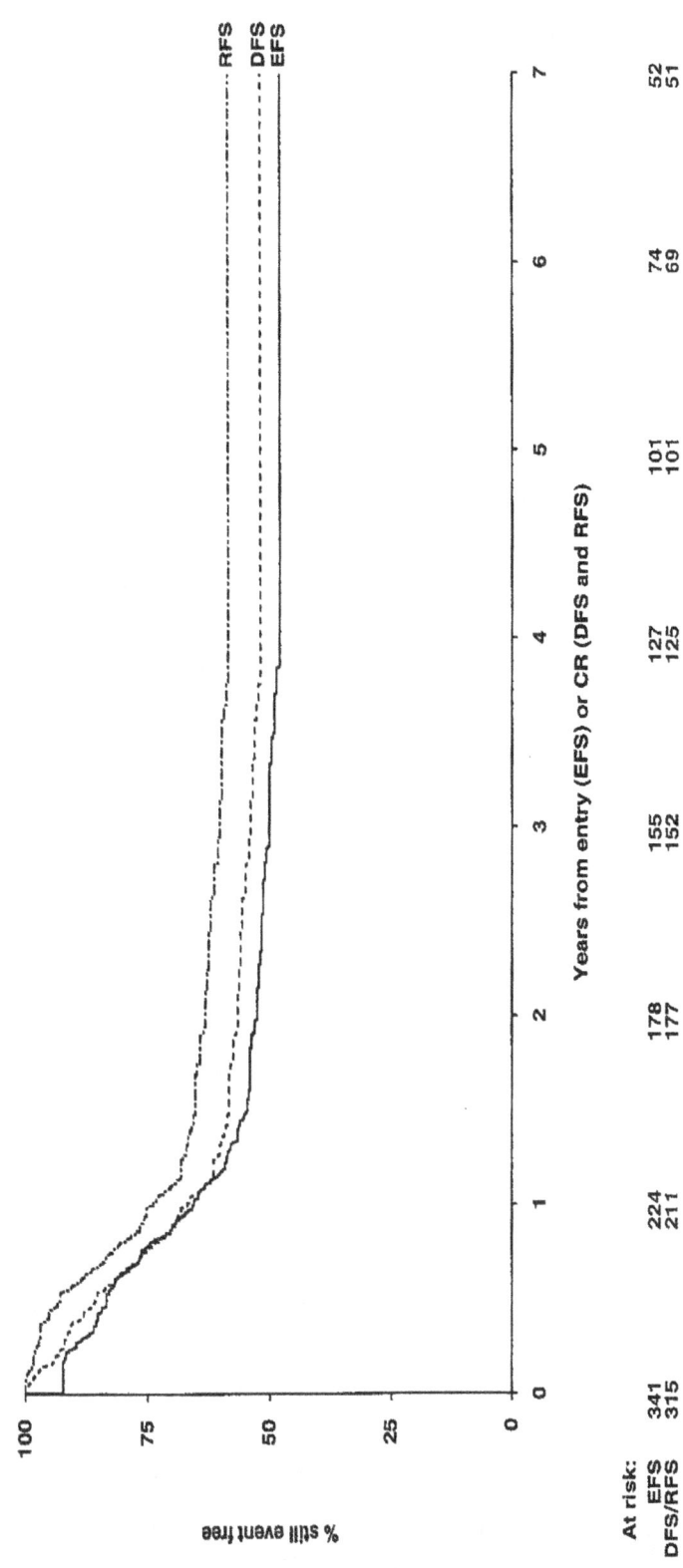

**Fig. 2.** Event-free survival, disease-free survival and relapse-free survival. At 7 years event-free (EFS) was 48%, disease-free (DFS) was 52% and relapse-free survival (RFS) was 58%.

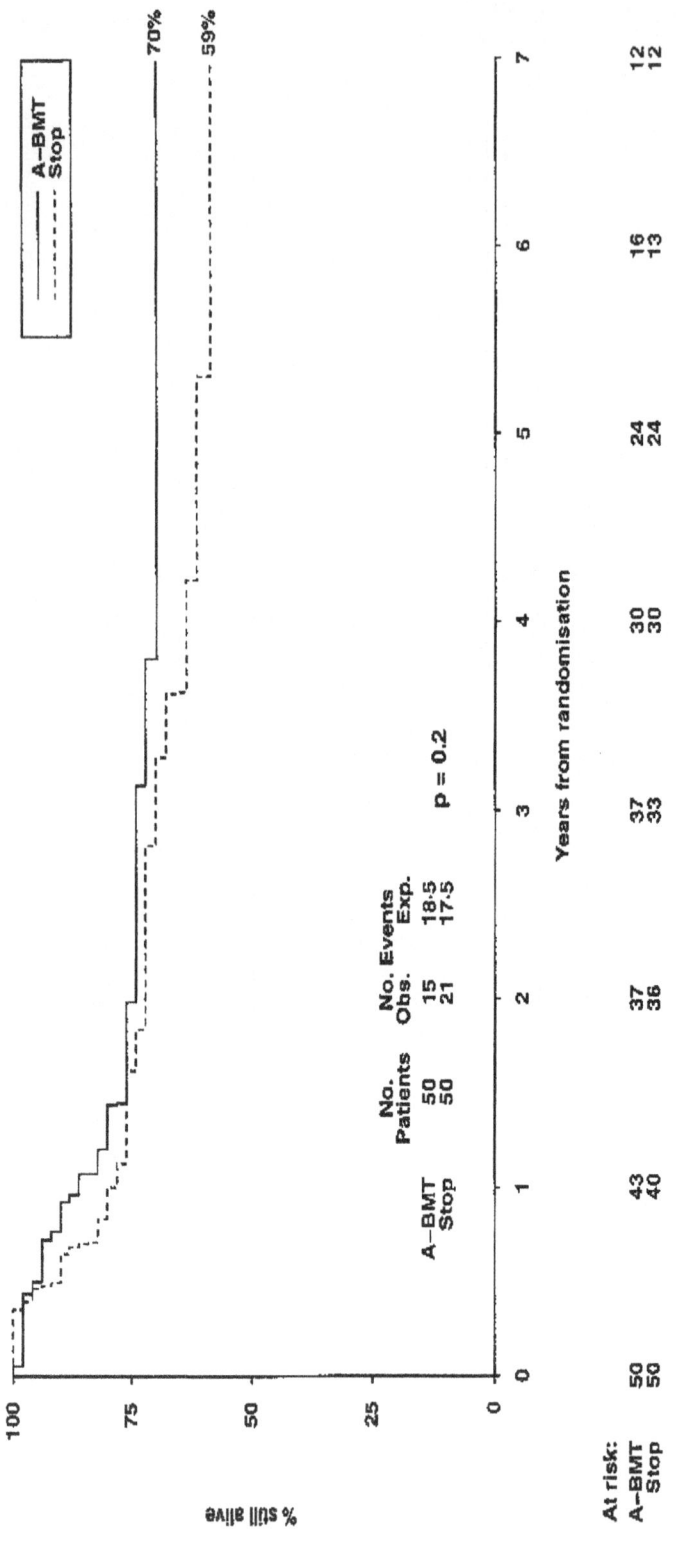

At risk:

| | 0 | 1 | 2 | 3 | 4 | 5 | 6 | 7 |
|---|---|---|---|---|---|---|---|---|
| A–BMT | 50 | 43 | 37 | 37 | 30 | 24 | 16 | 12 |
| Stop | 50 | 40 | 36 | 33 | 30 | 24 | 13 | 12 |

Fig. 3. Survival by autograft versus stop randomisation. Under numbers of events Obs. Is the observed number of deaths in each arm and Exp. is the expected number.

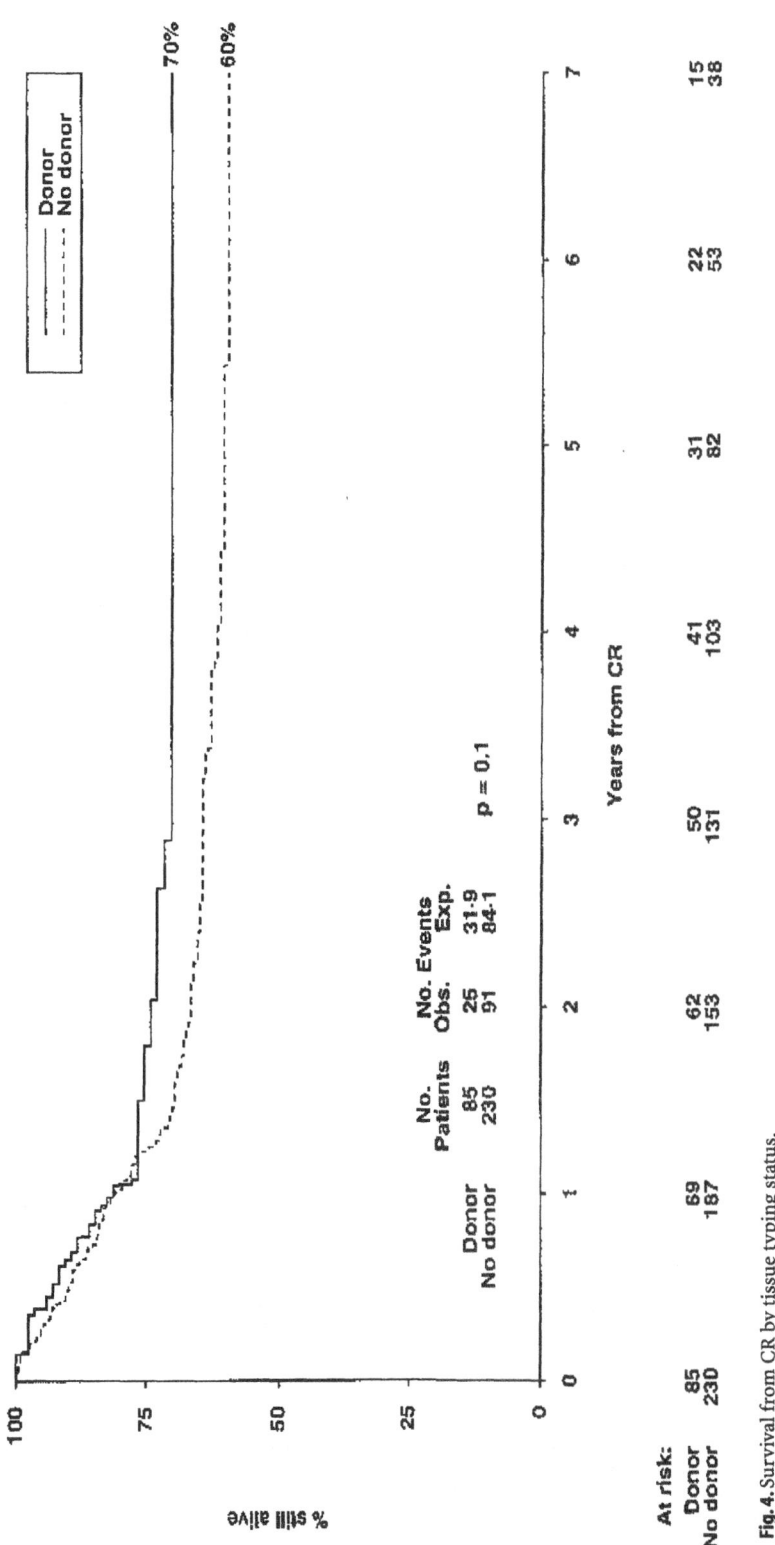

**Fig. 4.** Survival from CR by tissue typing status.

**Table 3.** Type of event by whether sibling donor available

| Matched sibling donor | No.of patients | Deaths in first CR during consolidation | Deaths in first CR after BMT | Relapses | Total events |
|---|---|---|---|---|---|
| No | 230 | 13 (6%) | 3 (1%) | 96 (42%) | 114 (50%) |
| Yes | 85 | 3 (4%) | 8 (9%) | 22 (26%) | 33 (39%) |

karyotype (more than 4 abnormalities). Standard risk patients made up the remainder. Good, standard and poor risk children constitute 28%, 52% and 20% of the population respectively. Outcome by risk group is shown in Table 4. Survival of the good- risk group is 18% better than that of the standard risk group, which in turn is 27% better than that of poor risk children.

## Discussion

The chemotherapy regimens used in MRC AML 10 appear to be very effective with the likelihood that greater than 50% of children entered into the trial are cured. When comparing the results of AML 10 with other studies it is important to remember that such non-randomised comparisons must be interpreted with great caution because of substantial differences between patients entered into the various studies. It is better to concentrate on the incontrovertible end point of survival. Table 5 summarises results from some of the larger trial groups.

The intensity of chemotherapy in AML 10 was greater than that used by most other groups, both in terms of duration, total dosage and number of courses given. This increased total therapy may be the main reason for the superior outcome seen in AML 10. This theory that more therapy may be beneficial is being tested in the current AML 12 trial where children are randomised between four versus five courses with the addition of high dose Ara-C and Asparaginase. At three years follow-up, the overall survival in AML 12 is 74% which compares favourably with AML 10 (59%) at the same time point.

In AML 10 the median time to completion of chemotherapy was relatively short at 19

**Table 4.** Outcome from CR by risk group.

| Endpoint | Risk group Good (n = 89) | Standard (n = 165) | Poor (n = 62) | p value |
|---|---|---|---|---|
| Deaths in first CR (%) | 9 | 12 | 10 | 0.5 |
| RFS (% at 7 years) | 65 | 62 | 36 | <0.0001 |
| DFS (% at 7 years) | 59 | 54 | 32 | 0.0001 |
| Survival from relapse (% at 3 tears) | 61 | 17 | 0 | <0.0001 |
| Survival from CR (% at 7 years) | 78 | 60 | 33 | <0.0001 |

**Table 5.** Comparison of the results of MRC AML 10 with other paediatric AML studies.

| Group/study | No.of patients | CR rate (%) | DFS %(time) | EFS %(time) | Survival %(time) |
|---|---|---|---|---|---|
| MRC AML10 | 341 | 92 | 53(5yr) | 49(5yr) | 59(5yr) |
| BFM-87 (Creutzig et al, 1996) | 307 | 75 | 54(5yr) | 43(5yr) | – |
| EORTC (Behar et al, 1996) | 108 | 77 | 52(5yr) | 41(3yr) | 56(3yr) |
| AIEOP 87 (Amadori et al, 1993) | 161 | 79 | 31(5yr) | 25(5yr) | 42(5yr) |
| POG-8821 (Ravindranath et al, 1996) | 649 | 85 | – | 34(3yr) | 42(3yr) |
| CCG-2891 (Woods et al, 1996) | 589 | 74 | 46(3yr) | 35(3yr) | 45(3yr) |
| NOPHO-88 (Lie et al, 1996) | 118 | 85 | 56(5yr) | 42(5yr) | – |

weeks. In children without CNS disease at presentation, craniospinal prophylaxis consisted of 4 separate intrathecal doses of triple therapy with each course of systemic therapy. The CNS relapse rate is very low with only one isolated and four combined CNS relapses representing only 4% of all relapses.

The number of deaths in CR during consolidation in AML 10 is relatively high at 6%, presumably related to the intensity of chemotherapy. It may be that a small excess of deaths in CR is an unavoidable consequence of intensive therapy which is more than counterbalanced by improved long-term survival. Continuing improvements in supportive care will hopefully reduce further the number of deaths in CR.

Although the randomised comparison in AML 10 between A-BMT and stopping therapy has shown that A-BMT reduces the risk of relapse, there is no evidence that this results in a substantial long term survival advantage. This appears to be related to inferior survival from relapse after BMT. With only 50 children in each arm of AML 10, it is difficult to come to any reliable conclusions as to the value of A-BMT. However, other randomised paediatric studies (Amadori et al, 1993; Ravindranath et al, 1996; Woods et al, 1996) have also not shown any survival benefit for A-BMT. Thus, on the randomised evidence currently available, A-BMT does not appear to have a major role as therapy for paediatric AML in first remission.

In the absence of randomised trials of allo-BMT, selection bias can be overcome if analysis is by genetic ("Mendelian") randomisation whereby patients with a matched sibling donor (most of whom receive an allo-BMT) are compared to those with no donor who cannot receive an allo-BMT. Such an analysis has been performed here and there is no significant difference in survival between patients with and without a donor. This finding in AML 10 is at odds with several other reports (Michel et al, 1992; Nesbit et al, 1994; Ravindranath et al, 1996; Woods et al, 1996) which have suggested that allo-BMT is an effective treatment for paediatric AML. However the numbers of patients in AML 10 are relatively small and the very intensive chemotherapy used prior to transplant has highly effective anti-leukaemia action, thereby reducing the potential benefit of allo-BMT. More unbiased evidence is needed to confirm or refute the place of allo-BMT in paediatric AML since this procedure would require a substantial survival benefit to justify the associated acute toxicity, long term sequelae and financial cost.

## Prognostic Factors

Prognostic factors cannot automatically be transferred from one trial to another. Nevertheless, they can assist with therapeutic decision making. Analysis of AML10 has identified a good risk group of children, with a 7-year survival of 78%, for whom any possible benefit of BMT in terms of reduced relapse is likely to be outweighed by the toxicities, both short and long term, of the procedure. There is also a small group of patients whose outcome on standard therapy is very poor. These children may constitute a group with disease that is unresponsive to any currently available therapeutic options, and in whom new therapies must be sought.

## Conclusions

It now appears that over half the children in AML 10 will be cured of their leukaemia. However, continuing improvement is still necessary. Preliminary results from AML 12 appear to suggest that this improvement may be maintained possibly with the aid of even further intensive chemotherapy. A-BMT at present seems to have little to offer and the place of allo-BMT in children is still not entirely clear. Paediatric AML is a rare disease and it may be difficult for individual trial groups to recruit sufficient patient numbers to identify reliably more effective treatments. The best way of achieving further progress may be for greater collaboration between trial groups in developing common, or parallel, protocols addressing important therapeutic questions.

## References

Amadori,S., Testi, A. M., Arico, M., Comelli, A., Giuliano, M., Madom, E., Masera, G., Rondelli, R., Zanesco, L., and Mandelli, F. (1993) Prospective comparative study of bone marrow transplantation and post remission chemotherapy for childhood acute myelogenous leukaemia. Journal of Clinical Oncology. 11, 1046-1054.

Behar, C., Suciu, S., Benoit, Y., Robert, A., Vilmer, E., Boutard, P., Bertrand, Y., Lutz, P., Ferster, A., Tokaji, E., Manel, A. M., Solbu, G., and Otten, J. (1996) Mitoxantrone containing regimen for treatment of childhood acute leukaemia (AML) and analysis of prognostic factors: results of the EORTC Children Leukaemia Cooperative Study 58872. Medical and Pediatric Oncology. 26, 173-179

Creutzig, U., Harbott, J., Sperling, C., Ritter, J., Zimmerman, M., Loffler, H., Riem, H., Schellong, G., and Ludwig, W. (1996) Clinical significance of surface antigen expression in children with acute myeloid leukaemia: results of Study AML-BFM-87. Blood. 86, 3097-3108.

Lie, O. E., Jonmundsson, G., Mellander, L., Siimes, M. A., Yssing, M., and Gustafsson, G. (1996) A population bases study of 272 children with acute myeloid leukaemia treated on two consecutive protocols with different intensity: best outcome in girls, infants and children with Down's syndrome. British Journal of Haematology. 94, 82-88.

Michel, G., Gluckman, E., Blaise, D., Esperou-Bourdeau, H., Vermant, J. P., Kuentz, M., Bordigoni, P., Milpied, N., Rubie, H., and Thuret, I. (1992) Improvement in outcome for children receiving allogeneic bone marrow transplantation in first remission of acute myeloid leukaemia: a report from the Groupe d'Etude des Greffes de Moelle Osseuse. Journal of Clinical Oncology. 10, 1865-1869.

Nesbit, M.E., Buckley, J. D., Feig, S. A., Anderson, J. R., Lampkin, B., Bernstein, I. D., Kim, T. H., Piomelli, S.,

Kersey, J. H., Coccia, P. E. (1994) Chemotherapy for induction of remission of childhood acute myelogenous leukaemia followed by marrow transplantation or multiagent chemotherapy: a report from the Childrens Cancer group. Journal of Clinical Oncology. 12, 127-135.

Ravindranath, Y., Yeager, A. M., Chang, M. N., Steuber, C. P., Krischer, J., Graham Pole, J., Carroll, A., Inoue, S., Camitta, B., and Weinstein, H. J. (1996) Autologous bone marrow transplantation versus intensive consolidation chemotherapy for acute myeloid leukaemia in childhood. New England Journal of Medicine. 334, 1428-1434.

Wheatley, K., Burnett, A., Goldstone, A., Hann, I., Stevens, R. F., Rees, J., and Gray, R. (1995) A simple, robust and highly predictive prognostic index for the determination of risk directed therapy in acute myeloid leukaemia (AML) derived from the United Kingdom Medical Research Council (MRC) AML 10 trial. Blood, 86, (Suppl. 1), 598a (Abstract 2381).

Woods, W. G., Kobrinsky, N., Buckley, J. D., Lee, J. W., Sanders, J., Neuborf, S., Gold, S., Barnard, D. R., DeSwarte, J., Dusenbery, K., Kalousek, D., Arthur, D. c., and Lange, B. J. (1996) Timed-sequential induction therapy improves postremission outcome in acute myeloid leukaemia: a report from the children's cancer group. Blood, 87, 4979-4989.

Woods, W. G., Neudorf, S., Gold, S., Sanders, J., Kobrinsky, D., Barnard, J., DeSwarte, D., Lange, A., and Lange, B. J. (1996) Aggressive post-remission (REM) chemotherapy is better than autologous bone marrow transplantation (BMT) and allogeneic BMT is superior to both in children with acute myeloid leukaemia (AML). Proceedings of the American Society of Clinical Oncology, 15, 368 (Abstract 1091).

# Preliminary Results of a Multicentre Therapy Study for the Treatment of Children and Adolescents with AML in the Ukraine

O. Ryzhak [1], S. Donska [1], I. Korenkova [2], E. Karamanesht [2], R. Polyschuk [3], and V. Usatchenko [4]

## Introduction

Modern intensified chemotherapeutical protocols for the treatment of children and adolescents with AML offered the possibility to achieve cure in 50-60% of patients [Ritter J., 1993]. Modern multicentre trials demonstrated a remission rate of 80-90% and a 4-5-year EFS of 47-50% [Creutzig U. et al., 1999; Schaison J. et al, 1999, Stevens R.F. et al., 1999]. At the same time, only 10 years ago, in the former Soviet Union less than 10% of children with ALL achieved long-term remission,and practically none of the children and adolescents with AML had a chance to survive.

The Cooperative Ukrainian Group for treating Pediatric Leukemias and Lymphomas (PGLLU), after introducing modern chemotherapy for ALL and gaining some experience, have organized a therapy study for patients with de novo AML.

The therapy protocol of the study AML-PGLLU-95/97 (with an initial pilot phase from Dec.1995 to June 1997 followed by the main phase) is a modification of the protocol AML-BFM-93. (Creutzig,U. et al., 1999). The main objective of the modifications was to decrease the general toxicity of the therapy without compromising the outcome in patients of the different prognostic groups.

## Therapy Protocol

1. Patients were allocated to three risk groups instead of two in the original BFM-protocol:

SRG: identical to AML-BFM stratification;

HRG 1: patients with FAB variants M0, M1 and M2 without Auer rods, M4, M5, M6, and M7, but with $\leq$ 5% BM blasts on day 15 of 1st induction;

HRG 2: all patients with >5% of BM blasts on day 15 of 1st induction.

2. For patients of HRG 2, the original 2nd induction AME was introduced, consisting of:

AraC    100mg/$m^2$/24h as continuous 72h infusion on days 1–3
          100mg/$m^2$ every 12h as short infusion on days 4–7
Mito-    10mg/$m^2$/day on days 4–5
xanthrone
Etoposide 150mg/$m^2$/day on days 6–7

3. Etoposide was excluded from the 1st induction: AD instead of ADE.

4. Cyclophosphamide was excluded from the 2nd phase of consolidation.

5. The dose of AraC in both intensifications was reduced from 3g/$m^2$ to 1g/$m^2$.

## Patients

From 01.12.95 to 13.11.98 (35 months) 61 non-selected patients from 4 Pediatric Hematologic Centers of the Ukraine entered the study (including the pilot phase) as protocol patients.The diagnosis was made on the basis of the internationally accepted morphocyto-chemical FAB-criteria.

---

AML – Study of PGLL – Ukraine
[1] Department of Pediatric Oncology–Hematology, Regional Oncologic Dispensary, Kiev
[2] Department of Intensive Hematology, Republican Pediatric Hematologic Center, Kiev
[3] Department of Hematology, Lviv Regional Children's Hospital
[4] Department of Hematology, Krym Republican Children's Hospital, Sympheropol

**Table 1.** General Characteristics of the 61 Patients

| Age | Range | 1y-18y |
|---|---|---|
| | Median | 9y |
| Sex | Boys | 31 |
| | Girls | 30 |
| FAB-variants | M0 | 2 |
| | M1 | 8 |
| | M2 | 8 |
| | M3 | 5 |
| | M4 | 19 |
| | M5 | 13 |
| | M6 | 4 |
| | M7 | 2 |
| Risk Groups | SRG | 13 (21%) |
| | HRG 1 | 30 (49%) |
| | HRG 2 | 18 (30%) |

## Results

As of Jan. 1st ,1999, the median time of observation for our group of 61 protocol patients was 18 months (range: 1.5–35 months). 3 children (5%) died before achieving remission because of bleeding and/or infections; another 3 patients (5%) were evaluated as »nonresponders« as they had more than 5% myeloid blasts in the bone marrow even after the second induction course. 55 children (90%) achieved complete remission. Two patients died in remission due to infections, and three were »lost to follow-up«; 12 relapsed till the time of analysis, and 41 were in CCR. The probabilityof event-free survival (pEFS) at 35 months is 63% (SD=6%), (Figure 1) and of event free interval (pEFI) 75% (SD=7%).

## Discussion

Our modification of the original protocol AML-BFM-93 is aimed at adapting the intensive chemotherapy to the conditions of Ukrainian pediatric hematologic centers with their limited material resources and lack of experience in intensive AML-treatment.

3 years of experience using the adapted protocol in 4 centers showed that the propo-

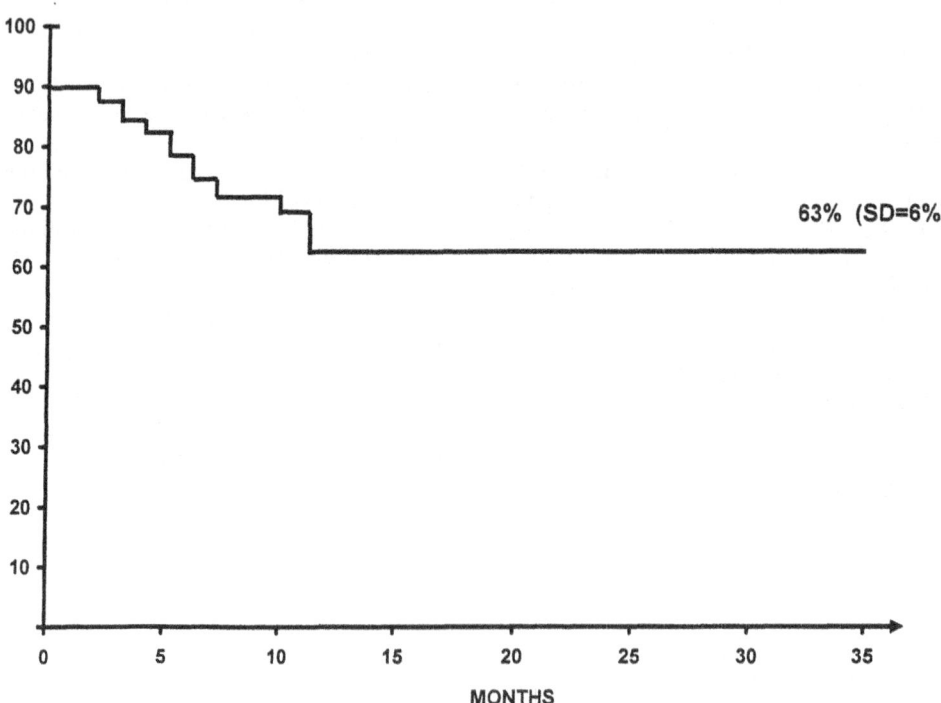

**Fig. 1.** Kaplan-Meier curve of probability of event-free survival for the total group of 61 AML-patients.

sed therapeutical strategy was appropriate. Reduced toxicity after omitting etoposide from induction I and cyclophosphamide from consolidation, and using 1 g/m$^2$ instead of 3 g/m$^2$ AraC in intensification resulted in a rather low level of therapy-associated morbidity and mortality.

Stratifying patients into three risk groups rather than two, and introducing the original second Induction AME for patients in HRG 2 led to a higher CR rate: 67.5% of all patients achieved remission after the 1$^{st}$ induction and another 22.5% after the 2$^{nd}$ induction.

*Acknowledgement.* We are very thankful to Professor Dr. med. Günther Schellong, Professor Dr. med. Ursula Creutzig and Professor Dr. med. Jörg Ritter for help in working out the therapy protocol and for permanent consultation and advice.

We would like to thank our donors, Dr. med. Martin Friedrichs, Manfred Bäurle, Irmgard Buhr and Dr. med. Friedeman Snigula for unfailing support supplying drugs and material for treating patients with AML.

## References

1. Creutzig U, Ritter J (1999) AML-BFM 93: Risk –adapted therapy and randomization in children with AML: Preliminary results. Ann Hematol 78 (Suppl II): S 12.
2. Ritter J (1993) Therapie der akuten myeloischen Leukämien (AML) bei Kindern und Jugendlichen. Onkologie Forum 3 (1): 2-8.
3. Schaison J, Aurignon A (1999) Acute myeloblastic leukemia in children. Results of the French LAME 98/91 Protocol. Ann Hematol 78 (Suppl II): S 12.
4. Stevens R.F., Hann I.M. (1999) Marked improvements in outcome with chemotherapy alone in pediatric acute myeloid leukemia: Results of the MRC 10$^{th}$ AML trial. Ann Hematol 78 (Suppl II): S 12.

# IDA-FLAG – An Effective Reinduction Therapy for Poor Prognosis AML of Childhood – Report of a Multicenter Phase II Trial

G. Fleischhack[1], C. Hassan[1], N. Graf[2], G. Mann[3] and U.Bode[1]

## Summary

The prognosis of refractory, relapsed or secondary AML is poor and effective reinduction regimens are rare. Allogeneic or autologous bone marrow transplantation (BMT or ABMT) offers a chance for long-term survival in these cases. Thus, a phase II trial of a combination therapy with fludarabine, HD-ARA-C, idarubicin and G-CSF was designed to study the feasibility and efficacy in the treatment of poor prognosis AML of childhood as a possible option prior to BMT or ABMT.

Thirty-six patients aged 1.2 to 17.5 years with refractory (n=3), relapsed (first relapse: n=29, second relapse: n=3) or secondary (n=1) AML were treated with the IDA-FLAG regimen. This regimen includes idarubicin (day 2-4, 12 mg/m_.d), fludarabine (day 1-4, 30 mg/m_.d), cytarabine (day 1-4, 2000 mg/m_.d) and G-CSF (day 0 up to ANC > 1000/μl, 400 μg/m_.d). Patients aged 1,2 to 17,5 years (median 7,7 years) were classified as having AML (n=33), a biphenotypical leukemia (n=1) and a MDS in leukemic transformation (n=2). They received a total of 55 courses of IDA-FLAG and/or FLAG.

24 of 36 patients (67 %) achieved a complete remission (CR) with a median duration of 11 months (1 to 51 months), two patients showed a partial remission and 10 were nonresponders. 17 patients in CR were transplanted by bone marrow or PBSC (4 autologous, 13 allogeneic). Overall, 14 patients (12 following BMT or PBSCT) are in continuous complete remission with a median duration of 20,2 months (1 to 51 months). The main toxicities were both a marked neutropenia and thrombocytopenia and severe pneumonia (7 of 36 patients).

IDA-FLAG is an efficient reinduction therapy of resistent and intensively pretreated AML with a moderate toxicity. The induction rate is dependent on both duration of first remission and futile previous therapies. The second CR lasted longer than the first one in more than half of patients. BMT as consolidation therapy has to follow in order to achieve long-term remissions.

## Introduction

In pediatric patients with newly diagnosed acute myelogenous leukemia (AML) complete remissions were reported in 70 % to 85 % of patients in clinical studies of the late 1970s and the 1980s. An intensive postremission therapy with or without maintenance therapy led to 35% to 55% longterm survival (Weinstein et al, 1992; Ritter et al, 1992; Grier et al, 1992; Wells et al, 1994b; Hurwitz et al, 1995; Behar et al, 1996; Hann et al, 1997). 15 to 20 percent of patients are refractory to firstline induction therapy and one fourth to one third of patients will relapse mostly within 12 months after achieving CR (Ritter et al, 1992; Hurwitz et al, 1995; Behar et al, 1996; Hann et al, 1997). The prognosis of refractory, relapsed or secondary AML is poor and effective reinduction regimens are rare. Allogeneic or autologous bone marrow transplantation (BMT or ABMT) offers a chance for longterm survival in cases of poor prognosis AML (Dini et al, 1996; Gale et al, 1996). Thus, the development of newer therapeutic strategies

---

[1] Department of Pediatric Haematology/Oncology of University Bonn, Germany
[2] Department of Pediatric Haematology/Oncology of University Homburg/Saar, Germany
[3] Department of Pediatric Haematology/Oncology of St. Anna Kinderspital Wien, Austria

as reinduction therapy prior to BMT or ABMT are needed.

In different leukemic models a synergistic activity between the new cytostatic drug fludarabine and cytarabine, anthracyclines and G-CSF could be documented regarding the inhibition of several cellular pathways in DNA synthesis, DNA repair and RNA synthesis and the induction of apoptosis (Rayappa & McCulloch, 1993; Gandhi et al, 1993a; Plunkett et al, 1993; Tosi et al, 1994; Loughlin et al, 1996). These were the rationales to initiate several trials of combination therapies of fludarabine, HD-ARA-C with or without G-CSF and with or without anthracyclines in the treatment of relapsed, refractory, secondary and finally de novo AML (Estey et al, 1993; Estey et al, 1994; Visani et al, 1994; Huhmann et al, 1996; Clavio et al, 1996; Leahey et al, 1997; Dinndorf et al, 1997).

On the basis of these pharmacokinetical and clinical studies and of the results of our pilot study (Fleischhack et al, 1996) a phase II trial of a combination therapy with fludarabine, HD-ARA-C, idarubicin and G-CSF was designed to study the feasibility and efficacy in the treatment of poor prognosis AML in childhood as a possible option prior to BMT or ABMT.

## Patients and Methods

### Patient eligibility

The study was designed as an open cooperative multicenter investigation and was started in February 1994. The histological diagnosis was confirmed in all patients by bone marrow aspiration. Patients with refractory, relapsed or secondary AML were eligible. Excluded were patients showing preexisting severe life-threatening organ insufficiencies (renal, cardiac, pulmonary or hepatic failure) or infections (septic shock or multiorgan failure, WHO scale 4).

### Study conduct

The study was conducted in accordance with the updated declaration of Helsinki and approved by the local ethic committee of the University Bonn. Prior to enrollment in the study all patients' parents and/or the patients, respectively, were informed about the investigational character of the study, the potential risks of this regimen as well as the poor prognosis of relapsed, refractory or secondary AML and gave their consent to treatment. A patient insurance was in effect. Regulatory approval was given by the participating institutions of Germany and Austria. The data of the patients were collected and documented in a database at the University Bonn.

### Patients characteristics

In the study between January 1994 and December 1998 36 patients were entered from 13 departments of pediatric haematology/oncology in Germany and Austria. Patients baseline characteristics at study entry are listed in Table 1. Of the 36 patients aged 1,2 to 17,5 years (median = 7,7 years) 29 had a first

**Table 1.** Patient characteristics

| Characteristics | n / range |
|---|---|
| n | 36 |
| age | 1·2 to 17·5 years (median 7·7 years) |
| sex (female/male) | 13/23 |
| FAB type/morphological classification | |
| – M1 | 4 |
| – M2 | 6 |
| – M4 | 9 |
| – M5 | 11 |
| – M6 | 1 |
| – M7 | 2 |
| – biphenotypic leukemia | 1 |
| – MDS (CMML, RAEBt) | 2 |
| Cytogenetics | |
| – evaluable | 27/36 |
| – abnormalities | 18/27 |
| Disease stage | |
| – refractory | 3 |
| – relapse first | 30 |
| second | 3 |
| – secondary | 1 |
| – CNS involvement | 5 |
| Duration | |
| first remission | 1 to 39 months (median 8 months) |
| ≤ 6 months | n = 14 |
| > 6 ; 18 months ≤ | n = 14 |
| > 18 months | n = 5 |
| second remission | n = 3 (2-3 months) |

relapse, three patients had a second relapse, one patient had a secondary AML and three patients had a refractory AML. Besides bone marrow infiltration 5 patients also had CNS involvement. Cytogenetic analysis performed on pretreatment bone marrow samples showed abnormalities in 17 of 27 patients but was not included in statistical evaluation because of limited data.

The relapses had occurred 1 to 39 months (median = 8 months) after achieving a first complete remission. In three patients with a second relapse the relapses occurred 2 to 3 months after achieving second complete remission. Most of the patients had a very early relapse (duration of first or second remission was 6 months or shorter; n = 14) or an early relapse (duration of first remission was 6 to 18 months; n = 14). The duration between the initial diagnosis and the diagnosis of first relapse was less than 12 months in 21 of 36 patients and less than 18 months in 30 of 36 patients.

35 of 36 patients had received firstline treatment polychemotherapy regimens according to the AML-BFM-studies (AML-BFM-87-study: n = 4, AML-BFM-93-study: n = 31) (Ritter et al, 1992; Ritter et al, 1993). One patient had a secondary AML 17 months after completion of treatment for a germ cell tumor (MAKEI-89-study) (Göbel et al, 1993). 12 of 36 patients received other relapse chemotherapies prior to IDA-FLAG or FLAG regimen. These were mostly combination therapies of HD-ARA-C with VP16 or mitoxantrone (n=12) (Stahnke et al, 1992) (Table 2). Patients had received a cumulative equivalent dose of anthracyclines of 100 to 680 mg/m$^2$ (median = 400 mg/m$^2$) prior to the IDA-FLAG regimen and showed no clinical and echocardiographic evidence of cardiomyopathy.

**Table 2.** Cytostatic pretreatment.

|  | study | n |
|---|---|---|
| first-line treatment | AML-BFM-87 | 4 |
|  | AML-BFM-93 SR/HR | 9/22 |
|  | *MAKEI-89* | 1 |
| relapse treatment (n=12) | AML-REZ-BFM-93 (MXN/VP16, HD-ARA-C/MXN) | 8 |
|  | AML-REZ-BFM-97 | 3 |
|  | HD-ARA-C/MXN | 4 |
|  | HD-ARA-C/VP16 | 2 |
|  | Ifosfamide/VP16 | 1 |
|  | ARA-C/IDA | 1 |

Abbreviations: MXN, mitoxantron; HD-ARA-C, high dose cytarabine; ARA-C, cytarabine; VP16, etoposide; IDA, idarubicin

## Treatment

Treatment with IDA-FLAG involved the application of (1) 30 mg/m$^2$/d of fludarabine by a 30 minutes intravenous infusion daily for four consecutive days from day 1 to day 4, (2) 2000 mg/m$^2$/d of cytarabine by three hours intravenous infusion daily for four consecutive days from day 1 to day 4 starting four hours after the beginning of fludarabine, (3) 12 mg/m$^2$ of idarubicin by an one hour intravenous infusion daily for three consecutive days from day 2 to day 4 starting one hour prior to cytarabine and (4) 400 µg/m$^2$ of G-CSF subcutaneously daily from day 0 to the day of absolute neutrophil count (ANC) of more than 1,0 x 10$^9$/l (Table 3). The FLAG course was a combination chemotherapy of fludarabine, cytarabine and G-CSF as in the IDA-FLAG regimen but without idarubicin.

16 patients received only one IDA-FLAG course and two patients only one FLAG course. 18 patients were treated with a second

**Table 3.** Treatment scheme of the IDA-FLAG regimen.

| Medicament |  | day 0 | day 1 | day 2 | day 3 | day 4 |
|---|---|---|---|---|---|---|
| G-CSF | 400 µg/m$^2$, s.c. up to ANC > 1,0x10$^9$/µl | ▽ | ▽ | ▽ | ▽ | ▽ |
| Fludarabine | 30 mg/m$^2$, i.v. 30 min |  | ▽ | ▽ | ▽ | ▽ |
| ARA-C | 2000 mg/m$^2$, i.v. 3 h 4 h after Fludarabine |  | ▽ | ▽ | ▽ | ▽ |
| Idarubicin | 12 mg/m_, i.v. 1 h after Fludarabine |  |  | ▽ | ▽ | ▽ |

FLAG ... IDA-FLAG without idarubicin

or a third course as [IDA-FLAG]-[IDA-FLAG] in 3 patients, as [IDA-FLAG]-[FLAG] in 14 patients and as [IDA-FLAG]-[FLAG]-[FLAG] in one patient. The second or third course was only started if patients had achieved a second complete (CR) or partial (PR) remission and the ANC was more than $1,0 \times 10^9/l$.

Prophylactic or therapeutic CNS therapy was administered in 20 of 36 patients in an age-dependent dose. 5 patients received an intrathecal monotherapy with cytarabine and 15 patients were treated with an intrathecal triple therapy consisting of cytarabine, methotrexate and prednisolon on day 0 or day 1 of each course.

### Response evaluation and statistical methods

Antileukemic response, i.e. the definition of complete remission (CR), partial remission (PR) and nonresponse (NR), and the treatment failure were classified according to previously published guidelines (Fleischhack et al. 1998).

CR duration was calculated from the initial date of documented response to relapse, to death by any cause or to the last day of follow-up (31.12.1998) and overall survival duration from the first day of treatment with IDA-FLAG/FLAG to death or to the last day of follow-up.

The haematological toxicity was evaluated for all patients who achieved CR or PR and was documented as duration of neutropenia less than $0,5 \times 10^9/l$, duration of leukopenia less than $1,0 \times 10^9/l$ and as duration of thrombocytopenia less than $30 \times 10^9/l$. Nonhaematological toxicities were stated according to the World Health Organization (WHO) grading system and were tabulated for all patients (World Health Organization, 1979).

The data of this study were analyzed using descriptive statistics for the evaluation of pretreatment and treatment patient characteristics as well as life table analysis according to Kaplan Meyer and log rank tests for the evaluation of the event free survival (EFS) and the overall survival (OS) (Bühl and Zöfel 1994).

## Discussion

Patients refractory to firstline treatment as well as early relapsed patients and patients with a secondary AML are poor responders to classical salvage reinduction therapy (Kantarjian et al, 1993; Stahnke et al, 1992). At the beginning of the 1990s several trials were based on the experience that HD-ARA-C was one of the most effective drugs in reinduction therapy of poor prognosis AML and that fludarabine administered prior to ARA-C enhances the ARA-CTP accumulation in the blast cells and acts synergistically with ARA-C, anthracyclines and G-CSF (Avramis et al, 1990; Gandhi et al, 1993b; Rayappa & McCulloch, 1993; Tosi et al, 1994; Loughlin et al, 1996). Combination therapies of fludarabine and HD-ARA-C with or without G-CSF tested in relapsed and refractory AML of adults produced CR rates of 50 % to 66 % (Estey et al, 1994; Visani et al, 1994; Clavio et al, 1996). Using idarubicin in combination with continuous infusion of fludarabine and cytarabine CR rates of 67 % (n=15) and 80 % (n=10) were reported in pediatric patients with a refractory or relapsed AML (Leahey et al, 1997; Dinndorf et al, 1997). In our study, with the IDA-FLAG regimen as single course reinduction treatment, a CR rate of 67 % was documented although the firstline or previous reinduction therapy according to the BFM protocols already contained idarubicin in 42 % of patients and HD-ARA-C/mitoxantrone in 75 % of patients.

Previous studies documented a relationship between the duration of first remission and both the rate and the duration of second CR. First remission duration longer than 18 months is related with a higher CR rate and a more favourable outcome of relapsed AML in adults and children. In contrast, both rate and duration of second CR is poor in patients with refractory or very early relapsed (within 6 months) leukemia (Kantarjian et al, 1988; Keating et al, 1989; Hiddemann et al, 1990; Archimbaud et al, 1995). However, the IDA-FLAG regimen achieved a CR with a duration of 1 to 34 months (median 12 months) in 9 of 17 patients with refractory AML or with very early relapses. 4 of them are alive in CCR, three after BMT or PBSCT. Despite an apparently higher response rate in patients with early and late relapses in our series no significant differences could be documented, probably because of limited numbers. Overall, the median duration of second CR was longer than of the first one (11 versus 8,5 months) for all responders.

In our study previous futile relapse therapy was a poor prognostic factor. One third of patients (12 of 36) were treated prior to the IDA-FLAG regimen with a futile relapse therapy, predominantly according to BFM protocols. Five of them achieved a CR following the IDA-FLAG regimen but only one is still alive.

In the absence of a postremission therapy most of patients will relapse again within the next 12 months after achieving a second CR. Thus, allogeneic or autologous BMT or PBSCT is considered as a therapeutic option (Hurwitz et al, 1995; Gale et al, 1996; Dini et al, 1996). The comparison of the different postinduction approaches in our study showed, as well, a significant better outcome for patients who received a BMT or PBSCT as consolidation therapy. Overall, 14 of 36 patients are in CCR. However, only 2 of 17 patients with conventional postremission consolidation and maintenance therapy are still in CCR.

The main toxicity of the IDA-FLAG regimen was a longterm myelosuppression associated with a high incidence of infections, predominantly bacteremia and pneumonia. As causes for the high rate of pulmonary infections a toxic injury of the lung epithelial cells by the cytostatic drugs and the longterm neutropenia involving a risk for fungal infection may be discussed (Anderlini et al, 1996). The neutropenia of the FLAG courses was clearly shorter than for the IDA-FLAG courses and was associated with a lower infection rate. A second IDA-FLAG course given in 3 patients seems to be more toxic with a prolonged myelosuppression and led to one toxic death. A relationship between the pretreatment residual haematopoiesis and the time of haematopoietic recovery after the IDA-FLAG could not be detected and needs further evaluation in a larger number of patients. The reinduction/consolidation regimen [IDA-FLAG]-[FLAG] was tolerated well and the advised option in the later phase of the trial. The other side effects were mild and reversible, but no severe neurotoxicity or hemolytic anemia, as reported in previous studies, were observed (Kornblau et al, 1993; Di Raimondo et al, 1993). Persistent T-cell depletion led to a pulmonary tuberculosis in one patient. Purine analogues as fludarabine or cladribine produce long-term T-helper-cell depletion involving a high risk of opportunistic infections (Goodman et al, 1996). Thus a longterm antimicrobial prophylaxis following the IDA-FLAG regimen was given and is essential.

Based on our data, [IDA-FLAG]-[FLAG] as double reinduction course is an efficient relapse therapy of resistant and intensively pretreated AML. Allogeneic or autologous BMT/PBSCT has to follow in order to achieve longterm remissions. With regard to the unfavourable prognosis of refractory or relapsed AML of childhood the toxicity of the IDA-FLAG reinduction regimen is acceptable. Further evaluation in a phase III trial is needed to determine the efficacy and toxicity in comparison to other reinduction therapies, especially such contaning high-dose ARA-C.

## Results

35 of 36 patients entering the study received the planned dose of IDA-FLAG or FLAG courses without dose reduction. One course of IDA-FLAG had to be interrupted on day 3 due to a progressive respiratory failure. Two patients considered at risk for cardiomyopathy received only one FLAG course without further anthracyclines as induction therapy.

### Treatment response

All 36 patients were evaluable for response (Table 4). 24 of 36 patients (67%) achieved a CR, two patients showed a PR and 10 patients were nonresponders. Using IDA-FLAG as induction therapy 24 of 34 patients (71%) achieved a CR. Both patients who were treated with only one FLAG course were nonresponders.

The complete remission rate showed a correlation with the duration of first remission and with futile previous relapse therapy. 9 of 17 patients (53%) with a refractory disease or a very early relapse (duration of first CR ≤ 6

**Table 4.** Response rates of the IDA-FLAG regimen.

| All | CR 24/36 | CCR+ 14/36 | OS 16/36 |
|---|---|---|---|
| First remission | | | |
| - ≤ 6 m | 9/17 | 5/17 | 6/17 |
| - ≥ 6 m; 18 m≤ | 10/14 | 5/14 | 6/14 |
| - ≥ 18 m | 5/5 | 4/5 | 4/5 |
| Relapse within 12 months after diagnosis* | | | |
| - yes | 13/21 | 5/21 | 6/21 |
| - no | 11/15 | 9/15 | 10/15 |
| Previous futile relapse therapy* | | | |
| - yes | 5/12 | 1/12 | 3/12 |
| - no | 19/24 | 13/24 | 13/24 |
| BMT/PBSCT* | | | |
| - yes | 17/19 | 12/19 | 13/19 |
| - no | 7/17 | 2/17 | 3/17 |

\* Mann Whitney U-test, significant difference, p = 0,005
+ Two CCR were achieved following BMT.

months), 10 of 14 patients (71%) with an early relapse (duration of first CR > 6 months and ≤ 18 months) and 5 of 5 patients (100%) with a late relapse (duration of first CR > 18 months) achieved a CR. Patients with resistant disease defined as induction failure of firstline treatment or relapse within 12 months after diagnosis of AML achieved a CR in 13 of 21 patients (62 %). Of the three patients with a second relapse prior to IDA-FLAG regimen one was a nonresponder and two showed a short third CR for 1 and 7 month. 5 of 12 patients in which a previous relapse therapy had failed went into a second or third CR by IDA-FLAG. However, only one of them is still alive in continuous complete remission (CCR).

Most of patients who achieved a second CR with an IDA-FLAG course as first reinduc-

tion therapy were treated with a second (n=17) or third (n=1) course as an IDA-FLAG or FLAG course or were rapidly transplanted with bone marrow (BMT) or peripheral blood stem cells (PBSCT) (n=6). Overall, 17 of 36 patients (47%) were transplanted in CR and one patient each in PR and NR following the IDA-FLAG/FLAG regimen. 4 patients got an autologous and 15 patients an allogeneic transplantation (matched unrelated donor BMT/PBSCT, n=9; matched related donor BMT, n=5; haploidentical BMT, n=1).

There was no treatment failure caused by early death. 5 patients died therapy-related. One patient died in CR by a fulminant aspergillus sepsis during aplasia following a second IDA-FLAG course and four patients died from allogeneic BMT associated complications.

### Duration of remission and survival

Duration of remission and survival following reinduction therapy with the IDA-FLAG/ FLAG regimen are shown in Table 5. In more than half of the responders to the reinduction therapy the second CR lasted longer than the first one with a median duration of 11 and 8,5 months, respectively. Overall, 14 patients are in CCR, 12 of them following BMT or PBSCT, with a median duration of 20,2 months (range 1 to 51 months). The median duration of overall survival for all 36 patients was up to the last day of follow-up (31.12.1998) 6,7 months (range 1 to 52 months).

Both, the rate of remission and the probability of EFS and OS following the IDA-FLAG regimen depended on the duration of first

**Table 5.** Duration of remission and survival following reinduction therapy with the IDA-FLAG regimen.

| Duration [months] | All patients BMT/PBSCT | | | Patients treated with | | |
|---|---|---|---|---|---|---|
| | n | median | (range) | n | median | (range) |
| First CR of responders to IDA-FLAG | 24 | 8.5 | (0–39) | 17 | 9 | (3 - 39) |
| Second CR after reinduction with | | | | | | |
| IDA-FLAG/FLAG | 24 | 11 | (1–51) | 17 | 13.5 | (1,5–51) |
| CCR | 14 | 20.25 | (1–51) | 12 | 20.25 | (1–51) |
| OS | 36 | 6.75 | (1–52) | 19 | 15 | (3,5–52) |

CR, complete remission; CCR, continuous complete remission; OS, overall survival

remission, a previous relapse therapy and the consolidation therapy by BMT/PBSCT. Life table analysis for EFS and OS demonstrates a better but not significantly different outcome of patients with a first remission duration longer than 6 months (log-rank test, $p_{EFS}$=0,1249, $p_{OS}$= 0,1582) and a significant better outcome for patients without previous relapse therapy (log-rank test, $p_{EFS}$=0,0012, $p_{OS}$=0,0035) and with consolidation therapy by BMT or PBSCT (log rank test, $p_{EFS}$=0,0014, $p_{OS}$=0,001), respectively (Figures 1 to 4).

### Haematological toxicity

After exclusion of nonresponders and of the patient who died therapy-related 32 of 37 IDA-FLAG courses and 16 of 18 FLAG courses were evaluable for haematological toxicity. All patients experienced as main toxicity bone marrow aplasia with a profound neutropenia and thrombocytopenia (Table 6). For the FLAG courses the duration of myelosuppression was clearly shorter than for the IDA-FLAG courses. For IDA-FLAG courses the median duration of
1. ANC less than 0,5 x10⁹/l was 21 days (range 14 to 70 days),
2. leukocytes less than 1,0 x 10⁹/l was 20,5 days (range 13 to 70 days) and
3. platelets less than 30 x 10⁹/l was 27,5 days (range 5 to 150 days).

The median duration of neutropenia, leukopenia and thrombocytopenia for the FLAG courses were 13 days (range 3 to 22 days), 13 days (range 0 to 22 days) and 16 days (range 2 to 31 days), respectively. G-CSF was administrated for a median time of 25,5 days (range 20 to 70 days) in the IDA-FLAG courses and of 21 days (range 6 to 34 days) in the FLAG courses. The time of haematopoietic recovery in responders was not significantly influenced by the pretreatment degree of residual normal haematopoiesis comparing patients with less than 50 percent (17 of 24 responders) and with more than 50 percent haematopoiesis (7 of 24 responders).

**Table 6.** Hematological toxicity of the IDA-FLAG/FLAG regimen.

| Number of evaluable courses | | IDA-FLAG 32/37 | | FLAG 16/18 | |
|---|---|---|---|---|---|
| Median duration (range) [days] | | | | | |
| neutropenia | < 0,5 x 10⁹/l | 21 | (14–70) | 13 | (3–22) |
| leukopenia | < 1,0 x 10⁹/l | 20,5 | (13–70) | 13 | (0–22 |
| thrombocytopenia | < 30 x 10⁹/l | 27,5 | ( 5–150) | 16 | (2–31) |
| G-CSF application | | 25,5 | (20–70) | 21 | (6–34) |

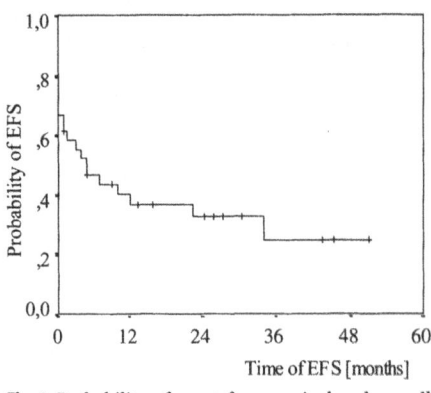 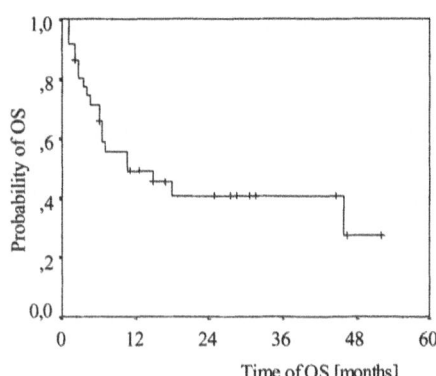

**Fig. 1.** Probability of event-free survival and overall survival of all patients
EFS: n=36 (0,25 ± 0,09, 24 events)
OS: n= 36 (0,27 ± 0,13, 20 events)

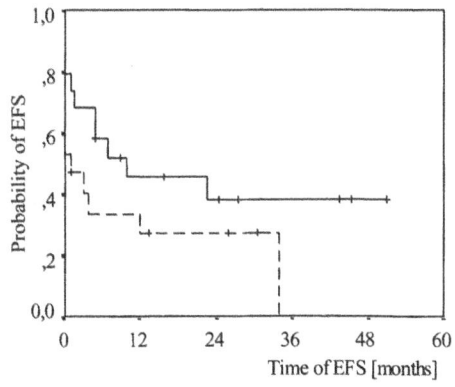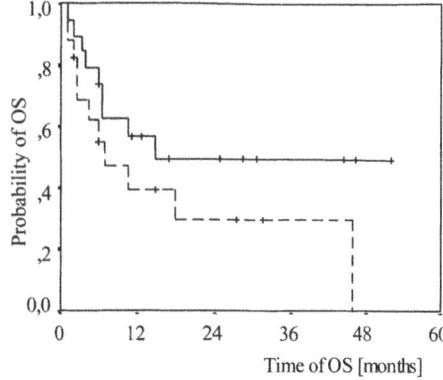

**Fig. 2.** Probability of event-free survival and overall survival dependent on duration of first remission
— > 6 months: EFS: n=19 (0,38 ± 0,12, 10 events) OS: n=19 (0,50 ± 0,12, 9 events)
--- ≤6 months: EFS: n=17 (0,00 , 12 events) OS: n= 17 (0,00 , 11 events)
    log-rank test: $p_{EFS}$=0,1249        $p_{OS}$ = 0,1582

## Nonhaematological toxicity

Nonhaematological toxicities using the WHO scale system are shown in Table 7. All patients and treatment courses (including patients with treatment failure and nonresponders) were evaluated for nonhaematological toxicities.

Side effects as nausea, haemorrhage, neurological symptoms, skin, cardiac, renal or hepatic disturbances were rare and mild. Ten patients showed a transient increase of hepatic transaminases (WHO grade I to III). Mucositis or diarrhea were observed follow-ing 20 IDA-FLAG courses and 7 FLAG courses and were more severe in patients who were treated with IDA-FLAG. The documented severe renal and cardiac complications were associated with septic or pulmonary infections. No persistent cardiomyopathy was seen at a median cumulative equivalent dose of anthracyclines of 580 mg/m² (range 280 to 860 mg/m²) after the treatment with the IDA-FLAG regimen in survivors.

The most common regimen-related toxicity were infections during bone marrow aplasia, predominantly with pulmonary involvement. Infectious complications were

**Table 7.** Nonhematological toxicity of the IDA-FLAG/FLAG regimen.

| Toxicity | | IDA-FLAG (n=35) WHO grade | | FLAG (n=18) | |
|---|---|---|---|---|---|
| | | I/II | III/IV | I/II | III/IV |
| Nausea/vomiting | | 19 | 4 | 12 | – |
| Fever | - during chemotherapy | 6 | - | 4 | – |
| | - during aplasia | 20 | 13 | 8 | 1 |
| Infection | | 18 | 15 | 7 | 2 |
| Mucositis | | 15 | 5 | 2 | – |
| Diarrhea | | 13 | 5 | 5 | – |
| Skin | - exanthema | 2 | 1 | 2 | – |
| | - alopecia | 30 | – | 13 | – |
| Renal | | – | 1 | – | – |
| Pulmonary | | 6 | 7 | – | – |
| Cardiac | | 1 | 3 | – | – |
| Hepatic | | 8 | 2 | 2 | – |
| Neurological | | 2 | – | – | – |
| Mortality | | 1 (IDA-FLAG complication) 4 (BMT complications) | | | |

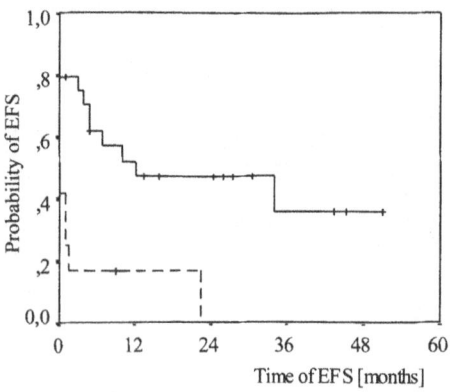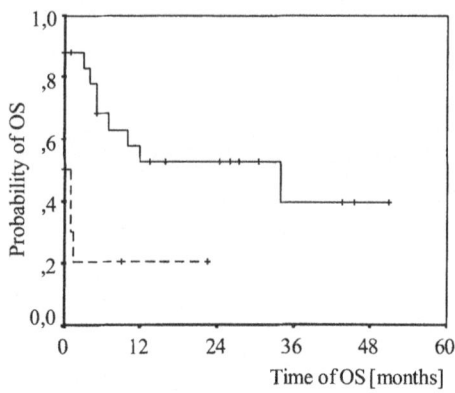

**Fig. 3.** Probability of event-free survival and overall survival dependent on futile previous relapse therapy
— no: EFS: n=24 (0,35 ± 0,13, 11 events)  OS: n= 24 (0,40 ± 0,14, 11 events)
--- yes: EFS: n=12 (0,00 , 11 events)  OS: n= 12 (0,20 ± 0,12, 9 events)
log-rank test:  $p_{EFS}$=0,0012  $p_{OS}$=0,0035

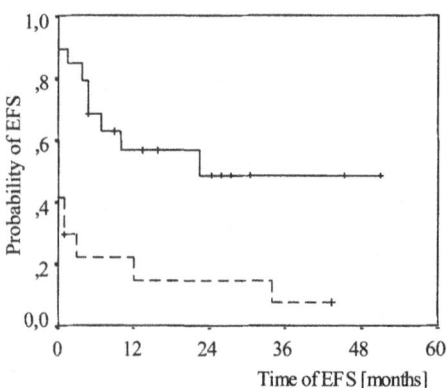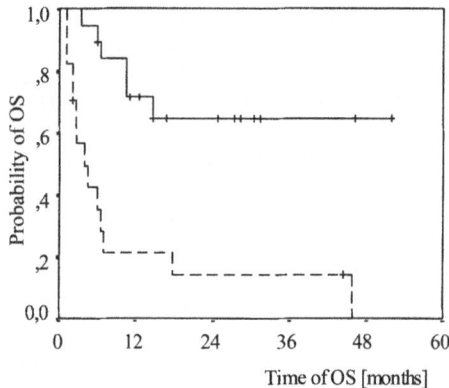

**Fig. 4.** Probability of event-free survival and overall survival dependent on consolidation therapy by BMT/PBSCT
— yes: EFS: n=19 (0,48 ± 0,12, 7 events)  OS: n= 19 (0,64 ± 0,12, 6 events)
--- no: EFS: n=17 (0,07 ± 0,07, 15 events)  OS: n= 17 (0,00 , 14 events)
log rank test:  $p_{EFS}$=0,0014  $p_{OS}$=0,001

more frequent and severe in IDA-FLAG than in FLAG courses. In 15 of 35 IDA-FLAG courses and only 2 of 18 FLAG courses clinically, radiologically or microbiologically documented severe infections were observed. 13 patients showed pulmonary involvement with fatal pneumonia in two patients, of whom one patient was a nonresponder and died from progressive disease and another patient developed a lethal aspergillus sepsis following a second IDA-FLAG course. Of the other patients with severe pneumonia three episodes were suspicious of fungal infections, too.

Microbiologically documented infections without pulmonary involvement were seen in 9 patients (4 grampositive bacteremia, 2 gramnegative bacteremia, 1 meningitis, 1 candidemia, 1 parvovirus B 19 infection). All of them were treated successfully. As a late complication one patient developed a pulmonary tuberculosis in CR 7 months after treatment with two IDA-FLAG courses.

*Acknowledgements.* We thank the following collegues entering patients in this study: S. Müller-Weihrich (München, Germany), W.

Scheurlen (Mannheim, Germany), J. Kühl (Würzburg, Germany), H. Breu (Dortmund, Germany), W. Dörffel (Berlin, Germany), W. Havers (Essen, Germany), K. Welte (Hannover, Germany), U. Göbel (Düsseldorf, Germany), J. D. Beck (Erlangen, Germany), J. Herrmann (Jena, Germany).

# References

1. Anderlini P, Luna M, Kantarjian HM, O'Brien S, Pierce S, Keating MJ, Estey EH (1996) Causes of initial remission induction failure in patients with acute myeloid leukemia and myelodysplastic syndromes. Leukemia 10: 600-608
2. Behar C, Suciu S, Benoit Y, Robert A, Vilmer E, Boutard P, Bertrand Y, Lutz P, Ferster A, Tokaji E, Manel AM, Solbu G, Otten J (1996) Mitoxantrone-containing regimen for treatment of childhood acute leukemia (AML) and analysis of prognostic factors: results of the EORTC Children Leukemia Cooperative Study 58872. Med Pediatr Oncol 26: 173-179
3. Bühl A, Zöfel B (1994) SPSS für Windows. Version 6.1.3. 1. edn. Addison-Wesley, Bonn, Paris, Reading, Mass.
4. Clavio M, Carrara P, Miglino M, Pierri I, Canepa L, Balleari E, Gatti AM, Cerri R, Celesti L, Vallebella E, Sessarego M, Patrone F, Ghio R, Damasio E, Gobbi M (1996) High efficacy of fludarabine-containing therapy (FLAG-FLANG) in poor risk acute myeloid leukemia. Haematologica 81: 513-520
5. Dini G, Cornish JM, Gadner H, Souillet G, Vossen JM, Paolucci P, Manfredini L, Miano M, Niethammer D (1996) Bone marrow transplant indications for childhood leukemias: achieving a consensus. The EBMT Pediatric Diseases Working Party. Bone Marrow Transplant 18: Suppl 2, 4-7
6. Dinndorf PA, Avramis VI, Wiersma S, Krailo MD, Liu MW, Seibel NL, Sato JK, Mosher RB, Kelleher JF, Reaman GH (1997) Phase I/II study of idarubicin given with continuous infusion fludarabine followed by continuous infusion cytarabine in children with acute leukemia: a report from the Children's Cancer Group. J Clin Oncol 15: 2780-2785
7. Di Raimondo F, Giustolisi R, Cacciola E, O'Brien S, Kantarjian H, Robertson LB, Keating MJ (1993) Autoimmune hemolytic anemia in chronic lymphocytic leukemia patients treated with fludarabine. Leuk Lymphoma 11: 63-68
8. Estey E, Thall P, Andreeff M, Beran M, Kantarjian H, O'Brien S, Escudier S, Robertson LE, Koller C, Kornblau S, Pierce S, Freireich EJ, Deisseroth A, Keating M (1994) Use of granulocyte colony-stimulating factor before, during, and after fludarabine plus cytarabine induction therapy of newly diagnosed acute myelogenous leukemia or myelodysplastic syndromes: comparison with fludarabine plus cytarabine without granulocyte colony-stimulating factor J Clin Oncol 12: 671-678
9. Fleischhack G, Graf N, Hasan C, Ackermann M, Breu H, Zernikow B, Bode U (1996) IDA-FLAG (idarubicin, fludarabine, high dosage cytarabine and G-CSF) - an effective therapy regimen in treatment of recurrent acute myelocytic leukemia in children and adolescents. Initial results of a pilot study. Klin.Pädiatr 208: 229-235
10. Fleischhack G, Hasan C, Graf N, Mann G, Bode U (1998) IADA-FLAG (idarubicin, fludarabine, cytarabine, G-CSF) an effective remission-induction therapy for poor -prognosis AML of childhood prior to allogeneic or autologous bone marrow transplantation: experiences of a phase II trial. Br J Haematol 102: 647-655
11. Gale RP, Horowitz MM, Rees, JK, Gray RG, Oken MM, Estey EH, Kim KM, Zhang MJ, Ash RC, Atkinson K, Champlin RE, Dicke KA, Gajewski JL, Goldman JM, Helbig W, Henslee Downey PS, Hinterberger W, Jacobsen N, Keating A, Klein JP, Marmont AM, Prentice HG, Reiffers J, Rimm AA, Rowlings PA, Sobocinski KA, Speck B, Wingard JR, Bortin MM (1996) Chemotherapy versus transplants for acute myelogenous leukemia in second remission. Leukemia 10: 13-19
12. Gandhi V, Estey E, Keating MJ, Plunkett W (1993) Fludarabine potentiates metabolism of cytarabine in patients with acute myelogenous leukemia during therapy. J Clin Oncol 11: 116-124
13. Goodman ER, Fiedor PS, Fein S, Athan E, Hardy MA (1996) Fludarabine phosphate: A DNA synthesis inhibitor with potent immunosuppressive activity and minimal clinical toxicity. Am Surg 62: 435-442
14. Göbel U, Bamberg M, Calaminus G, Gnekow AK, Herrmann HD, Lenard HG, Spaar HJ, Niethammer D, Kühl J, Harms D (1993) Improved prognosis of intracranial germ cell tumors by intensified therapy: results of the therapy protocol MAKEI 89. Klin Pädiatr 205: 217-224
15. Hann IM, Stevens RF, Goldstone AH, Rees JK, Wheatley K, Gray RG, Burnett AK (1997) Randomized comparison of DAT versus ADE as induction chemotherapy in children and younger adults with acute myeloid leukemia. Results of the Medical Research Council's 10th AML trial (MRC AML10). Adult and Childhood Leukaemia Working Parties of the Medical Research Council. Blood 89: 2311-2318
16. Hiddemann W, Martin WR, Sauerland CM, Heinecke A, Büchner T (1990) Definition of refractoriness against conventional chemotherapy in acute myeloid leukemia: a proposal based on the results of retreatment by thioguanine, cytosine arabinoside, and daunorubicin (TAD 9) in 150 patients with relapse after standardized first line therapy. Leukemia 4: 184-188
17. Huhmann IM, Watzke HH, Geissler K, Gisslinger H, Jäger U, Knobl P, Pabinger I, Korninger L, Mannhalter C, Mitterbauer G, Schwarzinger I, Kalhs P, Haas OA, Lechner K (1996) FLAG (fludarabine, cytosine arabinoside, G-CSF) for refractory and relapsed acute myeloid leukemia. Ann Hematol 73: 265-271
18. Hurwitz CA, Mounce KG, Grier HE (1995) Treatment of patients with acute myelogenous leukemia: review of clinical trials of the past decade. J Pediatr Hematol Oncol 17: 185-197
19. Kantarjian HM, Keating MJ, Walters RS, McCredie KB, Freireich EJ (1988) The characteristics and

outcome of patients with late relapse acute myelogenous leukemia. J Clinl Oncol 6: 232-238

20. Kantarjian HM, Estey EH, Keating MJ (1993) Treatment of therapy-related leukemia and myelodysplastic syndrome. Hematol Oncol Clin North Am 7: 81-107

21. Keating M, Kantarjian H, Gandhi V, O'Brien S, Koller C, Kornblau S, Beran M, Andreeff M, Plunkett W, Freireich E (1998) FLAG-Ida, an effective regimen for high risk AML. In: Hiddemann W et al. (eds.) Acute Leukemias VII. Experimental approaches and novel therapies. Springer-Verlag Heidelberg, pp 828-833

22. Kornblau SM, Cortes Franco J, Estey E (1993) Neurotoxicity associated with fludarabine and cytosine arabinoside chemotherapy for acute leukemia and myelodysplasia. Leukemia 7: 378-383

23. Leahey A, Kelly K, Rorke LB, Lange B (1997) A phase I/II study of idarubicin (Ida) with continuous infusion fludarabine (F-ara-A) and cytarabine (ara-C) for refractory or recurrent pediatric acute myeloid leukemia (AML). J Pediatr Hematol Oncol 19: 304-308

24. Plunkett W, Gandhi V, Huang P, Robertson LE, Yang LY, Gregoire V, Estey E, Keating MJ (1993) Fludarabine: pharmacokinetics, mechanisms of action, and rationales for combination therapies. Semin Oncol 20: 2-12

25. Rayappa C, McCulloch EA (1993) A cell culture model for the treatment of acute myeloblastic leukemia with fludarabine and cytosine arabinoside. Leukemia 7: 992-999

26. Ritter J, Creutzig U, Schellong G (1992) Treatment results of three consecutive German childhood AML trials: BFM-78, -83, and -87. AML-BFM-Group. Leukemia 6: Suppl 2, 59-62

27. Ritter J, Creutzig U, Gadner H, Fink FM, Herrmann J (1993) [Therapiestudie AML-BFM-93 für die akute myeloische Leukämie bei Kindern]. University Münster, Germany, pp 1-54

28. Stahnke K, Ritter J, Schellong G, Beck JD, Kabisch H, Lampert F, Creutzig U (1992) Treatment of recurrence of acute myeloid leukemia in childhood. A retrospective analysis of recurrence in the AML-BFM-83 study. Klin Pädiatr 204: 253-257

29. Tosi P, Visani G, Ottaviani E, Manfori S, Zinzani PL, Tura S (1994) Fludarabine + Ara-C + G-CSF: cytotoxic effect and induction of apoptosis on fresh acute myeloid leukemia cells. Leukemia 8: 2076-2082

30. Visani G, Tosi P, Zinzani PL, Manfroi S, Ottaviani E, Testoni N, Clavio M, Cenacchi A, Gamberi B, Carrara P, Gobbi M, Tura S (1994) FLAG (fludarabine + high-dose cytarabine + G-CSF): an effective and tolerable protocol for the treatment of 'poor risk' acute myeloid leukemias. Leukemia 8: 1842-1846

31. World Health Organization (1979) WHO Handbook for reporting results of cancer treatment. WHO Offset Publication 38: 1-41

# Acute Promyelocytic Leukemia

# APL Biology

B. Cassinat, S. Chevret, N. Balitrand, F. Zassowski, C. Barbey, L.Degos, P. Fenaux
and C. Chomienne for the European APL trials

*Abstract.* Acute promyelocytic leukemia (APL) is a specific type of acute myeloid leukemia (AML) characterized by the morphology of the blast cells, a specific t(15;17) translocation and risks of definite coagulopathy. Recently this leukemia was further characterized by an exquisite sensitivity to all-trans retinoic acid's differentiation effect and the production of a fusion gene altering the gene of RARa and a novel gene PML. In vivo differentiation therapy with retinoids in APL patients follows strict guidelines related both to the APL cell and the biodisposal of all-trans retinoic acid (ATRA).

## Introduction

Acute promyelocytic leukemia (APL) is a specific type of acute myeloid leukemia (AML) characterized by the morphology of blast cells (M3 in the French American British classification of AML) [1], the t(15;17) chromosomal translocation [2] which fuses the PML gene on human chromosome 15 to the retinoic acid receptor (RARa) alpha gene on chromosome 17 [3, 4], and by a coagulopathy combining disseminated intravascular coagulation (DIC) and fibrinolysis [5].

In recent years, discovery of the in vitro and in vivo differentiation of APL blasts by all-trans retinoic acid (ATRA) has modified the therapeutic approach of APL and also has lead to important advances in understanding the biology of APL, and opened new perspectives for differentiation therapy in cancer [6-10].

## The PML-RAR transcripts

Through the t(15;17) translocation [2], AML3 leukemic cells harbour PML/RARα fusion transcripts.. Each APL patient is characterized by a specific fusion transcript termed bcr1, bcr2 or bcr3. These transcripts are observed in all APL cases by reverse transcriptase polymerase chain reaction (RT-PCR) and used as a tool for molecular diagnosis and detection of minimal residual disease [11-13]. Other cases of cytologically defined APL have been reported in which cells harbour chromosomal translocations resulting in rearrangements of the RARα gene but involve chromosomes other than chromosome 15, such as t(11;17) and t(5;17). These translocations disrupt the RARα gene, in the same intron as the t(15;17) translocation, the fusion pattern being respectively PLZF or NPM genes, which encode for novel potential transcriptional by active proteins [14-16].

The fact that RA and its receptor RARα are implicated in the physiological process of granulocytic differentiation [17-19] suggested that the alteration of RARa blocked transactivation of RA responsive genes [3, 4, 20-23]. Identification of APL variants which affect chromosome 17 and the RARα gene, but not chromosome 15, strongly implicate RARα gene alteration in leukemogenesis. Furthermore, PML-RARα transfected cells are blocked in their differentiation towards granulocytes in the case of HL-60 cells [20], towards monocytes in U-937 cells [23], and towards erythrocytes in K562 cells [24, 25].

[1] Hopital Saint-Louis, Paris, Institute of Hematology, France;
[2] Centre Hospitalier Universitaire, Lille, France

## Differentiation induction of APL cells by RA

APL cells are successfully induced to differentiate in vitro to polymorphonuclear cells in the presence of retinoids [7]. Differentiation along the granulocytic pathway leads to the modulation of myeloid differentiation associated parameters such as decrease of expression of the Cathepsin G gene [28], increased GM-CSF receptors (26), and adhesion molecules (CD11b, CD15, CD45RO) [7], and decreased IL-8 secretion [27]. Though neutrophils are known to be eliminated from the peripheral blood by apoptosis, and HL-60 cells treated by ATRA produce up to 40% of apoptotic cells [29], ATRA fails to induce apoptosis in vitro in APL cells [30, 31]. However a topoisomerase II inhibitor, etoposide, induces apoptosis in APL cells, implying that other apoptotic features are functional in those cells [31]. These surprising data suggest that anti-apoptotic features in APL cells, such as the PML-RARα protein [23] or growth factors [32], may prevent effective induction of apoptosis in vitro by ATRA.

Pharmacologic studies of ATRA in APL patients have shown that the plasma concentrations of all-trans RA achieved was within the in vitro concentration range giving differentiates. Inter-patient variations were linked to an increased clearance rate of ATRA and to the leukemic cell burden [33, 34]. Intracellular concentrations of ATRA predict ATRA response equally well in vitro and in vivo [35, 36]. A significant decrease of the area under the plasma ATRA concentration curve is found very early after onset of ATRA treatment

Little is known about the exact physiological outcome of ATRA in normal or APL patients. Different enzymes are implicated in the conversion of the exogenous vitamin A to retinoic acid and its various metabolites. Reduction of RA sensitivity in APL cells after RA therapy may be linked to increased ATRA catabolism [33], mutations in the RARa gene and may be monitored by CRABPII levels [37, 38].

The differentiation of leukemic cells by retinoids is enhanced by the addition of cytokines. We have shown that APL cells express and secrete cytokines such as TNFα, IL-6, IL-8, IL-1β. The absence of TNFα or presence of IL-3, G-CSF or GM-CSF significantly reduced the efficacy of all-trans RA to differentiate APL cells [27, 32]. Interestingly, these cytokines are implicated in leucocyte activation and may be related to the ATRA syndrome occurring in APL patients during differentiation therapy with ATRA.

## ATRA syndrome and other side effects of ATRA

The ATRA syndrome is not due to leukostasis and/or thrombosis. Because its clinical signs are reminiscent of those observed in the endotoxic shock syndrome and in the adult respiratory distress syndrome (ARDS), a possible stimulatory effect of ATRA treatment on cytokine expression by APL cells has been envisaged. Induction of IL-1β and G-CSF secretion by APL cells under ATRA may contribute to hyperleukocytosis in vivo. On the other hand, the secretion of IL-1β, IL6, TNFα and IL-8, all of which are involved in leucocyte activation and adherence, and are implicated in the development of ARDS, could have a pathogenetic role in the ATRA syndrome [27, 32].

### Coagulopathy and thrombosis

In the European APL 91 trial, the median time to disappearance of significant coagulopathy was 6 days after chemotherapy alone and 3 days in the ATRA group (p=0.001) [39]. ATRA therapy may be especially important in reducing the severity of the bleeding tendency in hyperleucocytic APL patients, a population still at a relatively high risk of early death with chemotherapy alone.

In APL patients treated with ATRA alone, primary fibrinogenolysis disappears during the first five days of treatment, while DIC and leukocyte-mediated proteolysis seem to persist during the two or to three first weeks of ATRA therapy [40, 41]. This could lead to a transient period of hypercoagulability, which could explain the few well documented cases of thromboembolytic events in APL patients treated with ATRA.

## Resistance to ATRA

In spite of the progress made in the treatment of APL since the advent of ATRA, some patients still relapse because APL blasts acquire resistance to chemotherapy and to ATRA. Secondary resistance to ATRA is related to a feed back mechanism that progressively reduces plasma concentrations of ATRA. After ATRA withdrawal, this hypercatabolic state persists for a period of several months. Patients who relapse during this interval have clinical resistance to ATRA. CRABPII levels return to undetectable levels 3 months after ATRA withdrawal and patients may then become sensitive again to ATRA in vivo, as seen above .

Since the removal of ATRA as soon as CR is obtained, secondary resistance has no longer been observed in patients. This is also confirmed by the fact that patients who relapse are now again sensitive to ATRA and second CR can be achieved, and that reintroduction of ATRA in the maintenance therapy is also beneficial.

## Assessment of minimal residual disease

RT-PCR of PML-RARa transcripts [12, 13, 42-45] has proven a rapid and extremely sensitive technique for the diagnosis of APL. Accurate diagnosis of APL is now essential as all-trans retinoic acid therapy may only induce complete remission in leukemic cells harbouring a t(15;17) translocation resulting in PML- RARα transcripts. After CR induced by ATRA, PML-RAR transcripts remain detectable in all cases. At though the presence of a PML-RAR product after differentiation therapy may be attributed to residual differentiated leukemic cells with no leukemogenetic potential, constant relapse is observed if CR is not consolidated by chemotherapy. This implies that continuous ATRA therapy alone cannot eliminate the leukemic clone, and justifies the addition of chemotherapy to consolidation therapy. So far controversial reports.

Indeed, ATRA therapy followed by consolidation chemotherapy courses results in RT-PCR negativity for PML-RAR in more than 80% of cases. Thus, even if at CR induced by

ATRA significant amount of minimal residual disease (MRD) may remain, subsequent consolidation or intensification chemotherapy leads to absence of detectable MRD in most cases. Persistant positive RT-PCR results at the end of consolidation chemotherapy, or after a negative period, is highly correlated with a subsequent relapse. The time between a positive result and the hematological relapse is variable, generally within months (related to the sensitivity of the technique, the frequency of sampling and probably the leukemic potential of PML-RARα). RT-PCR of PML-RAR therefore provides a useful tool to monitor and compare the efficacy of currently proposed regimens of consolidation and maintenance chemotherapy

## References

1. Bennett, J.M., Catovsky. D., Daniel, M.T., Flandrin, G., Galton, D., Gralnick, M., Sultan, C. (1976) Proposals for the classification of the acute leukemias. *Br.J.Haematol*, 33, 451
2. Larson, R.A., Kondo, K., Vardiman, J.W., Butler, A.R.E., Golomb, H.M., Rowley, J.D. (1984) Evidence for a 15;17 translocation in every patient with acute promyelocytic leukemia. *Am.J.Med.*, 76, 827
3. De The, H., Lavau, C., Marchio, A., Chomienne, C., Degos, L., Dejean, A. (1991) The PML-RAR alpha fusion mRNA generated by the t(15;17) translocation in acute promyelocytic leukemia encodes a functionally altered RAR. *Cell*, 66, 675
4. Kakizuka, A., Miller, W.H., Umesono, K., Warrell, R., Frankel, S., Dmitrovsky, E., Evans, R. (1991) Chromosomal translocation t(15;17) in human acute promyelocytic leukemia fuses RAR alpha with a novel putative transcription factor, PML. *Cell*, 66, 663
5. Dombret, H., Sutton, L., Duarte, M., Daniel, M.T., Leblond, V., Castaigne, S., Degos, L. (1992) Combined therapy with all-trans retinoic acid and high-dose chemotherapy in patients with hyperleukocytic acute promyelocytic leukemia and severe visceral hemorrhage. *Leukemia* 6, 1237
6. Huang, M., Yu-Chen, Y., Shu-Rong, C., Lu, M.X., Zhoa, L., Gu, L.J., Wang, Z.Y. (1988) Use of all-trans retinoic acid in the treatment of acute promyelocytic leukemia. *Blood* 72, 567
7. Chomienne, C., Ballerini, P., Balitrand, N., Daniel, M.T., Fenaux, P., Castaigne, S., Degos, L. (1990) All trans retinoic acid in promyelocytic leukemias. II. In vitro studies structure function relationship. *Blood*, 76, 1710
8. Castaigne, S., Chomienne, C., Daniel, M.T., Berger, R., Fenaux, P., Degos, L. (1990) All-trans retinoic acid as a differentiating therapy for acute promyelocytic leukemias. I. Clinical results. *Blood*, 76, 1704
9. Grignani, F., Fagioli, M., Alcalay, M., Longo, L., Pandolfi, P., Donti, E., Biondi, A., Lo Coco, F., Pellici,

P.G. (1994) Review : acute promyelocytic leukemia : from genetics to treatment. *Blood,* 83, 10-25

10. Warrell, R. Jr., de The, H., Wang, Z.Y., Degos, L. (1993) Acute promyelocytic leukemia. *N.Engl.J. Med.,*329: 177

11. Castaigne, S., Balitrand, N., de The, H., Dejean, A., Degos, L., Chomienne, C. (1992) A PML/RARa fusion transcript is constantly detected by RNA-based polymerase chain reaction in acute promyelocytic leukemia. *Blood.* 79, 3110

12. Miller, W.H., Levine, K., DeBlasio, A., Frankel, S.R., Dmitrovsky, E., Warrell, R.P. (1993) Detection of minimal residual disease in acute promyelocytic leukemia by a reverse transcription polymerase chain reaction assay for PML-RARa fusion mRNA.*Blood* 82, 1689-1694

13. Diverio, D., Pandolfi, P.P., Rossi, V., Biondi, A., Pelicci, P.G., Lo Coco, F. (1994) Monitoring of treatment outcome in acute promyelocytic leukemia by RT-PCR. *Leukemia* 8, 1105-1107

14. Licht J.D, Chomienne, C., Goy, A., Chen, A., Scott, A.A, Head, D.R., Michaux, J.L., Wu, Y., Deblasio, A., Miller, W.H. (1995) Clinical and molecular characterization of a rare syndrome of acute promyelocytic leukemia associated with translocation (11;17). *Blood,* 85:1083-94

15. Guidez, F., Huang, W., Tong, J.H., Dubois, C., Balitrand, N., Waxman, S., Michaux, J.L., Martiat, P., Degos, L., Chen, Z., Chomienne, C. (1994) Poor response to all-trans retinoic acid therapy in a t(11;17) PLZF/RARa patient. *Leukemia,* 8:312-317

16. Redner, R.L., Rush, E.A., Faas, S., Rudert, W.A., Corey, S.J. (1996) The t(5;17) variant of acute promyelocytic leukemis expresses a nucleophosmin-retinoic acid receptor fusion. *Blood* 87, 882-886

17. Gratas, C., Menot, M.L., Dresch, C., Chomienne, C. (1993) Retinoic acid supports granulocytic but not erythroid differentiation of myeloid progenitors in normal bone marrow cells. *Leukemia,* 7: 1156-1162.

18. Van Bockstaele, D.R., Lenjou, M., Snoeck, H.W., Lardon, F., Stryckmans, P., Peetermans, M.E. (1993) Direct effects of 13-cis and all-trans retinoic acid on normal bone marrow (BM) progenitors: comparative study on BM mononuclear cells and on isolated CD34+ BM cells. *Ann Haematol.,* 66: 61-66

19. Collins S.J., Roberton K.A., Le Moyne Mueller. (1990) Retinoic acid-induced granulocytic differentiation of HL-60 myeloid leukemia cells is mediated directly through the retinoic acid receptor (RAR-a). *Mol. cell. Biol.,* 10 (5), 2154-2163

20. Rousselot, P., Hardas, B., Castaigne, S., Dejean, A., De Thé, H., Degos, L., Farzaneh, F., Chomienne. C. (1994). The PML-RARa gene product of the t(15;17) translocation inhibits retinoic acid induced granulocytic differentiation. *Oncogene,* 9, 545-551

21. Chen, Z., Guidez, F., Rousselot, P., Agadir, A., Chen, S. J., Wang, Z.Y., Degos, L., Waxman, S., Zelent, A., Chomienne, C. (1994) PLZF-RAR fusion protein generated from the translocation t(11;17) (q23;q21) displays altered transactivation properties against the wild-type retinoic acid receptors. *PNAS,* 91: 1178-1182

22. Koken, M.H.M., Puvion-Dutilleuil, F., Guillemin, M.C., Viron, A., Linares-Cruz, G., Stuurman, N., De Jong, L., Szostecki , C., Calvo, F., Chomienne, C., Degos, L., Puvion, E., De The, H. (1994) The t(15; 17) translocation alters a nuclear body in a retinoic acid-reversible fashion. *The EMBO Journal,* 13, 1073-1083

23. Grignani, F., Ferrucci, P.F., Testa, U., Talamo, G., Fagioli, M., Alcalay, M., Mencarelli, A., Grignani, F., Peschle, C., Nicoletti, L., Pellici P.G. (1993) The acute promyelocytic leukemia-specific PML-RARa fusion Protein Inhibits differentiation and promotes survival of myeloid precursor cells. *Cell,* 74, 423-431

24. Grignani, F., Testa, U., Mascuilli, R., Mariani, G., Fagioli, M., Barberi, T., Peschle, C., Pelicci, P.G. (1995) Promyelocytic leukemia -specific PML-retinoic acid alpha receptor fusion protein interferes with erythroid differentiation of human erythroleukemia K562 cells. *Cancer Research,* 55 (2) 440-443

25. Turhan, A.G., Lemoine, F.M., Debert, C., Bonnet, M.L., Baillou, C., Picard, F., Macintyre, E.A., Varet, B. (1995) Highly purified primitive hematopoietic stem cells are PML-RARa negative and generate monoclonal progenitors in acute promyelocytic leukemia. *Blood,* 85 (8), 2154-61

26. De Gentile, A., Toubert, M.E., Dubois, C., Krawice, I., Schlageter, M.H., Balitrand, N., Castaigne, S., Degos, L., Rain. J.D., Najean, Y., Chomienne, C. (1994) Induction of high-affinity GM-CSF receptors during all trans retinoic acid treatment of acute promyelocytic leukemia *Leukemia,* 8, 1758-1762

27. Dubois, C., Schlageter, M.H., De Gentile, A., Guidez, F., Balitrand, N., Toubert, M.E., Krawice, I., Fenaux, P., Castaigne, S., Najean, Y., Degos, L., Chomienne, C. (1994) Modulation of Il-6 and Il-1b and G-CSF secretion by all-trans retinoic acid in Acute Promyelocytic leukemia *Leukemia,* 8: 10, 1750-1757

28. Seale, J, Delva L., Renesto P., Balitrand, N., Dombret, H., Scrobohaci, M.L., Degos. L., Paul, P., Chomienne, C. (1996) All-trans retinoic acid rapidly decreases Cathepsin G synthesis and mRNA expression in acute promyelocytic leukemia. *Leukemia,* 10, 95-101

29. Martin, S.J., Bradley, J.G., Cotter, T.G. (1990) HL-60 cells induced to differentiate towards neutrophils subsequently die via apoptosis. *Clin Exp Imm.,* 79, 448-453

30. Tosi, P., Visani, G., Gibellini, D., Zauli, G., Ottoviani, E., Cenacchi A., Gamberi B., Manfrois S., Marchisio M.,Turas, S. (1994) All-trans retinoic acid and induction of apoptosis in acute promyelocytic leukemia cells. *Leukemia & Lymphoma,* 14 (5-6), 503-507

31. Calabresse, C., Barbey, S., Venturini, L., Balitrand, N., Degos, L., Fenaux, P., Chomienne, C. (1995) In vitro treatment with retinoids or the topoisomerase inhibitor, VP16, evidences different functional apoptotic pathways in acute promyelocytic leukemic cells. *Leukemia* 9, 2049-2057

32. Dubois, C., Schlageter, M.H., De Gentile, A., Guidez, F., Balitrand, N., Toubert, M.E., Krawice, I., Fenaux, P., Castaigne, S., Najean, Y., Degos, L., Chomienne, C. (1991) Hematopoietic growth factor expression and ATRA sensitivity in Acute Promyelocytic Leukemia. *Blood,* 83, 3264-3270

33. Lefebvre, P., Thomas, G,, Gourmel, B., Dreux, C., Castaigne, S., Chomienne, C. (1991) Pharmacokinetics of all-trans RA in patients with acute promyelocytic *Leukemia* 5, 1054

34. Muindi, J., Frankel, S.R., Miller, W.H., Jakubowski, A., Scheinberg, D.A., Young, C.W., Dimitrovsky, E. (1992) Continuous treatment with all-trans RA progressively decreases plasma drug concentrations: implications for relapse and resistance in acute promyelocytic leukemia. *Blood, 79*, 299

35. Agadir, A., Cornic, C., Lefebvre, P., Gourmel, B., Balitrand, N., Degos, L., Chomienne, C. (1995) Differential uptake of all-trans retinoic acid by acute promyelocytic leukemic cells : Evidence for its role in retinoic acid efficacity. *Leukemia, 9*, 139-145

36. Agadir, A., Cornic, M., Lefebvre, P., Gourmel, B., Jerome, M., Degos, L., Fenaux, P., Chomienne, C. (1995) All-trans retinoic acid pharmacokinetics and bioavailability in acute promyelocytic leukemia : Intracellular concentrations and biologic response relationship. *Journal of Clinical Oncology*, 13, 2517-2523

37. Delva, L., Cornic, M., Balitrand, N., Guidez, F., Miclea, J.M., Delmer, A., Teillet, F., Fenaux, P., Castaigne, S., Degos, L., Chomienne, C. (1993) Resistance to All-trans Retinoic Acid Therapy in Relapsing Acute Promyelocytic Leukemia. *Blood, 82*, 2175-2181

38. Cornic, M., Delva, L., Castaigne, S., Balitrand, N., Degos, L., Chomienne, C. (1994) In vitro all-trans retinoic acid (ATRA) sensitivity and cellular retinoic acid binding protein (CRABP) levels in relapse leukemic cells after remisssion induction by ATRA in acute promyelocytic leukemia. *Leukemia 8* (6), 914-7

39. Fenaux, P., Le Deley, M.C., Castaigne, S., Archimbaud, E., Chomienne, C., Link, H., Guerci, A., Duarte, M., Daniel, M.T., Bowen, D., Huebner, G., Bauters, F., Fegueux, N., Fey, M., Sanz, M., Lowenberg, B., Maloisel, F., Auzanneau, G., Sadoun, A., Gardin, C., Bastion, Y., Ganser, A., Jacky, E., Dombret, H., Chastang, C., Degos, L. (1993) Effect of all trans retinoic acid in newly diagnosed acute promyelocytic leukemia. Results of a multicenter randomized trial. *Blood 82*, 3241

40. Dombret, H., Scrobohaci, M.L., Ghorra, P., Zini, J.M., Daniel, M.T., Castaigne, S., Degos, L. (1993) Coagulation disorders associated with acute promyelocytic leukemia : Corrective effect of all-trans retinoic acid treatment. *Leukemia 7*, 2

41. Runde, V., Aul, C., Sudhoff, T., Heyll, A., Schneider, W. (1993). Retinoic acid in the treatment of acute promyelocytic leukemia : Inefficacy of the 13-cis isomer and induction of complete remission by the all-trans isomer complicated by thromboembolic events. *Ann. Hematol, 64*, 270

42. Huang, W., Sun, G.L., Li, X.S., Cao, Q., Lu, Y., Jang, G.S., Zhang, F.Q., Chai, J.R., Wang, Z.Y., Waxman, S. (1993) Acute promyelocytic leukemia: clinical relevance of two major PML-RAR alpha isoforms and detection of minimal residual disease by retrotranscriptase/polymerase chain reaction to predict relapse. *Blood, 82* (4): 1264-1269

43. Vadhat, L., Maslak, P., Miller, W.H., Eardley, A., Heller, G., Scheinberg, D.A., Warrell, R.P. (1994) Early mortality and the retinoic acid syndrome in acute promyelocytic leukemia. Impact of leucocytosis, low dose chemotherapy, PML-RARa isoform and CDB expression in patients treated with all-trans retinoic acid. *Blood 84*, 3843-3849

44. Fukutani, H., Naoe, T., Ohno, R., Yoshida, H., Kiyooi, H., Miyawaki, S., Morishita, H., Sano, F., Kmibayashi, H., Matsue, K. (1995) Prognostic significance of the RT-PCR assay of PML-RARa transcripts in acute promyelocytic leukemia. The Leukemia Study Group of the Ministry of Health and Welfare (Kouseisho). *Leukemia, 9* (4) 588-93

45. Chomienne, C. (1995) RT-PCR in Acute Promyelocytic Leukemia. Second Workshop of the European Retinoic Group. Paris, France, December 17-18, 1994. *Leukemia 10*, 368-371

# Molecular Diagnosis and Monitoring of Acute Promyelocytic Leukemia: Updated Results of the Italian Gimema Group

F. Lo Coco[1], D. Diverio[1], S. De Santis[1], G. Avvisati[1], G. Saglio[2], A. Biondi[3] and F. Mandelli[1]

## Rationale and Background

Long before the advent of all-trans retinoic acid (ATRA) acute promyelocytic leukemia was recognised as a distinct subset of acute myeloid leukemia (AML) with peculiar clinico-biological features and treatment requirements. These include the frequent association at diagnosis of a life threatening hemorrhagic syndrome, the presence in leukemic blasts of a unique t(15;17) translocation and a striking sensitivity to anthracyclines even if used as single agents [1].

Two paramount discoveries, i.e. the capability of APL blasts to undergo differentiation in vitro and in vivo following treatment with vitamin A derivatives such as all-trans retinoic acid (ATRA), and the cloning of genes involved in the t(15;17), paved the way in the early 90's to modern treatment strategies, refined diagnosis and disease monitoring at the molecular level [2-6]. Besides providing a rapid detection of the PML/RARα fusion underlying the t(15;17), the use of reverse-transcriptase polymerase chain reaction (RT-PCR) allow sensitive monitoring of minimal residual disease (MRD), therefore representing a powerful toll to better assess response to treatment in these patients. Using conventional RT-PCR assays with sensitivity levels of $10^3$-$10^4$, several retrospective studies showed that persistence or reappearance of PCR-detectable MRD during hematologic remission correlate with subsequent relapse, whereas patients in long-term survival have no detectable PML/RARα transcripts [6].

Following early reports on the efficacy of ATRA treatment and the superiority of an ATRA plus chemotherapy (CHT) combination over CHT alone [7], the Italian group GIMEMA designed in 1993 a protocol including ATRA and idarubicin (AIDA) for newly diagnosed PML/RARα-positive APL. Apart from considering genetically confirmed diagnosis as a mandatory criterion for patient enrollment, we planned to prospectively monitoring MRD at pre-established time intervals in all patients, with the aim of identifying during hematologic remission patients at highest risk of relapse. Preliminary results of this trial, published in 1997 showed that:

i) virtually 100% of genetically diagnosed APL patients obtain hematologic complete remission with such treatment;

ii) early death due to hemorrhage or ATRA syndrome is considerably reduced by the simultaneous combination;

iii) 98% of patients achieve negativization of the RT-PCR test after a polychemotherapy consolidation [8].

While these results were extremely encouraging, it appeared that post-consolidation PCR evaluation was poorly informative on patient outcome, as a relapse rate of approximately 15-20 % was documented in patients who tested negative at the end of therapy. By contrast, successive monitoring results showed that conversion from PCR-negative to PCR-positive for PML/RARα was uniformly associated with subsequent hematologic relapse, leading to consider the early institution of salvage therapy in these cases at the time of molecular relapse [9].

We report here an update of the molecular studies carried out in patients enrolled in the

---

[1] Department of Cellular Biotechnologies and Hematology, University La Sapienza of Rome;
[2] Department of Clinical and Biological Sciences, University of Turin;
[3] Clinica Pediatrica, Ospedale S. Gerardo, University of Milano-Monza, Italy.

front line AIDA protocol, as well as preliminary data on a series of 15 patients who received salvage treatment for molecular relapse.

## Updated Molecular Results

As of January 1999, 669 patients were evaluable for eligibility. Of these, 69 (10%) were excluded from the study due to erroneous diagnosis or clinical contra-indications to receive the AIDA scheme. All the remaining 600 patients had genetic documentation of t(15;17) in leukemic cells at presentation. Since early 1998, an anti-PML monoclonal antibody (PG-M3) was employed in conjunction with routine karyotyping and RT-PCR to rapidly confirm diagnosis at the genetic level [10]. This allows distinction of the typical microparticulate nuclear distribution of the PML protein (also referred to as "microspeckled") in APL cells, as opposite to the so-called nuclear bodies pattern present in normal as well as in non-APL leukemic cells. Using either immunohistochemistry or immunofluorescence as revelation system, this technique provides rapid, easy and low-cost specific diagnosis extremely useful for prompt patient enrollment in APL-tailored protocols [10].

The diagnostic characterization of PML/RARα isoforms disclosed bcr1, bcr2 and bcr3 trancript types in 55%, 6% and 39% of patients, respectively. As also reported in our preliminary analysis [8], no correlations were found among fusion gene isoforms and response to induction, overall survivall (OS) event-free survival (EFS) and disease-free survival (DFS), although a trend (not statistically significant) towards inferior outcome was observed for patients with the bcr3 fusion type.

A total of 322 patients in hematologic remission were analysed by RT-PCR at completion of induction before initiating consolidation. Of these, 134 (42%) tested PCR-positive and 188 (58%) PCR-negative at this time point. No correlation was found between PML/RARα breakpoint type and PCR status after induction therapy. After the end of consolidation therapy, 411 were analysed. Of these, 15 (3.6% ) tested PCR-positive and 396 (96.3%) PCR-negative. Finally, PCR status after induction had no influence on either EFS or DFS.

## Therapy of Molecular Relapse: Preliminary Results

Recently reported results of prospective monitoring in patients enrolled in our trial showed that virtually all patients who converted to PCR-positive after the end of consolidation underwent subsequently hematologic relapse within a median time of 3 months. By contrast, the relapse rate for patients who tested $\geq 2$ times PCR-negative was below 10% after a median follow-up of 18 months postconsolidation [9]. As a result of these findings, patients who converted to PCR-positive in two successive marrow samples after the end consolidation were considered as having molecular relapse and given anticipated salvage therapy.

At present, 15 patients who received the AIDA induction and consolidation as front line therapy were treated at the time of first molecular relapse. The median duration of first molecular remission was 7 months (range 2–23). Salvage therapy consisted of oral ATRA for 30 days followed by 4 daily courses of chemotherapy (CHT) with cytarabine 1g/m²/d and mitoxantrone 6 mg/m²/d.

After reinduction, a status of second molecular remission was obtained in 12/15 patients (80%). Nine of these 15 (60%) converted to PCR-negative after ATRA alone. Of the 3 patients who persisted PCR-positive after ATRA and CHT, one died in remission and two progressed to hematologic relapse. Of 12 patients PCR-negative after salvage therapy, 8 received consolidation with autologous bone marrow transplantation (ABMT), and 4 received ATRA-containing maintenance. Ten patients in this group remained in prolonged second molecular remission at a median time of 13.5 months (range 7-35+). Two patients underwent hematologic recurrence at 6 and 12 months after transient second molecular remission. The actuarial probability of remaining in 2nd MR was 77% at 35 months.

Given the small patient number and limited follow-up in this series, conclusive statements on the advantage of anticipating salvage treatment in APL at the time of molecular relapse might be premature. However, this study represents, to the best of our knowledge, the first report on the treatment of molecular recurrence in acute leukemia and some preliminary observations are worth of note.

Despite having high probability of entering second remission, APL patients treated for hematologic relapse are at high risk of early death [3-6]. Early treatment of relapse at the time of minimal disease recurrence minimizes the most serious treatment-related risks such as hemorrhage and ATRA syndrome. Moreover, we obtained a second molecular remission in 90% of patients after ATRA + CHT reinduction, and in 60% after ATRA alone. The actuarial OS and EFS rates of 87% and 61%, respectively, are quite encouraging, particularly considering that these patients relapsed at the molecular level after receiving optimal front line therapy. Finally, the median duration of second molecular remission already exceeds that of first molecular remission in this cohort.

Given the relatively low frequency of relapse in APL, it is presumable that comparison studies aimed at establishing the advantage of anticipating therapy at the time of molecular relapse will require cooperation at the multi-national level.

# References

1. Bernard J (1994) History of promyelocytic leukemia. Leukemia 8 (Suppl.2): 1-5.
2. Chen S-J, Wang Z-Y, Chen Z (1995) Acute promyelocytic leukemia: from clinic to molecular biology. Stem Cells 13:22-31.
3. Wiernik PH, Gallagher RE, Tallman MS (1996) Diagnosis and treatment of acute promyelocytic leukemia. In: Wiernik PH, Canellos GP, Dutcher JP, Kyle RA (eds): Neoplastic diseases of the blood. 3rd edition, New York: Churchill Livingstone 1996: pp 353-380.
4. Fenaux P, Chomienne C, Degos L (1997) Acute promyelocytic leukemia: Biology and treatment. Sem Oncol 24: 92-102.
5. Warrell RP Jr (1996) Pathogenesis and management of acute promyelocytic leukemia. Annu Rev Med 47: 555-65.
6. Lo Coco F, Nervi, Avvisati G, Mandelli F (1998) Acute promyelocytic leukemia: a curable disease. Leukemia 12:1866-80.
7. Fenaux P, Le Deley MC, Castaigne S, Archimbaud E, Chomienne C, Link H, Guerci A, Duarte M, Daniel MT, Bowen D, Huebner G, Bauters F, Fegueux N, Fey M, Sanz MA, Lowenberg B, Maloisel F, Auzanneau G, Sadoun A, Gardin C, Bastion Y, Gansr A, Jacky E, Dombret H, Chastang C, Degos L, for the European APL 91 Group (1993) Effect of All-trans retinoic acid in newly diagnosed acute promyelocytic leukemia. Blood 82:3241-49.
8. Mandelli F, Diverio D, Avvisati G, Luciano A, Barbui T, Bernasconi C, Broccia G, Cerri R, Falda M, Fioritoni G, Leoni F, Liso V, Petti MC, Rodeghiero F, Saglio G, Vegna ML, Visani G, Jehn U, Willemze R, Muus P, Pelicci PG, Biondi A, Lo Coco F (1997) Molecular remission in PML/RARα-positive acute promyelocytic leukemia by combined all-trans retinoic acid and idarubicin (AIDA) therapy. Blood 90:1014-21.
9. Diverio D, Rossi V, Avvisati G, De Santis S, Pistilli A, Pane F, Saglio G, Martinelli G, Petti MC, Santoro A, Pelicci PG, Mandelli F, Biondi F, Lo Coco F (1998) Early detection of relapse by prospective RT-PCR analysis of the PML/RARα fusion gene in patients with acute promyelocytic leukemia enrolled in the GIMEMA-AIEOP multicenter "AIDA" trial. Blood 92:784-89.
10. Falini B, Flenghi L, Fagioli M, Lo Coco F, Cordone I, Diverio D, Biondi A, Raganelli D, Liso A, Martelli MF, Pileri S (1997) Immunocytochemical diagnosis of acute promyelocytic leukemia (M3) with the anti-PML monoclonal antibody PG-M3. Blood 90: 4046-53.

# All-Trans-Retinoic Acid Maintenance for Acute Promyelocytic Leukemia

M. S. Tallman[1], J. W. Andersen[2], Ch. A. Schiffer[3], F. R. Appelbaum[4], J. H. Feusner[5], A. Ogden[6], L. Shepherd[7], Ch. Willman[8], C. D. Bloomfield[9], J. M. Rowe[10] and P. H. Wiernik[11]

## Introduction

Acute promyelocytic leukemia (APL) is now the most curable subtype of acute myeloid leukemia (AML) in adults. Studies including prospective randomized trials have definitively established that all-trans-retinoic acid (ATRA), given alone or with chemotherapy for induction, significantly improves outcome.(1-8) The event-free survival (EFS) at 2 to 4 years is 55%-85%, and the overall survival (OS) is 70%-80% (Table 1). This improvement is generally attributable to a decrease in relapse rather than an increase in the complete remission (CR) rate or a decrease in the early deaths.

Despite these excellent results, approximately 10% of patients die early and 10%-30% of patients relapse, which has prompted evaluation of the role of maintenance therapy with ATRA. A role for maintenance chemotherapy in APL has been suggested in nonrandomized studies conducted before the introduction of ATRA. [9-11] In a study by Kantarjian and colleagues, the 3-year CR duration was statistically significantly better among patients receiving maintenance chemotherapy with prednisone, vincristine, 6-mercaptopurine (6-MP) and methotrexate than among patients not receiving maintenance [9]. In a report by

Fenaux and colleagues, the actuarial DFS was significantly shorter among a small cohort of patients not receiving maintenance with 6-MP and methotrexate compared to that among patients receiving such maintenance [10]. Therefore, interest in exploring the potential benefits of maintenance ATRA either alone or combined with chemotherapy is well founded.

## Prospective Randomized Trials

The North American Intergroup study (INT0129) was a prospective trial in which adults and children with newly diagnosed APL were randomly assigned to receive either ATRA alone or chemotherapy with daunorubicin plus cytarabine for induction.(3) After two cycles of consolidation chemotherapy, patients still in complete remission (CR) were then randomly assigned to either a maintenance regimen of daily ATRA (45 mg/m$^2$) for 1 year or observation, stratified by induction assignment. Patients randomly assigned to ATRA maintenance therapy had a significantly (P<0.001) better outcome than did patients assigned to observation alone with no maintenance therapy (Table 2). The 3-year disease-free survival (DFS) from the date of

---

[1] Northwestern University Medical School, Robert H. Lurie Comprehensive Cancer Center, Chicago IL, Eastern Cooperative Oncology Group
[2] Dana-Farber Cancer Institute, Division of Biostatistics, Boston MA, Eastern Cooperative Oncology Group
[3] Wayne State University, Karmanos Cancer Center, Detroit MI, Cancer and Leukemia Group B
[4] University of Washington, Fred Hutchinson Cancer Research Center, Seattle WA, Southwest Oncology Group
[5] Children's Hospital-Oakland, Oakland CA, Children's Cancer Group
[6] Texas Childrens Hospital, Houston TX, Pediatric Oncology Group
[7] National Cancer Institute of Canada Clinical Trials Group, Kingston, Ontario
[8] University of New Mexico, Albuquerque, New Mexico
[9] The Ohio State University, Comprehensive Cancer Center, Columbus, OH, Cancer and Leukemia Group B
[10] Technion, Israel Institute of Technology, Haifa, Israel
[11] Albert Einstein Cancer Center, Montefiore Medical Center, Bronx NY, Eastern Cooperative Oncology Group

**Table 1.** Prospective Trials of ATRA in APL

| Trial | N | Induction | % CR | % ED | %DFS/EFS |
|---|---|---|---|---|---|
| **Randomized** | | | | | |
| APL91 (Europe)[1] | 54 | ATRA (+ Chemo) | 97 | 9 | 79 (1 year) |
| | 47 | Chemo | 81 | 8 | 50 |
| APL93 (Europe)[2] | 109 | ATRA → Chemo | 95 | 8 | 75 (2 years) |
| | 99 | ATRA + Chemo | 94 | 7 | 86 |
| No. Am. Intergroup[3] | 172 | ATRA | 72 | 11 | 67 (3 years) |
| | 174 | Chemo | 69 | 14 | 32 |
| UK MRC (England)[4] | 119 | ATRA (5d) → Chemo | 70 | 23 | 59 (3 years) |
| | 120 | ATRA + Chemo | 87 | 12 | 78 |
| **Nonrandomized** | | | | | |
| GIMEMA (Italy)[5] | 240 | ATRA + Chemo | 95 | 5 | 79 (2 years) |
| JALSG (Japan)[6] | 196 | ATRA ± Chemo | 88 | 9 | 62/54 (4 years) |
| PETHEMA (Spain)[7] | 100 | ATRA + Chemo | 87 | 11 | Too Early |
| German AMLCG[8] | 43 | ATRA + Chemo | 91 | 9 | 85 (2 years) |

CR = Complete Remission
ED = Early Death
DFS = Disease-Free Survival
EFS = Event-Free Survival

randomization to maintenance therapy or observation was 65% for patients randomized to ATRA compared to 40% for patients assigned to observation. Patients assigned to receive ATRA for both induction and maintenance had the best outcome; however, the study was not powered to test differences between the induction maintenance combinations, and differences between the three induction maintenance sequences with any exposure to ATRA were not significant. In the APL93 trial, patients in CR after 2 cycles of consolidation chemotherapy were randomized to either intermittent ATRA (45 mg/m$^2$ per day, given for 15 days every 3 months), or chemotherapy (6-mercaptopurine 90 mg/m$^2$ per day and methotrexate 15 mg/m$^2$ per week), or both ATRA and chemotherapy for 2 years or no maintenance [2]. The fewest relapses occurred among patients who received concurrent maintenance ATRA and chemotherapy compared to either maintenance ATRA or chemotherapy alone, both of which were associated with fewer relapses than among patients not receiving maintenance (Table 2).

## Toxicities of atra Maintenance Therapy

Maintenance ATRA appears to be reasonably well tolerated. In the North American Intergroup Study, no patients developed hyperleukocytosis or retinoic acid syndrome during maintenance. Sixty-four patients (68%) receiving maintenance completed one full year of therapy. The causes for discontinuing ATRA early included relapse in 12 patients, toxicities in 14 patients, withdrawal of consent in 2 patients, complicating disease in 1 patient, and withdrawal from the study in 1 patient. Thirty-six percent of the patients receiving ATRA maintenance sustained severe or life-

**Table 2.** Prospective Maintenance Therapy in APL

| Trial | N | Maintenance | Relapse Rate (%) |
|---|---|---|---|
| APL93 (Europe)[2] | 63 | ATRA | 20 |
| | 64 | ATRA + CT | 9 |
| | 63 | CT | 22 |
| | 67 | Observation | 32 |
| No. Am. Intergroup[3] | 94 | ATRA | 32 |
| | 105 | Observation | 57 |
| GIMEMA (Italy)[28] | 172 | ATRA | 10 |
| | 157 | Observation | 18 |

threatening toxicities including neurotoxicity in 11 patients, 5 of whom had headache, 3 had pseudotumor cerebri (2 children, 1 adult), 2 had hearing loss, and 1 had depression. Seven patients developed infections, although these were primarily catheter-related. There were 5 patients who sustained hepatotoxicity, generally manifested by transient elevation in the hepatic transaminases or serum bilirubin. In the APL93 trial, there were no cases of retinoic acid syndrome seen on any of the maintenance arms.

## Prognostic Variables

Now that studies with large numbers of patients evaluating ATRA therapy have been completed, factors predictive of success or failure with the current approach can be identified. Such factors may prove useful in identifying cohorts of patients who may benefit the most from maintenance therapy. The Japan Adult Leukemia Study Group (JALSG) analyzed the prognostic factors for predicting CR, EFS, and DFS [6]. In this trial, patients with newly diagnosed APL underwent differentiation therapy with ATRA alone or in combination with chemotherapy followed by intensive postremission chemotherapy. These investigators found that an initial white blood cell count (WBC) less than 10,000/µL was a favorable prognostic factor for EFS and DFS. This study also demonstrated that age less than 30 years was an important predictor of CR and EFS. In the APL93 trial, patients ages 66 to 75 as well as patients presenting with a white blood cell count of more than 10,000/µL had a significantly lower EFS than in patients less than 65 years of age and those presenting with a WBC of less than 5,000/µL [2]. Patients in the high WBC group had more relapses than the patients presenting with a lower WBC.

## Future Directions

Although preliminary studies suggest that maintenance therapy with ATRA, chemotherapy or both improves outcome, any evaluation of the benefits of maintenance therapy must take into account both remission induction and consolidation intensity. More intensive remission induction with higher doses of anthracyclines may yield the same benefit as maintenance therapy [12]. SWOG reported excellent outcome (61% survival at 9 years and no relapse after 3 years) with APL patients treated with high-dose daunorubicin induction (210 mg/m$^2$ per course) and consolidation (420 mg/m$^2$). Earlier studies conducted by the same group with lower doses of daunorubicin did not yield this same survival advantage.

There may be subsets of patients, as suggested above, who may benefit from maintenance therapy more than others. Given pharmacokinetic data indicating an early decrease in plasma retinoid levels with daily ATRA exposure and recovery to higher levels with a drug holiday, continued evaluation of an intermittent ATRA maintenance schedule may be warranted [13-16]. A limited exposure to ATRA following chemotherapy-induced CR may be beneficial in eliminating minimal residual disease [16]. Seiter and colleagues administered ATRA for 10 weeks to 8 patients with APL in CR after intensive induction chemotherapy which included mitoxantrone (75-80 mg/m$^2$) and high-dose cytarabine (3 g/m$^2$ daily for 5 days). Seven remained in CR after a median follow-up of 29 months. Two patients with evidence of minimal residual disease after chemotherapy by RT-PCR converted to a negative status. However, the high doses of mitoxantrone may have accounted for the favorable outcome, and the contribution of the limited ATRA exposure is difficult to evaluate. Alternatively, these patients may have had delayed clearance of blasts.

Recent reports showing the remarkable activity of arsenic trioxide in patients with both relapsed/refractory and newly diagnosed APL have paved the way for the next generation of studies [17-23]. Preliminary results from the first US experience of arsenic trioxide in patients with relapsed and refractory of APL have preliminarily confirmed the high response rates reported by investigators from China [24]. Arsenic trioxide induces apoptosis although the exact mechanism(s) has not been established [25]. Preliminary reports suggest that bcl-2 is down-regulated and caspases are activated [26]. However,

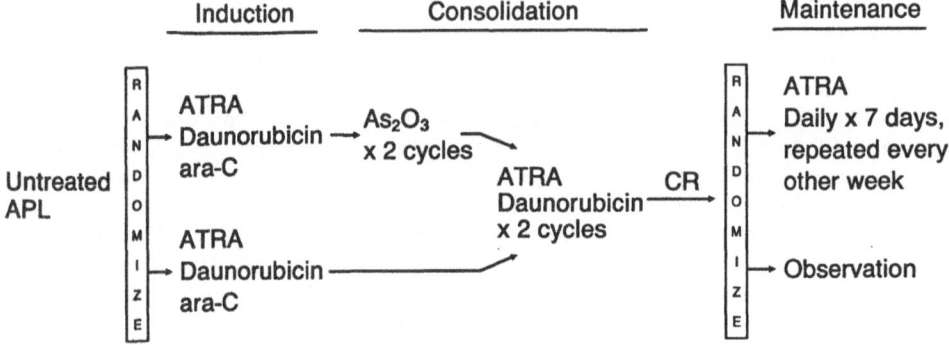

Induction | Consolidation | Maintenance

**Fig. 1.** Schema for proposed NCI-sponsored North American Intergroup Trial

both of these phenomena are generally observed in the process of apoptosis.

The North American Intergroup has proposed to examine the benefit of a course of arsenic trioxide as part of consolidation in one arm of a prospective randomized trial in which all patients are induced with anthracycline/cytarabine (Figure 1). All patients will receive two cycles of consolidation with anthracycline alone with seven days of ATRA, preceded in one arm by two courses of arsenic trioxide. Patients will undergo a second randomization to compare an intermittent schedule of seven days of ATRA repeated every other week for 12 months to observation. This trial will examine not only the role of arsenic trioxide as part of consolidation in improving long-term outcome, but will also evaluate its impact in minimal residual disease as identified by molecular studies. The role of arsenic trioxide as induction therapy for previously untreated patients will need to be explored. Finally, the combination of ATRA and arsenic trioxide to induce differentiation and apoptosis will be an important direction to pursue.(27)

Historically, APL has been described as the only form of AML in which marrow aplasia was not a prerequisite for the achievement of CR. In a similar way, one can speculate that APL may be the first subtype of AML that does not require treatment with any myelosuppressive agents.

# References

1. Fenaux P, Le Deley MC, Castaigne S, et al. (1993) Effect of all-trans retinoic acid in newly diagnosed acute promyelocytic leukemia. Results of a multicenter randomized trial. Blood 82(11):3241-3249.
2. Fenaux P, Chastang C, Sanz M, et al. (1997) ATRA followed by chemotherapy (CT) vs ATRA plus CT and the role of maintenance therapy in newly diagnosed acute promyelocytic leukemia. First interm results of the APL93 trial. Blood 90(suppl 1):533 (abstr).
3. Tallman MS, Andersen JW, Schiffer CA, et al. (1997) All-trans retinoic acid in acute promyelocytic leukemia. N Engl J Med 337:1021-1028.
4. Burnett AK, Goldstone AH, Gray RG, Wheatley K. (1997) All trans-retinoic acid given concurrently with induction chemotherapy improves the outcome of APL: Results of the UK MRC ATRA trial. Blood 90 (suppl 1):1474a(abstr).
5. Mandelli F, Diverio D, Avvisati G, et al. (1997) Molecular remission in PML/RARα-positive acute promyelocytic leukemia by combined all-trans retinoic acid and idarubicin (AIDA) therapy. Blood 90:1014-1021.
6. Asou N, Adachi K, Kanamaru TA, et al. (1998) Analysis of prognostic factors in newly diagnosed acute promyelocytic leukemia treated with all-trans retinoic acid and chemotherapy. J Clin Oncol 16:78-85.
7. Sanz MA, Martin G, Gonzalez M, et al. (1998) High molecular remission (MR) rate and low toxicity with a modified AIDA protocol omitting cytarabine and etoposide from treatment of newly diagnosed PML/RARα positive acute promyelocytic leukemia (APL). Blood 92 (supple 1):1662a.
8. Lengfelder E, Reichert A, Schoch C, et al. (1998) Molecular remission of PML/RARα after TAD/HAM double induction therapy combined with all-trans retinoic acid, TAD consolidation and monthly maintenance in patients with acute promyelocytic leukemia. Blood 92 (suppl 1):1661a.
9. Kantarjian HM, Keating MJ, Walters RS, Smith TL, McCredie KB, Freireich EJ. (1987) Role of maintenance chemotherapy in acute promyelocytic leukemia. Cancer 59:1258-1263.

10. Fenaux P, Pollet JP, Vandenbossche-Simon L, Morel P, Zandecki M, Jouet JP, Bauters F. (1990) Treatment of acute promyelocytic leukemia: A Report of 70 cases. Leukemia Lymphoma 4:239-2448.

11. Marty M, Ganem G, Fisher J, et al. (1984) Leucemie aigue promyelocytaire: etude retrospective de 11a malades traites par daunorubicine. Nous Rev Fr Hematol 24:40-54.

12. Head D, Kopecky KJ, Weick J, et al. (1995) Effect of aggressive daunomycin therapy on survival in acute promyelocytic leukemia. Blood 86:1717-1728.

13. Lefebvre P, Thomas G, Gourmel B, et al. (1991) Pharmacokinetics of oral all-trans retinoic acid in patients with acute promyelocytic leukemia. Leukemia 5:1054-1058.

14. Muindi JRF, Frankel SR, Huselton C, et al. (1992) Clinical pharmacology of oral all-trans retinoic acid with acute promyelocytic leukemia. Cancer Res 52:2138-2142.

15. Adamson PC, Boylan JF, Balis FM, et al. (1993) Time course of induction of metabolism of all-trans retinoic acid and the up-regulation of cellular retinoic acid-binding protein. Cancer Res 53:472-476.

16. Seiter K, Miler WH, Feldman EJ, Ahmed T, Arlin Z. (1995) Pilot study of all-trans retinoid acid as postremission therapy in patients with acute promyelocytic leukemia. Leukemia 9:15-18.

17. Sun HD, Ma L, Hu XC, Zhang TD. (1992) Treatment of apoptosis by ailing-1 therapy with use of syndrome differentiation of traditional Chinese medicine. Chin J Comb Trad Chin Med West Med 12:170-1.

18. Zhang P, Wang SY, Hu XH. (1996) Arsenic trioxide treated 72 cases of acute promyelocytic leukemia. Chin J Hematol 17:58-62.

19. Chen G-Q, Zhu J, Shi X-G, et al. (1996) In vitro studies on cellular and molecular mechanisms of arsenic trioxide ($As_2O_3$) in the treatment of acute promyelocytic leukemia: $As_2O_3$ induces NB4 cells apoptosis with down-regulation of Bcl-2 expression and modulation of PML-RARα/Pml proteins. Blood 88:1052-1061.

20. Chen G-Q, Shi X-G, Tang W, et al. (1997) Use of arsenic trioxide ($As_2O_3$) in the treatment of acute promyelocytic leukemia (APL): I, ($As_2O_3$) Exerts dose-dependent dual effects on APL cells. Blood 89:3345-3353.

21. Shen ZX, Chen GQ, Ni JH, et al. (1997) Use of arsenic trioxide ($As_2O_3$) in the treatment of acute promyelocytic leukemia (APL): II. Clinical efficacy and pharmacokinetics in patients at relapse. Blood 89:3354-3360.

22. Chen G-Q, Zhu J, Shi X-G, et al. (1996) In vitro studies on cellular and molecular mechanisms of arsenic trioxide ($As_2O_3$) in the treatment of acute promyelocytic leukemia: $As_2O_3$ induces NB4 cell apoptosis with down-regulation of Bcl-2 expression and modulation of PML-RARα/Pml proteins. Blood 88:1052-1061.

23. Zhu J, Koken M, Quignon F, Chelbi-Alix, et al. (1997) Arsenic-induced PML targeting onto nuclear bodies: Implications for the treatment of acute promyelocytic leukemia. Proc Natl Acad Sci 84:3978-3983.

24. Warrell RP, Soignet S, Maslak P, et al. (1998) Initial Western study of arsenic trioxide ($As_2O_3$) in acute promyelocytic leukemia (APL). Proc Am Soc Clin Oncol 17:19a.

25. Shao W, Fanelli M, Ferrara F, et al. (1998) Arsenic trioxide as an inducer of apoptosis and loss of PML-RARα protein in acute promyelocytic leukemia cells. J Nat Cancer Inst 90:124-133.

26. Akao Y, Mizoguchi H, Kojima S, et al. (1998) Arsenic induces apoptosis in B-cell leukaemic cell lines in vitro: activation of caspases and down-regulation of Bcl-2 protein. Br J Haemat 102:1055-1060.

27. Gianni M, Koken M, Chelbi-Alix M, et al. (1998) Combined arsenic and retinoic acid treatment enhances differentiation and apoptosis in arsenic-resistant NB4 cells. Blood 91:4300-4310.

28. Avvisati G. Personal communication.

569

# Treatment of Acute Promyelocytic Leukemia with Arsenic Trioxide

J. Hu, H.-P. Sun, C. Niu, H. Yan, T. Yu, G.-Q. Chen, Z.-X. Shen, S.-J. Chen, Z.-Y. Wang and Z. Chen

Supported in part by the Chinese Climbing Project, National Natural Sciences Foundation of China, Shanghai Municipal Commission for Sciences and Technologies, and Clyde Wu Foundation of Shanghai Institute of Hematology.

The authors thank all members of Shanghai Institute of Hematology for their support and Prof. Dao-Pei LU from Beijing Medical University, Beijing, China, Prof. Samuel Waxman from Mount Sinai Medical Center, New York, USA, Prof. Laurent Degos from Saint-Louis Hospital, Paris, France and Prof. Ryuzo Ohno from Hamamatse University School of Medicine, Japan for constructive discussion.

*Abstract.* Fifty three cases of acute promyelocytic leukemia (APL) patients, including 43 relapsed and 10 primary cases, were evaluated as to the effectiveness of As2O3 treatment. Clinical complete remission (CR) was obtained in 40 out of 43 (93%) patients in the relapsed group. Two of the three non-responders studied showed clonal evolution at relapse. In a follow-up of 33 cases for 1 to 42 months, the estimated disease-free survival (DFS) rates for 1- and 2- years were 62.4% and 36.7%, respectively and the actual median DFS was 11 months. Patients presenting white blood cells (WBC) count below $10 \times 10^9$/L at relapse showed better survival than those with WBC count over $10 \times 10^9$/L (p=0.044). Clinical outcome was related to post-remission therapy, since there was only 2 relapse out of 11 cases in combination therapy group, compared to 11 out of 18 with As2O3 treatment alone (p=0.01). Meanwhile, eight out of 10 (80%) primary cases achieved clinical CR. However, six out of 10 primary patients had elevated plasma liver transaminase levels and two died with severe hepatic toxicity, in contrast to the mild liver dysfunction in one fourth of the patients with relapsed APL. RT-PCR analysis in both relapsed and de novo groups showed that induction using As2O3 over short period of time was not sufficient to eliminate minimal residual disease. Long-term use of the drug could, nevertheless, lead to a molecular remission at least in some patients. We thus recommend that ATRA should be used as first line remission induction in de novo APL, while As2O3 can be either used as a rescue for relapsed cases, or included into multi-drug consolidation/maintenance clinical trials.

## Introduction

Acute promyelocytic leukemia (APL) is characterized by chromosome translocation t(15;17) with resultant PML-RARα fusion gene [1-3], which determines both the pathogenesis of APL and the specific response to the differentiation inducer, all-trans retinoic acid (ATRA). It is now well established that ATRA together with chemotherapy allows not only a very high complete remission rate (>90%) but also an overall 5 year disease-free survival in 60~70% APL patients, the best result ever obtained in the treatment of AML without bone marrow transplantation [4-6]. This breakthrough has thus opened a new approach in cancer differentiation therapy.

In spite of this progress, however, 30-40% of APL patients still relapsed within 5 years

From Shanghai Institute of Hematology, Department of Hematology/Oncology, Rui Jin Hospital, Shanghai Second Medical University, Shanghai, China.

after CR. The majority of these patients lose the sensitivity to ATRA and chemotherapy, necessitating new treatment rescue. In early 1970s, a group from Harbin Medical University in Northeast China suggested that intravenous administration of As2O3, with relatively small dose of 10mg/day, was effective in treating patients with APL, lymphoma and hepatic cancer [7–9]. In 1996, we confirmed the therapeutic effect of this drug in APL by reporting a successful use of As2O3 in a group of 16 relapsed APL patients with a CR rate of 96% [10]. These results mainly obtained in Chinese population were very recently confirmed by Soignet et al in Western population because 11 out of 12 relapsed APL patients in their series obtained CR with As2O3 treatment [11]. In vitro studies showed that As2O3 may exert biphasic actions on APL cells, induction of apoptosis at high concentrations (0.5-2 µM) and induction of partial differentiation at low concentrations (0.1-0.5µM). Of note, both high and low concentrations of As2O3 are able to trigger the degradation of PML-RARα fusion protein [12]. Recent studies of our group showed that the main in vivo therapeutic effect of As2O3 is the induction of APL cell differentiation. As2O3 may trigger granulocytic differentiation in a similar way as ATRA does (CHEN GQ et al, in preparation).

In this paper, we report on the updated data of the As2O3 treatment in 43 relapsed APL, especially those concerning the possible prognostic parameters and suitable post-remission treatment in relapsed APL patients rescued with As2O3, we also report experiences of arsenic treatment in 10 de novo APL cases, which is important to define the position of As2O3 in the comprehensive treatment of APL. Finally, we examined the minimal residual disease status in patients under treatment of As2O3.

## Patients and Methods

### Patients

Two groups of patients, de novo and relapsed APL, diagnosed according to French-American-British classification, cytogenetic analysis and RT-PCR for PML-RARα, were entered into this study between December, 1994 and April, 1998. All 43 relapsed cases (2 at the second relapse, 2 at the third relapse, and 39 at the first relapse) had received ATRA and chemotherapy for the previous remission induction and consolidation/maintenance therapy. 10 cases of newly diagnosed APL were not exposed to any anti-leukemia treatment. Informed consent was obtained for every patient entering into this study. The main clinical and hematological characteristics of these patients were shown on Table 1.

### Induction therapy

As2O3 solution was prepared by the Pharmacy of Traditional Chinese Medicine in the First Hospital affiliated to Harbin Medical University of China. Patients were treated with daily dose of 10 mg As2O3 (10 ml, 0.1%

**Table 1.** Characteristics of Patients with APL in the Present Study

|  | De novo APL | Relapsed APL |
|---|---|---|
| Number of cases | 10 | 43 |
| Sex (male/female) | 3/7 | 26/17 |
| Mean age (range, years) | 41(24-60) | 36(7-55) |
| Median WBC (range, X10^9/L) | 2.15 (1.1-40.0) | 3.4 (0.6-31.9) |
| <2 | 0 | 5 |
| 2-10 | 8 | 29 |
| 10-20 | 0 | 3 |
| >20 | 2 | 6 |
| Median RBC (range, (10^12/L) | 2.17 (1.03-2.95) | 3.65 (1.78-5.31) |
| Median hemoglobin(range, g/L ) | 70.0 (51-94) | 109 (56-180) |
| Median platelet (range, X10^9/L) | 20.0 (10-50) | 38.5 (4.0-186) |
| Median percentage of blast cells in BM (range) | 84.5 (38.0-95.5) | 64.0 (12.5-90) |

solution) diluted in 500 ml of 5% glucose-normal saline solution for intravenous drip over 2 to 3 hours. One course is of six weeks. If necessary, a second course was carried out after an interval of 7 days. Patients not entering CR after 2 courses were considered as non responders (NR) and the treatment was shifted to chemotherapy.

## Supportive care

Circulating blood cell count (every other day), bone marrow (BM) cytology, renal and hepatic functions (every 1-2 weeks) were performed during the remission induction treatment. Measurement of coagulation and fibrinolysis parameters, including fibrinogen, DD dimers, fibrin degradation product (FDP), prothrombin time, and activated partial thromboplastin time were carried out by standard methods for each patient prior to and during the As2O3 treatment. Coagulopathy was treated using low dose heparin, platelet suspension and fresh plasma. Patients with white blood cell (WBC) count over $20 \times 10^9$/L prior or during arsenic course were treated with hydroxyurea or moderate DA protocol (DNR: 40mg/m2/dayX3day; Ara-C: 100mg/M$^2$/dayX3-5day). In relapsed patients, ATRA (20 mg/ M$^2$/day) was added when WBC count was less than $2.0 \times 10^9$/L. Symptomatic therapy was performed without discontinuation of As2O3 when moderate side effects occurred while As2O3 was withdrawn in the case of serious toxic effects.

## Cytogenetic studies and reverse transcription PCR (RT/PCR)

Metaphase chromosomes were prepared from BM cells after short-term culture(24hrs.). RHG-banding technique was used and karyotype analysis was carried out according to ISCN nomenclature [18]. RT/PCR analysis for PML-RARα transcripts was performed according to our previously described methods [13].

## Follow-up

Disease-free survival (DFS) was defined as the time from CR to relapse, death from any cause, or censoring of the data on the patients. After CR achieved with As2O3, relapsed patients were divided into three groups according to therapeutic protocols:

1. chemotherapy group: continuous treatment with chemotherapy DA/MA monthly (DNR 40-80 mg per day on day 1-3 or MTN 8 mg per day on day 1-3, and Ara-C 200 mg per day on day 1-7);
2. As2O3 group: 10mg As2O3 daily continuing 28-30 days as a course with 30 days interval between two courses;
3. chemotherapy and As2O3 combination group. The termination of following-up was Sep 30,1998.

## Statistical analysis

Association between pairs of patients' covariates, including individual characteristics and the treatment indicator, were evaluated using Fisher's exact test and generalized exact test. Analysis of DFS and overall survival (OS) were performed with Kaplan-Meier product-limit estimation.

## Results

### Relapsed Patient Group

#### Remission induction
Among 43 evaluable patients, 27 were treated with As2O3 alone, 11 with combination of As2O3 and moderate chemotherapy, and 5 with As2O3 and ATRA. 40 (93%) had a CR and 3 were resistant to As2O3. The CR rate was 96% (26/27) when 27 patients receiving As2O3 alone were analyzed. The overall median time for getting CR was 31 days, with a median total As2O3 dosage of 310 mg.

#### Hyperleukocytosis
During As2O3 treatment, 25 out of 43 relapsed patients (58%) showed increased WBC from $11.9 \times 10^9$/L to $167 \times 10^9$/L (median $37 \times 10^9$/L), after 1 to 43 days (median 17 days). The WBC counts in 11/25 patients

returned to the normal range after undertaking chemotherapy, while those in other 14 cases were normalized spontaneously. There was no evidence of BM suppression during the therapy.

## Side effects

The major As2O3-related toxicities in this group, as listed on Table 2, were skin reaction (rash, itching, erythema) (12/43), gastrointestinal reaction (vomiting, nausea, diarrhea) (10/43), liver dysfunction (11/43), cardiac dysfunction (8/43), facial edema and neuropathy (5/43). Most of these manifestations were modest and could be recovered after symptomatic treatment, further confirming our previous report (10). One patient had high WBC count over 21.3X10$^9$/L at relapse, and developed adult respiratory distress syndrome (ARDS) on day 22 when WBC count was 67.0X10$^9$/L. After the treatment with chemotherapy and dexamethasone, this case recovered and entered into CR. There was no difference in frequency or in extent of side effects between patients treated with As2O3 alone and those with combination therapy (As2O3+ chemotherapy or As2O3 +ATRA).

## Disease-free survival

The estimated DFS rates at 1- and 2- years among 33 evaluable patients were 62.3% and 36.7%, respectively, and the median DFS was 11 months (Fig 1). The estimated 1- and 2-year rates were 75.0% and 51.3%, respectively, while the actual median OS was 13 months (Fig 1). Among possible prognostic factors the disease status prior to As2O3-induced CR

was noted, in that 3/4 patients at advanced stage (the second or third relapse) relapsed again, compared to 13/29 at the first relapse. More importantly, WBC counts at relapse were statistically significantly associated with the clinical outcome, patients with WBC lower than 10X10$^9$/L having DFS curve better than those with higher WBC (P<0.044). For post-remission therapy after As2O3-induced CR, 4 were treated with chemotherapy alone (follow-up: 8-17 months), 18 with As2O3 alone (follow-up: 1-42 months), and 11 with combination therapy (follow-up: 5-38 months). Disease recurrence developed in 3/4 cases treated with chemotherapy alone, 11/18 with As2O3 alone and 2/11 with combination, respectively. The combination therapy thus gave better DFS compared with As2O3 alone (p=0.01).

Among the 16 relapsed cases, two (case 24 and 35) received re-induction with chemotherapy alone due to As2O3 shortage but failed to get CR. Two patients received As2O3 alone and failed. Two abandoned treatment. Among the remaining 10 cases, eight received As2O3 and chemotherapy for re-induction, 4 showed no response and 4 regained CR. Unfortunately, the latter 4 cases also showed poor outcome in that 1/4 censored, 2/4 patients relapsed again within 4 months after remission while an overt relapse occurred in the other one after 15 months. Two cases received ATRA for re-induction. One had no response while the other regained CR. The latter case has been in non-disease survival for 14 months with combined chemotherapy and ATRA as the maintenance treatment.

**Table 2.** Side Effects of As2O3

|  | De novo APL (10 cases)(%) | Relapsed APL (43 cases)(%) | P value |
|---|---|---|---|
| Skin reaction | 2 (20.0%) | 12 (27.9%) | NS |
| Gastrointestinal | 4 (40.0%) | 10 (23.3%) | NS |
| Liver dysfunction | 6 (60.0%) | 11 (25.6%) | <0.05 |
| SGPT (u/L)# | 266 (82-918) | 114 (60-223) | =0.051 |
| SGOT (u/L)# | 109 (58-934) | 65 (45-120) | =0.068 |
| Cardiovascular | 1(10.0%) | 8 (18.6%) | NS |
| ARDS | 0 | 1 (2.32%) | NS |
| Neurological | 0 | 2 (4.65%) | NS |
| Others | 0 | 3 (6.70%) | NS |
| Death due to toxicity | 2 (20.0%) | 0 | <0.05 |

# medium ; NS, not significant

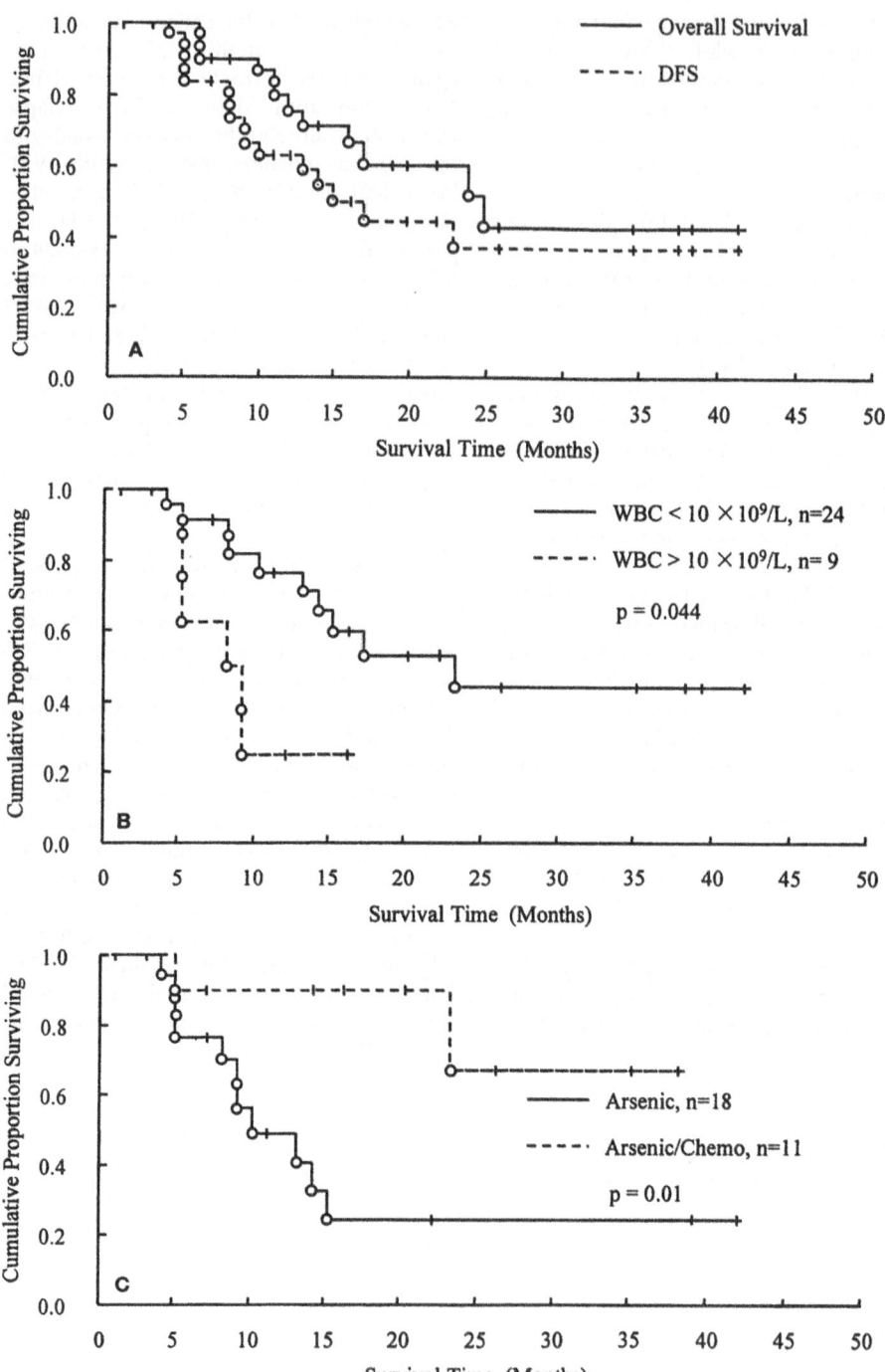

**Fig. 1a–c. a** Kaplan-meier product-limit estimate of disease-free survival (DFS) and overal survival from the time of CR for relapsed patients. **b** DFS in relapsed APL patients with regard to WBC count at relapse. **c** DFS in relapsed APL patients between arsenic group and combination therapy group. Open circles represent completed cases, + represents cencored cases.

Among patients without leukemia relapse, one died of infection while 16 remained in continuous CR.

## Cytogenetics and molecular genetics

Karyotyping was performed and successful in 22 cases at diagnosis. 19 had t(15;17) while only normal Karyotype was found in 3 cases, 29 cases had RT/PCR results at relapse. Among them, one was PCR negative for PML-RARα in spite of the fact that fusion gene transcript was positive at first disease presentation. In another case, both PML-RARα and AML1-ETO were amplified by RT/PCR, but AML1-ETO was the only fusion gene detected by FISH. These two patients showed no response to As2O3 induction, as described above. Among other patients, 4 cases had S-type fusion genes, 1 of whom remained in CR till now, 2 died and the other was out of follow-up. The remaining 23 cases all showed RT/PCR positivity for L-type transcript, among whom 14 remained in CR, 8 cases died whereas the follow-up data were unavailable in the remaining 2 cases. RT-PCR data immediately after hematological CR were available only in 15 cases. Positive PML-RARα fusion transcripts were observed in 14 out of 15 cases, indicating that As2O3 induction of short period was unable to induce a molecular CR in the great majority of patients. It is worthnoting, however, that RT-PCR negative results were obtained in two patients after long time maintenance therapy (41 and 37 months, respectively) with As2O3 alone.

## Newly Diagnosed Patient Group

### Complete remission

Out of 10 patients with newly diagnosed APL, 7 cases were treated with As2O3 and 3 with combined As2O3 and chemotherapy. 8 entered into CR, and the median time to obtain CR was 35 days (range from 30-44 days) with a median dosage of 295 mg. The other two patients died on day 15 after As2O3 treatment.

### Toxic effects

Hyperleukocytosis developed in seven of the 10 de novo patients (70%) with WBC count from $26 \times 10^9$/L to $111.6 \times 10^9$/L (median

$32.9 \times 10^9$/L) after a median of 15 days (range: 5 to 20 days) without any sign of BM suppression. The hyperleukocytosis was declined with moderate chemotherapy in 2 cases and spontaneously in 4 cases. In one case hyperleukocytosis co-developed with liver damage and may be one of the causes leading to treatment failure. Other side effects included skin reaction, nausea and diarrhea, and cardiac effect, as in relapsed patients. However, the hepatic damage occurred in 6/10 patients with elevation of the SGPT ranged from 82-918 u/L (median 266u/L) and SGOT 58-920 u/L (median 114u/L). Among these 6 patients, symptomatic medication was administered and withdrawal of As2O3 was indicated when severe liver dysfunction occurred. 4 patients recovered and the other 2 failed.

### Disease-free survival

5 newly diagnosed patients received chemotherapy for maintenance treatment after CR whereas 2 patients received As2O3 as maintenance therapy. With a median follow-up of 5 months, these 8 patients are still alive (range: 1-13 months).

### Cytogenetics and molecular genetics data

t(15;17) was found in 8 cases when diagnosed whereas cytogenetic analysis failed in 2 cases due to lack of metaphase. All of the 10 de novo APL patients were PML-RARα positive by RT/PCR when diagnosed. RT/PCR remained positive in 4/5 patients when CR was obtained, while it began to convert to negative after 1-3 months' consolidation with chemotherapy in 3 cases.

## Discussion

In this study, we present a clinical research on the use of As2O3 among 43 relapsed APL patients. 93% (40/43) of them achieved CR whereas 3 cases were non-responders. Among these three patients, one had no available cytogenetic and molecular data, the other two had altered genotype of leukemic cells at relapse, as compared with those at first diagnosis, one losing PML-RARα and the other had emergence of a new leukemic clone with AML1-ETO fusion gene. This suggests that the in vivo response to As2O3 could be related to the expression of PML-RARα. In APL cells, PML and/or nuclear body (NB) functions are lost since PML-RARα displaces PML and other NB antigens onto nuclear microspeckles while arsenic could target PML and PML-RARα onto NB and induce them to degradation (14). We found recently that in vitro differentiation-inducing effects at low dose (0.1~1μM) of As2O3 was specific and decisive for APL cells. The hyperleukocytosis comprising partially differentiated granulocytes during in vivo treatment with As2O3 was in strong support to this concept.

The outcome of relapsed APL patients after CR achieved with As2O3 was studied in order to find out possible prognostic factors and what could be the best post-remission treatment. Among 33 evaluable relapsed APL patients, the median DFS time was 11 months, while relapse occurred in 16 patients. As expected, patients at the second or third relapse before As2O3-induced CR seemed to relapse more frequently (3/4) than those at the first relapse before As2O3-induced CR (13/29), although more cases should be studied. More importantly, patients with lower tumor burden as reflected by WBC below $10 \times 10^9$/L showed statistically better DFS than those with higher tumor burden (WBC>$10 \times 10^9$/L). When three different treatment protocols, i.e., chemotherapy alone, As2O3 alone, or chemotherapy/As2O3 combination were compared, clinical outcome seems also to be associated with post-remission therapy, since there was only 2 relapse out of 11 cases in combination therapy group, compared to 11 out of 18 with As2O3 treatment. These results indicate that the combination therapy may be the treatment of choice to prolong the patients' survival.

Eight out of 10 de novo patients achieved CR. This result was comparable to that in relapsed patients or to that achieved by ATRA in de novo patients. An unexpected finding was that toxic effects, especially the liver damage, were much higher in de novo patients than those in relapsed ones. None of the 6 de novo patients with liver toxicity presented abnormal liver functional tests or hepatitis B or C viral antigens and/or antibodies prior to As2O3. The significant difference between the two subgroups could be ascribed to their distinct sensitivity towards the toxic

effects of the drug. Recent data suggested that intracellular anti-oxidant levels may be involved in the defense of cells against arsenite genotoxicity [15]. One possibility could be that in relapsed patients, long-term treatment with ATRA and/or chemotherapeutic drugs could induce or modify some anti-oxidant enzymatic system and enhance the antioxidant ability, so they had better tolerance to arsenic than de novo patients. Another possibility is that patients with higher susceptibility to As2O3 may belong to a special group with reduced ability of drug detoxication and could be already selected out through previous ATRA/chemotherapy. Since remission induction with ATRA in de novo APL patients never gives rise to such a severe liver toxic effect and the retinoic acid syndrome now can be easily handled, we believe that ATRA should be used as the first line drug for remission induction while As2O3 can be incorporated into a multi-drug consolidation/maintenance therapy during remission or as a rescue in relapsed patients.

The previously reported long-time remission in a series of APL patients treated with As2O3 as single therapeutic agent suggested that As2O3 may induce molecular remission. In the present work, we analyzed this issue by using RT-PCR before and after As2O3 induced CR. It was found that immediately after CR, the leukemic clone persisted in 14/15 relapsed patients and 4/5 de novo patients investigated. Therefore, As2O3 induction is not sufficient to induce a molecular remission. Nevertheless, a relatively long DFS (42 and 38 months) with negative RT/PCR was observed in 2 cases in relapsed group, indicating that long-term use of As2O3 alone could indeed lead to a molecular remission in some patients. This result suggests that As2O3 may be more potent than ATRA with regard to maintaining molecular/clinical remission and justifies the including of As2O3 into multidrug post remission treatment in the future clinical trials.

In conclusion, As2O3 treatment can lead to a high CR rate in most relapsed APL patients. The As2O3/chemotherapy combination after As2O3-induced CR in relapsed patients yielded better DFS than As2O3 or chemotherapy alone. Although the therapeutic effect of As2O3 was also confirmed in de novo APL cases, the severe hepatic adverse effects do not support As2O3 to be used as a first line remission induction drug. Finally, long-term use of As2O3 alone is able, at least in a part of the patients, to induce a molecular remission, justifying the investigation of its use in a more appropriate way, so as to further improve DFS in APL patients.

# References

1. Larson RA, Kondo K, Vardiman JW, Butler AE, Colomb HM, Rowley JD: Evidence for a 15;17 translocation in every patient with acute promyelocytic leukemia. Am J Med 76:827,1984
2. de The H, Chomienne, Lanotte M, Degos L, Dejean A: The t(15;17) translocation of acute promyelocytic leukemia fuses the retinoic acid receptor ? gene to a novel transcribed locus. Nature 347:558,1990
3. Tong JH, Dong S, Geng JP, Huang W, Wang ZY, Sun GL, Chen SJ, Chen Z, Larsen CJ, Berger R: Molecular rearrangements of the MYL gene in acute promyelocytic leukemia (APL, M3) define a breakpoint cluster region as well as some molecular variants. Oncogene 7:311,1992
4. Warrell RP Jr, de The H, Wang ZY, Degos L. Acute promyelocytic leukemia. N Engl J Med 329:177,1993
6. Chen Z, Wang ZY, Chen SJ. Acute promyelocytic leukemia: cellular and molecular basis of differentiation and apoptosis. Pharmacol Ther 76:141,1997
7. Zhang TD, Li YS, HuYS, Li MX, Rong FX, Zhang PF, Shun HD, Li HR, Wu YX . Summary of Arsenic trioxide in treating 73 cases of acute promyelocytic leukemia. Meeting Discussion of treating hematological disorders. 1982
8. Li YS, Zhang TD, Li CHW, Zhao XL, Wei ZHR, Tan W, Li RL, Mao YY: Traditional Chinese and Western Medicine in the treatment of 27 patients with malignant lymphoma. Chin J Oncol 10:61, 1988
9. Sun HD, Ma L, Hu XC, Zhang TD: Ai-Lin I treated 32 cases of acute promyelocytic leukemia. Chin J Integrat Chin & West Med 12:170,1992
10. Chen GQ, Zhu J, Shi XG, Ni JH, Zhong HJ, Si GY, Jin XL, Tang W, Li XS, Xong SM, Shen ZX, Sun GL, Ma J, Zhang P, Zhang TD, Gazin C, Naoe T, Chen SJ, Wang ZY, Chen Z. In vitro studies on cellular and molecular mechanisms of arsenic trioxide (As2O3) in the treatment of acute promyelocytic leukemia: As2O3 induces NB4 cell apoptosis with downregulation of Bcl-2 expression and modulation of PML-RAR alpha/PML proteins. Blood 88: 1052,1996
11. Soignet SL, Maslak P, Wang ZG, Jhanwar ,Calleja E, Dardashti LJ, Corso D, Deblasio A, Gabrilove J, Scheinberg DA, Pandolfi PP, Warrell RP: Complete remission after treatment of acute promyelocytic leukemia with arsenic trioxide. The New England Journal of Medicine 339: 6, 1998
12. Chen GQ, Shi XG, Tang W, Xiong SM, Zhu J, Cai X, Han ZG, Ni JH, Shi GY, Jia PM, Liu MM, He KL, Niu C, Ma J, Zhang P, Zhang TD, Paul P, Naoe T, Kitamura K, Miller W, Waxman S, Wang ZY, de The H, Chen SJ, Chen Z: Use of Arsenic Trioxide (As2O3) in the Treatment of Acute Promyelocytic Leukemia (APL) : I. As2O3 Exerts dose-Dependent Dual Effects on APL Cells. Blood 89:3345,1997
13. ISCN Guidelines for cancer cytogenetics (1995) Supplement to an international system for human cytogenetic nomenclature. Basel:S.Karger AG.
14. Zhu J, Koken MH, Quignon F, Chelbi-Alix MK, Degos L, Wang ZY, Chen Z, de The H. Arsenic-inducing PML targeting onto nuclear bodies: implications for the treatment of APL. Proc Natl Acad Sci USA 94:3978,1997
15. Lee TC, Ho IC: Modulation of cellular antioxidant defense activities by sodium arsenite in human fibroblasts. Arch Toxicol 69: 498,1995

# Randomized Comparison of Sequential High-Dose Cytosine Arabinoside and Idarubicin (S-HAI) with or without Chemo-Modulation by Fludarabine in Refractory and Relapsed Acute Myeloid Leukemia

W. Kern[1], A. Matylis[2], T. Grüneisen[3], C. Huber[4], A. Grote-Metke[5], B. Wörmann[6], T. Büchner[7], J. Ohnesorge[1], W.D. Ludwig[2] and W. Hiddemann[1] for the German AML Cooperative Group

*Abstract.* In order to assess the value of the addition of fludarabine as a chemo-modulator to a high-dose AraC based salvage regimen for patients with refractory and relapsed acute myeloid leukemia the German AML Cooperative Group initiated a prospective randomized comparison between fludarabine q 12 hours on days 1, 2, 8, and 9 in addition to the S-HAI regimen, consisting of high-dose AraC q 12 hours on days 1, 2, 8, and 9 and idarubicin on days 3, 4, 10, and 11, as compared with S-HAI alone. Ninety-one patients have entered the ongoing study, 66 of whom are fully evaluable at the present time (median age 54 years, range 20-75). Twenty-five patients had refractory disease or early relapses, 39 patients had relapses after a preceding CR of more than six months duration and two patients had a second relapse. The response rates are CR 45%, PR 3%, NR 32%, ED 20%. Patients with an unfavorable karyotype at diagnosis or at relapse tended to have lower CR rates than other patients, mainly due to a higher NR rate. Autologous peripheral blood stem cell transplantation has been performed in three patients 20 to 70 days after achievement of CR using asservates with 2.9 to 5.5 x $10^6$/kg CD34+ cells. Neutropenia laseted for less than two weeks. Non-hematologic toxicity and infectious complications were acceptable.

## Introduction

Cytosine arabinoside (AraC) is the most active single agent in the treatment of adults with acute myeloid leukemia (AML) and provides the basis for most currently used regimens [35]. A substantial improvement of the antileukemic efficacy of the drug has been achieved both in patients receiving first line combination regimens and in cases undergoing salvage therapy by applying higher than conventional doses of AraC [9,41,48]. Fludarabine has been shown, mediated by pharmacologic interactions with the intracellular metabolism of AraC, to augment the intracellular levels of the main cytotoxic AraC metabolie, AraC triphosphate (AraCTP), in AML blasts both ex vivo and in vivo [25,26]. Following promising results in previous phase II studies applying the combination of fludarabine and AraC [17,22,23,38,51,53,54, 62,69], the current study evaluates this chemo-modulating effect of fludarabine on the metabolism of AraC in way of a prospective randomized comparison of the sequential high-dose AraC and idarubicin (S-HAI) regimen plus fludarabine with S-HAI alone in patients with refractory and relapsed AML.

In previous studies, the incorporation of an myeloablative therapy followed by autologous bone marrow transplantation or by autologous stem cell transplantation into the first line therapy of patients with newly diagnosed de novo AML was evaluated and com-

[1] University Hospital Großhadern, Department of Medicine III, Ludwig-Maximilians-University, München;
[2] Robert-Rössle-Klinik, Charité, Humbolt-University, Berlin;
[3] Krankenhaus Neukölln, Berlin;
[4] Department of Medicine III, Johannes-Gutenberg-University, Mainz;
[5] Evangelisches Krankenhaus, Hamm;
[6] Department of Hematology and Oncology, Georg-August-University, Göttingen;
[7] Department of Hematology and Oncology, Westfälische-Wilhelms-University, Münster; Germany.

pared to conventional consolidation strategies [15,29,32,76]. Most outstanding, the recent results of the British MRC10 trial [15] suggest that the addition of an autologous transplantation to an intensive triple consolidation can significantly increase the disease free survival and might also have an impact on overall survival. Preliminary analyses in patients in second complete remission indicate that an autologous bone marrow transplantation might be feasible [49], however, studies on the mobilization of peripheral blood stem cells followed by myeloablative therapy and stem cell retransfusion in patients having achieved a complete remission after intensive salvage therapy have not yet been reported. The current study therefore addresses the feasibility of mobilizing stem cells and of performing a stem cell transplatation in patients in complete remission after S-HAI ± fludarabine salvage therapy.

The analyses of karyotype abnormalities have yielded further insights into the differential biology of different subtypes of AML and now serve the basis for substantially improved stratification models [11, 18, 19, 24, 31, 39, 46, 52, 58-61, 63, 65, 75]. Hence, the patients' prognosis can be more accurately estimated than on the basis of the FAB subtype and of the possibly not independent factors like WBC count and level of LDH alone and treatment modalities can be evaluated for biologically more homogeneous groups of patients in order to define the most appropriate therapy for the individual case. However, only limited data are available on the impact of cytogenetic abnormalities on the prognosis of patients undergoing salvage chemotherapy [21,27,34]. The most useful stratification model for patients with refractory and relapsed AML is based mainly on the duration of the first complete remission [37] and could recently be refined by the incorporation of karyotype aberrations which had a negative impact on the achievement of a second complete remission and on survival [45]. To improve the prognostic impact of this model and to more accurately characterize the biology and its evolution of the disease in these patients, in the current study cytogenetics are performed both at diagnosis and at relapse.

## Patients and Methods

### Patients

Consecutive patients at ages 18 or older with relapsed and refractory AML who were admitted at the participating centers between april 1996 and february 1999 were eligible for the study. The diagnosis of AML was based on the revised French-American-British (FAB) Group criteria [6]. Refractoriness against standard chemotherapy was defined according to previously established criteria [37]: These included

a) primary resistance against two cycles of induction therapy;
b) first early relapse with a remission duration of less than 6 months;
c) second and subsequent relapse.

Patients with first relapses after six months remission duration were not considered refractory to standard therapy and were included as relapsed AML.

All patients were recruited from the first line trials of the German AML Cooperative Group and had thus received a standardized first line treatment. In patients less than 60 years of age first line therapy consisted in double induction therapy with the sequential application of the nine-day-regimen of thioguanine, AraC, daunorubicin (TAD-9) followed by high-dose AraC and mitoxantrone (HAM). Older patients all received one course of TAD-9 and were treated by a HAM course only upon inadequate response to TAD-9. Patients of all ages who achieved a complete remission (CR) subsequently received TAD-9 for consolidation and monthly maintenance therapy for three years [13,14].

Patients with a preceding allogeneic bone marrow transplantation were excluded from the study. Further exclusion criteria comprized coronary heart disease; heart failure; cardiomyopathy; severe arterial hypertension; abnormal liver function tests (aspartate aminotransferase [AST], alanine aminotransferase [ALT], or alkaline phosphatase [AP] more than three times the upper normal limits; total bilirubin > 2.0 mg/dl); impaired renal function (serum creatinine > 2.0 mg/dl); severe infections; or pregnancy.

## Antileukemic Therapy

Patients meeting the entry criteria were enrolled into the current study and were treated by S-HAI [43] comprizing AraC every 12 hours by a 3-hour infusion on days 1, 2, 8, and 9 and idarubicine 10 mg/m²/day as a 30-min infusion on days 3, 4, 10, and 11, respectively (figure 1). Based on the results of a previous study comparing two dose levels of high-dose AraC [41], patients younger than 60 years with refractory disease, early relapse following a first CR of less than six months, or second and subsequent relapses received AraC at doses of 3.0 g/m² per application while all other patients were treated with 1.0 g/m² AraC per single dose. All patients were randomly assigned to receive fludarabine in addition to S-HAI or S-HAI alone. Patients randomized for fludarabine received the drug at 15 mg/m² as a 30-min infusion four hours prior to each AraC administration, i.e. twice daily on days 1, 2, 8, and 9. To avoid imbalances in the patients´ risk profile randomization was stratified for the following criteria:

a) primary resistance against two cycles of induction therapy,
b) first early relapse with a remission duration of less than 6 months,
c) first relapse with a remission duration of more than 6 months but less than 18 months,
d) first relapse with a remission duration of more than 18 months,
e) second and subsequent relapse.

Based on prior evaluations of supportive growth-factor administration [55], all patients received G-CSF 5 µg/m² subcutaneously starting on day 14, i.e. two days following the completion of chemotherapy. G-CSF was stopped in case of persistance of more than 5% leukemic blasts on a day 18 bone marrow examination or upon recovery of granulocytes to more than 1500/µl. To prevent high-dose AraC induced photophobia and conjunctivitis all patients received glucocorticoid eye drops every 6 hours starting before the first dose and continuing for 24 hours after the last dose of high-dose AraC. Antimicrobial prophylaxis consisted of co-trimoxazol 960 mg po three times daily, colistine sulphate two million units po four times daily, and amphotericin B suspension 40 mg po six times daily.

Patients in CR after S-HAI ± fludarabine therapy were scheduled to undergo an attempt to mobilze peripheral blood stem cells if no related or unrelated donors were available. Stem cells were mobilized within six weeks after achievement of CR with cyclophosphamide 2 g/m² intravenously daily on two consecutive days followed by G-CSF 10 µg/kg subcutaneously twice daily. A minimum of 2x10⁶/kg CD34-positive cells and of 2x10⁵/kg CFU-GM were required to perform myeloablative therapy, which was applied within two months of mobilization. The conditioning regimen consisted of busulfan 4 mg/kg orally daily on days -6 to -3 and cyclophosphamide 60 mg/kg intravenously daily on days -2 and -1. Following the retransfusion of stem cells the patients received G-CSF 5 µg/kg subcutaneously daily until recovery of neutrophiles.

## Study Parameters

Bone marrow examinations were carried out on day 18, i.e. one week after the end of chemotherapy, and upon full recovery of peripheral blood counts. Response to therapy was assessed according to CALGB criteria [74]. CR was defined as a normal cellular bone marrow with normal erythroid and myeloid elements and less than 5% myeloblasts, and with peripheral blood counts of more than 100,000/µl platelets and more than 1,500/µl granulocytes for at least four weeks. Patients with regenerated peripheral blood values but more than 5% and less than 25% myeloblasts were considered to be in partial remission (PR), as were patients fulfilling the bone marrow criteria of CR but without full recovery of peripheral blood platelet and/or white blood cell counts. Patients with persisting leukemic blasts in the bone marrow or blood or with leukemic regrowth within four weeks after initial response were considered as non-responders (NR). Patients dying within six week after the end of antileukemic therapy without evidence of leukemic regrowth were classified as early deaths (ED).

The duration of critical neutropenia was evaluated by the time for granulocyte recovery to more than 500/µl from the onset of S-HAI treatment. The time to CR was measured from the onset of treatment to the date of documented CR and disease free survival from the date of documented CR to relapse or death during remission. Survival and time to treatment failure were measured by the time from the beginning of treatment to death, documentation of persisting leukemia, or relapse, respectively.

Toxicity was evaluated according to the World Health Organization (WHO) grading system [73]. Infectious complications were classified according to the Consensus Report of the Immunocompromised Host Society as reported previously [42].

Cytogenetic evaluations were performed both at diagnosis and at relapse. Karyotype abnormalities were classified according to definitions previously established for the German AML Cooperative Group first line trilas [12,65-67]. Favorable aberrations included t(8;21), t(15;17), and inv(16)/t(16;16) while unfavorable karyotypes were inv(3)/t(3;3), -5/5q-, t(6;9), -7/7q-, 11q23 abnormalities, 17p abnormalities, and complex chromosomal changes ($\geq 3$ numeric and/or structural changes). All other karyotypes, including normal cases, were considered intermediate.

## Statistics

The primary end point of the present study was the impact of the addition of fludarabine to S-HAI on the time to treatment failure as compared to a randomly assigned control group receiving S-HAI alone. The comparison of both study arms was designed to test whether S-HAI + fludarabine could decrease the one-year treatment failure rate of 75% expected for S-HAI by 15%. On this basis a one-sided sequential test with a working significance level of 0.05 was applied [71]. This procedure allowed to detect the assumed superiority of S-HAI + fludarabine over S-HAI with a probability of 90%. The test statistics were calculated after entry of every evaluable patient.

Secondary end points were the rates of CR, NR, and ED, the disease free and overall survival as well as the incidence of hematologic and non-hematologic side effects. Numerical values were compared by the Fisher's-exact-test. Response to antileukemic therapy was compared by an ordinal $C^2$-test. Remission duration and survival was calculated according to Kaplan Meier estimates. Comparisons were carried out using the log-rank test.

## Study Conduct

Prior to therapy all patients gave their informed consent for participation in the current evaluation after having been advised about the purpose and investigational nature of the study as well as of potential risks. The study design adhered to the declaration of Helsinki and was approved by the ethics committees of the participating institutions prior to its initiation.

## Results

### Patient Characteristics

Ninety-one patients were entered into the ongoing study from 24 centers in Germany, 66 of whom were fully evaluable at the time of analyses. Thirty-five patients were randomized to fludarabine in addition to S-HAI while 31 patients were randomized to S-HAI alone. The patients' ages ranged from 20 to 75 years (median 54 years) and did not differ between the respective groups (Table 1). All patients had received prior chemotherapy for their disease as indicated above. Overall, 10 (15%) patients had primary refractory disease and 15 (23%) had early relapses after a first CR of less than six months duration. In 24 (36%) and 15 (23%) cases the relapses occured after a CR of more than six but less than 18 months and of more than 18 months duration, respectively; 2 (3%) patients suffered from second or subsequent relapses (Table 1). The comparison of the profile of disease status revealed a similarity for the two study groups. AML subtypes were predominantly M1, M2, M4, and M5. Karyotypes were classified intermediate at diagnosis in 19 and 18 patients in the fludarabine and control groups, respectively, while the corresponding figure at relapse was 10 and 18 cases. Also, both at diagnosis and at relapse the were no

**Table 1.** Patient characteristics

| | Fludarabine (n=35) | Control (n=31) |
|---|---|---|
| Sex (male/female) | 19/16 | 17/14 |
| Age | | |
| Median/Range (years) | 50/20-75 | 56/24-73 |
| <60 years | 22 | 19 |
| >60 years | 13 | 12 |
| FAB-Subtype | | |
| M0 | 1 | 5 |
| M1 | 13 | 1 |
| M2 | 11 | 12 |
| M3 | 1 | - |
| M4 | 4 | 7 |
| M5 | 3 | 5 |
| M6 | – | 1 |
| n.d. | 2 | - |
| Disease Status | | |
| Refractory AML | 5 | 5 |
| Duration of CR1 | | |
| <6 months | 9 | 6 |
| Duration of CR1 | | |
| ≥6 <18 months | 13 | 11 |
| Duration of CR1 | | |
| ≥18 months | 6 | 9 |
| ≥2$^{nd}$ relapse | 2 | - |
| Karyotype at diagnosis | | |
| Favorable | 4 | 1 |
| Normal / intermediate | 19 | 18 |
| Unfavorable | 3 | 3 |
| n.d. | 9 | 9 |
| Karyotype at relapse | | |
| Favorable | 4 | - |
| Normal / intermediate | 10 | 18 |
| Unfavorable | 5 | 5 |
| n.d. | 16 | 8 |

**Table 2.** Antileukemic efficacy of S-HAI ± Fludarabine

| | n (%; 95% confidence interval) |
|---|---|
| Complete remission | 30 (45%; 33%-59%) |
| Partial remission | 2 (3%; 0%-11%) |
| Non-response | 21 (32%; 21%-44%) |
| Early death | 13 (20%; 11%-31%) |

differences between the two groups with regard to favorable and unfavorable cytogenetic abnormalities (Table 1). All 66 patients received one course of S-HAI therapy only.

## Antileukemic Activity

A bone marrow examination on day 18 was evaluable in 48 cases, in 46 (96%) of whom an adequate reduction of leukemic blasts to less than 5% was achieved. Overall, 30 (45%) and 2 (3%) of the 186 evaluable patients achieved a CR and a PR, respectively, while 21 (32%) cases were NR. Thirteen (20%) patients suffered from ED (Table 2). The sequential analyses of the log-rank test has not yet decided to stop patient recruitment, i.e. it has not yet decided either for superiority of the fluarabine arm or for equal efficacy of both arms. The recruitment of patients is still ongoing.

## Impact of karyotype and remission duration on response rate

Patients with unfavorable karyotypes at diagnosis tended to have a lower CR rate following salvage therapy as compared with other cases (17% versus 49% to 60%), mainly due to a higher rate of NR (67% versus 20% to 30%, Table 3). A similar trend was observed for unfavorable karyotypes at relapse (Table 3). With regard to the duration of the first remission, for patients with a short remission of less than six months duration and for patients with refractory disease the CR rate was lower as compared with other patients (27% to 40% versus 47% to 58%), also mainly due to a higher rate in NR (40% to 60% versus 13% to 25%, Table 4).

**Table 3.** Antileukemic efficacy according to karyotype

| | Karyotype | | | | | |
|---|---|---|---|---|---|---|
| | favorable | at diagnosis intermediate/ normal | unfavorable | favorable | at relapse intermediate/ normal | unfavorable |
| | n=5 | n=37 | n=6 | n=4 | n=28 | n=10 |
| Complete remission | 60% | 49% | 17% | 50% | 46% | 20% |
| Partial remission | - | 5% | - | - | 4% | 10% |
| Non-response | 20% | 30% | 67% | 25% | 36% | 40% |
| Early death | 20% | 16% | 17% | 25% | 14% | 30% |

**Table 4.** Antileukemic efficacy according to duration of first remission

|  | refractory n=10 | CR1 <6 months n=15 | CR1 >6<18 months n=24 | CR1 >18 months n=15 | 2. relapse n=2 |
|---|---|---|---|---|---|
| Complete remission | 4 (40%) | 4 (27%) | 14 (58%) | 7 (47%) | 1 (50%) |
| Partial remission | 1 (10%) | – | 1 (4%) | – | – |
| Non-response | 4 (40%) | 9 (60%) | 6 (25%) | 2 (13%) | – |
| Early death | 1 (10%) | 2 (13%) | 3 (13%) | 6 (40%) | 1 (50%) |

## Hematologic Side Effects

The additional administration of fludarabine resulted in a longer recovery time of granulocytes to more than 500/µl, which amounted to a median of 38 vs. 32 days (p=0.03). In patients achieving a CR the time till CR was longer in patients receiving fludarabine (median, 62 vs. 49 days; p=0.07).

## Non-hematologic Side Effects

Overall, the most frequent non-hematologic side effects were nausea/vomiting, diarrhea, mucositis, elevation of bilirubin levels, and bleeding with no significant differences in toxicity according to WHO grade III/IV. Nausea/vomiting (p<0.01), diarrhea (p<0.01), and CNS toxicity (p<0.05) according to WHO grade I/II/III/IV occured more frequently during fludarabine plus S-HAI. There were no major differences in the freuquency and the severity of the remaining toxicities.

## Infectious Complications

The infectious complications encountered were predominantly fever of unknown origin (FUO, 53%), pneumonia (48%), and bacteremia (33%). Bacteremias were more frequently detected in patients receiving fludarabine plus S-HAI (49% vs. 16%, p<0.01). There were no siginficant differences in the frequency of other documented infections or FUO. However, there were slightly more episodes of pneumonia in patients receiving fludarabine plus S-HAI. Only minor differences occured in the frequency of FUO, sepsis syndrome, septic shock, perianal infections, catheter-related infections, and other infections.

## Autologous stem cell transplantation in second CR

Four patients underwent autologous stem cell transplantation 20 to 99 days after achievement of second CR. The CD34-positive cells, which were harvested in first remission in most cases, amounted to 2.9 to 9.3x10⁶/kg. Neutropenia recovered above 500/µl 8 to 11 days after retransfusion of stem cells and thrombocytopenia lasted for 10 to 35⁺ days. The non-hematologic side-effects encountered during transplantation included WHO III° liver toxicity (1 patient), sepsis syndrome (2), bacteremia (1), and pneumonia (1).

## Discussion

Despite of the addition of novel compounds to AraC-based regimens [3,5,7,8,10,47,56,57, 70,72] and of applying AraC at high doses [9,11,16,36,41,48,50,64], resulting in an improved outcome of patients receiving first line therapy, the prognosis of cases with refractory and relapsed AML remains inferior and warrants the analyses of new treatment strategies [20]. The sequential high-dose AraC and idarubicin (S-HAI) therapy applied in the current study resulted in a 48% response rate, which compares favorably with other intermediate-dose and high-dose AraC based salvage regimens [1,2,4,33,40-42,44,51, 68,69]. On the basis of these results, an analysis of the efficacy of fludarabine as a chemomodulator is performed, however, patient recruitment has not yet been completed.

In order to more specifically assign the individual patient to the most appropriate treatment, the current study aims at improving the stratification model for patients with refractory and relapsed AML, which has been based on the duration of the first remission only, by cytogenetic analyses both at diagnosis and at relapse. As has been demonstrated recently in a multivariate analysis of prognostic factors in 254 patients having received sequential high-dose AraC and mitoxantrone (S-HAM) salvage treatment for refratory and relapsed AML, an unfavorable karyotype at diagnosis seems to have a negative impact on the achievement of a second remission, mainly due to a higher rate of non-response. This might also be true for unfavorable cytogenetic aberrations at relapse, although overall the numbers are quite small. Interestingly, however, these patients are not identical to those with refractory disease and early relapses, which is in accordance to previous results indicating that karyotype and reission duration are independent prognostic indicators for patients undergoing salvage therapy [20,45].

Four patients who achieved a complete remission following S-HAI treatment and who did not have a related or unrelated donor received a myeloablative therapy and an autologous stem cell transplantation. In this preliminary analysis, the encountered side effects were acceptable and, in particular, the hematologic toxicity in this setting was comparable to the autologous transplantation of patients with lymphomas and solid tumors [28,30]. More patients have to be evaluated in large scale studies, however, to specify the role of autologous stem cell transplantation in second complete remission.

# References

1. Amadori S, Meloni G, Petti MC, Papa G, Miniero R, Mandelli F. (1989) Phase II trial of intermediate dose ARA-C (IDAC) with sequential mitoxantrone (MITOX) in acute myelogenous leukemia. Leukemia 3: 112-114.
2. Archimbaud E, Fenaux P, Reiffers J, Cordonnier C, Leblond V, Travade P, Troussard X, Tilly H, Auzanneau G, Marie JP, et al. (1993) Granulocyte-macrophage colony-stimulating factor in association to timed-sequential chemotherapy with mitoxantrone, etoposide, and cytarabine for refractory acute myelogenous leukemia. Leukemia 7: 372-377.
3. Archimbaud E, Leblond V, Michallet M, Cordonnier C, Fenaux P, Travade P, Dreyfus F, Jaubert J, Devaux Y, Fiere D. (1991) Intensive sequential chemotherapy with mitoxantrone and continuous infusion etoposide and cytarabine for previously

4. Archimbaud E, Thomas X, Leblond V, Michallet M, Fenaux P, Cordonnier C, Dreyfus F, Troussard X, Jaubert J, Travade P, et al. (1995) Timed sequential chemotherapy for previously treated patients with acute myeloid leukemia: long-term follow-up of the etoposide, mitoxantrone, and cytarabine-86 trial [see comments]. J Clin Oncol 13: 11-18.
5. Arlin Z, Case DC, Jr., Moore J, Wiernik P, Feldman E, Saletan S, Desai P, Sia L, Cartwright K. (1990) Randomized multicenter trial of cytosine arabinoside with mitoxantrone or daunorubicin in previously untreated adult patients with acute nonlymphocytic leukemia (ANLL). Lederle Cooperative Group. Leukemia 4: 177-183.
6. Bennett JM, Catovsky D, Daniel MT, Flandrin G, Galton DA, Gralnick HR, Sultan C. (1985) Proposed revised criteria for the classification of acute myeloid leukemia. A report of the French-American-British Cooperative Group. Ann Intern Med 103: 620-625.
7. Berman E, Wiernik P, Vogler R, Velez Garcia E, Bartolucci A, Whaley FS. (1997) Long-term follow-up of three randomized trials comparing idarubicin and daunorubicin as induction therapies for patients with untreated acute myeloid leukemia. Cancer 80: 2181-2185.
8. Bishop JF, Lowenthal RM, Joshua D, Matthews JP, Todd D, Cobcroft R, Whiteside MG, Kronenberg H, Ma D, Dodds A, et al. (1990) Etoposide in acute nonlymphocytic leukemia. Australian Leukemia Study Group. Blood 75: 27-32.
9. Bishop JF, Matthews JP, Young GA, Szer J, Gillett A, Joshua D, Bradstock K, Enno A, Wolf MM, Fox R, et al. (1996) A randomized study of high-dose cytarabine in induction in acute myeloid leukemia. Blood 87: 1710-1717.
10. Bjorkholm M, Liliemark J, Gahrton G, Grimfors G, Gruber A, Hast R, Juliusson G, Jarnmark M, Killander A, Kimby E, et al. (1995) Mitoxantrone, etoposide and ara-C vs doxorubicin-DNA, ara-C, thioguanine, vincristine and prednisolone in the treatment of patients with acute myelocytic leukaemia. A randomized comparison. Eur J Haematol 55: 19-23.
11. Bloomfield CD, Lawrence D, Byrd JC, Carroll A, Pettenati MJ, Tantravahi R, Patil SR, Davey FR, Berg DT, Schiffer CA, Arthur DC, Mayer RJ. (1998) Frequency of prolonged remission duration after high-dose cytarabine intensification in acute myeloid leukemia varies by cytogenetic subtype. Cancer Res 58: 4173-4179.
12. Büchner T, Hiddemann W, Wörmann B, et al. (1997) Threapeutic outcome in AML is mainly determined by cytogenetics, LDH in serum, early response and, in a poor risk subgroup, by intensified induction treatment. Blood 90: 504a
13. Büchner T, Hiddemann W, Wörmann B, Löffler H, Maschmeyer G, Hossfeld D, Ludwig WD, Nowrousian M, Aul C, Schaefer UW, Sauerland C, Heinecke A. (1992) Longterm effects of prolonged maintenance and of very early intensification chemotherapy in AML: data from AMLCG. Leukemia 6 Suppl 2: 68-71.
14. Büchner T, Urbanitz D, Hiddemann W, Ruhl H, Ludwig WD, Fischer J, Aul HC, Vaupel HA, Kuse R,

Zeile G, Nowrousian MR, Konig HJ, Walter M, Wendt FC, Sodomann H, Hossfeld DK, von Paleske A, Löffler H, Gassmann W, Hellriegel KP, Fulle HH, Lunscken C, Emmerich B, Pralle H, Pees HW, Pfreundschuh M, Bartels H, Koeppen KM, Schwerdtfeger R, Donhuijsen-Ant R, Mainzer K, Bonfert B, Koppler H, Zurborn KH, Ranft K, Thiel E, Heinecke A. (1985) Intensified induction and consolidation with or without maintenance chemotherapy for acute myeloid leukemia (AML): two multicenter studies of the German AML Cooperative Group. J Clin Oncol 3: 1583-1589.

15. Burnett AK, Goldstone AH, Stevens RM, Hann IM, Rees JK, Gray RG, Wheatley K. (1998) Randomised comparison of addition of autologous bone-marrow transplantation to intensive chemotherapy for acute myeloid leukaemia in first remission: results of MRC AML 10 trial. UK Medical Research Council Adult and Children's Leukaemia Working Parties. Lancet 351: 700-708.

16. Cassileth PA, Andersen JW, Bennett JM, Harrington DP, Hines JD, Lazarus HM, Mazza JJ, McGlave PP, O'Connell MJ, Paietta E, et al. (1992) Escalating the intensity of post-remission therapy improves the outcome in acute myeloid leukemia: the ECOG experience. The Eastern Cooperative Oncology Group. Leukemia 6 Suppl 2: 116-119.

17. Clavio M, Carrara P, Miglino M, Pierri I, Canepa L, Balleari E, Gatti AM, Cerri R, Celesti L, Vallebella E, Sessarego M, Patrone F, Ghio R, Damasio E, Gobbi M. (1996) High efficacy of fludarabine-containing therapy (FLAG-FLANG) in poor risk acute myeloid leukemia. Haematologica 81: 513-520.

18. Cuneo A, Ferrant A, Michaux JL, Boogaerts M, Demuynck H, Van Orshoven A, Criel A, Stul M, Dal Cin P, Hernandez J, et al. (1995) Cytogenetic profile of minimally differentiated (FAB M0) acute myeloid leukemia: correlation with clinicobiologic findings [see comments]. Blood 85: 3688-3694.

19. Dreyling MH, Schrader K, Fonatsch C, Schlegelberger B, Haase D, Schoch C, Ludwig W, Löffler H, Büchner T, Wörmann B, Hiddemann W, Bohlander SK. (1998) MLL and CALM are fused to AF10 in morphologically distinct subsets of acute leukemia with translocation t(10;11): both rearrangements are associated with a poor prognosis. Blood 91: 4662-4667.

20. Estey E. (1996) Treatment of refractory AML. Leukemia 10: 932-936.

21. Estey E, Keating MJ, Pierce S, Stass S. (1995) Change in karyotype between diagnosis and first relapse in acute myelogenous leukemia. Leukemia 9: 972-976.

22. Estey E, Plunkett W, Gandhi V, Rios MB, Kantarjian H, Keating MJ. (1993) Fludarabine and arabinosylcytosine therapy of refractory and relapsed acute myelogenous leukemia. Leuk Lymphoma 9: 343-350.

23. Estey E, Thall P, Andreeff M, Beran M, Kantarjian H, O'Brien S, Escudier S, Robertson LE, Koller C, Kornblau S, et al. (1994) Use of granulocyte colony-stimulating factor before, during, and after fludarabine plus cytarabine induction therapy of newly diagnosed acute myelogenous leukemia or myelodysplastic syndromes: comparison with fludarabine plus cytarabine without granulocyte colony-stimulating factor. J Clin Oncol 12: 671-678.

24. Ferrant A, Labopin M, Frassoni F, Prentice HG, Cahn JY, Blaise D, Reiffers J, Visani G, Sanz MA, Boogaerts MA, Lowenberg B, Gorin NC. (1997) Karyotype in acute myeloblastic leukemia: prognostic significance for bone marrow transplantation in first remission: a European Group for Blood and Marrow Transplantation study. Acute Leukemia Working Party of the European Group for Blood and Marrow Transplantation (EBMT). Blood 90: 2931-2938.

25. Gandhi V, Estey E, Keating MJ, Plunkett W. (1993) Fludarabine potentiates metabolism of cytarabine in patients with acute myelogenous leukemia during therapy. J Clin Oncol 11: 116-124.

26. Gandhi V, Estey E, Keating MJ, Plunkett W. (1993) Biochemical modulation of arabinosylcytosine for therapy of leukemias. Leuk Lymphoma 10 Suppl: 109-114.

27. Garson OM, Hagemeijer A, Sakurai M, Reeves BR, Swansbury GJ, Williams GJ, Alimena G, Arthur DC, Berger R, de la Chapelle A, et al. (1989) Cytogenetic studies of 103 patients with acute myelogenous leukemia in relapse. Cancer Genet Cytogenet 40: 187-202.

28. Goldman JM, Schmitz N, Niethammer D, Gratwohl A. (1998) Allogeneic and autologous transplantation for haematological diseases, solid tumours and immune disorders: current practice in Europe in 1998. Accreditation Sub-Committee of the European Group for Blood and Marrow Transplantation. Bone Marrow Transplant 21: 1-7.

29. Gorin NC. (1998) Autologous stem cell transplantation in acute myelocytic leukemia. Blood 92: 1073-1090.

30. Gratwohl A, Passweg J, Baldomero H, Hermans J. (1998) Blood and marrow transplantation activity in Europe 1996. European Group for Blood and Marrow Transplantation (EBMT). Bone Marrow Transplant 22: 227-240.

31. Grimwade D, Walker H, Oliver F, Wheatley K, Harrison C, Harrison G, Rees J, Hann I, Stevens R, Burnett A, Goldstone A. (1998) The importance of diagnostic cytogenetics on outcome in AML: analysis of 1,612 patients entered into the MRC AML 10 trial. The Medical Research Council Adult and Children's Leukaemia Working Parties. Blood 92: 2322-2333.

32. Harousseau J, Cahn J, Pignon B, Witz F, Milpied N, Delain M, Lioure B, Lamy T, Desablens B, Guilhot F, Caillot D, Abgrall J, Francois S, Briere J, Guyotat D, Casassus P, Audhuy B, Tellier Z, Hurteloup P, Herve P. (1997) Comparison of autologous bone marrow transplantation and intensive chemotherapy as postremission therapy in adult acute myeloid leukemia. The Groupe Ouest Est Leucemies Aigues Myeloblastiques (GOELAM). Blood 90: 2978-86

33. Harousseau J, Reiffers J, Hurteloup P, et al. (1989) Treatment of relapsed acute myeloid leukemia with idarubicin and intermediate-dose cytarabine. Journal of Clinical Oncology 7: 45-9

34. Hayashi Y, Raimondi SC, Behm FG, Santana VM, Kalwinsky DK, Pui CH, Mirro J, Jr., Williams DL. (1989) Two karyotypically independent leukemic clones with the t(8;21) and 11q23 translocation in acute myeloblastic leukemia at relapse [published erratum appears in Blood 1989 Aug 15;74(3): 1180]. Blood 73: 1650-1655.

35. Hiddemann W. (1991) Cytosine arabinoside in the treatment of acute myeloid leukemia: the role and place of high-dose regimens. Ann Hematol 62: 119-128.

36. Hiddemann W, Kreutzmann H, Straif K, Ludwig WD, Mertelsmann R, Donhuijsen Ant R, Lengfelder E, Arlin Z, Büchner T. (1987) High-dose cytosine arabinoside and mitoxantrone: a highly effective regimen in refractory acute myeloid leukemia. Blood 69: 744-749.

37. Hiddemann W, Martin WR, Sauerland CM, Heinecke A, Büchner T. (1990) Definition of refractoriness against conventional chemotherapy in acute myeloid leukemia: a proposal based on the results of retreatment by thioguanine, cytosine arabinoside, and daunorubicin (TAD 9) in 150 patients with relapse after standardized first line therapy. Leukemia 4: 184-188.

38. Huhmann IM, Watzke HH, Geissler K, Gisslinger H, Jäger U, Knobl P, Pabinger I, Korninger L, Mannhalter C, Mitterbauer G, Schwarzinger I, Kalhs P, Haas OA, Lechner K. (1996) FLAG (fludarabine, cytosine arabinoside, G-CSF) for refractory and relapsed acute myeloid leukemia. Ann Hematol 73: 265-271.

39. Keinanen M, Griffin JD, Bloomfield CD, Machnicki J, de la Chapelle A. (1988) Clonal chromosomal abnormalities showing multiple-cell-lineage involvement in acute myeloid leukemia. N Engl J Med 318: 1153-1158.

40. Kern W, Aul C, Maschmeyer G, Kuse R, Kerkhoff A, Grote-Metke A, Eimermacher H, Kubica U, Wörmann B, Büchner T, Hiddemann W, for the German AML Cooperative Group. (1998) Granulocyte colony-stimulating factor shortens critical neutropenia and prolongs disease free survival after sequential high-dose cytosine arabinoside and mitoxantrone (S-HAM) salvage therapy for refractory and relapsed acute myeloid leukemia. Ann Hematol 77: 115-122.

41. Kern W, Aul C, Maschmeyer G, Schönrock-Nabulsi R, Ludwig WD, Bartholomaus A, Bettelheim P, Wörmann B, Büchner T, Hiddemann W, for the German AML Cooperative Group. (1998) Superiority of high-dose over intermediate-dose cytosine arabinoside in the treatment of patients with high-risk acute myeloid leukemia: results of a age-adjusted prospective randomized comparison. Leukemia 12: 1049-1055.

42. Kern W, Behre G, Rudolf T, Kerkhoff A, Grote-Metke A, Eimermacher H, Kubica U, Wörmann B, Büchner T, Hiddemann W, for the German AML Cooperative Group. (1998) Failure of fluconazole prophylaxis to reduce mortality and the requirement of systemic amphotericin B therapy during treatment for refractory acute myeloid leukemia: results of a prospective randomized phase III study. Cancer 83: 291-301.

43. Kern W, Matylis A, Gruneisen T, Huber C, Grote-Metke A, Wörmann B, Büchner T, Ohnesorge J, Ludwig WD, Hiddemann W, for the German AML Cooperative Group. (1999) Modulation of arac by fludarabine: results of salvage therapy by AMLCG. Ann Hematol 78: S5

44. Kern W, Schleyer E, Unterhalt M, Wörmann B, Büchner T, Hiddemann W. (1997) High antileukemic activity of sequential high dose cytosine arabinoside and mitoxantrone in patients with refrac-tory acute leukemias. Results of a clinical phase II study. Cancer 79: 59-68.

45. Kern W, Schoch C, Haferlach T, Braess J, Unterhalt M, Wörmann B, Büchner T, Hiddemann W. (1998) Significance of cytogenetic abnormalities in a multivariate analysis of prognostic factors in patients with refractory and relapsed acute myeloid leukemia. Blood 92: 78a

46. Leith CP, Kopecky KJ, Godwin J, McConnell T, Slovak ML, Chen IM, Head DR, Appelbaum FR, Willman CL. (1997) Acute myeloid leukemia in the elderly: assessment of multidrug resistance (MDR1) and cytogenetics distinguishes biologic subgroups with remarkably distinct responses to standard chemotherapy. A Southwest Oncology Group study. Blood 89: 3323-3329.

47. Lowenberg B, Suciu S, Archimbaud E, Haak H, Stryckmans P, de Cataldo R, Dekker AW, Berneman ZN, Thyss A, van der Lelie J, Sonneveld P, Visani G, Fillet G, Hayat M, Hagemeijer A, Solbu G, Zittoun R. (1998) Mitoxantrone versus daunorubicin in induction-consolidation chemotherapy – the value of low-dose cytarabine for maintenance of remission, and an assessment of prognostic factors in acute myeloid leukemia in the elderly: final report. European Organization for the Research and Treatment of Cancer and the Dutch-Belgian Hemato-Oncology Cooperative Hovon Group. J Clin Oncol 16: 872-881.

48. Mayer RJ, Davis RB, Schiffer CA, Berg DT, Powell BL, Schulman P, Omura GA, Moore JO, McIntyre OR, Frei E. (1994) Intensive postremission chemotherapy in adults with acute myeloid leukemia. Cancer and Leukemia Group B. N Engl J Med 331: 896-903.

49. Meloni G, Vignetti M, Avvisati G, Capria S, Micozzi A, Giona F, Mandelli F. (1996) BAVC regimen and autograft for acute myelogenous leukemia in second complete remission. Bone Marrow Transplant 18: 693-698.

50. Mitus AJ, Miller KB, Schenkein DP, Ryan HF, Parsons SK, Wheeler C, Antin JH. (1995) Improved survival for patients with acute myelogenous leukemia [see comments]. J Clin Oncol 13: 560-569.

51. Montillo M, Mirto S, Petti MC, Latagliata R, Magrin S, Pinto A, Zagonel V, Mele G, Tedeschi A, Ferrara F. (1998) Fludarabine, cytarabine, and G-CSF (FLAG) for the treatment of poor risk acute myeloid leukemia. Am J Hematol 58: 105-109.

52. Mrozek K, Heinonen K, Lawrence D, Carroll AJ, Koduru PR, Rao KW, Strout MP, Hutchison RE, Moore JO, Mayer RJ, Schiffer CA, Bloomfield CD. (1997) Adult patients with de novo acute myeloid leukemia and t(9; 11)(p22; q23) have a superior outcome to patients with other translocations involving band 11q23: a cancer and leukemia group B study. Blood 90: 4532-4538.

53. Nokes TJ, Johnson S, Harvey D, Goldstone AH. (1997) FLAG is a useful regimen for poor prognosis adult myeloid leukaemias and myelodysplastic syndromes. Leuk Lymphoma 27: 93-101.

54. Parker JE, Pagliuca A, Mijovic A, Cullis JO, Czepulkowski B, Rassam SM, Samaratunga IR, Grace R, Gover PA, Mufti GJ. (1997) Fludarabine, cytarabine, G-CSF and idarubicin (FLAG-IDA) for the treatment of poor-risk myelodysplastic syndromes and acute myeloid leukaemia. Br J Haematol 99: 939-944.

55. Patt YZ, Peters RE, Chuang VP, Wallace S, Mavligit G. (1983) Effective retreatment of patients with colorectal cancer and liver metastases. Am J Med 75: 237-240.

56. Pavlovsky S, Gonzalez Llaven J, Garcia Martinez MA, Sobrevilla P, Eppinger Helft M, Marin A, Lopez Hernandez M, Fernandez I, Rubio ME, Ibarra S, et al. (1994) A randomized study of mitoxantrone plus cytarabine versus daunomycin plus cytarabine in the treatment of previously untreated adult patients with acute nonlymphocytic leukemia. Ann Hematol 69: 11-15.

57. Reiffers J, Huguet F, Stoppa AM, Molina L, Marit G, Attal M, Gastaut JA, Michallet M, Lepeu G, Broustet A, Pris J, Maraninchi D, Hollard D, Faberes C, Mercier M, Hurteloup P, Danel P, Tellier Z, Berthaud P. (1996) A prospective randomized trial of idarubicin vs daunorubicin in combination chemotherapy for acute myelogenous leukemia of the age group 55 to 75. Leukemia 10: 389-395.

58. Rowley JD. (1988) Chromosome abnormalities in leukemia. J Clin Oncol 6: 194-202.

59. Rowley JD, Alimena G, Garson OM, Hagemeijer A, Mitelman F, Prigogina EL. (1982) A collaborative study of the relationship of the morphological type of acute nonlymphocytic leukemia with patient age and karyotype. Blood 59: 1013-1022.

60. Rowley JD, Golomb HM, Vardiman JW. (1981) Nonrandom chromosome abnormalities in acute leukemia and dysmyelopoietic syndromes in patients with previously treated malignant disease. Blood 58: 759-767.

61. Russell NH. (1997) Biology of acute leukaemia. Lancet 349: 118-122.

62. Russo D, Candoni A, Grattoni R, Bertone A, Zaja F. (1998) Fludarabine and cytosine-arabinoside for poor-risk acute myeloid leukemia [letter]. Haematologica 83: 281-282.

63. Schiffer CA, Lee EJ, Tomiyasu T, Wiernik PH, Testa JR. (1989) Prognostic impact of cytogenetic abnormalities in patients with de novo acute nonlymphocytic leukemia. Blood 73: 263-270.

64. Schiller G, Gajewski J, Territo M, Nimer S, Lee M, Belin T, Champlin R. (1992) Long-term outcome of high-dose cytarabine-based consolidation chemotherapy for adults with acute myelogenous leukemia. Blood 80: 2977-2982.

65. Schoch C, Haase D, Fonatsch C, Haferlach T, Löffler H, Schlegelberger B, Hossfeld DK, Becher R, Sauerland MC, Heinecke A, Wörmann B, Büchner T, Hiddemann W. (1997) The significance of trisomy 8 in de novo acute myeloid leukaemia: the accompanying chromosome aberrations determine the prognosis. German AML Cooperative Study Group. Br J Haematol 99: 605-611.

66. Schoch C, Haase D, Haferlach T, Freund M, Link H, Lengfelder E, Löffler H, Büchner T, Fonatsch C. (1996) Incidence and implication of additional chromosome aberrations in acute promyelocytic leukaemia with translocation t(15;17)(q22; q21): a report on 50 patients. Br J Haematol 94: 493-500.

67. Schoch C, Haase D, Haferlach T, Gudat H, Büchner T, Freund M, Link H, Lengfelder E, Wandt H, Sauerland MC, Löffler H, Fonatsch C. (1996) Fifty-one patients with acute myeloid leukemia and translocation t(8;21)(q22;q22): an additional deletion in 9q is an adverse prognostic factor. Leukemia 10: 1288-1295.

68. Spadea A, Petti MC, Fazi P, Vegna ML, Arcese W, Avvisati G, Aloe Spiriti MA, Latagliata R, Meloni G, Testi AM, et al. (1993) Mitoxantrone, etoposide and intermediate-dose Ara-C (MEC): an effective regimen for poor risk acute myeloid leukemia. Leukemia 7: 549-552.

69. Visani G, Tosi P, Zinzani PL, Manfroi S, Ottaviani E, Testoni N, Clavio M, Cenacchi A, Gamberi B, Carrara P, et al. (1994) FLAG (fludarabine + high-dose cytarabine + G-CSF): an effective and tolerable protocol for the treatment of 'poor risk' acute myeloid leukemias. Leukemia 8: 1842-1846.

70. Vogler WR, Velez Garcia E, Weiner RS, Flaum MA, Bartolucci AA, Omura GA, Gerber MC, Banks PL. (1992) A phase III trial comparing idarubicin and daunorubicin in combination with cytarabine in acute myelogenous leukemia: a Southeastern Cancer Study Group Study. J Clin Oncol 10: 1103-1111.

71. Whitehead J. AnonymousNew York: Ellis Horwood, (1992) The design and analysis of sequential clinical trials (second edition).

72. Wiernik PH, Banks PL, Case DC, Jr., Arlin ZA, Periman PO, Todd MB, Ritch PS, Enck RE, Weitberg AB. (1992) Cytarabine plus idarubicin or daunorubicin as induction and consolidation therapy for previously untreated adult patients with acute myeloid leukemia. Blood 79: 313-319.

73. World Health Oraganization. AnonymousA handbook for reporting results of cancer treatment. Geneva: WHO publications, (1979)

74. Yates J, Glidewell O, Wiernik P, Cooper MR, Steinberg D, Dosik H, Levy R, Hoagland C, Henry P, Gottlieb A, Cornell C, Berenberg J, Hutchison JL, Raich P, Nissen N, Ellison RR, Frelick R, James GW, Falkson G, Silver RT, Haurani F, Green M, Henderson E, Leone L, Holland JF. (1982) Cytosine arabinoside with daunorubicin or adriamycin for therapy of acute myelocytic leukemia: a CALGB study. Blood 60: 454-462.

75. Yunis JJ, Brunning RD, Howe RB, Lobell M. (1984) High-resolution chromosomes as an independent prognostic indicator in adult acute nonlymphocytic leukemia. N Engl J Med 311: 812-818.

76. Zittoun RA, Mandelli F, Willemze R, de Witte T, Labar B, Resegotti L, Leoni F, Damasio E, Visani G, Papa G, et al. (1995) Autologous or allogeneic bone marrow transplantation compared with intensive chemotherapy in acute myelogenous leukemia. European Organization for Research and Treatment of Cancer (EORTC) and the Gruppo Italiano Malattie Ematologiche Maligne dell'Adulto (GIMEMA) Leukemia Cooperative Groups [see comments]. N Engl J Med 332: 217-223.

# Acute Promyelocytic Leukemia and Pregnancy

A.A.N. Giagounidis, A.S. Giagounidis, M. Beckmann*, M. Aivado, T. Emde, A. Heyll and C. Aul

## Introduction

Observations that vitamin- A- deficient rats develop premalignant epidermal lesions that are reversible with repletion of retinoids (Wolbach et al. 1925) first suggested that vitamin A derivatives might play a substantial role in the differentiation of cells. In 1982, Flynn et al. first introduced 13- *cis*- retinoic acid in the therapy of a patient with refractory acute promyelocytic leukemia. Nowadays, All- *trans*- retinoic acid (ATRA) has become part of the standard induction therapy in APL. However, retinoids are well known to cause severe embryopathy in the first trimester of pregnancy (Lammer et al 1985) and little is known about their effects in later stages of pregnancy.

We report the case of a 23-year- old woman in the 21st week of pregnancy with APL who was successfully treated with ATRA and combination chemotherapy.

## Case report

A 23 year old woman (gravida I, para 0) presented with exertional dyspnea and minor bruising to her gynecologist in her 21st week of pregnancy. Full blood count revealed an anemia (hemoglobin 3,2 g/dl), leucopenia (white blood cell count 800/ul) and thrombocytopenia (20.000/ ul). The differential count showed 68% of lymphocytes, 20% polymorphonuclears, 8% metamyelocytes and 4% promyelocytes. Coagulation studies were consistent with disseminated intravascular coagulation. Electrolytes, renal and liver fun-

ction, uric acid, and lactate dehydrogenase were within normal limits. Bone marrow puncture showed a 60% infiltration with promyelocytes, several of them displaying bundels of Auer rods. Cytogenetic analysis of 23 metaphases showed a normal female karyotype in two, the translocation t(15;17) (q22;q21) and a trisomy 21 in 21 metaphases. These findings were confirmed by fluorescence in-situ hybridisation. Unfortunately, the PML- RARa fusion transcript could not be demonstrated by reverse transcriptase- PCR, as the amount of RNA isolated from the initial bone marrow aspiration was not enough.

Treatment was started with all- trans retinoic acid (ATRA) 45mg/m2/d orally in two doses. Thrombocyte transfusions were used to maintain a thrombocyte count of about 50. 000/ ul. Within ten days the white blood cell count rose to 1800/ ul and the FDP and D-dimers had nearly come back to normal levels. Fibrinogen had risen to 350 mg/dl. Chemotherapy was commenced according to standard induction chemotherapy at day ten of ATRA administration.

Herpes simplex genitalis appeared shortly after the beginning of therapy and was treated wih acyclovir 500 mg tid and tonsillitis due to anaerobes unresponsive to piperacilline plus tazobactam 4,5 g tid was treated by imipenem 500 mg tid. On day 16 after chemotherapy commencement, a repeat bone marrow examination showed a complete remission morphologically, cytogenetically and a negativity for the PML-RARa fusion transcript. However, fever persisted and on day 19 after begin of chemotherapy G- CSF admini-

---

Clinic for Hematology, Oncology and Clinical Immunology
*Clinic of Gynecology and Obstetrics, Heinrich- Heine- Universität Düsseldorf, Germany

stration was started for two days. Leucocyte recovery was prompt and temperatures disappeared at once. We discharged the patient for a week. WBC rose to 12.000/ ul, thrombocytes to 453.000/ ul. On day 30 after the start of chemotherapy and day 40 after beginning of ATRA treatment (26th gestational week), she was readmitted for a further chemotherapy including cytarabine at 1000 mg/m2 bd over 3 days. ATRA treatment was stopped.

This chemotherapy was complicated by *Strep. mitis* septicemia, but treatment with Penicillin G rapidly controlled the situation.

Labour was induced in the 35th week of pregnancy. The vaginal delivery was uneventful. A healthy girl of 47 cm and 2500 g was born. Apgar score was 8 after 1 min and 10 after 5 min.

Cord blood was collected and screened for PML/RARa, which was negative.

9 weeks post partum the patient started with a second course of high dose cytarabine chemotherapy. Bone marrow aspiration at the beginning of this course of chemotherapy still showed complete remission in terms of morphology, cytogenetics and PML/RARa fusion transcript. So far, 4 months later, the development of the child has been without any complications.

## Discussion

Increasing evidence has accumulated over the last decade suggesting that pregnant women with acute leukemia should be treated in the same way than non- pregnant subjects (Aviles A et al. 1988).

In acute promyelocytic leukemia, the introduction of ATRA as an effective, non-myelotoxic drug has dramatically improved the short term prognosis of patients. In pregnancy, however, retinoids have been associated with an increased risk of cranial neural crest defects, and the use of ATRA during the first trimester has been reported to lead to major malformations in about 20% of cases (Lammer EJ et al. 1985, Rosa et al. 1993).

In the case presented here, the patient was 21 weeks pregnant and therefore at the end of her second trimester. Induction of birth was impossible due to the strikingly low survival chances of the child and the unacceptable risk of bleeding to the mother. Reviewing the literature, we identified 13 cases of children born to mothers with APL treated with ATRA. The details are outlined in Table 1. ATRA administration varied from 1 to more than 200 days. Dosage was either 45 mg/m2, or 70 mg per day. Delivery of the children took place between the 29th and 40th week, mothers' ages varied between 18 and 37 years. Three mothers suffered from retinoic acid syndrome and emergency cesarean section was performed. Out of all children treated with ATRA none was born with malformations. In one case ATRA treatment probably induced labour and a non- viable infant was delivered (Sham et al., 1996) This child had previously diagnosed Potter's syndrome. Two children had cardiac symptoms at birth: One had atrial arrythmia which resolved quickly without medication (Terada et al., 1997), while one child had sustained cardiac arrest immediately following birth, but survived without sequelae (Harrison et al., 1994). Two newborn delivered by cesarean section had Apgar scores of 1 at 1 minute and of 9 at five minutes, indicating respiratory suppression due to anesthetic drugs applied to the mother (Maeda et al., 1997, Nakamura et al., 1995). In one case, a patient with relapsed APL was given ATRA as early as in the 3rd week of pregnancy and went into complete remission. ATRA treatment was maintained during the whole pregnancy, while other chemotherapy was not administered. The patient relapsed again in the 30th week, and a normal premature infant was born in the 32nd week. Unfortunately, this patient later failed to respond to further chemotherapy and eventually died of infectious complications (Simone MD et al., 1995). 5 children were born without any complications.

Considering the risk of recidive on ATRA treatment alone and taking into account the available evidence for feasibility of conventional chemotherapy treatment during pregnancy, we opted for a combination treatment of both ATRA and chemotherapy in our patient.

In our case the patient received ATRA for 40 days in a dosage of 45 mg/m2, beginning from the 21st week of gestation. Chemotherapy was commenced ten days later after

**Table 1**

| Author | Mother's age | Week of At diagnosis | pregnancy At delivery | Method of delivery | ATRA dose (mg/m2)/days | CT | Out-Fetal | come Maternal |
|---|---|---|---|---|---|---|---|---|
| Terada | 37 | 29 | 34 | CS | 45/ 19 | none | cardiac arrythmia | CR |
| Lipovsky | 34 | 34 | 38 | ISB | 45/28 | none | uneventful | CR |
| Watanabe | 30 | 28 | 31 | CS | 45/23 | none | respiratory distress | CR |
| Maeda | 29 | 29 | 32 | CS | 70mg/d/13 | mPSL | Apgar1/9, recidivating apnoea | RAS/CR |
| Nakamura | 30 | 30 | 32 | CS | 70 mg/d/12 | none | Apgar1/9 | RAS/CR |
| Simone | 18 | 3 | 32 | CS | 45/>100 | PSN | small for date | relapse |
| Stentoft | 34 | 23 | 32 | SB | 45(22,5)/63 | none | twins/ uneventful | CR/excessive bleeding at delivery |
| Lin | 28 | 14 | 40 | CS | 45/60 | rhG-CSF erythropoetin | uneventful | CR |
| Sham | 29 | 29 | 29 | SB | 45/1 | none | death | Induction of labour |
| Heistinger | n/a | 31 | 34 | CS | n/a | none | uneventful | CR |
| Incerpi | 29 | 24 | 33 | ISB | 45/>30 | daunorubicin | bilat. subependymal hemorrhages | RAS/CR |
| Harrison | 22 | 26 | 30 | CS | 45/30 | none | sustained cardiac arrest | CR |
| Morton | 27 | 13 | 32 | SB | 45/>40 | none | uneventful | CR (PML-RARa negative) |
| present case | 23 | 21 | 35 | ISB | 45/45 | TAD-9/ iHAM | uneventful | CR (PML-RARa negative) |

CS: cesarean section; SB: spontaneous birth; ISB: induced spontaneous birth; mPSL: methyl- prednisolone; PSN: prednisone; rhG- CSF: recombinant human granulocyte colony- stimulating factor; iHAM: intermediate dose cytarabine/ mitoxantrone; numbers after APGAR: index after 1 and 5 minutes respectively; CR: morphological complete remission; RAS: retinoic acid syndrome;

Patient characteristics, treatment results and materno- fetal outcome in 14 published cases of APL in pregnancy and ATRA use.

significant reduction of fibrinogen degradation products and circulating d-dimers. This patient achieved a complete remission in terms of morphology, cytogenetics and molecular analysis of the PML- RARa fusion transcript after 16 days of chemotherapy and 26 days of ATRA. A second course of chemotherapy was applied on day 40 of ATRA administration. Seeing that the patient had achieved complete remission, we stopped ATRA treatment at that point. Regular gynecological control examinations both clinically and by ultrasound revealed no growth abnormalities or malformtions in the fetus. The induced delivery during the 35th week of pregnancy was completely uneventful.

This report shows that aggressive chemotherapy in combination with ATRA is a possible mode of therapy in pregnant patients with APL. Presently, at the age of three months the child does not show any psychomotor abnormality in its development. Further longitudinal studies of children born to mothers who underwent ATRA treatment during pregnancy are needed to clearly assess the risk of long term sequelae.

# References

1. Aviles A, Diaz- Maqueo JC, Talavera A, Guzman R, Garcia EL. Growth and development of children of mothers treated with chemotherapy during pregnancy: current status of 43 children. Am J Hematol 36: 243- 248, 1991
2. Flynn PJ, Miller WJ, Weisdorf, DJ, Arthur DC, Brunning R, Branda RF: Retinoic acid treatment of acute promyelocytic leukemia: In vitro and in vivo observations. Blood 62: 1211- 1217, 1983
3. Harrison P, Chipping P, Fothergill GA: Successful use of all- trans- retinoic acid in acute promyelocytic leukaemia presenting during the second trimester of pregnancy. Br J Haematol 86: 681- 682, 1994
4. Heistinger M, Schumer J, Isak E, van Trostenburg M, Preglau F, Kuen- Kuckenburger B, Karlic H, Geissler D: Acute promyelocytic leukemia (APL) in late pregnancy: Successful treatment with all- trans- retinoic acid (ATRA)- a case report. Onkologie 18 (Suppl 2): 137, 1995
5. Incerpi MH, Miller DA, Posen R, Byrne JD: All- trans- retinoic acid for the treatment of acute promyelocytic leukemia. Obstet Gynecol 89: 826- 828, 1997
6. Lammer KJ, Chen DT, Hour RH, Agnish ND, Benke PJ, Braun JT, Curry CJ, Fernhoff PM, Grix AW, Lott JT, Richard JM, Sun SC Retinoic acid embryopathy. New England Journal of Medicine 313: 837- 841, 1985
7. Lin C-P, Huang M-J, Liu H-J, Chang IY, Tsai C-H: Successful treatment of acute promyelocytic leukemia in a pregnant Jehovah's witness with all- trans- retinoic acid, rhG- CSF, and erythropoetin. Am J Hematol 51: 251, 1996
8. Lipovsky MM, Biesma DH, Christiaens GCML, Petersen EJ: Successful treatment of acute promyelocytic leukaemia with all- trans- retinoic- acid during late pregnancy. Br J Haematol 97: 699- 701, 1996
9. Maeda M, Tyugu H, Okubo T, Yamamoto M, Nakamura K, Dan K: A neonate born to a mother with acute promyelocytic leukemia treated by all- trans- retinoic acid
10. Morton J, Taylor K, Wright S, Pitcher L, Wilson F, Tudehope D, Savage J, Williams B, Taylor D, Wiley J, Tsoris D, O'Donnell A: Successful maternal outcome following the use of ATRA for the induction of APML late in the first trimester. Blood 86 (Suppl 1) 772a, 1995
11. Nakamura K, Dan K, Iwakiri R, Gomi S, Nomura T: Successful treatment of acute promyelocytic leukemia in pregnancy with all- trans- retinoic acid. Ann Hematol 71:263- 264, 1995
12. Rosa FW. Retinoid emryopathy in humans. In: Koren G, ed. Retinoids in clinical practice. The risk- benefit ratio. New York: M Dekker, 1993: 77- 109
13. Sham RL All- trans- retinoic acid- induced labor in a pregnant patient with acute promyelocytic leukemia. Am J Hematol 53: 145, 1996
14. Simone MD, Stasi R, Venditti A, Del Poeta G, Aronica G, Bruno A, Masi M, Tribalto M, Papa G, Amadori S: All- trans- retinoic acid (ATRA) administration during pregnancy in relapsed acute promyelocytic leukemia. Leukemia 9: 1412-1413, 1995
15. Stentoft J, Lanng Nielsen J, Hvidman LE: All- trans- retinoic acid in acute promyelocytic leukemia in late pregnancy. Leukemia 8: 1585- 1588, 1994
16. Terada Y, Shindo T, Endoh A, Watanabe M, Fukaya T, Yajima A: Fetal arrhythmia during treatment of pregnancy- associated acute promyelocytic leukemia with all- trans- retinoic acid and favorable outcome. Leukemia 11: 454-455, 1997
17. Watanabe R, Okamoto S, Moriki T, Kizaki M, Kawai Y, Ikeda Y: Treatment of acute promyelocytic leukemia with all-trans- retinoic acid during the third trimester of pregnancy. Am J Hematol 48: 210-211, 1995
18. Wolbach SB, Howe PR: Tissue changes following deprivation of fat soluble A vitamin. J Exp Med 42: 753, 1925

# Severe Laryngeal Edema in Acute Promyelocytic Leukemia under All-Trans Retinoic Acid

M. Aivado, A.A.N. Giagounidis, A. Rong, T. Emde, A. Grust, A. Heyll and C. Aul

*Abstract.* All-trans retinoic acid (ATRA) has become a valuable agent in the treatment of acute promyelocytic leukemia (APL). However, administration is complicated by the frequently observed "Retinoic Acid Syndrome" (RAS), which occurs in approximately 20-25% of the patients. It is characterized by fever, dyspnea, weight gain, pleural or pericardial effusions, pulmonary infiltrates and hypotension. Given the potentially lethal nature of this syndrome, an early intervention with corticosteroids is imperative.

We report the case of a 24-year-old woman with APL and a hitherto unknown complication of ATRA-treatment: a life-threatening edema of the larynx. She received ATRA (Vesanoid®) 45mg/m_/day combined with standard induction chemotherapy (TAD-9). On day 20 of ATRA medication our patient developed dyspnea and fever. At the same time, there were progressive, painful nodular swellings mainly on the distal part of the extremities.

A computed tomography of the neck disclosed a prominent laryngeal, pharyngeal and parapharyngeal swelling of the soft tissues, which led to a displacement of midline structures and severe narrowing of the trachea.

After discontinuation of ATRA and administration of prednisolon iv. (625mg cumulative dose) the dyspnea almost completely subsided within the next 48 hours. A repeated computed tomography of the neck, one week later, revealed complete resolution of the swelling. We conclude that ATRA can evoke severe, even life-threatening soft tissue swellings in patients with APL.

## Introduction

Acute promyelocytic leukemia (APL) is a rare subtype of acute myelogenous leukemia representing only 5 to 10% of AML cases [1,2]. It is characterized by specific morphological features [3,4] and the presence of the specific translocation t(15;17) [5], which results in two new chimeric genes (RARα /PML and PML/RARα) consisting of the gene for the retinoic acid receptor-α localized on chromosome 17 and *pml*-gene on chromosome 15 [6,7]. The typical clinical presentation is dominated by hemorrhage, due to severe coagulopathy and thrombocytopenia [8].

The abbreviation ATRA stands for all-trans retinoic acid (tretinoin, Vesanoid®), a differentiating agent, which is a member of the vitamin A family (carotenes and retinoids). All-trans retinoic acid induces maturation of the leukemic cells, resulting in a switch to polyclonal hemopoiesis and remission in most cases [9,10,11,12]. A rapid increase in the blood leukocyte count in the first weeks of therapy has been associated with the "Retinoic Acid Syndrome" (RAS), a potentially lethal syndrome, occuring in about 25% of patients with APL and ATRA treatment [13,14]. However RAS is not uniformly accompanied by peripheral blood leukocytosis: A suspicion of RAS should therefore lead to prompt corticosteroid treatment and discontinuation of ATRA treatment [14].

Clinic for Hematology, Oncology and Clinical Immunology, Heinrich-Heine-University of Düsseldorf, Germany

## History

A 23-year-old female patient with acute promyelocytic leukemia was admitted to our hospital in January, 1998. She presented with several hematomas and fatigue, but without any fever, weight loss or night sweats.

On admission, we found pancytopenia (leukocytes 900/μl, hemoglobin 8,5g/dl, platelets 36.000/μl), hypofibrinogenemia (81 mg/dl) and increased fibrin-fibrinogen degradation products (D-dimers 7,7 mg/dl).

## Clinical Course

**Day 1:** Immediately after the diagnosis of an acute promyelocytic leukemia had been confirmed, we initiated the administration of ATRA (Vesanoid®) 45 mg/m$^2$ per day, divided in two doses orally. After normalization of coagulation studies we administered chemotherapy, i.e. a protocol consisting of cytosine arabinoside, daunorubicin and 6-thioguanine (TAD-9) as cytotoxic induction therapy.

**On day 16** of ATRA treatment a bilateral efflorescence developed mainly on the distal extremities. The reddish, nodular papules were about 1 cm (0.5 inch) in diameter, slightly raised and somewhat painful. At this time, the leukocytes were 6500/μl, decreasing from a maximum of 13100/μl the day before, while C-reactive protein (CRP) increased within the same time from 7.5 to 9.5 mg/dl (no fever).

On **day 20** the patient developed, an inspiratory stridor and a mild swelling on the left side of the neck, at the level of the hyoid bone. The leukocyte count dropped to 4900/μl and the CRP rose to 23,6 mg/dl. At this time neither auscultation of the lungs nor a chest-X-ray revealed any pathological findings. We discontinued the administration of ATRA. An exacerbation of symptoms particularly of the dyspnea followed on **day 21**. Therefore a computed tomography of the neck, from petrous bone to the upper thoracic outlet (with application of contrast medium) was performed, which disclosed a prominent laryngeal, pharyngeal and parapharyngeal swelling of the soft tissues (Fig. 1a,b). Its space-occupying effect led to a displacement of the midline structures and severe narrowing of the trachea. The remaining lumen was approximately 1 cm (0.5 inch) in diameter. There was no evidence of an abscess, a phlegmonous inflammation or an extensive hemorrhage as a cause of the stenosis. Therefore, we had to

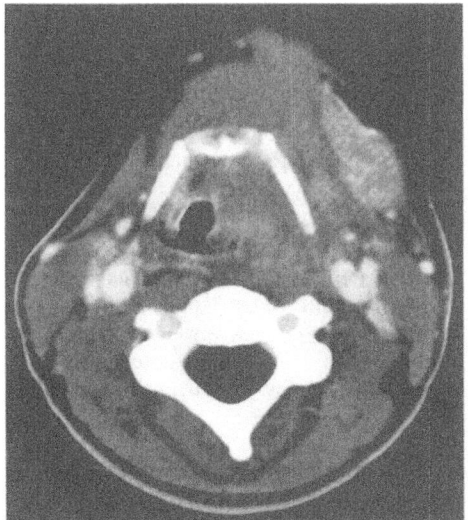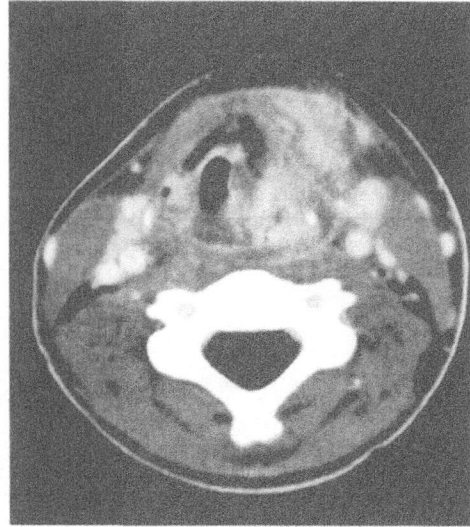

**Fig. 1a,b.** Left-sided, diffuse swelling of the cervical soft tissue with space-occupying effect at the height of the hyoid bone, leading to a deviation of the larynx and hypopharynx. Recessus piriformis is not discernible, the edema of the plica aryepiglottica leads to stenosis of the supraglottic larynx with a diameter less than 1 cm (0.5 inch).

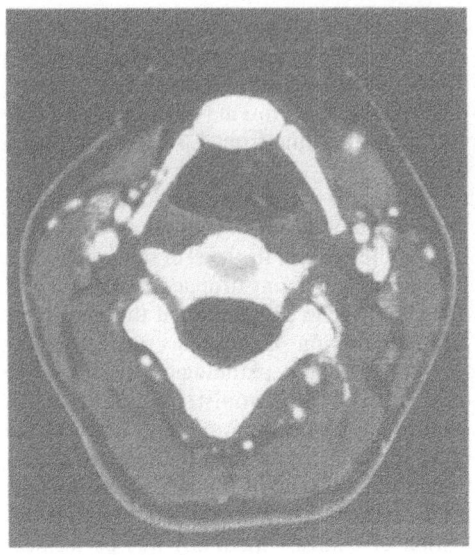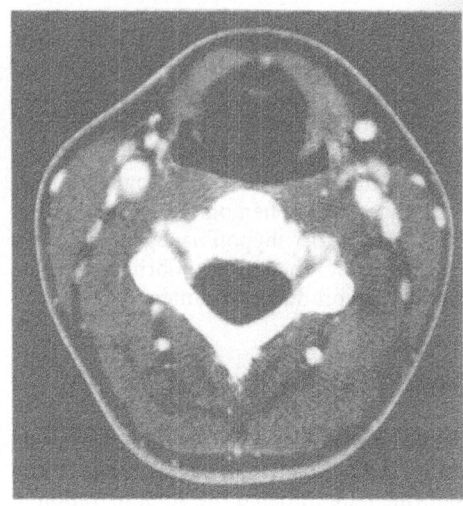

**Fig. 1c,d.** One week later complete restitution after discontinuation of ATRA and administration of Prednisolon 625 mg i.v. (cumulative dose).

consider a leukemic infiltration or a serious side effect of ATRA in our differential diagnosis. We immediately administered Prednisolon (Solu-Decortin H ) 500 mg i.v. and repeated Prednisolon with 125 mg i.v. the next day. The patient began to recover promptly and in particular the dyspnea almost disappeared within 48 hours (**day 23**) after the first administration of corticosteroids. At the same time, the skin rash was virtually gone. The leukocytes (700/μl) and the CRP (14 mg/dl) decreased.

On **day 28** another computed tomography of the neck (Fig. 1c,d) showed a rapid and complete restitution. At this time, leukocytes were 500/μl and CRP 4.6 mg/dl. As the patient recovered quickly, there was no need for further corticosteroid treatment.

## Discussion

During the maintenance chemotherapy, an ATRA-re-challenge was tried out about 5 months after the first ATRA-administration. Treamtment with ATRA was again complicated by fever, a dorsal swelling of the left hand and pain at the right costal arch. All these symptoms immediately disappeared after discontinuation of ATRA and treatment with

corticosteroids (dexamethasone 20 mg i.v., twice a day for three days).

A major problem of remission induction therapy with ATRA is the development of a potentially lethal syndrome called "Retinoic Acid Syndrome", which is usually accompanied by peripheral blood leukocytosis. However, some authors also reported the occurence of RAS in patients with low leukocyte counts and in patients who were in complete remission [14,16]. The syndrome has been described by European and American investigators in about 25% of the cases, whereas in the Chinese experience it has been observed only in a minority of patients (<2%) [15].

Clinical features of the "Retinoic Acid Syndrome" are:

| | |
|---|---|
| – fever | – dyspnea |
| – pulmonary infiltrates | – pleural effusions |
| – pericarditis | – weight gain |
| – edema | – hypotension |
| – lymphadenopathy | – hyperbilirubinemia |
| – renal, liver or multi-organ insufficiency | |

The cause of this syndrome is speculative. Clinically, the symptom complex most closely resembles the "capillary leak" syndrome associated with administration of various (vasoactive) cytokines, particularly interleukin-2

[17]. The ATRA-induced acquisition of migratory capabilities of previously undifferentiated leukemic cells has been discussed as well as integrins, up-regulated by retinoic acid, which mediate leukocyte adherence to capillary endothelial cells and extracellular matrix [15,18,19].

In the prevention and treatment of RAS early onset of chemotherapy has been successful [16]. Several cases were reported, where early administration of dexamethasone alone was sufficient [13,14].

In the presented case the severe larynx edema must be considered as an ATRA-side effect, because it immediately responded to corticosteroid treatment. We conclude, that ATRA can evoke severe, life-threatening soft tissue swellings in patients with APL.

# References

1. Groopman J, Ellman L (1979) Acute promyelocytic leukemia. Am J Hematol 7:395-408
2. Haferlach T, Gassman W, Löffler C, Jürgensen J, Noack J, Ludwig WD, Thiel E, Haase D, Fonatsch C, Becher R, Schlegelberger B, Nowrousian MR, Lengfelder E, Eimermacher H, Weh HJ, Braumann D, Maschmeyer G, Koch P, Heinecke A, Sauerland MC, and Büchner T for the AML cooperative group (1993) Clinical aspects of acute promyelocytic leukemias of the FAB types M3 and M4 Eo. Ann Hematol 66:165-170
3. Bennett JM, Catovsky D, Daniel MT, Flandrin G, Galton D, Gralnick HR, Sultan C (1976) Proposals for the classificatian of acute leukemias. Br J Haematol 33:451-458
4. Bennett JM, Catovsky D, Daniel MT, Flandrin G, Galtan D, Gralnick HR, Sultan C (1980) A variant form of hypergranular promyelocytic leukemia. Br J Haematol 44:169-170
5. Larson RA, Kondo K, Vardiman JW, Butler AE, Golomb HM, Rowley JD (1984) Evidence for a 15;17 translocation in every patient with acute promyelocytic leukemia. Am J Med 76:827-841
6. De The H, Chomienne C, Lanotte M, Degos L, Dejean A (1990) The t(15;17) translocation of acute promyelocytic leukemia fuses the retinoic acid receptor α-gene to a novel transcribed locus. Nature 347:558-651
7. Kakizuka A, Miller, Jr, WH, Umesono K, Warrell, Jr, RP, Frankel SR, Murty VS, Dimitrovsky E, Evans RE (1991) Chromosomal translocation t(15;17) in human acute promyelocytic leukemia fuses *RAR* with a novel putative transcription factor, *PML*. Cell 66:663-674
8. Tallman S, Kwaan HC (1992) Reassessing the hemostatic disorder associated with acute promyelocytic leukemia. Blood 79:543-553
9. Castaigne S, Chomienne C, Daniele MT, Ballerini P, Berger R, Fenaux P, Degos L (1990) All-trans retinoic acid as a differentiation therapy for acute promyelocytic leukemia. 1. Clinical results. Blood 76:1704-1709
10. Chomienne C, Ballerini P, Balitrand N, Daniele MT, Fenaux P, Castaigne S, Degos L (1990) All-trans retinoic acid in acute promyelocytic leukemias. II. In vitro studies: Structure-function relationship. Blood 76:1710-1717
11. Elliott S, Taylor K, White S, Rodwell R, Marlton P, Meagher D, Wiley J, Taylor D, Wright S, Timms P (1992) Proof of differentiation mode of action of all-trans retinoic acid in acute promyelocytic leukemia using x-linked clonal analysis. Blood 79:1916-1919
12. Meng-er H, Yu-chen YS, Shu-rong C, Jin-ren C, Jia-xiang L, Lin Z, Long-jun G, Zhen-yi W (1988) Use of all-trans retinoic acid in the treatment of acute promyelocytic leukemia. Blood 72:567-572
13. Frankel SR, Eardley A, Heller G, Berman E, Miller WH, Dimitrowsky E, Warrell RP (1994) All-trans retinoic acid for acute promyelocytic leukemia. Results of the New York study. Ann Intern Med 120:278-286
14. Frankel SR, Eardley A, Lauwers G, Weiss M, Warrell RP (1992) The retinoic acid syndrome in acute promyelocytic leukemia. Ann Intern Med 117:292-296
15. Sacchi S, Russo D, Avvisati G, Dastoli G, Lazzarino M, Pelicci PG, Regazzi Bonora M, Visani G, Grassi C, Iacona I, Luzzi L, Vanzanelli P (1997) All-trans retinoic acid in hematological malignancies. An update. Haematologica 82:106-121
16. Fenaux P, Le Deley MC, Castaigne S, Archimbaud E, Chomienne C, Link H, Guerci A, Duarte M, Daniele MT, Bowen D, Huebner G, Bauters F, Fegueux N, Fey M, Sanz M, Lowenberg B, Maloisel F, Auzanneau G, Sadoun A, Gardin C, Bastion Y, Ganser A, Jacky E, Dombret H, Chastang C, Degos L and the European APL 91 Group (1993) Effect of all-trans retinoic acid in newly diagnosed acute promyelocytic leukemia. Results of a multicenter randomized trial. Blood 82:3241-3249
17. Margolin KA, Raynor AA, Hawkins MJ, Atkins MB, Dutcher JP, Fisher RI (1989) Interleukin-2 and lymphokine-activated killer cell therapy of solid tumors: analysis of toxicity and management guidelines. J Clin Oncol 7:486-498
18. Springer TA (1990) Adhesion receptors of the immune system. Nature 346:425-434
19. Hickstein DD, Hickey MJ, Collins SJ (1988) Transcriptional regulation of the leukocyte adherence protein beta subunit during human myeloid cell differentiation. J Biol Chem 263:13863-13867

# Extramedullary Acute Promyelocytic Leukemia

G. Specchia, E.M. Pogliani°, D. Pastore, D. Mininni, V. Rossi°, A. Mestice, I. Attolico, and V. Liso

Acute promyelocytic leukemia (APL) is a distinct type of acute myelogenous leukemia (AML) with peculiar morphologic, cytogenetic and molecular characteristics. Although the most common site of relapse observed in APL patients is the bone marrow (BM), extramedullary disease (EMD) is occasionally observed in these patients. Some debate has arisen as to whether treatment of APL with ATRA predisposes patients to extramedullary relapse.

We report 8 patients with extramedullary APL documented by cytologic, phenotypic and molecular analyses among 128 APL adult patients referred to two different hematological Institutions over a period of 10 years. Of 128 patients 69 were treated with ATRA plus chemotherapy (CT) and 59 with CT alone. In this APL series EMD occurred in 8 of 128 cases (6,2%). The extramedullary sites were the skin in five patients, the central nervous system (CNS) in two and the lymph nodes in one. Molecular analysis of the PML/RARa rearrangement was performed on four skin and two CSF samples. All patients exhibited the same molecular pattern in the BM and EMD sites. Relapse was observed in 40 patients, 7 of whom had EMD: 3 had received ATRA plus CT and 4 had received CT alone; 1 patient had developed EMD at the onset of APL. Further studies in large series of patients are needed to establish whether ATRA is in fact responsible for EMD in APL.

## Introduction

Acute Promyelocytic Leukemia (APL) is a distinct type of acute myelogenous leukemia (AML) characterized by peculiar morphological, cytogenetic and molecular findings [1,2].

From 1970-85, Anthracyclines [daunorubicin (DNR) or idarubicin (IDA)] with or without associated cytosine arabinoside (ARA-C) were commonly employed in the treatment of this Acute Leukemia (AL) type [3]. More recently, a high percentage (80-95%) of complete remission (CR) and low incidence of early death in APL has been reported using all-*trans* retinoic acid (ATRA) alone or associated with chemotherapy [4].

Although the most common site of relapse observed in APL is the bone marrow, 44 cases of extramedullary disease (EMD) have been reported in literature [5-17]. Some debate has arisen as to whether treatment of APL with ATRA predisposes patients to the development of extramedullary relapse [9].

In this paper we report 8 cases of extramedullary APL documented by cytologic, phenotypic and molecular analysis among 128 APL cases referred to two different Institutions over a period of nine years.

## Methods

### Morphology

Diagnosis was made according to French-American-British (FAB) criteria [18].

### Cytogenetic analysis

Cytogenetic analyses were performed on bone marrow cells and on cultured fibroblasts

---

Hematology - University of Bari - Italy; °Hematology - University of Monza - Italy

for constitutional karyotype. GTG-banded chromosomes were studied according to the ISCN nomenclature [19].

## Immunophenotypic analysis

Leukemic cell analysis was performed on bone marrow and peripheral blood cells by standard direct or indirect immunofluorescence methods using monoclonal antibodies (MoAbs) directed against CD2, CD3, CD4, CD5, CD7, CD8, CD10, CD11b, CD13, CD14, CD15, CD19, CD33, CD34, CD45, CD56 and HLA-DR (Becton Dickinson). Isotype-matched myeloma murine immunoglobulin was used as negative control at the same concentration as the test antibodies. In selected experiments, double-fluorescent immuno-labelling was performed using the following combination of MoAbs: CD33-PE/CD2-FITC and CD33-PE/CD3-FITC. Flow cytometric analysis was performed on a FACScan flow cytometer (Becton Dickinson Immunocytometry System, Mountain View, CA) equipped with a 0.5 W argon laser emitting 250 mW at 488 nm. The percentage of positive cells was compared to the gated blast cell population; a sample was considered antigen-positive if >20% of the leukemic cells reacted with a particular MoAb.

## PCR amplification of PML/RARa junction

Mononuclear cells were isolated from bone marrow cells by Ficoll-Hypaque centrifugation. RNA was extracted by guanidium thyocyanate cell lysis and caesium chloride ultracentrifugation. PCR amplification of PML/RARa and RARα/PML transcripts was performed as described previously in detail [20]. The primers used were: M2: 5'-AGTGTACGCCTTCTCCATCA-3', M4: 5'-AGCTGCTGGAGGCTGTGGACGCGCGGTAC C-3' as 5' primers and R8: 5'-CAGAACTGCT-GCTCTGGGTCTCAAT-3' and R5: 5'-CCAC-TAGTGGTAGCCTGAGGACT-3' as the 3' primers to amplify the PML/RARα fusion transcript primer. After an initial denaturation at 95°C for 3 min., denaturation, annealing and extension were performed on an automated heat block (DNA Thermal Cycler:

Perkin Elmer-Cetus) at 95°C for 20 s. 65°C for 20 s. and 72°C for 20 s., respectively, for a total of 30 cycles. For detection of the PML/RARα fusion gene, 2 μl of the first PCR product were used in a second round of amplification for a further 30 cycles using nested primer (R8). Finally, 10 μl of PCR mixture was run on a 2% Nusieve agarose gel stained with ethidium bromide and visualized under a UV lamp.

## Case 1

A 17-year-old male presented in December 1987 with acute promyelocytic leukemia (APL) (BM was hypercellular with 88% hypergranular promyelocytes). Cytogenetic analysis confirmed the presence of t(15;17) translocation. CR was obtained after IDA 10 mg/m²/day administered for 6 days. The patient received three consolidation courses according to the GIMEMA Protocol [21]. Ten months later, in October 1988, he underwent a first hematologic relapse (bone marrow). Second CR was obtained after one course of Mitoxantrone (MTZ) 10 mg/m²/day (5 days). In January 1990 the patient presented with tumescence of the left forearm and homolateral axillary adenopathy. Lymph-node biopsy confirmed extramedullary APL relapse. Bone marrow evaluation also showed hematologic relapse. He was treated with DNR plus ARA-C and he achieved CR. The patient underwent autologous bone marrow trasplantation. Hematologic relapse was observed after 3 months and he died in April 1990 of progression of the disease.

## Case 2

A 48-year-old man presented in September 1991. Bone marrow examination confirmed the diagnosis of hypergranular APL with 92% promyelocytes. Cytogenetic analysis confirmed the presence of the t(15;17) and RT-PCR revealed the bcr3 pattern breakpoint in the PML/RARα fusion mRNA. CR was obtained after IDA 10 mg/m²/day administered for 6 days. The patient received three consolidation courses according to the GIMEMA Protocol [21]. He underwent hematologic relapse (bone marrow) 8 months later, in June 1992. Treatment with MTZ 10 mg/m²/day for 4 days was administered and second CR was obtained. He received three consolidation courses with MTZ 6 mg/m² and ARA-C 1g/m² for 4 days. In November 1992, the patient developed multiple erythematous skin lesions, featuring brownish-red papules (2-3 cm in diameter) on the back and abdomen. Biopsy specimens were taken and histopathology showed promyelocyte infiltration; cytogenetic analysis confirmed the presence of t(15;17). Bone marrow examination also showed hematologic relapse. The patient received two courses of DNR 45mg/m²/day for 3 days and ARA-C 200 mg/m²/day for 7 days achieving a partial response. Severe spreading of the skin lesions occurred and in January 1993 he died of CNS bleeding due to progression of the disease.

### Case 3

A 22-year-old woman presented in July 1992. Bone marrow examination confirmed the diagnosis of APL with 93% hypogranular promyelocytes (FAB: M3v). Cytogenetic analysis confirmed the presence of t(15;17), and RT-PCR revealed the bcr3 pattern of PML-RARα fusion transcripts. CR (cytologic and molecular) was obtained after induction therapy with IDA 12 mg/m² for four days and ARA-C 200 mg/m² for seven days. The patient received three consolidation chemotherapy courses according to the GIMEMA Protocol [21]. In March 1994, fourteen months after the beginning of the maintenance course with Methotrexate (MTX) plus 6- Mercaptopurine (6-MP) she developed a single purplish skin lesion in the sacral region. Magnetic Resonance Imaging (MRI) showed dishomogeneous echogenicity with an anechogenous central area and bioptic samples revealed promyelocyte infiltration: evaluation by RT-PCR confirmed the presence of PML/RARα fusion mRNA. There was no cytologic evidence of disease in the BM but RT-PCR analysis revealed the presence of the PML/RARα fusion mRNA (bcr-3). She received treatment with ATRA 45 mg/m² for 50 days combined with ARA-C 1 g/m² and MTZ 6 mg/m² for 6 days. During treatment with ATRA (20th day), cytologic examination of skin lesion in the sacral region showed differentiation of leukemic promyelocytes. She achieved CR; MRI revealed fibrotic residues of the previous lesion and RT-PCR was negative for PML/RARα mRNA. After 2 months the patient underwent allogenic bone marrow

transplantation; she died after 6 months due to non-engraftment and severe infections.

### Case 4

A 25-year-old female affected by APL was observed in August 1992. RT-PCR revealed the bcr1 pattern of PML-RARα fusion mRNA. The patient achieved CR after a chemotherapy regimen including DNR 45 mg/m² for 3 days plus ARA-C 200 mg/m² for 7 days. After one year of CR, she suddenly developed multiple large (>3 cm in diameter) raised skin lesions located on the anterior and posterior thoracic regions, the neck and abdomen. Skin biopsy showed patchy and/or dense promyelocyte infiltration of the dermis and of the sub-cutaneous layer. Cytogenetic analysis of the skin biopsy showed the classical t(15;17) translocation thus confirming extramedullary APL involvement. Nevertheless, there was no cytologic or molecular disease in the bone marrow. We began treatment with DNR 45 mg/m2 for 3 days plus ARA-C 200 mg/m² for 7 days without obtaining significant regression of the skin lesions. Four months after the skin manifestation, relapse occurred in the bone marrow. The patient's clinical conditions deteriorated progressively and she died of cerebral hemorrhage, with concomitant disseminated intravascular coagulation.

### Case 5

A 30-year-old man presented in December 1994. BM was hypercellular with 87% hypogranular promyelocytes (M3v). Cytogenetic analysis confirmed the presence of t(15;17) in all metaphases and RT-PCR demonstrated the presence of bcr1 pattern breakpoint in the PML-RARα fusion mRNA. CR was obtained with ATRA 45 mg/m²/day and IDA 12 mg/m² for four days. The patient received three consolidation courses according to the GIMEMA Protocol [4]. In September 1995, he complained of headache and double-vision. MRI revealed subependymal infiltration of the right frontal lobe. Cerebro-spinal fluid (CSF) cytologic examination demonstrated hypogranular promyelocytes and RT-PCR CSF evaluation confirmed the presence of PML-RARα fusion m-RNA (bcr3). Notably, there was no cytologic or molecular disease in the bone marrow. The patient was treated with

MTX, ARA-C, Prednisone (PDN) intrathecally and high dose ARA-C (3 g/m$^2$ x 2 for 4 days). By the following month, there were no signs of leptomeningeal infiltration at brain MRI and there were no promyelocytes in the CSF. The patient received consolidation therapy with three courses of ARA-C 1 g/m$^2$ plus MTZ 6 mg/m$^2$ for 4 days; MTX, ARA-C, PDN intrathecal therapy monthly and cranial radiotherapy (total dose 18 Gy). In October 1996, seven months after the beginning of maintenance therapy with MTX plus 6-Mercaptopurine (6-MP), he underwent hematologic relapse with negative (cytologic and molecular) CSF findings. CR was achieved after treatment with IDA 12 mg/m$^2$ for four days. He received consolidation therapy with IDA 5 mg/m$^2$ plus ARA-C 1 g/m$^2$ for four days. After 2 months the patient underwent mismatched bone marrow transplantation and he died after 8 months due to severe infections.

## Case 6

A 44-year-old woman presented in April 1995 with APL (BM with 90% hypergranular promyelocytes). Cytogenetic analysis confirmed the presence of t(15;17), and RT-PCR revealed the bcr3 pattern of PML-RARα fusion mRNA. The patient achieved CR with AIDA Protocol (ATRA 45 mg/m$^2$ for 40 days and IDA 12 mg/m$^2$ for four days); she received three consolidation courses according to the GIMEMA Protocol [4]. In February 1996 we observed the appearance of 13 purplish-red tender skin lesions (0.5 cm in diameter) only in the abdominal region. Biopsy of the skin lesions revealed the presence of promyelocytes. RT-PCR showed the presence of PML-RARα fusion mRNA in the skin and BM specimens (bcr3). No cytologic evidence of BM relapse was observed. The patient was treated according to the MEC protocol (MTZ 6 mg/m$^2$ plus Etoposide 80 mg/m$^2$ plus ARA-C 1 g/m$^2$ for six days). After the first course of treatment we observed a marked reduction in the skin lesions (3 lesions of 0.1 cm in diameter). We performed biopsy of the residual skin lesions, which showed no PML-RARα fusion mRNA. The patient was treated with a second course of MEC and she has been in continuous complete remission (CCR) (cytologic and molecular) since May 1996.

## Case 7

In March 1995, a 45-year-old man presented with anemia, leukopenia, thrombocytopenia, fever and rash featuring erythematous multiple plaques with raised borders and hyperpigmentation. Bone marrow aspirate revealed a diffuse homogeneous pattern of blast granular cells with Auer Rods; cytogenetic analysis demonstrated t(15;17) and RT-PCR revealed the bcr-3 of PML/RAR fusion transcripts. A skin biopsy was performed and histologic, immunophenotypic and PCR analyses confirmed extramedullary APL involvement. After treatment with the AIDA Protocol the patient achieved complete hematologic and molecular remission with complete disappearance of the skin infiltration. He received three consolidation courses (4). He is now on maintenance treatment with MTX plus 6-MP (4) and the most recent BM examination confirmed CCR at cytologic and molecular levels.

## Case 8

A 36-year-old man presented in February 1997. Bone marrow examination confirmed the diagnosis of APL with 93% promyelocytes. Cytogenetic analysis demonstrated the presence of the t(15;17) and RT-PCR revealed the bcr2 pattern breakpoint in the PML/RARα fusion mRNA. CR was obtained after induction therapy with AIDA Protocol; then the patient received three consolidation courses according to the GIMEMA Protocol [4]. In July 1998 he complained moderate paresthesias. Cerebrospinal fluid cytologic examination demonstrated hypergranular promyelocytes RT-PCR confirmed the presence of PML/RARα fusion mRNA (bcr2). Bone marrow examination showed only molecular relapse. The patient was treated with MTX, ARA-C, PDN intrathecally and with HAM and he achieved CR at cytologic and molecular levels. Then he underwent mismatched bone marrow transplantation and he is still alive.

## Results and Discussion

Extramedullary involvement in AML is most frequently associated with monocytic leukemia [22[. Extramedullary leukemia (EML) is a rarer observation in the other cytotypes and

**Table 1.** Clinical and laboratory features of APL patients with extramedullary involvement

| Case | Age/Sex | WBC x 10⁹/l | FAB | Evidence of t(15;17) | Immunophenotype | | | | | | Extra-medullary disease (EMD) site | Conco-mitant hematological relapse | RT-PCR detection of t(15;17) | | Interval (months) | Induction Protocol | Disease status |
|---|---|---|---|---|---|---|---|---|---|---|---|---|---|---|---|---|---|
| | | | | | CD34 | CD13 | CD33 | CD2 | CD56 | CD11b | | | BM | EM specimen | | | |
| 1 | 17/M | 32,2 | M3 | 46,XY, t((15;17) | nd | 99 | 93 | nd | nd | nd | LN | yes | nd | nd | 24 | IDA | died |
| 2 | 48/M | 18 | M3 | 46,XY,(15;17) PCR (bcr3) | 83 | 99 | 99 | 20 | 12 | 83 | Skin | yes | + | nd | 14 | IDA | died |
| 3 | 22/F | 39.8 | M3v | 46,XX, t(15;17) PCR (bcr3) | nd | 99 | 99 | 72 | 95 | 7 | Skin | no | + | + | 20 | IDA+ARA-C | died |
| 4 | 25/F | 3.2 | M3 | 46,XX, t(15;17) PCR (bcr1) | nd | 50 | 48 | 20 | 5 | 10 | Skin | no* | - | + | 12 | DNR+ARA-C | died |
| 5 | 30/M | 6.2 | M3v | 46,XY, t((15;17) PCR (bcr1) | 95 | 97 | 97 | 86 | 2 | nd | CNS | no* | - | + | 9 | AIDA | died |
| 6 | 44/F | 4 | M3 | 46,XX, t(15;17) PCR (bcr3) | 39 | 96 | 100 | 19 | 5 | 5 | Skin | no | + | + | 11 | AIDA | alive |
| 7 | 45/M | 10,4 | M3 | 46,XY, t(15;17) PCR (bcr3) | nd | 62 | 54 | nd | 8 | 15 | Skin | - | + | + | - | AIDA | alive |
| 8 | 36/M | 80.7 | M3 | 46,XY, t((15;17) PCR (bcr2) | 2 | 69 | 100 | 7 | 15 | 3 | CNS | yes | + | + | 17 | AIDA | alive |

* cytologic and molecular remission

is particularly associated with chromosomal abnormalities [t(8;21); inv16], cell surface marker positivity to CD2, CD56, CD4, age and high WBC count at presentation [23]. EMD is only occasionally observed in patients with APL. In literature, 44 well documented cases have been reported [5-17, 24-43], 17 of which were evaluated using cytogenetic or molecular methods to demonstrate t(15;17) or PML/RARa rearrangement.

Extramedullary relapse in patients with APL has been said to occur more frequently after treatment with ATRA than after treatment with cytotoxic drugs [9, 38, 40]. Ko [16] suggests that the occurrence of RA syndrome during the treatment is a risk factor. Several biological effects modulated by ATRA have been suggested to play a role in extramedullary leukemic infiltration, such as increased expression of adhesion molecules [45, 46].

In the present series we report eight patients with extramedullary APL among 128 observed patients (Table 1). EM involvement occurred in our APL series in 6.2% of patients, at diagnosis (one) or at relapse (seven); four of these seven cases showed a bcr3 pattern of PML/RARα transcript as detected by RT-PCR, an apparently higher incidence than that observed in the recent prospective series of Italian APL patients [44].

Continuous complete remission in APL patients is now well assessed with molecular evaluation by RT-PCR of PML/RARa negativity in bone marrow aspirates [44]. It is important to note that PML/RARα may be negative in the bone marrow in some patients with EMD of APL, as observed in two patients of our series (cases n.4 and n.5).

In agreement with previous reports [9], the site of EMD most frequently observed was the skin (in 5 of 8 cases). No significant differences in antigen profile were found in APL cases with extramedullary involvement as compared to those relapsed only in BM. We did not in fact observe any clinical or laboratory characteristics of APL at diagnosis which could distinguish patients that recurred with extramedullary disease from those that recurred in the bone marrow only.

In our series of 128 APL patients, 69 received induction therapy at onset of disease including anthracyclines and ATRA and 59 were treated with anthracyclines (IDA - DNR)

with or without ARA-C. We observed 40 relapses of 128 APL patients; 7/40 (17.5%) had EMD: 3 who had received ATRA plus chemotherapy and 4 treated only with chemotherapy.

The Fisher test was used in order to assess any differences between the patients in our series treated with chemotherapy and the patients treated with ATRA; no statistical difference was observed. In none of the patients with EMD and treated with ATRA we observed retinoic acid (RA) syndrome during induction therapy.In a recent review of EMD in APL Wiernik et al. [9] reported the clinical and laboratory characteristics of 26 patients: 7/26 (30%) had received ATRA before the development of EMD; these data suggest but do not prove that EMD in APL may occur more frequently after ATRA than after other therapy. EMD does not seem to have a particular prognostic significance in APL. In our experience, patients with extramedullary relapse have the same chance of achieving a second CR and the same survival rate as patients who relapse in the bone marrow only. In our series of seven patients who relapsed in extramedullary sites, five achieved CR, one a PR and one failed to respond. Of the five patients who achieved a second CR, three are still alive in CR at 34, 28 and 7 months, one died of allogenic bone marrow transplantation (BMT)-related mortality and one died of refractory relapse, three months after autologous BMT.

The data obtained with our series do not provide evidence that EMD APL may occur more frequently after ATRA than any other therapy. Careful surveillance and additional experience in a large series of patients treated with ATRA are needed to establish whether ATRA may be responsible for extramedullary disease in APL.

## References

1. Castoldi GL, Liso V, Specchia G, Tomasi P. Acute Promyelocytic Leukemia: Morphological Aspects. Leukemia 1994;8:1441-6.
2. Grignani F, Fagioli M, Alcalay M, Longo L, Pandolfi PP, Donti E, et al. APL: from genetic to treatment. Blood 1994;83:10-25.
3. Kantarajian H.M., Keating M..J., Waltser R.S. Acute promyelocytic leukemia: MD Anderson Hospital Experience. Am J Med 1986;89:789-97.

4. Avvisati G, Lo Coco F, Diverio D, Falda M, Ferrara F, Lazzarino M, et al. AIDA (All-Trans Retinoic Acid + Idarubicin) in newly diagnosed acute promyelocytic leukemia: a Gruppo Italiano Malattie Ematologiche Maligne dell'Adulto (GIMEMA) pilot study. Blood 1996;88:1390-8.
5. Solano Vercet C, Escudero A, Fernandez-Ranada JM. Meningeal relapse in acute promyelocytic leukemia. Acta Haemat 1982;70:137-8.
6. Pogliani ME, Fowst C, Marozzi A, Salvatore M, Polli EE. Cerebral parenchymal involvement in acute promyelocytic leukemia. Haematologica 1988;73:71-3.
7. Marra R, Storti S, Pagano L. Central nervous system acute promyelocytic leukemia: a report of three cases. Haematologia 1989;22:195-9.
8. Santillana S, Kohatt C, Argumanis E, Vallejos C, Otero J. Double extramedullary relapse in acute promyelocytic leukemia (APL) following treatment with ATRA and chemotherapy. Blood 1996;88 (suppl.1),abstract 3402.
9. Wiernik PH, De Bellis R, Muxi P, Dutcher JP. Extramedullary acute promyelocytic leukemia. Cancer 1996;78:2510-4.
10. Maloisel F, Kurtz JE, Oberling F. Extramedullary acute promyelocytic leukemia. Cancer 1997;79: 2263-4.
11. Evans G, Grimwade D, Prentice HG and Simpson N. Central nervous system relapse in acute promyelocytic leukaemia in patients treated with all-trans retinoic acid. Br J Haemat 1997;98:437-9.
12. Molero T, Valencia JM, Gomez-Casares MT. Central nervous system (CNS) infiltration in a case of promyelocytic leukemia. Haematologica 1997;82: 637.
13. Chen Z, Mostafavi HS, Shevrin DH, Morgan R, Vye MV. Stone JF, Sandberg AA. A case of therapy related extramedullary acute promyelocytic leukemia. Cancer Genet Cytogenet 1996;86:29-30.
14. Kishimoto S, Ishii E, Murakami Y, Takeshita M, Watanabe M, Sakai R, Miyazaki S. Cutaneous infiltration by leukemic cells in acute promyelocytic leukemia of a child after treatment with all-trans retinoic acid. Pediatr Hematol Oncol 1997;14:169-75.
15. Tobita T, Shinjyo K, Yanagi M, Takeshita A, Ohnishi K, Ohno R. Relapse in the external auditory canal of acute promyelocytic leukemia after treatment with all-trans retinoic acid. Intern Med 1997; 36:484-6.
16. Ko BS, Tang JL, Yao M, Wang CH, Chen YC, Shen MC, Tien HF. Extramedullary relapse after all-trans retinoic acid treatment in acute promyelocytic leukemia. The occurrence of retinoic acid syndrome is a risk factor. Blood (ASH 98)
17. Ferrari D, Migliorini L, Cazzaniga M, Brunati S, Copia C, Ferrara F. Extramedullary relapse of acute promyelocytic leukemia (APL) occurring at middle ear level. Blood (ASH 98)
18. Bennet JM, Catovsky D, Daniel MT, Flandrin G, Galton DAG, Gralnick HR, et al. Proposal for the classification of the acute leukemias (FAB cooperative group). Br J Haematol 1976;33:451-8.
19. ISCN (1991) Mitelman F (ed). Guidelines for Cancer Cytogenetics, Supplement to an International System for Human Cytogenetic Nomenclature. Karger: Basel, 1991.
20. Biondi A, Rambaldi A, Pandolfi PP, Rossi V, Giudici G, Alcalay M, et al. Molecular monitoring of the myl/retinoic acid receptor-a fusion gene in acute promyelocytic leukemia by polymerase chain reaction. Blood 1992;80:492-7.
21. Avvisati G, Mandelli F, Petti MC, Vegna ML, Spadea A, Liso V, et al. Idarubicin (4-demethoxydaunorubicin) as single agent for remission induction of previously untreated acute promyelocytic leukemia: a Pilot study of the Italian cooperative group GIMEMA. Eur J Haemat 1990;44:257-60.
22. Baer MR, Barcos M, Farrell H, Raza A, Preisler HD. Acute myelogenous leukemia with leukemia cutis. Cancer 1989;63:2192-200.
23. Krishnan K, Ross CW. Neural cell-adhesion molecule (CD56)-positive, t(8;21) acute myeloid leukemia (AML, M-2) and granulocytic sarcoma. Ann Hematol 1994;69:321-3.
24. Uematsu I. A case of promyelocytic leukemia with leukemia cutis. Intern Med 1970;26:357-62.
25. Bernego MG, Leigheb G, Zina G. A case of acute promyelocytic leukemia with bullous, haemorrhagic and necrotic skin lesions. Dermatologica 1975;151:184-90.
26. Belasco JB, Bryan JH, McMillan CW. Acute promyelocytic leukemia presenting as pelvic mass. Med Pediatr Oncol 1978;4:289-95.
27. Matsumoto K. A case of acute promyelocytic leukemia with skin nodules and mammary tumors during hematologic remission. Jpn J Clin Hematol 1978;19:1211-6.
28. Kubonishi I, Ohtsuki Y, Machida KI, Agatsuma Y, Tokuoka H, Iwata K, et al. Granulocytic sarcoma presenting as a mediastinal tumor. Am J Clin Pathol 1984;82:730-4.
29. Nihei K, Terashima K, Nito T, Imai Y, Aoyama K, Takahashi K. An electron microscopic study of acute promyelocytic leukemia with chloroma. Acta Pathol Japan 1984;34:159-68.
30. Kanakura Y, Yonezawa T, Hamaguchi Y, Otsuka A, Matayoshi Y, Kondoh H, et al. Acute promyelocytic leukemia with an intracerebral mass and meningeal involvement after treatment of non Hodgkin's lymphoma. Cancer 1987;59:94-8.
31. Sawartari T, Kawano F, Akahoshi Y, Asou N, Fujimoto K, Murai C. Relapse of gingival tumor during hematological remission in APL. Rinsho Ketsueki 1989;30:2020-3.
32. Zuiable A, Aboud H, Nandi A, Powles R, Treleaven J. Extramedullary disease initially without bone marrow involvement in acute promyelocytic leukemia. Clin Lab Hematol 1989;11:288-9.
33. Ajarim DS, Santhosh-Kumar CR, Higgj KE, el Saghir NS, Almomen AK, Shipkey FD. Granulocytic sarcoma of the thymus in acute promyelocytic leukemia. Clin Lab Haematol 1990;12:97-9.
34. Rush M, Toth BB, Pinkel D. Clinically isolated mandibular relapse in childhood leukemia. Cancer 1990;66:369-72.
35. Niazi Z, Molt P, Mittelman A, Arlin ZA, Ahmed T. Leukemic dermal infiltrates at permanent indwelling central venous catheter sites. Cancer 1991;68:2281-3.
36. Brown DM, Kimura AE, Ossoinig KC, Weiner GJ. Acute promyelocytic infiltration of the optic nerve treated by oral trans retinoic acid. Ophthalmology 1992;99:1463-7.

37. Longacre T, Smoller B. Leukemia cutis. Am J Clin Pathol 1993;100:276-84.
38. Giralt S, O'Brien S, Weeks E, Luna M, Kantarjian H. Leukemia cutis in acute promyelocytic leukemia: report of three cases after treatment with all-trans retinoic acid. Leukemia and Lymphoma 1994;14:453-6.
39. Thomas X, Fiere D, Archimbaud E. Persistence of retinoic acid sensitivity in relapsed acute promyelocytic leukemia with extramedullary involvement. Leukemia 1994;8:520-1.
40. Weiss MA, Warrel RP Jr. Two cases of extramedullary acute promyelocytic leukemia. Cancer 1994;74:1882-6.
41. Haznedaroglu IC, Ustundag Y, Benekli M, Savas MC, Safali M, Dundar SV. Isolated gingival relapse during complete hematological remission in acute promyelocytic leukemia. Acta Haematol 1995;93:54-5.
42. Lederman CA, Weisberger J, Seiter K, Feldman EJ. Differentiation of extramedullary acute promyelocytic leukemia by all-trans-retinoic acid. Leukemia and Lymphoma 1995;18:189-3.
43. Selleri C, Pane F, Notaro R, Catalano R, Santoro LEF, Luciano L, et al. All-trans retinoic acid (ATRA) responsive skin relapses of acute promyelocytic leukemia followed by ATRA-induced pseudotumor cerebri. Br J Haematol 1996;92:937-40.
44. Mandelli F, Diverio D, Avvisati, Luciano A, Barbui T, Bernasconi C et al. Molecular remission in PML/RARa positive acute promyelocytic leukemia by combined all-trans retinoic acid and Idarubicin (AIDA) therapy. Blood 1997;90:1014-21.
45. Saiki I, Fujii H, Yoneda J, Abe A. Role of aminopeptidase N (CD13) in tumor cell invasion and extracellular matrix degeneration. Int J Cancer 1993;54:137-40.
46. Marchetti M, Falanga A, Giovannelli S, Oldani E, Barbui T. All-trans retinoic acid increases adhesion to endothelium of the human APML cell line NB4. Br J Haemat 1996;93:360-6.

# Chemotherapy and All-Trans Retinoic Acid in Patients >60 Years with Acute Myeloid Leukemia: First Results of the Multicenter Treatment Trial AML HD98-B

S. Fröhling[1], R.F. Schlenk[1], F. Del Valle[2], F. Hartmann[3], A. Glasmacher[4], J.T. Fischer[5], W. Grimminger[6], C. Weber[7], W. Weber[8], U. Gunzer[9], K. Götze[10], K. Döhner[1], R. Haas[1], A.D. Ho[1] and H. Döhner[1]

## Introduction

More than half of the cases of acute myeloid leukemia [AML] occur in patients over the age of 60 (Brincker 1985, Stone and Mayer 1993). In contrast to younger patients, AML in the elderly is frequently resistant to chemotherapy and overall outcome remains poor. The probability of entering complete remission [CR] averages 30 to 50%, median disease-free survival [DFS] is 9 to 12 months, and only 15 to 20% of the patients survive beyond 2 years (Bishop et al. 1996, Dombret et al. 1995, Löwenberg et al. 1997, Mayer et al. 1994, Rowe et al. 1995, Stone et al. 1995, Taylor et al. 1995).

The inferior prognosis results in part from reduced tolerance of myelosuppressive chemotherapy (Champlin et al. 1989, Johnson and Liu Yin 1993, Löwenberg et al. 1989, Rees et al. 1986, Stone and Mayer 1993, Tilly et al. 1990). On the other hand, there are more and more data indicating that AML in the elderly is biologically different from AML in younger patients. The frequency of AML evolving from myelodysplastic syndrome [MDS] increases with age (Aul et al. 1992, Foucar et al. 1985). Additionally, AML in the elderly is often associated with unfavorable cytogenetic abnormalities (Dastugue et al. 1995, Fenaux et al. 1989, Leith et al. 1997, Schiffer et al. 1989, Swansbury et al. 1994, Yunis et al. 1988) and with a high incidence of intrinsic drug resistance of the leukemic blasts, mediated by expression of the multidrug resistance glycoprotein MDR1 or alternative mechanisms (Leith et al. 1997).

All-trans retinoic acid [ATRA] given as induction or maintenance treatment results in improved DFS and overall survival [OS], as compared with chemotherapy alone, in patients with newly diagnosed acute promyelocytic leukemia [APL] (Avvisati et al. 1996, Fenaux et al. 1993, Tallman et al. 1997). In vitro studies have demonstrated that ATRA increases the sensitivity of AML blasts to cytarabine or anthracyclines by down-regulation of the antiapoptotic protein bcl-2 (Benito et al. 1995, Bradbury et al. 1996, Hu et al. 1995, Hu et al. 1996, Hu et al. 1998, Ketley et al. 1997, Yang et al. 1993, Yang et al. 1994). The results of 2 clinical trials indicate that ATRA is effective in patients with AML other than APL (Estey et al. 1997, Venditti et al. 1995).

In April 1998, we initiated a multicenter treatment trial for AML in patients over the age 60 years. The objectives of this study are
i) to evaluate the influence of ATRA given during double induction and early consolidation therapy on the rate of CR, DFS and OS,
ii) to assess the toxicity of ATRA, and
iii) to evaluate efficacy and toxicity of a second intensive consolidation versus a one-year oral maintenance therapy.

[1] Medizinische Klinik und Polklinik, Universität Heidelberg, Germany
[2] Städtische Kliniken Oldenburg, Germany
[3] Universitätskliniken des Saarlandes, Homburg/Saar, Germany
[4] Medizinische Klinik, Universität Bonn, Germany
[5] Städtisches Klinikum Karlsruhe, Germany
[6] Bürgerhospital Stuttgart, Germany
[7] Zentrum für Innere Medizin, Universität Gießen, Germany
[8] Krankenhaus der Barmherzigen Brüder Trier, Germany
[9] Medizinische Klinik, Universität Würzburg, Germany
[10] Medizinische Klinik und Poliklinik, Technische Universität München, Germany

## Methods

### Eligibility criteria

Eligibility was limited to patients 61 years of age or older with the diagnosis of AML or refractory anemia with excess blasts in transformation [RAEB-T] on the basis of bone marrow morphology, cytochemical staining and immunophenotypic analysis. Patients with secondary leukemias after previous chemotherapy or previous MDS were also included. Cytogenetic evaluation of all patients was mandatory. Patients were not enrolled in the study if they were in poor general condition with severe cardiac, pulmonary, hepatic or renal disease.

### Study design

The study design is shown in Figure 1. Randomized induction chemotherapy consisted of two cycles of ICE (idarubicin 12 mg/m² i.v. on days 1 and 3; cytarabine 100 mg/m² i.v. per continuous infusion on days 1 through 5; etoposide 100 mg/m² i.v. on days 1 and 3) with or without ATRA (45 mg/m² p.o. on days 3 through 5, 15 mg/m² p.o. on days 6 through 28) followed by early consolidation therapy with HAM (cytarabine 0.5 g/m² i.v. every 12 hours on days 1 through 3; mitoxantrone 10 mg/m² i.v. on days 2 and 3) with or without ATRA (15 mg/m² p.o. on days 3 through 28). For further postremission therapy, patients were randomized to intensive late consolidation therapy (idarubicin 12 mg/m² i.v. on days 1 and 3; etoposide 100 mg/m² i.v. on days 1 through 5) or 12 monthly courses of outpatient maintenance therapy (idarubicin 5 mg p.o. on days 1, 4, 7, 10, 13; etoposide 100 mg p.o. on days 1 and 13). Patients who failed to achieve CR after ICE I/A-ICE I received one cycle of A-HAE (cytarabine 0.5 g/m² i.v. every 12 hours on days 1 through 3; etoposide 250 mg/m² i.v. per continuous infusion on days 4 and 5; ATRA 45 mg/m² p.o. on days 3 through 5, 15 mg/m² p.o. on days 6 through 28).

## Results

### Accrual

At present, 49 patients (median age, 65 years; range, 61 to 83) from 10 centers have been registered. Twelve patients were excluded from analysis: 3 had diagnoses other than AML, 8 patients were in poor clinical condition, and 1 patient refused written informed consent. In a pilot phase, 15 patients were treated with the ATRA-containing regimen. Thus, 22 patients were randomly assigned to receive either A-ICE or ICE. Five patients were randomized between intensive late consolidation and maintenance therapy; 4 patients have completed treatment.

### Induction therapy

#### Toxic Effects of ATRA
Toxicity was mild. Side effects occurred during the first course of A-ICE and included

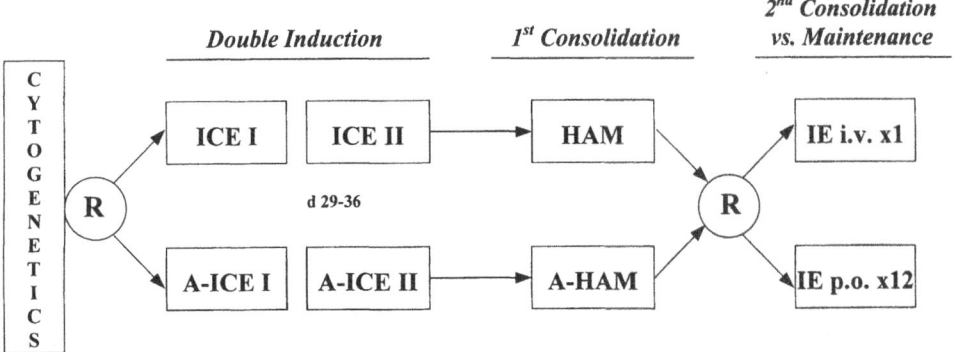

**Fig. 1.** Design of the treatment trial AML HD98-B

unexplained fever (n=1) and headache (n=1). Bone pain required dose reduction in 1 patient. One patient developed cutaneous vasculitis. One patient with several risk factors for coronary artery disease (cigarette smoking, family history of coronary heart disease) died of myocardial infarction. Signs or symptoms suggestive of the retinoic acid syndrome (defined as unexplained fever, weight gain, respiratory distress, interstitial pulmonary infiltrates, and pleural or pericardial effusions; Frankel et al. 1992) were not observed.

### Complete Remission and Induction Failures

Fourteen of the 37 eligible patients (38%) achieved a CR. Nineteen patients (51%) had resistant disease [RD]. There were 4 deaths (11%) within 28 days among the 37 patients who could be evaluated. One patient died of myocardial infarction, 2 patients died of bacterial pneumonia, and 1 of progressive leukemia.

## Discussion

The preliminary results of this ongoing trial show that the addition of ATRA to induction and consolidation chemotherapy is feasible and not associated with excess toxicity. Of the 26 patients assigned to an ATRA-containing regimen, 4 (15%) experienced minor toxic effects (fever, headache, bone pain, cutaneous vasculitis). One patient without a documented history of coronary artery disease died of myocardial infarction. Although this patient had preexisting cardiovascular risk factors, the administration of ATRA may have contributed to the coronary event. Several reports indicate that ATRA increases the frequency of thromboembolic events in patients with APL (Hashimoto et al. 1994, Pogliani et al. 1997). In one study, thrombotic events were more common in patients suspected of having ATRA syndrome (Escudier et al. 1996). The incidence of toxic effects we observed with ATRA, particularly with regard to the retinoic acid syndrome, is lower than the rates reported in several studies of the drug in APL (Avvisati et al. 1996, de Botton et al. 1998, Tallman et al. 1997). Intrinsic biologic differences between APL and non-APL AML, silmultaneous administration of ATRA and chemo-

therapy (Avvisati et al. 1996), and the strategy of using a lower dose of ATRA might be responsible for this effect. In a randomized trial, Chen and colleagues treated 27 cases of newly diagnosed APL with low-dose ATRA (15 mg/m$^2$ p.o.). Twenty-four of the 26 evaluable patients (92%) achieved a CR. Cases of the retinoic acid syndrome were not observed (Chen et al. 1996).

Two clinical trials have previously addressed the question whether the addition of ATRA to conventional chemotherapy improves outcome (i.e. CR rate, DFS and OS) in patients over 60 years of age with AML other than APL. Venditti and co-workers observed a CR rate of 48% in patients with 'poor prognosis' AML (advanced age, poor clinical condition, other severe diseases associated with organ failure) treated with ATRA and low-dose cytarabine (Venditti et al. 1995). The median duration of CR was 34.4 weeks. Mild to moderate hematologic toxicity was the most common adverse effect. In 1997, Estey and colleagues reported that the addition of ATRA ± granulocyte colony-stimulating factor [G-CSF] to fludarabine, cytarabine and idarubicin [FAI] resulted in longer DFS and OS in patients with 'poor prognosis' non-APL AML or MDS (age >70 years, history of abnormal blood counts, secondary AML or MDS, failure to respond to one course of anthracycline + cytarabine, abnormal hepatic or renal function) (Estey et al. 1997). However, after a longer follow-up period and randomization of a total of 215 patients the addition of ATRA ± G-CSF to FAI had no effect on CR rate, DFS and OS (Estey et al. 1999). In the latter study, ATRA (45 mg/m$^2$ p.o.) was given over 10 days starting on day -2 prior to chemotherapy. Based upon the observation that ATRA increases chemosensitivity of AML blast cells to cytarabine or anthracyclines when it is given after these drugs (Hu et al. 1995, Hu et al. 1996, Yang et al. 1993, Yang et al. 1994), we administered ATRA on days 3 through 5 (45 mg/m$^2$ p.o.) and on days 6 through 28 (15 mg/m$^2$ p.o.), respectively.

The median follow-up period in our study is too short to provide an analysis of DFS and OS. We plan to enroll 200 patients to answer the question whether the addition of ATRA to conventional chemotherapy will result in an improvement of CR rate, DFS and OS in patients over 60 years of age with AML. Cytogenetic analysis may help to identify patients who benefit from this novel therapeutic approach and those who do not.

# References

1. Aul C, Gattermann N, Schneider W (1992) Age-related incidence and other epidemiological aspects of myelodysplastic syndromes. Br J Haematol 82: 358-367
2. Avvisati G, Lo-Coco F, Diverio D, Falda M, Ferrara F, Lazzarino M, Russo D, Petti MC, Mandelli F (1996) AIDA (all-*trans* retinoic acid + idarubicin) in newly diagnosed acute promyelocytic leukemia: a Gruppo Italiano Malattie Ematologiche Maligne dell'Adulto (GIMEMA) pilot study. Blood 88: 1390-1398
3. Benito A, Grillot D, Nunez G, Fernandez-Luna JL (1995) Regulation and function of Bcl-2 during differentiation-induced cell death in HL-60 promyelocytic cells. Am J Pathol 146: 481-490
4. Bishop JF, Matthews JP, Young GA, Szer J, Gillett A, Joshua D, Bradstock K, Enno A, Wolf MM, Fox R, Cobcroft R, Herrmann R, van der Weyden M, Lowenthal RM, Page F, Garson OM, Juneja S (1996) A randomized study of high-dose cytarabine in induction in acute myeloid leukemia. Blood 87: 1710-1717
5. de Botton S, Dombret H, Sanz M, Miguel JS, Caillot D, Zittoun R, Gardembas M, Stamatoulas A, Conde E, Guerci A, Gardin C, Geiser K, Makhoul DC, Reman O, de la Serna J, Lefrere F, Chomienne C, Chastang C, Degos L, Fenaux P (1998) Incidence, clinical features, and outcome of all-*trans* retinoic acid syndrome in 413 cases of newly diagnosed acute promyelocytic leukemia. The European APL Group. Blood 92: 2712-2718
6. Bradbury DA, Aldington S, Zhu YM, Russell NH (1996) Down-regulation of bcl-2 in AML blasts by all-*trans* retinoic acid and its relationship to CD34 antigen expression. Br J Haematol 94: 671-675
7. Brincker H (1985) Estimate of overall treatment results in acute nonlymphocytic leukemia based on age-specific rates of incidence and of complete remission. Cancer Treat Rep 69: 5-11
8. Champlin RE, Gajewski JL, Golde DW (1989) Treatment of acute myelogenous leukemia in the elderly. Semin Oncol 16: 51-56
9. Chen GQ, Shen ZX, Wu F, Han JY, Miao JM, Zhong HJ, Li XS, Zhao JQ, Zhu J, Fang ZW, Chen SJ, Chen Z, Wang ZY (1996) Pharmacokinetics and efficacy of low-dose all-*trans* retinoic acid in the treatment of acute promyelocytic leukemia. Leukemia 10: 825-828
10. Dastugue N, Payen C, Lafage-Pochitaloff M, Bernard P, Leroux D, Huguet-Rigal F, Stoppa AM, Marit G, Molina L, Michallet M, et al. (1995) Prognostic significance of karyotype in *de novo* adult acute myeloid leukemia. The BGMT Group. Leukemia 9: 1491-1498
11. Dombret H, Chastang C, Fenaux P, Reiffers J, Bordessoule D, Bouabdallah R, Mandelli F, Ferrant A, Auzanneau G, Tilly H, Yver A, Degos L (1995) A controlled study of recombinant human granulocyte colony-stimulating factor in elderly patients after treatment for acute myelogenous leukemia. N Engl J Med 332:1678-1683
12. Escudier SM, Kantarjian HM, Estey EH (1996) Thrombosis in patients with acute promyelocytic leukemia treated with and without all-*trans* retinoic acid. Leuk Lymphoma 20: 435-439
13. Estey E, Beran M, Pierce S, Kantarjian H, Keating M (1997) All-*trans* retinoic acid (ATRA) may improve results of chemotherapy in poor prognosis non-APL AML and MDS: a randomized study. Blood 90 (Suppl 1): 416a (abstract)
14. Estey EH, Thall PF, Pierce S, Cortes J, Beran M, Kantarjian H, Keating MJ, Andreef M, Freireich E (1999) Randomized phase II study of fludarabine + cytosine arabinoside + idarubicin ± all-*trans* retinoic acid ± granulocyte-colony stimulating factor in poor-prognosis newly-diagnosed non-APL AML and MDS. Blood, in press
15. Fenaux P, le Deley MC, Castaigne S, Archimbaud E, Chomienne C, Link H, Guerci A, Duarte M, Daniel MT, Bowen D, et al. (1993) Effect of all-*trans* retinoic acid in newly diagnosed acute promyelocytic leukemia. Results of a multicenter randomized trial. European APL 91 Group. Blood 82: 3241-3249
16. Fenaux P, Preudhomme C, Lai JL, Morel P, Beuscart R, Bauters F (1989) Cytogenetics and their prognostic value in *de novo* acute myeloid leukaemia: a report on 283 cases. Br J Haematol 73: 61-67
17. Foucar K, Langdon RM, Armitage JO, Olson DB, Carroll TJ (1985) Myelodysplastic syndromes. A clinical and pathologic analysis of 109 cases. Cancer 56: 553-561
18. Frankel SR, Eardley A, Lauwers G, Weiss M, Warrell AP (1992) The "retinoic acid syndrome" in acute promyelocytic leukemia. Ann Intern Med 117: 292-296
19. Hashimoto S, Koike T, Tatewaki W, Seki Y, Sato N, Azegami T, Tsukada N, Takahashi H, Kimura H, Ueno M, et al. (1994) Fatal thromboembolism in acute promyelocytic leukemia during all-*trans* retinoic acid therapy combined with antifibrinolytic therapy for prophylaxis of hemorrhage. Leukemia 8: 1113-1115
20. Hu ZB, Minden MD, McCulloch EA (1995) Direct evidence for the participation of bcl-2 in the regulation by retinoic acid of the Ara-C sensitivity of leukemic stem cells. Leukemia 9: 1667-1675
21. Hu ZB, Minden MD, McCulloch EA (1996) Post-transcriptional regulation of bcl-2 in acute myeloblastic leukemia: significance for response to chemotherapy. Leukemia 10: 410-416
22. Hu ZB, Minden MD, McCulloch EA (1998) Phosphorylation of BCL-2 after exposure of human leukemic cells to retinoic acid. Blood 92: 1768-1775
23. Johnson PR, Liu Yin JA (1993) Acute myeloid leukaemia in the elderly: biology and treatment. Br J Haematol 83: 1-6
24. Ketley NJ, Allen PD, Kelsey SM, Newland AC (1997) Modulation of idarubicin-induced apoptosis in human acute myeloid leukemia blasts by all-*trans* retinoic acid, 1,25(OH)$_2$ vitamin D3, and granulocyte-macrophage colony-stimulating factor. Blood 90: 4578-4587

25. Leith CP, Kopecky KJ, Godwin J, McConnell T, Slovak ML, Chen IM, Head DR, Appelbaum FR, Willman CL (1997) Acute myeloid leukemia in the elderly: assessment of multidrug resistance (MDR1) and cytogenetics distinguishes biologic subgroups with remarkably distinct responses to standard chemotherapy. A Southwest Oncology Group study. Blood 89: 3323-3329

26. Löwenberg B, Suciu S, Archimbaud E, Ossenkoppele G, Verhoef GEG, Vellenga E, Wijermans P, Berneman Z, Dekker AW, Stryckmans P, Schouten H, Jehn U, Muus P, Sonneveld P, Dardenne M, Zittoun R (1997) Use of recombinant granulocyte-macrophage colony-stimulating factor during and after remission induction chemotherapy in patients aged 61 years and older with acute myeloid leukemia (AML): final report of AML-11, a phase III randomized study of the Leukemia Cooperative Group of European Organisation for the Research and Treatment of Cancer (EORTC-LCG) and the Dutch Belgian Hemato-Oncology Cooperative Group (HOVON). Blood 90: 2952-2961

27. Löwenberg B, Zittoun R, Kerkhofs H, Jehn U, Abels J, Debusscher L, Cauchie C, Peetermans M, Solbu G, Suciu S, et al. (1989) On the value of intensive remission-induction chemotherapy in elderly patients of 65+ years with acute myeloid leukemia: a randomized phase III study of the European Organization for Research and Treatment of Cancer Leukemia Group. J Clin Oncol 7: 1268-1274

28. Mayer RJ, Davis RB, Schiffer CA, Berg DT, Powell BL, Schulman P, Omura GA, Moore JO, McIntyre OR, Frei E (1994) Intensive postremission chemotherapy in adults with acute myeloid leukemia. N Engl J Med 331: 896-903

29. Pogliani EM, Rossini F, Casaroli I, Maffe P, Corneo G (1997) Thrombotic complications in acute promyelocytic leukemia during all-*trans* retinoic acid therapy. Acta Haematol 97: 228-230

30. Rees JKH, Gray RG, Swirsky D, Hayhoe FGJ (1986) Principal results of the Medical Research Council's 8th acute myeloid leukaemia trial. Lancet 2: 1236-1241

31. Rowe JM, Andersen JW, Mazza JJ, Bennett JM, Paietta E, Hayes FA, Oette D, Cassileth PA, Stadtmauer EA, Wiernik PH (1995) A randomized placebo-controlled phase III study of granulocyte-macrophage colony-stimulating factor in adult patients (>55 to 70 years of age) with acute myelogenous leukemia: a study of the Eastern Cooperative Oncology Group (E1490). Blood 86: 457-462

32. Schiffer CA, Lee EJ, Takafumi T, Wiernik PH, Testa JR (1989) Prognostic impact of cytogenetic abnormalities in patients with de novo acute nonlymphocytic leukemia. Blood 73: 263-270

33. Stone RM, Mayer RJ (1993) The approach to the elderly patient with acute myeloid leukemia. Hematol Oncol Clin North Am 7: 65-79

34. Stone RM, Berg DT, George SL, Dodge RK, Paciucci PA, Schulman P, Lee EJ, Moore JO, Powell BL, Schiffer CA (1995) Granulocyte-macrophage colony-stimulating factor after initial chemotherapy for elderly patients with primary acute myelogenous leukemia. N Engl J Med 332: 1671-1677

35. Swansbury GJ, Lawler SD, Alimena G, Arthur D, Berger R, van den Berghe H, Bloomfield CD, de la Chapelle A, Dewald G, Garson OM, et al (1994) Long-term survival in acute myelogenous leukemia: a second follow-up of the Fourth International Workshop on Chromosomes in Leukemia. Cancer Genet Cytogenet 73: 1-7

36. Tallman MS, Andersen JW, Schiffer CA, Appelbaum FR, Feusner JH, Ogden A, Shepherd L, Willman C, Bloomfield CD, Rowe JM, Wiernik PH (1997) All-*trans* retinoic acid in acute promyelocytic leukemia. N Engl J Med 337: 1021-1028

37. Taylor PR, Reid MM, Stark AN, Brown N, Hamilton PJ, Proctor SJ (1995) De novo acute myeloid leukaemia in patients over 55-years-old: a population-based study of incidence, treatment and outcome. Northern Region Haematology Group. Leukemia 9: 231-237

38. Tilly H, Castaigne S, Bordessoule D, Casassus P, Le Prise PY, Tertian G, Desablens B, Henry-Amar M, Degos L, et al. (1990) Low-dose cytarabine versus intensive chemotherapy in the treatment of acute nonlymphocytic leukemia of the elderly. J Clin Oncol 8: 272-279

39. Venditti A, Stasi R, del Poeta G, Buccisano F, Aronica G, Bruno A, Pisani F, Caravita T, Masi M, Tribalto M, Domenica Simone M, Avvisati G, Amadori S, Papa G (1995) All-*trans* retinoic acid and low-dose cytosine arabinoside for the treatment of 'poor prognosis' acute myeloid leukemia. Leukemia 9: 1121-1125

40. Yang GS, Minden MD, McCulloch EA (1993) Influence of schedule on regulated sensitivity of AML blasts to cytosine arabinoside. Leukemia 7: 1012-1019

41. Yang GS, Minden MD, McCulloch EA (1994) Regulation by retinoic acid and hydrocortisone of the anthracycline sensitivity of blast cells of acute myeloblastic leukemia. Leukemia 8: 2065-2075

42. Yunis JJ, Lobell M, Arnesen MA, Oken MM, Mayer MG, Rydell RE, Brunning RD (1988) Refined chromosome study helps define prognostic subgroups in most patients with primary myelodysplastic syndrome and acute myelogenous leukaemia. Br J Haematol 68: 189-194

# AML in Elderly Patients

# Treatment of Older Patients with Acute Myeloid Leukemia (AML)

T. Büchner, W. Hiddemann, C. Schoch, T. Haferlach, H. Eimermacher, P. Staib, L. Balleisen, H.E. Reis, H.J. Pielken, A. Reichle, H.J. Schmoll, F. Griesinger, A. Grüneisen, M.-C. Sauerland and A. Heinecke for the AMLCG

*Abstract.* The inferior outcome in the older patients with AML when compared with that in younger patients can be explained, in part, by a traditional undertreatment in most of the published series. In correspondence to the benefit of patients under age 60 from high-dose AraC there are dose effects in the over 60es in particular for daunorubicin in the induction treatment, and for the quantity in terms of duration of postremission treatment. The use of these effects can partly overcome the mostly unfavorable disease biology in older age AML as expressed by the absence of favorable and the overrepresentation of adverse chromosomal abnormalities as well as the expression of drug resistance. We recommend an adequate dosage of 60 mg/m$^2$ daunorubicin on three days in a combination with standard dose AraC and 6-thioguanine given for induction and consolidation and followed by a prolonged monthly maintenance chemotherapy for an at least one year duration. Further improvements in supportive care may help delivering additional antileukemic cytotoxicity. As a novel approach, non-myeloablative preparative regimens may open allogeneic transplantation for older patients with AML. Given the actual median age in this disease being more than 60 years the management of older age AML remains as the major challenge.

## Introduction

Dealing with AML in older patients is a two fold challenge. 1. These patients do not participate in the increasing cure rates seen in younger patients. While their diseases are more resistant against common chemotherapy their treatment is generally less intensive. And 2. patients of 60 years and over represent only 1/3 of the patients in the large multicenter studies but may actually account for the majority of our AML patients.

1. When compared with AML in younger patients the disease more often emerges secondary to myelodysplasia [1] or treatment of a previous cancer [2], and even without such a history karyotype changes associated with secondary AML [3-5] occur more frequently in the older patients [6-10]. The observed abnormalities of chromosomes 5 and 7 and complex abnormalities are known to predict an unfavorable outcome [5-11]. In elderly patients with AML different from younger patients clonality markers of the leukemic cells were also positive in all hematopoietic cells [12]. It has been suggested that neutropenia after chemotherapy lasts longer in older patients [13] and a defective pool of hematopoietic stem cells could prolong myelosuppression [14]. The age-related differences in the disease biology explain in part why patients 60 years of age and older do not achieve the same remission rates [15-25] and remission duration [18, 19, 21, 23-25] as achieved in younger patients. To another part, however, inadequate antileukemic treatment might have contributed to the inferior results since chemotherapy intensity commonly has been reduced in the older patients.

2. As from relevant population based evaluations the incidence of AML increases to more than 10 fold between the age of 20 and 65 years [26]. On the other hand, in

Dept. of Medicine, University of Münster, Germany

the 1992 study of the German AMLCG patients of 60+ years typically contributed 35 % of the entire adult patients included, but they contributed 63 % of the patients excluded from the study according to various protocol criteria. Supposing similar proportions in the unknown number of patients not referred to the study centers and not registered patients over age 60 may well represent 50 % or more of our AML patients.

By present analysis of published trials and contribution of our own data we here address the questions:
- What kinds of treatment intensification may improve outcome in older patients?
- Has an age-related hematotoxicity to be taken into account?
- What can growth factors contribute?
- What are the further directions according to supportive treatment and antileukemic options?

## Age and trends in chemotherapy

The trends in modern chemotherapy for AML in patients of all ages are best exemplified by the multicenter randomized trials and their results published since 1981 [15, 17-24, 27, 28]. In these trials a total of 6757 patients were treated. The average complete remission (CR) rate is 62 % and the probability to remain in CR after 4-5 years is 21 %. These representative results can serve as a standard for the relative ranking of specific results. Comparing publications from the 1980ies with those from the 1990ies there is no difference in the CR rates (62 % vs 63 %) but the 5-year CR rates have increased from 16 % to 25 %.

The age related study results are listed in Table 1 in the order of increasing age in the groups of patients treated [14-25, 27-41]. The standard CR rate (see above) of 62 % is frequently exceeded in younger but not in older patients with one exception [29]. The same is true for the 21 % standard 5-year CR rate which is exceeded in older patients in only three trials [17, 34, 39]. Within the same trials markedly inferior CR rates and 5-year continuous CR rates were found in the older when

compared with the younger groups of patients.

The impact of special treatment modalities in younger and older patients is also shown in Table 1 as far as documented by significant differences in randomized comparisons. Important are the effects of high-dose AraC, of the daunorubicin (DNR) dosage and of prolonged maintenance treatment. Thus, high-dose AraC either in induction [36, 37] or in postremission [2] treatment significantly improved the 5-year CR rate in younger patients while older patients treated in only one trial [21] did not benefit from postremission high-dose AraC. In contrast, DNR and its dosage showed a significant impact in the CR rate of patients over age 60 [23]. Table 2 summarizes the results from studies using different doses of DNR. As demonstrated by the German AMLCG 60 mg/m$^2$ DNR induced significantly more remissions than the traditional dose of 30 mg/m$^2$ (54 vs 43 %, p=.038). Importantly, in the 60 mg arm more remissions were induced by only one course (38 %) when compared to the 30 mg arm (20 %, p=.002).

As from Table 1 prolonged maintenance significantly improved the 5-year CR rate in two trials [17, 41] both of them treating older patients. The AMLCG showed that prolonged maintenance resulted in a 25 % 5-year survival for the responders (Fig. 1). Thus, the gain in remission induced by the higher DNR dosage translated into a gain in longterm survival. Figure 2 illustrates the relapse free survival of older patients receiving prolonged maintenance or no maintenance or high-dose AraC/Mitoxantrone in sequential trials of the AMLCG. While the identical maintenance treatment produced a consistent 5-year relapse free survival of around 20 %, inferior results are found with no maintenance or high-dose AraC/Mitoxantrone instead of maintenance.

While Table 1 provides a synopsis of different treatment modalities, differences between the trials must be interpreted with caution. Since children were included [15, 16, 18, 30, 31, 33] or various proportions of patients became excluded at the occasion of randomizations in remission [15, 17, 19, 21, 32, 33, 35] fair inter-study are certainly compromized by comparisons unknown selection factors.

**Table 1.** Therapeutic outcome in multicenter randomized trials in the order of patients age

| Publication | Age | No. of Patients | % CR | % CCR at 4-5 Y |
|---|---|---|---|---|
| Hann et al. 1997 [30], | | | | |
| Burnett et al. 1998 [3] | 0-55 | 1857 | 82 | 42[1] |
| Mandelli et al. 1992 [32] | 15-55 | 448 | 68 | 24 |
| Rai et al. 1981 [15] | 0-60 | 247 | 36-59[2] | 22[3] (not age specific) |
| Yates et al. 1982 [16] | 1-60 | 427 | 57-72[4] | not given |
| Büchner et al. 1985 [17] | 16-60 | 255 | 68 | 8-24[5] |
| Rees et al. 1986 [18] | 0-60 | 740 | 73 | 18 |
| Hayat et al. 1986 [33] | 10-60 | 257 | 66 | 17 (not age specific) |
| Preisler et al. 1987 [19] | 14-60 | 564 | 65 | 17 |
| Hansen et al. 1991 [34] | 17-60 | 135 | 60 | 34 |
| Dillman et al. 1991 [20] | 15-60 | 226 | 69 | 10 (not age specific) |
| Cassileth et al. 1992 [35] | 15-60 | 449 | 71 | 16-27 (not age specific) |
| Mayer et al. 1994 [21] | 16-60 | 742 | 71 | 24-44[6] |
| Bishop et al. 1996 [36] | 15-60 | 301 | 73 | 23-41[7] |
| Weick et al. 1996 [37] | < 65 | 665 | 54 | 19[8] |
| Büchner et al. 1999 [24] | 16-60 | 725 | 68 | 32 |
| Büchner et al. 1999 [25] | 16-60 | 450 | 74 | 36 |
| Hayat et al. 1986 [33] | 60-65 | 30 | 47 | no age specific data |
| Hansen et al. 1991 [34] | 60-65 | 39 | 46 | 30 |
| Cassileth et al. 1992 [35] | 60-65 | 73 | 52 | no age specific data |
| Rowe et al. 1995 [38] | 55-70 | 117 | 61 | not given |
| Witz et al. 1998 [39] | 55-75 | 132 | 62 | 23[9] |
| Goldstone et al. 1999 [40] | 56+ | 1314 | 50-62[10] | 18-26 |
| Rai et al. 1981 [15] | 60+ | 105 | 16-45[11] | no age specific data |
| Yates et al. 1982 [16] | 60-84 | 226 | 31-47[12] | not given |
| Büchner et al. 1985 [17] | 60-78 | 79 | 39 | 0-28[13] |
| Rees et al. 1986 [18] | 60-83 | 305 | 48 | 9 |
| Preisler et al. 1987 [19] | 60+ | 104 | 41 | 17 |
| Dillman et al. 1991 [20] | 60-83 | 100 | 41 | no age specific data |
| Mayer et al. 1994 [21] | 60-86 | 346 | 47 | 15 |
| Stone et al. 1995 [14] | 60+ | 388 | 53 | not given |
| Büchner et al. 1997 [23] | 60+ | 340 | 42-54[14] | 22 |
| Dombret et al. 1995 [29] | 65+ | 172 | 47-70[15] | not given |
| Rees et al. 1996 [22] | 1-79 | 923 | 63[16] | 26[16] (not age specific) |
| Löwenberg et al. 1998 [41] | 60-88 | 489 | 38-47[17] | 8[18] |

[1] Autologous bone marrow transplantation better than no further treatment (p=.04)
[2] AraC infusion better than bolus (p<.05) and 7+3 better than 5+2 (p<.01)
[3] AraC in maintenance s.c better than i.v. (p<.01)
[4] DNR 45 better than DNR 30 or ADR 30 (p<.05)
[5] Maintenance better than no maintenance (p<.05)
[6] Relapse-free survival positively correlated to post-remission AraC dosage (p=.002)
[7] High-dose better than standard dose AraC (p=.007)
[8] High-dose better than standard dose AraC (p=.049)

[9] GM-CSF during and after chemotherapy better than no GM-CSF in 2-year relapse free survival (p=.003)
[10] 6-Thioguanine better than etoposide (p=.002)
[11] 7+3 better than 5-2
[12] DNR 30 better than DNR 45 or ADR 30 (p<.05)
[13] Maintenance better than no maintenance (p=.002)
[14] DNR 60 better than DNR 30 (p=.026)
[15] G-CSF better than no G-CSF (p=.002)
[16] Mitoxantrone better than DNR (p=.069)
[17] Low dose AraC for maintenance better than no maintenance (p=.006)

## Treatment attenuation in older patients

As alternative approaches treatment attenuation strategies for older patients have been investigated in four major studies (Table 3). The attenuated or oral regimens showed some advantages in survival and CR rate in two of the studies [43, 45] and relapse free survival in one study [45] with no improvement on common results.

## Age-related disease biology and treatment intensity

Prognostic features could be compared between younger and older patients by the AMLCG within the same trial involving 1065 patients [23, 24]. There was a striking difference in the occurrence of favorable karyotypes with 22 % in younger and 2 % in older patients (p=.001) and the unfavorable com-

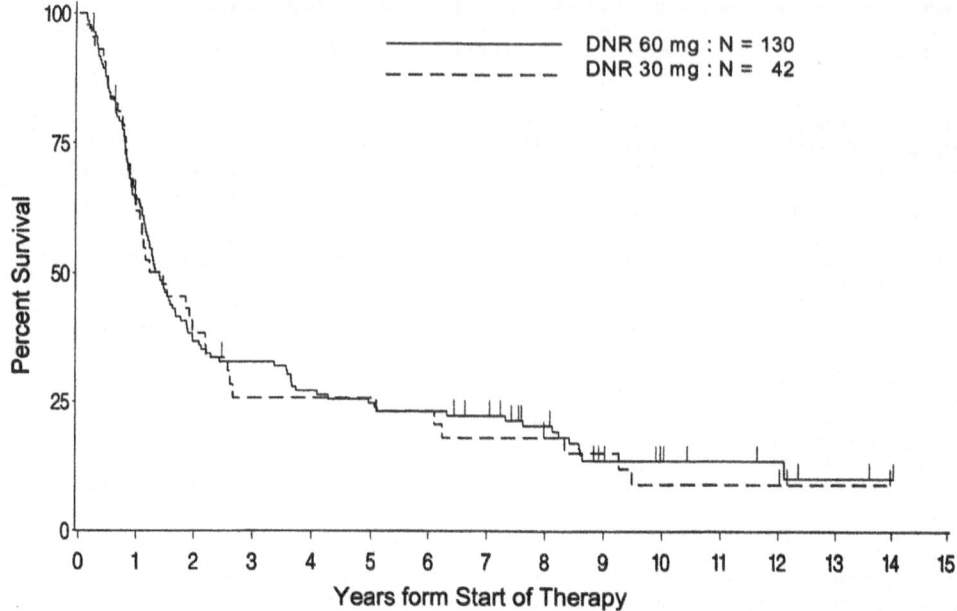

**Fig. 1.** Survival in patients 60 years of age and older who attained complete remission after induction therapy with TAD containing DNR either 60 or 30 mg/m² x 3. The remission rate was 54 vs 43 % (p=.038). The higher number of patients in the 60 mg arm is explained by closing the 30 mg arm when a significantly superior response rate to the higher dose became obvious.

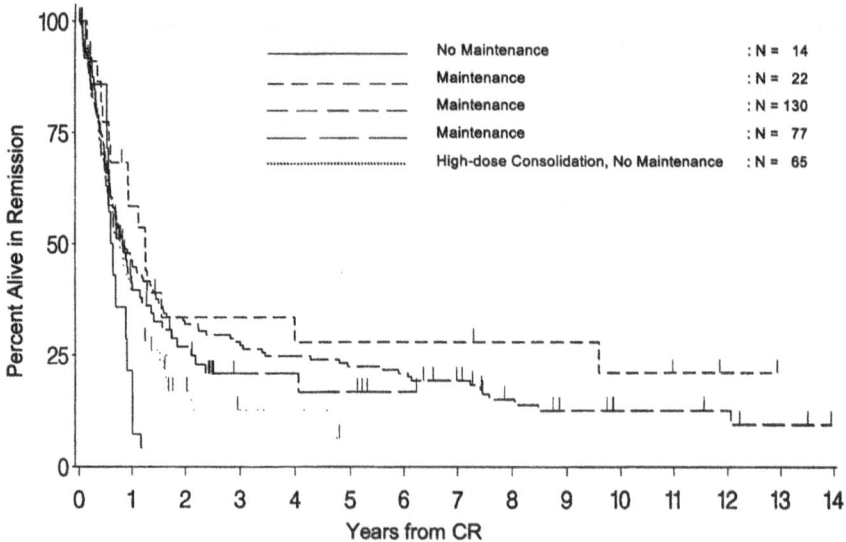

**Fig. 2.** Relapse free survival in patients 60 years of age and older who received or did not receive prolonged maintenance treatment in sequential trials of the German AMLCG.

**Table 2.** DNR Dosage and Outcome in Older Patients

| Publication | DNR mg/m² | Age (Y) | Patients No. | Overall survival (5 Y) | CR | Relapse free survival (5 Y) |
|---|---|---|---|---|---|---|
| Rees et al. 1986 [18] | 50 x 1 | 60-83 | 305 | 9 % | 48 % | 9 % |
| Yates et al. 1982 [16] | 30 x 3 | 60+ | 72 | | 47 % | |
| Preisler et al. 1987 [19] | 30 x 3 | 60+ | 104 | 10 % | 41 % | 17 % |
| Löwenberg et al. 1989 [42] | 30 x 3 | 65-85 | 31 | 13 % | 58 % | 17 % |
| Dillman et al. 1991 [20] | 30 x 3 | 60-83 | 100 | 3 % | 41 % | < 10 % |
| Mayer et al. 1994 [21] | 30 x 3 | 60-86 | 346 | 9 % | 47 % | 15 % |
| Büchner et al. 1997 [23] | 30 x 3 | 60-83 | 103 | 10 % | 42 % | 17 % |
| Löwenberg et al. 1998 [41] | 30 x 3 | 60-88 | 489 | 6 % | 38 % | 8 % |
| Yates et al. 1982 [16] | 45 x 3 | 60+ | 68 | | 31 % | |
| Stone et al. 1995 [14] | 45 x 3 | 60-> 80 | 388 | | 53 % | |
| Dombret et al. 1995 [29] | 45 x 4 | 64-83 | 172 | | 47-70 % | |
| Büchner et al. 1997 [23] | 60 x 3 | 60-83 | 240 | 16 % | 54 % | 22 % |

**Table 3.** Full-dose versus Attenuated or Low-dose Chemotherapy in Older Patients with AML

| Publication | Treatment | Age (Y) | Patients No. | Overall survival (median) | p | CR | p | Relapse free survival (median) | p |
|---|---|---|---|---|---|---|---|---|---|
| Kahn et al. 1984 [43] | Full[1] versus attenuated[2] dose DAT | 70+ | 40 | 29 vs 159 days | <.02 | 25 vs 30 % | n.s. | | |
| Löwenberg et al. 1989 [42] | Immediate intensive induction chemothera-py[3] vs wait and see[4] | 65-85 | 60 | 21 vs 11 weeks | .015 | 58 vs 0 % | | | |
| Tilly et al. 1990 [44] | Intensive chemo-therapy[5] vs low-dose AraC[6] | 65-83 | 87 | 12.8 vs 8.8 months | n.s. | 52 vs 32 % | .001 | 13.8 vs 8.3 months | n.s. |
| Ruutu et al. 1994 [45] | TAD[7] vs oral ETI[8] | 65-87 | 51 | 3.7 vs 9.9 months | .042 | 23 vs 60 % | .007 | 2.7 vs 7.2 months | n.s. |

[1] DNR 60 mg/m²/d x 3; AraC 200 mg/m²/d x 5; thioguanine 200 mg/m²/d x 5

[2] DNR 50 mg/m²/d x 1; AraC 100 mg/m²/d x 5; thioguanine 200 mg/m²/d x 5

[3] DNR 30 mg/m²/d x 3; VCR 1 mg/m²/d x 1; AraC 200 mg/m²/d x 7

[4] Cytoreduction by HU 3 g/d x 2; AraC 200 mg/m²/d x 4

[5] Rubidazone 100 mg/m²/d x 4; AraC 200 mg/m²/d x 7

[6] AraC 20 mg/m²/d x 21

[7] Thioguanine 200 mg/m²/d x 5; AraC 200 mg/m²/d x 5; DNR 60 mg/m² x 1

[8] Etoposide 160 mg/m²/d orally x 5; thioguanine 200 mg/m²/d orally x 5; Idarubicin 15 mg/m²/d orally x 3

plex karyotype abnormalities with 6 % vs 20 % (p=.001). These data explain a 35 % disadvantage for the older patients. As additional cellular features predicting poor prognosis the South-West Oncology Group detected a CD34+ phenotype in 65 %, MDR1 expression in 71 % and active drug efflux in 58 % of their older AML patients [46, 47]. While those cell biologic features explain the general experi- ence of a greatly unfavorable and chemoresistant disease, the few older patients with favorable karyotypes apparently share a good prognosis with the related younger patients [48]. In contrast to the general prognosis not different between the younger and older patients was the recovery time of neutrophils and platelets after the identical chemotherapy, shown in Figure 3. Suggestions of a

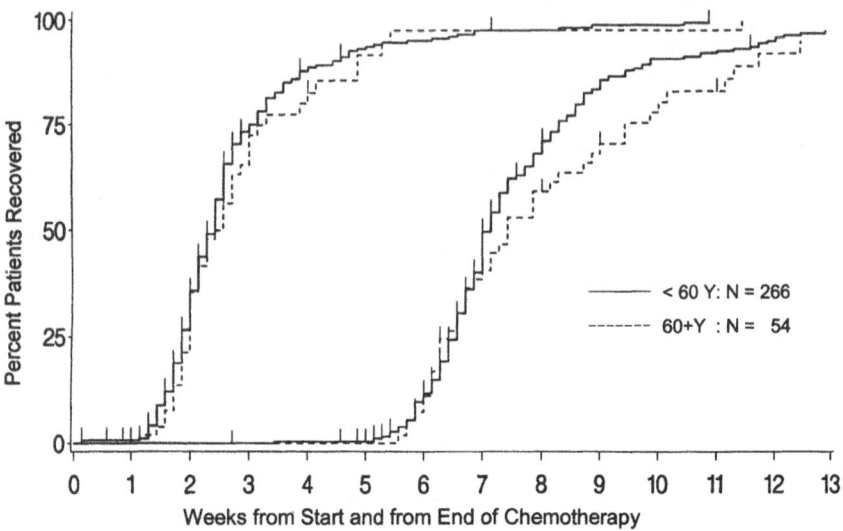

**Fig. 3.** Recovery time to 500 neutrophils/μl and 50.000 platelets/μl after the start (right hand side) and end (left hand side) of chemotherapy comparing patients under and over age 60. The patients were treated within the same trial. The data shown are restricted to patients receiving two identical courses of TAD with daunorubicin 60 mg/m[2]. The splitting of the right hand curves is explained by some longer delay of the second induction course in the older patients.

defective hematopoiesis in older patients [13, 14] could thus not be confirmed. As Figure 3 also shows the neutrophil and platelet recovery time calculating from the start of the induction treatment does not show a major delay in the delivery of induction treatment for older compared with younger patients. In the same trial of the AMLCG patients under age 60 were randomized to receive double induction either at standard dosage or with the inclusion of high-dose AraC. While there was no difference in outcome in the patients overall, those with poor risk according to karyotype, LDH and slow response had a significantly superior response and survival in the high-risk arm not seen in the good risk patients [24]. This first evidence that a poor prognosis can be improved by more intensive treatment appears confirmed by the dose effects of daunorubicin and the effect of prolonged maintenance in the older patients, again a poor prognostic group.

## Growth factors in older patients

The effect of GM-CSF [14, 38, 39, 49, 50] or G-CSF [29] given after [14, 29, 38, 49], during

and after [39], or before, during and after [50] chemotherapy for older patients with AML has now been explored in six studies (Table 4). There were benefits in the recovery of neutrophils in all studies, in mortality and survival in two studies [38, 49], remissions in one [29] and relapse free survival in one [39] study. Except for some toxicity of GM-CSF in one study [50] no adverse effects were observed.

## Conclusions and recommendations

Present evaluation strongly suggests that patients 60 years of age and older receive their best chance of achieving a remission and surviving disease free, by the administration of full dose induction treatment containing DNR 60 mg/m[2]/d x 3 and of prolonged maintenance chemotherapy. This strategy is persued in the studies of the German AMLCG using the regimens described in Figure 4. Needles to say, that up to date supportive care such as adequate platelet support, early empiric prophylactic antimicrobial treatment and protective programs are indispensable prerequisites for delivering an intensive antileu-

**Table 4.** Synopsis of Clinical Studies on Growth-factors in Induction Treatment for Older Patients with AML:

| Publication | Special Risk | Growth Factor Product | Growth Factor Daily Dose | Growth Factor Start | Controls | Chemotherapy Dose | Patients No. | Growth Factor Benefit | No Difference | GF Worse |
|---|---|---|---|---|---|---|---|---|---|---|
| Büchner et al. 1991 [49] | early/mult. relapse or age 65+ | GM-CSF (yeast) | 250 µg/m² | day four after chemo | historic | relapses high-dose age 65+ standard | 112 | - neutropenia (p=.02)<br>- mortality (p=.009) | - disease-free-survival<br>- leukemic regrowth | |
| Rowe et al. 1995 [38] | age 55-70 | GM-CSF (yeast) | 250 µg/m² | day four after chemo | placebo | standard | 124 | - neutropenia (p=.001)<br>- grade 4/5 infections (p=.002)<br>- survival (p=.048) | - disease-free-survival | |
| Stone et al. 1995 [14] | age 60+ | GM-CSF (E. coli) | 5 µg/kg | day one after chemo | placebo | standard | 388 | - neutropenia (p=.02) | - mortality<br>- remissions<br>- leukemic regrowth<br>- survival<br>- hospitalisation | |
| Witz et al. 1998 [39] | age 55-75 | GM-CSF (E. coli) | 5 µg/kg | with start of chemo | placebo | standard | 240 | - neutropenia (p=.0001)<br>- disease-free-survival (p=.003) | - mortality<br>- remissions<br>- infections<br>- survival<br>- hospitalisation | |
| Löwenberg et al. 1997 [50] | age 60+ | GM-CSF (E. coli) | 5 µg/kg | day one before chemo | random | standard | 318 | - neutropenia (p=.0002)<br>- disease-free-survival (p=.003) | - remissions<br>- infections<br>- survival<br>- disease-free-survival | - fever<br>- chills<br>- hypotension<br>- fluid retention |
| Dombret et al. 1995 [29] | age 65+ | G-CSF | 5 µg/kg | day two after chemo | placebo | standard | 172 | - neutropenia (p<.001)<br>- remissions (p=.002) | - mortality at 8 weeks<br>- infections<br>- leukemic regrowth<br>- survival | |

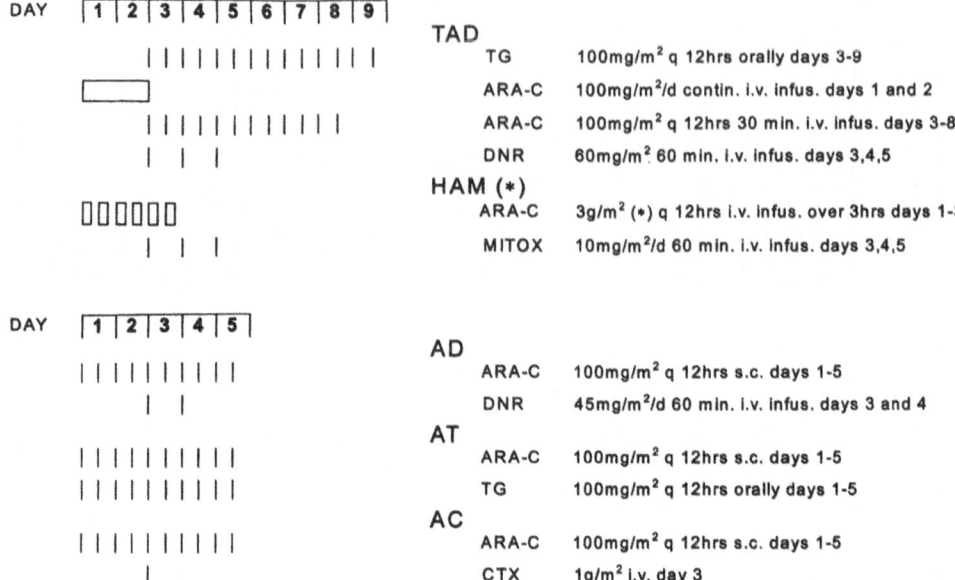

**Fig. 4.** Therapeutic regimens used by the German AML Cooperative Group. TAD and HAM are used for induction treatment with HAM starting on day 21 of treatment. After attaining remission patients receive an additional TAD for consolidation. Subsequent maintenance treatment is given for three years and consists of AD or AT or AC rotatingly every month. The only age adaptation is AraC in HAM 1 instead of 3 g/m² for patients over age 60.

kemic therapy to older patients. The additional individual use of G- or GM-CSF as an adjunct to supportive care appears justified and reasonable, as well.

## New perspectives

Beyond the above recommendations it remains open whether further intensification of chemotherapy such as by high-dose AraC in induction treatment as investigated in a current trial of the AMLCG will further improve the outcome in older AML patients. New approaches to supportive care like granulocyte transfusion [5] or mucous membrane protection by IL11 [52] may facilitate delivering the intensive treatment. Novel anti-leukemic principles like an antibody targeted cytotoxic treatment [53] or MDR modifiers [54] may help overcoming the chemoresistance in higher age AML. Finally, the allogeneic cell therapy using non-myeloablative

conditioning is on a promising way to be offered even to older patients with AML [55].

## References

1. Hamblin TJ: The treatment of acute myeloid leukemia preceded by the myelodysplastic syndrome. Leukemia Research 1992;16:4101-8
2. Hoyle CF, de Bastos M, Wheatley K, et al. AML associated with previous cytotoxic therapy. MDS or myelo-proliferative disorders: results from the MRC's 9th AML trial. British Journal of Haematology 1989;72:45-53.
3. Second International Workshop on Chromosomes in Leukemia. Cancer Genetics and Cytogenetics 1980;2:89-113.
4. Rowley J. Annotation: Chromosome changes in acute leukaemia. British Journal of Haematology 1980;44:339-46.
5. Yunis JJ, Lobell M, Arnesen MA et al.Refined chromosome study helps define prognostic subgroups in most patients with primary myelodysplastic syndrome and acute myelogenous leukaemia. British Journal of Haematology 1988;68:189-94.
6. Fourth International Workshop on Chromosomes in Leukemia. Cancer Genetics and Cytogenetics 1984;11:332-50.

7. Keating MJ, Smith TL, Kantarjian H et al. Cytogenetic pattern in acute myelogenous leukemia: a major reproducible determinant of outcome. Leukemia 1988;2:403-12.
8. Schiffer CA, Lee EJ, Tomiyasu T et al. Prognostic impact of cytogenetic abnormalities in patients with de novo acute nonlymphocytic leukemia. Blood 1989;73:263-70.
9. Swansbury GJ, Lawler SD, Alimena G et al. Longterm survival in acute myelogenous leukemia: A second follow-up of the Fourth International Workshop on chromosomes in leukemia. Cancer Genetics and Cytogenetics 1994;73:1-7.
10. Dastugue N, Paven C., Lafage-Pochitaloff M et al. Prognostic significance of karyotype in de novo adult acute myeloid leukemia. Leukemia 1995;9:1491-8.
11. Yunis JJ, Brunninng RD, Howe RB et al. High-resolution chromosomes as an independent prognostic indicator in adult acute nonlymphocytic leukemia. New England Journal of Medicine 1984;311:812-8.
12. Fialkow PJ, Singer JW, Raskind WH et al. Clonal development, stem-cell differentiation, and clinical remissions in acute nonlymphocytic leukemia. New England Journal of Medicine 1987;317:468-73.
13. Hamblin TJ. Meeting report: 1st International Conference on reversal of multidrug resistance in cancer. Leukemia Research 1995;19: 509-14.
14. Stone RM, Berg TB, George SL et al. Granulocyte-macrophage colony-stimulating factor after initial chemotherapy for elderly patients with primary acute myelogenous leukemia. New England Journal of Medicine 1995;332:1671-7.
15. Rai KR, Hollannd JF, Glidewell OJ et al. Treatment of acute myeloid leukemia: A study by Cancer and Leukemia Group B. Blood 1981;58:1203-12.
16. Yates J, Glidewell O, Wiernik P et al. Cytosine arabinoside with daunorubicin or adriamycin for therapy of acute myelocytic leukemia: A CALGB study. Blood 1982;60:454-62.
17. Büchner T, Urbanitz D, Hiddemann W et al. Intensified Induction and Consolidation with or without maintenance chemotherapy for acute myeloid leukemia (AML): Two multicenter studies of the German AML Cooperative Group. Journal of Clinical Oncology 1985;3:1583-9.
18. Rees JKH, Gray RG, Swirsky D, Hayhoe FGJ. Principal results of the Medical Research Council's 8th acute myeloid leukaemia trial. The Lancet 1986;332:1236.
19. Preisler H, Davis RB, Kirshner J et al. Comparison of three remission induction regimens and two postinduction strategies for the treatment of acute nonlymphocytic leukemia: A Cancer and Leukemia Group B Study. Blood 1987;69:1441-9.
20. Dillman RO, Davis RB, Green MR et al. A comparative study of two different doses of cytarabine for acute myeloid leukemia: A phase III trial of Cancer and Leukemia Group B. Blood 1991;78:2520-6.
21. Mayer RJ, Davis RB, Schiffer CA et al. Intensive postremission chemotherapy in adults with acute myeloid leukemia. New England Journal of Medicine 1994;6:896-942.
22. Rees JKH, Gray RG, Weathley K: Dose intensification in acute myeloid leukaemia: greater effectiveness at lower cost. Principal report of the Medical Research Council's AML9 study. British Journal of Haematology 1996;94:89-98.
23. Büchner T, Hiddemann W, Wörmann B et al. Daunorubicin 60 instead of 30 mg/sqm improves response and survival in elderly patients with AML. Blood 1997;90 (Suppl 1):583a.
24. Büchner T, Hiddemann W, Wörmann B. et al. Double Induction Strategy for Acute Myeloid Leukemia: The Effect of High-Dose Cytarabine with Mitoxantrone instead of Standard-Dose Cytarabine with Daunorubicin and 6-Thioguanine. A Randomized Trial by the German AML Cooperative Group. Blood 1999;93:4116-24.
25. Büchner T, Hiddemann W, Wörmann B et al. One single course of sequential highdose AraC/Mitoxantrone (S-HAM) has the same long-term effect as three years of maintenance in AML patients after TAD-HAM double induction. Randomized trial by the German AMLCG. Blood 1999; 94 (Suppl 1): 383a
26. McNally, RJQ, Rowland D, Roman E et al. Age and sex distributions of hematological malignancies in the U.K. Hematological Oncology 1997;15:173-89.
27. Vogler WR, Winton EF, Gordon DS et al. A randomized comparison of postremission therapy in acute myelogenous leukemia. A Southeastern Cancer Study Group trial. Blood 1984;63:1039-45.
28. Vogler WR, Velez-Garcia E, Weiner RS et al. A phase III trial comparing idarubicin and daunorubicin in combination with cytarabine in acute myelogenous leukemia: A Southeastern Cancer Study Group Study. Journal of Clinical Oncology 1992;10:1103-11.
29. Dombret H, Chastang C, Fenaux P et al. A controlled study of recombinant human granulocyte colony-stimulating factor in elderly patients after treatment for acute myelogenous leukemia. New England Journal of Medicine 1995;332:1678-83.
30. Hann IM., Stevens RF, Goldstone AH et al. Randomized comparison of DAT versus ADE as induction chemotherapy in children and younger adults with acute myeloid leukemia. Results of the Medical Research Council's 10th AML Trial (MRC AML10). Blood 1997;89:2311-8.
31. Burnett AK, Goldstone AH, Stevens RM et al. Randomised comparison of addition of autologous bone-marrow transplantation to intensive chemotherapy of acute myeloid leukaemia in first remission: results of MRC AML10 trial. The Lancet 1998;351:700-8.
32. Mandelli F, Vegna ML, Avvisati G et al. A randomized study of the efficacy of postconsolidation therapy in adult acute nonlymphocytic leukemia: a report of the Italian Cooperative Group GIMEMA. Annals of Hematology 1992;64:166-72.
33. Hayat M, Jehn U, Willemze R et al. A randomized comparison of maintenance treatment with androgens, immunotherapy, and chemotherapy in adult acute myelogenous leukemia. Cancer 1986;58:617-23.
34. Hansen OP, Pedersen-Bjergaard J, Ellegaard J et al. Aclarubicin plus cytosine arabinoside versus daunorubicin plus cytosine arabinoside in previously untreated patients with acute myeloid leukemia: a Danish National Phase III Trial. Leukemia 1991;5:510-6.

35. Cassileth PA, Lynch E, Hines JD et al. Varying intensity of postremission therapy in acute myeloid leukemia. Blood 1992;79:1924-30.

36. Bishop JF, Matthews JP, Young GA et al. A randomized study of high-dose cytarabine in induction in acute myeloid leukemia. Blood 1996;87:1710-7.

37. Weick JK, Kopecky KJ, Appelbaum FR et al. A randomized investigation of high-dose versus standard dose cytosine arabinoside with daunorubicin in patients with previously untreated acute myeloid leukemia: A Southwest Oncology Study Group. Blood 1996;88:2841-51.

38. Rowe JM, Andersen JW, Mazza JJ et al. A randomized placebo-controlled phase III study of granulocyte-macrophage colony-stimulating factor in adult patients (>55 to 70 years of age) with acute myelogenous leukemia: A study of the Eastern Cooperative Oncology Group (E1490). Blood 1995;86:457-62.

39. Witz F, Sadoun A, Perrin MC et al. A placebo-controlled study of recombinant human granulocyte-macrophage colony-stimulating factor administered during and after induction treatment for de novo acute myelogenous leukemia in elderly patients. Blood 1998;91:2722-30.

40. Goldstone AH, Burnett AK. Wheatly K et al. Superior CR rates with DAT induction compared to ADE or MAC in older patients with AML, but three additional courses of consolidation chemotherapy and maintenance with interferon do not improve survival: Results of the MRC, AML 11 Trial. Proceedings of the American Society of Clinical Oncology 1999;18:6a.

41. Löwenberg B, Suciu S, Archimbaud E et al. Mitoxantrone versus daunorubicin in induction-consolidation chemotherapy - The value of low-dose cytarabine for maintenance of remission, and an assessment of prognostic factors in acute myeloid leukemia in the elderly: Final report of the Leukemia Cooperative Group of the European Organization for the Research and Treatment of Cancer and the Dutch-Belgian Hemato-Oncology Cooperative Hovon Group randomized phase III study AML-9. Journal of Clinical Oncology 1998;16:872-81.

42. Löwenberg B, Zittoun R, Kerkhofs H et al. On the value of intensive remission-induction chemotherapy in the elderly patients of 65+ years with acute myeloid leukemia: A randomized phase III study of the European Organization for Research and Treatment of Cancer Leukemia Group. Journal of Clinical Oncology 1989;7:1268-74.

43. Kahn SB, Begg CB, Mazza JJ et al.: Full dose versus attenuated dose daunorubicin, cytosine arabinoside and 6-thioguanine in the treatment of acute nonlymphocytic leukemia in the elderly. Journal of Clinical Oncology 1984;2:865-70.

44. Tilly H, Castaigne S, Bordessoule D et al. Low-dose cytarabine versus intensive chemotherapy in the treatment of acute nonlymphocytic leukemia in the elderly. Journal of Clinical Oncology 1990; 8:272-9.

45. Ruutu R, Almqvist A, Hallmann H et al. Oral induction and consolidation of acute myeloid leukemia with etoposide, 6-thioguanine, and idarubicin (ETI) in elderly patients. a randomized comparison with 5-day TAD. Leukemia 1994;8:11-5.

46. Leith CP, Chen I, Kopecky KJ. Correlation of multidrug resistance (MDR1) protein expression with functional Dye/Drug efflux in acute myeloid leukemia my multiparameter flow cytometry: Identification of discordant MDR-/Efflux+ and MDR1+/Efflux- cases. Blood 1995;86:2329-42.

47. Leith CP, Kopecky KJ, Godwin J et al. Acute myeloid leukemia in the elderly: Assessment of multidrug resistance (MDR1) and cytogenetic distinguishes biologic subgroups with remarkable distinct response to standard chemotherapy. A Southwest Oncology Group study. Blood 1997; 89:3323-9.

48. Hiddemann W, Kern W, Schoch E et al. Management of acute myeloid leukemia in elderly patients. Journal of Clinical Oncology 1999; 17:3569-76.

49. Büchner T, Hiddemann W, Koenigsmann M et al. Recombinant human granulocyte-macrophage colony-stimulating factor after chemotherapy in patients with acute myeloid leukemia at higher age or after relapse. Blood 1991;78:1190-7.

50. Löwenberg B, Suciu S, Archimbaud E et al. Use of recombinant granulocyte-macrophage colony-stimulating factor during and after remission induction chemotherapy in patients aged 61 years and older with acute myeloid leukemia (AML): Final report of AML-11, a phase III randomized study of the Leukemia Cooperative Group of European Organisation for the Research and Treatment of Cancer (EORTC-LCG) and the Dutch Belgian Hemato-Oncology Cooperative Group (HOVON). Blood 1997;90:2952-61.

51. Peters C, Minkov M, Matthes-Martin S et al. Leucocyte transfusions from rhG-CSF or prednisolone stimulated donors for treatment of severe infecitons in immunocompromised neutropenic patients. British Journal of Haematology 1999;106:689-96.

52. Keith CR, Albert L, Sonis ST et al. IL-11, a pleiotropic cytokine: exciting new effects of IL-11 on gastrointestinal mucosal biology. Stem Cells (Dayt.) 1994;12:79-90.

53. Sievers EL, Appelbaum FR, Spielberger RT et al. Selective ablation of acute myeloid leukemia using antibody-targeted chemotherapy: A phase I study of an anti CD33 calicheamicin immunoconjugate. Blood 1999;93:3678-84.

54. List AF, Kopecky KJ, Willman CL et al. Benefit of cycloporine (CsA) modulation of anthracycline restistance in high-risk AML: A Southwest Oncology Group (SWOG) Study. Blood 1998;92 (Suppl1):312a

55. Xun CQ, McSweeney PA, Boeckh M et al. Successful nonmyeloablative allogeneic hematopoietic stem cell transplantation in an acute leukemia patient with chemotherapy-induced marrow aplasia and progressive pulmonary aspergillosis. Blood1999; :3273-6

# AML in the Elderly

E. Estey, J. Cortes, M. Beran, Ch. A. Koller and M. J. Keating

*Abstract.* It is commonly accepted that elderly patients with AML have much worse outcomes than younger patients due to increased risk of both early death and resistant disease. Beyond this truism several points should be addressed. First, because other variables (e.g. performance status, organ function) besides age predict these outcomes, it may not be advisable to include age as the sole eligibility criterion for a study; rather use of multivariate models should be considered for this purpose. Second, use of martingale residual graphics illustrate that age itself behaves as a continuous rather than categorical variable and so might be treated as such in such models. Third, these graphics illustrate that the effect of increasing age on survival is limited to the first weeks after beginning therapy; beyond this time older and younger patients should be regarded identically. These matters aside, our efforts at improving outcome in older patients have included
1. use of laminar air flow rooms,
2. use of prophylactic granulocyte transfusions from donors given G-CSF,
3. prophylactic use of fluconazole + itraconazole vs liposomal amphotericin (randomized study), and
4. administration of new anti-AML regimens (e.g. those containing topotecan ± ATRA) aimed at patients with abnormal karyotypes, prior MDS.

While all these strategies will be discussed, the most successful one has been use of laminar flow rooms (PE), treatment in which have been shown to be an independent predictor of better outcome in several studies published from our hospital. An example of such data are shown for patients age β 65 with Zubrod performance status treated at M.D. Anderson since 1991.

It is well-known that the incidence of AML rises with age [1]. Therefore, as the risk of death from cardiovascular disease decreases, it is highly likely that the number of elderly adults with AML will increase. At M.D. Anderson Hospital a median of 20% of adults with newly diagnosed AML (APL excepted) were over age 65 years during the 1980s. In contrast, the corresponding figure has been 34% during the 1990s. Since 1991, our practice has been to treat patients with RAEB-t or RAEB as if they had AML [2]. Given the strong association between MDS and increasing age, it is not surprising that the median age of our newly-diagnosed patients with AML (again excepting APL), RAEB-t, or RAEB was 62 years for the 1995 through 1998 period, with 25% of the patients being at least 70 years old. This aging of our population is a direct result of an increase in the number of elderly patients referred to us.

It is also well-known that older age predicts for worse outcome in AML [3]. This reflects both the tendency of older patients to die before the outcome of induction chemotherapy is known, and the high incidence of resistance to treatment in those surviving long enough to be evaluated for response. Here we review such issues as the definition of elderly AML, the length of time over which the age effect is manifested, and the rationale for assigning to patients to treatment solely on the basis of age. We also review our results in older patients with AML over the past 16 years, focusing on a reduction in early death rate in such patients.

The Department of Leukemia, Division of Medicine
The University of Texas M.D. Anderson Cancer Center Houston, Texas

## Definition of Elderly AML

Eligibility for studies of new therapies in elderly patients with AML is typically limited to patients above a certain age. Different studies select different ages. For example, in studies exploring colony-stimulating factors in older patients, the age cut-off was > 55 years in the study of Rowe et al. [4], >59 years in the study of Stone et al. [5], > 61 years in Lowenberg et al.'s trial [6], and > 64 years in Dombret et al.'s study [7]. This variation implies uncertainty in the exact relationship between age and outcome. One way to examine this relationship uses martingale residual plots [8]. In these plots, the variable of interest, here age in years, is plotted on the X-axis, one value for each patient in the data set. On the Y-axis is the corresponding martingale residual. These are numerical values that quantify the excess risk (e.g. of death) not explained by a baseline Cox model that includes only a hazard function derived from all patients without attention to any prognostic variables. A large positive martingale residual indicates that the baseline model underestimates the risk associated with (in this case) a particular age; a large negative residual indicates that the model overestimates this risk. In other words, large positive martingale residuals correspond to relative risks > 1.0, while large negative residuals correspond to relative risks < 1.0. By examining the plot over its full domain (e.g. ages 16-90), using an automatic smoother to create a line through the scattergram, one can visually examine the effect of variable of interest (here age) on the outcome of interest (here death). Figure 1 is such a plot derived from published M.D. Anderson data [2] obtained in trials in newly-diagnosed AML/MDS. The shape of the smoothed line indicates that the relationship between increasing age and risk of death is direct and continuous. Thus our data do not support the practice of selecting an age cut-off as a criterion for eligibility in clinical trials. In short, there can be no true definition of elderly AML.

## Length of the Age Effect

The Cox model assumes that the effect of a given prognostic factor such as age does not vary over time [9]. This assumption, at least with respect to age, appears counter-intuitive.

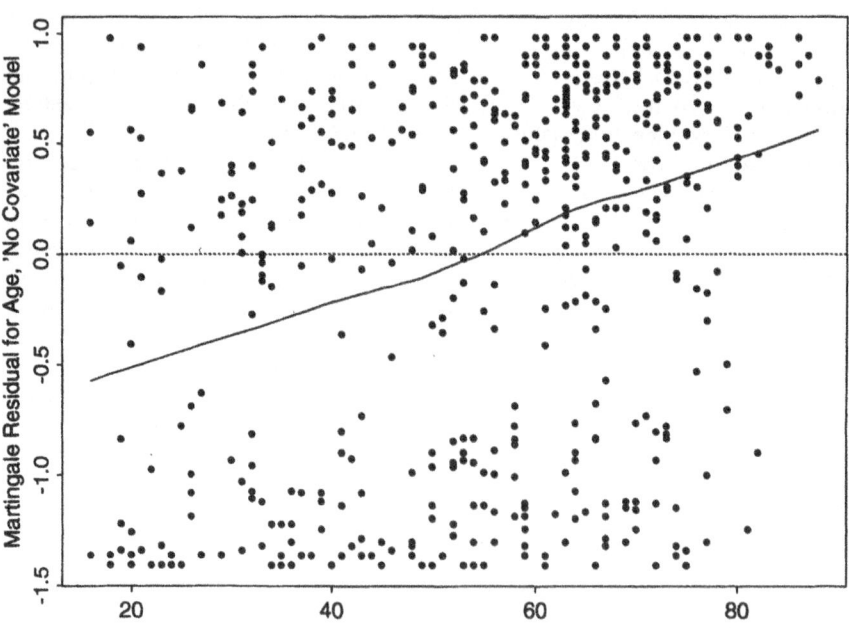

**Fig. 1.** Martingale residual plot showing that relationship between age and risk of death is direct and continuous.

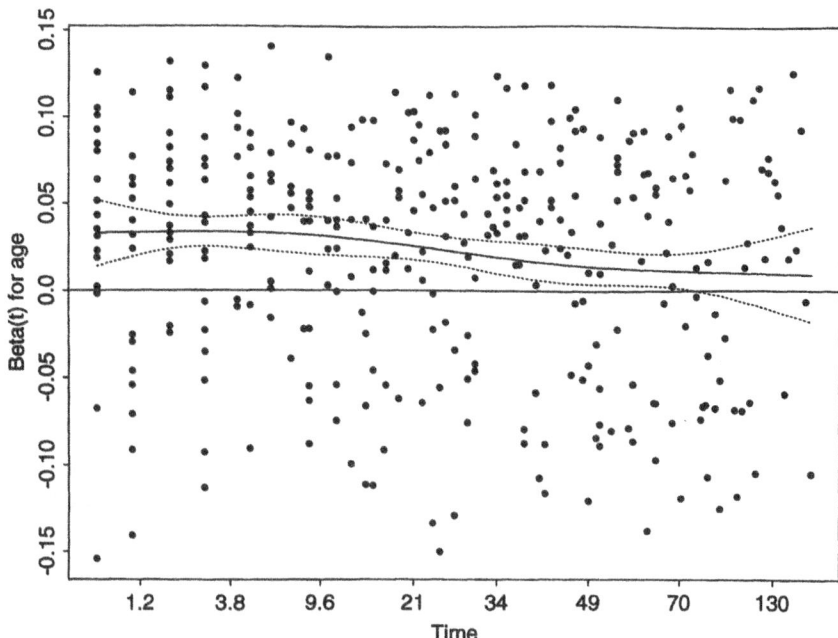

**Fig. 2.** Plot demonstrating that age effect becomes insignificant after about one year from start of therapy. Dashed lines are the 95% confidence intervals.

For example, clinicians might suspect that the unfavorable prognosis associated with advanced age results from the tendency of elderly patients to die relatively early during remission induction. A Grambsch-Therneau-Schoenfeld plot (Fig. 2), similar to the martingale residual plot, is a method to examine the effect of a prognostic factor such as age as a function of time (10). On the X-axis is time in weeks. On the Y-axis is a number, denoted β, analogous to the slope of a line relating the age on the X-axis to the risk of death associated with that age. β= 0 indicates no relationship between age and survival; β> 0 indicates a positive association between increasing age and death, β< 0 indicates a negative association. Figure 2 based on the same data base as Figure 1, shows that increasing age increases the risk of death for about the first 9 months after initiation of therapy. The majority of the effect occurs during the first 3 months. Hence, increasing age predisposes to early death, failure to enter CR despite surviving induction therapy, and early, but not late, relapse. In the remainder of this paper, we will focus on the effect of age on early death.

## Use of Variables other than Age

In 1987, we reported that the risk of death in newly-diagnosed AML was greatest in the first 4 weeks after treatment begins [11]. This led to an attempt to identify those variables independently predictive of death in the first 4 weeks after beginning chemotherapy [11]. These were shown to include pretreatment performance status, bilirubin, albumin, fibrinogen, creatinine, hemoglobin, and neutrophil count, in addition to age. The implication is that assignment of patients to a treatment regimen solely on the basis of age ignores the independent contribution of these other variables to outcome. This applies regardless of the outcome in question; for example interpatient variability in achieving CR would best be explained by accounting for cytogenetics, history of abnormal blood counts etc, in addition to age. From the above it follows that eligibility for a protocol or treatment should not depend on only a single variable, unless no other variable contributes prognostic information to the clinical outcome the study is designed to achieve. For example, eligibility for trials of a csf in newly-diagnosed AML, where a principal objective is to prevent early death, could be determined by a score computed from a model relating values for various prognostic factors to risk of early death. Factors included would be those mentioned above. Consistent with the earlier discussion, age would be considered as a continuous variable; for example, the patient's actual age would be used rather than whether she/he was older than some arbitrarily defined age. Likewise, other factors would be considered according to the form indicated by the relevant martingale residual plot.

## Reduction in Early Death Rate

With the above as background, Table 1 examines the proportion of patients considered at high risk for death in weeks 1-4 after the start of chemotherapy who died during that time. Patients were considered at high risk of early death thus defined if their early risk of mortality (ERM) score was > .1. The ERM was computed using the variables noted above. A value of .1 corresponds to a 10% risk of death in weeks 1-4. This value was selected for this analysis because it was the median value for newly-diagnosed patients presenting to M.D. Anderson during the 1980s. Of course, the same objections to selecting an arbitrary cut-off value for age apply to selecting such a value, e.g. .1, for ERM. Table 1 illustrates that there has been a 5-6-fold increase in the proportion of patients with ERM scores > .1 over the last 12 years. Furthermore, the median ERM score of this high-risk group has increased. Nonetheless, there has been a decrease in the early death rate. The same is true if early death is considered to be one that occurs in the first 35 days. Furthermore, there has been an increase in the CR rate and survival of

patients with ERM scores > .1. The data are essentially the same if attention is restricted to patients age 65 and over regardless of ERM score (Table 2).

**Table 2.** Early Deaths and CR Rates in Pts Age ≥65

| Years | Pts | Median Age/ Median ERM | 28-Day Mortality Rate | CR Rate |
|-------|-----|------------------------|----------------------|---------|
| 83-86 | 60  | 71/.17                 | 22%                  | 47%     |
| 87-90 | 113 | 70/.26                 | 35%                  | 38%     |
| 91-94 | 172 | 73/.28                 | 19%                  | 56%     |
| 95-98 | 278 | 71/.38                 | 20%                  | 50%     |

## Role of Laminar Air Flow Rooms in Reduction in Early Death Rate

Laminar air flow rooms ("protected environment" = PE) have been in use at M.D. Anderson since the early 1970s. Initially, younger patients were placed in these rooms on the assumption that they were most likely to benefit from chemotherapy. However, in the 1990s our practice changed (Table 3). Now patients over age 50 were treated in these rooms, with younger patients largely treated as outpatients. Given the temporal relationship between this change in practice and the fall in early death rate noted in Tables 1 and 2, the relationship between site of treatment (in or out of the PE) and early death rate becomes of interest. Table 4 summarizes the data. To be admitted to the PE, patients must be able to assume a certain amount of self-care. Obviously then, it is possible that death rates are lower in the PE not because of the PE itself but because of the patients that are placed in the PE. One way to examine this issue is via multivariate analysis that examines other relevant factors besides treatment in the PE. We have done several such analyses, with each

**Table 1.** Early Death and CR Rates in Pts with ERM Values >.1

| Years | Pts | Median ERM Value | 28-Day Mortality Rate | CR Rate |
|-------|-----|------------------|----------------------|---------|
| 83-86 | 43  | .24              | 28%                  | 35%     |
| 87-90 | 98  | .32              | 37%                  | 40%     |
| 91-94 | 137 | .38              | 23%                  | 50%     |
| 95-98 | 241 | .43              | 17%                  | 49%     |

**Table 3.** % of Older Patients and Patients with ERM values >.1 in PE by Year

| Years | Pts with Age $65 | In PE | Pts with ERM >.1 | In PE |
|-------|------------------|-------|------------------|-------|
| 83-86 | 60               | 33%   | 43               | 21%   |
| 87-90 | 113              | 28%   | 98               | 26%   |
| 91-94 | 172              | 63%   | 137              | 61%   |
| 95-98 | 278              | 79%   | 241              | 73%   |

**Table 4.** Results by PE Status in Pts with ERM Values >.1

|  | No PE | PE |
|---|---|---|
| Pts | 208 | 287 |
| 28-Day Mortality Rate | 44% | 11% |
| CR Rate | 30% | 60% |

concluding that treatment in the PE predicts a higher CR rate and longer survival even after accounting for age, performance status, cytogenetics, history of abnormal blood counts etc [2, 12, 13].

## Role of Prophylactic Amphotericin

Since 1992, all our patients, whether treated inside or outside the PE, have received antibacterial prophylaxis (generally trimethoprim/sulfamethoxasole, less often a quinolone) and anti-fungal prophylaxis (fluconazole + itraconazole). The availability of liposomal associated amphotericin (lipoAmpho) preparations has made it possible to assess the usefulness of amphotericin in preventing early death, without the risk of renal failure seen following use of standard amphotericin. We have recently begun a study randomizing patients with ERM values > .1 to receive fluconazole/itraconazole or lipoAmpho (ABLC). Table 5 shows results in the first 68 patients. There appears to be slight advantage for lipoAmpho, but the data are obviously incomplete.

## Prophylactic Granulocyte Transfusions

We have taken advantage of another new treatment modality, G-CSF, to examine the role of prophylactic granulocyte (PMN) transfusions. Prior to beginning the fluconazole/itraconazole vs. amphotericin trial, we conducted a trial in which patients with ERM scores > .1 and two donors (family or friends) willing to donate PMNs were randomly assigned to receive PMNS prophylactically (beginning once the WBC count fell below 500) or therapeutically (after failure of a febrile episode to resolve within 3 days of beginning antibiotics for the episode). The donors received G-CSF (300 micrograms) one day before each PMN donation, with donations scheduled QOD; males could donate 4 times and females 3 times. Table 6 shows that there was no difference in CR rates among patients in the prophylactic arm, patients in the therapeutic arm, and patients with < 2 donors, some of whom did receive PMNs when infection developed. The same is true considering early death rates. One possible explanation for the failure of prophylactic PMN transfusion may have been the general inability to identify more than 2 donors per patient. Accordingly, patients usually could receive no more than 8 days of prophylactic transfusions, whereas the period of neutropenia was usually 3-4 weeks. It is interesting to note that fewer patients in the prophylactic group had pneumonia or fungal infections (Table 7). Alt-

**Table 6.** CR Rates in Prophylayactic Granulocyte Transfusion Study

| Group | Pts | CR |
|---|---|---|
| Prophylactic PMNS | 26 | 50% |
| Therapeutic PMNS | 29 | 56% |
| <2 Donors | 43 | 51% |

**Table 7.** Rates of Pneumonia or Fungal Infection

| Group | Pts | Pneumonia or Fungal Infection | |
|---|---|---|---|
| Prophylactic PMNS | 26 | 8% | P = .08 |
| No Prophylactic PMNS[a] | 72 | 25% | |

[a]Therapeutic PMNS + pts with <2 donors.

**Table 5.** Comparison of Patients Given Prophylaxis with Liposomal Amphotericin vs Fluconazole/Itraconazole

| RX | Pts | Median Values | | Treated in PE | 28-Day Mortality Rate | CR Rate |
|---|---|---|---|---|---|---|
|  |  | ERM | Age |  |  |  |
| L-Ampho | 37 | .17 | 61 | 21/32 | 5% | 65% |
| FI | 31 | .15 | 60 | 22/29 | 10% | 48% |

**Table 8.** Death Rates According to Development of Pneumonia or Fungal Infection

| Group | Pneumonia or Fungal Infection | | | No Pneumonia or Fungal Infection | | |
|---|---|---|---|---|---|---|
| | Pts | Deaths | | Pts | Deaths | |
| Prophylactic PMNS | 2 | 100% | | 24 | 21% | |
| | | | $P = .11$ | | | |
| No Prophylactic PMNS[a] | 18 | 28% | | 54 | 11% | $P = .29$ |

[a]Therapeutic PMNS + pts with < 2 donors

hough such episodes predisposed to induction death, the likelihood of death after acquiring such an infection was higher in the prophylactic group; furthermore, among patients who did not have such episodes, the death rate was higher in the prophylactic group (Table 8). This suggests either that prophylactic PMN transfusions can themselves predispose to death, e.g. via lung injury, or that the criteria for pneumonia or fungal infection are not totally objective.

## Improvements in Anti-AML Therapy

Clearly, reduction in early death rates are ultimately meaningless unless accompanied by use of anti-AML therapy capable of producing substantial remissions. Because elderly patients with AML frequently have abnormal karyotypes, long histories of abnormal blood counts, high MDR levels and probably other features associated with resistance to standard regimens, it is unlikely that improvements in supportive care will translate into long remissions if such patients continue to receive such regimens. Here "standard" includes regimens containing high-dose ara-C, as well as 3+7 type therapies. On the other hand, results with investigational regimens, e.g. those containing topotecan have also been poor. We have investigated such regimens in phase II studies, i.e. those accruing > 50 patients. While we continue to believe that new investigational regimens remain the best option for elderly patients whose AML, RAEB-t, or RAEB is characterized by abnormal cytogenetics etc, we believe that the optimal statistical design for trials with such regimens is one that accrues a smaller number (up to 20) of patients per treatment, therefore allowing more treatments to be tested. As accrual pro-

ceeds, treatments that so not meet a certain minimum acceptability criterion are terminated before 20 patients are entered. If no early termination occurs, 20 patients are treated, and the regimen that has the highest response rate is selected for further, i.e. phase II testing. Although the false negative rate associated with such a design may approach 20-25%, this rate is still lower than that associated with the arbitrary selection of one of, say, three regimens for phase II testing in a trial accruing > 50 patients. In this circumstance the effective false negative rate is 67%, assuming that there is no scientifically valid for choosing one regimen over the others, and that, given limitations in patient numbers, it is impossible to test all three regimens in full scale phase II studies. We believe these conditions frequently apply. Further discussion can be found in reference 14.

## References

1. Brincker H: Population-based age- and sex-specific incidence rates in the 4 main types of leukaemia. Scand J Haematol 29:241-249, 1982.
2. Estey E, Thall P, Beran M, Kantarjian H, Pierce S, Keating M: Effect of diagnosis (RAEB, RAEB-t, or AML) on outcome of AML-type chemotherapy. Blood 90:2969-2977, 1997.
3. Clinical Annotation. "Acute myeloid leukemia in the elderly: biology and treatment." Brit J Haemat 83:1-6, 1993.
4. Rowe JM, Andersen JW, Mazza JJ, Bennett JM, Paietta E, Hayes FA, Oette D, Cassileth PA, Stadtmauer EA, Wiernik PH: A randomized placebo-controlled phase III study of granulocyte-macrophage colony-stimulating factor in adult patients (>55 to 70 years of age) with acute myelogenous leukemia: a study of the Eastern Cooperative Oncology Group (E1490). Blood 86:457-462, 1995.
5. Stone RM, Berg DT, George SL, Doge RK, Paciucci PA, Schulman P, Lee EJ, Moore JO, Powell BL, Schiffer CA: Granulocyte-macrophage colony-stimulating factor after initial chemotherapy for elderly patients with primary acute myelogenous leukemia. N Engl J Med 332:1671-1677, 1995

6. Löwenberg B, Suciu S, Archimbaud E, Ossenkoppele G, Verhoef GEG, Vellenga E, Wijermans P, Berneman Z, Dekker AW, Stryckmans, P, Schouten H, Jehn U, Muus P, Sonneveld P, Dardenne M, Zittoun R: Use of recombinant granulocyte-macrophage colony-stimulating-factor (GM-CSF) during and after remission induction chemotherapy in patients aged 61 years and older with acute myeloid leukemia: final report of AML-11, a phase III randomized study of the EORTC-LCG and HOVON Groups. Blood 90:2952-2961, 1997

7. Dombret H, Chastang C, Fenaux P, Reiffers J, Bordessoule D, Bouabdallah R, Mandellli F, Ferrant A, Auzanneau G, Tilly H, Yver A, Degos L: A controlled study of recombinant human granulocyte colony-stimulating factor in elderly patients after treatment for acute myelogenous leukemia. N Engl J Med 332:1678-1683, 1995

8. Therneau TM, Grambsch PM, Fleming TR: Martingale-based residuals for survival models. Biometrika 77:147-160, 1990.

9. Fleming TR, Harrington DP: Counting Processes and Survival Analysis. New York, Wiley, 1991

10. Grambsch PM, Therneau TM: Proportional hazards tests and diagnostics based on weighted residuals. Biometrika 81:515-526, 1994.

11. Estey E, Smith TL, Keating MJ, McCredie KB, Gehan EA, and Freireich EJ: Prediction of survival during induction therapy in patients with newly diagnosed acute myeloblastic leukemia. Leukemia 3:257-263, 1989.

12. Estey E, Thall P, Andreeff M, Beran M, Kantarjian H, O'Brien S, Escudier S, Robertson LE, Koller C, Kornblau S, Pierce S, Freireich EJ, Deisseroth A, Keating M: Use of granulocyte colony-stimulating factor before, during, and after fludarabine plus cytarabine induction therapy of newly-diagnosed acute myelogenous leukemia or myelodysplastic syndromes: comparison with fludarabine plus cytarabine without granulocyte colony-stimulating factor. J Clin Oncol 12:671-678, 1994.

13. Estey EH, Thall PF, Pierce S, Cortes J, Beran M, Kantarjian H, Keating MJ, Andreeff M, Freireich E: Randomized phase II study of fludarabine + cytosine arabinoside + idarubicin ± all-trans retinoic acid ± granulocyte-colony stimulating factor in poor prognosis newly-diagnosed non-APL AML and MDS. Blood. In press.

14. Thall PF, Estey EH: A Bayesian strategy for screening cancer treatments prior to phase II clinical evaluation. Stat Med 12:1197-1211, 1993.

# The EORTC-HOVON Approach to the Older Patient with AML: The Use of GM-CSF

B. LÖWENBERG on behalf of the EORTC Leukemia and HOVON Co-operative Group, University Hospital Rotterdam and Erasmus University Rotterdam, The Netherlands

The approach to the older patient with AML has been subject of investigation in two recently completed studies involving a total of more than 800 patients conducted by the EORTC and HOVON Leukemia co-operative Groups (AML-9 and AML-11). In AML-9 two induction schedules (mitoxantrone – Ara-C versus daunomycin – Ara-C) and in AML-11 two schedules of daunomycin – Ara-C with or without GM-CSF were compared. In this presentation the emphasis will be on the AML-11 study: the use of GM-CSF did not reveal improvements of response, relapse rate following remission or survival in relation to the addition of GM-CSF to treatment, although granulocyte recovery was significantly enhanced in the GM-CSF treatment group. The principal results of the study will be presented. For future developments in the older patient group, it appears useful to invest in the identification of older patients with variable risks. The analysis revealed poor prognostic indicators for survival: poor performance status at diagnosis, high white blood cell count, older age, secondary AML, and the presence of cytogenetic abnormalities.

## Introduction

The incidence of death due to bacterial and fungal infections during episodes of neutropenia during and after remission induction therapy may range up to 30% among adults of 60+ yrs of age with acute myeloid leukemia. In various studies the application of G-CSF or GM-CSF in association with induction or consolidation chemotherapy has been evaluated in recent years. The EORTC HOVON co-operative Groups designed a study in which GM-CSF was applied concomitantly with the induction chemotherapy as well as post chemotherapy. The rationale for the design was that GM-CSF would not only accelerate myeloid recovery, but in addition it might activate AML blasts and as a result enhance susceptibility of AML to the cytotoxic effects of chemotherapy. Here the results of the latter study are summarised.

## Study design

Patients aged 61 yrs and older were entered to be randomised to receive either Daunomycin 30 mg/m$^2$ on days 1, 2 and 3 and Cytarabine 200 mg/m$^2$ per continuous infusion on days 1–7 or the same chemotherapy for induction combined with GM-CSF. GM-CSF (Molgrastim, Novartis, Basel, Switzerland) was an Escherichia coli derived CM-CSF and was applied at 5 µg/kg/day per continuous infusion, starting at day 1 prior to the beginning of chemotherapy. It was continued until day 28 or until granulocyte recovery to 0.5 x 10$^9$/l. The details of the design of the study have been described (Löwenberg 1997).

## Results

157 eligible and evaluable patients were assigned to receive chemotherapy with GM-CSF (experimental group) and 161 patients were assigned to the control chemotherapy with no GM-CSF (control group). The median age of each of the two treatment groups were 68 yrs of age and the patients were well balanced for FAB cytology, cytogenetics, performance status and secondary and de novo AML. The CR rates were 56% (GM-CSF group) and 55% (control group), respectively. There was no difference in the probability of response after cycle I between the two groups

**Table 1.** Use of GM-CSF in adjunct to remission induction chemotherapy in AML (large randomized studies)

| study | age (median) | comparative treatment arms | number of cases | days to neutrophil recovery 0.5x10⁹/l | fewer documented infections | better survival |
|---|---|---|---|---|---|---|
| Godwin et al 1998 | 67 | G-CSF 400 µg/m²/d<br>placebo | (n=106)<br>(n=105) | 24<br>27<br>(p=0.014) | no | no |
| Löwenberg et al*1997 | 68 | GM-CSF 5 µg/kg/d<br>controls | (n=161)<br>(n=157) | 23<br>25<br>(p=0.0002) | no | no |
| Rowe et al 1995 | 64 | GM-CSF 250 µg/m²/d<br>placebo | (n=60)<br>(n=57) | 13<br>17<br>(p=0.001) | – | 10.6 mo(median)<br>4.8 mo (median)<br>(p=0.048) |
| Stone et al 1995 | 69 | GM-CSF 5 µg/kg/d<br>placebo | (n=193)<br>(n=195) | 15<br>17<br>(p=0.02) | no | no |
| Witz et al 1998 | 66 | GM-CSF 5 µg/kg/d<br>placebo | (n=114)<br>(n=126) | 24<br>29<br>(p=0.0001) | no | no |

Randomized studies including at least 100 patients
* GM-CSF was administered not only during the aplastic phase; but it was also administered on the days concomitantly with the chemotherapy

nor were there any differences in the causes of induction deaths. Response did not differ, although neutrophil recovery was significantly enhanced in patients of the GM-CSF treatment series. Median times to granulocyte recovery of 0.5 x 10⁹/l after induction cycle I in GM-CSF treated patients and control patients were 23 and 25 days, respectively (p=0.0002). The median times of platelet recovery and the median number of days spent in the hospital did not differ between the two groups.

## Survival and disease free survival

Patients have been followed for a median of 36 months after diagnosis and probabilities of overall survival at two years after randomisation were identical, i.e., 22% in the GM-CSF and the control groups. Also the disease free survival probabilities after randomisation

were not significantly different between the two groups: 14% in the GM-CSF and 19% in the control series.

## Prognostic factors for response and survival

Only 4% of cases presented with specific cytogenetic abnormalities of favourable type so that this subset of patients clearly is underrepresented among the older individuals with AML. Unfavourable type abnormalities were seen in 19% of cases. Especially patients with hyperleucocytosis (white blood cells of 100 x 10⁹/l or more), a poor performance status at diagnosis and abnormal cytogenetics showed a significantly reduced probability of attaining complete remission. Also patients with unfavourable type cytogenetics had reduced CR rates. As regards overall survival, abnormal cytogenetics and poor risk cytogenetic abnormalities again had significant adverse impact. The latter two prognostic factors also predicted for poor disease free survival.

## Discussion

In this randomised study we evaluated the role of GM-CSF in elderly patients with AML (Löwenberg 1997). We assume that the use of GM-CSF in parallel to the chemotherapy might sensitise the leukemic cells for the cytotoxic effects of chemotherapy and enhance treatment effect. In this large study no evidence for in vivo sensitisation of AML for chemotherapy was apparent. In patients assigned to GM-CSF treatment the response nor disease free survival were better than those in patients treated with standard chemotherapy with no addition of GM-CSF. Thus, the current study does not support the hypothesis of growth factor induced chemotherapy modulation. In the same study GM-CSF was continued post chemotherapy in an attempt to reduce complications during neutropenia and improve outcome. Although a slight reduction of the duration of granulocytopenia was seen, this difference did not translate into an advantage of response or survival. Again, the response to treatment, overall survival and disease free survival were identical in the two comparative treatment groups. As a matter of fact, this would suggest that the standard use of GM-CSF in treatment of patients with AML is not warranted. A few other studies have evaluated the use of GM-CSF in patients with AML of comparatively older age. In the study of Rowe (Rowe 1995) a better survival was seen, but survival of the placebo treated control patients was extremely poor and survival outcome of GM-CSF treated patients did not improve above usual. Three other phase III studies in older patients with AML (Stone 1995, Witz 1998, Godwin 1998) also produced negative results, even though granulocyte recovery was consistently enhanced in each of these studies.

For future treatment development it appears important to distinguish subsets of older individuals with clearly distinct prognosis. The current study would indicate that patients with high white blood cell counts (hyperleucocytosis), poor performance status and unfavourable cytogenetics, represent particularly poor groups of patients for which entirely new treatments would be required. One such approach might be the use of multidrug resistance modulation in an effort to overcome treatment resistance that is so prominent in older patients with AML. The HOVON group is currently participating into an intergroup co-operative study that addresses the use of PSC833 as a drug resistance modifier in the context of a detailed analysis of prognostic factors.

## References

Godwin JE, Kopecky KJ, Head, DR, et al (1998) A double-blind placebo-controlled trial of granulocyte colony-stimulating factor in elderly patients with previously untreated acute myeloid leukemia: a Southwest Oncology Group Study (9031). Blood 91:3607-15

Löwenberg B, Suciu S, Archimbaud E, et al on behalf of EORTC-LCG and HOVON (1997) Use of recombinant granulocyte-macrophage colony stimulating factor during and after induction chemotherapy in patients aged 63 years and older with acute myeloid leukemia (AML): a final report of AML-11, a phase III randomized study of the Leukemia Cooperative Group of the European Organization for Research and Treatment of Cancer (EORTC-LCG) and the Dutch-Belgian Hemato-Oncology Group (HOVON). Blood 90:2952-61

Rowe JM, Andersen J, Mazza JJ, et al (1995) A randomized placebo-controlled study of granulocyte-macrophage colony-stimulating factor in adult patients (>55-70 years of age) with acute myeloid myelogenous leukemia (AML): a study of the Eastern Cooperative Oncology Group (E1490). Blood 86:457-62

Stone RM, Berg DT, George SL, et al (1995) Granulocyte-macrophage colony-stimulating factor after initial chemotherapy for elderly patients with primary acute myelogenous leukemia. N Engl J Med 332:1671-7

Witz F, Sadoun A, Perrin MC, et al (1998) A placebo-controlled study of recombinant human granulocyte-macrophage colony-stimulating factor administered during and after induction treatment for de novo acute myelogenous leukemia in elderly patients. Blood 91:2722-30

# Therapy of Older Adults with AML: CALGB Studies

R. M. STONE

*Abstract.* Successive CALGB studies have sought to overcome the intrinsic disease resistance and poor tolerance of myelosuppression in older adults with AML. Although CALGB 8525 demonstrated that post-remission high dose ara-C was superior to lower doses, no benefit was noted in patients (pts) over the age of 60. Similarly, of the 201 pts ≥60 years old who achieved complete remission (CR) in CALGB 8923 two cycles of an intensive ara-C/mitoxantrone combination led to the same disease-free survival time (10.5 months) as four cycles of lower dose ara-C. GM-CSF failed to decrease induction-related mortality in the same study. Since cytokine support during induction and intensive post-remission therapy have not been proven beneficial in the older age cohort, the CALGB is now determining the value of drug resistance modulation (DRM) and immunostimulation. Because of the effect of multi-drug resistance gene inhibition on the metabolism of chemotherapeutic agents, a Phase I trial (CALGB 9420) was conducted to develop equitoxic ara-C/daunorubicin/etoposide (ADE) induction regimens in older pts with and without PSC-833 for DRM. 50% and 60% higher doses of D and E, respectively, could be given in the non-PSC cohort. The ongoing CALGB study (9720) for pts ≥60 years old involves randomization to either ADE or ADE + PSC-833 at the previously derived doses. Pts who achieve CR and receive a cycle of consolidation therapy are randomized to receive either no therapy or subcutaneous IL-2 with intermittent boluses. Given the rarity of cure (only 19/388 pts enrolled on CALGB 8923 were long-term disease-free survivors), it is hoped that one of the newer strategies will change the natural history of AML in older pts.

Patients over the age of 60 who develop acute myeloid leukemia (AML) fare much more poorly than do younger patients with the same disease. Large cooperative group studies, in which patients are probably more selected than a representative community based sample, report complete remission rates in the 45-50% range for older adults with AML compared with 70-80% from those under the age of 60 [1]. The difference in disease free survival is similarly striking: 30-40% of those patients in CR in the younger age cohort can expect to achieve long-term disease free survival, a rate at least twice that reported for those greater than 60 years of age. Given the small chance of cure at disease outset (5-10%) for an older patient with AML it can reasonably asked whether the myelosuppressive therapy considered standard treatment is worthwhile. However, randomized studies that compared either observation [2] or low-dose chemotherapy [3] to immediate standard induction therapy suggested that a slight, but significant benefit was associated with prompt administration of myelosuppressive chemotherapy.

Leaving aside for the moment the probity of treatment of an elderly individual who is diagnosed with AML, the reasons for the inferior outcome relative to that obtained in younger adults are fairly well understood. First, and probably of least importance, is the frequent occurrence of co-morbid diseases, such as diabetes, hypertension, congestive heart failure, chronic obstructive pulmonary disease, and osteoporosis, in the older adult thereby making the poor tolerance of myelosuppressive chemotherapy more likely. For example, the hypotension associated with gram negative sepsis is more likely to be a fatal complication in a 70 year old with base-

Dana-Farber Cancer Institute, 44 Binney Street, Boston, MA 02115, Phone: 617-632-2214, Fax: 617-632-2933

line cardiovascular disease than in an otherwise healthy 35 year old. Myelosuppression may be somewhat more prolonged in an older person due to the intrinsically lowed stem cell tolerance. However, the most important issue is the inherent degree of disease resistance characteristic of AML in the older patient.

The evidence that AML in the older adult is intrinsically more resistant comes from several sources. The 50% failure rate in the older patient is accounted for by an almost equal contribution of treatment-related mortality, and resistant disease. The percentage of those not achieving CR due to resistant disease, therefore is comparable to the rate in younger adults. The difference in overall CR rates, then, is accounted for by a much higher rate of early and hypoplastic death during induction in the elderly (20-30%) compared with 5-15% in the younger age cohort. However, it is presumed that the inability to clear enough leukemia cells to allow for restoration of normal hematopoiesis in a timely enough fashion accounts in part for the delayed recovery and a longer neutropenic period. The fairly direct reasons that AML in the older patient is less likely to respond to chemotherapy are

a) expression of genes that confer resistance is relatively common [4],
b) higher incidence of chromosomal abnormalities associated with poor prognosis [5], and
c) frequent occurrence of real or presumed antecedent hematologic disease, usually primary or secondary myelodysplasia.

In summary, the leukemia progenitor cells in the older patient are believed to emanate from a stem cell more proximal (and more resistant) in the hematopoietic hierarchy than those from younger individuals with AML.

The CALGB has attempted to improve the therapeutic outcome in older adults with AML in a successive series of studies which have focused on both reducing treatment-related mortality and enhancing antineoplastic efficacy. CALGB 8525 [6] demonstrated the effectiveness of intensive post-remission therapy, but only in patients under the age of 60. 1088 adults with newly diagnosed primary AML 16 years of age or older received an induction regimen (»3+7«) consisting of cytarabine (200 mg/m² by continuous intravenous infusion for seven days), with daunorubicin given as a bolus on the first three days of cytarabine therapy (45 mg/m² for patients 60 years of age or younger and 30 mg/m² for patients older than 60). Patients received a second course of induction therapy consisting of five days of cytarabine and two days of daunorubicin at a dose identical to the initial treatment if a significant amount of residual leukemia was noted when a bone marrow examination was performed 14 days after the start of therapy or later. Establishing the baseline for subsequent CALGB studies, the CR rate for those 60 years of age or younger was 73% (with one-third requiring two courses of induction therapy) compared with 47% for older adults (26% requiring a second course). Early death or death during hypoplasia accounted for treatment failure in (31%) of older adults, but only 13% in those under 60 years of age (Table 1). The problem of excess induction-related deaths in the older age cohort would be dealt with in a subsequent CALGB study, one specifically designed for older adults with AML.

Of the 693 patients enrolled in CALGB 8525 who achieved remission 596 were randomized to receive four courses of cytarabine at a dose of

a) 100 mg/m² by continuous intravenous infusion for 5 days,
b) 400 mg/m² by continuous intravenous infusion for 5 days or
c) 3.0 gm/m² over 3 hours twice daily every other day for 6 doses.

Patients still in CR at the conclusion of the aforementioned treatment were to receive 4 courses of cytarabine (100 mg/m² subcuta-

**Table 1.** CALGB 8525: Results According to Age n=1088

|  | age ≤60 | age >60 |
|---|---|---|
| n | 742 | 346 |
| CR% | 73% | 47% |
| (CR in one course) | (67%) | (74%) |
| ED/hypoplastic death | 13% | 31% |
| Resistant disease | 15% | 22% |
| DFS (5yr) | 30% | 13% |
| O.S. (5yr) | 30% | 8% |

Daunorubicin/cytarabine induction (»3+7« ± »2+5«; dauno dose 45 mg/m² [age ≤60]; 30 mg/m² [age >60]

neously bid for 5 days) plus daunorubicin (45 mg/m$^2$ in a single intravenous push). The major finding of the study was the documentation of the superiority of high dose ara-C in the post-remission setting, with a 42% likelihood of 5 year disease free survival for those 60 years of age or younger. However, dose intensification in the older patient was not beneficial; the likelihood of 5 year disease free survival was 14% or less in each of the ara-C dose arms with a 8% likelihood of survival after 5 years (Table 2).

**Table 2.** CALGB 8525: Results According to Age and Assigned Post-CR Treatment

| | 5 year DFS (median F/U=63.5 months) | |
| | age ≤60 n=467 | age >60 n=129 |
| --- | --- | --- |
| 100 | 19% | 14% |
| 400 | 29% | 14% |
| 3gm | 42% (62%)* | 14% (29%)* |

p=.002    * receiving all 4 courses of planned therapy

Post-remission randomization to 4 courses of ara-C @ a) 100 mg/m$^2$/d CIVI x 5d; b) 400 mg/m$^2$/d x 5d; c) 3gm/m$^2$/3h q12h d1, 3, 5

The failure of high dose ara-C to yield better results in older patients was possibly due in part to an inability to receive planned therapy. Only 29% of patients over the age of 60 received all four courses of high-dose cytarabine (compared with approximately 60% of younger patients). Older patients had a higher risk of high dose ara-C associated cerebellar toxicity, but the likelihood of this devastating complication was also related to renal insufficiency and increased levels of alkaline phosphatase. Patients over the age of 60 who had a serum creatinine less than 1.2 gm/dl and a normal alkaline phosphatase had only a 1% risk of such a problem [7]. A study correlating cytogenetic status with cytarabine dose response showed that favorable prognostic karyotypic abnormalities (e.g. t(8;21) or inv 16) were less common in those over the age 60 [8] (Table 3). Although age was a significant factor for CR duration (univariate analysis), a regression analysis suggested that cytogenetic risk group and cytarabine dose were most important in predicting cure [8].

Only patients 60 years of age or older with previously untreated primary AML were eli-

**Table 3.** CALGB 8525: Frequency of Cytogenetic Abnormalities according to Age Randomized CR patients with adequate cytogenetics

| | CBF* | NL | Other |
| --- | --- | --- | --- |
| age >60 (n=67) | 18% | 43% | 39% |
| age ≤60 (n=133) | 26% | 38% | 36% |

*t(8:21) or inv 16 (and related abnormalities)

Note: Multivariate regression analysis showed that cytogenetic risk group and cytarabine dose were the most important factors for long term disease-free survival (Bloomfield, et al. Canc Res, 1998)

gible for CALGB 8923, which focused on improving supportive care and on evaluating a tolerable yet effective myelosuppressive post-remission therapy program. The goals of this study were to determine if E. coli-derived granulocyte-macrophage colony stimulating factor (GM-CSF) would provide supportive care benefits during induction and if a myelosuppressive yet hopefully tolerable and effective post-remission therapy could be developed. When the study was designed one of the concerns was that GM-CSF might promote leukemic proliferation, thereby increasing the likelihood of disease resistance. However, an uncontrolled trial reported by Büchner [9] suggested that GM-CSF was both safe and effective in reducing duration of neutropenia compared to historical controls in patients with high risk AML. Furthermore, the CALGB 8923 study design included the administration of growth factor only after the completion of induction chemotherapy, thus eliminating the potential confounding issue of »priming« in which leukemic cells would be stimulated to grow, thereby potentially becoming more sensitive to cell cycle specific therapeutic agents such as cytarabine. It was felt that it would be optimal to test »full dose« daunorubicin in the older age cohort in the setting of a trial designed to determine the efficacy of a hemopoietic growth factor. In fact, results from CALGB 8525 using the 30 mg/m$^2$ dose of daunorubicin were essentially no different from that in an earlier CALGB trial [10] in older adults in which the 45 mg/m$^2$ dose had been employed.

383 patients with primary AML age 60 years of age or older were enrolled onto CALGB 8923 [11] and received the identical

»3+7« daunorubicin/cytarabine induction given to younger patients on CALGB 8525. They were randomized to receive, in a double-blind fashion, either GM-CSF at a dose of 5µg/kg over 6 hours daily beginning on the eighth day after the initiation of chemotherapy (the day after the conclusion of the infusional cytarabine). The GM-CSF was continued until the neutrophil count exceeded 1000 per µl. The GM-CSF was discontinued before such neutrophil recovery was achieved if there were signs of leukemic regrowth manifested by an increase in the number of circulating myeloblasts or if, in the opinion of investigator on site, there was felt to be intractable toxicity due to the growth factor. As in CALGB 8525, a second course of two days of daunorubicin and five days of cytarabine could be administered if there was post-therapeutic evidence of leukemic involvement of the bone marrow. However, only the bone marrow exam done 21 days after initiation of therapy (or later) was used to justify the administration of a second course of chemotherapy in comparison to day 14 on the previous CALGB study. If a second course of chemotherapy was needed, then GM-CSF was discontinued during the period of chemotherapy administration, but restarted the day following its completion. The results showed a significant but probably clinically meaningless reduction in the duration of neutropenia (15 days for patients assigned to the GM-CSF arm versus 13 days for those assigned to the placebo infusion). The complete remission rates were essentially identical (Table 4). There was no reduction in treatment related mortality or in serious infections associated with the administration of GM-CSF. Fully one-third of the patients had their experimental infusion discontinued prematurely due to the apparent appearance of growth factor-associated toxicity. However, half the time that severe GM-CSF-associated toxicity was believed to be occurring, the patient was actually receiving placebo. While this phenomenon stressed the difficulty of assigning toxicity to a specific drug in a very ill group of patients, even in those patients who received a »full course« of GM-CSF no major benefit could be discerned. One interesting result from CALGB 8923 was that the CR rate was similar to that seen in previous

**Table 4.** CALGB 8923: Results According to Induction Randomization

|  | GM-CSF n=187 | Placebo n=189 |  |
| --- | --- | --- | --- |
| CR rate | 51%* | 54%* |  |
| neutropenic duration | 15 days | 17 days | p.02 |
| hospital stay duration | 28 days | 30 days | p.11 |
| ED/hypoplastic death | 27% | 23% |  |
| severe infection | 18% | 18% |  |
| CR duration, median | 8.2 mo | 10.4 mo |  |
| O.S. duration | 8.4 mo | 10.8 mo |  |

*one course of induction used in 88%

studies, even though only about one-seventh of the patients required a second dose of induction chemotherapy. The lower numbers requiring a more prolonged induction were probably due to the fact that the decision to retreat was made at day 21, rather than day 14. Certainly some of the patients who had been treated in prior studies based on the residual appearance of leukemic cells did not »need« this therapy and therefore some degree of toxicity could have been saved without compromising therapeutic efficacy.

Although the results of CALGB 8923 with regard to GM-CSF administration were disappointing, almost all of the many similar trials of growth factor administration for supportive care of older adults with AML [12-18] also failed to document a significant benefit in terms of improving CR rate, reducing infectious deaths, or improving overall survival. The one major study that came to a different conclusion was performed by the Eastern Cooperative Oncology Group [18]. In the ECOG trial the major differences compared to CALGB 8923 were that a higher dose (60 mg/m² per day) of daunorubicin was used, yeast-derived (glycosylated) GM-CSF was used and patients were required to have bone marrow hypoplasia on day 10 prior to the start of GM-CSF. While design considerations could have accounted for the apparent improvement in CR rate associated with GM-CSF administration in the ECOG trial, it is also possible that the salutory results were noted by chance, especially in so far as the ECOG trial was relatively smaller (124 patients).

The second goal of CALGB 8923 was the evaluation of a novel post-remission intensification regimen consisting of a combination of mitoxantrone and ara-C developed at Mt. Sinai Hospital's Neoplastic Disease Division. Of the 198 patients who achieved remission, 169 were deemed medically fit e87ugh to be randomized to one of the two post-remission therapy arms. 79 patients were randomized to receive two courses of ara-C/mitoxantrone (ara-C 250 mg/m$^2$ over 30 minutes followed by 250 mg/m$^2$ over three hours plus mitoxantrone 5 mg/m$^2$ beginning 6 hours after the start of ara-C every 12 hours for 6 doses) with the second course being administered no sooner than 56 days after the first course. 82 patients were randomized to receive four courses of ara-c 100mg/m$^2$ per day by continuous intravenous infusion for 5 days. Each course was to be given no sooner than 28 days after the first course. There was no difference in disease-free or overall survival based on randomization to either arm and/or induction randomization to GM-CSF or placebo (Table 5). However, those patients receiving ara-C/mitoxantrone experienced a higher likelihood of treatment-associated toxicities (Table 6). The most striking result was the relatively poor overall disease-free survival (9 months) and overall survival (10 months) in both arms [19]. Relatively low dose ara-C may be considered the 'standard' post-remission therapy for the older adult with AML given these results plus those of a recent trial demonstrating the benefit of such an approach compared with observation [20].

In CALGB 8923, even those few individuals whose blasts harbored »favorable« chromosomal abnormalities did not enjoy a superior outcome in either post-remission arm. Most patients whose blasts expressed the natural killer cell antigen CD56 favored even more poorly than those whose blasts did not express this marker. The overall results in

**Table 6.** CALGB 8923: Toxicities According to Post-CR Randomization

| Toxicity | Grade | Randomized Arm | | P |
|---|---|---|---|---|
| | | Ara-C | Ara-C+M | |
| Hemorrhage | <4 | 80 | 78 | .03 |
| | ≥4 | 0 | 6 | |
| Infection | <4 | 74 | 70 | .10 |
| | ≥4 | 6 | 14 | |
| Diarrhea | <3 | 79 | 73 | .005 |
| | ≥3 | 1 | 11 | |
| Dysrhythmias | <4 | 80 | 78 | .03 |
| | 4 | 0 | 6 | |
| Malaise | <3 | 79 | 74 | .01 |
| | 3 | 1 | 10 | |

CALGB 8923 suggested that avenues other than supportive care with GM-CSF or postremission intensification with an ara-C/mitoxantrone containing regimen needed to be considered for older patients with AML.

A significant proportion of older patients with AML express the gp170 multidrug resistance protein that is responsible for an energy dependent drug efflux preventing accumulation of chemotherapeutic agents such as etoposide, anthracyclines, and vinca alkaloids. The Southwest Oncology Group has shown that expression of this protein is an independent adverse prognostic factor in older patients with AML [2]. Preliminary results from a SWOG study [21] have suggested that the administration of cyclosporine, an inhibitor of PGP function, can improve the therapeutic response in patients with relapsed AML [20]. However, cyclosporine has immunosuppressive effects and also influences the metabolism of anthracyclines and epipodophylotoxins. PSC 833, an alternative MDR inhibitor does not have the immunosuppressive effects of cyclosporine nor the effects on calcium metabolism characteristic

**Table 5.** CALGB 8923: Results in CR Patients Randomized to Post-Remission Therapy

| | Results | | | |
|---|---|---|---|---|
| Induction Randomization | GM-CSF | | Placebo | |
| Postremission Randomization | Ara-C | Ara-C+M | Ara-C | Ara-C+M |
| Number of patients | 37 | 42 | 45 | 45 |
| Median DFS (months) | 8.7 | 8.8 | 11.1 | 10.2 |
| Overall survival (months) | 19.1 | 16.2 | 20.0 | 17.5 |
| Number (%) of relapses | 30 (81%) | 33 (79%) | 35 (78%) | 34 (76%) |
| Number of deaths in CR | 4 | 5 | 3 | 6 |
| Total number of events | 34 (92%) | 38 (90%) | 38 (84%) | 40 (89%) |

of verapamil another agent capable of blocking the drug efflux mediated by GP 170 [22]. However, PSC 833 does block hepatic metabolism of daunorubicin and etoposide. Consequently, in order to effectively test the ability of drug resistance modulation to specifically enhance therapeutic efficacy (rather than just pharmacologically increase drug levels) it was necessary to design equitoxic induction regimens with and without the drug resistance modulator. The addition of etoposide to the standard daunorubicin/cytarabine induction was included in order to provide another therapeutically useful drug that might also be affected by MDR modulation in this resistant cohort of patients.

CALGB 9420 was a phase I trial in which 111 patients with previously untreated AML greater than 60 years of age were enrolled [23]. Sequential cohorts of at least three patients were entered to receive an induction regimen consisting of ara-C/daunorubicin/etoposide with (ADEP) or without (ADE) the drug resistance modulator PSC 833. The dose of daunorubicin was escalated in successive cohorts of patients. As expected the dose of daunorubicin that could be given in association with the drug resistance modulator was considerably lower than that possible without PSC 833. All patients received cytarabine at a dose of 100 mg/m$^2$ by continuous infusion for seven days, etoposide at a dose of 100 mg/m$^2$ per day on days 1, 2, 3 and daunorubicin at a starting dose of 30 mg/m$^2$ per day by intravenous push on the first three days of therapy. At a daunorubicin dose of 40 mg/m$^2$ per day in association with PSC 833 seven out of eight patients experienced a dose limiting toxicity (DLT) which was defined as grade three or greater non-hematological toxicity. Rather than further compromise the dose of daunorubicin, the dose of etoposide was lowered to 60 mg/m$^2$ per day. As such, the maximum tolerated dose of ADEP was found to be cytarabine at a dose of 100 mg/ m$^2$ by continuous infusion, daunorubicin at a dose of 40 mg/m$^2$ per day and etoposide at 60 mg/m$^2$ per day. At this dose seven out of twenty-four evaluable patients experienced DLT. In the non-PSC containing arm the maximum dose of daunorubicin was 60mg/m$^2$ per day (with etoposide at 100 mg/m$^2$ per day). Even though less than one-

**Table 7.** CALGB 9420: Development of Induction regimens for Phase III n=111 (60M/51F) median age 69 (60-84)

| Max dose ADE | Gr>3 non-heme tox (early death) |
|---|---|
| ara-C 100 x 7 | |
| etop 100 x 3 | 5/24 (3) |
| dauno 60 x 3 | |
| Max dose ADEP | |
| ara-C 100 x 7 | |
| etop 60 x 3 | 9/29 (7) |
| dauno 40 x 3 | |
| ADEP | |
| ara-C 100 x 7 | |
| etop 100 x 3 | 7/8 (5) |
| dauno 40 x 3 | |

99 evaluable for response 46% CR, 22% ED, 31% NR

third (5/25) patients experienced DLT, it was felt best not to further escalate the daunorubicin given the potential risk of cardiotoxicity in this older group of patients (Table 7). The incidence of stomatitis, esophagitis, and hyperbilirubinemia was more common in patients who received PSC-833 (Table 8).

Because of the failure of myelointensive chemotherapy to be effective in older patients with AML, a novel approach is required. The effects of the immunostimulatory molecule interleukin-2 (IL-2), include activation of T-cells, activation and mitogenesis of natural killer cells. Natural killer cells are believed to be one of the mediators of the so-called graft-vs-leukemia effect after allogeneic bone marrow transplant which is one of the reasons why this approach has potent anti-leukemic efficacy. Preliminary studies conducted at Roswell Park Cancer Institute [24] and the Dana-Farber Cancer Institute [25] documented the feasibility and biological efficacy of

**Table 8.** Toxicity According to Induction Without and With PSC-833 Gr≥3 Toxicity of induction chemo by regimen

| | ADE | ADEP |
|---|---|---|
| stomatitis | 11% | 56% |
| esophagitis | 14% | 36% |
| bilirubin | 35% | 57% |
| neurological toxicity (all grades) | | |
| cortical | 20% | 32% |
| cerebellar | 6% | 2% |

relatively low doses of interleukin-2 administered either post intensification chemotherapy or post bone marrow transplant. Therefore, patients on CALGB 9420 who remained in remission after a single cycle of post-remission therapy were assigned to receive subcutaneous interleukin 2 at a starting dose of $1\times10^6$ /m$^2$ units per day for a total of 90 days. To further stimulate natural killer cell activity subcutaneous bolus doses of interleukin 2 were administered at regular intervals during this 90 day period. Although the final analysis of toxicity and biological effects of interleukin 2 administered in this older cohort of patients is underway, a preliminary analysis (Table 9) suggested that the approach is feasible.

**Table 9.** CALGB 9420: Toxicities of Post-Remission IL-2 35/50 patients achieving CR received IL-2*

| Gr≥2 Toxicities occuring in >10 patients (Gr 3/4) | |
|---|---|
| Fever: | 19 (3) |
| Anemia: | 20 (3) |
| Lymphopenia: | 20 (15) |
| Thrombocytopenia: | 12 (7) |

* reasons for not receiving IL-2: relapse (4); toxicity (3); withdraw/refused (4); other (4)

Based on the results of CALGB 9420 a pivotal phase III study in patients with AML older than age 60 is now being carried out. In this phase III trial (CALGB 9720) patients are randomized to receive either the ADE or ADEP induction regimens developed in CALGB 9420. Those patients who achieve remission are given an abbreviated course of ADE or ADEP according to their induction randomization. Those remaining in remission and fully recovered after post-remission chemotherapy will be randomized to either observation or interleukin 2 at the doses developed in the phase I study. Currently at 117 patients after one year of accrual, the 400 patient target should be met by 2002. It is hoped that the approach of drug resistance modulation and/or immunostimulation with interleukin-2 will prove to favorably alter the therapeutic outcome in this difficult group of patients. Unless major strides can be made, older patients with AML will remain good subjects for evaluation of novel concepts in the therapy of AML including new drugs such as topoisomerase I inhibitors (e,g. topotecan) [26], novel biologically active molecules (e.g. the protein kinase C active agent bryostatin 1 [27]; angiogenesis inhibitors [28]), or new immunotherapeutic approaches such as myeloid-specific monoclonal antibodies (e.g. humanized anti-CD33 coupled with the anthracycline like toxin calicheamicin [29]), or vaccines [30].

*Acknowledgments.* The author would like to thank Marcella E. Hussey for expert secretarial assistance, Richard K. Dodge for statistical guidance, as well as Robert J. Mayer, and Edward J. Lee for sharing updated and/or preliminary results of the CALGB studies they chaired. Finally, the thoughtful leadership provided by the successive CALGB Leukemia Core Committee Chairs Charles Schiffer and Richard Larson is greatly appreciated.

# References

1. Stone RM, Mayer RJ (1993) The approach to the elderly patient with acute myeloid leukemia. Hematology/Oncology Clinics of North America 7: 65-79
2. Löwenberg B, Zittoun R, Kerkhofs H, et al (1989) On the value of intensive remission-induction chemotherapy in elderly patients of 65+ years with acute myeloid leukemia: A randomized phase III study of the European Organization for Research and Treatment of Cancer Leukemia Group. J Clin Oncol 7:1268-74
3. Tilly H, Castaigne S, Bordessoule D, et al (1990) Low-dose cytarabine versus intensive chemotherapy in the treatment of acute nonlymphocytic leukemia in the elderly. J Clin Oncol 8:272-9
4. Leith CP, Kopecky KJ, Godwin J, et al (1997) Acute myeloid leukemia in the elderly: Assessment of multidrug resistance (MDR) and cytogenetics distinguishes biologic subgroups with remarkably distinct responses to standard chemotherapy. A Southwest Oncology Group study. Blood 89: 3323-29
5. Swansbury GJ, Lawler SD, Alimena G, et al (1994) Long-term survival in acute myelogenous leukemia: A second follow-up of the Fourth International Workshop on Chromosomes in Leukemia. Cancer Genet Cytogenet 7:1-7
6. Mayer RJ, Davis RB, Schiffer CA, et al (1994) Intensive postremission chemotherapy in adults with acute myeloid leukemia. N Engl J Med 331: 896-942
7. Rubin EH, Adersen JW, Berg DT, Schiffer CA, Mayer RJ, Stone RM (1992) Risk factors of high-dose cytosine arabinoside neurotoxicity: analysis of a CALBG trial of post-remission cytosine arabinoside in patients with acute myeloid leukemia. J Clin Oncol 10: 948-953

8. Bloomfield CD, Lawrence D, Byrd JC, et al (1998) Frequency of prolonged remission duration after high-dose cytarabine intensification in acute myeloid leukemia varies. Cancer Res 58: 4173-4179

9. Büchner T, Hiddemann W, Koenigsman M, et al (1991) Recombinant human granulocyte-macrophage colony-stimulating factor after chemotherapy with acute myeloid leukemia at higher age or after relapse. Blood 78: 1190-7

10. Preisler H, Davis RB, Krishner J, et al (1998) Comparison of three remission induction regimens and two post-induction strategies for the treatment of acute nonlymphocytic leukemia: A Cancer and Leukemia Group B Study. Blood 69:1441-1449

11. Stone RM, Berg DT, George SL, et al (1995) Granulocyte-macrophage colony-stimulating factor after initial chemotherapy for elderly patients with primary acute myelogenous leukemia. N Engl J Med 332: 1672-7

12. Dombret H, Chastang C, Fenaux P, et al (1995) A controlled study of recombinant human granulocyte colony-stimulating factor in elderly patients after treatment for acute myelogenous leukemia. N Engl J Med 332: 1678-83

13. Heil G, Hoelzer D, Sanz MA, et al (1997) A randomized double-blind, placebo-controlled phase III study of filgastrim in remission induction and consolidation for adults with de novo acute myeloid leukemia. Blood 90: 4710-8

14. Goodwin JE, Kopecky KJ, Head DR, et al (1998) A double-blind placebo controlled trial of granulocyte colony-stimulating factor in elderly patients with previously untreated acute myeloid leukemia: A Southwest Oncology Group Study (9031). Blood 91: 3607-3615

15. Zittoun R, Suciu S, Mandelli F, et al (1996) Granulocyte-macrophage colony-stimulating factor associated with induction treatment of acute myelogenous leukemia: A randomized trial by the European Organization for research and treatment of Cancer Leukemia Cooperative Group. J Clin Oncol 14: 2150-2159

16. Lowenberg B, Suciu S, Archimbaud E, et al (1997) Use of recombinant granulocyte-macrophage colony-stimulating factor during and after remission induction chemotherapy in patients aged 61 years and older with acute myeloid leukemia (AML): Final report of AML-11, a phase III randomized study of the Leukemia Cooperative Group of European Organization for the Research and Treatment of Cancer (EORTC-LCG) and the Dutch Belgian Hemato-Oncology Cooperative Group (HOVON). Blood 90:2952-2961

17. Witz F, Sadoun A, Perrin M, et al (1998) A placebo-controlled study of recombinant human granulocyte-macrophage colony-stimulating factor administered during and after induction treatment for de novo acute myelogenous leukemia in elderly patients. Blood 91:2722-2730

18. Rowe JM, Andersen JW, Mazza JJ, et al (1995) A randomized placebocontrolled phase III study of granulocyte-macrophage colony-stimulating factor in adult patients (>55 to 70 years of age) with acute myelogenous leukemia: A study of the Eastern Cooperative Oncology Group (E1490). Blood 86: 457-62

19. Stone RM, Berg DT, George SL, et al (1997) Post-remission therapy in older patients with de novo acute myeloid leukemia: a randomized trial of mitoxantrone/intermediate dose cytarabine 'v' standard dose cytarabine (CALGB 8923). Blood 90 (suppl. 1): 2255a

20. Löwenberg B, Suciu S, Archimbaud, et al (1998) Mitoxantrone versus daunorubicin in induction-consolidation chemotherapy-The value of low-dose cytarabine for maintenance of remission, and an assessment of prognostic factors in acute myeloid leukemia in the elderly: Final report of the Leukemia Cooperative Group of the European Organization for the Research and Treatment of Cancer and the Dutch-Belgian Hemato-oncology Cooperative Hovon Group Randomized Phase III Study AML-9. J Clin Oncol 16: 872-881

21. List AF, Kopecky, Wilman CL, et al (1998) Benefit of cycloporine (CsA) modulation of anthracycline resistance in high-risk AML: A Southwest Oncology Group (SWOG) study. Blood 92 (suppl. 1): 1281a

22. Kornblau SM, Estey E, Madden T, et al (1997) Phase I study of mitoxantrone plus etoposide with multidrug blockade by SDZ PSC-833 in relapsed or refractory acute myelogenous leukemia. J Clin Oncol 15: 1796-1802

23. Lee E, George S, Caligiuri, et al (1997) A phase I study of induction chemotherapy for older patients with acute myeloid leukemia using ara-C, daunorubicin, and etoposide with and without the MDR modulator PSC-833: Cancer and Leukemia Group B study 9420. Blood 90 (suppl. 1): 2256a

24. Frankel SR, Porter M, Nagel G, et al (1994) Low dose interleukin-2 as post-remission therapy for AML increases NK cell populations. Proc Am Assoc Cancer Res 35: A1344

25. Soiffer RJ, Murray C, Cochran K, et al (1992) Clinical and immunologic effects of prolonged infusion of recombinant interleukin-2 after autologous and T-cell depleted allogeneic bone marrow transplantation. Blood 79: 517

26. Beran M, Kantarjian H (1998) Topotecan in the treatment of hemotologic malignancies. Semin Hematol 35 (Suppl 4): 26-31

27. Stone RM, Galinsky, Berg D, et al (1998) Protein kinase C (PKC)-based antileukemic therapy: A randomized phase II trial of all-trans retinoic acid (ATRA) and bryostatin 1 (BRYO) in patients (PTS) with myelodysplastic syndromes (MDS) and acute myeloid leukemia (AML). Blood 92: 2602a

28. Shami PJ, Hussong JW, Rogers GM (1998) Evidence of increased angiogenesis in the bone marrow of patients with acute nonlymphocytic leukemia. Blood 92 (suppl. 1): 2105

29. Sievers EL, Larson RA, Estey E, et al (1998) Interim analysis of the efficacy and safety of CMA-676 in patients with AML in first relapse. Blood 92 (suppl.1): 2527

30. Kohler T, Mohr B, Brendel C, et al (1998) Dendritic cells generated out of blasts from patients with acute leukemia. Blood 92 (suppl. 1): 2523

# Treatment of Older Adults with Acute Myelogenous Leukemia: Studies of the Eastern Cooperative Oncology Group (ECOG)

M. S. Tallman[1], P. A. Cassileth[2], P. H. Wiernik[3], and J. M. Rowe[4]

## Introduction

The treatment of older adults with acute myeloid leukemia (AML) remains unsatisfactory. There are several reasons why the outcome remains poor for this group of patients. One explanation is that older adults do not tolerate intensive chemotherapy as well as younger adults. Indeed for patients over the age of 55 years, the treatment-related early mortality rate ranges between 20%-40% [1-5]. In addition, older adults with AML have inherently more resistant disease. This is attributable in part to the increased incidence of unfavorable and complex karyotype abnormalities compared to younger adults [6]. Furthermore, older adults present more often with multi-lineage dysplasia and have more frequent expression of the MDR1 gene at diagnosis [6,7].

The Eastern Cooperative Oncology Group (ECOG) recently examined the long-term outcome of patients treated on six previous clinical trials for patients with newly diagnosed AML [8] The five-year survival for 508 patients ages 55 years of age or older was approximately 10%. To improve the treatment of older adults with AML, the ECOG has conducted a series of studies designed to improve supportive care by exploring the benefits of both myeloid and thrombopoietic growth factor support, to identify the best induction regimen, and to determine the benefits of modulating multidrug resistance. In addition, a variety of new studies are planned as described below.

## Improving Supportive Care

Eastern Cooperative Oncology Group Protocol E1490 was designed primarily to determine the benefits of granulocyte-macrophage colony-stimulating factor (GM-CSF) for older adults with newly diagnosed AML [1]. Either GM-CSF or placebo was administered to patients with aplastic bone marrows after induction chemotherapy. In this prospective, double-blind randomized trial, 124 adults older than 55 years entered the study, and remission induction included one or two courses of daunorubicin at a dose of 60 $mg/m^2$/day intravenously one days 1-3 and cytarabine 100 $mg/m^2$/day by continuous infusion on days 1-7. A bone marrow was examined on day 10. If the bone marrow was aplastic, the GM-CSF or placebo was administered beginning on day 11. Either yeast-derived recombinant GM-CSF or placebo was administered until the absolute neutrophil count was $\geq 1,500/\mu L$ for three consecutive days or a maximum of 42 days. The overall complete remission rate was 52%; 60% for the patients in the GM-CSF arm and 44% for patients in the placebo arm (p=.08). The median times to neutrophil recovery were significantly shortened among patients receiving GM-CSF. The overall treatment-related toxicity from the time of administration of GM-CSF or placebo was reduced among patients receiving GM-CSF (p=.049). Infectious toxicity was also reduced for patients on the GM-CSF arm (p=.015). The median survival for all patients was modestly better for patients receiving GM-CSF (10.6 months)

[1] Northwestern University Medical School, Robert H. Lurie Comprehensive Cancer Center, Chicago, IL
[2] Sylvester Cancer Center, University of Miami, Miami, FL
[3] Albert Einstein Cancer Center, Montefiore Medical Center, Bronx, NY
[4] Technion, Israel Institute of Technology, Haifa, Israel

compared to patients receiving placebo (4.8 months) (p=.048). Improvement was also seen in the mortality rate from pneumonia and fungal infection by patients receiving GM-CSF. Importantly, no simulation of leukemic cells was observed. This trial established the safety of GM-CSF in this setting and benefits with respect to infectious toxicity and overall survival.

## Improving the Complete Remission Rate

In order to identify the best induction regimen for older adults, the ECOG has recently completed a prospective, randomized comparison of daunorubicin, idarubicin, and mitoxantrone, each combined with cytarabine for induction in patients over the age of 60 years [9]. This study was prompted by the fact that there continues to be debate as to the best anthracycline for induction in AML. In younger adults, several randomized studies suggested that idarubicin, mitoxantrone, amsacrine, and aclacinomycin may be superior to daunorubicin at a dose of 45 mg/m$^2$ [10-15] However, whether this is true for older adults is not clear [16,17]. ECOG Protocol E3993 was a trial in which patients received either daunorubicin 45 mg/m$^2$ for three days or idarubicin at a dose of 12 mg/m$^2$ or mitoxantrone at a dose of 12 mg/m$^2$, each with cytarabine at a dose of 100 mg/m$^2$ given by continuous infusion for seven days. All patients achieving complete remission (CR) then received consolidation chemotherapy with high-dose cytarabine at a dose of 1.5 g/m$^2$ given every 12 hours for 12 doses (a total of only six doses were given for patients age 70 years or older). Three-hundred-forty-nine patients were analyzed. At the time of study entry, patients underwent a randomization between GM-CSF or placebo as priming. The overall CR rate for all 349 patients was 42%: 40% for daunorubicin, 43% for idarubicin, and 43% for mitoxantrone. The median disease-free survival for all 147 patients achieving CR was seven months (5.7 months for daunorubicin, 9.7 months for idarubicin, and 6.9 months for mitoxantrone, p=0.43). The median survival for all patients achieving CR was 14 months. The treatment-related mortality was 16% for daunorubicin, 22% for idarubicin, and 14% for mitoxantrone, and no statistical differences were observed. In patients less than 70 years of age, the overall CR rate was 51% (46% for daunorubicin, 52% for idarubicin, and 51% for mitoxantrone, with no statistically significant differences). For patients 70 years of age or older, the overall complete remission rate was 29% (30% for daunorubicin, 24% for idarubicin, and 33% for mitoxantrone, with no statistically significant differences observed). In an analysis of the first 113 patients on the study, the overall complete remission rate was 50% compared to 38% among the subsequent 236 patients in whom induction therapy was delayed 2-5 days because of the priming randomization (p=0.03). Therefore, in this study, there were no clear differences in response or toxicity between the three induction regimens and the doses used. Furthermore, the delay in induction therapy because of priming in older adults appeared to result in a lower CR rate.

## Modulating Multidrug Resistance

One of the best understood mechanisms of drug resistance is that which is mediated by the multidrug transporter P-glycoprotein (P-gp) which is encoded by the MDR1 gene. The MDR1 P-gp functions as a transmembrane efflux pump which leads to reduced intracellular retention of chemotherapeutic drugs. The drugs involved in multidrug resistance include the anthracyclines, vinca alkaloids, and the epipodophyllotoxins. Several agents including cyclosporin, the potent immunosuppressive agent routinely used for organ transplantation, are capable of reversing multidrug resistance in vitro. In a preliminary study, the ECOG tested the efficacy and toxicity of mitoxantrone, etoposide, and intermediate-dose cytarabine (MEC) with cyclosporine as an MDR modulator in patients with recurrent or refractory AML [18]. In this trial, attempts were made to correlate P-gp expression in leukemia cells with response. Among 38 patients who were either in first relapse after less than six months of CR (11 patients), refractory to initial induction therapy or to one attempted reinduction after recurrence (18 patients), in second relapse (4 patients), or in relapse after either allogeneic or autologous bone marrow transplantation (5 patients), 3 of the 13 patients (23%) who received MEC achieved CR as did 6 of the 25 patients (24%) who received MEC plus cyclosporin. The median remission duration for all patients who achieved CR was 149 days (range 26 to 466 days), 91 days (range 81 to 172 days) for the few patients who received MEC, and 189.5 (range 26 for 466 days) for the patients treated with MEC plus cyclosporine. The median survival for patients treated with MEC and MEC plus cyclosporine was 104 and 72 days, respectively. No significant association was found between P-gp expression on leukemic cells and response. Although no apparent benefit of the CR rate, remission duration, or survival was observed with the addition of the putative MDR modulator cyclosporin, the cyclosporin derivative, PSC-833, appears to be a more potent MDR modulator and was shown to be non-immunosuppressive [19,20] Therefore, several ECOG institutions carried out a multicenter phase II clinical trial combining MEC chemotherapy with PSC-833 [21]. The doses of mitoxantrone and etoposide were substantially reduced in this trial compared to the previous trial to compensate for pharmacokinetic interactions of these two agents with PSC-833. PSC-833 was administered as a pre-treatment loading dose at 2 mg/kg over four hours with a concomitant continuous infusion at 10 mg/kg/day for 120 hours (5 days). Induction chemotherapy began immediately after completion of the four-hour loading dose of PSC-833. Two dose levels of chemotherapy were used. In the first cohort of patients, mitoxantrone at a dose of 5 mg/m$^2$ per day by intravenous bolus on Days 1-5, etoposide 150 mg/m$^2$ per day on Days 1-5, and cytarabine 1 gm/m$^2$ per day on Days 1-5 were administered as a short intravenous infusion over one hour. Because of excessive toxicity in this first group of patients, the subsequent group of patients received a dose of mitoxantrone at 4 mg/m$^2$ and etoposide at 40 mg/m$^2$. Among 37 patients, 12 (32%) achieved CR, and four achieved a partial remission. Responses were evenly distributed among disease categories. Three of 13 patients (23%) over 60 years of age achieved CR compared with 9 of 24 patients (38%) who were age 60 years or less.

Significant grade III or IV mucositis occurred in the first group of patients (50%), and this incidence was substantially reduced (19%) among patients receiving the lower doses of mitoxantrone and etoposide. Transient hyperbilirubinemia was observed in 34 of the 37 patients (92%). The hyperbilirubinemia was transient in the majority of patients and generally resolved in the median of 10 days (range 4 to 19 days). P-glycoprotein function and expression as well as CD34 expression were evaluated. No correlation was observed between P-gp expression and response to therapy. Although the majority of patients treated on this study had poor-risk characteristics, 32% of patients achieved CR. These results were encouraging enough to proceed to a prospective, randomized trial, which is currently underway (E2995). In this trial, patients with relapsed or refractory AML are randomized to MEC chemotherapy or MEC plus PSC-833. If differences in response exist among MDR-positive patients compared to MDR-negative patients, therapy will subsequently be targeted to patients whose leukemia cells express MDR.

## Future Directions

CMA-676 is a conjugate of an anti-CD33 monoclonal antibody linked to a potent toxin, calicheamicin. A preliminary study has suggested significant activity in patients with relapsed AML [22] A subsequent study suggested a relationship between CD33 site saturation and dye efflux of 3.3% diethyloxacarbocyanine iodide as a measure of functional drug resistance with antileukemic effect [23]. In an initial phase II trial, 10 of 23 patients (43%) with AML in first relapse with at least a six-month first remission duration achieved a second CR by morphologic evaluation [24]. It will be of interest to determine whether this agent has a role either alone or in combination with a standard induction chemotherapy program for patients with previously untreated AML. If CMA-676 proves to be effective in previously untreated patients, a prospective comparison with a conventional induction program will be of interest. A variety of immunotherapeutic agents have been studied in AML. The most well studied has been interleukin-2 (IL-2) [25-28]. Recent studies suggest that among patients with relapsed and refractory AML who have minimal disease burden (≤ 30% bone marrow blasts), CR was achieved in 11 of 20 patients (55%) [26]. A new immunotherapeutic agent under current investigation is Flt3 Ligand (Flt3L) [29]. This agent is capable of significantly increasing peripheral blood dendritic cells which have the ability to present antigen for primary specific T-lymphocyte responses *in vitro* and *in vivo*. Dendritic cells are relatively rare hematopoietic cells that express high levels of both Class I and Class II major histocompatibility complex antigens and adhesion and co-stimulatory molecules. Recombinant human Flt3L increases peripheral blood dendritic cells in healthy volunteers and is safe [30]. Based on these data, the ECOG currently plans to do a randomized trial for patients in second remission who will receive either Flt3L or observation to test whether immunologic enhancement can contribute to the outcome of treatment.

Hematopoietic growth factors effectively shorten the duration of neutropenia following induction chemotherapy in AML. There is, however, no clear evidence that hematopoietic growth factors have a beneficial effect on survival. Such agents do appear to have a beneficial effect in supportive care of patients receiving intensive induction chemotherapy, particularly for older adults or those who at high risk for treatment-related morbidity and mortality. Thrombopoietin (TPO) is a primary regulator of megakaryocytopoiesis and thrombopoiesis [31]. Although the therapeutic role of TPO in AML is not established, it has been safely administered in AML. Therefore, the ECOG plans a prospective, randomized trial for older adults with newly diagnosed AML which will randomize patients who achieve marrow aplasia to receive the GM-CSF with either TPO or placebo during induction and consolidation therapies. Subsequently, all patients who achieve CR will then be randomized to receive either one or two cycles of high-dose cytarabine consolidation using 1.5 $g/m^2$ every 12 hours for 12 doses.

# References

1. Rowe JM, Andersen JW, Mazza JJ, et al. A randomized placebo-controlled phase III study of granulocyte-macrophage colony-stimulating factor in adult patients (>55 to 70 years of age) with acute myelogenous leukemia: a study of the Eastern Cooperative Oncology Group (E1490). Blood 86:457, 1995.
2. Sebban C, Archimbaud E, Coiffier B, Guyotat D, Treille-Ritouet D, Maupas J, Fiere D: Treatment of acute myeloid leukemia in elderly patients. A retrospective study. Cancer 61:227, 1998.
3. Yates J, Glidewell O, Wiernik P, et al. Cytosine-arabinoside with daunorubicin or adriamycin for therapy of acute myelocytic leukemia: A CALGB study. Blood 60:454, 1982.
4. Rees JK, Gray R: Comparison of 1 + 5 DAT and 3 + 10 DAT followed by COAP or MAZE consolidation therapy in the treatment of acute myeloid leukemia: MRC ninth AML trial. Semin Oncol 14:32, 1987 (suppl 1).
5. Preisler H, Davis RB, Kirshner J, Dupre E, Richards F III, Hoagland HC, Kopel S, Levy RN, Carey R, Schulman P, Gottlieb AJ, McIntyre OR, and the Cancer and Leukemia Group B: Comparison of three remission induction regimens and two post-induction strategies for the treatment of acute nonlymphocytic leukemia: a Cancer and Leukemia Group B study. Blood 69:1441, 1987.
6. Taylor PRA, Reid MM, Stark AN, Brown N, Hamilton PJ, Proctor SJ. De novo acute myeloid leukaemia in patients over 55-years-old: A population-based study of incidence, treatment and outcome. Leukemia 9, 231, 1995.
7. Leith CP, Kopecky KJ, Godwin J, et al. Acute myeloid leukemia in the elderly: assessment of multidrug resistance (MDR1) and cytogenetics distinguishes biologic subgroups with remarkable distinct responses to standard chemotherapy. A Southwest Oncology Group study. Blood 89:3323, 1997.
8. Bennett JM, Young ML, Andersen JW, et al. Long-term survival in acute myeloid leukemia: The Eastern Cooperative Oncology Group Experience. Cancer 80:2205, 1997.
9. Rowe JM, Neuberg D, Friedenberg W, et al. Phase III study of daunorubicin vs idarubicin vs mitoxantrone for older adult patients (>55 yrs) with acute myelogenous leukemia (AML): a study of the Eastern Cooperative Oncology Group (E3993). Blood 22(10; suppl 1):1284a, 1998.
10. Berman E, Heller G, Santorsa J, et al. Results of a randomized trial comparing idarubicin and cytosine arabinoside with daunorubicin and cytosine arabinoside in adult patients with newly diagnosed acute myelogenous leukemia. Blood 77:1666, 1991.
11. Wiernik PH, Banks PLC, Case DC, et al. Cytarabine plus idarubicin and daunorubicin as induction and consolidation therapy for previously untreatable adult patients with acute myeloid leukemia. Blood 79:313, 1992.

12. Arlin Z, Case DC, Moore J, et al. Randomized multicenter trial of cytosine arabinoside with mitoxantrone or daunorubicin in previously untreated adult patients with acute nonlymphocytic leukemia (ANLL). Leukemia 4:177, 1990.
13. Hansen OP, Pedersen-Bjergaard J, Ellegaard J, et al. Idarubicin plus cytosine arabinoside versus daunorubicin plus cytosine arabinoside in previously untreated patients with acute myeloid leukemia: a Danish National phase III trial. Leukemia 5:510, 1991.
14. Berman E, Arlin ZA, Gaynor J, et al. Comparative trial of cytarabine and thioguanine in combination with amsacrine or daunorubicin in patients with untreated acute nonlymphocytic leukemia. Results of the L-16M protocol. Leukemia 3:115, 1989.
15. Vogler WR, Velez-Garcia E, Weiner RS, et al. A phase III trial comparing idarubicin and daunorubicin in combination with cytarabine in acute myelogenous leukemia: a Southeastern Cancer Study Group study. J Clin Oncol 10:1103, 1992.
16. Mandelli F, Petti MC, Ardia A, et al. A randomised clinical trial comparing idarubicin and cytarabine to daunorubicin and cytarabine in the treatment of acute nonlymphoid leukemia. Eur J Cancer 27:750, 1991.
17. Lowenberg B, Suciu S, Archimbaud E, et al. Mitoxantrone versus daunorubicin in induction consolidation chemotherapy: the value of low-dose cytarabine for maintenance of remission, and an assessment of prognostic factors in acute myeloid leukemia in the elderly: final report of the Leukemia Organization for the Research and Treatment of Cancer and the Dutch-Belgian Hemato-Oncology Cooperative Hovon Group randomized phase III study AML-9. J Clin Oncol 16:872, 1998.
18. Tallman MS, Lee S, Sikic BI, Paietta E, Wiernik PH, Bennett JM, Rowe JM: Mitoxantrone, etoposide, and cytarabine plus cyclosporine for patients with relapsed or refractory acute myeloid leukemia: an Eastern Cooperative Oncology Group pilot study. Cancer 85:358-367.
19. Boesh D, Gaveriaux C, Jachez B, Pourtier-Manzanedo A, Bollinger P, Loor F. In vitro circumvention of P-glycoprotein-mediated multidrug resistance of tumor cells with SDZ PSC 833. Cancer Res 51:4226, 1991.
20. Twentyman PR, Bleehen NM. Resistance modification y PSC-833, a novel non-immunosuppressive cyclosporin. Eur J Cancer 27:1639, 1991.
21. Advani R, Saba HI, Tallman MS, et al. Treatment of refractory and relapse acute myelogenous leukemia with combination chemotherapy plus the multidrug resistance modulator PSC 833 (Valspodar). Blood 93:787, 1999.
22. Sievers EL, Bernstein ID, Spielberger RT, Forman SJ, Berger MS, Shannon-Dorcy K, Appelbaum ER. Dose escalation phase I study of recombinant engineered human anti-CD33 antibody-calicheamicin drug conjugate (CMA-676) in patients with relapsed and refractory acute myeloid leukemia (AML). Proc Am Soc Clin Oncol 16:8, 1997 (abstr).
23. Sievers EL, Appelbaum FA, Spielberger RT, et al. Selective ablation of acute myeloid leukemia using an anti-CD33 calicheamicin immunoconjugate. Blood 10:504a, 1997.
24. Sievers EL, Larson RA, Estey E, Stadtmauer EA, Berger MA, Eten C, Bernstein I, Appelbaum F. Interim analysis of the efficacy and safety of CMA-676 in patients in first relapse. Blood 92 (10, suppl 1):2527, 1998 (abstr).
25. Maraninchi D, Blaise D, Viens P, et al. High-dose recombinant interleukin-2 and acute myeloid leukemias in relapse. Blood 78:2182, 1991.
26. Meloni G, Vignetti M, Andrizzi C, Capria S, Foa R, Mandelli F. Interleukin-2 for the treatment of advanced acute myelogenous leukemia patients with limited disease: Updated experience with 20 cases. Leukemia and Lymphoma 21:429, 1996.
27. Foa R. Does interleukin-2 have a role in the management of acute leukemia? J of Clin Oncol 11:1817, 1993.
28. Blaise D, Maraninchi D. Interleukin 2 in the treatment of acute leukemia. Leukemia Res 22:1165, 1998.
29. Lynch DH, Andreasen A, Maraskovsky E, et al.: Flt3 Ligand in duces tumor regression and anti-tumor immune responses in vivo. Nature Medicine 3:625-633, 1997.
30. Maraskovsky E, Roux E, Terpe M, et al. Flt3 Ligand increases peripheral blood dendritic cells in healthy volunteers. Blood 90(suppl 6):2585, 1997 (abstr).
31. Kaushansky K, Lok S, Holly RD, et al.: Promotion of megakaryocyte progenitor expansion and differentiation by the c-Mpl ligand thrombopoietin. Nature 369:568-571, 1994.
32. Cripe L, Tallman MS, Neuberg D, Saba H, Wiernik P, Gordon M. A pilot study of thrombopoietin (rh-TPO) and GM-CSF following induction and consolidation therapy in patients greater than 55 years with acute myeloid leukemia. Blood 92 (10, suppl 1):2539, 1998.

# A Landmark Analysis of Survival by Response Category in Elderly Patients with Acute Myeloblastic Leukemia

F. Marmont, B. Allione, E. Audisio, C. Boccomini, V. Ciocca, S. D'Ardia, M. Falda, F. Locatelli and E. Gallo

## Introduction

The achievement of complete remission (CR) after an aplastic phase induced by intensive chemotherapy (ICT) is considered a prerequisite for prolonged survival in patients with Acute Myeloblastic Leukemia (AML). However, no general agreement exists on the treatment of choice for elderly patients [1]. They may suffer from associated co-morbidities that could independently influence survival or prevent the use of ICT. Moreover, the prognostic significance of the response to chemotherapy has been questioned [2]. In fact, a patient must survive enough to be able to enter CR (the so called "guarantee time") and therefore CR itself could be a marker of a less aggressive disease and not only the result of an effective treatment. The aim of our work was to assess the possible survival advantage induced by the achievement of CR in the elderly AML patients treated with ICT. We have analysed the survival according to the response to chemotherapy in a consecutive series of patients observed in the last ten years at our Institution and accrued in aggressive chemotherapy protocols. To avoid the bias inherent to the "guarantee time" of responders, we have applied the "Landmark Method" in the survival analysis by response category [3].

## Patients and Methods

From January 1988 to April 1998 , 93 consecutive elderly patients with "de-novo" AML were observed in our Institution and treated with ICT. Their median age was 68 years (range 61-

86). The FAB classification was: 15 M1, 15 M2, 4 M3, 41 M4, 13 M5, 4 M6, 1 M7. During the same time period additional 25 patients (21.2%) were observed but were not considered eligible for ICT because of very poor performance status and/or associated severe co-morbidities. They were treated with palliative and supportive therapy, showed a poor survival (median 1.2 months) and were not considered in the present study. Treatment schedules varied with time : 64 patients were treated from 1988 to 1994 with Mitoxantrone 6 mg/m$^2$/day plus Ara-C 1 g/m$^2$/day for 6 consecutive days. Twenty-nine patients were treated from 1995 to 1998 with Idarubicin 8 mg/m$^2$ days 1,3,5 plus Ara-C 100 mg/m$^2$/day for 7 days continuous perfusion and Etoposide 100 mg/m$^2$ days 1,2,3. No differences were observed in terms of CR (35.9% vs. 37.9% ; p=1) and survival (2.2 months vs. 3.6 months; p=0.89). Therefore all the patients were considered together in the survival and landmark analyses. CR was defined according to standard criteria [4] and time to CR was calculated from the start of chemotherapy. In the landmark analysis, survival was credited from the time of the landmark, arbitrarily placed at 45 days from the start of treatment. The median time to CR was 34.8 days (range 25–66). 90% of responders could qualify for CR within 45 days. We therefore regarded as acceptable the defined landmark even if 4 more patients obtained CR beyond the landmark (2 at day +50 , 1 at +63, 1 at +66). The patients in CR at the landmark time were considered at risk in the CR category. the non-responders (NR) and the few patients obtaining CR beyond the landmark were considered at risk in the NR category. The

Dept. of Hematology, San Giovanni Battista Hospital, Torino, Italy.

patients dying before the landmark were excluded from the analysis. All calculations were made with BMDP computer programs [5].

## Results

### Response to therapy

Thirty-four patients entered CR with an overall CR rate of 36.6%. The incidence of CR decreased with age (45.6% in patients < 70 yrs. vs. 22.3% in patients ≥70 yrs.; p=0.03). An higher incidence of early deaths both in the first seven days from the start of treatment and during the aplastic phase was observed in the more aged patients. In addition, 70.2% of the patients < 70 yrs. survived the induction phase compared with 44.4% of the patients ≥70 yrs. (p=0.02). (Table 1)

**Table 1.** Response to intensive chemotherapy

|                  | < 70 yrs. N° (%) | ≥70 yrs. N° (%) | Total N° (%) |
|------------------|------------|------------|------------|
| CR               | 26 (45.6)  | 8 (22.2)   | 34 (36.6)  |
| NR               | 14 (24.6)  | 8 (22.2)   | 22 (23.7)  |
| Died in induction | 2 (3.5)   | 5 (13.9)   | 7 (7.5)    |
| Died in aplasia  | 15 (26.3)  | 15 (41.7)  | 30 (32.3)  |
| Total            | 57 (61.3)  | 36 (38.7)  | 93 (100)   |

### Survival analysis

The overall median survival was 2.8 months. The median survival was significantly longer

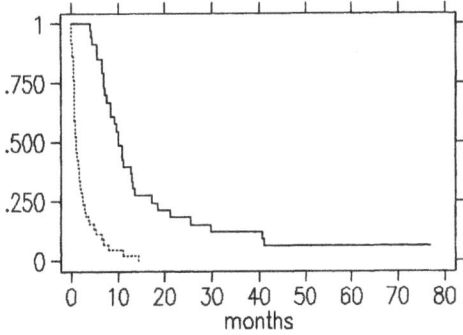

**Fig. 1.** Survival CR (solid line) vs. NR (dotted line); p=0.000

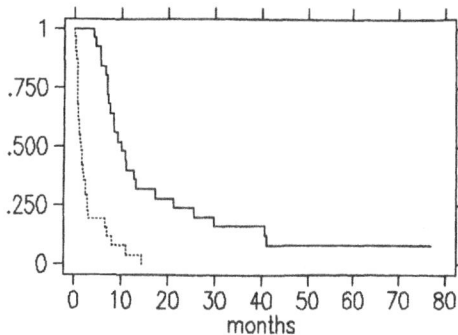

**Fig. 2.** Survival CR (solid line) vs. NR (dotted line) in patients < 70 yrs.; p=0.000

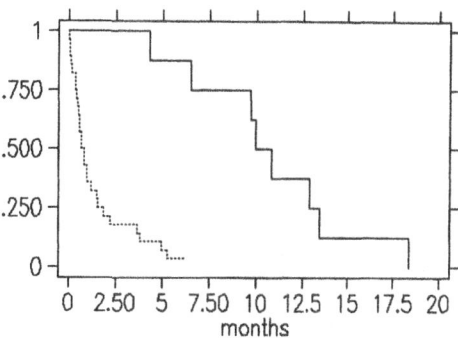

**Fig. 3.** Survival CR (solid line) vs. NR (dotted line) in patients ≥70 yrs.; p=0.000

in patients < 70 yrs. then in those ≥70 yrs. (5.5 months vs. 1.2 months; p=0.003). Patients entering CR survived longer then NR (10.2 months vs. 1.2 months; p=0.000) (Fig.1). The same was observed both in patients < 70 yrs. (CR 9.3 months vs. NR 1.5 months; p=0.000) (Fig.2) as well as in patients ≥70 yrs. (CR 10 months vs. NR 0.6 months; p=0.000) (Fig.3). The event-free survival was not different in the two age groups (<70 yrs. 6.3 months vs. ≥70 yrs. 7 months; p=0.85).

### Landmark analysis

Sixty-one patients (44 < 70 yrs. and 17 ≥70 yrs.) could be submitted to the landmark analysis because the remaining 32 patients who died within 45 days from the start of chemotherapy were excluded. The landmark analysis confirmed a survival advantage for responders as a whole (CR 9.74 months vs. NR 3.0 months; p= 0.001) (Fig.4) and in patients < 70 yrs. (CR 10.15 months vs. NR 3.0 months; p=0.005) (Fig.5). Only 17 out of 36 patients ≥70 yrs. were analysed with the landmark method, showing a trend towards significance in favor of responders (CR 9.7 months vs. NR 3.8 months; p=0.08) (Fig.6).

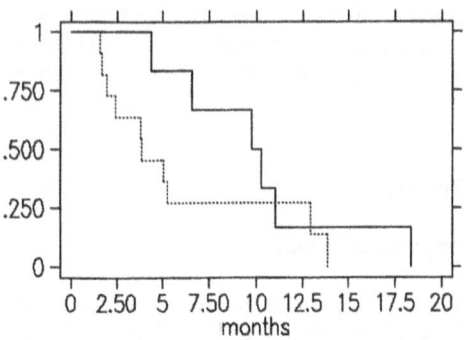

**Fig. 6.** Landmark analysis CR (solid line) vs. NR (dotted line) in patients ≥70 yrs. ; p=0.08

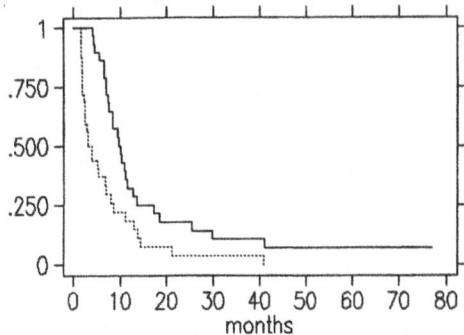

**Fig. 4.** Landmark analysis CR (solid line) vs. NR (dotted line); p=0.001

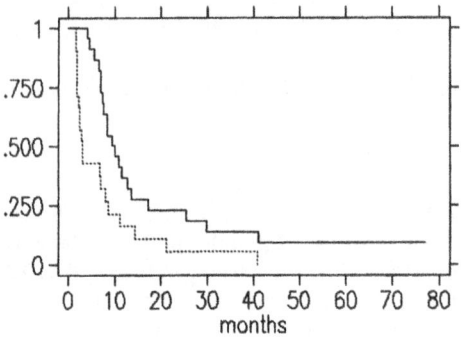

**Fig. 5.** Landmark analysis CR (solid line) vs. NR (dotted line) in patients < 70 yrs. ; p=0.005

## Conclusion

The landmark analysis performed in the present series of elderly AML patients would support the indication to use ICT for induc-

tion therapy in patients up to 70 years of age, if they are fit enough to undergo an aggressive regimen. The use of ICT is questionable in the more advanced decades due to the high incidence of early mortality, even in patients eligible for aggressive therapy. However, a few patients with more advanced age may survive the induction phase and experience a prolonged survival. Prospective studies addressing the issue of intensive treatment in very old and frail patients are warranted.

## References

1. Löwenberg B (1996) Treatment of elderly patients with acute myeloid leukemia. Baillières Clin Haematol 9:147-160
2. Anderson JR, Cain KC, Gelber RD (1983) Analysis of survival by tumor response. J Clin Oncol 1:710-719
3. Anderson JR, Cain KC, Gelber RD, Gelman RS (1985) Analysis and interpretation of the comparisons of survival by treatment outcome variables in cancer clinical trials. Cancer Treat Rep 69:1139-1144
4. Cheson BD, Cassileth PA, Head DR, et al.(1990) Report of the national cancer institute-sponsored workshop on definitions of diagnosis and response in acute myeloid leukemia. J Clin Oncol 8:813-819
5. Dixon WJ, Brown MB, Engelman L et al. (eds). (1985) BMDP statistical software. Berkeley, CA, University of California.

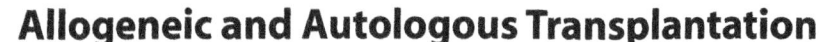

**Allogeneic and Autologous Transplantation**

# Intensive Chemotherapy Followed by Stem Cell Transplantation for the Treatment of Myelodysplastic Syndromes

T. DE WITTE, S. SUCIU, G. VERHOEF, B. LABAR, E. ARCHIMBAUD, C. AUL, D. SELLESLAG, A. FERRANT, P. WIJERMANS, F. MANDELLI, S. AMADORI, U. JEHN, P. MUUS, H. DEMUYNCK, M. DARDENNE, R. ZITTOUN, R. WILLEMZE, A. GRATWOHL and J. APPERLEY

*Abstract.* Most patients with MDS are treated with supportive care only, mainly in view of the average advanced age in MDS and the poor response to more intensive therapy. Allogeneic stem cell transplantation is today the treatment of choice in the majority of young patients with histocompatible siblings. The results of treatment with allogeneic stem cell transplantation depend on the stage of disease at the time of transplantation and various clinical factors, such as the presence of cytogenetic abnormalities, age, and the percentage of blasts in the bone marrow at time of transplantation. Most patients may benefit optimally from an allogeneic stem cell transplantation when the transplant is performed as soon as an HLA-identical family member has been identified. Progression to more advanced leukemic conditions is associated with a higher failure rate mainly due to an increased incidence of relapse after transplantation. Delay of the transplant may be justified in a minority of patients with refractory anemia without cytopenias or complex cytogenetic abnormalities.

Conventional, multidrug chemotherapy, such as that applied to induce complete remission (CR) in de novo AML, has been demonstrated to be effective in MDS with CR rates varying from 15% to 64%. CR rates of patients with MDS or sAML appear lower than those of patients with de novo AML treated with similar chemotherapy regimens. Prolonged survival rates are disappointingly low and less than 10 per cent at 4 years after chemotherapy. The experience with ABMT in patients with MDS or sAML is limited. Until now 144 recipients of autologous marrow grafts with MDS or AML following MDS have been reported to the registries of the EBMT. The overall survival at 2 years of the 79 patients transplanted in first CR was 39%, the DFS was 34% and the actuarial relapse rate was 64%. Patients younger than 40 years had a significantly (p=0.04) better DFS compared to patients with age ≥40 years. This difference could be explained by the significantly higher relapse rate of 72% in the older age group compared to the 59% in the patients younger than 40 years (p=0.05). Sixteen patients received autologous peripheral blood SCT in a prospective study of the EORTC Leukemia Cooperative Group and the EBMT. Peripheral stem cells were collected during the recovery phase of the first consolidation course using 300 µg of Filgrastim daily until completion of PBSC collections. Repopulation was much faster compared to autologous bone marrow transplantation.

Both allogeneic and autologous stem cell transplantation have emerged as treatment options for patients with myelodysplastic syndromes. About one third of the patients transplanted with stem cells from histocompatible siblings and about one quarter of the patients with stem cells from other sources may be free of disease for three years or longer.

## Introduction

The prognosis of the myelodysplastic syndromes (MDS) varies from a few months to many years. Refractory anemia (RA) and RA with ringsideroblasts (RARS) are characterized by

Department of Haematology, University Hospital St. Radboud, 8 Geert Grooteplein, 6525 GA Nijmegen, The Netherlands

a low risk of transformation to acute myeloid leukemia (AML) and a median survival usually in excess of 30 months [1]. In contrast the median survival of patients with refractory anemia and excess of blasts (RAEB) or RAEB in transformation (RAEBt) is less than 12 months [2,3]. The karyotype is an additional prognostic factor for survival in MDS [4-6]. A recent international workshop has proposed a scoring system based on cytogenetic abnormalities, marrow blasts, and peripheral blood cytopenias, which identifies patients in whom median survival is <1 year [7].

Most patients with MDS receive supportive care only [3], mainly in view of the average advanced age in MDS and the poor response to therapy. Allogeneic BMT is the treatment of choice for young patients with histocompatible siblings. The first cases were transplanted more than ten years ago [8,9]. Subsequent publications have addressed the role of allogeneic transplantion for MDS in adults [10-12] and children [13,14]). National and international bone marrow transplant registries have collected data on patients transplanted for myelodysplasia [15]. Results of allogeneic BMT depend on the same risk factors as defined for conventional treatment, such as the presence of cytogenetic abnormalities [15,16], age [15,16], and the percentage of blasts in the bone marrow [10,11,16]. Recently, donors other than HLA-identical siblings and autologous cells have been used as alternative sources of stem cells.

## Allogeneic bone marrow transplantation with HLA-identical sibling donors: the role of chemotherapy prior the transplant procedure

Young patients with RA and RARS are considered good candidates for allogeneic BMT. Relapses are rare, provided that the pretransplant conditioning includes a marrow ablative regimen [11, 16]. Disease-free survival is usually higher than 50 percent [10, 15, 16]. T-cell depletion of the graft may be beneficial in patients with RA and RARS as there is a low risk of relapse and a relatively high treatment-related mortality. Eleven patients with RA were transplanted with marrow from matched siblings, depleted of T-lymphocytes by counterflow centrifugation [17]. The DFS was 73 percent and the relapse risk was 11 percent similar to the relapse risk of 13 percent observed in a recent analysis of the EBMT [18]. The high treatment-related mortality suggests early transplantation is indicated before there is sensitization due to transfusion of blood products, before the development of iron overload and opportunistic infections and before transformation to more advanced stages of MDS or AML. The TRM was significantly lower for patients transplanted within 3 months in a multivariate analysis of the EBMT [18]. Postponement of allogeneic stem cell transplantation may be justified in patients with a relatively good prognosis. These patients are characterized by an absence of profound cytopenias, and an absence of poor prognostic cytogenetic characteristics [7].

An increase in the proportion of marrow blasts to more than 5 percent has a negative impact on disease-free survival after transplantation, mainly due to an increased risk of relapse. A recent analysis by the EBMT on 131 MDS patients treated by HLA-identical sibling BMT confirmed that bone marrow blast count is the most important risk factor for increased relapse, and decreased survival [18]. One of the analyses from Seattle [10] showed a cumulative relapse risk of 45 percent in 30 patients transplanted with RAEB or RAEBt.

The results of allogeneic BMT as primary therapy appeared worse for patients with overt AML after MDS as compared to patients transplanted at earlier stages of MDS [15,16, 18,19]. Disease-free survival was approximately 20 percent when patients were transplanted for MDS-AML [15,18,19]. The remission duration of patients treated with AML-type chemotherapy is usually short [6,20,21]. Allogeneic BMT may be offered to these patients as consolidation therapy in complete or partial remission. The two-year disease-free survival was 42 percent for 116 patients transplanted in complete remission after chemotherapy. Patients not in first remission after chemotherapy responded less well and showed a three-year DFS of 24 percent. The issue as to whether patients with sAML should receive remission-induction therapy prior to the transplant procedure is controversial. Some patient categories may be identified who are unlikely to enter CR after intensive chemotherapy. These patients are characterized by a prolonged history of MDS, hypocellular marrow or multiple chromosomal abnormalities. In these cases allogeneic BMT may be considered as first line therapy [19,22]. Only large prospective studies may resolve this issue. In the report from Seattle [19] no significant difference in outcome was observed between patients treated with immediate transplantation and patients treated after remission-induction therapy. However, the numbers were limited and only six of the 20 patients treated with chemotherapy prior to the transplant procedure received the transplant in first CR [19].

## Intensive chemotherapy

Conventional, multidrug chemotherapy, such as that applied to induce complete remission (CR) in de novo AML, has been demonstrated to be effective in MDS with CR rates varying from 15% to 64% [6,21,23,24]. CR rates of patients with MDS or sAML appear lower than those of patients with de novo AML treated with similar chemotherapy regimens. The higher failure rate of remission-induction therapy can be explained partly by the longer duration of hypoplasia after chemotherapy [6,24,25], but also by a higher intrinsic biological drug-resistance of the leukemic clone [26,27]. Addition of drugs that are less dependant on P-glycoproteine, such as idarubicine or induction into proliferation of leukemic stem cells by G-CSF may overcome this higher drug resistance [28-29]. Some patients with MDS in CR after combination chemotherapy may achieve prolonged, disease-free survival [21], but overall median remission duration appeared to be short and usually less than 12 months [6,32]. Prolonged survival rates are disappointingly low and were reported to be 8% at 4 years after chemotherapy [34] and 7% after after 3 years [6]. The use of G-CSF after remission-induction chemotherapy may increase the response rate, but does not prolong remission duration and survival [28].

## Prognostic factors on outcome after intensive chemotherapy

Patients with the morphological picture of RAEB and RAEBt [21], appeared to respond favourably to intensive chemotherapy, approaching remission rates of de novo AML. Auer rod positive patients, regardless of karyotype, appeared to have a better prognosis than auer rod negative patients when treated with intensive chemotherapy [34]. Patients with secondary AML evolved from MDS respond less well to chemotherapy than do those with de novo leukaemias and long-term remissions are rare [6,32]. The clinical outcome after intensive chemotherapy for therapy-related MDS and AML (t-MDS/t-AML) is usually poor with only an exceptional patient surviving beyond one year [35]. A minority of the patients with specific cytogenetic rearrangements of de-novo AML or no cytogenetic abnormalities who presented with AML not preceded by MDS seemed to have a high remission rate and a more prolonged CR duration compared to the average patient with MDS [35-37].

Children with myelodysplastic syndrome respond poorly to intensive chemotherapy. The proportion of complete remission in 20 patients with MDS was 35% compared to 74% in 35 children with AML treated with the same protocols [38]. Patients younger than 45 to 50 years appeared to respond better to combination chemotherapy than older patients. CR rates in patients less than 45 to 50 years old ranged from 71% to 86% in several studies and the remission rates in the older patients ranged from 25% to 43% [6,23,32,39].

The presence of cytogenetic abnormalities specific for MDS, such as abnormalities of chromosomes 5 or 7, has a major negative impact on the prognosis after combination chemotherapy. Fenaux observed a CR rate of 57% in MDS patients with a normal karyotype [21], contrasting with a CR rate of 31% in patients with rearrangements of chromosomes 5 or 7. None of the five patients with multiple chromosomal abnormalities achieved complete remission in a Leukemia Cooperative Group study of the EORTC [30]. Remission duration is short in patients with cytogenetic abnormalities of chromosomes 5 and/or 7 with all patients relapsing within 5 months [21].

## Autologous bone marrow transplantation

Maintaining remission after remission induction-chemotherapy is a difficult issue. Some patients may achieve prolonged, disease-free survival if treated with post-remission chemotherapy, but overall median remission duration was usually less than 12 months [6,21,33]. The feasibility to collect normal polyclonal hematopoietic stem cells in patients with MDS has been challenged until recently. However, the majority of patients with MDS who reach remission after intensive chemotherapy appeared to achieve a cytogenetic remission [30, 31]. Moreover, the remission appeared to be polyclonal when tested with X-linked polymorphic genes [40]. Polyclonality was also observed in marrow progenitor cells of patients with MDS in remission [41]. The experience with ABMT in patients with MDS or sAML is limited and the literature contains only case-reports [42,43]. Until now 114 recipients of autologous marrow grafts with MDS or AML following MDS have been reported to the registries of the EBMT [44]. The overall survival at 2 years of the 79 patients transplanted in first CR was 39%, the DFS was 34% and the actuarial relapse rate was 64%. Nineteen patients were transplanted for MDS which had not progressed to AML prior to ABMT. The actuarial DFS at 2 years after ABMT was 40% and the relapse rate 58%. Thirty-nine MDS patients had progressed to AML prior to chemotherapy and ABMT. DFS of these patients was 30% and the relapse rate 68%. Twenty-one patients were transplanted for MDS or AML which had developed after treatment with chemotherapy for other malignancies or auto-immune diseases. Actuarial DFS of these patients was 36% and the relapse rate 60%. Patients younger than 40 years had a significantly (p=0.04) better DFS compared to patients with age ≥40 years. This difference could be explained by the significantly (p=0.05) higher relapse rate of 72% in the older age group compared to the 59% in the patients younger than 40 years [50]. The results were compared with a matched control group of 110 patients with de novo AML. The DFS at two years was 28% for the cohort of 55 patients transplanted for MDS/sAML and 51% for those transplanted for de novo AML (p = 0.025). ABMT for MDS or sAML resulted in a lower DFS due to a higher relapse rate [44].

Transplant-related mortality and death due to regeneration failure did not appear to occur more often than after ABMT for de novo AML. The haematopoietic engraftment was slower despite the sufficient number of CFU-GM collected per kilogram body weight (5 x 10$^4$/kg), similar to that observed in de novo AML patients [43]. The median time to engraftment was 37 days for the white blood cells and 75 days for the platelets in the first retrospective analysis of the EBMT on 17 autografted MDS patients [44]. Laporte reported the results of ABMT with mafosfamide treated marrow in 7 patients with AML following MDS. The haematopoietic engraftment was also slower in these 7 patients, but all patients engrafted except for one patient who died early before engraftment of treatment-related causes. Two patients were alive and well at 10, and 28 months following ABMT [43]. Demuynck et al investigated the feasibility to collect peripheral stem in eleven patients with myelodysplasia [51]. This resulted in seven patients in an adequate yield (>1 x 10$^6$/kg b.w.) of CD34-cells [51]. Three patients with a normal to excellent stem cell harvest were demonstrated to be polyclonal by PCR techniques based on X-chromosome inactivation patterns (40). Six patients received autologous peripheral blood SCT in a prospective study of the EORTC Leukemia Cooperative Group and the EBMT (47). Peripheral stem cells were collected during the recovery phase of the first consolidation course using 300 μg of Filgrastim (s.c.) daily until completion of PBSC collections. Preliminary data indicate that the repopulation was much faster compared to autologous bone marrow transplantation [40,45-47].

Patients without a donor who achieve CR and maintain CR after intensive consolidation may benefit from a consolidation by autologous stem cell transplantation. The hematopoietic recovery after transfusion of mobilized blood stem cells is significantly faster than after ABMT. A prospective randomized trial is needed to show that autologous stem transplantation improves the outcome compared to treatment with chemotherapy only. This study (EORTC and EBMT cooperative trial 06961: CRIANT) has started in December 1996.

# References

1. Mufti GJ, et al. Myelodysplastic syndromes: a scoring system with prognostic significance. Br. J. Haematol. 1985; 59: 425-433.
2. Bennett JM, et al. (FAB Cooperative Group) Proposals for the classification of the myelodysplastic syndromes. Br. J. Haematol. 1982; 51: 189-199.
3. Kantarjian HM, et al. Therapy-related leukemia and myelodysplastic syndrome: clinical, cytogenetic, and prognostic features. J. Clin. Oncol. 1986; 4: 1748-1757.
4. Yunis JJ, et al. Refined chromosome analysis as an independent prognostic indicator in de novo myelodysplastic syndrome. Blood 1986; 67: 1721-1730.
5. Geddes A, et al. A. Clonal karyotypic abnormalities and clinical progress in the myelodysplastic syndromes. Br. J. Haematol. 1990; 76: 194-202.
6. De Witte T, et al. Intensive antileukemic treatment of patients younger than 65 years with myelodysplastic syndromes and secondary acute myelogenous leukemia. Cancer 1990; 66: 831-837.
7. Greenberg P, et al. International Workshop risk analysis system for evaluating prognosis in myelodysplastic syndromes. Blood 1997; 89: 2077-2088.
8. De Witte T, et al. Allogeneic bone marrow transplantation in a patient with acute myeloid leukemia secondary to Hodgkin's disease. Cancer 1984; 53:1507-1508.
9. Appelbaum FR, et al. Allogeneic transplantation in the treatment of preleukemia. Ann. Int. Med. 1984; 100: 689-693.
10. Appelbaum FR, et al. Bone marrow transplantation for patients with myelodysplasia. Ann. Int. Med. 1990; 112: 590-597.
11. Anderson JE, et al. Allogeneic bone marrow transplantation for 93 patients with myelodysplastic syndrome. Blood 1993; 82: 677-681.
12. O'Donnell MR, et al. Busulphan/cyclophosphamide as conditioning regimen for bone marrow transplantation for myelodysplasia. J. Clin. Oncol. 1995; 13: 2973-2977.
13. Guinan EC, et al. Bone marrow transplantation for children with myelodysplastic syndromes. Blood 1989; 73: 919-922.
14. Locatelli F, et al. Allogeneic bone marrow transplantation for chronic myelomonocytic leukemia in childhood: a report from the European Working Group on Myelodysplastic Syndrome in Childhood. J. Clin. Oncol. 1997; 15: 566-573.
15. De Witte T, et al. Allogeneic bone marrow transplantation for secondary leukaemia and myelodysplastic syndrome: a survey by the Leukaemia Working Party of the European Bone Marrow Transplantation Group (EBMTG). Br. J. Haematol. 1990; 74: 151-157.
16. Sutton L, al. Factors influencing outcome in de novo myelodysplastic syndromes treated by allogeneic bone marrow transplantation: a long-term study of 71 patients. Blood 1996; 88: 358-365.
17. Mattijssen V, et al. Outcome of allogeneic bone marrow transplantation with lymphocyte depleted marrow grafts in adult patients with myelodysplastic syndromes. Bone Marrow Transplant. 1997; 19: 791-794.
18. Runde V, et al. Bone marrow transplantation from HLA-identical sibling as first-line treatment in patients with myelodysplastic syndromes: early transplantation is associated with improved outcome. Bone Marrow Transplant. 1998; 21: 255-261.
19. Anderson JE, et al. Stem cell transplantation for secondary acute myeloid leukemia: evaluation of transplantation as initial therapy or following induction chemotherapy. Blood 1997; 89: 578-585.
20. Armitage O, et al. Effect of chemotherapy for the dysmyelopoietic syndrome. Canc. Treatm. Rep. 1981; 65: 601-605.
21. Fenaux P, et al. Prognostic factors in adult de novo myelodysplastic syndromes treated by intensive chemotherapy. Br. J. Haematol. 1991; 77: 497-501.
22. Marmont AM, Tura S. Bone marrow transplantation for secondary leukemia. Report of two cases. Bone Marrow Transplant. 1986; 1(suppl. 1):191-192.
23. Michels SD, et al. Refractory anemia with excess of blasts in transformation. Hematologic and clinical study of 52 patients. Cancer 1989; 64: 2340-2346.
24. Preisler HD, et al High-dose cytosine arabinoside in the treatment of preleukemic disorders: A leukemia intergroup study. A. J. Hematol. 1986; 23: 131-134.
25. Richard C, et al. Therapy of advanced myelodysplastic syndrome with aggressive chemotherapy. Oncology 1989; 46: 6-8.
26. Holmes J, et al. Multidrug resistance in haematopoietic cell lines, myelodysplastic syndromes, and acute myeloblastic leukaemia. Br. J. Haematol. 1989; 72: 40-44.
27. Sonneveld P, et al. High expression of the multidrug resistance P-glycoprotein in high risk myelodysplasia is associated with immature phenotype. Leukemia 1993; 7: 963-969.
28. Bernasconi C, et al. Randomized clinical study comparing aggresssive chemotherapy with or without G-CSF support for high-risk myelodysplastic syndromes or secondary acute myeloid leukaemia evolving from MDS. Br. J. Haematol. 1998; 102: 678-683.
29. Ruutu T, et al. Intensive chemotherapy of poor prognosis myelodysplastic syndromes (MDS) and acute myeloid leukemia following MDS with idarubicin and cytarabine. Leukemia Res. 1997; 21:133-138.
30. De Witte T, et al. Intensive chemotherapy for poor prognosis myelodysplastia (MDS) and secondary acute myelogenous leukemia following MDS of more than 6 months duration. A pilot study by the Leukemia Cooperative Group of the European Organisation for Research and Treatment in Cancer. (EORTC-LCG). Leukemia 1995; 9: 1805-1810.
31. Parker JE, et al. Fludarabine, cytarabine, G-CSF and idarubicin (FLAG-IDA) for the treatment of poor-risk myelodysplastic syndromes and acute

myeloid leukaemia. Br. J. Haematol. 1997; 99: 939-944.

32. Tricot G, et al. The role of aggressive chemotherapy in the treatment of myelodysplastic syndromes. Br. J. Haematol. 1986; 63: 477-483.

33. Mertelsmann R, et al. Morphological classification, response to therapy, and survival in 263 adult patients with acute nonlymphoblastic leukemia. Blood 1980; 56: 773-781.

34. Seymour JF, Estey EH. The prognostic significance of auer rods in myelodysplasia. Br. J. Haematol. 1993; 85: 67-76.

35. Vaughan WP, et al. Effective chemotherapy of acute myelocytic leukemia occurring after alkylating agent or radiation therapy for prior malignancy. J. Clin. Oncol. 1983; 1: 204-207.

36. Fenaux P, et al. Therapy-related myelodysplastic syndrome and leukemia with no unfavourable cytogenetic findings have a good response to intensive chemotherapy: a report on 15 cases. Leukemia and Lymphoma 1991; 5: 117-125.

37. Estey E, et al. Treatment of myelodysplastic syndromes with AML-type treatment. Leukemia and Lymphoma 1989; 11: 59-65.

38. Hasle H, et al. Intensive chemotherapy in childhood myelodysplastic syndrome. A comparison with the results in acute myeloid leukemia. Leukemia 1996; 10: 1269-1273.

39. Gajewsky JL, et al. Efficacy of intensive chemotherapy for acute myelogenous leukemia associated with preleukemic syndrome. J. Clin. Oncol. 1989; 7: 1637-1645.

40. Delforge M, et al. Polyclonal primitive hematopoietic progenitors can be detected in mobilized peripheral blood from patients with high-risk myelodysplastic syndromes. Blood 1995; 86: 3660-3667.

41. Delforge M, et al. Patients with high-risk myelodysplastic syndrome can have polyclonal or clonal haemopoiesis in complete haematological remission. Br. J. Haematol. 1998; 102: 486-494.

42. Öberg G, et al. Is haematological reconstitution seen after ABMT in MDS patients? Bone Marrow Transplant. 1989; 4 (suppl 2): 52.

43. Laporte JP, et al. Autologous bone marrow transplantation with marrow purged by Mafosfamide in seven patients with myelodysplastic syndromes in transformation (AML-MDS): a pilot study. Leukemia 1993; 7: 2030-2033.

44. De Witte T, et al. Autologous bone marrow transplantation for patients with myelodysplastic syndrome (MDS) or acute myeloid leukemia following MDS. Blood 1997; 10: 3853-3857.

45. Demuynck H, et al. Feasibility of peripheral blood progenitor cell harvest and transplantation in patients with poor-risk myelodysplastic syndromes. Br. J. Haematol. 1996; 92: 351-359.

46. T. De Witte, et al. Autologous or allogeneic stem cell transplantation (SCT) for high risk MDS and aml secondary to MDS (sAML) in patients <60 years. A joint study of the EORTC and the EBMT leukaemia groups (#2458). Blood 1995; 86 (suppl. 1): 618a.

47. Carella AM, et al. In vivo mobilization of karyotypically normal peripheral blood progenitor cells in high-risk MDS, secondary or therapy-related acute myelogenous leukaemia. Br. J. Haematol. 1996; 95: 127-130.

# Secondary Leukemia or Myelodysplasia Treated by Bone Marrow Transplantation

R. P. Witherspoon, H. J. Deeg, R. Storb, F. R. Appelbaum and F. Hutchinson

Supported in part by HL36444 of the National Heart, Lung and Blood Institute, CA 18029, 18221 and NO1-CP51027 of the National Cancer Institute of the National Institutes of Health, Bethesda, MD, USA and the Gabriella Rich Foundation.

## Introduction

Patients who develop secondary leukemia face a poor prognosis for survival. Chemotherapy to induce a remission has been complicated by prolonged leukopenia, infection, and a low likelihood of achieving a complete remission. Once achieved, the remissions are of short duration [1]. Combination chemotherapy with cytosine arabinoside and fludarabine, or treatment with topotecan show promise to increase the remission rate and duration of remission [2,3]. However, long-term survival is not likely for patients with secondary leukemia. Treatment of secondary acute leukemia by bone marrow transplantation from a family member or unrelated donor suitably matched for HLA has resulted in long term disease free survival for less than 30 % of patients due to a high relapse rate and significant non-relapse mortality [4,5,6]. We previously reported no statistically significant improvement in outcome whether patients with secondary acute myeloid leukemia (AML) were transplanted as initial therapy or following induction chemotherapy [4]. The data reviewed here are taken from patients transplanted after a diagnosis of secondary myelodysplasia or acute leukemia. The results suggest a role for transplantation at earlier stages of disease and use of busulfan blood level concentration at steady state to achieve lower non-relapse mortality and better long-term disease-free survival.

## Methods

The records were reviewed of 108 patients who were transplanted with allogeneic marrow consecutively at the Fred Hutchinson Cancer Research Center for secondary leukemia or myelodysplasia from December 1971 to through July 1998 with follow up based on the date of last contact through January 1999. The age range was 5.4–61 (median 42.3) years. Before leukemia or myelodysplasia developed, the original diseases and the number of patients each were Hodgkin's disease 36, non-Hodgkin lymphoma 14, breast cancer 7, acute lymphocytic leukemia 6, polycythemia vera 4, multiple myeloma 2, ovarian carcinoma 2, aplastic anemia 5, and other miscellaneous individual diagnosis 33. Ninety-nine patients had treatment of the original disease consisting of chemotherapy alone 36, radiation alone 9, chemoradiotherapy 50, immunosuppressive therapy 4, and in 9 treatment details were not known. At the time of transplantation 54 had AML, 15 refractory anemia with excess blasts in transition (RAEB-T), 22 refractory anemia with excess blasts (RAEB), 15 refractory anemia (RA), 1 refractory anemia with ringed sideroblasts (RARS), and 1 whose stage was not classified. Chromosome analyses were completed on 84 of the patients, and the results were classified into 3 chromosome risk categories. Risk level 1 consisted of normal chromosomes, or deletions of Y, 5q minus or 20q

Cancer Research Center and University of Washington Seattle, Washington, USA

minus. Risk level 3 consisted of abnormalities of chromosome 7, or a total of 3 or more chromosome abnormalities. Risk level 2 consisted of all other chromosome abnormalities. Fifty-two patients were classified in risk level 3, 18 in risk level 2, and 14 in risk level 1. Among the 16 patients in the RA or RARS stage, 7 had risk level 3, 4 had risk level 2, 3 had risk level 1, and 2 had no chromosome analyses. The donors consisted of 53 HLA A, B, and D locus matched siblings, 2 phenotypically matched family members, 9 haploidentical family members, 4 syngeneic siblings and 40 HLA phenotypically matched or minor mismatched unrelated donors. Conditioning regimens for grafting were chemoradiotherapy consisting of cyclophosphamide and 9.6-15.75 Gy total body irradiation (TBI) in 38 patients, chemotherapy consisting of busulfan 14-16 mg/kg and cyclophosphamide 120 mg/kg (BuCy) in 27 patients, busulfan 16 mg/kg with dose adjustment to achieve a concentration at steady state of 600-900 ng/10$^{-6}$L and cyclophosphamide 120 mg/kg in 22 patients (BuCy[t]) (7), miscellaneous chemoradiotherapy regimens usually busulfan 7 mg/kg and 12 Gy TBI in 19 patients, and miscellaneous chemotherapy regimens in 2 patients. The prophylactic treatment for acute GVHD employed various regimen of methotrexate, cyclosporine, FK506, or a combination of these over the 27 years. Kaplan-Meier probabilities were used to analyze the data.

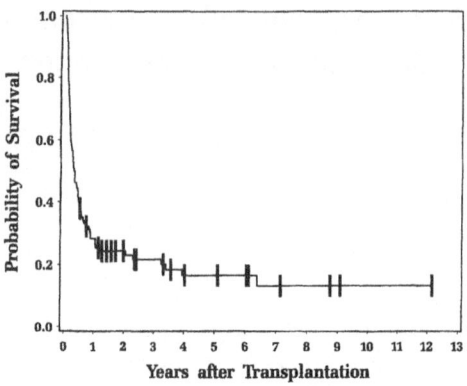

**Fig. 1.** Probability of overall survival by time after allogeneic bone marrow transplantation. The probability of survival was 13.3% at 6.4 years. Tic marks indicate data censored by date of last contact.

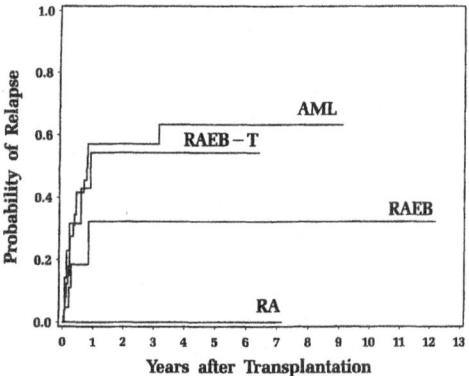

**Fig. 2.** Probability of relapse by disease stage at transplantation. The probability of relapse was 63.3% for AML, 54.3% for RAEB-T, and 32.1% for RAEB. None of the 16 patients transplanted at the RA stages have relapsed. (RA includes the RARS patient. See text for abbreviations)

## Results

One patient failed to engraft, and the remaining 107 patients engrafted. The median time to reach a peripheral blood neutrophil count of 500/10$^{-9}$L was 19 days. The median time and probability to develop acute graft versus host disease (GVHD) grade 2 or greater was 15 (range 6-74) days and 67.5%, respectively. Overall twenty-one patients survived. The Kaplan-Meier (KM) probability of survival overall when the curve reached a plateau at 6.4 years was 13.3% (Fig.1).

Relapse developed in 31 patients. The overall KM probability of relapse was 48.5%. The probabilities of relapse for patients transplanted with AML, RAEB-T, or RAEB were 63.3%, 54.3%, and 32.1% respectively. None of the 16 patients transplanted at the RA or RARS stages relapsed with follow up between 1.0 and 8.2 years (Fig. 2).

The causes of death were relapse in 30 patients and non-relapse mortality in 57 patients. The 100 day non-relapse mortality was 38.6%, and the overall non-relapse mortality was 76.1%. Organ failure accounted for 17 of the non-relapse deaths. The types of organ failure and number of deaths each were hepatic venocclulusive disease 5, multiple organ failure 3, idiopathic pneumonia or diffuse alveolar damage 4, respiratory failure syndrome 4, and cardiomyopathy 1. The probability of organ failure death was 42.3% for patients transplanted at the RA or RARS stage, 9% for RAEB, 14.4% for RAEB-T, and 25.7% for AML. Infection accounted for 20 of the non-relapse deaths. The types of infection and number of deaths each were disseminated aspergillus 9, candida septicemia 3, bacterial septicemia or pneumonia 5, cytomegalovirus pneumonia 2, and disseminated varicella 1. The probability of death from infection was 23.4% for patients transplanted at the RA or RARS stage, 47.1% for RAEB, 12.5% for RAEB-T, and 26.7% for AML. Five patients died of acute and 3 of chronic GVHD. Four died of central nervous system hemorrhage. One died of graft failure. Secondary cancer resulted in 3 deaths, and 4 died of unknown causes.

The disease-free survival was 33.3% for patients transplanted at the RA or RARS stage, 18.2% for the RAEB stage, 17.8% for the RAEB-T stage, and 9.5% for the AML stage. The patient with RAEB-T who had the longest follow-up died of chronic GVHD and infection at 6.4 years after transplantation (Fig. 3).

Chromosome abnormality risk groups 1, 2, and 3 were associated with a probability of survival of 21.4%, 22.2%, and 13.4%, respectively.

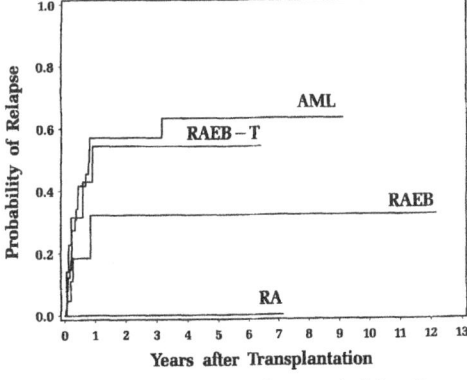

**Fig. 3.** Probability of disease-free survival by disease stage at transplantation. The disease-free survival was 33.3% for RA or RARS, 18.2% for RAEB, 17.8 % for RAEB-T, and 9.5% for AML. The patient with RAEB-T with the longest follow-up died of chronic GVHD complicated by infection. Tic marks indicate data censored by date of last contact. (See text for abbreviations)

Because of the high mortality seen in this group of patients, an analysis was done of the correlation of the conditioning regimens with survival, relapse, non-relapse mortality and death due to organ failure. BuCy[t] was used in 22 patients, BuCy in 27 patients, and regimens containing TBI in 57 patients. The probabilities of survival in the BuCy[t], BuCy, and TBI grouups were 32.2%, 13.9%, and 9.0%, respectively. The probabilities of relapse in the BuCy[t], BuCy, and TBI groups were 37.4%, 48.7% and 52.5%, respectively. The probabilities of non-relapse mortality for BuCy[t], BuCy, and TBI groups were 53.5%, 72.9%, and 83.8% respectively. Among the deaths due to non-relapse causes, the probability of death due to organ failure was 10.5% among the patients who received BuCy[t]. The probability of death due to organ failure was 30.4% for patients who received BuCy, and 23.1% for patients who received regimens containing TBI.

## Discussion

These data review the results of marrow transplantation for a group of predominantly treatment-related secondary myelodysplasia or leukemia. During the 27 year span of time, varied regimens of supportive care to prevent and treat acute GVHD and infection or organ toxicity were used. The data suggest that when allogeneic hematopoietic stem cell transplantation is used for treatment of secondary myelodysplasia or AML, substantial advantage is gained by transplantation early in the evolution of the disease at the RA or RARS stage. The long-term disease-free survival in these patients was 33%. None of these patients have relapsed with substantial follow up ranging from 1 to 8 years. Transplantation still has the potential to cure the disease when it has advanced to the RAEB, RAEB-T or AML stage with 18.2, 17.8, and 9.5 percent disease-free survival, respectively, with follow up ranging from 1.2 to 9.1 years. Relapse is a major cause of death after transplantation for patients with these more advanced stages of disease.

Unfortunately, non-relapse mortality accounted for the highest probability of death after transplantation. These deaths resulted primarily from organ failure or infection. Of the patients transplanted at the RA or RARS stage, death from organ failure or infection reduced the long-term disease-free survival considerably from the 46-50% actuarial 3 year disease-free survival seen for patients transplanted with spontaneous RA or RARS, which is not related to previous treatment for cancer or other hematologic malignancy (8).

Because of the high non-relapse mortality, we retrospectively examined the potential indicators of prognosis for myelodysplasia based on chromosome risk factor levels. It is not clear whether chromosome risk factor levels correlate with prognosis in treatment related leukemia. Indeed, most of the patients in this report had chromosome risk level 3 abnormalities often associated with previous treatment for malignancy. Even among the patients with RA or RARS, nearly half had risk level 3 abnormalities. Because the RA or RARS patients were believed to have a malignant clone, they were transplanted without undue delay. Therefore, any potential advantage of normal chromosomes or lower risk chromosome abnormalities on the clinical course before transplantation could not be determined. There was no significant correlation between chromosome risk level and survival after transplantation. Therefore, it is not clear from these data how chromosome risk factors could be used to identify patients who might have a particularly good prognosis in whom transplantation could be delayed or not done at all.

Since organ failure was a significant cause of non-relapse mortality, we retrospectively examined the conditioning regimens used for transplantation. The use of the BuCy[t] regimen with busulfan administered to achieve a concentration at steady state of between 600 and 900 ng/10⁻⁶L resulted in the best overall survival (32.2%) and was substantially better than the result using either BuCy without targeting the busulfan blood level (13.9%), or TBI containing regimens (9.0%). There was very little difference in the relapse rate with any of these three regimens (BuCy[t] 37.4%, BuCy 48.6%, and TBI 52.5%). The difference in overall survival was primarily due to non-relapse mortality which occurred in 53.5% for the BuCy[t] group, 72.9% for the BuCy group, and 83.3% for the TBI group. Among

the causes of non-relapse mortality, death due to organ failure was lowest in the BuCy[t] group. These data are difficult to interpret because the groups receiving BuCy or the TBI regimens contained a higher proportion of patients transplanted at more advanced stages of disease. The stage of disease may interact with the regimens used for transplantation as cofactors affecting the outcome of death due to organ failure. A multivariable analysis is needed to definitively clarify the roles of these competing factors on the outcome. Nevertheless, there appeared to be an advantage in reduction of death due to organ failure by use of busulfan dosing targeted to achieve a blood level which is associated with less toxicity and mortality. Further study of this approach, especially in those patients transplanted at the RA stage, is warranted to reduce the mortality of transplantation at early stages of disease. In addition, the role of remission induction prior to transplantation, especially for patients with more advanced disease should be explored anew, to determine whether it leads to lower mortality after transplantation.

We conclude that both relapse and non-relapse mortality are significant impediments for long-term disease-free survival after allogeneic marrow transplantation for patients with treatment-related secondary myelodysplasia or leukemia. The lowest relapse rate was seen among patients transplanted at early stages of disease. Patients who are at risk to develop treatment-related secondary leukemia should be followed closely for the development of myelodysplasia, and transplantation should be considered at the RA stage to achieve the best long-term disease-free survival. Innovative approaches to transplantation are warranted to reduce non-relapse mortality.

*Acknowledgement.* The authors are grateful to Gary Schoch of the Fred Hutchinson Cancer Research Center for assistance in data analysis and preparation of the figures.

# References

1. Kantarjian HM, Estey EH, Keating MJ (1993) Treatment of therapy-related leukemia and myelodysplastic syndrome. Hamatol Oncol Clin North Am 7:81–107.

2. Estey EH, Kantarjian HM, O'Brien S, Kornblau S, Andreef M, Beran M, Pierce S, Keating M (1995) High remission rate, short remission duration in patients with refractory anemia with excess blasts (RAEB) in transformation (RAEB-t) given acute myelogenous leukemia (AML)-type chemotherapy in combination with granulocyte-CSF (G-CSF). Cytokines & Molecular Therapy 1:21–8.

3. Beran M, Kantarjian H, O'Brien S, Koller C, al-Bitar M, Arbuck S, Pierce S, Moore M, Abbruzzese JL, Andreeff M, Keating M, Estey E (1996) Topotecan, a topoisomerase I inhibitor, is active in the treatment of myelodysplastic syndrome and chronic myelomonocytic leukemia. Blood 88:2473–9.

4. Anderson JE, Gooley TA, Schoch G, Anasetti C, Bensinger W, Clift R, Hansen JA, Sanders JE, Storb R, Appelbaum FR (1997) Stem cell transplantation for secondary acute myeloid leukemia: Evaluation of transplantation as initial therapy or following induction chemotherapy. Blood 89:2578–85.

5. Runde V, de Witte T, Arnold R, Gratwohl A, Hermans J, van Biezen A, Niederwieser D, Labopin M, Walter-Noel MP, Bacigalupo A, Jacobsen N, Ljungman P, Carreras E, Kolb HJ, Aul C, Apperley J (1998) Bone marrow transplantation from HLA-identical siblings as first-line treatment in patients with myelodysplastic syndromes: early transplantation is associated with improved outcome. Chronic Leukemia Working Party of the European Group for Blood and Marrow Transplantation. Bone Marrow Transplantation 21:255–61.

6. Ballen KK, Gilliland DG, Guinan EC, Hsieh CC, Parsons SK, Rimm IJ, Ferrara JL, Bierer BE, Weinstein JH, Antin JH (1997) Bone marrow transplantation for therapy-related myelodysplasia: comparison with primary myelodysplasia. Bone Marrow Transplantation 20:737–43.

7. Slattery JT, Clift RA, Buckner CD, Radich J, Storer B, Bensinger WI, Soll E, Anasetti C, Bowden R, Bryant E, Chauncey T, Deeg HJ, Doney KC, Flowers M, Gooley T, Hansen JA, Martin PJ, McDonald GB, Nash R, Petersdorf EW, Sanders JE, Schoch G, Stewart P, Storb R, Sullivan KM, Thomas ED, Witherspoon RP, Appelbaum FR (1997) Marrow transplantation for chronic myeloid leukemia: the influence of plasma busulfan levels on the outcome of transplantation. Blood 89:3055–60.

8. Anderson JE, Appelbaum FR, Schoch G, Gooley T, Anasetti C, Bensinger WI, Bryant E, Buckner CD, Chauncey TR, Clift RA, Doney K, Flowers M, Hansen JA, Martin PJ, Matthews DC, Sanders JE, Shulman H, Sullivan KM, Witherspoon RP, Storb R (1996) Allogeneic marrow transplantation for refractory anemia: a comparison of two preparative regimens and analysis of prognostic factors. Blood 87:51–8.

# Comparison of Intensive Chemotherapy and Autologous Transplantation as Post Remission Therapy in Adult Acute Myeloid Leukemia. Update of the GOELAM 1 Trial

J. L. Harousseau, B. Pignon, M. P., Chevalier and J. Y. Cahn on behalf of the GOELAM Group

Three strategies are currently used to prevent relapse in younger patients with acute myeloid leukemia (AML) in first complete remission (CR). In most centers, patients under 50 years of age with an HLA identical sibling are offered allogeneic bone marrow transplantation. For all other patients up to the age of 60, two other options can be proposed, either intensive consolidation chemotherapy (ICC) or autologous stem cell transplantation (ASCT). In the past 10 years, several cooperative groups have prospectively compared these two strategies in patients lacking an HLA identical sibling. The French GOELAM group conducted such as study between November 1987 and May 1994. Out of 367 patients in first CR, 164 were randomly assigned to receive after a first course of ICC, either a myeloablative regimen followed by ASCT, or a second course of ICC. The first analysis of this study was performed as of June 1996. With a median follow-up of 62 months, there was no significant difference in the 4 year disease-free survival (DFS) and overall survival (OS) between 86 patients in the ASCT arm and 78 in the ICC arm. The results of this study were updated as of January 1998. We herein report this updated analysis of the GOELAM 1 trial and discuss the place of ASCT in AML by comparing our data to those published by other groups.

## Patients and Methods

Patients 15 to 50 years of age with previously untreated primary AML were eligible for entry into the trial. Patients with a previous myelodysplasia diagnosed for more than 3 months were excluded, whereas patients with antecedent of unexplained cytopenia were included. We also excluded patients with a myeloproliferative disorder in blast crisis, patients who had previously received cytotoxic chemotherapy or radiotherapy (or both), patients with clinical or electrocardiographic signs of heart failure or coronary disease, and patients with hepatic or renal disturbances (hepatic enzymes levels over 4 times the normal values, creatinine level over 130 µmol/L). The induction treatment consisted of a continuous infusion of ARA-C (200 mg/m$^2$/d) for consecutive days (days 1 through 7) with either idarubicin (IDR) administered intravenously on days 1 through 5 at a daily dose of 8 mg/m$^2$ or rubidazone (RBZ) administered intravenously on days 1 through 4 are a daily dose of 200 mg/m$^2$. Central randomization was stratified by center. A BM aspiration was performed on day 17. If the marrow was hypoplastic and nonblastic, no further treatment was administered. If the marrow was hypoplastic and contained less than 50% blasts, a second induction course was administered with a combination of ARA-C over 3 days and of the anthracycline initially allocated over 2 days. If the marrow was normocellular and blastic or contained more than 50% blasts, the result was estimated as a failure and the patient was withdrawn from the study. All patients in CR after one or two courses of induction treatment were scheduled to receive an intensive consolidation therapy. A search for an HLA identical sibling was performed on each patient 40 years of age or younger and an allogeneic BMT was proposed to all these patients having an HLA identical sibling. All other

Department of Hematology, Nantes, France.

patients were assigned to receive a first course of ICC consisting of HD-ARA-C (3 g/m$^2$) administered on a 3 hour infusion every 12 hours, days 1 through 4 (total dose, 24 g/m$^2$), combined with either IDR administered intravenously on days 5 and 6 at a daily dose of 10 mg/m$^2$ or RBZ administered intravenously on days 5 and 6 at a daily dose of 200 mg/m$^2$, according to the initial randomization. The first course of ICC was to be administered as soon as possible after remission achievement and no later than 75 days after induction treatment initiation. BM was harvested after the first course of ICC without any in vitro manipulation. Patients still in CR with at least 1 x 108 nucleated cells/kg in the collected marrow were randomly assigned to receive either a second course of ICC or an ABMT. The second course of ICC consisted of amsacrine administered as a 1 hour Infusion on 5 consecutive days (days 1 through 5) at a daily dose of 150 mg/m$^2$ and etoposide administered as a 2 hour Infusion on days 1 through 5 at a daily dose of 100 mg/m$^2$. Before ABMT, the conditioning regimen was the combination of busulfan administered orally at a daily dose of 4 mg/kg for 4 consecutive days (days 9 through 6 before transplantation) and cyclophosphamide administered intravenously at a daily dose of 50 mg/kg for 4 consecutive days (days 5 through 2 before transplantation).

## Results

### Feasibility of Postremission Treatment

Out of 535 patients included by 16 centers, 517 were eligible and 504 were evaluable for induction treatment. The CR rate was 73% (367/504). Of the 367 patients in CR, 146 did not undergo the assigned intensive postremission therapy for a variety of reasons (extrahematologic toxicity 27, protocol violation 26, refusal 24, relapse 22, poor hematopoietic reconstitution 21, infectious complications 19, toxic death 7). Two patients were lost for follow-up. Only 219 patients did actually receive the intensive treatment as scheduled in the protocol (59,5% of the patients in CR). 73 allogeneic BMT, 75 ABMT, 71 ICC. The feasibility of the protocol is shown in Figure 1.

### Comparison of ICC and ASCT

With a median follow-up of 80 months, the 6 year DFS was 44% for the 75 patients who actually underwent ASCT versus 38% for the 71 patients who received the second course of ICC (P = 0,47). The 6 year OS was 52% in the ASCT arm and 55% in the ICC arm with again no significant difference (p = 0,67). However, because 11 patients randomized in the ASCT arm and 7 patients randomized in

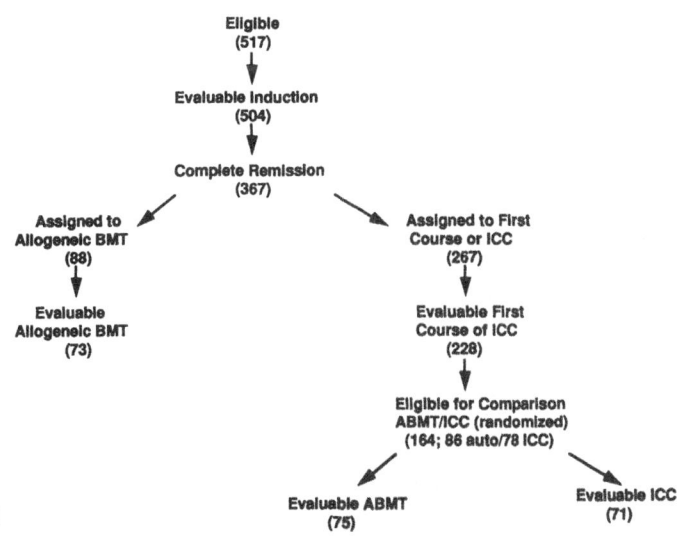

**Fig. 1.** Feasibility of the protocol

the ICC arm did not undergo the assigned treatment, the comparison between the 2 groups was also performed according to the intention to treat participle. The toxic-death rate was 13% in the ASCT arm and 3% in the ICC arm and the relapse rate was 45% in the ASCT arm and 59% in the ICC arm Kaplan-Meier plots showed that the 6 year probability of relapse was 47,5% +/– 5,5% in the ICC arm (Fig. 2). Although the difference was not significant, there was a trend in favor of ABMT

(p = 0,11). The 6 year DFS was 44% +/– 5% in the ABMT arm versus 38% +/– 5% in the ICC arm (p=0,47) (Fig 3). Finally the 6 year OS was 50% +/– 5% in the ABMT arm versus 51% +/– 5% in the ICC arm (p = 0,75) (Fig 4).

## Discussion

This updated analysis of the GOELAM 1 trial confirms the previously published results [1].

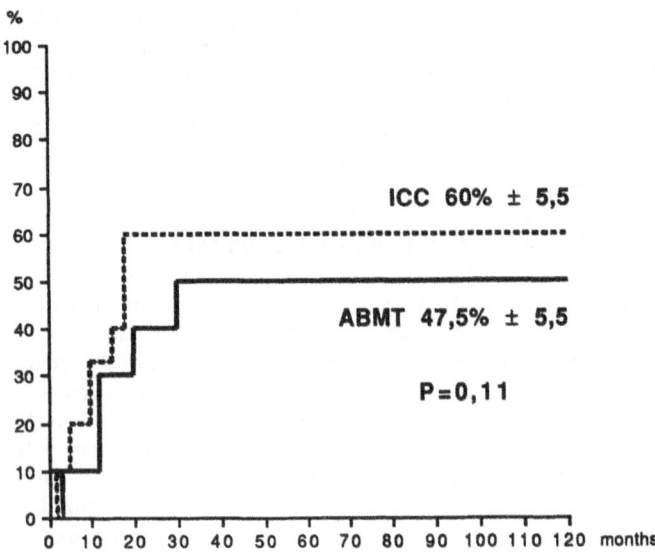

Fig. 2. Actuarial relapse rate (Intention to treat analysis)

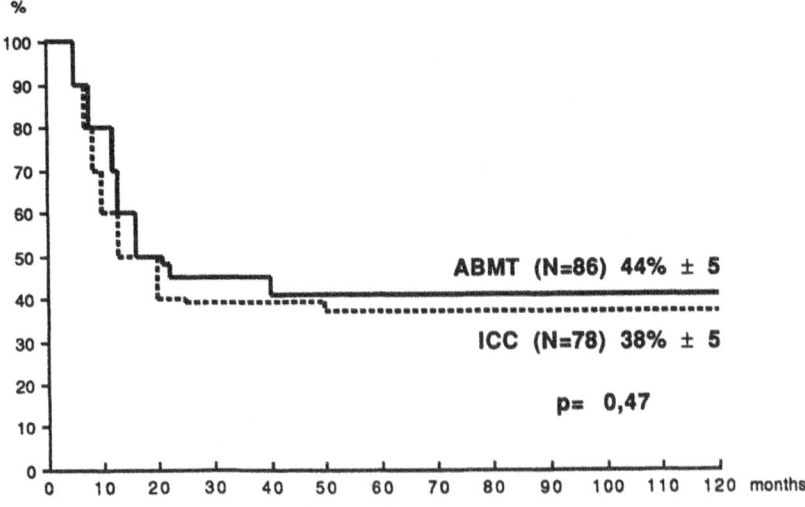

Fig. 3. Disease free survival (intention to treat analysis)

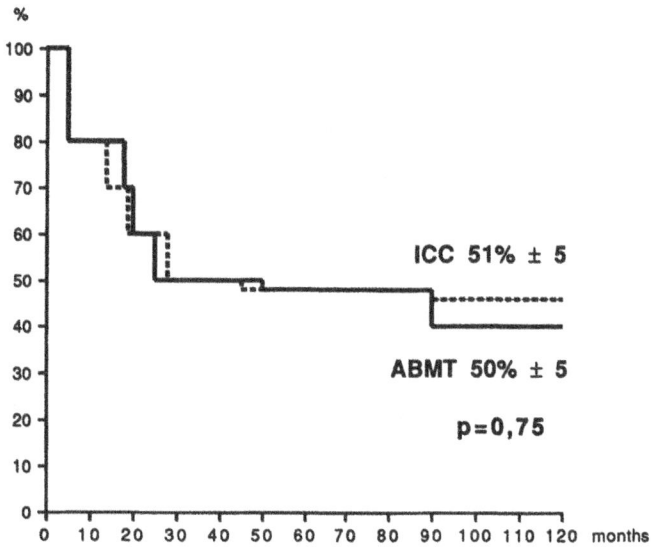

%

Fig. 4. Overall survival (intention trial analysis)

ICC 51% ± 5

ABMT 50% ± 5

p=0,75

With a median follow-up of 6 years, after a first course of ICC, there is no difference in the outcome between ABMT and a second course of ICC. These results are in line with those published by other cooperative groups [2–3].

Both the Pediatric Oncology Group for children and the US Intergroup (SWOG, ECOG and CALGB) for adults also failed to demonstrate a significant superiority of ASCT as compared to ICC. The EORTC/ GMEMA study showed that ABMT resulted in significantly better 4 year DES than ICC (48% versus 30%) [4]. However, the 4 years was not significantly different (56% versus 46%) since patients relapsing after ICC were more readily salvaged than patients relapsing after ABMT. Moreover, the results of the ICC arm in the EORTC/GIMEMA study were lower than those achieved in other comparable studies and lower than those previously published by the CALGB with 4 courses of HD ARA-C [5]. Therefore, one can assume that the chemotherapy are in the EORTC/GIMEMA trial was not optimal.

Finally, the MRC trial demonstrated that the addition of ASCT to 4 cycles of intensive chemotherapy reduced the risk of relapse [6]. In this large randomized multicenter study, the number of relapses was significantly lower in the group of 190 patients allocated to receive ABMT, than in the group of 191

patients assigned to no further treatment (37% versus 58%, p = 0,0007). Although there were more deaths in remission in the ABMT arm (12% versus 4%), the 7 year DES was superior in this arm (53% versus 40%, p = 0,04). However, the design of this study does not allow a direct comparison of ABMT and ICC. Therefore, the current analysis of published studies suggests that, in terms of DFS, the benefit of ABMT as compared to the best available ICC is only marginal and that the demonstration of a statistical significant would need a very large study or a metaanalysis of randomized trials. However, it is important to underline the fact that in all studies, the relapse rate after ICC was round 60% and was superior to that observed after ABMT. The absence of significant difference in DFS curves was explained by a higher toxic-death rate after ABMT (Table 1). In the only study showing a significant advantage for ABMT,

Table 1. Comparison ABMT/ICC in published trials. Relapsed rate and toxic-death rate (percentages)

|  | Relapse | | Toxic death | |
|  | ABMT | ICC | ABMT | ICC |
|---|---|---|---|---|
| Zittoun | 40,5 | 57 | 9 | 7 |
| Ravindranath | 31 | 58 | 15 | 3 |
| Burnett | 37 | 58 | 12 | 4 |
| Cassileth | 48 | 61 | 14 | 3 |
| GOELAM | 45 | 59 | 13 | 3 |

the toxic-death rates were comparable in the two arms.

Therefore, one could conclude that a myeloablative regimens followed by ABMT is a more effective antileukemic therapy than repeated courses of ICC, but at the expenses of a more severe toxicity. Moreover, in all studies the issue of feasibility of these intensive programs was critical, since 33 to 50% of patients in CR did not receive the assigned treatment. This was mainly observed in the ABMT arms since only 54 to 87% of patients randomly assigned to ABMT underwent the scheduled therapy, compared to 83 to 97% of patients assigned to ICC. The objectives of future trials should be to increase the feasibility and decrease the toxicity of ASCT. This could be achieved thanks to the use of growth factors and of peripheral blood progenitors instead of some marrow.

# References

1. Harousseau JL, Cahn JY, Pignon B et al. (1995) Comparison of autologous bone marrow transplantation and intensive chemotherapy as postremission therapy in adult acute myeloid leukemia. Blood 90: 2978–2986
2. Ravindranath Y, Yeager AM, Chang MN et al. (1996) Autologous bone marrow transplantation versus intensive consolidation chemotherapy for acute myeloid leukemia in childhood. N Engl J Med 334: 1428–1434
3. Cassileth PA, Harrington DP, Appelbaum FR et al. (1998) Chemotherapy compared with autologous or allogeneic bone marrow transplantation in the management of acute myeloid leukemia in first remission. N Engl J Med 339: 1649–1656
4. Zittoun RA, Mandelli F, Willemze R et al. (1995) Autologous or allogeneic bone marrow transplantation compared with intensive chemotherapy in acute myelogenous leukemia. N Engl J Med 332: 217–223
5. Mayer RJ, Davis RB, Schiffer CA et al. (1994) Intensive postremission chemotherapy in adults with acute myeloid leukemia. N Engl J Med 331: 896–903
6. Burnett A, Goldstone AH, Stevens RMF et al. (1998) Randomised comparison of addition of autologous bone-marrow transplantation to intensive chemotherapy for acute myeloid leukemia in first remission: results of MRC AML 10 trial. Lancet 351: 700–707

# Adoptive Immunotherapy of Acute Leukemia and Acute Phase Chronic Myeloid Leukemia after Allogeneic Bone Marrow Transplantation

C. SCHMID[1], A. MUTH[1], M. HUMANN[1], G. LEDDEROSE[1], C. SALAT[1], R. MUNKER[1], M. SCHLEUNING[1], E. HOLLER[3] and H.-J. KOLB[1,2] for the EBMT Chronic Leukemia Working Party.

*Abstract.* Recurrence of leukemia after allogeneic hematopoietic transplantation presents a serious therapeutic problem. Chemotherapy and second transplants have been of limited value. In contrast, transfusion of lymphocytes from the original donor has induced remissions in more than 70% of patients with recurrent chronic myelogenous leukemia (CML) in chronic phase or cytogenetic relapse, in about 30% of patients with acute myeloid leukemia (AML) or myelodysplastic syndrome (MDS), and in about 10–15% of patients with acute lymphoid leukemia (ALL). In most CML patients remissions were lasting without further therapy, but in most patients with AML/MDS or ALL remissions were of limited duration. The differences in the response of CML, AML/MDS and ALL could best be explained by differences in antigen presentation. Indeed in CML dendritic cells are of leukemic origin as shown by FISH analysis. AML blasts may differentiate to dendritic cells in culture, but ALL blasts do not produce dendritic cells. More than 80% of fresh AML blasts do not express the co-stimulatory molecules B7.1 and B 7.2 and fail to stimulate allogeneic cells. However after culture in the presence of granulocyte-monocyte-colony stimulating factor (GM-CSF) and interleukin-4 (IL-4) cells of AML patients express co-stimulatory molecules and stimulate allogeneic cells. Another possibility to improve antigen presentation is the substitution of deficient antigen presenting by donor stem cells along with T-cells. Therefore we studied the transfusion of donor blood stem cells including T-cells and the treatment with GM-CSF after transfusion of donor cells in patients with recurrent AML, ALL and acute phase CML. Complete remissions could be induced in the majority of AML and some acute phase CML patients without intensive chemotherapy. Several patients remained in remission for a prolonged period of time. In ALL intensive chemotherapy was required for remission induction. Patients treated with intensive chemotherapy had a high risk of acute and chronic GVHD. These results confirm an allogeneic graft versus leukemia effect in acute leukemia and acute phase CML. They indicate an improvement of the response rate by the combination of PBSC and GM-CSF.

## Introduction

The term *adoptive immunotherapy* was coined by G. Mathé who showed convincingly that leukemia may be eliminated by allogeneic bone marrow transplantation. However the prize to be paid was severe graft-versus-host disease [1]. Patients surviving the first five months had a lesser risk of leukemic relapse, if they had acute or chronic graft-versus-host disease [2]. The role of T-cells in the control of leukemia became apparent following a high relapse rate after transplantation of marrow from which T-cells were depleted [3]. In a retrospective study of the IBMTR the graft-versus-leukemia effect of T-cells was demonstrated even after adjustment to the occurrence of graft-versus-host disease [4]. However transfusion of donor lymphocytes early after transplantation did not improve survival nor decrease the relapse incidence

Hematopoietic Cell Transplantation, Med. Dept. III, Klinikum Großhadern, Ludwigs-Maximilians-University Munich, and GSF – National Research Center for Environment and Health, Germany (1); Div. Hematology and Oncology, Klinikum University Regensburg, Germany (3)

significantly [5]. Animal experiments demonstrated that donor lymphocytes can be given safely in tolerant chimeras [6, 7], they would convert mixed chimerism into complete chimerism [6] and eliminate leukemia [7]. Donor lymphocyte transfusions were introduced into the clinic as a form of adoptive immunotherapy in patients with CML [8,9]. The effect of donor lymphocyte transfusions on leukemic relapse was subsequently evaluated in multicenter studies in Europe [10] and the USA [11].

## Graft-versus-Leukemia Activity of Donor Lymphocyte Transfusions

Donor lymphocyte transfusions have been used for the treatment of a great variety of recurrent hematological malignancies after allogeneic bone marrow transplantation. These included chronic myelogenous leukemia (CML), acute myeloid leukemia (AML), acute lymphoid leukemia (ALL), myelodysplastic syndromes (MDS), multiple myeloma (MMY), Hodgkin's disease (HD), Non-Hodgkin lymphoma (NHL), polycythemia vera and other diseases. The largest experience and the best results have been obtained in CML [10, 11], an intermediate response rate was seen in AML and MDS [10] and a low response rate in ALL [10]. Complete remissions (CR) were

**Table 1.** Overall remission rate after therapy with donor lymphocyte transfusion for relapsed hematologic malignancies after allogeneic bmt

| Diagnosis | number of patients | | |
| --- | --- | --- | --- |
| | studied | evaluable* | complete remission (%) |
| CML | | | |
| molecular relapse | 57 | 50 | 40 (80%) |
| hematological relapse | 124 | 114 | 88 (77%) |
| transformed relapse | 42 | 36 | 13 (36%) |
| PV/MPS | 2 | 1 | 1 |
| AML | 97 | 59 | 15 (25%) |
| ALL | 55 | 18 | 2 (11%) |
| MM | 24 | 17 | 5 (29%) |

*Patiens surviving more than 30 days after DLT were considered eligible. Patients with chemotherapy including 14 patients with recurrent CML were excluded because of unknown relapse state. 7 patients with other diagnosis were excluded (2 NHL, 1 juvenile CML and 3 unknown)

also observed in patients with recurrent MMY, but the number of patients treated is still limited (Table 1; Figure 1).

## Chronic myelogenous leukemia

In CML response rates were highest in patients with relapse in chronic phase or cytogenetic rsp. molecular evidence of relapse, intermediate in advanced phase and

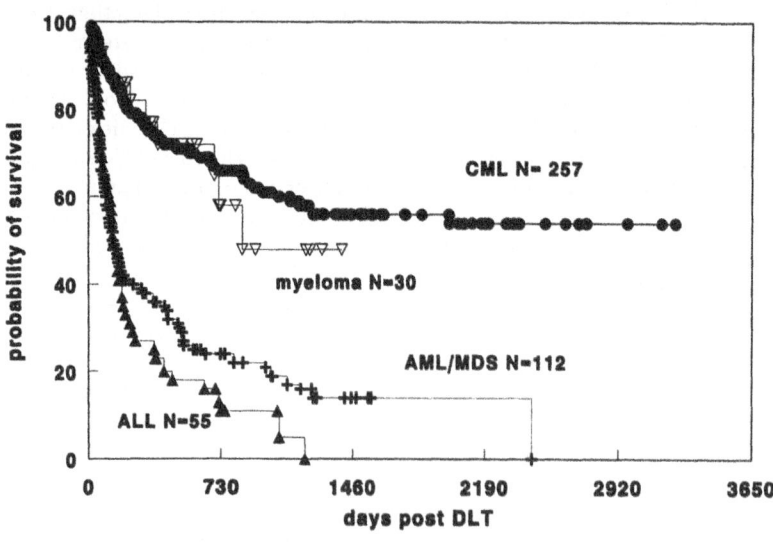

**Fig. 1.** DLT for Leukemia and Myeloma-Survival – EBMT 2/99

blast crisis. In chronic phase rsp. cytogenetic relapse remissions were durable in most patients, they were brief in patients with advanced phase relapses. Factors influencing the response to donor lymphocyte transfusions besides form of relapse were stage of the disease at time of transplantation, i.e. chronic phase, accelerated phase or blast phase, the time to relapse after transplantation, and a history of chronic GVHD. Patients who had previously experienced chronic GVHD were less likely to respond to donor lymphocyte transfusions. Interestingly donor lymphocytes failed to induce remissions in four patients with syngeneic twin donors. The graft-versus-leukemia effect correlated significantly with the severity of GVHD after DLT. This result together with the finding of the elimination of host T-cells [12; 13] which are usually not part of the leukemic clone in CML indicates a graft-versus-host reaction including leukemic cells. However it is remarkable that in 50% of the patients without any sign of GVHD CML did respond to the treatment with DLT. This indicates a high sensitivity of leukemic cells to the GVH-reaction or even a GVL effect separable from GVHD. The time until a complete cytogenetic and/or molecular remission is achieved ranges from a few weeks [14] to many months. The median time is between 4 and 6 months, and some responses occur after more than a year [15].

Major complications of the treatment of CML relapse with donor lymphocyte transfusions were GVHD and myelosuppression. GVHD occurred in about 60% of patients, 40% of patients required immunosuppressive treatment. These rates are not different from those seen after transplantation and during postgrafting immunosuppression. Most patients respond to immunosuppression and the treatment can be discontinued. Risk factors for GVHD include T-cell depletion of the prior transplant. GVHD may be prevented by the depletion of CD-8 positive cells from DLT [16] or the application in a dose escalating schedule starting with very small doses and escalating the doses only, if GVHD does not develop prior to the disease response [13]. Myelosuppression is less frequent, it occurs in between 10% and 20% of patients. It is more frequent in patients with hematological relapse than in patients with cytogenetic

relapse. Presumably it is the consequence of an insufficient number of donor stem cells present in the patient. Transfusion of donor marrow without further conditioning has been sufficient to reconstitute hemtatopoiesis in these patients.

## Results in Acute Leukemia

The results of donor lymphocyte transfusions may be summarized in two major groups, acute myeloid leukemia including myelodysplastic syndromes and acute lymphoid leukemia. There has been a significantly better response rate and survival of patients with AML/MDS as compared to ALL. However the results of donor lymphocyte transfusions can only be interpreted with caution. Many patients did not survive more than 30 days, others were treated additionally with chemotherapy. Recurrent AML did respond to lymphocyte transfusion without chemotherapy or after chemotherapy had failed, and remissions were of prolonged duration in several cases, but response rate was better if CR was induced by prior chemotherapy or if chemotherapy and lymphocyte transfusion were given at one time (Table 2). In 40 evaluable patients the FAB subtype was given, in 29 patients cytogenetic analyses were available. However there was no clear correlation to the response. The duration of remission was not different whether or not remissions were induced by chemotherapy. Obviously the graft-versus-leukemia effect of donor lym-

**Table 2, 3.** Response rate of patients with Acute Leukemia to donor lymphocyte transfusion for relapse after allogeneic BMT. Influence of chemotherapy induced CR on longterm disease free survival. Induction of long lasting remission is possible in AML even without CR achieved by prior chemotherapy.

| Chemotherapy | Response to DLT (%) | Remission Duration (days) |
|---|---|---|
| No | 9/37 (24%) | 112+, 155+, 244, 301, 436, 598+, 969, 1014, 2374 |
| Yes - CR | 14/15 (93%) | 59, 96+, 159+, 237, 312, 324, 372+, 438+, 527+, 1245, 1417+, 1453+, 1547+, 1563+ |
| Yes - no CR | 6/22 (27%) | 30, 346, 621+, 800, 977, 1263+ |

**Table 3**

| Chemo- therapy | Response to DLT (%) | Remission Duration (days) |
|---|---|---|
| No | 1/6 (17%) | 417 |
| Yes - CR | 15/29 (75%) | 21, 32, 47, 59+, 71, 122+, 158+, 164, 185+, 200, 255, 701+, 721, 1053, 1197 |
| Yes - no CR | 1/12 (8%) | 371 |

phocyte transfusions influences the duration of remission independently from the induction chemotherapy. In 15 patients with relapsed ALL cytogenetic analyses were available, 6 patients had Philadelphia-chromosome positive ALL. Only two patients responded to DLI without successful prior chemotherapy (Table 3). In contrast to chronic phase CML acute leukemia and acute phase CML may be rapidly progressive, not allowing the time for a graft-versus-leukemia effect to build up. So chemotherapy may be required to control leukemic proliferation before DLT can be initiated. The rapidly growing tumor mass of undifferentiated blasts may escape alloimmunity. However the difference between ALL and AML/MDS may give a hint for the understanding graft-versus-leukemia reactions in acute leukemia. We hypothesized that myeloid forms of leukemia may be more sensitive to immune mechanisms than lymphoid forms, because leukemic cells may differentiate towards dendritic cells which are physiologically derived from myeloid precursors. We and others have demonstrated dendritic cells of leukemic origin in patients with CML [17, 18].

## Immune escape of leukemia by deficient antigen presentation

Several mechanisms have been discussed, by which leukemic blasts might escape from immunosurveillance or adoptive immunotherapy. They include down-regulated expression of HLA-antigens and insufficient processing of the relevant peptides, diminished expression of adhesion molecules and of costimulatory molecules like B7.1 and B7.2 [19], resulting in an inadequate presentation of tumor antigens to T-cells [20]. Inadequate cytokine responses with diminished produc-

tion of proinflammatory cytokines as TNF-$\alpha$ and IFN-$\gamma$ or elevated production of inhibitory cytokines as IL-10 and TGF-$\beta$ have also been reported. Induction of apoptosis of leukemic cells may fail because of insufficient expression of FAS or inadequate transduction of the signal. Expression of FAS-ligand by the leukemic cell may inhibit the donor lymphocyte from killing.

## The role of GM-CSF

Hematopoietic growth factors have been commonly used for the treatment of neutropenia induced by chemotherapy. Their role in the treatment of hematological malignancies has been controversial. Stimulation of leukemic cells into proliferation may render them more sensitive to antiproliferative chemotherapy. This goal may be achieved in some patients with low proliferative leukemia (Hiddemann, W. et al. personal communication). The hope for the induction of terminal differentiation of blasts has not been fulfilled yet. Neither has the concern been justified by clinical studies that mobilization of leukemic cells by hematopoietic growth factors deteriorates the course of the leukemia. G-CSF has been used with success for the treatment of relapse after allogeneic transplantation [20]. Durable remissions were induced in three of seven patients with leukemic relapse, but follow up reports have been less enthusiastic [22]. GM-CSF has not been studied systematically for the treatment of relapse after allogeneic transplantation, but experience in single patients has not been promising (Kolb et al. personal communication). GM-CSF not only stimulates proliferation and differentiation of myelopoiesis, but it has also has strong immunomodulatory properties. Large numbers of dendritic cells can be produced from stem cells in human blood and bone marrow, if CD34-positive cells are stimulated with GM-CSF, IL4 and one ore more other cytokines (TNF$\alpha$, FLT-3 ligand) [23]. Recently, GM-CSF has been used in culture assays showing that dendritic cells can be developed from leukemic cells as well in CML [24] as in AML [25], thereby upregulating the expression of costimulatory molecules and regaining their stimulatory capacity on T-cells.

Based on these data there are two ways to improve antigen presentation of leukemic blasts by the treatment with GM-CSF. Firstly leukemic blasts may be differentiated into DC-like cells expressing all relevant antigens in vivo (Figure 2), and secondly, donor dendritic cells may be derived from stem cells transfused together with the T-cells. Healthy dendritic cells of the donor are able to pick up the antigen in question from the patient's deficient leukemic DC's and present it to donor T-cells [26].

## Results of the treatment of recurrent acute leukemia after allogeneic BMT with donor cells and GM-CSF

Ten patients with relapsed AML, three patients with CML in transformed phase and five patients with recurrent ALL have been treated with donor cells and GM-CSF. Donor cells consisted of leukocyte concentrates enriched for stem cells. Donors were treated with G-CSF for 4–6 days prior to collection.

AML patients were treated with non-myeloablative chemotherapy (mostly low dose cytosine-arabinoside) for at least 2 cycles to control leukemic proliferation. In case of progressive disease, idarubicine or AMSA were added to the treatment. Similarly patients with CML in transformed phase were treated with low dose cytosine-arabinoside

and interferon-α. In ALL patients leukemia could not be controlled by mild chemotherapy but patients required intensive chemotherapy. They were treated with high dose cisplatinum, VP-16 and ifosfamide.

Eight out of 10 patients with relapsed AML responded to the treatment with complete remissions, in two patients remission could not be induced. Remissions were prolonged in 4 patients without maintenance treatment, they were short in two patients requiring immunosuppressive treatment because of GVHD. Two patients died in remission with pulmonary failure due to veno-occlusive disease. Two patients are still in complete remission more than 2 years after treatment, one of these had a relapse in form of a leukemic infiltrate in her ovary which could be treated successfully by radiation and another course of low dose cytosine-arabinoside, donor cells and GM-CSF. In ALL complete remissions were induced in 3 out of 4 patients, in CML in one out of 4 patients.

## Complications

The major complication following treatment with donor cells and GM-CSF was GVHD of grade >I. It occurred in patients given more intensive chemotherapy prior to donor cells and in patients given higher doses of GM-CSF. In particular attaints treated with a larger dose of GM-CSF showed pulmonary

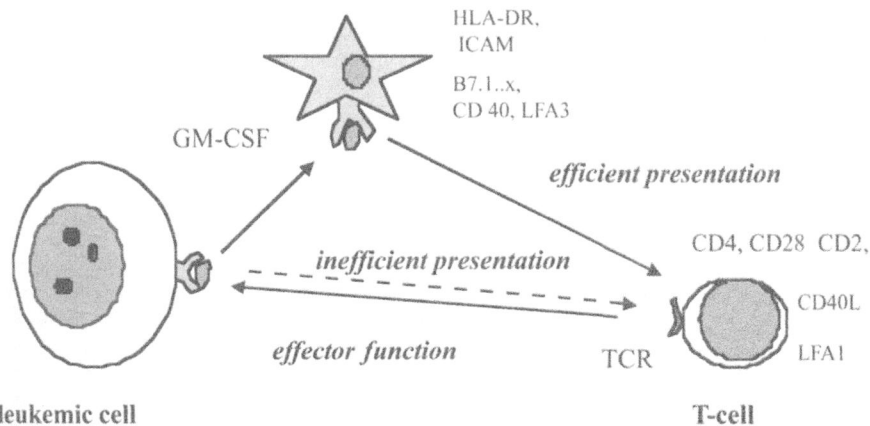

**Fig. 2.** AML Cells May Develop to Antigen Presenting Cells

669

complications. Reduction of the dose of GM-CSF to between 60 and 100 μg/m² was successful in the prevention of pulmonary complications in subsequent patients.

## Discussion and Outlook

Leukemic relapse after allogeneic bone marrow transplantation remains the most frequent cause of treatment failure and often has a poor prognosis. Donor lymphocyte transfusion (DLT) has shown to be a powerful tool for remission induction in chimeric patients, particularly in cytogenetic or hematological relapse of CML. However, results in acute leukemia are still unsatisfying, requiring new approaches in order to improve remission rate and disease free survival. Defects in antigen presentation resulting in insufficient stimulation of transfused donor T-lymphocytes are thought to be an important mechanism of immune escape of leukemic blasts. Experimental data from FACS analysis and culture assays suggest, that it might be possible to improve the ability of leukemic cells to effectively stimulate T-cell response and to upregulate co-stimulatory molecule expression by using GM-CSF. Furthermore it has been shown that AML blasts can be differentiated into dendritic cells in vitro. On the other hand, it has been shown, that normal stem cells from peripheral blood of healthy individuals can be differentiated into dendritic cells in presence of GM-CSF and IL4. Dendritic cells of donor origin may present leukemic antigens to donor T-cells, if T-cell stimulation by the leukemic cells themselves is not effective.

Based on this results a treatment protocol for relapsed acute leukemia and relapse of CML in accelerated phase was initiated including chemotherapy to control leukemic proliferation, transfusion of G-CSF stimulated peripheral blood stem cells from the original bone marrow donor and GM-CSF given by daily intravenous infusion. Patients with AML and acute phase CML received low dose AraC alone or in combination with idarubicine or AMSA if disease progression could not be controlled by AraC alone. Patients with relapsed ALL required high dose chemotherapy, and the regimen administered was the combination of cisplatinum, VP-16 and ifosfamide or chosen according to the patient's individual history.

Rapidly progressive myeloid leukemia and ALL required more intensive chemotherapy to control leukemic proliferation in order to give the graft-versus-leukemia effect time to develop. Intensive chemotherapy carries an increased risk of severe GvHD. Abrogation of tolerance in these patients might be due to release of pro-inflammatory cytokines by the effect of high dose chemotherapy or the elimination of potential suppressor cells that maintain tolerance. In several patients immunosuppressive treatment was required to control GvHD thereby counteracting the graft-versus-leukemia effect.

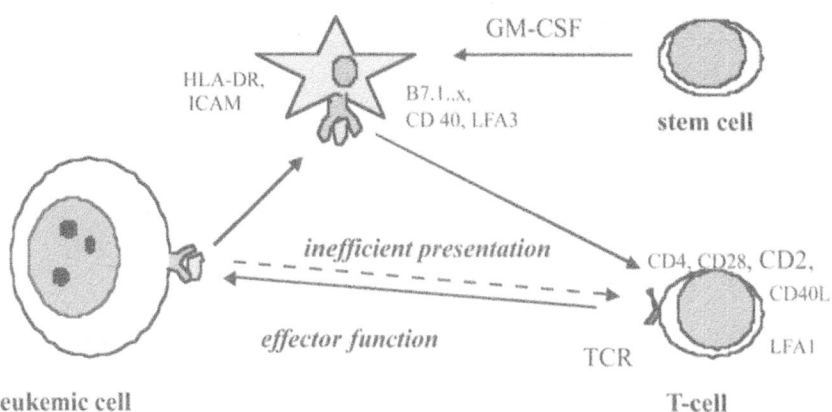

**Fig. 3.** PBSC Contain T-Cells and Develop Antigen Presenting Cells

Effective immunotherapy should be able to kill leukemic cells without causing severe GVHD. Improving the graft-versus-leukemia effect has been possible by improving antigen presentation with the use of GM-CSF or substituting antigen-presenting cells from the donor. Dendritic cells are the most potent antigen presenting cells, they are derived from stem cells stimulated with GM-CSF with and without IL-4, SC, Flt3-ligand and TNF-α. Improvement of antigen-presentation by treatment with GM-CSF and transfusion of stem cells has been chosen by us in this study. Another way may be the stimulation of T-cells by the treatment with IL-2 [23]. The reactivity of T-cells may be improved by supplying IL-2 as the most important growth factor. Unfortunately improving antigen presentation and proliferation of T-cells may increase the risk of GVHD. Prevention of GVHD has been attempted by depleting CD8-positive T-cells from the leukocyte concentrate [16; 24], but the reports have included only patients with CML in chronic phase or multiple myeloma. There have been no reports on acute phase leukemia. Similarly the treatment with escalating doses may be limited to patients with CML in cytogenetic or hematological relapse [13]. A more promising approach is the treatment of established GVHD inducing suicide of the T-cells. This technology is still in an developmental stage, a few patients have been treated with T-cells transduced with the thymidine kinase gene of herpes simplex virus that allows suicide of transduced cells by ganciclovir [25]. Animal experiments are needed to improve suicide technology [26,27]. However this technology provides safety against the deleterious effects of GVH. The graft-versus-leukemia effect may also be inhibited, if it does not occur earlier than GVHD. Only vaccination of donor cells to antigens on leukemic cells may improve treatment of acute phase leukemia. There is a number of leukemia specific antigens resulting from products of chromosomal rearrangements such as the bcr/abl fusion protein and its peptides [29]. Strong cytotoxic T-cell responses could elicited in vitro by co-culturing dendritic cells with the patients T-cells [30]. Recent reports describe CTL generated against peptide -loaded dendritic cells to recognize CML cells [31]. According to this report CML-reactive CTL were found in 5 of 21 CML-patients studied. Other candidates of leukemia-specific antigens are peptides coded by the Wilms tumor gene 1(WT1) which are overexpressed on acute myeloid leukemia cells [32]. These peptides may generate potent CTL when loaded to dendritic cells [33]. More universal tumor antigens may be derived from telomerase subunits [34]. These peptides may be valuable for adoptive immunotherapy, but the question remains why they fail to induce a potent graft-versus-leukemia naturally. In our analysis strong graft-versus-leukemia reactions were limited to allogeneic donor recipient combinations. Therefore histocompatibility antigens may play a major role in the GVL effect. A mismatch for HLA-C between donor and host decreases the relapse risk [34], whereas other HLA class I differences have no impact on the relapse rate. In HLA-identical donor-recipient combinations minor histocompatibility antigens (mHA) are responsible for alloimmune reactions. Some of the mHA derived peptides are preferentially located on hematopoietic cells which gives a chance to eliminate leukemia together with the host's hematopoietic system [36]. The generation of cytotoxic T-cells sufficient in number and function appears feasible [37]. It can be anticipated that adoptive immunotherapy will be successful also for acute phase leukemia within the next years.

# References

1. Mathé G, Amiel JL, Schwarzenberg L, Cattan A, Schneider M: Adoptive immunotherapy of acute leukemia: Experimental and clinical results. Cancer Res. 25:1525, 1965
2. Weiden PL, Sullivan KM, Flournoy N, Storb R, Thomas ED, The Seattle Marrow Transplant Team: Antileukemic effect of chronic graft-versus-host disease. Contribution to improved survival after allogeneic marrow transplantation. N Engl J Med 304:1529, 1981
3. Apperley JF, Mauro FR, Goldman JM, et al.: Bone marrow transplantation for chronic myeloid leukemia in first chronic phase: importance of a graft-versus-leukemia effect. Br J Haematol 69:239, 1988
4. Horowitz MM, Gale RP, Sondel PM, Goldman JM, Kersey J, Kolb HJ, Rimm AA, Ringden O, Rozman C, Speck B, et al: Graft-versus-leukemia reactions after bone marrow transplantation. Blood 75:555, 1990
5. Sullivan KM, Storb R, Buckner CD, Fefer A, Fisher L, Weiden PL, Witherspoon RP, Appelbaum FR,

Babaji M, Hansen J, Martin P, Sanders JE, Singer J, Thomas ED: Graft-versus-host disease as adoptive immunotherapy in patients with advanced hematologic neoplasms. N Engl J Med 320:828, 1989

6. Kolb HJ, Günther W, Schumm M, Holler E, Wilmanns W, Thierfelder S: Adoptive immunotherapy in canine chimeras. Transplantation 63:1, 1997

7. Johnson BD, Drobyski WR, Truitt RL: Delayed infusion of normal donor cells after MHC-matched bone marrow transplantation provides an antileukemia reaction without graft-versus-host disease. Bone Marrow Transplant 11:329, 1993

8. Kolb HJ, Mittermueller J, Clemm C, Ledderose G, Brehm G, Heim M, Wilmanns W: Donor leukocyte transfusions for treatment of recurrent chronic myelogenous leukemia in marrow transplant patients. Blood 76:2462, 1990

9. Slavin S, Ackerstein A, Weiss L, Nagler A, Or R, Naparstek E: Immunotherapy of minimal residual disease by immunocompetent lymphocytes and their activation by cytokines. Cancer Invest. 10:221, 1992

10. Kolb HJ, Schattenberg A, Goldman JM, Hertenstein B, Jacobsen N, Arcese W, Ljungman P, Ferrant A, Verdonck L, Niederwieser D, van Rhee F, Mittermüller J, De Witte T, Holler E, Ansari H: Graft-versus-leukemia effect of donor lymphocyte transfusions in marrow grafted patients. Blood 86:2041, 1995

11. Collins RH, Shpilberg O, Drobyski WR, Porter DL, Giralt S, Champlin R, Goodman SA, Wolff SN, Hu W, Verfaillie C, List A, Dalton W, Ognoskie N, Chetrit A, Antin JH, Nemunaitis J: Donor leukocyte infusions in 140 patients with relapsed malignancy after allogeneic bone marrow transplantation. J Clin Oncol 15:433, 1997

12. Mackinnon S, Papadopoulos EB, Carabasi MH, Reich L, Collins NH, O'Reilly RJ: Adoptive immunotherapy using donor leukocytes following bone marrow transplantation for chronic myeloid leukemia: is T cell dose important in determining biological response? Bone Marrow Transplant 15:591, 1995

13. Mackinnon S, Papadopoulos EB, Carabasi MH, Reich L, Collins NH, Boulad F, Castro-Malaspina H, Childs BH, Gillio AP, Kernan NA, Small TM, Young JW, OReilly RJ: Adoptive immunotherapy evaluating escalating doses of donor leukocytes for relapse of chronic myeloid leukemia after bone marrow transplantation: separation of graft-versus-leukemia responses from graft-versus-host disease. Blood 86:1261, 1995

14. Baumrann H, Nagel S, Binder T, Neubauer A, Siegert W, Huhn D: Kinetics of the graft-versus-leukemia response after donor leukocyte infusions for relapsed chronic myeloid leukemia after allogeneic bone marrow transplantation. Blood 92:3582, 1998

15. van Rhee F, Goldman JM: Donor lymphocyte therapy in bone marrow transplantation., in Morstyn G, Sheridan W (eds): Cell Therapy - Stem Cell Transplantation, Gene Therapy, and Cellular Immunotherapy., Cambridge, Cambridge University Press, 1996, p 550

16. Giralt S, Hester J, Huh Y, Hirsch-Ginsberg C, Rondon G, Seong D, Lee M, Gajewski J, Van Besien K,

Khouri I, Mehra R, Przepiorka D, Körbling M, Talpaz M, Kantarjian H, Fischer H, Deisseroth A, Champlin R: CD8-depleted donor lymphocyte infusion as treatment for relapsed chronic myelogenous leukemia after allogeneic bone marrow transplantation. Blood 86:4337, 1995

17. Eibl B, Ebner S, Duba Ch, Böck G, Romani N, Gächter A, Nachbaur D, Schuler G, Niederwieser D: Philadelphia-chromosome positive dendritic cells (DC) of chronic myelocytic leukemia (CML) patients induce primary cytotxoc T-cell responses to CML cells. Bone Marrow Transplant 19:S33, 1997 (abstr.)

18. Smit WM, Rijnbeck M, van Bergen CAM, de Paus RA, Willemze R, Falkenburg JHF: Dendritic cells generated from FACS sorted chronic myeloid leukemia (CML) precursor cells express BCR/ABL, and are potent stimulators for allogeneic T cells. Br J Haematol 93:313, 1996 (abstr.)

19. Hirano, N, Takahashi T, et al: Expression of costimulatory molecules in human leukemias: Leukemia 10: 1168, 1996

20. Guinan, E.C., Gribben, J.,G., et al.: Pivotal role of the B27:CD28 pathway in transplantation tolerance and tumor immunity. Blood 84 : 3261, 1994

21. Giralt S, Escudier S, Kantarijan H, et al.: Preliminary results of treatment with filgrastim for relapse of leukemia and myelodysplasia after allogeneic bone marrow transplantation. N.Engl.J. Med. 329:757, 1993

22. Giralt SA, Champlin RE: Leukemia relapse after allogeneic bone marrow transplantation: A review. Blood 84:3603, 1994

23. Romani, N, Gruner, S, Brang D, et al. : Proliferating dendritic cell progenitors in human blood. J Exp Med 180: 83, 1994

24. Smit, W, Rijnbeek, M, van Bergen, C A, et al.: Generation of dendritic cells expressing bcr/abl from CD34+ chronic myeloid leukemia precursor cells. Hum Immunol 53(2), 216, 1997

25. Choudhury BA, Liang J, Thomas EK, Flores-Romo L, Xie QS, Agusala K, Sutaria S, Sinha I, Champlin RE, Claxton D: Dendritic cells derived in vitro from acute myelogenous leukemia cells stimulate autologous anti-leukemic T-cell responses. Blood 93:780, 1999

26. Huang AYC, Golumbek P, Ahmadzadeh M, Jaffee E, Pardoll D, Levitsky H: Role of bone marrow-derived cells presenting MHC class I- restricted tumor antigens. Science 264:961, 1994

27. Slavin S, Naparstek E, Nagler A, Ackerstein A, Samuel S, Kapelushnik J, Brautbar C, Or R: Allogeneic cell therapy with donor peripheral blood cells and recombinant human interleukin-2 to treat leukemia relapse after allogeneic bone marrow transplantation. Blood 87:2195, 1996

28. Alyea EP, Soiffer RJ, Canning C, et al.: Toxicity and efficacy of defined doses of CD4+ donor lymphocytes for treatment of relapse after allogeneic bone marrow transplantation.. Blood 91:3671, 1998 (abstr.)

29. Bonini C, Ferrari G, Verzelletti S, Servida P, Zappone E, Ruggieri L, Ponzoni M, Rossini S, Mavilio F, Traversari C, Bordignon C: HSV-TK gene transfer into donor lymphocytes for control of allogeneic graft-versus-leukemia. Science 276:1719, 1997

30. Georges GE, Storb R, Brunvand MW, Kiem HP, Moore PF, Malik P, Ennist D, Nash RA: Canine T cells transduced with herpes simplex virus thymidine kinase gene: a model to study effects on engraftment and control of graft-versus-host disease. Transplantation 66:540, 1998

31. Georges GE, Nash RA, Storb R: Canine CTL transduced with HS-thymidine kinase gene maintain cytotoxic activity and are eliminated by ganciclovir: A model to enhance engraftment, control GVHD and decrease preparative regimen intensity in allogeneic blood stem cells transplantation. Blood 88:245a, 1996 (abstr.)

32. Weissinger EM, Franz M, Grammer C, Braakmann E, Bonini C, Kolb HJ: Transduction of primary T cells of the dog using retroviral vectors expressing marker and suicide genes. Onkologie 20:653, 1997 (abstr.)

33. Bocchia M, Korontsvit T, Xu Q, Mackinnon S, Yang SY, Sette A, Scheinberg DA: Specific human cellular immunity to bcr-abl oncogene-derived peptides. Blood 87:3587, 1996

34. Choudhury A, Gajewski JL, Liang J, Popat U, Claxton DF, Kliche KO, Andreeff M, Champlin RE: Use of leukemic dendritic cells for the generation of antileukemic cellular cytotoxicity against Philadelphiachromosome positive chronic myelogenous leukemia . Blood 89:1133, 1997

35. Yotnda P, Firat H, Garcia-Pons F, Garcia Z, Gourru G, Vernant JP, Lemonnier FA, Leblond V, Langlade-Demoyen P: Cytotoxic T cell response against the chimeric p210 BCR-ABL protein in patients with chronic myelogenous leukemia. J.Clin.Invest. 101:2290, 1998

36. Inoue K, Ogawa H, Sonoda Y, Kimura T, Sakabe H, Oka Y, Miyake S, Tamaki H, Oji Y, Yamagami T, Tatekawa T, Soma T, Kishimoto T, Sugiyama H: Aberrant overexpression of the Wilms tumor gene (WT1) in human leukemia. Blood 89:1405, 1997

37. Yasukawa M, Ohminami H, Hasegawa A, Arai J, Yakushijn Y, Fujita S: HLA class I-restricted lysis of leukemia cells by a CD8+ cytotoxic T-lymphocyte cone directed against WT1 peptide. Blood 92:#2541, 1998 (abstr.)

38. Vonderheide RH, Hahn WC, Schultze J, Nadler LM: Search for universal tumor antigens: potential of the catalytic telomerase subunit. Blood 92:1998 (abstr.)

39. Sasazuki T, Juji T, Morishima Y, Kinukawa N, Kashiwabara H, Inoko H, Yoshida T, Kimura A, Akaza T, Kamikawaji N, Kodera Y, Takaku F: Effect of matching of class I HLA alleles on clinical outcome after transplantation of hematopoietic stem cells from an unrelated donor. N.Eng.J.Med. 339:1177, 1998 (abstr.)

40. Goulmy E: Human minor histocompatibility antigens: New concepts for marrow transplantation and adoptive immunotherapy. Immunol.Rev. 157:125, 1997

41. Mutis T, Verdijk R, Schrama E, Esendam B, Brand A, Goulmy E: Feasability of immunotherapy of relapsed leukemia with ex vivogenerated cytotoxic T lymphocytes specific for hematopoietic system-restricted minor histocompatibility antigens. Blood 93:2336, 1999

# Shifting Towards Better Immunotherapy Rather Than More Intensive Chemoradiotherapy Using a Non-Myeloablative Approach in Patients with Leukemia

S. Slavin, A. Nagler, S. Panigrahi, G. Varadi, A. Ackerstein, S. Samuel and R. Or

## Introduction

Allogeneic cell therapy, or donor lymphocyte infusion (DLI), following allogeneic bone marrow or blood stem cell transplantation (BMT) introduced at Hadassah in Jerusalem in early 1987 was already shown to be effective for treatment and prevention of relapse following maximally tolerated doses of chemoradiotherapy (1-3). Starting more than 5 years ago, these observations led to developing the concept of non-myeloablative stem cell transplantation (NST) as a new modality for the treatment of hematologic malignancies and more recently, metastatic solid tumors based on the use of alloreactive donor lymphocytes, rather than more aggressive chemoradiotherapy, for elimination of tumor cells resistant to conventional anti-cancer modalities (4-8). Optimal use of NST depends on induction of transplantation tolerance to donor alloantigens, which can be accomplished by a 'window of immunosuppression', using well tolerated immunosuppresive rather than myeloablative conditioning, followed by donor stem cell infusion (step 1). The concept of using NST for induction of host vs graft transplantation tolerance through the induction of a transient stage of mixed chimerism was developed in the 70s, first in rodents conditioned with non-myeloablative total lymphoid irradiation (TLI) (9-11). Following induction of host vs graft tolerance by donor stem cells, donor T-cells present in the graft can induce effective graft versus leukaemia, graft versus lymphoma, graft versus myeloma, graft versus genetically abnormal stem cells or graft versus autoimmunity

effects (step 2), which can eliminate residual stem cells of host origin (1-3). Graft vs tumor effects could be further amplified with DLI given on an outpatient basis, preferably as graded increments for safer control of graft vs host disease (GVHD), while eliminating residual hematopoietic cells of host origin (step 3) by in vivo and/or in vitro activation of donor cells with rIL-2 (3). By using NST in steps 1-3, engraftment appears consistent with eventual replacement of host with donor hematopoietic cells. Several versions of NST regimen are currently being examined in patients with hematologic malignancies and metastatic solid tumors (11-14). The following report summarises the results of NST at Hadassah in Jerusalem.

## Results of the first cohort of NST recipients

NST protocols based on the use of fludarabine with either busulfan, cytoxan or single low dose total body irradiation (TBI) were used for accomplishing stable engraftment of donor blood stem cells mobilised with G-CSF (Neupogen) 5µg/kg twice daily for 5 days collected on days 4 and 5. Step 1 consisted of immunosuppression induced with fludarabine 30mg/m²/day x6; ATG 5-10mg/kg x4 (Fresenius, AG) and mild tumor cytoreduction with busulfan 4mg/kgx2 or cytoxan 60mg/kg x2 or single dose TBI 200cGy, followed by infusion of mobilized blood stem cells from siblings (single locus mismatched allowed) or marrow cells from matched unrelated donors (MUD) to establish host vs graft chimerism and specific transplantation tole-

Department of Bone Marrow Transplantation and the Cancer Immunotherapy & Immunobiology Research Laboratory, Hadassah University Hospital, Jerusalem 91120, Israel.

rance (step 2). Low dose cyclosporine A (CSA) 3mg/kg for 30-100 days was used as the sole anti-GVHD prophylaxis. The busulfan based protocol was given to over 100 patients, hence our discussion will focus on the results obtained with busulfan based regimen, following analysis of the first 70 patients with hematologic malignancies with sufficiently long observation period. A total of 16 patients underwent NST with MUD, and 9 patients received an allograft following failure of autologous BMT. Patients age ranged 3-63 (median 38) including CML (n=19); AML (n=17); ALL (n=10); NHL (n=15); MDS & 2$^{nd}$ leukemia (n=6); Hodgkin's disease (n=2) and multiple myeloma (n=1). Patients received fully matched (n=66) or single locus mismatched (n=4) stem cells on day 0. Patients of all age groups very well tolerated the protocol. Day 100 mortality was 4%; 0% in patients with non-malignant diseases and 7% in patients with malignancy. Fast and durable engraftment was observed in all patients with a matched sibling. Similarly, patients with poor general condition or with pulmonary complications were treated with TBI based protocol, also resulting in consistent engraftment in all 10 patients. Patients with severe aplastic anemia or Fanconi's anemia were conditioned with cytoxan based regimen (patients with Fanconi's anemia received a cytoxan dose of 5mg/kg on 2 occasions). Persistent evidence of disease or recurrent disease in mixed chimeras was treated by discontinuation of CSA or by graded increments of DLI with 10 of 15 responders. After 3 years, with an observation period of 3-39 months (median 24 months) actuarial probability of survival was 68% and disease-free survival was 48%. Corresponding numbers for MUD at 12 months were 75% and 70%, and at 18 months was 48%, respectively. However, GVHD remained the single major problem with half of the 10 that developed advanced GVHD developing grade IV disease while on CSA, while the other half developing severe GVHD after discontinuation of CSA or shortly after administration of DLI. Based on our preliminary data, clinical application of NST appears most promising, especially in patients in poor general condition or at high risk of procedure related toxicity and mortality, including elderly individuals. However,

larger cohorts of patients and longer observation periods will be required to confirm the overall advantage of NST compared with conventional BMT at an early and at later stages of the disease.

## Discussion and relevance of NST to the future of cellular therapies in medicine

Myeloablative chemoradiotherapy for conditioning of BMT recipients was considered mandatory until recently (16), the aim being to eliminate resistant tumor cells or other abnormal stem cells of host origin, in genetic diseases or other life-threatening non-malignant diseases.

The recent introduction of NST, especially those regimen focusing on the use of fludarabine based protocols instead of standard myeloablative chemoradiotherapy for conditioning of BMT recipients appears to be most effective for engraftment of MHC compatible stem cell allografts with reduced procedure-related toxicity and mortality (4-8,15). Based on our preliminary experience with an observation period of approximately 5 years, we anticipate lower incidence of late complications as well, but larger number of patients and longer observation period is required to fully assess the overall benefits of NST in comparison with standard BMT regimen.

Following induction of graft vs host transplantation tolerance additional GVL (1-3) and most likely GVT effects in experimental animals (17-19) and man (15,20,21) may be accomplished by alloreactive donor lymphocytes introduced with donor stem cells or later following BMT or NST with DLI. Based on our original observations, now confirmed by cumulative international experience, it appears that alloreactive donor lymphocytes can effectively eliminate malignant or otherwise abnormal host stem cells, regardless of resistance to chemoradiotherapy, hence, DLI may be applied for both treatment (1-3) as well as for prevention of relapse (22). We reasoned, therefore, that the standard myeloablative conditioning, associated with immediate and late procedure-related toxicity and mortality, could be replaced with well tolerated non-myeloablative conditioning, thus focusing on cell-mediated immunotherapy following induction of host vs graft tolerance inducible by the stem cell transplantation procedure. Consequently, induction of transplantation tolerance has been accomplished by a 'window of immunosuppression', using well tolerated immunosuppresive rather than myeloablative conditioning followed by donor stem cell infusion (steps 1). By using NST (steps 1–3), engraftment appears consistent with eventual replacement of all host with donor hematopoietic cells. Our new protocol design, based on our working hypothesis, provides an option for rational treatment of otherwise incurable malignant and non-malignant diseases for any patient in need with a matched sibling or matched unrelated donor, with no upper or lower age limit. NST minimises procedure-related toxicity and mortality and most likely late complications as well. The use of NST may therefore open new therapeutic horizons for a broad spectrum of clinical indications with potential indications for stem cell transplantation for malignant and non-malignant disorders, including immunoregulation of autoimmune diseases, as well as inducing transplantation tolerance to organ and tissue allografts. It is not yet clear which of the NST regimen is superior. Using chemotherapy alone offers many advantages, since patients may eventually receive he entire preparatory regimen on an outpatient basis. The use of low dose TBI (200cGy) was previously shown to be sufficient for induction of bilateral transplantation tolerance and durable engraftment in heavily immunosuppressed mice pre-treated with low dose TLI, suggesting that in well immunosuppressed recipients, even a single fraction of low dose TBI may be sufficient to tip the balance towards durable engraftment (23) with the mechanism of unresponsiveness being most likely a combination of central clonal deletion, with additional antigen dependent clonal anergy/deletion (24).

In the future, more sophisticated approaches are likely to be applied, using specifically immune donor lymphocytes rather than naïve donor peripheral blood lymphocytes to amplify the anti-cancer potential inducible by DLI while trying to minimise anti-host responses resulting in GVHD (Ji, Weiss & Slavin; submitted for publication). The use of alloreactive and tumor reactive lymphocytes may provide a platform for innovative immunotherapeutic procedures in an attempt to maximise desirable anti-cancer effects while minimising untoward anti-host responses (Slavin et al., submitted for publication). The use of NST may therefore open new horizons for a broader spectrum of clinical indications for stem cell transplantation for the treatment of malignant and non-malignant diseases as well as for organ transplantation.

*Acknowledgement.* We would like to thank the following for their ongoing support: Baxter International Corporation; Ryna & Melvin Cohen; The Szydlowsky Foundation; The Gabriella Rich Foundation; the Himmelfarb Foundation and The German-Israel Foundation. The work was done at The Danny Cunniff Leukemia Research Laboratory.

# References

1. Slavin S, Or R, Naparstek E, Ackerstein A, Weiss L. Cellular – mediated immunotherapy of leukemia in conjunction with autologous and allogeneic bone marrow transplantation in experimental animals and man. Blood 72: (suppl 1) 407a, 1988.
2. Slavin S, Naparstek E, Nagler A, Ackerstein A, Kapelushnik Y, Or R: Allogeneic cell therapy for relapsed leukemia following bone marrow transplantation with donor peripheral blood lymphocytes. Exp Hematol 1995; 23:1553-1562.
3. Slavin S, Naparstek E, Nagler A, Ackerstein A, Samuel S, Kapelushnik J, Brautbar C, Or R. Allogeneic cell therapy with donor peripheral blood cells and recombinant human interleukin-2 to treat leukemia relapse post allogeneic bone marrow transplantation. Blood 1996; 87:2195-2204.
4. Slavin S, Nagler A, Naparstek E, Ackerstein A, Kapelushnik Y, Varadi G, Kirschbaum M, Ben-Yosef R, Samuel S, Or R. Immunotherapy of leukemia in conjunction with non-myeloablative conditioning: engraftment of blood stem cells and eradication of host leukemia with non-myeloablative conditioning based on Fludarabine and anti-thymocyte globulin (ATG). Blood 1996;88(10) 614a.
5. Slavin S, Nagler A, Naparstek E, Kapelushnik J, Varadi G, Kirschbaum, Hussein A, Ackerstein A, Or R. Non-myeloablative conditioning in preparation for allogeneic stem cell transplantation: the future treatment of choice of hematologic malignancies and genetic diseases. Exp Hematol 1997; 25(8) 787.
6. Khouri I, Keating MJ, Przepiorka D, et al: Engraftment and induction of GVL with fludarabine-based non-ablative preparative regimen in patients with chronic lymphocytic leukemia. Blood 88(suppl l):301a, 1996.

7. Giralt S, Estey E, Albitar M, et al: Engraftment of allogeneic hematopoietic progenitor cells with purine analog-containing chemotherapy: Harnessing graft-vs-leukemia without myeloablative therapy. Blood 89:4531-4536, 1997.

8. Slavin S, Nagler A, Naparstek E, Kapelushnik Y, Aker M, Cividalli G, Varadi G, Kirschbaum M, Ackerstein A, Samuel S, Ben-Tal O, Eldor A, Or R. Nonmyeloablative stem cell transplantation and cell therapy as an alternative to conventional bone marrow transplantation with lethal cytoreduction for the treatment of malignant and non-malignant hematologic diseases. Blood 1998; 91(3): 756-763.

9. Slavin S, Strober S, Fuks Z, Kaplan HS. Long-term survival of skin allogafts in mice treated with fractionated total lymphoid irradiation. Science 1976;193:1252-1254.

10. Slavin S, Strober S, Fuks Z, Kaplan HS. Induction of specific tissue transplantation tolerance using fractionated total lymphoid irradiation in adult mice: Long-term survival of allogeneic bone marrow and skin grafts. J Exp Med 1977;146:34-48.

11. Slavin S. Total lymphoid irradiation (TLI). Immunol Today 1987;8:88-92.

12. Or R, Mehta J, Naparstek E, Okon E, Cividalli G, Slavin S. Successful T cell-depleted allogeneic bone marrow transplantation in a child with recurrent multiple extramedullary plasmacytomas. Bone Marrow Transplant 1992;10:381-382.

13. Lokhorst HM, Schattenberg A, Cornelissen JJ, et al: Donor leukocyte infusions are effective in relapsed multiple myeloma after allogeneic bone marrow transplantation. Blood 90:4206-4211, 1997.

14. Or R, Nagler A, Ackerstein A, Naparstek E, Samuel S, Drakos P, Kapelushnik Y, Amar A, Slavin S : Allogeneic cell-mediated cytokine-activated immunotherapy of non-Hodgkin lymphoma for eradication of minimal residual disease in conjunction with autologous bone marrow transplantation (ABMT). Blood 82: (suppl 1) 171a, 1993.

15. Successful Treatment of Metastatic Renal Cell Carcinoma With a Nonmyeloablative Allogeneic Peripheral-Blood Progenitor-Cell Transplant: Evidence for a Graft-Versus-Tumor Effect Childs, R. W., Clave, E., Tisdale, J., Plante, M., Hensel, N., Barrett, J. J Clin Oncol 1999 17: p. 2044-2044

16. Horowitz MM, Gale RP, Sondel PM, et al: Graft-vs-leukemia reactions after bone marrow transplantation. Blood 75:555-562, 1990.

17. Moscovitch M, Slavin S. Anti-tumor effects of allogeneic bone marrow transplantation in (NZB x NZW)F1 hybrids with spontaneous lymphosarcoma. J Immunol 1984;132:997-1000.

18. Morecki S, Moshel Y, Gelfend Y, Pugatsch T, Slavin S. Induction of graft vs tumor effect in a murine model of mammary adenocarcinoma. International Journal of Cancer 1997;71:59-63.

19. Morecki S, Yacovlev E, Diab A, Slavin S. Allogeneic cell therapy for a murine mammary carcinoma. Cancer Research. 1998;58:3891-5.

20. Eibl B, Schwaighofer H, Nachbaur D, Marth C, Gächter A, Knapp R, Böck G, Gassner C, Schiller L, Petersen F, Niederwieser D. Evidence for a graft-versus-tumor effect in a patient treated with marrow ablative chemotherapy and allogeneic bone marrow transplantation for breast cancer. Blood 1996, 88:1501-1508.

21. Ben-Yosef R, Or R, Nagler A, Slavin S. Graft vs tumor and graft vs leukemia in patient with concurrent breast cancer and acute myelocytic leukemia. The Lancet. 1996; 348:1242-1243.

22. Naparstek E, Or R, Nagler A, Cividalli G, Engelhard D, Aker M, Gimon Z, Manny N, Sacks T, Tochner Z, Weiss L, Samuel S, Brautbar C, Hale G, Waldmann H, Steinberg S M, Slavin S : T-cell-depleted allogeneic bone marrow transplantation for acute leukaemia using Campath-1 antibodies and post-transplant administration of donor's peripheral blood lymphocytes for prevention of relapse. Brit J Haematol 89: 506-515, 1995.

23. Slavin S, Fuks Z, Weiss L, Morecki S. Mechanisms of tolerance in chimeric mice prepared with total lymphoid irradiation (TLI). In: Gale RP, Fox CF, eds. Biology of Bone Marrow Transplantation. ICN- UCLA Symposia on Molecular and Cellular Biology. New York: Academic Press 1980;17:383-394.

24. Morecki S, Leshem B, Weigensberg M, Bar S, Slavin S. Functional clonal deletion versus active suppression in transplantation tolerance induced by total lymphoid irradiation (TLI). Transplantation 1985;40:201-210.

# Long-Term Results of Autologous Bone Marrow Transplantation as Late Intensification in AML

C. Annaloro, G. Lambertenghi Deliliers, E. Pozzoli, V.G. Bertolli, S. Saviano, A. Della Volpe and D. Soligo

## Summary

Thirty-four AML patients (17 male, 17 female; median age 44 years, range 20-57) underwent unpurged autologous bone marrow transplantation (BMT) as late intensification. The conditioning regimen included HD Ara-C, HD CTX and fractionated TBI at a dosage of 10 Gy. As of 31 October 1998, 11 patients had relapsed, 3 had died in CR and 20 were alive and in CCR. The median EFS had not been reached: the 10 y chance was 53.1%. In 19 patients previously treated with an idarubicin-based protocol, the median EFS had not been reached and the 10 y chance was 56.2%; all of the six relapses occurred within 18 months. In 15 patients referred for autologous BMT as late intensification of other protocols, the median EFS was 65 months, with a 10 y chance of 48.1%; two of the five relapses occurred more than two years after autologous BMT. Another 17 patients treated with the idarubicin-based protocol received HD Ara-C instead of autologous BMT as late intensification; ten of them relapsed (four more than two years and two more than five years after the end of late intensification); the median EFS was 60 months and the 10 y EFS chance was 41%. Autografting is generally regarded as an outdated late intensification therapeutic strategy in AML and it can be held that the rather high long-term EFS merely reflects the cure chance of conventional treatment. However, the patients included in the idarubicin protocol not only had a somewhat better EFS, but none of them experienced a late relapse; the patients not undergoing autologous BMT after the same protocol had a worse outcome. Autologous BMT still has a place among the post-CR options for late intensification.

## Introduction

Most of the current strategies in the post-CR treatment of AML favour the use of intensive short-term consolidation followed by early intensification (Heil et al. 1995, Zittoun et al. 1995, Keating et al. 1998, Mitus et al. 1995). Allogeneic bone marrow transplantation (BMT) as early intensification has proved to be superior to autologous BMT or chemotherapy in many experiences, including some controlled trials (Mitus et al. 1995, Zittoun et al. 1997, Zittoun et al. 1995), although autologous BMT seems to offer a limited advantage over chemotherapy in terms of event free survival (EFS) (Zittoun et al. 1995). Furthermore, use of autografting as early intensification makes »ex-vivo« purging advisable in order to minimize the burden of residual leukemic cells in bone marrow harvesting (Gorin 1992), which implies a significant delay in engraftment and an increased risk of transplant-related mortality (Bishop et al. 1997, Damon et al. 1996, Löwenberg 1996). These negative considerations raise the question as to whether early intensification is really the best location for autologous BMT in the treatment of AML.

This paper presents single-institution results on autologous BMT as late intensification for AML in first CR.

Centro Trapianti di Midollo, Università degli Studi and Ospedale Maggiore IRCCS, Milano Italy.

## Materials and Methods

Between 1978 and 1988, thirty-four AML patients (17 male, 17 female: median age 44 years, range 20-57) underwent autografting as late intensification during first CR. The previous treatments had been heterogeneous but all of them had been referred to our institution at the end of treatment programs including remission induction and standard dose consolidation/early intensification. Remission induction had been achieved after 1-2 cycles of an anthracycline/standard dose Ara-C combination; as post-remission treatment, at least four cycles were scheduled. Nineteen patients had received the same idarubicin-based protocol (Lambertenghi et al. 1993); the others had received different therapies. In all cases, the source of hematopoietic stem cells was unpurged bone marrow that had been harvested and cryopreserved after the end of the conventional therapeutic program. The median time interval between the achievement of CR and autologous BMT was 10 months (range 7-12). The conditioning regimen included Ara-C, 3 g/sqm/12 h on days -9/-8, CTX 60 mg/kg/die on days -6/-5 and TBI at a total dosage of 10 Gy fractionated in three equal doses on days -3 through -1.

Only the patients with a minimum follow-up of six months after autologous BMT were evaluated. Furthermore, the outcome of the 19 autografted patients previously treated with the idarubicin protocol was compared with that of another 17 patients who had been treated using the same protocol, had achieved CR exceeding 10 months and had received HD Ara-C instead of autologous BMT as late intensification.

Relapses, deaths during CR and drop-outs were considered events. Starting from the date of autologous BMT, event free survival (EFS) curves were calculated according to Kaplan & Meier and compared by means of the log-rank test.

## Results

The total number of infused mononucleate cells ranged from 0.86 to 13.7 x $10^8$/kg (median 1.56), and CFU-GM cells from 0.53 to 15.6$^5$/kg (median 5.76). All of the patients achieved peripheral neutrophil recovery, 13-84 days (median 28) after autologous BMT. Three patients failed to achieve platelet recovery, one of whom relapsed 6 months after autologous BMT, one died of reactivated

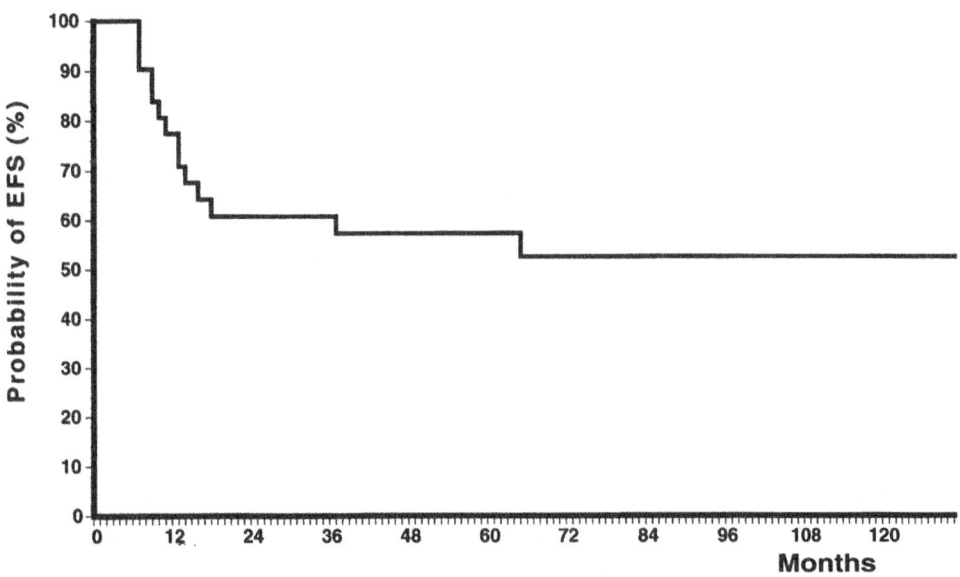

**Fig. 1.** EFS curve of 34 AML patients treated with autologous BMT as late intensification during first CR.

HBV infection and one developed secondary MDS. In the other patients, platelet recovery occurred after 22-418 days (median 65).

As of 31 October 1998, the median follow-up for the censored patients was 89 months, range 6-132; 11 patients had relapsed 6-68 months after autologous BMT, three had died during CR 6-12 months after autologous BMT, and 20 were alive and in CCR. The median EFS had not been reached, and the 10 y chance was 53.1% (Figure 1). Among the 19 patients treated with the above-mentioned idarubicin protocol, the median EFS had not been reached and the 10 y chance was 56.2%; all of the six relapses in this group occurred within 18 months. In the 15 patients referred for autologous BMT as late intensification of other protocols, the median EFS was 65 months, with a 10 y chance of 48.1%; two of the five relapses in this group occurred more than two years after autologous BMT (after 36 and 64 months, respectively) (Figure 2). Seventeen other patients treated with the idarubicin-based protocol achieved a CR lasting more than 10 months but had received HD Ara-C instead of autologous BMT as late intensification, most because of their refusal to undergo autografting. They were comparable with the patients undergoing autologous BMT in terms of clinical and hematological variables, but their median age was older although this difference was not statistically significant. Ten of them relapsed (four more than two years, and two more than five years after the end of late intensification); their median EFS was 60 months, with a 10 y chance of 41% (Figure 3).

## Discussion

This paper describes the results of autologous BMT as late intensification in AML patients during their first CR; this is generally regarded as an outdated therapeutic strategy because the observed long-term EFS may be due to the fact that the patients are already cured (Imrie et al. 1996). Nevertheless, experiences with autologous BMT as late intensification are still reported in the literature and the long-term EFS observed in uncontrolled studies compare favourably even with that found in allogeneic BMT patients (Martin et al. 1998, Miggiano et al. 1996); furthermore, our own EFS results can be described as encouraging. It can be argued that these favourable long-term EFS rates merely reflect the chance of cure following conventional tre-

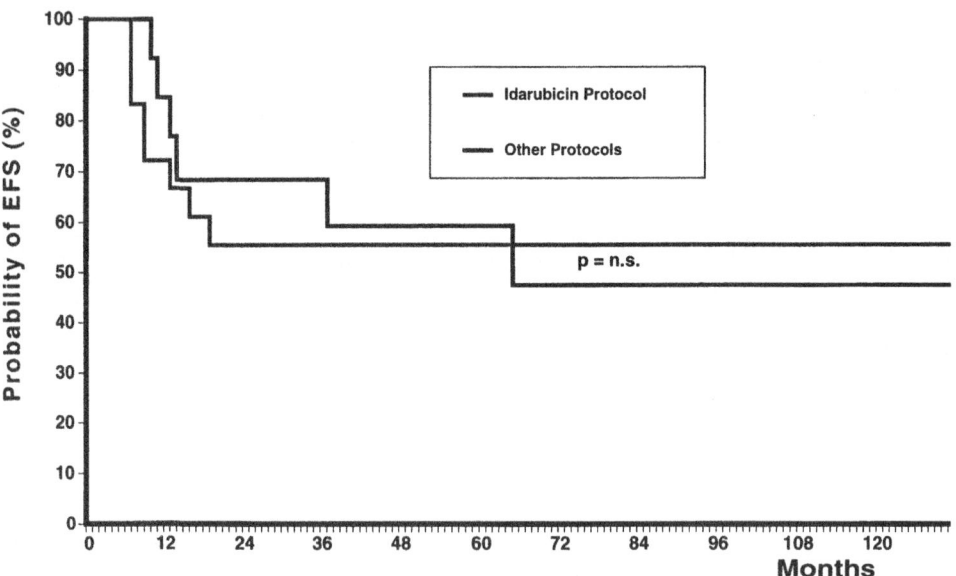

**Fig. 2.** EFS curves of 19 patients treated with idarubicin protocol compared with 15 patients treated with other protocols before ABMT.

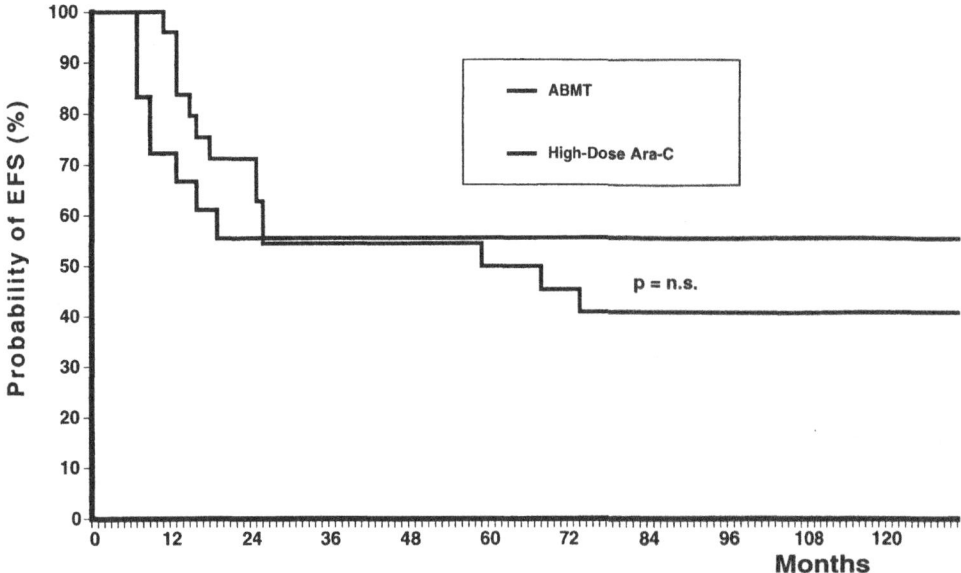

**Fig. 3.** EFS curves of 19 patients submitted to ABMT compared with 17 patients who underwent HD Ara-C as late intensification.

atment in patients achieving CR durations exceeding 6-12 months. However, unlike in patients receiving chemotherapy alone, most of the relapses in autografted patients occur within 18 months and these different behaviours seem to be attributable to therapy-related factors (Dann 1995).

In the present study, patients undergoing autologous BMT as late intensification of an idarubicin-based protocol were compared with other patients treated with the same protocol, but who received high-dose Ara-C as late intensification. The patients not undergoing autologous BMT had a worse outcome characterized by late relapses, although this difference was not statistically significant. These results are quite similar to those reported by Miggiano et al. (1996), and speak in favour of an advantage of autologous BMT over chemotherapy as late intensification.

The autografted patients were also subdivided according to the type of previous chemotherapy. The patients receiving the idarubicin protocol not only had a somewhat better EFS, but there were also no late relapses unlike in the patients referred for autologous BMT as late intensification of different treatment protocols. This observation underlines the antileukemic activity of idarubicin

and is in line with the results of other studies suggesting that previous chemotherapy may play a role in the outcome of autologous BMT patients (Mehta et al. 1995).

In terms of conditioning treatment, our favourable data support other experiences showing a better outcome in patients receiving TBI-containing regimens (Vignetti et al. 1996). Furthermore, prolonged or more intensive pre-transplant chemotherapy may have an »in vivo« purging activity (Schiller et al. 1997, Stein et al. 1996) that allows autologous BMT to be safely performed using unpurged bone marrow (Martin et al. 1998, Miggiano et al. 1996).

It is worth mentioning that the advantage of allogeneic over autologous BMT in terms of EFS is partially counterbalanced by the worse quality of life revealed by objective indicators (Zittoun et al. 1997); moreover, in the setting of first CR, autologous BMT has been proved to be significantly superior to allogeneic BMT from unrelated donors, also in terms of EFS (Ringden et al. 1997). Autologous BMT should therefore not be regarded merely as a minor option for patients unsuitable for allogeneic BMT.

In conclusion, autologous BMT as late intensification still has a place among post-

CR options; idarubicin may have an »in vivo« antileukemic activity that allows the use of unpurged autologous BMT.

## References

Bishop MR et al. (1997) Ex-vivo treatment of bone marrow with phosphorothioate oligonucleotide OL(1)p53 for autologous transplantation in acute myelogenous leukemia and myelodysplastic syndrome. J Hematother 6:441-6

Damon LE et al. (1996) Delayed engraftment of 4-hydroperoxy-cyclophosphamide purged autologous bone marrow after induction treatment containing mitoxantrone for acute myelogenous leukemia. Bone Marrow Transplant 17:93-9

Dann EJ et al. (1995) Late relapse following autologous bone marrow transplantation for acutemyelogenous leukemia: case report and review of the literature. Leukemia 9: 1072-4,

Gorin NC (1992) Marrow purging for autologous bone marrow transplantation and its role in acute myelocytic leukemia. European Cooperative Group for Bone Marrow Transplantation (EBMT). Leukemia 6:96-101

Heil G et al. (1995) High-dose cytosine arabinoside and daunorubicin post remission therapy in adults with de novo acute myeloid leukemia. Long-term follow-up of a perspective multicenter trial. Ann Hematol 71:219-25

Imrie K et al. (1996) Autologous bone marrow transplantation for acute myeloid leukemia. Stem Cells 14:69-78

Keating S et al. (1998) The influence of HLA-matched sibling donor availability on treatment outcome for patients with AML: an analysis of the AML 8 A study of the EORTC Leukaemia Cooperative Group and GIMEMA. Br J Haematol 102:1344-53

Lambertenghi Deliliers G et al. (1993) Idarubicin in the therapy of acute myeloid leukemia: final analysis in 57 previously untreated patients. Semin Oncol 20 (Suppl 8):27-33

Lowenberg B (1995) Post-remission treatment of acute myelogenous leukemia. N Engl J Med 332:260-2

Martin C et al. (1998) Autologous peripheral blood stem cell transplantation (PBSCT) mobilized with G-CSF in AML in first complete remission. Role of intensification therapy in outcome. Bone Marrow Transplant 21:375-82

Mehta J et al. (1996) Factors affecting engraftment and hematopoietic recovery after unpurged autografting in acute leukemia. Bone Marrow Transplant 18:319-24

Miggiano MC et al. (1996) Autologous bone marrow transplantation in late first complete remission improves outcome in acute myelogenous leukemia. Leukemia 10:402-9

Mitus AJ et al. (1995) Improved survival for patients with acute myelogenous leukemia. J Clin Oncol 13:560-9

Ringden O et al. (1997) Donor search or autografting in patients with acute leukaemia who lack an HLA-identical sibling? A matched-pair analysis. Acute Leukaemia Working Party of the European Cooperative Group for Blood and Marrow Transplantation (EBMT) and the International Marrow Unrelated Search and Transplant (IMUST) Study. Bone Marrow Transplant 19:963-8

Schiller G et al. (1997) Transplantation of autologous peripheral blood progenitor cells procured after high-dose cytarabine based consolidation chemotherapy for adults with acute myelogenous leukemia in first remission. Leukemia 11:1533-9

Stein AS et al. (1996) In vivo purging with high-dose cytarabine followed by high-dose chemoradiotherapy and reinfusion of unpurged bone marrow for adult acute myelogenous leukemia in first complete remission. J Clin Oncol 14:2206-16

Vignetti et al. (1996) Autologous bone marrow transplantation in children with acute myeloblastic leukemia: report from the Italian National Pediatric Registry (AIEOPBMT). Bone Marrow Transplantation 18 (Suppl 2):59-62

Zittoun RA et al. (1995) Autologous or allogeneic bone marrow transplantation compared with intensive chemotherapy in acute myelogenous leukemia. European Organization for Research and Treatment of Cancer (EORTC) and the Gruppo Italiano Malattie Ematologiche Maligne dell'Adulto (GIMEMA) Leukemia Cooperative Groups. N Eng J Med 332:217-23

Zittoun R et al. (1997) Quality of life in patients with acute myelogenous leukemia in prolonged first complete remission after bone marrow transplantation (allogeneic or autologous) or chemotherapy: a cross-sectional study of the EORTC GIMEMA AML 8 A trial. Bone Marrow Transplant 20:307-15

# Results of Allogeneic Hematopoietic Stem Cell Transplantation in Patients with High-Risk MDS

C. Aul, U. Germing, A. Niederste-Hollenberg, G. Meckenstock and A. Heyll

## Introduction

Myelodysplastic syndromes encompass a heterogenous group of cloncal stem cell disorders which are characterized by abnormal hematopoietic differentiation and blast cell accumulation in the bone marrow and reduced peripheral blood cell counts. Most patients with these disorders succumb to complications of bone marrow failure or transformation to AML within months or years of diagnosis. Life expectancy is particularly poor for patients with an increased medullary blast infiltration (RAEB and RAEB/T), profound pancytopenia and abnormal cytogenetics (particularly complex aberrations and chromosome 7 anomalies). Allogeneic stem cell transplantation offers a potential cure for younger patients with myelodysplastic syndromes. Although increasingly used during recent years, clinical experience with this treatment modality is still limited and most reports include only small patient series. In addition, it is unclear whether BMT should be performed as consolidation treatment after induction chemotherapy or whether patients should be transplanted immediately after diagnosis of MDS. In this paper, we report our own data of 20 patients with advanced primary MDS which were subjected to allogeneic stem cell transplantation over a period of 10 years.

## Patients And Methods

Between 1989 and 1998 20 patients with MDS underwent allogeneic BMT/PBSCT at the University of Düsseldorf. There were 3 patients with refractory anemia (RA), 1 patient with chronic myelomonocytic leukemia (CMML), 4 patients with RA with excess of blasts (RAEB), 10 patients with RAEB in transformation (RAEB/T) and 2 patients with AML evolving from MDS.

Median interval from diagnosis of MDS to transplantation was 14 months (range, 3–218 months). 7 patients were male, 13 patients were female. Median age at transplantation was 30 years (range, 16–53 years). All patients with a medullary blast count > 5% received conventional chemotherapy (TAD9, HAM, ICE protocols) prior to stem cell transplantation and were transplanted in complete remission. 2 patients presenting with a normal blast count (RA) received stem cells without previous chemotherapy. 16 patients received bone marrow and 4 patients received peripheral stem cells. In 5 cases bone marrow cells from matched unrelated donor were used.

Conditioning regimen consisted of myeloablative chemotherapy and TBI. Prophylaxis against GvHD included CSA and MTX. T cell depletion of stem cell sources to prevent graft-versus-host disease was not employed.

## Results

At the time of analysis, 10 patients were alive at a median follow-up of 14 months (range, 0–103 months). 10 patients died at a median interval of 2 months after transplantation (range, 0–25 months). The cumulative 3-year disease-free survival for the entire group of patients was 47%.

Heinrich-Heine-University of Düsseldorf, Germany

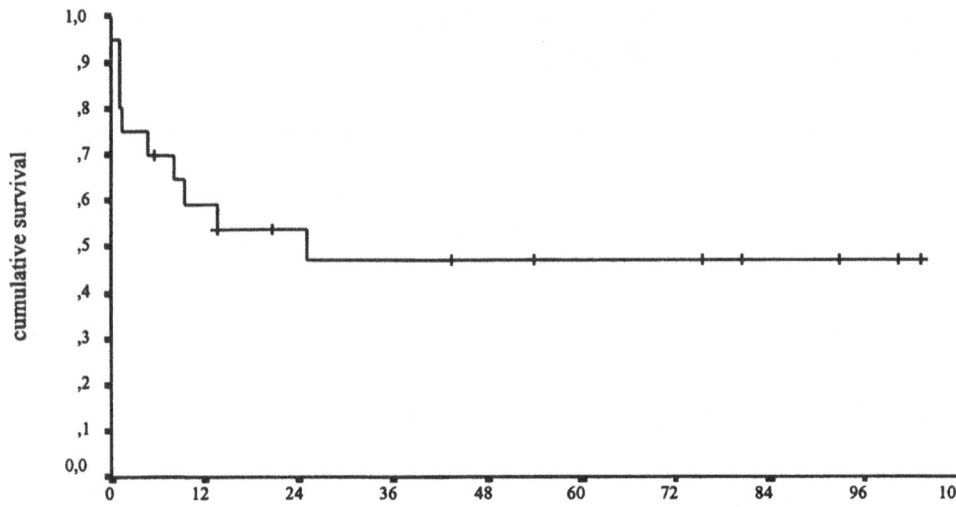

**Fig. 1.** Overall survival after BMT

8 patients (40%) succumbed to transplant-related complications and only one patient relapsed 21 months after transplantation. One patient died in CR because of a secondary neoplasia (pleural carcinosis).

Median cumulative survival of the entire group was 25 months (Fig. 1). The 1- and 3-year overall survival for the entire group of patients were 70% and 55%, respectively. Transplant-related mortality and relapse risk at 3 years after transplantation was 48% and 13% respectively.

## Conclusions

Our report confirms previous studies demonstrating the curative potential of allogeneic BMT/PBSCT for patients with myelodysplastic syndromes. The timing of transplant in the management of MDS remains largely controversial. Whereas most centers applied BMT as primary cytoreductive treatment, we used allogeneic MBT/PSCT as second-line treatment after successful remission induction with conventional chemotherapeutic regimens. This policy was followed strictly in our department for those patients who presented with an increased medullary blast cell infiltration. Our series differs from previous reports by a relatively low relapse risk of only 13% after 3 years. In other series employing allogeneic BMT/SCT as frontline-treatment of MDS, the risk of MDS relapse varied between 17% and 40%. Our data suggest that allogeneic stem cell transplantation should be performed as consolidation treatment to initial remission induction chemotherapy. However, a larger study is required for definitely answering the important question of optimal timing of allogeneic BMT/PSCT in the management of high-risk myelodysplastic syndromes.

## References

Anderson J, Appelbaum FR, Storb R (1995) An Update on allogeneic morrow transplantation for myelodysplastic syndromes. Leuk Lymphoma 17: 95

Runde V, de Witte T, Arnold R, et al. (1998) Bone marrow transplantation from HLA-identical siblings as firstline treatment in patients with myelodysplastic syndromes: early transplantation is associated with improved outcome. BMT 21: 255

# Dose Reduced Conditioning for Allogeneic Blood Stem Cell Transplantation from Sibling and Unrelated Donors in 51 Patients

M. Bornhäuser, C. Thiede, F. Kroschinsky, A. Neubauer* and G. Ehninger

*Abstract.* Between February 1998 and July 1999 fifty-one patients with progressed or refractory leukemia, lymphoma and solid tumors of whom most had a reduced performance status received either bone marrow (BM) or peripheral blood stem cells (PBSC) from sibling (n=18) and unrelated (n=33) donors after dose reduced conditioning therapy. Conditioning therapy consisted out of 3.3 mg/kg intravenous busulfan x 2 days, 30 mg/m² fludarabine x 5 days. In unrelated or mismatched transplants 2.5 mg/kg ATG x 4 days were added. GvHD prophylaxis was performed with cyclosporine A (CsA) and short course methotrexate or mycophenolate mofetil in patients receiving unmanipulated grafts. Low dose CsA was given after transplantation with CD34 positive selected grafts. The regimen was tolerable for all patients with only mild toxicity. The day 100 survival was 92% for the whole group. Primary engraftment was reached in 50 patients after 14 days (range, 9-24) and 18 days (range, 7-38) for neutrophils and platelets, respectively. The median time with a neutrophil count of < 0.5 x 10⁹/L was 8 days (range, 2 to 20). Secondary graft-failure was observed in 8 patients, all with unrelated donors and no prior intensive chemotherapy. In 6 patients autologous blood stem cells were reinfused as a rescue. Relapse of disease and toxicity associated with retreatment or second transplantation were the main causes of death. Symptoms of acute GvHD were observed in 17 patients. CMV antigenemia was detected in 9 patients. The actuarial 12 month overall/event-free survival is 57/23% for related transplants and 32/27% for unrelated transplants, respectively. Graft-versus-tumor responses were observed in patients with metastatic renal cell carcinoma and melanoma. Reduced-intensity conditioning is feasible without ATG in related transplants and leads to a reduction of transplant-related mortality.

## Introduction

Allogeneic hematopoietic stem cell transplantation after conditioning regimen with reduced doses of cytostatic drugs has been shown to combine the known antitumor effects of allogeneic immunotherapy with less toxicity. Especially older patients with reduced performance status and prior infectious complications might benefit from this treatment modality.

Significant graft-versus-leukemia effects have been demonstrated in patients with recurrent leukemia after allogeneic bone marrow transplantation (BMT). Prolonged remission can be achieved by donor leukocyte infusions in 70 to 80% of patients with relapsing chronic myeloid leukemia [1,2]. Therefore the success of allogeneic BMT seems to depend mostly on graft-versus-tumor effects which can also be obtained after less intensive preparative regimens when a persistent hematopoietic chimerism is achieved.

There are several reports in the literature on the establishment of mixed lymphohematopoietic chimerism after nonmyeloablative radio-/chemotherapy in animal models [3,4]. Encouraging clinical results have been achieved by using reduced doses of alkylating

Medizinische Klinik und Poliklinik I, Universitätsklinikum Carl Gustav Carus, Dresden
*Medizinische Klinik, Phillips Universität, Marburg, Germany

agents together with purine analogues for conditioning therapy [5,6]. Only recently, stable engraftment was achieved in patients after 200 rad total body irradiation (TBI) combined with immunosuppressive drugs [7]. Most of these studies have used blood stem cell grafts from HLA-identical sibling donors. Since there is evidence for graft-versus tumor reactions in solid tumors[8,9,10] we felt that allogeneic cell therapy with less toxic conditioning therapy might be one way to explore these effects in a greater proportion of patients with non-hematological malignancies in the near future.

In this study we observed successful engraftment in recipients of blood stem cell grafts from HLA identical siblings without ATG and from unrelated donors in most cases. Prolonged remissions were achieved in patients with limited tumor burden at the time of transplant. Graft-versus tumor effects were observed in patients with renal cell carcinoma and malignant melanoma.

## Patients and methods

*Fifty one patients* were included after having given informed consent from February 1998 to July 1999. The study had been approved by the local ethical board. Only patients not eligible for standard allogeneic BMT were included. Table 1 gives an overview on the whole patient population. The disease characteristics of the patients receiving grafts from unrelated donors (n=33) are summarized in Table 2, those of the related group (n=18) in Table 3. In brief, most patients belonged to a high-risk category with either a reduced performance status or extensive pretreatment

**Table 1.** Patient characteristics (n=51)

| | |
|---|---|
| Age: | 46 (r=16–63) |
| Sex: | 36 M/15 F |
| Months from diagnosis: | 18 (r=4–95) |
| Sibling/Unrelated: | 18/33 |
| After atologous Tx: | 7 |
| Prior aspergillosis: | 9 |
| Septic complication: | 3 |
| HLA-match unrelated: | 21 A, B, C + DRB1 ident |
| | 2 B + Cw Mismatch |
| | 10 Cw + DRB1 Micromismatch |

**Table 2.** Unrelated transplants (n=33)

| | | |
|---|---|---|
| AML: | 13 | 2 s-AML, 10 PR/Ref, 1 CR2$^{nd}$ |
| CML: | 7 | 1 1$^{st}$ CP, 4 AP, 1 BC, 1 2$^{nd}$ CP |
| ALL: | 3 | 2 Ref, 1 PR |
| MDS: | 3 | 1 Richter's Transformation |
| | | 1 Relapse after auto PBSCT |
| Multiple Myeloma | 1 | 1 Relapse after auto PBSCT |

**Table 3.** Related transplants (n=18)

| | | |
|---|---|---|
| AML: | 7 | 2 1$^{st}$ CR, 4 Ref |
| CML: | 2 | 1 BC 1$^{st}$ CP |
| MDS: | 2 | 1 CMMoL, 1 s-MDS |
| Hodgkin's Disease: | 2 | 2 relapsing after auto-PBSCT |
| SCLC: | 1 | |
| CLL | 1 | |
| Melanoma | 1 | |
| Renal-Cell Ca | 2 | |

including autologous PBSCT. Invasive aspergillosis or other severe infectious complications had occurred during pretreatment in 12 out of 51 patients. 4 patients with solid tumors were included (2 renal cell carcinoma, 1 small cell lung cancer and 1 melanoma).

*HLA matching.* All patients and donors were tested serologically for HLA-A and B and with high-resolution PCR-SSP typing for HLA-C, DRB1 and DQB1 according to standard procedures.[11] In the unrelated transplants complete matching was possible in 22 patients. DRB1/DQB1 micromismatches were detected in 9 transplants with an additional HLA-C mismatch in 5 patients. In three patient-donor pairs an one antigen mismatch in the HLA-A or B locus was accepted.

*Stem cell collection.* The sources of blood stem cells used are summarized in Table 4. Bone marrow was harvested after informed consent of the donors in general anesthesia. Mobilization of PBSC was performed using 7.5 µg/ml lenograstim or 10 µg/kg filgrastim for 5 days and two subsequent aphereses on days 5 and 6 of the stimulation period. The product was cryopreserved when indicated.

**Table 4.** Graft sources

| Related | | Unrelated | |
|---|---|---|---|
| BM: | 0 | BM: | 8 |
| PBSC: | 17 | PBSC: | 16 |
| CD34+PBSC: | 1 | CD34+PBSC: | 9 |

CD34 positive selection of PBSC from 9 unrelated donors was performed using an immunomagnetic device (CliniMACS®, Milteny Biotec, Bergisch Gladbach, Germany) according to the manufacturers instructions. Briefly, PBSC were washed once to reduce platelet contamination. The washed cells were incubated with QBEND-10 antibody (mouse antihuman CD34) for 30 minutes at room temperature. Two centrifugation steps followed to reduce unbound antibody. The labeled cells were loaded onto the CliniMACS column and a semiautomated separation process was started. Marked cells were bound in the column and flushed out with buffer after removing the column out of the magnetic field. The negative fraction was recovered and stored as was the CD34 positive fraction. Purity and content of CD3 positive T cells of each graft were measured by flow cytometric analysis using a FACSCAN (Becton Dickinson, San Jose). All patients who had received CD34 selected PBSC were infused with $1 \times 10^5$/kg CD3 positive donor T cells on day 14 and $1 \times 10^6$/kg on day 21 when no signs of GvHD were detectable. Those T cells had been collected and frozen before G-CSF stimulation. When $< 4 \times 10^6$ CD34 positive cells/kg were obtained with the first apheresis, unmanipulated PBSC were infused. Bone marrow was infused without prior manipulation.

*Chemotherapy.* Conditioning therapy started with 3.3 mg/kg busulfan (Sigma-Aldrich, Deisenhofen, Germany) dissolved in 10 ml of dimethyl sulphoxide and further diluted by 1000 ml saline. The daily dose was infused over 3 hours on day -6 and -5. Prior studies had shown 3.3 mg/kg iv to be equivalent to 4 mg/kg busulfan given orally in a single dose. The pharmacokinetic data for this formulation have been published.[12] Fludarabine (medak, Munich, Germany) was infused at 30 mg/m² over 30 minutes from day -6 to day -2. In the unrelated transplants, ATG (Rabbit, Pasteur Mérieux, Lyon, France) was administered at 2.5 mg/kg over 4 hours from day -5 to day -2. In four patients ATG Fresenius (Bad Homburg, Germany) was used at the same dose. No ATG was used in the related setting.

*Supportive care.* Patients were treated in single or double rooms. All patients received antibacterial and antifungal prophylaxis with ciprofloxacine at 500 mg twice daily and flu-conazole at 200 mg/d . Acyclovir was given at 1200 mg daily in patients with positive herpes simplex virus IgG titers. Patients with negative CMV IgG titers received blood products from CMV seronegative donors. Bacterial and fungal surveillance cultures were performed every second week. Broad spectrum antibiotics were begun whenever body-temperature increased beyond 38.5°C, C-reactive protein increased significantly or when a positive finding was made on chest x-ray. PCR for CMV DNA and pp65 antigen testing in peripheral blood were performed once weekly. Patients received filgrastim at 5 µg/kg/d from day + 6 to day +13. Hemoglobin was maintained at a level of > 5 mmol/l and the platelet count was maintained at $> 20 \times 10^9$/L with in-line filtered and irradiated blood products.

GvHD prophylaxis was performed with 3 mg/kg cyclosporine (CsA) starting one day before infusion of the graft. Further intravenous or oral dosage was adapted according to CsA trough blood levels. High-risk AML patients with > 30% blasts in the bone marrow received only CsA (n= 10). Additional Methotrexate (MTX) 5 mg/m² was administered in the first 11 recipients receiving unmanipulated grafts on days +1, +3 and +6. Mycophenolate mofetil (MMF) was given orally at 4 x 500 mg from day +1 to day +28 instead of MTX to the subsequent 20 patients because the rate of acute GvHD with MTX still seemed to be quite high (56%) and animal data supposed MMF also to be useful as graft rejection prophylaxis.[13] Patients developing GvHD were maintained at MMF and received 2 mg/kg/d prednisolone in addition which was tapered upon clinical response.

*Study endpoints* Engraftment defined as $> 0,5 \times 10^9$/L ANC for 3 days, $> 50 \times 10^9$/L platelets without transfusion and the toxicity of the protocol in this patient cohort were the primary endpoints. Secondary objectives had been the antileukemic effects and the rate of acute GvHD observed. Organ toxicity was documented according to WHO criteria. Acute and chronic GvHD were graded according to consensus criteria [14,15].

*Analysis of chimerism.* Chimerism analysis in peripheral blood was performed twice a week during hospital stay. The methods applied were either XY FISH in sex-mismatched donor-recipient pairs[16] or a quantitative multiplex PCR assay with amplification of nine tetranucleotide repeats and the amelogenin locus.[17]

*Statistical analysis.* Most quantitative parameters are provided as median with minimum and maximum. The actuarial overall and event-free survival was calculated as of October 1st, 1999 from the day of transplantation according to the methods of Kaplan and Meier [18].

## Results

The clinical results of both groups are summarized in Table 5.

*Toxicity.* The maximum WHO toxicity for non hematological parameters observed in 4 patients was grade 4 mucositis or diarrhea. Toxicity grade 3 was observed in additional 2 patients for bilirubine and creatinine, respectively. In 46 patients no toxicity >2 could be documented. No early deaths or severe infectious complications were observed. Only 7 patients experienced fever > 38.5°C for a median of 3 days. (range, 2 to 8 days)

**Table 5.** Results

| | |
|---|---|
| CD34+ x $10^6$/kg: | 5.3 (range, 1.0–16.1) |
| > 0.5 x $10^9$/l ANC: | 14 (range, 9–24) |
| > 50 x $10^9$/l plts: | 18 (range, 7–38) |
| < 0.5 x $10^9$/l ANC: | 8 (range, 2–20) |
| RBC Transfus.: | n=8 (r=2–28) |
| Plt. Transfus.: | n=6 (r=0–25) |
| Fever > 38.5 °C | n=7 (Median 3 days) |
| WHO 3–4 Tox. | n=6 3 Mucositis |
| | 1 Diarrhea |
| | 1 Hyperbilirubinemia |
| | 1 Creatinine |
| acute GvHD: | n=17 (14 I°+II°, 3 III°) |
| chronic GvHD: | n=10 (n=35 > day 100) |
| Graft-failure | |
| unrelated: | n=9/33 (3 CD34+, 2 PBSC, 4 BM) |
| | 5 CML, 1 MDS, 2 ALL, 1 AML |
| | 6 Rescue with auto Back-up |
| related: | n=0/18 |
| Relapse: | n=16 (10 AML, 1 ALL, 2 CML, |
| | 2 MH, 1 CMMoL) |
| Causes of death: | n=25 |
| | Relapse n=13 |
| | GvHD/MOF/Retransplantation |
| | n=6 |
| | Pneumonia n=6 |

*Engraftment.* Primary neutrophil engraftment with an absolute neutrophil count (ANC) of greater than 0.5 x $10^9$ /L was achieved in 50/51 patients at a median of 14 days posttransplantation (range, 9 to 24 days). Transfusion requirements were moderate with 8 units of RBC (range, 2 to 28) and 6 thrombapheresis products (range, 0 to 25) per patient. A platelet count of > 50 x $10^9$/L sustained without transfusion was reached 18 days (range, 7 to 38) after transplantation. The median number of days with an ANC below 0.5 x $10^9$ /L was 8 with a range from 2 to 20, dependent on the underlying disease and pretreatment. Non-engraftment was observed in one CML patient. He had received an adequate BM inoculum from a donor with an 1-antigen mismatch in the A-locus. Secondary graft-failure occurred in 8 patients (1 AML, 1 ALL, 2 MDS, 4 CML) receiving grafts from unrelated donors.

*GvHD.* Acute GvHD was observed in 17 patients. The median day of occurrence of clinical GvHD was + 17. In 15 patients grade I or II GvHD could be controlled with systemic steroids. Two patients experienced grade 3 GvHD of gut and liver and another patient eventually died from acute GvHD. Chronic GvHD was documented in 10 out of 35 patients evaluable after day 100, so far.

*Infections and other complications.* Varicella zoster reactivation with neuralgic symptoms involving the nervus trigeminus and the cornea occurred in one patient. The same patient had experienced sinusitis colonized by aspergillus fumigatus before. Preemptive therapy for CMV antigenemia had to be started in 9 patients with positive pp65 antigen testing. Invasive CMV pneumonitis was assumed as the cause of death in one patient who had experienced early graft-failure at day +28. All patients with CMV antigenemia or infection had had a positive testing for anti-CMV IgG prior to transplantation. None of the patients with negative CMV serology and a donor positive for anti-CMV IgG experienced CMV reactivation.

Delayed type immune hemolysis occurred in two cases of major blood group incompatibility. The donor isoagglutinin titers decreased spontaneously in one patient whereas the other patient with CML died with signs of relapsing disease. Immune mediated thrombocytopenia occurred in one patient on day +73. Prednisolone 1 mg/kg/d lead to an immediate increase in platelet counts.

*Chimerism.* Figure 1 compares the increase of donor chimerism in representative patients receiving either related PBSC transplants or unrelated PBSC, BM or CD34 selected PBSC. Although the speed of increase in donor signals was heterogeneous, all patients with stable engraftment eventually developed complete donor chimerism.

*Relapse and survival.* Intermittent clinical responses could be documented in most patients. The day 100 overall (OS) and event-free survival (EFS) for all patients is 92% and 75%, respectively. The Kaplan-Meyer Plots for OS and EFS of related and unrelated transplants are depicted in Figure 2A and 2B. With a median observation time of 7 months, the expected 12 months OS and EFS for related transplants is 57% and 23%, respectively. The respective figures are 32% and 25% for unrelated transplants. In both patients with progressed renal cell carcinoma and in the patient with metastatic melanoma regression

of size of the metastases was observed. The clinical responses were associated with acute GvHD in all 3 patients and the melanoma patient died from grade III-IV GvHD. Early evaluation of the patient with ewing's sarcoma revealed regression of pulmonary metastases due to the conditioning regimen. This patients follow-up is to short to comment on graft-versus tumor effects.

## Discussion

Although improvements of supportive treatment have been achieved during the last decade, conventional conditioning therapy and consecutive allogeneic stem cell transplantation is associated with significant toxicity and early morbidity [19,20]. The high rate of acute GvHD even increases the early toxicity especially for recipients of grafts from HLA mismatched or unrelated donors [21,22]. Only patients under the age of 50 with good performance status without prior infectious complications therefor meet the

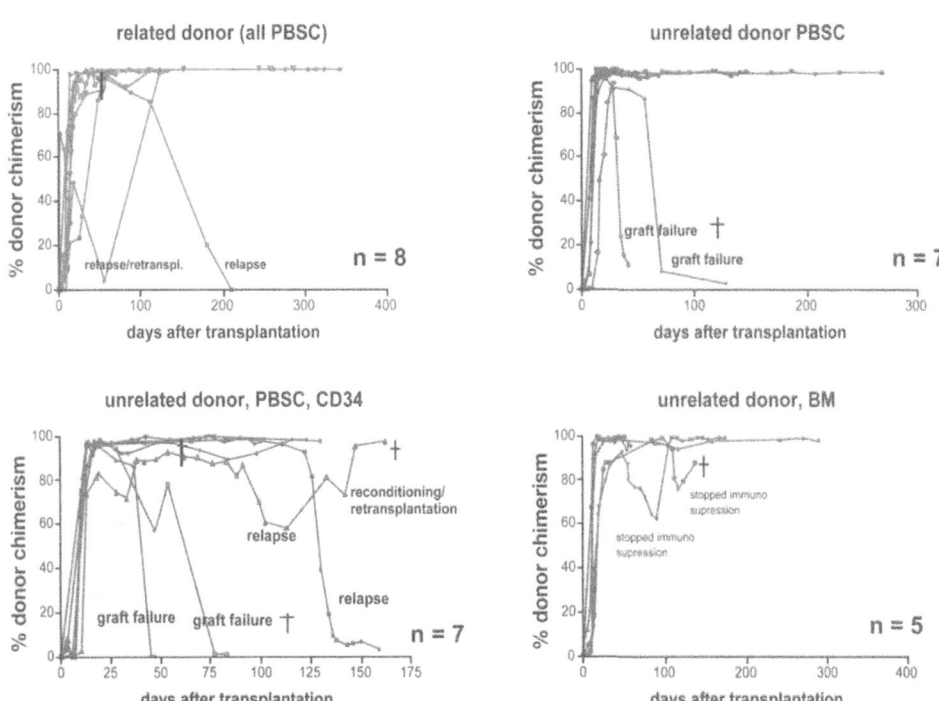

**Fig. 1.** Dynamics of chimerism according to graft source and clinical course

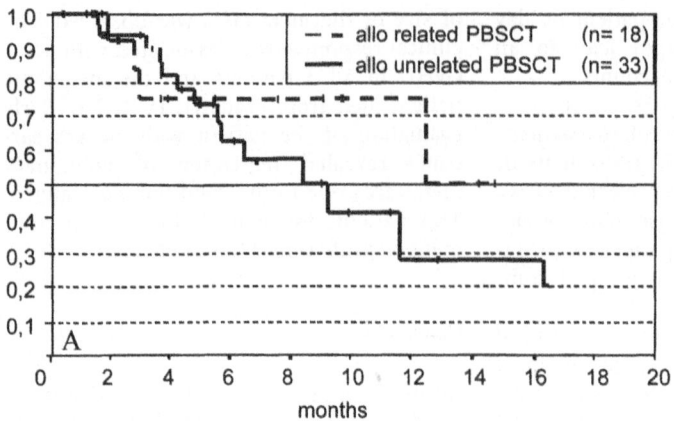

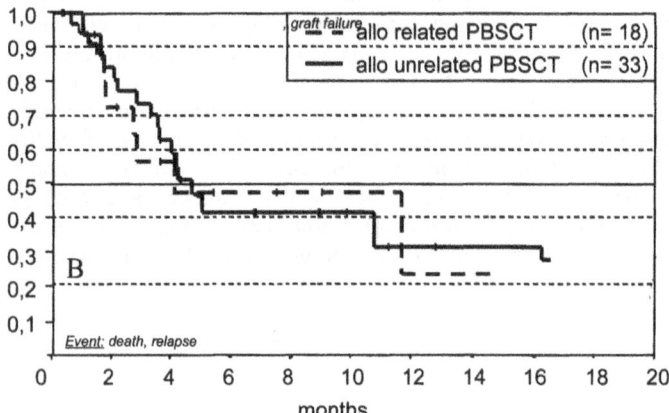

**Fig. 2a,b.** a Overall survival,
b Event-free Survival

inclusion criteria for most protocols of unrelated stem cell transplantation. Nevertheless, only one third of potential recipients have an HLA identical sibling donor. Therefore the other patients depend on HLA matched unrelated volunteer donors as alternative choice. Since the curative potential of allogeneic cell therapy is attractive for many patients with malignant hematological diseases, investigators have started to explore less toxic conditioning therapies as an option to treat patients with impaired performance status and progressed disease [5,23]. These trials have been preceded by animal models showing the possibility of sustained engraftment even after nonmyeloablative irradiation of the recipient [24].

The rate of graft failure increases, when an unrelated donor is chosen [25]. This may be mainly due to the high rate of HLA disparity which can be found by performing high resolution typing of the HLA class I alleles of donor/recipient pairs [21,26]. In our study, we saw graft-failure in 9 out of 33 patients receiving unrelated transplants with either BM or G-CSF mobilized PBSC. The secondary graft-failure observed after CMV antigenemia in 2 patients as well as the poor graft function in four CML and three MDS patients may be a sign of unstable hematopoiesis using unrelated stem cell donors after nonablative conditioning. When analyzing engraftment, one has to keep in mind that the leukemic burden had been significant in several patients when chemotherapy was started. Although not statistically definable, graft-failure seemed to occur more often in transplants with HLA-Class I mismatches (n=2) and in patients with myeloproliferative disease or MDS (n=6) where no induction chemotherapy had preceded the transplantation. No graft-failure was observed in the 18 related transplants although ATG had been omitted in contrast to the series reported by Slavin et al [5].

The dynamics of chimerism showed a somewhat slower increase of donor signals when compared with patients after myeloablative conditioning [27]. Predominating donor type chimerism for T and B cells as well as NK cells might be critical for tolerance of the graft [4,28]. Nevertheless, complete chimerism is obtained in several patients with stable long term engraftment. Infusion of higher doses of CD34 positive cells might possibly further improve engraftment. G-CSF mobilized PBSC have been used for allogeneic progenitor cell transplantation with increasing frequency during the last years. Faster engraftment and similar rates of acute GvHD have been observed [29]. Nevertheless, the amount of CD34 positive PBSC or BM cells available from volunteer donors may stay somewhat limited because the issues of donor safety have to be kept in mind.

Autologous PBSC or BM showed to be useful for rescue of patients with graft failure because there was a significant aplasia even in patients losing their grafts 2-3 months after transplantation. This aplasia may be caused by the occupation of marrow space by donor hematopoiesis when temporary engraftment is achieved [30]. These observations as well as the chimerism analyses showing complete donor chimerism even in CD34 positive progenitors underline the myeloablative nature of these transplants. Therefore we suppose to leave the term 'nonmyeloablative' in this context.

As expected, the low early toxicity of the chemotherapy allowed to treat older patients as well as patients with extensive pretreatment or prior infectious complications. There was no toxic death associated with the chemotherapy applied resulting in an 100 day survival of 92 percent. The dose intensity reached by the use of 3.3 mg/kg busulfan x 2 and 30 mg/m$^2$ fludarabine x 5 can be regarded to be about 50 percent of that known from conventional conditioning therapy. One has to keep in mind that intensive immunosuppression is induced for several months and acute GvHD might even necessitate intensified immunosuppression and thereby can lead to an increased risk for infectious complications.

The rate of acute GvHD observed was in the range expected. In the group of patients receiving CD34 selected PBSC and delayed T cell add-back only one case of acute GvHD 1 of the skin was observed. Stable engraftment could be reached in patients receiving > 4 x 10$^6$ CD34/kg positive selected PBSC passively depleted from T cells. It can be argued that the rate of engraftment could have been higher if all patients had received unmodified PBSC. The high rate of acute GvHD observed by Slavin at al. in a cohort of patients receiving PBSC from sibling donors lead us to explore T cell depleted PBSC transplantation with an add-back of a defined dose of T cells in the unrelated setting. Furthermore allogeneic PBSC transplantation was reported to be associated with a higher rate of chronic GvHD compared to BMT in the related setting [31]. So far, chronic GvHD has been observed in 10 patients who had received unmodified BM or PBSC.

CMV antigenemia was observed in 9 out of 51 patients. This rate is similar to the data reported after allogeneic BMT using intensive conditioning therapy [32]. All patients had a positive CMV serology. Subsequent ganciclovir treatment was associated with graft-failure in one patient. Another patient had experienced early graft failure after detection of CMV antigenemia. Residual recipient leukocytes might presumably be the origin of CMV antigenemia in patients receiving less intensive preparative regimens and subsequent immunosuppressive medication. Delayed immunological recovery has been observed after unrelated BMT in adults, especially in recipients of T cell depleted grafts [33]. The same data have to be collected prospectively in patients after less intense conditioning therapy. Whether these patients are at the same risk for invasive CMV infection like myeloablated hosts after T cell depletion is unknown. These knowledge would be important to have more rationales for preemptive treatment strategies like donor leukocyte infusions in this setting.

Although mixed lymphohematopoietic chimerism and subsequent tolerance is the goal of nonmyeloablative conditioning some immunological complications may theoretically occur especially in the unrelated setting. The persistence of recipient T and B cells might lead to delayed erythroid engraftment or pure red cell aplasia in the donor-recipient pairs with major blood group incompatibility [34]. High titers of recipient isoagglutines were observed in 2 patients of the study group. In one CML patient, plasmapheresis had no effect on transfusion requirements. This patient developed pancytopenia and subsequently died with multiorgan failure. A bone marrow aspiration had shown Philadelphia chromosome positive interphases shortly before death. In the second patient, isoagglutinin titers decreased spontaneously and the hemoglobin level increased thereafter. Sudden occurrence of thrombocytopenia was associated with a positive test for platelet associated antibodies (MAIPA). The platelet count rose after prednisolone had been given at a dose of 1 mg/kg/d. Steroids could be tapered subsequently without a second drop in platelet counts. Whether these findings are merely accidental or whether blood group incompatibilities and CMV serostatus are of prognostic importance in this setting has to be studied in a larger cohort.

Unrelated BMT after dose reduced or 'nonmyeloablative' preparative regimens has been described by two groups only recently [35,36]. The preparative regimen described by Giralt et al. contains melphalan doses of 140 to 180 mg/m$^2$ which are known to induce prolonged aplasia [37]. Stable allogeneic engraftment has been achieved after conditioning therapy with 240 mg/m$^2$ melphalan alone [38]. Our data obtained by sequential quantitative analysis of chimerism in cellular subsets show that myeloablation is induced in most patients after 50% of the usual dose of busulfan.

In summary, this study shows that purine analog-containing conditioning therapy can achieve allogeneic engraftment in recipients of stem cell grafts from unrelated volunteer donors. Nevertheless, the rate of secondary graft-failure is still too high (27%). Engraftment can be achieved in the related setting without ATG. The reduced toxicity of the regimen leads to a short hospital stay and a low early mortality compared to intensive conditioning therapy. Nevertheless significant acute and chronic GvHD may occur later

after transplantation. Engraftment is possible with BM, PBSC and CD34 positive selected PBSC. Further studies have to explore the leukemia-free survival obtained with this approach compared to standard conditioning therapy. In patients with high risk myeloid leukemia prophylactic donor leukocyte infusion is one way to improve the antileukemic effects of the procedure. Regular quantitative analysis of chimerism is important to detect imminent relapse earlier. As observed in two patients, cessation of immunosuppressive medication offers the possibility to reinduce remission at least in CML patients. Allogeneic immunotherapy seems to be most promising when performed at the stage of minimal residual disease. As described previously, patients with progressive or refractory leukemia are not likely to obtain durable remission [23].

Like other groups, we have observed antitumor responses associated with clinical GvHD in patients with renal cell carcinoma and melanoma [39]. Unfortunately, GvHD was severe in these patients and further attempts have to be undertaken to control GvHD without abrogating Graft-versus-tumor reactions.

Tolerance induction for subsequent organ transplantation might be another potential field of interest. For this purpose, engraftment of HLA mismatched hematopoietic progenitor cells has to be studied. Encouraged by the stable engraftment obtained in one patient with an 1-antigen mismatch, we think this goal might be reached perhaps by modifying the immunosuppressive strategies.

After all, we would like to stress the fact that there are still a lot of unanswered questions in this field which have to be studied in carefully designed trials including patients not eligible for conventional allogeneic blood stem cell transplantation.

*Acknowledgments.* We thank the 'Deutsche Krebshilfe' for supporting the Bone Marrow Transplantation Unit in Dresden.

# References

1. Kolb HJ, Schattenberg A, Goldman JM, et al (1995) Graft-versus-leukemia effect of donor lymphocyte transfusions in marrow grafted patients. European

Group for Blood and Marrow Transplantation Working Party Chronic Leukemia [see comments]. Blood 86:2041-2050

2. Slavin S, Naparstek E, Nagler A, et al (1996) Allogeneic cell therapy with donor peripheral blood cells and recombinant human interleukin-2 to treat leukemia relapse after allogeneic bone marrow transplantation. Blood 87:2195-2204

3. Colson YL, Wren SM, Schuchert MJ, et al (1995) A nonlethal conditioning approach to achieve durable multilineage mixed chimerism and tolerance across major, minor, and hematopoietic histocompatibility barriers. J Immunol 155:4179-4188

4. Kimikawa M, Sachs DH, Colvin RB, Bartholomew A, Kawai T, Cosimi AB (1997) Modifications of the conditioning regimen for achieving mixed chimerism and donor-specific tolerance in cynomolgus monkeys. Transplantation 64:709-716

5. Slavin S, Nagler A, Naparstek E, et al (1998) Nonmyeloablative stem cell transplantation and cell therapy as an alternative to conventional bone marrow transplantation with lethal cytoreduction for the treatment of malignant and nonmalignant hematologic diseases. Blood 91:756-763

6. Khouri I, Keating M, Korbling M, et al (1998) Transplant-lite: induction of graft-versus-malignancy using fludarabine-based nonablative chemotherapy and allogeneic blood progenitor-cell transplantation as treatment for lymphoid malignancies. J Clin Oncol 16:2817-2824

7. McSweeney PA, Wagner JL, Maloney DG, et al (1998) Outpatient PBSC allografts using immunosuppression with low-dose TBI before, and cyclosporine (CSP) and mycophenolate mofetil (MMF) after transplant. Blood 92 (suppl 1):519a

8. Ueno NT, Rondon G, Mirza NQ, et al (1998) Allogeneic peripheral-blood progenitor-cell transplantation for poor-risk patients with metastatic breast cancer. J Clin Oncol 16:986-993

9. Or R, Ackerstein A, Nagler A, et al (1998) Allogeneic cell-mediated immunotherapy for breast cancer after autologous stem cell transplantation: a clinical pilot study. Cytokines Cell Mol Ther 4:1-6

10. Eibl B, Schwaighofer H, Nachbaur D, et al (1996) Evidence for a graft-versus-tumor effect in a patient treated with marrow ablative chemotherapy and allogeneic bone marrow transplantation for breast cancer. Blood 88:1501-1508

11. Ottinger HD, Albert E, Arnold R, et al (1997) German consensus on immunogenetic donor search for transplantation of allogeneic bone marrow and peripheral blood stem cells. Bone Marrow Transplant 20:101-105

12. Ehninger G, Schuler U, Renner U, et al (1995) Use of a water-soluble busulfan formulation—pharmacokinetic studies in a canine model. Blood 85:3247-3249

13. Storb R, Yu C, Wagner JL, et al (1997) Stable mixed hematopoietic chimerism in DLA-identical littermate dogs given sublethal total body irradiation before and pharmacological immunosuppression after marrow transplantation. Blood 89:3048-3054

14. Przepiorka D, Weisdorf D, Martin P, et al (1995) Consensus conference on acute GvHD grading. Bone Marrow Transplant 15:825-828

15. Sullivan KM, Agura E, Anasetti C, et al (1991) Chronic graft-versus-host disease and other late complications of bone marrow transplantation. Semin Hematol 28:250-259

16. Najfeld V, Burnett W, Vlachos A, Scigliano E, Isola L, Fruchtman S (1997) Interphase FISH analysis of sex-mismatched BMT utilizing dual color XY probes. Bone Marrow Transplant 19:829-834

17. Thiede C, Florek M, Bornhäuser M, et al (1999) Rapid quantification of mixed chimerism using multiplex amplification of short tandem repeat markers and fluorescence detection. Bone Marrow Transplant 23:1055-1060

18. Kaplan E, Meier P (1958) Nonparametric estimation from incomplete observations. J Am Stat Assoc 53:457-462

19. deMagalhaes SM, Bloom EJ, Donnenberg A, et al (1996) Toxicity of busulfan and cyclophosphamide (BU/CY2) in patients with hematologic malignancies. Bone Marrow Transplant 17:329-333

20. Miralbell R, Bieri S, Mermillod B, et al (1996) Renal toxicity after allogeneic bone marrow transplantation: the combined effects of total-body irradiation and graft-versus-host disease. J Clin Oncol 14:579-585

21. Nademanee A, Schmidt GM, Parker P, et al (1995) The outcome of matched unrelated donor bone marrow transplantation in patients with hematologic malignancies using molecular typing for donor selection and graft-versus-host disease prophylaxis regimen of cyclosporine, methotrexate, and prednisone. Blood 86:1228-1234

22. Hansen JA, Gooley TA, Martin PJ, et al (1998) Bone marrow transplants from unrelated donors for patients with chronic myeloid leukemia [see comments]. N Engl J Med 338:962-968

23. Giralt S, Estey E, Albitar M, et al (1997) Engraftment of allogeneic hematopoietic progenitor cells with purine analog-containing chemotherapy: harnessing graft-versus-leukemia without myeloablative therapy. Blood 89:4531-4536

24. Colson YL, Li H, Boggs SS, Patrene KD, Johnson PC, Ildstad ST (1996) Durable mixed allogeneic chimerism and tolerance by a nonlethal radiation-based cytoreductive approach. J Immunol 157:2820-2829

25. Madrigal JA, Scott I, Arguello R, Szydlo R, Little AM, Goldman JM (1997) Factors influencing the outcome of bone marrow transplants using unrelated donors. Immunol Rev 157:153-166

26. Scott I, O'Shea J, Bunce M, et al (1999) Molecular typing shows a high level of HLA class I incompatibility in serologically well matched donor/patient pairs: Implications for unrelated bone marrow donor selection. Blood 92:4864-4871

27. Thiede C, Brendel C, Mohr B, et al (1998) Comparative analysis of chimerism in the early posttransplantation period in cellular subsets of patients undergoing myeloablative and nonmyeloablative allogeneic blood stem cell transplantation. Blood 92, Supplement 1:132a

28. Gyger M, Baron C, Forest L, et al (1998) Quantitative assessment of hematopoietic chimerism after allogeneic bone marrow transplantation has predictive value for the occurrence of irreversible graft failure and graft-vs.-host disease. Exp Hematol 26:426-434

29. Bacigalupo A, Zikos P, Van-Lint MT, et al (1998) Allogeneic bone marrow or peripheral blood cell transplants in adults with hematologic malignancies: a single-center experience. Exp Hematol 26:409-414

30. Stewart FM, Zhong S, Wuu J, Hsieh Cc, Nilsson SK, Quesenberry PJ (1998) Lymphohematopoietic engraftment in minimally myeloablated hosts. Blood 91:3681-3687

31. Storek J, Gooley T, Siadak M, et al (1997) Allogeneic peripheral blood stem cell transplantation may be associated with a high risk of chronic graft-versus-host disease. Blood 90:4705-4709

32. Bacigalupo A, Tedone E, Isaza A, et al (1995) CMV-antigenemia after allogeneic bone marrow transplantation: correlation of CMV-antigen positive cell numbers with transplant-related mortality. Bone Marrow Transplant 16:155-161

33. Small TN, Papadopulos EB, Boulad F, et al (1999) Comparison of immune reconstitution after unrelated and related T-cell-depleted bone marrow transplantation: Effect of patient age and donor leukocyte infusions. Blood 93:467-480

34. Mizon P, Jouet JP, Vanhaesbroucke C, Villard F, Wibaut B, Goudemand J (1994) Immunohematologic surveillance of patients treated with ABO incompatible bone marrow allografts. Transfus Clin Biol 1:271-277

35. Giralt S, Cohen A, Claxton D, et al (1998) Fludarabine/melphalan as a less intense preparative regimen for unrelated donor transplants in patients with hematologic malignancies. Blood 92 (suppl 1):289a

36. Nagler A, Or R, Naparstek E, Varadi G, Brautbar C, Slavin S (1998) Matched unrelated bone marrow transplantation (BMT) using a non-myeloablative conditioning regimen. Blood 92 (suppl 1):289a-289a

37. Tricot G, Jagannath S, Vesole D, et al (1995) Peripheral blood stem cell transplants for multiple myeloma: identification of favorable variables for rapid engraftment in 225 patients. Blood 85:588-596

38. Singhal S, Powles R, Treleaven J, Horton C, Swansbury GJ, Mehta J (1996) Melphalan alone prior to allogeneic bone marrow transplantation from HLA-identical sibling donors for hematologic malignancies: alloengraftment with potential preservation of fertility in women. Bone Marrow Transplant 18:1049-1055

39. Childs RW, Clave E, Tisdale J, Plante M, Hensel N, Barett J (1999) Sucessful treatment of metastatic renal cell carcinoma with nonmyeloablative allogeneic peripheral-blood progenitor-cell transplant: Evidence for a graft-versus-tumo effect. J Clin Oncol 17:2044-2049

# Analysis of Chimerism in the Early Posttransplantation Period in Cellular Subsets of Patients Undergoing Myeloablative and Non-Myeloablative (Metakine) Allogeneic Blood Stem Cell Transplantation (BSCT)

C. Brendel[1], C. Thiede[1], B. Mohr[1], M. Florek[1], U. Oelschlägel[1], M. Ritter[2], R. Naumann[1], G. Geissler[1], G. Ehninger[1], M. Bornhäuser[1] and A. Neubauer[2]

*Abstract.* Acute and chronic graft versus host disease (GvHD) is a life threatening problem for patients undergoing blood stem cell transplantation (BSCT). Graft engineering and novel treatment modalities, i.e. non-myeloablative (NMA, metakine) conditioning, have been introduced in order to avoid these complications. We analyzed chimerism in T-, B-, NK-, and myeloid cell subsets in the early post-transplantation period to investigate the effect of these different approaches on the kinetics of engraftment and the incidence of GvHD. After non-myeloablative (metakine) transplantation cellular engraftment kinetics were slower compared to the standard regimen. These differences in engraftment between myeloablative and non-myeloablative conditioning were observed in all subsets, but were most pronounced in T-cells, whereas myeloid and NK-cell engraftment showed similar kinetics. Rapid increase of donor type CD8+ cells (> 90% day 14) was associated with GHVD grade ≥ II in three patients, irrespective of the conditioning regimen chosen, whereas lack of donor NK-cells might be associated with graft failure. One patient with NMA conditioning experienced grade III GvHD at day 84, the same time when CD8+ T-cells reached 97% donor chimerism. A patient receiving a T-cell depleted graft from an unrelated donor experienced graft failure at day 28. In this patient, only CD14+ and CD15+ donor cells were found in significant number during the entire follow up. Whether differential monitoring of certain cellular subsets in the early transplantation period might be of some prognostic value remains to be determined during follow up analyses.

## Introduction

Allogeneic transplantation after non-myeloablative conditioning is a novel treatment approach intended to overcome treatment-related toxicity (Slavin, Blood 1998). The kinetic in the developement of chimerism in different cell compartments as well as the effects of persistent recipient hematopoiesis on engraftment, graft versus host disease (GvHD) and graft failure are under ivestiga-tioncurrent at the moment. The aim of the present study was to analyze the kinetics of donor chimerism in cellular subsets (T-, NK-, B-, myeloid and peripheral blood progenitor cells) in order to get a better understanding of the mutual influence of these subpopulations on engraftment and the incidence of GvHD. To address this question we applied fluores-cence activated cell sorting in combination with STR(short-tandem-repeat)-analysis, a method that has proven to be highly discriminative, sensitive and reproducible even with low cell numbers.

## Patients and Methods

We analyzed five patients with metakine conditioning regimen, two of them had matched related and three had matched unrelated donors. In comparison five patients after myeloablative conditioning regimen were investigated, one of them had matched related and four had matched unrelated donors. Of these ten patients three recieved bone marrow and seven received peripheral blood stem cells (PBSCs), three patients were T-cell

[1] Medizinische Klinik und Poliklinik I, Universitätsklinikum Carl Gustav Carus, Technische Universität Dresden, Germany
[2] Present adress: Zentrum für Innere Medizin, Klinikum der Philipps-Universität Marburg, Germany

depleted. The median age was 39.5 years with a range from 28 to 61 years. Five patients suffered from chronic myeloid leukemia (CML), three from acute myeloid leukemia (AML), one from myelodysplastic syndromes (MDS) and one patient had an acute lymphoblastic leukemia (ALL).

The conditioning regimen was as following: For myeloablative therapy patients received 4 x 3.3 mg/kg Busulfan i.v., 200 mg/kg Cyclophosphamide and 10 mg/kg ATG in case of an unrelated donor situation. The patients with metakine (NMA) conditioning received 2 x 3.3 mg/kg Busulfan i.v., 150 mg Fludarabine and eventually 10 mg/kg ATG for unrelated donor grafts. The patients were monitored for their development of subset chimerism from day 7 to 112 post transplantation. 30-60 ml peripheral blood were drawn from each patient for one complete subset analysis, followed by Ficoll-separation of mononuclear cells (MNC) (see Figure 1). After the immunomagnetic preenrichment of CD34+ cells (Mini-MACS, Miltenyi-Biotec, Bergisch Gladbach, Germany) from MNC-fraction, FACS-sorting of subpopulations was performed on a FACSVantage Cell Sorter (Becton Dickinson, Heidelberg) as following: CD3+/CD4+(MoAb obtained from Beckmann-Coulter-Immunotech/PharMingen), CD3+/CD8+ (Beckmann-Coulter-Immunotech/Becton Dickinson) and CD3+/CD4-/CD8- T-cells; CD56+/CD3- NK-cells (Becton Dickinson/Beckmann-Coulter-Immunotech); CD19+ B-cells (Becton Dickinson); CD14+ monocytes (Becton Dickinson); CD15+ granulocytes (Beckmann-Coulter-Immunotech) and CD34+ progenitor cells (PharMingen). 500-5000 cells were collected with a median purity of 98%. After DNA-extraction (QIAamp DNA Blood Kit, QIAGEN, Hilden, Germany) of sorted cells STR-PCR for quantitative determination of donor chimerism with subsequent polyacrylamide gel electrophoresis was performed on an ABI377 automatic sequencer with GeneScan™ (Perkin Elmar) software.(see Thiede et. al., Bone Marrow Transplantation 1999, in press).

## Results and Discussion

The majority of patients with non-myeloablative transplantations showed slower kinetics of engraftment compared to standard myeloablative transplantations (Figure 2). The differences were most pronounced in the T-cell subsets and lowest in the B-cells. However, additional factors like cell dose or kind of pretherapy might be important for interindividual differences. This is in keeping with clinical observations. It was observed that with metakine conditioning depletion of recipient cells and expansion of donor cells are over-

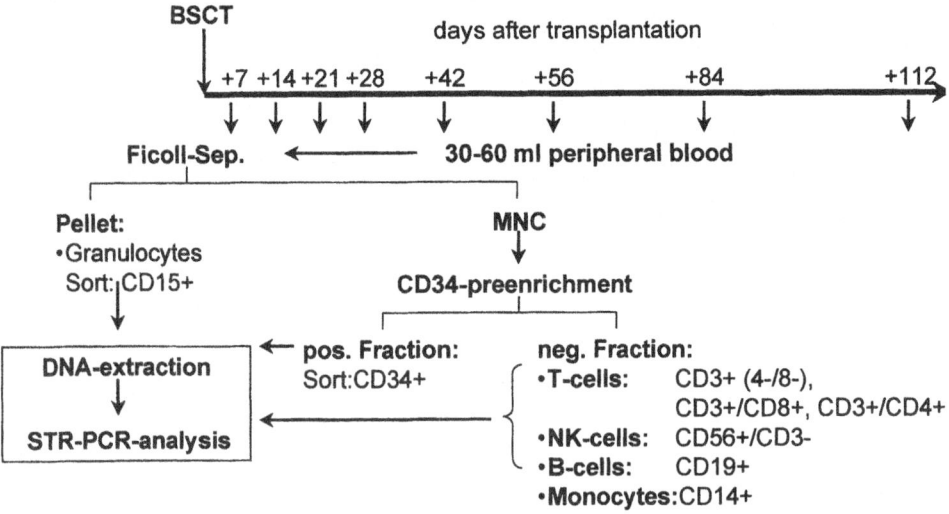

Fig. 1. The flow sheath explains the study design and processing of patients blood samples.

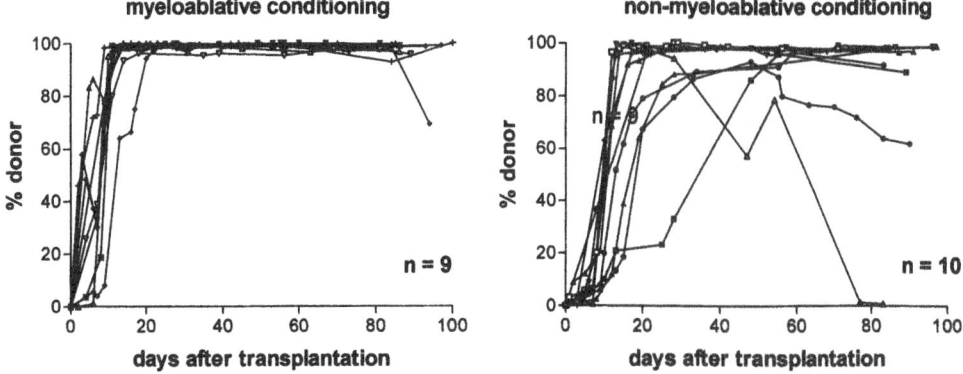

**Fig. 2.** The two diagrams depict the difference between chimerism development in the myeloablative versus the non-myeloablative (metakine) transplanted patients.

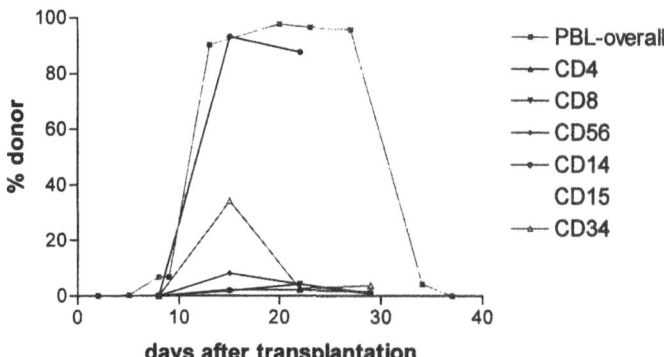

**Fig. 3.** This figure illustrates the analysis of cellular subsets in a patient with graft failure. The patient shown here had an metakine allogeneic BCST for refractory ALL.

lapping events so that the period of neutropenia and thrombocytopenia is much shorter than with standard myeloablative therapy.

Rapid development of T-cell chimerism was associated with grade II-III GVHD in two patients. A patient (NMA-group) developed grade III GvHD at day 84, the same time when the T-cells reached 100% donor chimerism. Therefore we conclude that rapid T-cell chimerism can be associated with acute GvHD, but is not necessarily associated with this complication. Delayed development of complete T-cell chimerism is not sufficient to induce tolerance.

Profound differences can be found in chimerism of cellular subpopulations in case of early graft failure as depicted in Figure 3. Monocytes and granulocytes in this patient showed almost complete chimerism within a short time and therefore overall chimerism analysis reveals high donor chimerism. But T-cell and NK-cell analysis were almost exclusively of recipient origin. CD34 progenitor cells showed a little increase in donor chimerism and a subsequent drop to almost zero in spite of persisting high overall donor chimerism. Some days later overall chimerism dropped as a consequence of declining chimerism in granulocytes and monocytes. At the same time the graft failure became obvious.

In all patients with engraftment, complete donor NK-cell chimerism developed rapidly. These results are in keeping with other observations (Gyger et al., Exp. Hematol. 1998). In summary, NK-cell chimerism seems to be important for engraftment, supporting earlier reports from the literature.

CD34-chimerism shows instability in both groups. More patients and longer follow up is needed to assess the relevance of these findings for patient outcome.

# Somnolence Syndrome after Total Body Irradiation in Children with Bone Marrow Transplantation

U. Zimmermann*, J. Hermann, D. Fuchs and F. Zintl

## Summary

The somnolence syndrome is a transient cerebral disorder well-known in children with acute leukemia after prophylactic cranial irradiation. In 1986 we observed identical clinical symptoms in a patient after bone marrow tranplantation (BMT). The aim of the study was to identify the frequency and symptoms of somnolence syndrome in children after BMT.

Between 1980 and 1995, 200 children were transplanted at the pediatric center of BMT at the University of Jena. Ninety of 200 children received total body irradiation and chemotherapy, 91 of 200 children were treated with chemotherapy and additional prophylactic cranial irradiation. In 19 of 200 children conditioning regimen consisted of total nodal irradiation and chemotherapy. Following BMT, 25 of 200 children developed a somnolence syndrome. Twenty-three of these were conditioned with total body irradiation and chemotherapy, whereas 2 children received chemotherapy and additional prophylactic cranial irradiation. No child with total nodal irradiation developed a somnolence syndrome. The somnolence syndrome occurred 33.8 days $\pm$ 8.1 SD (range 14 to 50 days) after BMT. Somnolence and fever were the predominant symptoms. Fever occurred in 88% of the patients and somnolence in 68% of the patients, respectively. Other frequent symptoms were irritability, nausea and vomiting, headache and anorexia. The symptoms lasted for 6.2 days $\pm$ 4.2 SD (range 1 to 14 days) and disappeared spontaneously or after therapy with dexamethasone. The EEG of these children showed uniform but unspecific abnormal activity, characterized by decreased electroencephalographic background frequencies. There was no evidence for bacterial or viral infections.

The somnolence syndrome is a temporary cerebral disorder possibly caused by elevated intracranial pressure due to irradiation of the central nervous system. Up to now, precise pathophysiological or histopathological causes are not known. It is more frequent in children than in adults. It is an important differential diagnosis in irradiated patients after BMT who develop fever about 4 weeks after transplantation. There is no evidence for neuropsychological long term sequelae.

## Introduction

Firstly, Druckmann [8] observed a syndrome associated with strong drowsinesss, apathy, anorexia and headache in 30 out of 1100 children treated for ringworm of the scalp by irradiation with X-rays. The symptoms occurred within 6 to 8 weeks after cranial irradiation and persisted for 4 to 14 days. They disappeared spontaneously and completely without mental or physical sequelae [8].

In 1970, prophylactic central nervous system (CNS) irradiation was introduced as part of treatment of acute lymphoblastic leukemia in children. Its purpose was to eradicate residual CNS leukemia [17]. Since this time the same symptoms as described by Druckmann [8] have been observed again and were called somnolence syndrome. Now the somnolence syndrome is a well-known and common neurologic complication after prophylactic craniospinal irraditon given to

---

University of Jena, Department of Pediatrics and *Department of Internal Medicine II Jena, Germany

prevent meningeosis in children with acute leukemia [9].

Up to now, there are only three reports of somnolence syndrome after bone marrow transplantation (BMT). Firstly, Daute et al. [6] studied the EEG changes in children with somnolence syndrome after BMT at the Department of Pediatrics of the Universitiy of Jena. Goldberg et al. [10] published a case report of an adult women. Christie et al. [5] described the occurrence of the somnolence syndrome in children after BMT, too.

Therefore, the aim of our retrospective study was to identify the frequency and symptoms of somnolence syndrome after BMT at the Department of Pediatrics of the Universitiy of Jena since 1980.

## Patients and methods

From October 1980 to February 1995, 200 children with different hematologic and oncologic malignancies were transplanted at the centre of BMT for children at the University of Jena. Among them, there were 128 boys and 72 girls (aged 8.5 years, range, 0.3 to 40.3 years). Eightee-five patients received autologous and 115 patients allogeneic BMT.

For conditioning, patients were treated with a combination of cytostatic drugs and irradiation. Additional cranial irradiation was given as part of central nervous system prophylaxis in children with leukemia. Ninety of 200 children received total body irradiation and chemotherapy and 91 of 200 children chemotherapy and additional prophylactic cranial irradiation. Moreover, 19 children were treated with total nodal irradiation and chemotherapy without cranial irradiation. Total body irradiation was given as a single dose of 10 Gy one day before BMT or fractionated with a dose of 6 fractions of 2 Gy. Total nodal irradiation was administered with 7.5 Gy.

The cumulative dose of cranial irradiation consisted of: prophylactic cranial irradiation as a part of primary therapy after diagnosis, boost irradiation before BMT and the total body irradiation.

The following clinical data were recorded: occurrence of fever, somnolence, irritability, anorexia, nausea, vomiting and headache;

beginning and duration of the symptoms; diagnostic parameters (EEG-findings); therapy of somnolence syndrome and occurrence of bacterial, fungal and viral infections, especially infections with cytomegalovirus.

## Statistical analysis

Statistical analysis was performed using the Statistical Package for Social Science (SPSS). The data were expressed as mean ± standard deviation (SD). If the distribution of these variables differed substantially from the normal, they were expressed as medians. For comparisons the U-Test of Mann-Withney and Fisher's exact test were used. Significance was defined at the 0.05 level.

## Results

Following BMT, 25 out of 200 children developed a somnolence syndrome. Among them, there were 13 boys and 12 girls aged 2 to 16 years (mean 8.0 years ± 3.9 SD). Seventeen patients underwent autologous and 8 patients received allogeneic BMT. The diagnoses of patients are shown in Table 1.

**Table 1.** Diagnoses of patients

| Diagnosis | Number of patients |
|---|---|
| Acute lymphoblastic leukemia | 13 |
| Acute myeloid leukemia | 6 |
| Neuroblastoma | 2 |
| Non Hodgkin's lymphoma | 2 |
| Chronic myeloid leukemia | 1 |
| Primitive neuroectodermal tumor | 1 |
| Patients with somnolence syndrome | 25 |

## Conditioning regimens

Twenty-three of the 25 children with somnolence syndrome were conditioned with total body irradiation and chemotherapy. One patient received total body irradiation as a single dose of 10 Gy. In 22 patients it was administered fractionated with a dose of 12 Gy. In 17 of these children boost irradiation of the CNS was applied before beginning of the total body irradiation.

Two children received chemotherapy and prophylactic cranial irradiation. Both children were irradiated prophylactically during primary therapy after diagnosis and with a 6 Gy boost before BMT.

No child of the 19 children with total nodal irradiation without cranial irradiation developed somnolence syndrome.

The cumulative dose of cranial irradiation of patients with total body irradiation and patients with additional cranial irradiation is shown in Figures 1 and 2. For comparison we used the cumulative dose of cranial irradiation of patients without somnolence syndrome.

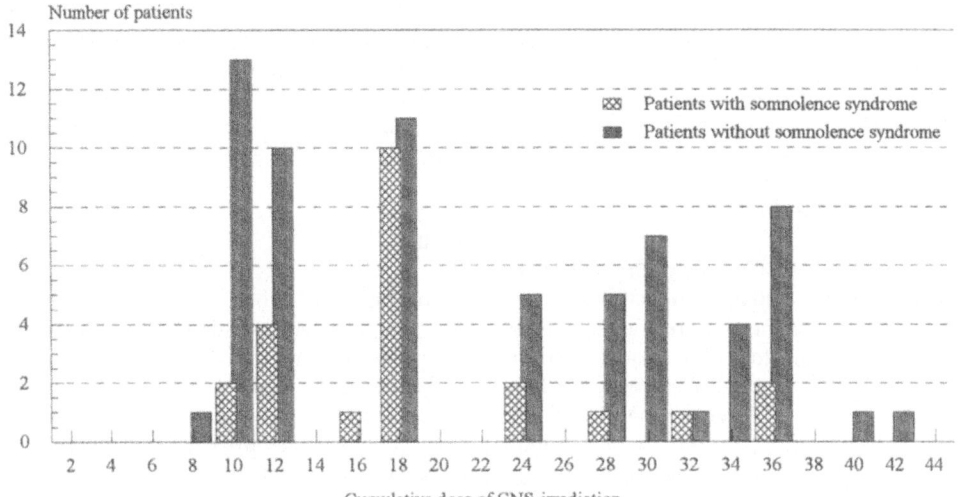

**Fig. 1.** Cumulative CNS doses of patients with total body irradiation and chemotherapy (n=90). It was distinguished between patients with and without somnolence syndrome (p=0.52).

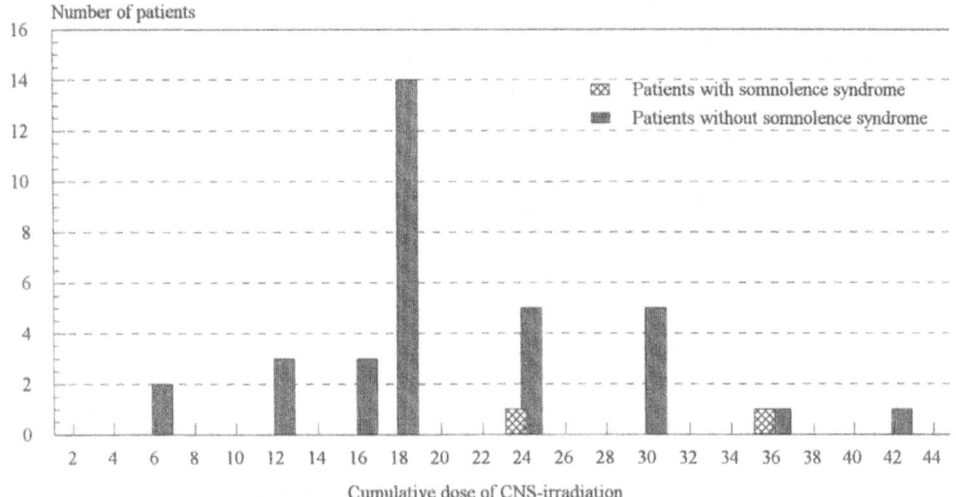

**Fig. 2.** Cumulative CNS doses of patients with chemotherapy and additional cranial irradiation (n=91). It was distinguished between patients with and without somnolence syndrome (p=0.01).

### Symptoms, beginning and duration of somnolence syndrome

The following symptoms were found: in 88% of the patients fever over 38°C, in 68% somnolence, in 56% psychical irritability, in 56% nausea and vomiting, in 16% headache and in 4% anorexia.

Fever and somnolence were the predominant and first symptoms. In the mean, fever of 38.8 °C ± 0.5 SD (maximum 40.0 °C) occurred and lasted between 2 and 6 days. The somn-

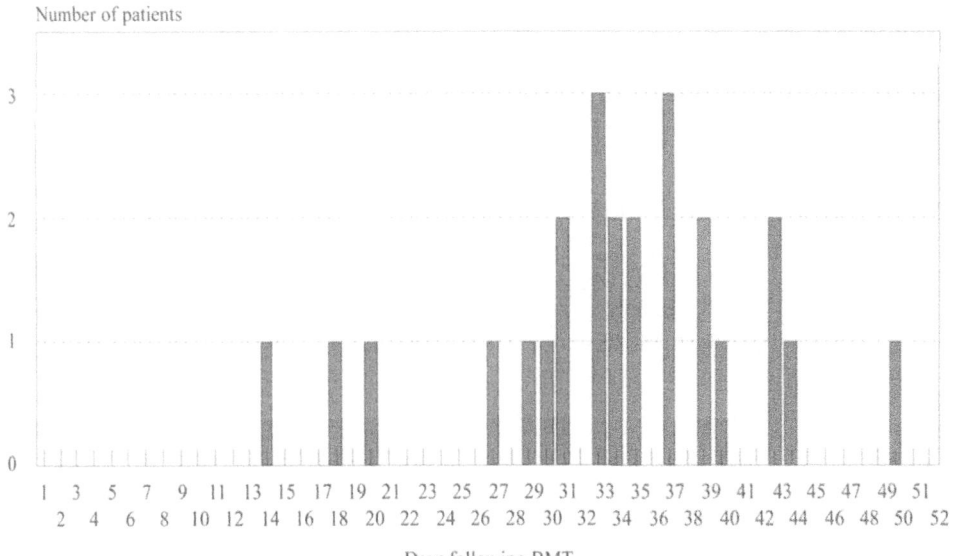

**Fig. 3.** Onset of the somnolence syndrome in 25 patients after BMT.

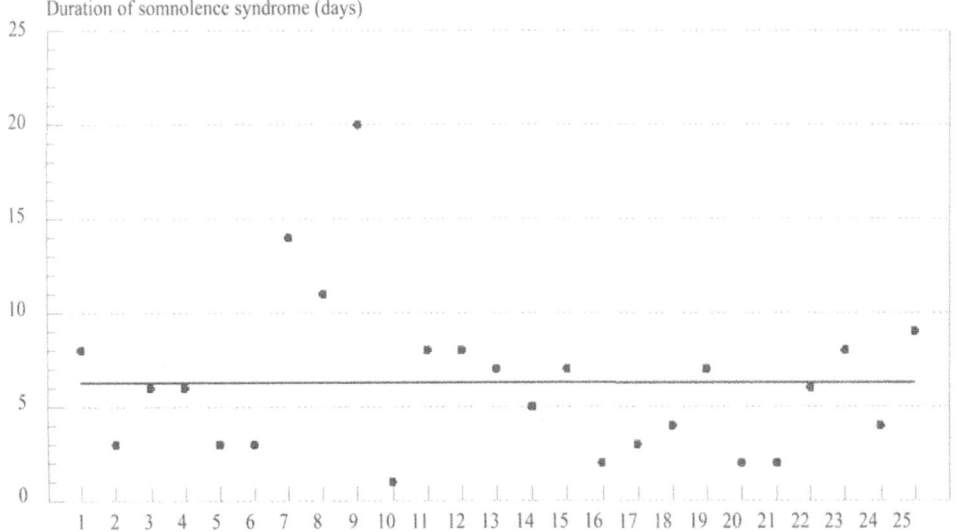

**Fig. 4.** Duration of symptoms in patients with somnolence syndrome.

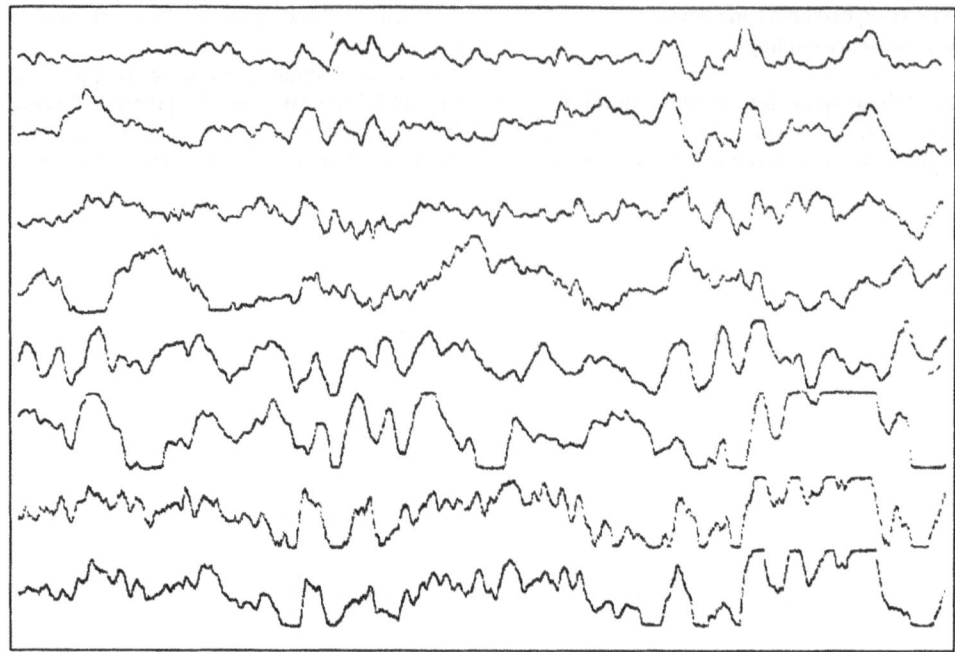

**Fig. 5.** EEG-findings of eight years old boy with T-cell-lymphoma. The EEG was performed +51 days after BMT. The boy was drowsy, tearful and intolerable. The EEG shows a severe generalized decrease of background frequencies.

olence varied from mild drowsiness to prolonged periods of sleep. In most cases a combination of different symptoms was found. The symptoms appeared between 14 and 50 days (mean 33.8 days ± 8.1 SD) after BMT (Figure 3) and lasted from one to 20 days (median 6.0), (Figure 4). In one girl somnolence syndrome lasted for 20 days and was followed by graft versus host disease.

### EEG-findings as diagnostic parameters

Before BMT and during the somnolent phase in all children an EEG was performed. It was repeated after full recovery.

Uniform but non specific EEG changes occurred in 22 of 25 children with somnolence syndrome (Figure 5). The most frequent finding was a generalized decrease of electroencephalographic background frequencies (12 of 25 patients). Between normal waves the following activities were found: an alpha-rhythm between 6 and 9 Hz, a slow theta-activity between 3 and 6 Hz and a delta-activity between 2 and 3 Hz.

There were no differences between the two hemispheres and there was no evidence for a local change. Moreover, there were no spikes.

### Therapy of somnolence syndrome

The therapy of the somnolence syndrome consisted of corticosteroids (dexamethasone) as monotherapy. The duration of the therapy with dexamethasone depended on the clinical symptoms of the patients. Table 2 shows an overview of the doses of dexamethasone, duration of the therapy and duration of the somnolence syndrome after onset of therapy. Using this therapy the symptoms of patients resolved rapidly. Eight patients improved within one day. In 3 patients the symptoms disappeared spontaneously without any therapy.

In 10 patients the decrease of electroencephalographic background frequencies normalized.

**Table 2.** Therapy of somnolence syndrome

| | Dose of dexamethasone mg / day | | Duration of therapy with dexamethasone in days | Duration of somnolence syndrome after beginning of therapy |
|---|---|---|---|---|
| | single dose | dose / day | | |
| Patient 1 | 3 x 4 | 12 | 26 | 5 |
| Patient 2 | 4 x 2 | 8 | 17 | 6 |
| Patient 3 | 4 x 3 | 12 | 14 | 1 |
| Patient 4 | 1 x 8 | 8 | 23 | 4 |
| Patient 5 | 1 x 4 | 4 | 14 | 1 |
| Patient 6 | 4 x 4 | 16 | 15 | 3 |
| Patient 7 | 4 x 4 | 16 | 14 | 6 |
| Patient 8 | 1 x 3 | 3 | 4 | 1 |
| Patient 9 | 3 x 6 | 18 | not evaluated | not evaluated |
| Patient 10 | 3 x 4.5 | 13.5 | not evaluated | 3 |
| Patient 11 | 2 x 4.5 | 9 | not evaluated | 2 |
| Patient 12 | 4 x 4 | 16 | not evaluated | 7 |
| Patient 13 | no therapy | | | |
| Patient 14 | 1 x 7 | 7 | 10 | 1 |
| Patient 15 | 3 x 4 | 12 | 11 | 3 |
| Patient 16 | 1 x 8 | 8 | 9 | 1 |
| Patient 17 | 1 x 6 | 6 | 15 | 1 |
| Patient 18 | no therapy | | | |
| Patient 19 | 1 x 8 | 8 | 24 | 1 |
| Patient 20 | 4 x 4 | 16 | not evaluated | 2 |
| Patient 21 | 3 x 7.5 | 22.5 | 18 | 1 |
| Patient 22 | 3 x 4 | 12 | 12 | 6 |
| Patient 23 | 3 x 4.5 | 13.5 | not evaluated | 7 |
| Patient 24 | 2 x 4 | 8 | not evaluated | 3 |
| Patient 25 | no therapy | | | |
| Mean | | 11.2 ± 4.8 | 15 ± 5.9 | 3 ± 2.2 |

**Table 3.** CMV-antibody titers

| | Days after BMT | Anti-CMV-Ig G | Anti-CMV-Ig M | CMV-early-antigen |
|---|---|---|---|---|
| Patient 1 | + 1 | 1 : 2500 | 1 : 40 | |
| Patient 2 | + 1 | 1 : 2500 | 1 : 320 | 1 : 320 |
| Patient 3 | + 1 | 1 : 40000 | 1 : 40 | 1 : 320 |
| Patient 4 | + 75 | 1 : 2500 | 1 : 40 | |

## Infections as differential diagnosis of somnolence syndrome

In order to exclude bacterial, fungal or viral infections blood and urine samples were analyzed. In addition, X-ray of the thorax was performed. In two children, pseudomonas aeruginosa and streptococcus were found in the urine. No patient had an evidence for inflammation or sepsis and there was no association with the somnolence syndrome.

In 4 of 25 patients with somnolence syndrome primary infections with cytomegalovirus (CMV) were observed. A primary infection was defined as an increase of anti-CMV-IgG and anti-CMV-IgM following seronegativity prior BMT. In 3 patients, increased anti-CMV antibody titers were detected one day after BMT. In the other patient, anti-CMV antibody titers increased on day + 75 after BMT (Table 3). In all four children no correlation could be observed between CMV infection and onset of somnolence syndrome.

## Discussion

Since the application of prophylactic central nervous system irradiation as an important part of the treatment of acute lymphoblastic leukemia in children the somnolence syndrome is well-known and often described [9]. The data about the incidence of somnolence syndrome after CNS irradiation are very different. Freeman et al. [9] reported an incidence of somnolence syndrome of 79% in 28 patients. Hustu et al. [11] found an incidence of 10% in 298 patients and Zippel et al. [21] of 66% in 50 patients, respectively.

Surprisingly, the only reports of somnolence syndrome after BMT are published by Daute et al. [6], Goldberg et al. [10] and Christie et al. [5]. Christie et al. [5] reported an incidence of somnolence syndrome of 64% after prophylactic cranial irradiation and of 25% after total body irradiation in 14 patients.

In contrast to the studies of Christie et al. [5] in the present trial the somnolence syndrome was mainly found following total body irradiation and chemotherapy. Only in two children the somnolence syndrome occurred after chemotherapy and additional cranial irradiation.

According to our data the somnolence syndrome is the consequence of irradiation of the CNS as a part of total body irradiation or the additional cranial irradiation. In the group of patients with total nodal irradiation without cranial irradiation no child developed a somnolence syndrome. There was no association between the cumulative dose of cranial irradiation and the occurrence of the somnolence syndrome in patients conditioned with total body irradiation. But there was an association between the cumulative dose of cranial irradiation and the occurrence of the somnolence syndrome in patients with chemotherapy and additional cranial irradiation.

The clinical symptoms in our children are comparable to the observation of Freeman et al. [9] and Terheggen et al. [18]. However, there are differences in the frequencies of various symptoms. In some studies the somnolence was described as the primary symptom [3, 7, 11, 12, 15]. In contrast to our study, the most frequent symptom was fever followed by somnolence and the other symptoms. Because in most cases only one symptom occurred, often the somnolence syndrome was difficult to diagnose.

Littman et al. [13] proposed a system for the severity of the somnolence syndrome.

The beginning of the somnolence syndrome in our children is in agreement with the data of the literature [9, 11, 12, 14, 18]. These authors observed the somnolence syndrome 4 to 6 weeks after the end of the CNS-irradiation. Our results showed the beginning of the somnolence syndrome 5 to 6 weeks after BMT. An earlier or later onset, between 2 and 7 weeks is also possible. The duration of the somnolence syndrome was not comparable with the data of the literature, because our children were treated with dexamethasone. Freeman et al. [9] reported the duration of the somnolence syndrome without therapy between 10 and 38 days. Other periods given by Terheggen et al. [18] were 3 to 49 days or 7 to 14 days [14]. In our children treated with dexamethasone the somnolence syndrome lasted between 6 and 7 days.

Twenty-two patients showed unique but unspecific EEG findings. The most frequent alteration was a generalized decrease of electroencephalographic background frequencies. These changes were also described in patients after prophylactic cranial irradiation [1, 9, 16, 18]. Terheggen et al. [18] and Zippel et al. [21] observed a focal or paroxysmal dysrhythm as well as irregular spikes and waves. We did not find spikes and waves in the EEG's of our patients.

Based on the assumption that the somnolence syndrome occurred due to an elevated intracranial pressure our children were treated with dexamethasone. Parameters demonstrating the success of our therapy were an improvement in clinical symptoms and the disappearance of EEG-alterations. Neither in the reports of Freeman et al.[9] and Terheggen et al. [18] or in the reports of Goldberg et al.[10] and Christie et al. [5] there were data about therapy of somnolence syndrome.

At time of recovery of marrow graft infections are life threatening complications of the patients. Fever which occured in 88% of our patients is the most common clinical manifestation of infection in immunocompromised children [19]. In 23 patients there was no evidence for bacterial, fungal or viral infections. Only in 2 children, at the onset of somnolence syndrome bacteria were found in urine.

The most important infection during the time of somnolence syndrome is the CMV-infection [20]. The somnolence syndrome mostly occurred between day +30 and +40 after BMT and the CMV-infection between +27 and +44 after BMT [20]. In our patients there was no evidence for an active CMV-infection during the somnolent phase.

Up to now precise pathophysiological or histopathological reasons of somnolence syndrome are not known. It is thought to be a result of either myelin dysfunction [9] or direct microvascular damage with possible interruption of cell membrane [14] or a radiation-induced edema of the CNS [3].

The somnolence syndrome is a transient cerebral disorder without any neuropsychological long term sequelae [2, 4].

*Acknowledgement.* The authors thank Dr. Bernd Gruhn and Dr. Ralf Schiel for critically reading this manuscript.

## References

1. Aronson S, Elmquist D, Garwicz S (1974) Somnolence in children with acute leukemia. Br Med J 3 (5926):344
2. Berg RA, Ch'ien LT, Lancaster W, Williams S, Cummins J (1983) Neuropsychological Sequelae of postradiation somnolence syndrome. Dev Behav Pediatr 4(2):103-107
3. Bode U (1982) Nebenwirkungen antineoplastischer Therapie auf das kindliche Nervensystem. Klinische Pädiatrie 194:351-358
4. Ch'ien LT, Aur RJA, Stagner S, Cavallo K, Wood A, Goff J, Pitner S, Hustu HO, Seifert MJ, Simone JV (1980) Long-term neurological implications of somnolence syndrome in children with acute lymphocytic leukemia. Ann Neurol 8:273-277
5. Christie D, Battin M, Leiper AD, Chessells J, Vargha-Khadem F, Neville BGR (1994) Neuropsychological and neurological outcome after relapse of lymphoblastic leukemia. Arch Dis Child 70:275-280
6. Daute KH, Hermann J, Rieger B, John K (1989) Das EEG-Bild des Somnolenzsyndroms nach Ganzkörperbestrahlung zur Knochenmarktransplantation. 5. Symposium für Elektroenzephalographie im Kindesalter:13-16
7. Dritschilo A, Cassady JR, Camitta B, Jaffe N, Furman L, Traggis D (1976) The role of irradiation in central nervous system treatment and prophylaxis for acute lymphoblastic leukemia. Cancer 37:2729-2735
8. Druckmann A (1929) Schlafsucht als Folge der Röntgenbestrahlung. Strahlentherapie 33:382-384
9. Freeman JE, Johnston PGB, Voke JM (1973) Somnolence after prophylactic cranial irradiation in children with acute lymphoblastic leukemia. Br Med J 4:523-525
10. Goldberg SL, Tefferi A, Rummans TA, Chen MG, Solberg LA, Noel P (1992) Post-irradiation somnolence syndrome in an adult patient following allogeneic bone marrow transplantation. Bone marrow tranplantation 9:499-501
11. Hustu H O, Aur R JA, Verzosa MS, Simone JV, Pinkel D (1973) Prevention of central nervous system leukemia by irradiation. Cancer 32:585-597
12. Lampert F (1975) Leukämie im Kindesalter. Medizinische Welt 26(4):133-136
13. Littman P, Rosenstock J, Gale G, Krisch RE, Meadows A, Sather H, Coccia P, DeCamargo B (1984) The somnolence syndrome in leukemic children following reduced daily dose fractions of cranial irradiation. Int J Radiat Oncol Biol Phys 10:1851-1853
14. Mandell LR, Walker RW, Steinherz P, Fuks Z (1989) Reduced incidence of the somnolence syndrome in leukemic children with steroide coverage during prophylactic cranial radiation therapy. Cancer 63:1975-1978
15. Maurer AM, Simone JV (1976)The current status of the treatment of childhood acute lymphoblastic leukemia. Cancer Treatm Rev 3:17-41
16. Ochs J, Mulhern R, Fairclough D, Parvey L, Withaker J, Ch'ien L, Mauer A, Simone J (1991) Comparison of neuropsychologic functioning and clinical indicators of neurotoxicity in long-term survivors of childhood leukemia given cranial radiation or parenteral methotrexate: a prospective study. J Clin Oncol 9(1):145-151
17. Simone J, Aur RJA, Hustu HO, Pinkel D (1972) "Total therapy" studies of acute lymphocytic leukemia in children. Current results and prospects for cure. Cancer 30:1488-1494
18. Terheggen HG, Rado M (1978) Cerebrale Komplikationen der Leukämiebehandlung. I. Das Apathiesyndrom. Monatszeitschrift Kinderheilkunde 126:693-695
19. Viscoli C, Castagnola E, Rogers D (1991) Infections in the compromised child. Bailliere's Clin Haematol 4(2):510-543
20. Wingard JR (1990) Advances in the management of infectious complications after bone marrow transplantation. Bone marrow transplantation 6:371-383
21. Zippel RM, Sack H (1979) Nebenwirkungen und Spätfolgen der kombinierten Strahlen- und Chemotherapie des Gehirnschädels bei Kindern mit akuter Lymphoblastischer Leukämie (ALL). Strahlentherapie 155(3):165-170

# Ten Years of Autologous Stem Cell Transplantation in Acute Leukemia: Single Center Experience in 46 Patients

U. Kaiser, M. Hinz, B. Reckzeh, C. Faoro, G. Zugmaier and M. Wolf

*Abstract.* Autologous stem cell transplantation with subsequent high dose therapy (HDT) is controversial in acute leukemia. We analysed the data of 46 patients (pts) who received autotransplants for acute leukemia in one center, 31 pts.with AML (acute myeloid leukemia), 15 pts with ALL (acute lymphoblastic leukemia). 41 pts (89%) were in CR 1, 5 pts in CR 2 at the time of HDT. We reach the follwing conclusions using a chemotherapy based conditioning regimen:

HDT for acute leukemia is associated with a higher treamtment related mortality than HDT for lymphoma and breast cancer (11% versus 4% versus 3%).

Among AML patients overall survival is 42%, event free survival 32%. All five patients who received tandem transplantations are free of disease after a median observation period of 62 months. Among ALL patients overall survival is 64%, event free survival 36%.

HDT with cyclophosphamide, etoposide and cytarabine is feasible, however with a considerable relapse rate. Tandem transplantation may improve results.

## Introduction

Autologous stem cell transplantation after high dose therapy (HDT) has evolved as one treatment option in pts with acute leukemia besides conventional therapy and allogeneic stem cell trans-plantation.

In ALL several non-randomized studies have been performed that evaluated autologus bone marrow transplantation (ABMT) in first CR [1-3]. An analysis of 15 studies with more than 1000 pts who were tranplanted in 1.CR revealed the relapse probability to be 27-68%, the leukemia-free survival 15-65% [4]. Hence, it is not yet established if autologous stem cell transplantation can extend survival for patients who cannot be cured by chemotherapy alone.

ABMT has been widely used as a means of consolidation therapy for patients with AML in first remission. Registry data and numerous single center studies suggest an expected survival of 45 to 55% [5]. However, mortality rates up to 15% have been reported.

We reviewed the long term results of 46 pts treated with autolo-gous stem cell transplantation for acute leukemia in one center.

## Material and Methods

Between 1987 and 1998 autologous stem cell transplantations were performed in 46 patients with acute leukemia, among them 31 pts with AML, 15 pts with ALL.

Pts with **AML** were diagnosed with the follwing subtypes according to the FAB classification : M1 (n=2), M2 (n=8), M4 (n=14), M5 (n=7). Median age was 47 years (24-63). 15 pts were female, 16 male. Clinical characteristics of the patients are listed in Table 1. Induction therapy was either the combination of idarubicin and cyto-sine arabinoside [6] or daunorubicine, 6-thioguanine and cytosine arabinoside [7]. Patients reaching complete remission after the first induction course received the same course as reinduction before the autotransplantation. Patients who reached complete remission after the second course received a consolidation with high

Abt. Hämatologie/Onkologie, Philipps-Universität Marburg, Baldinger Str., 35033 Marburg

**Table 1.** clinical characteristics of pts with AML

| induction therapy | n | % |
|---|---|---|
| IDA/ARA C | 14 | 45 |
| TAD | 15 | 48 |
| hAM | 2 | 6 |
| **cycles prior to HDT** | | |
| 2 cycles | 19 | 61 |
| ≥ 3 cycles | 12 | 39 |
| **status prior to HDT** | | |
| CR 1 | 28 | 90 |
| CR 2 | 3 | 10 |
| **HDT** | | |
| ABMT | 29 | 94 |
| PSCT | 1 | 3 |
| ABMT + PSCT | 1 | 3 |

Clinical characteristics of pts with ALL

| status prior to HDT | n | % |
|---|---|---|
| CR 1 | 13 | 86 |
| CR 2 | 2 | 14 |
| **HDT** | | |
| ABMT | 5 | 36 |
| PSCT | 10 | 64 |

dose cytarabine/mitoxantrone (cumulative dose of 24 g cytarabine). Conditioning regimen was CEA (cyclophosphamide 2x60 mg/kg, etoposide 4x700mg/m² and cytarabine 6x 1000mg/m²) in all cases. All but two pts received autologous bone marrow that was harvested prior to the conditioning regimen. No purging procedures were undertaken. Five patients (16%) received tandem transplants (with the same conditioning regimen).

Pts with ALL were diagnosed with the following subtypes: T ALL (n=3), c ALL (n=5), prepreB ALL (n=3), preB ALL (n=3), B ALL (n=1).Median age was 28 years [17-43]. 2 patients were female, 13 male. 11 patients (71%) were classified as high risk, 4 patients (29%) as standard risk (according to cytogenetics, leukocyte counts and achievement of CR). Clinical characteristics of the patients are listed in Table 2. Patients received the standard induction course of the German ALL study group followed by a consolidation course with high dose cytarabine/mitoxantrone (1-3 g/m², generally for 6-8 doses) [8].

In ten pts peripheral stem cells (PSCT) were collected after stimulation with G-CSF 5µg/kg given after the consolidation course. In five pts autologous bone marrow was harvested prior to the high dose regime. In two of these pts prior attempt to collect peripheral stem cells had been unsuccessful. No purging procedures were undertaken. Con-ditioning regimen was CEA in all cases. Two patients received tandem transplantation.

## Results

### AML

Among the pts with AML the time to *neutrophil recovery* (neutro-phils>500/µl ) was 16 days (range 13-57), the time to *platelet recovery* (platelets >20.000/µl) 13.6 days (8->100). G-CSF (300 µg/day) was generally given starting from day 5 after transplan-tation until recovery of neutrophils.

The *treatment related mortality* was 13% (n=4). ARDS, septic shock, VOD and capillary leakage syndrome were the causes.

The *treatment results* were as follows: With a median observation time of 60 months for surviving patients the relapse incidence is 54%, the relapse free survival 32% and the overall survival 42%. Median disease free survival is 11 months, median survival 30 months.Three patients received allogeneic bone marrow trans-plantation for relapse.

### ALL

Among the pts with AML the time to *neutrophil recovery* (neutro-phils>500/µl )

was 13 days (range 10-19), the time to *platelet recovery* (platelets >20.000/µl) 13 days [7-22]. G-CSF (300 µg/day) was generally given starting from day 5 after autologous bone marrow trans-plantaion until recovery of neutrophils, but not after PSCT.

The *treatment related mortality* was 13% (n=2). One patient died of ARDS, one of septic shock. The *treatment results* were as follows: With a median observation time of 50 months for surviving patients the relapse incidence is 54%, the relapse free survival 36% and the overall survival 64%.Median

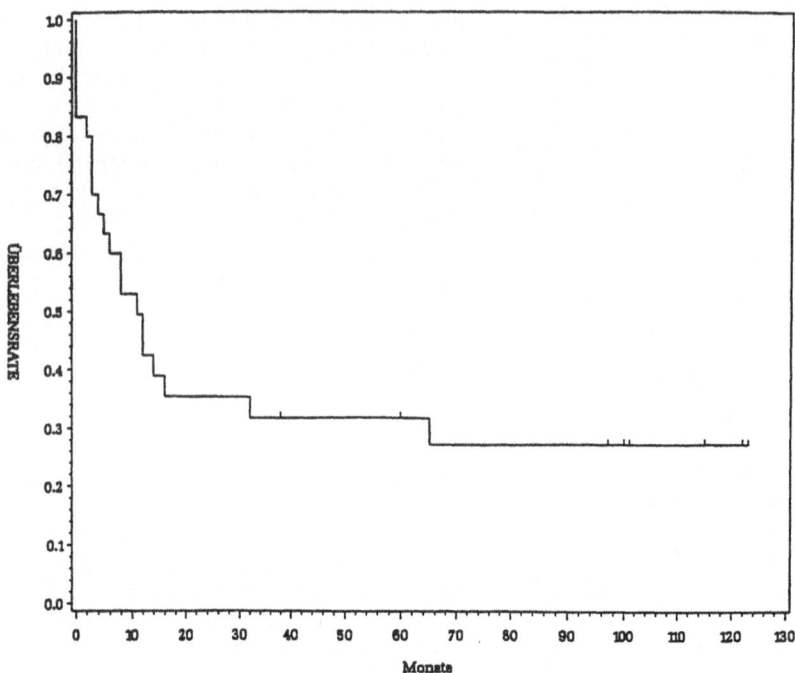

**Fig. 1.** Probability of relapse free survival in pts with AML (n=30) treated with autologous bone marrow transplantation

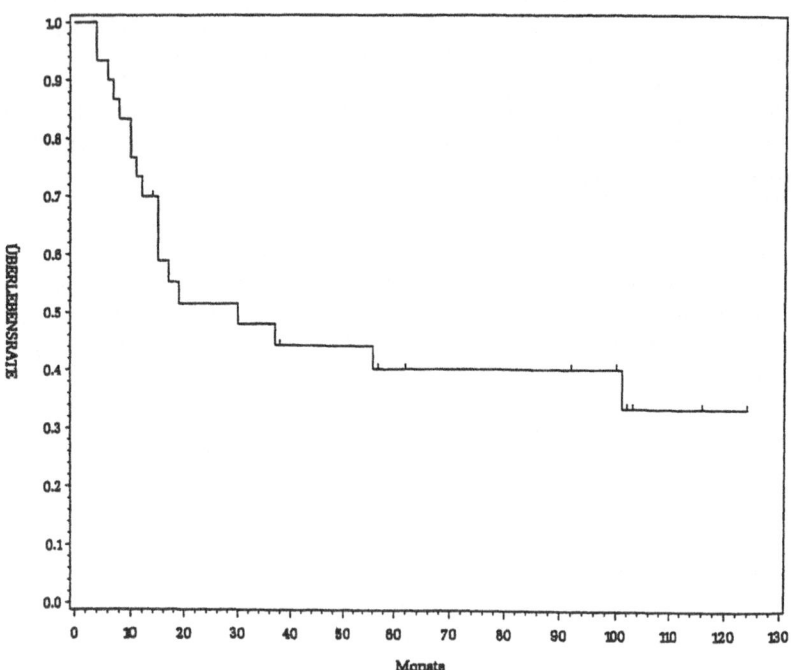

**Fig. 2.** Probability of survival in pts with AML (n=30) treated with autologous bone marrow transplantation

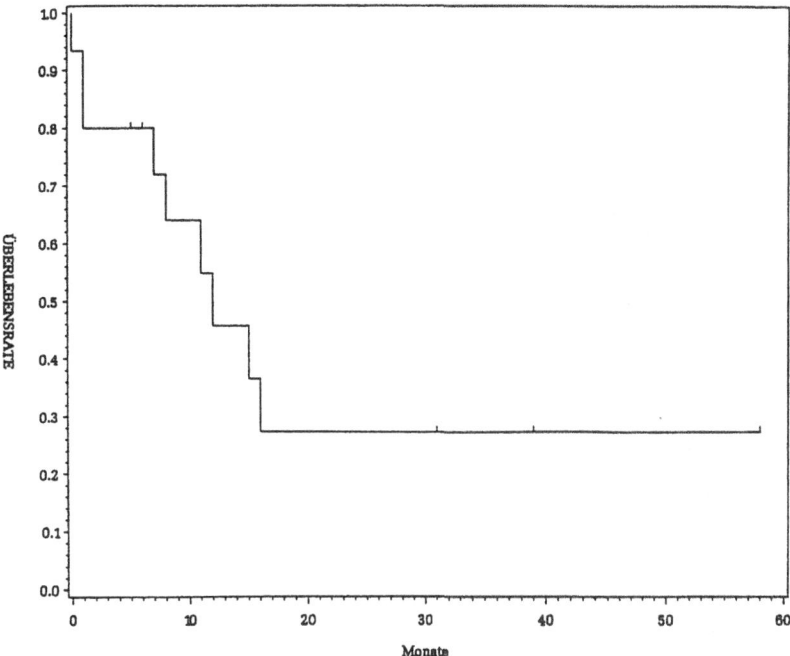

**Fig. 3.** probability of relapse free survival in pts with ALL (n=14) treated with autologous stem cell transplantation

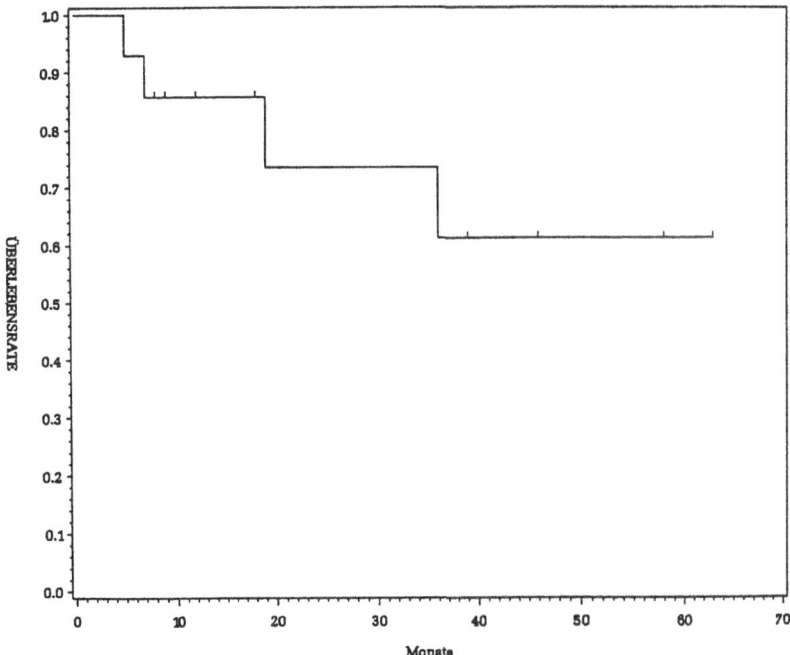

**Fig. 4.** probability of survival in pts with ALL (n=14) treated with autologous stem cell transplantation

disease free survival is 12 months, median survival has not been reached. Three patients received allogeneic bone marrow transplantation for relapse.

## Discussion

Autologous stem cell transplantation for acute myeloid leukemia has been studied in three major randomized trials: In the GOELAM study [9] patients in the ABMT arm received one course of con-solidation after having achieved CR followed by ABMT after cyclophosphamide/busulfan as conditioning regimen. Among the patients who actually received ABMT the 4-years disease free survival was 48% the overall survival 52%. In the MRC AML10 trial [10] patients assigned to ABMT received four courses of intensive chemotherapy prior to ABMT. In the whole trial 205 patients received an autologous BMT (by randomisation or by choice). The disease free survival at 7 years was 53%, the overall survival 58% on an intent to treat basis. In the US intergroup trial [11] patients received one consolidation cycle after having achieved CR. Patients assigned to autologous bone marrow transplantation received myeloablative therapy with busulfan/cyclophosphamide. Disease free survival at four years on an intent to treat basis was 35%. Our results with autologus bone marrow transplantation support the hypothesis that autologous stem cell transplantation may best be used after effective postremission therapy. Early ABMT as the only consolidation regime is associated with a considerable risk of relapse. However, tandem transplantation in pts with CR 1 deserves further notice.

In acute lymphoblastic leukemia autologus stem cell transplan-tation is less well established than in AML. Our results confirm the previous study that suggested a beneficial effect of maintenance therapy after autologous transplantation [12]: all four patients who received maintenance therapy are free of relapse.

In the same time period 33 pts with breast cancer and 81 pts with malignant lymphoma received autologus transplantation with a treatment related mortality of 3%, respective 4%. Treatment re-lated mortality of 11% among all transplants for acute leukemia is considerably higher. Toxicities of the conditioning regimens used as well as intensities of prior chemotherapy are comparable. Our data therefore suggest that the observed higher risk of fatal toxicities in acute leukemia may be associated with the disease itself.

## References

1. Rowe JM. Bone marrow transplantation in first remission. *Leukemia* 11 (Suppl4): 12-14 (1997)
2. Doney K, Buckner CD, Fisher L, Petersen FB, Sanders J, Appelbaum FR et al. Autologous bone marrow transplantation for acute lymphoblastic leukemia. *Bone Marrow Transplantation* 12:315-321 (1993).
3. Vey N, Blaise D, Stoppa AM, Bouabdallah R, Lafage M et al. Bone marrow transplantation in 63 adult patients with acute lymphoblastic leukemia in first complete remission. *Bone Marrow Transplantation* 14:383-388 (1994)
4. Hoelzer D. Acute lymphoblastic leukemia in adults. in: Textbook of malignant Haematology. ed Degos L, Linch DC, Löwenberg B. Martin Dunitz Ltd, London 1998, pp538
5. Gorin NC, Labopin M, Meloni G et al. Autologous bone marrow transplantation for acute myeloid leukemia in Europe: further evidence of the role of marrow purging by mafosfamide. *Leukemia* 5:896-904 (1997)
6. Berman E, Heller G, Santorsa J, McKenzie S, Gee T et al. Results of a randomised trial comparing idarubicin and cytosine arabinoside with daunorubicin and cytosine arabinoside in adult patients with newly diagnosed acute myologenous leukeimia. *Blood* 77:1666-1674 (1991)
7. Büchner T. Acute leukemia. *Curr Opinion Hematol* 1:172-182 (1993)
8. Hoelzer D. Treatment of acute lymphoblastic leulemia. *Semin Hematol* 31:1-15 (1994).
9. Harousseau J-L, Cahn J-Y, Pignon B, Witz F, Milipied N et al. Comparison of autologus bone marrow transplantation and intensive chemotherapy as post-remission therapy in adult acute myeloid leukemia. *Blood* 8:2978-2986 (1997).
10. Burnett AK, Goldstone AH, Stevens RMF, Hann IA, Rees JKH et al. Randomised comparison of addition of autologous bone-marrow transplantation for acute myeloid leukeima in first remission: results of MRC AML 10 trial. *The Lancet* 351:700-708 (1998).
11. Cassileth PA, Harrington DP, Appelbaum FR, Lazarus HM, Rowe JM et al. Chemotherapy compared with autologous or allogeneic bone marrow transplantation in the management of acute myeloid leukemia in first remission. *The New England Journal of Medicine* 339:1649-1656 (1998).
12. Powles R, Mehta J, Singhal S et al. Autologous bone marrow transplantation or peripheral blood stem cell transplantation followed by maintenance chemotherapy for adult acute lymphoblastic leukemia in first remission: 50 cases from a single center. *Bone Marrow Transplantation* 16:241-247 (1995)

# Transplant Characteristics: Minimal Residual Disease and Impaired Megakaryocytic Colony Growth as Sensitive Parameters for Predicting Relapse in Acute Myeloid Leukemia

A. Reichle, G. Rothe, S. Krause, M. Zaiss, H. Ullrich and R. Andreesen

*Abstract.* Dose-escalation during induction and consolidation therapy of de novo AML, including myeloablative chemotherapy supported with autologous peripheral blood stem cell transplantation, continuously improve outcome. Therefore, quality control of transplants is getting increasing interest. We studied leukapheresis products (LPs), consecutively collected during postremission treatment of 20 patients (pts) with de novo AML for minimal residual disease (MRD) by 5-parametric flow cytometry and for myelodysplasia (MDS)-associated alterations, within the non-leukemic hematopoietic progenitor cells (HPCs), by paired lineage-selected colony assays for colony-forming units-megakaryocytes (CFU-mega) and burst-granulocytes-monocytes colony-forming units (CFU) to evaluate the predictive value of these transplant-associated parameters on outcome.

We defined the leukemic immunophenotype at diagnosis and studied the impact of MRD detection in LPs collected after double induction with TAD (thioguanine, daunorubicin, cytarabine) and HAM (mitoxantrone, high-dose cytarabine, n=18 pts) and TAD consolidation treatment (n=20 pts) on relapse-free survival of 19 pts with AML entering morphologically complete remission. The level of MRD in the transplants correlated with the relapse-free survival (RFS) using a cut-off level of 0.1% MRD (p=0.003). Five of 14 pts (35%) with < 0.1% MRD (median 0.02%, range 0.0 to 0.06%) relapsed within 12 months and all 5 pts with >0.1% MRD (median 0.42%, range 0.15 to 0.63 %) within 18 months. By using the same cut-off level a weak correlation could also be demonstrated between MRD in the pregraft bone marrow and RFS (p=0.04). Quantitatively abnormal megakaryocytic colony growth in the back-up LPs collected after dopple-induction and in the transplant LPs was characterized by the ratio CFU-mega/CFU. In the group of relapsing patients the ratio CFU-mega/CFU was significantly lower than in the group of pts with CCR (p= 0.004), both in the back-ups and in the transplants. All patients with CFU-mega/CFU ratios <0.12 relapsed with AML and five of seven pts had a preceding MDS. Using the optimized cut-off level for the ratio CFU mega/CFU (< 0.12), seven of ten relapsing patients (70%) could be identified to be at risk of relapse, whereas MRD in the transplants identified only 50% of the relapses and MRD in the pregraft bone marrow 25%. In conclusion, the study could identify two pretransplant risk-factors predicting relapse in patients with AML receiving aPBSCT in first CR: MRD in transplants as well as MDS-like alterations within the non-leukemic HPCs of the transplants. These results may have multifold implications on the design of risk-adapted chemotherapy as well as on purging techniques and may contribute to a better understanding of leukemogenesis.

## Introduction

Myeloablative chemotherapy combined with autologous peripheral blood stem cell transplantation (aPBSCT) is nowadays a standard therapy of de novo AML in postremission. Analysis of the tranplants in correlation with outcome offers new insights into the biology of the disease. We used 5-parametric flow

From the Department of Hematology and Oncology and the Institute of Clinical Chemistry, University of Regensburg, Germany

cytometry to monitor minimal residual disease (MRD) in transplants and CFU assays to determine lineage-selected colony growth in the transplants [1].

## Material and Methods

### Patients: Patient selection and treatment

Twenty-seven patients aged 15 to 60 years with de novo AML entering consecutively our institution were enrolled in the study protocol on the basis of intent to treat. Diagnosis of AML was made according to French-American-British (FAB) group revised criteria [2]. In none of the patients cytogenetic aberrations at diagnosis were suggestive of a preexisting myelodysplastic syndrome (MDS). Twenty patients (69%) without a HLA-identical sibling who achieved CR after double induction chemotherapy were considered eligible to receive consolidation chemotherapy followed by an intensive postremission chemotherapy with a myeloablative conditioning regimen and aPBSCT. One transplantation-associated death was observed. Nineteen patients were followed over a median time of 35 months (range 13 to 54 months).

Leukemia-specific aberrant immunophenotypes were determined at diagnosis (n=20 pts) and could be followed in the leukapheresis products (LPs) of 20 pts. MRD studies were performed during first morphological CR in all available leukapheresis products (n=30 LPs) following double induction treatment (18 pts), in the transplants (n=46 LPs) collected after TAD consolidation (n= 13 pts) or after an additional mobilization cycle with CY (7 pts), respectively, in the pregraft bone marrow (n= 18 pts) and in the postgraft bone marrow (19 pts), 4 to 10 weeks after aPBSCT when criteria for CR were assessed in the peripheral blood (hemoglobin >10.0g/dl, leukocytes >3.0/nl, platelets >100/nl). Colony growth was studied with paired lineage-selected CFU-mega und CFU assay in 76 LPs of 38 apheresis cycles: following double induction (18 pts) and in the transplants (n= 20 pts) collected during TAD consolidation treatment (n = 13pts) or following CY (n = 7pts). Pregraft follow-up data were reported for 20 pts, transplant-associated characteris-

tics were correlated with the outcome of the 19 pts being available for follow-up. Median relapse-free survival (RFS) was 30 months at 4 years, with the overall survival of 31 months at 4 years.

### Treatment

Double-induction chemotherapy consisted of one cycle TAD, daunorubicin (60 mg/m$^2$ day 1 to 3), AraC (100 mg/m$^2$ day 1 and 2, twice daily 100 mg/m$^2$ day 3 to 8) and thioguanine (twice daily 100 mg/m$^2$ day 3 to 9) and one cycle of HAM, cytarabine (twice daily 3g/m$^2$ day 1 to 3) combined with mitoxantrone (20 mg/m$^2$ day 3 to 5) [3]. When complete remission was achieved, patients received a TAD consolidation cycle. A further mobilization course with 2 g/m$^2$ cyclophosphamide (CY) day 1 was applied when enough CD34 positive cells could not be harvested during HAM and TAD mobilization (n=7 pts). As intensive consolidation therapy, high-dose busulfan (4mg/kg day -9 to -6) combined with CY (60 mg/kg day -5 to -2) was given followed by aPBSCT on day +1 [4]. The median time intervall from first complete remission (CR) to aPBSCT was 8 weeks (range 5 to 12 weeks).

### Stem cell mobilization

G-CSF (Neupogen®) was given after HAM and TAD consolidation chemotherapy to mobilize PBSCs. Daily G-CSF application was started on day 2 after end of chemotherapy (5µg/kg s.c.).

### Harvesting of PBSC

Stem cells were collected with a continous flow blood cell separator, either a Cobe Spectra Apheresis System or a Fenwal CS 3000. During leukapheresis a total volume of 8-12 l at a flow rate of 50-70 ml/min was processed. Leukaphereses were done during recovery following chemotherapy when CD34 counts were >3x10$^3$/ml. Daily leukaphereses were necessary during 1 to 5 subsequent days within a mobilization cycle. A median of 2.0

leukaphereses per mobilization with HAM and TAD consolidation or CY, respectively.

## Cryopreservation, thawing and retransfusion of aPBSC

The apheresis product was mixed with an equal volume of minimal essential medium containing 20% dimethylsulfoxide (DMSO, Merck, Darmstadt, Germany) and immediately transfered into freezing bags and vials containing 1 ml cell suspension (Cryocyte freezing container, Fenwal) and frozen to –100°C with a computer-controlled cryopreservation device (Cryoson BV-6, Cryoson Deutschland GmbH, Schöllkrippen, Germany). The frozen bags and vials were stored in liquid nitrogen at 196°C until use.

The vials for MRD and paired lineage-selected CFU studies were thawed in a 40°C waterbath with addition of 1 ml DNAse stocksolution (final concentration of 3.6 µg/ml) and 8 ml PBS. Before plating mononuclear cells (MNC) of the LPs, cells were subjected to two successive low-speed centrifugations to remove platelets which could be a source of growth inhibiting factors (TNFα and TNFβ) [5,6].

The transplants were thawed in a 40°C waterbath. A mean of $1.33 \times 10^6$ CD34 positive cells per kg (range 0.1 to $2.9 \times 10^6$) and $1.38 \times 10^5$ CFU-GM/kg (range 0.14 to $2.8 \times 10^5$) were retransfused.

## Bone marrow morphology

Bone marrow aspirates were taken after each induction and consolidation cycle and every 3 months, following transplantation. The first posttransplant aspiration was performed directly after peripheral remission parameters were achieved, 4 to 10 weeks after transplantation.

Diagnosis of MDS was made according to typical morphological features [7]. Complete remission (CR) was defined according to the Cancer and Leukemia Group B [8].

## Immunophenotyping at diagnosis and for detection of minimal residual disease

Heparinized bone marrow aspirates for the initial diagnosis were analyzed for antigen coexpression by flow cytometric analysis of 20,000 to 50,000 cells for each of the following double and triple stainings fluorescein isothiocyanate (FITC), R-phycoerythrin (PE), and peridinin chlorophyll (PerCP) or tandem conjugates of PE with indodicarbocyanine (PE/Cy5) with directly fluorochrome-conjugated monoclonal antibodies (MoAB): HLA-DR/CD14/CD45, CD8/CD4/CD3, CD7/CD1a/CD2, CD10/CD5/CD19, CDw65/CD33, CD34/CD13/CD20, CD41/anti-glycophorin A, CD42b/CD15, anti-kappa/anti-lambda/CD19, anti-IgM/CD22, anti-terminal deoxynucleotidyl transferase (TdT)/CD22(CD79a upon availability)/CD3, anti-myeloperoxidase (MPO)/anti-IgM. Individual three-color combinations according to the malignant phenotype were analyzed for the detection of residual disease.

## Staining for cell surface immunofluorescence

For flow cytometric immunophenotyping of surface antigens unseparated bone marrow (100 µl) or apheresis product ($10^6$ cells/100 µl) was incubated for 15 min on ice with saturating concentrations of the fluorochrome-conjugated antibodies. Cells were washed three times (5 min, 425xg) with 3 ml of Dulbecco's phosphate-buffered saline without Ca++ or Mg++ (PBS, Biochrom, Berlin, Germany) prior to incubation with MoAB for staining of surface immunoglobulins. The MoAB CD1a (clone SFCI19Thy1A8), CD10 (J5), CD13 (366), CD14 (RMO52), CD33 (906), CD41 (P2), CD42b (SZ2), anti-glycophorin A (D2.10) and anti-HLA-DR (B8.12.2) were obtained from Coulter-Immunotech (Hamburg, Germany). MoAB against CD3 (SK7), CD4 (SK3), CD5 (L17F12), CD7 (4H9), CD20 (L27), CD22 (S-HCL-1), CD34 (8G12) and CD45 (2D1) were obtained as R-PE or PerCP conjugates from Becton Dickinson (Heidelberg, Germany). MoAB against CD15 (DU-HL60-3) and CD19 (SJ25-C1) were obtained as R-PE conjugates from Sigma (Deisenhofen, Germany). Antibodies against CD2 (G11) and

CD65 (VIM2) were obtained from Caltag (Burlingame, CA, USA). Anti-CD8 (OKT8) antibody, directly conjugated to FITC, was obtained from Ortho (Neckargmünd, Germany). R-PE conjugated anti-CD 79a antibody (HM 57) and FITC and R-PE conjugated rabbit F(ab')2-fragments of anti-human kappa and lambda, resp., immunoglobulin light chains were obtained from Dako (Hamburg, Germany). FITC and R-PE conjugates of goat F(ab')2-fragments of anti-human IgM were from Tago (Burlingame, CA). Anti-myeloperoxidase (H-43-5) was obtained as a FITC conjugate from Fix&Perm (Vienna, Austria) and anti-TdT as a mixture of three different FITC-conjugated MoAB from Supertech (WAK-Chemie Medical, Bad Homburg v.d.H., Germany). After the incubation, blood samples were treated for 10 min with the erythrocyte lysis solution from Becton Dickinson (FACSlyse), then washed twice (5 min, 425xg) with 3 ml of PBS. The cells were then stored on ice in the dark until analysis. Sample preparation and analysis were always performed within 4 hours of venipuncture.

## Staining for intracellular immunofluorescence

For simultaneous flow cytometric analysis of intracellular expression of the triple color combination of TdT, CD22 or CD79a, and CD3 or the dual color combination of anti-MPO and anti-IgM, unseparated bone marrow or apheresis product (50 µl) was first fixed for 5 min at room temperature using a commercial solution (Fix & Perm reagent A, Vienna, Austria). The cells were then washed once with PBS. The pellet was resuspended in 200 µl of a permeabilization medium (Fix & Perm reagent B, Vienna, Austria) and then incubated with saturating concentrations of fluorescent dye conjugated antibodies for 15 min on ice and finally washed with PBS. The cells were then stored on ice in the dark until analysis.

## Flow cytometric analysis

Following staining of the cells, the cellular light scatter signals and three fluorescence signals (20,000 to 50,000 nucleated cells per sample) were analyzed in list mode at 1,024 channel resolution using forward scatter as the trigger parameter on a FACScan flow cytometer (Becton Dickinson). The photomultiplier gains and compensation were adjusted using FITC and R-PE coated microbeads (Becton Dickinson) and peripheral blood lymphocytes triple-stained with antibodies against CD3, CD4, and CD8 as a biological control. Bivariate dot plots were produced for all combinations of the 5-parametric list mode data following pseudo-color coding for typical light scatter regions using CELLQuest (Becton Dickinson) for the visual detection of malignant phenotypes [27]. The percentage of abnormal cells was then calculated following multidimensional gating using Paint-a-Gate Pro software (Becton Dickinson).

## Clonogenic progenitor assay

Colony-forming units (CFU), ie, the total number of mixed colony-forming units (CFU-mix), granulocyte-macrophage colony-forming units (CFU-GM), erythroid burst-forming units (BFU-E) and erythroid colony-forming units (5 CFU-E correspond to 1BFU-E) were evaluated using commercially available media (Methocult H 4431, Stemcell Technologies INC Vancouver, Canada).

Briefly, 1ml aliquots of thawed MNC cells were plated at concentrations of $5x10^4$/ml, in triplicates, in 35 mm culture dishes (Falcon; Becton Dickinson Labware) and incubated at 37°C in a humidified incubator with 7% $CO_2$ and 5% $O_2$. After 14 days of culture the total number of CFUs was counted under an inverted microscope.

Megakaryocytic colony growth from hematopoietic progenitor cells was studied in a serum-free, semisolid collagen containing medium (EASY-MEGATM, Hemeris, Sassenage, France) with the addition of an optimized cytokine cocktail for human megakaryocytic progenitor culture. First, 0.8 ml human purified collagen (final concentration 0.1%) was added to 2.4 ml medium (final concentrations: 1,5% bovine serum albumin, 2mM L-glutamin, 100 µM 2 b mercaptoethanol, 0,1 mM Na pyruvate, 250 µM CaCl2, 4% lipid mixture, 10 µg/ml bovine pancreatic insulin, 300 μg/ml human transferrin in Iscoove's modified Dulbecco's Medium) and immediately vortexed. Finally, 20μl cell suspension, 20 μl RPMI and 60 μl cytokine cocktail (rhIL3 2.5 ng/ml, rhIL 6 10 ng/ml, R&D Systems, Abingdon, UK, rh MGDF 50 ng/ml, kindly provided by AMGEN) were added. After mixing, the solution was dispensed rapidly in three 35mm non-treated culture Petri dishes at 1 ml per dish. The gels were cultured for 14 days at 37°C in a humidified incubator with 7% CO2 and 5% O2.

Additional paired analysis were done with LPs collected from patients without bone marrow involvement of their malignant disease (n=10), receiving chemotherapy for the first time to validate the CFU-mega assay (control group). To exclude a significant impact of MRD on the lineage selection potential of normal hematopoietic progenitor cells, back-up leukapheresis samples of patients without detectable MRD in LPs and in CCR were mixed with 0.1 to 0.5% autologous leukemic blast cells for in vitro culture (paired lineage-selected colony assays).

For gel-dehydration and immunochemistry the gel was released from the culture dish with a plastic pipet. The culture dish was then covered with a glass slide and turned up side down. While shaking gently the gel slipped out of the culture dish and spread out on the slide. Afterwards a nylon sifting fabric was put on the gel (Serynel, NYHC, 37mm) and a blotting paper 3 mm (CW Whatman). For gentle pressing purpose a glass slide was applied. After removing blotting paper and nylon sifting fabric the collagen film was air dried. Slides were either stained immediately or stored dried and unfixed at –20°C until staining.

For staining, gels were fixed at room temperature with methanol-aceton for 5 minutes and subsequently incubated first with anti-CD41 MoAB (Hemeris, Sassenage, France) or an irrelevant control antibody (Dako, Glostrup, Denmark) and than with 300 μl diluted APAAP complex (Dianova, Hamburg, Germany) per slide for 30 minutes at room temperature. Finally, 400 μl alkaline phosphatase substrate (Dianova, Hamburg, Germany) per slide was added and incubated at room temperature for 20 minutes.

After staining gels were washed in PBS and counterstained with Mayer's Hematoxylin for 30 seconds. Colonies were evaluated by microscopy.

CFU-mega., ie, colonies of 5 to 20 CD41+ cells and BFU-mega, ie, colonies of >20 cells were evaluated after 14 days of culture. The ratio of BFU-mega to CFU-mega was relatively constant throughout our study (1 BFU-mega on 5 to 12 CFU-mega). Therefore, the number of total CFU-mega is reported as the sum of BFU-mega and CFU-mega. The ratio of CFU-mega and CFU was calculated to document changes in the proportion of clonogenic MPs in the LPs and to correct for the decreasing clonogenicity within consecutive apheresis cycles.

## Statistical methods

Kaplan-Meier life-tables were constructed for relapse-free survival and overall survival. Relapse-free survival for MRD positive and negative groups were compared by means of a one-sided log- rank test with surviving patients (actual follow-up).

The Mann-Whitney test (two-sided) was used to analyze the CFU mega/CFU ratio in the relapsing group, the survivors and the control group

## Results

### Phenotype of blast cell population

At diagnosis an aberrant leukemia-specific immunophenotype, as described by San Miguel et al [10], could be identified in 18 of 20 cases (90%). Two cases displayed immunophenotypes also found in low frequency within normal subpopulation of progenitor cells, however, expressed an aberrant light scatter and therefore be included in flow cytometric MRD analysis. The aberrant immunophenotypes are listed in Table 1. Cross-lineage antigen expression was detected in 11 cases (TdT, CD7, CD5, CD22, CD79a), antigen overexpression in 10 cases (CD4, CD 33, CD 34, CD 65, HLA-DR), antigen underexpression in 3 cases (CD 45), asynchronous coexpression of antigens in 7 cases (CD 33/CD65, CD13/CD34, CD13/ CD45, CD4/ CD45) and an aberrant light scatter in 6 cases

**Table 1.** Distribution of leukemia-associated phenotypes

| Leukemia-asociated phenotypes | No. of cases | % |
|---|---|---|
| **Crosslineage antigen expression (n=11)** | | |
| CD22/TdT | 1 | |
| CD7/TdT | 1 | |
| TdT | 3 | 55% |
| CD7 | 3 | |
| CD5 | 1 | |
| CD5/CD7 cyCD22/TdT | 1 | |
| cyCD79a/TdT | 1 | |
| | | |
| **Antigen overxpression (n=10)** | | |
| CD34 | 3 | |
| CD33 | 1 | |
| CD4 | 1 | |
| CD65/HLA-DR | 1 | |
| CD14/CD65 | 1 | 50% |
| CD4/CD65/HLA-DR | 1 | |
| CD34/HLA-DR | 1 | |
| CD4/CD34/HLA-DR | 1 | |
| | | |
| **Antigen underexpression (n=3)** | | |
| CD45 | | 15% |
| | | |
| **Aberrant light scatter (n=6)** | | |
| FSC high/ CD45 high/CD4+/HLA-DR | 1 | |
| SSC high/HLA-DR+ | 1 | |
| SSC low/ CD4 high | 1 | 30% |
| SSC high/CD14+/HLA-DR+ | 1 | |
| SSC high/CD45low | 1 | |
| SSC high/CD45 low/HLA-DR+ | 1 | |
| | | |
| **Asynchronous antigen expression (n=7)** | | |
| CD45 low/CD4 high | 1 | |
| CD33 high/CD65 high | 1 | 35% |
| CD33 low/CD65 high | 2 | |
| CD33 low/CD13 high | 1 | |
| CD33-/CD65+ | 1 | |
| CD13 high/CD34+ | 1 | |

(Table 1). In 13 of 20 patients (65%) two or three criteria could be used for the definition of the aberrant leukemia-associated phenotype.

## Detection of minimal residual disease and outcome

Residual blast cells were detected within a total number of 28 LPs (92%) collected during 15 mobilization cycles. The median number of residual leukemic cells within the LPs was $5.2 \times 10^{-3}$ (range $0.6 \times 10^{-3}$ to $27 \times 10^{-3}$), following HAM $8.4 \times 10^{-3}$ (range $1.6 \times 10^{-3}$ to $27 \times 10^{-3}$) and significantly less in the transplants collected following TAD or CY $3.2 \times 10^{-3}$ (range $4 \times 10^{-3}$ to $6.3 \times 10^{-3}$, p<0.02).

For further analysis of outcome we defined a threshold of $1 \times 10^{-3}$ residual blast cells as the median number of residual blast cells within consecutively collected LPs of a mobilization cycle. Using this cut-off level, the transplants of 15 pts (75%) with a median number of $1 \times 10^{-4}$ residual leukemic cells (range not detectable to $6 \times 10^{-4}$) were estimated MRD negative and the transplants of 5 pts (25%) with a median number of $4.2 \times 10^{-3}$ residual leukemic cells (range $1.5 \times 10^{-3}$ to $6.3 \times 10^{-3}$) were defined as MRD positive.

MRD positive cases (>$1 \times 10^{-3}$ residual leukemia cells) were more freqently observed following TAD consolidation (5 of 20, 25%) than following HAM (3 of 18, 17%). In four cases residual leukemia cells were primarily detected in the transplants but not in the corresponding back-up LPs following HAM. Two of these four patients with detectable residual blast cells in the transplant had levels of >$1 \times 10^{-3}$ residual leukemia cells and relapsed, the other two patients with levels <$1 \times 10^{-3}$ are still in continous CR (CCR).

Incidence of relapse and RFS correlated with the number of residual leukemic cells in the transplants. RFS was not correlated with the time interval between first CR and aPB-SCT. This interval was variable due to additional mobilization cycles with Cy (n=7) or the entrance of CR following TAD or HAM. In the group with less than $1 \times 10^{-3}$ residual cells 5 of 14 patients (35%) relapsed and in the group with >$1 \times 10^{-3}$ of residual leukemia cells all 5 pts relapsed (100%), with a corresponding median relapse-free survival for the MRD positive group of 6 months. The median survival of the MRD negative group has not been reached (p=0.003) (Fig.1). The diagnostic sensitivity and specifity to detect patients at risk of relapse by the leukemia-associated immunophenotype was 50% and 100%, respectively.

To determine the most suitable stem cell source to detect MRD by 5-parametric flow cytometry we compared the frequency and number of residual leukemia cells in the pre-transplant bone marrow and in the corre-

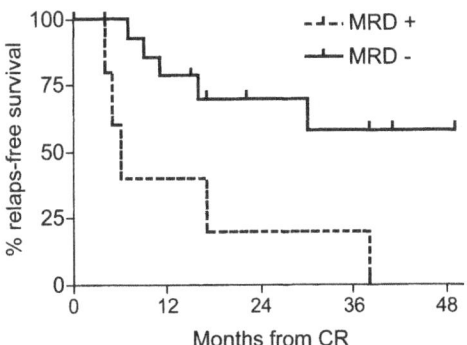

**Fig. 1.** Minimal residual disease and relapse-free survival

sponding transplant. Residual leukemia cells ($1.6 \times 10^{-3}$, range $2 \times 10^{-4}$ to $3.3 \times 10^{-3}$) could be detected in the bone marrow of five pts. For two relapsing MRD positive patients not enough bone marrow aspirate was available for immunophenotypical analysis due to sicca punctions. These two patients were excluded from further analysis. Two of the remaining eight relapsing patients (25%) were MRD positive ($> 1 \times 10^{-3}$ residual blast cells). On the basis of these MRD results, in the pretransplant bone marrow only a marginally significant difference in relapse-free survival between the MRD positive and negative group could be demonstrated using the same cut-off level of $1 \times 10^{-3}$ residual blast cells (p <0.04).

Posttransplant bone marrow analysis for MRD has shown low numbers of residual leukemia cells (range $2 \times 10^{-4}$ to $9 \times 10^{-4}$, median $6 \times 10^{-4}$) in 3 cases. All three patients are in CCR. Thus, posttransplant analysis of MRD in the bone marrow with 5-parametric flow cytometry has no prognostic value.

### Bone marrow morphology in follow-up

All 20 patients achieved morphological complete remission after double-induction treatment without any direct evidence of a myelodysplastically impaired bone marrow. Further bone marrow aspirates were taken every 3 months following aPBSCT, with the first aspirates being taken after peripheral complete remission, 4 to 10 weeks after aPBSCT. In the first postgraft aspirate, all pts met the criteria for morphological CR. At relapse morphological changes complied with the criteria for MDS in 5 pts. MDS (1x refractory anemia, RA, 3x refractory anemia with ringed sideroblasts, RARS, 1x refractory anemia with excess blasts, RAEB) was diagnosed 5 to 18 months after aPBSCT and 5 to 14 months before transition into a AML. The other five relapsing patients suffered from a primary AML relapse. Three patients relapsing with MDS have shown additional chromosomal aberrations.

### Colony growth in leukapheresis products

Colony growth was consecutively followed in single LPs. Megakaryocytic colony growth in a serum-free test system, supplied with rhIL3, rhIL6 and rhMGDF provided highly reproducible results. We observed stepwise decreasing median CFU- mega counts within consecutive mobilization cycles. Median CFU-mega counts in LPs following HAM were 18.5 (range 1 to 51), following TAD consolidation 16.0 (range 1 to 69) and following CY 11.2 (range 1 to 16) with a p value < 0.01 for CFU-mega HAM vs CFU-mega CY. These results were paralleled by a decreasing mean number of CFUs within consecutive mobilization cycles. The median number of CFUs following HAM was 122.9 (range 19 to 236) following TAD 109.8 (range 19 to 346) and 39 (range 10 to 68) following CY (p value <0.01).

To correct for the stepwise decreasing clonogenicity and for varying numbers of seeded CD34 positive cells, a ratio of CFU-mega to CFU was calculated to record differences in the proportion of megakaryocytic progenitors (MPs) within single LPs. The ratio was rather constant within single LPs of an apheresis cycle (maximal deviation + 21%).

In contrast to the invariably high ratio CFU-mega/CFU in the control group, ie, patients without bone marrow involvement by underlying solid tumors, the ratios CFU-mega/CFU in LPs of AML patients during first CR were highly variable and significantly lower than in the standard group (p<0.001).

Whereas clonogenicity decreased in both lineage-specific assays with the number of preceding chemotherapy cycles, the median ratios CFU-mega/CFU did not substantially change within consecutive mobilization

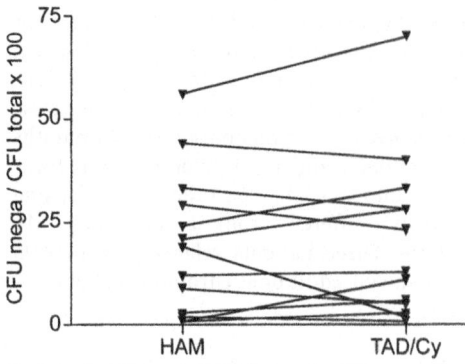

**Fig. 2.** Ratio CFU mega/CFU from paired lineage-selected colony assays in back-up and transplant

cycles (Fig. 2). Megacaryocytic colony growth was not disturbed by leukemic blast cells added to leukapheresis samples.

## CFU mega and outcome

Low CFU mega/CFU ratios were not correlated with a delayed entrance of remission or a delayed aPBSCT. Additional mobilization cycles with Cy were nessesary both, in the CCR group and in the relapsing group. Platelets recovered at a median time interval of 59 days (range 16 to 92 days) to >100/nl. Platelet recovery was not significantly different in the group of patients relapsing with MDS in comparison with patients being in CCR or relapsing with AML (p= 0.23).

To evaluate a possible pathophysiological impact of low and high proportions of MPs in the LPs, ratios CFU mega/CFU were correlated with the outcome and the type of relapse in 19 AML patients available for follow-up. The median ratio CFU mega/CFU was significantly lower in relapsing patients than in patients with CCR (p=0.004). The significant difference in the ratio CFU mega/CFU between the relapsing and CCR group was due to the high frequency of very low ratios CFU-mega/CFU in the relapsing group (Fig. 3). Whereas median CFU-mega counts (data not shown) and the median ratios CFU-mega/CFU were well correlated with outcome, the number of CFUs, CFU-GM, BFU-E or the ratio BFU-E/CFU-GM, were not predictive for relapse-free survival (data not shown in detail).

The pathophysiological relevance of a low ratio CFU-mega/CFU (<0.12) in the transplant is supported by the frequent (71%) occurence of a MDS at relapse in these pts. The cut-off level of 0.12 was chosen according to the observed relapse behavior: All patients with a ratio >0.12 relapsed with AML. Five patients relapsing with MDS (5 of 10 relapses) could be assigned to the group with low ratios CFU-mega/CFU (n=7 pts), the remaining two patients relapsed with AML. Thus, altered CFU-mega growth could be identified in the transplant, at times when no morphological, immunophenotypical or clinical evidence for MDS were available. Using the ratio

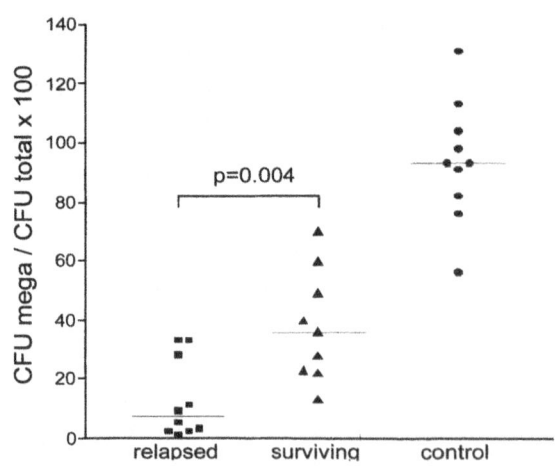

**Fig. 3.** CFU-mega growth depending on outcome

CFU-mega/CFU, 7 of 10 pts (70%) with a high risk of relapse could be detected. Additionally, the median time to relapse was significantly different between the group with low CFU mega/CFU ratios (< 0.12) and the group with higher CFU-mega/CFU ratios (>0.12), 17.3 months vs 8.0 months (p <0.01).

Combining both predictive variables in the transplant, MRD and ratio CFU-mega/CFU, five relapsing patients (50%) expressed both transplant-associated risk profiles, indicating a high coincidence. Two additional relapsing patients being MRD negative in the transplant, that means 20% more, could be detected to be at risk of relapse by a low ratio CFU-mega/CFU.

## Discussion

The study shows, for the first time, that different levels of MRD in the transplants significantly correlate with the probability of relapse.

Up to now, MRD in the pretransplant bone marrow has been considered to be the most important criteria defining stem cell quality in autologous transplants. Results from the paired lineage-selected CFU assays now give evidence that relapses in AML may also be related to a functionally altered remission hematopoiesis characterized by a highly decreased CFU-mega growth in the transplant. This defect in the lineage selection was shown not to be associated with an incomplete hematopoietic reconstitution or myelodysplastic features following aPBSCT. Therefore, altered pretransplant CFU-mega growth is indicative for a clinically inapparent preleukemic disposition of the remission hematopoiesis, ie a pre-MDS.

The presence of a clinically not detectable pre-MDS may have an important impact on therapeutic strategies in postremission: On the background of a pre-MDS maintenance therapy may get a new biological rationale. The cyclic application of relatively low doses of cytotoxic drugs could probably inhibit the regrowth of leukemic cells from a preleuke-

mic postremission hematopoiesis or could be able to eradicate such preleukemic cell clones. The presence of a pre-MDS in remission hematopoiesis should exclude aPBSCT as postremssion therapy. In those cases a new indication for allogeneic transplantation could be given besides cytogenetic risk profiles.

## References

1. Reichle A (1998). Transplant characteristics: Minimal residual disease and impaired megakaryocytic colony growth as sensitive parameters for predicting relapse in acute myeloid leukemia. Leukemia 13; 1227-1234
2. Bennett JM, Catovsky D, Daniel MT, Flandrin G, Galton DA, Gralnick HR, Sultan C (1985). Criteria for the diagnosis of acute leukemia of megakaryocyte lineage (M7). A report of the French-American-British Cooperative Group Ann Intern Med 103: 460-462.
3. Büchner T, Hiddemann W, Wörmann B, Löffler H, Maschmeyer G, Hossfeld D, Ludwig WD, Nowrousian M, Aul C, Schaefer UW, et al (1992). Longterm effects of prolonged maintenance and of very early intensification chemotherapy in AML: data from AMLCG. Leukemia; 6 Suppl 2: 68-71.
4. Tutschka PJ, Copelan EA, Klein JP (1997). Bone marrow transplantation for leukemia following a new busulfan and cyclophosphamide regimen. Blood; 70: 1382-1388.
5. Berthier R, Valiron O, Schweitzer A, Marguerie G (1993). Serum-free medium allows the optimal growth of human megakaryocyte progenitors compared with human plasma supplemented cultures: role of TGF beta. Stem Cells Dayt; 11: 120-129.
6. Zauli G, Vitale L, Brunelli MA, Bagnara GP (1992). Prevalence of the primitive megakaryocyte progenitors (BFU-meg) in adult human peripheral blood. Exp Hematol; 20: 850-854.
7. Goasguen JE; Bennett JM (1992). Classification and morphologic features of the myelodysplastic syndromes. Semin Oncol; 19: 4-13.
8. Yates J, Glidewell O, Wiernik P, Cooper MR, Steinberg D, Dosik H, Levy R, Hoagland C, Henry P, Gottlieb A, Cornell C, Berenberg J, Hutchison JL, Raich P, Nissen N, Ellison RR, Frelick R, James GW, Falkson G, Silver RT, Haurani F, Green M, Henderson E, Leone L, Holland JF (1982). Cytosine arabinoside with daunorubicin or adriamycin for therapy of acute myelocytic leukemia: a CALGB study. Blood; 60: 454-462.
9. Rothe G, Schmitz G (1996). Consensus protocol for the flow cytometric immunophenotyping of hematopoietic malignancies. Working Group on Flow Cytometry and Image Analysis. Leukemia; 10: 877-895.

# Subject Index